Neoplastic Diseases

Fundamentals of Clinical Oncology

Edited by
C. Julian Rosenthal, M.D., F.A.C.P.

Professor of Medicine and Oncology at State University of New York—Health Science Center at Brooklyn. Chief Executive Officer of the Cancer Consortium of the Community Clinical Oncology Program of the County of Kings, New York.

Precept Press, Inc., Chicago

© 1991 by Precept Press, Inc.
All Rights Reserved

Except for appropriate use in critical reviews or works of scholarship, the reproduction or use of this work in any form or by any electronic, mechanical or other means now known or hereafter invented, including photocopying and recording, and in any information storage and retrieval system is forbidden without the written permission of the publisher.

95 94 93 92 91   5 4 3 2 1

Library of Congress Catalog Card Number: 91-62100

International Standard Book Number: 0-944496-24-5

Precept Press, Inc.
160 East Illinois Street
Chicago, Illinois 60611

Printed in the United States of America

To my wife and children, who make my life meaningful.

To many generations of students and postgraduate trainees and to my colleagues who helped shape our concepts and presentations.

To our patients, from whom we learn and try to help.

C.J.R.

CONTENTS

48. Pediatric Malignancies   810
Sreedhar P. Rao, M.D.

**Appendix: Combination Chemotherapy and Supportive Therapy: Regimens
and Schedules of Administration   841**

PREFACE

Despite significant progress registered in many fields of medicine, neoplastic diseases—the object of study of clinical oncology—are still a group of disorders whose pathogenesis is poorly understood and treatment is curative in just a few of advanced cases. The large amount of information accumulated during the past 5 decades has been presented in most of the existing textbooks over the course of several volumes. These are difficult to use as an easy source of reference. The editor and authors of this book on neoplastic diseases have decided to present most of the information in a more concise form. This could be especially useful to postgraduate students in oncologic and nononcologic fields, and also to family physicians caring for cancer patients.

It is for this reason that we limited this book to about 891 pages and presented some important and frequently used information in 3 chapters. The first of these is a diagnostic imaging chapter focusing on the presentation of computerized tomographic images and other diagnostic radiologic tests recommended in the workup of the most common malignant tumors at various sites. Second, there is a pathology chapter containing histologic pictures of the most common neoplasms. Finally, there is a chemotherapy compendium presented as an appendix. It contains the commonly used chemotherapy regimens, some of which are considered to be standard therapy leading to the cure of advanced malignancies such as germ cell neoplasms and lymphomas. Others simply represent the best available treatment leading to responses in some of the most common advanced malignant tumors (e.g., carcinoma of the breast, lung, stomach, ovary). This is subject to constant change. Although the accuracy of the prescribed dosages of the drugs included in these various therapeutic regimens has been checked, it is imperative that they be administered only under the supervision of medical oncologists who are familiar with their numerous side effects and with the methods used to prevent and treat such side effects.

In view of recent progress made in understanding some aspects of the pathogenesis of malignant neoplasms, special chapters are devoted to the presentation of the genetics and viral etiology of malignant tumors, as well as to the most important aspects of tumor growth, tumor cell kinetics, and the enzymatic pathways of neoplastic cells. The principles of antineoplastic chemotherapy and radiation therapy are also succinctly presented. Chapters on clinical oncology that discuss neoplasms for which there are effective and complex therapies are presented in more detail (e.g., breast, lymphoma, leukemias).

In retrospect, I hope that this book has achieved its objective of serving as a useful reference source that conveniently provides information for trainees and physicians involved in the care of cancer patients.

C. Julian Rosenthal, M.D., F.A.C.P.

ACKNOWLEDGEMENTS

The editor is grateful to several people whose excellent help and commitment to the publication of this book he would like to acknowledge.

Rex Olsen provided valuable editorial assistance and contributed to the preparation and compilation of many of the manuscripts. His valuable help has contributed greatly to the publication of this book.

Sandra Amrani contributed to the typing and corrections of many of the manuscripts and to the expert preparation of their tables and reference lists.

ABOUT THE EDITOR

C. Julian Rosenthal, M.D., F.A.C.P., received his medical degree from the University of Rome. He completed his medical residency at the Albert Einstein College of Medicine. He trained in Hemato-Oncology at the Mount Sinai Hospital and Medical School and had a research fellowship in tumor immunology at New York University Medical Center. Dr. Rosenthal is currently Professor of Medicine and Oncology at State University of New York—Health Science Center at Brooklyn, Director of the Clinical Community Oncology Program of the County of Kings, a consortium of four medical centers' oncology clinical research programs and its principal investigator in the South West Oncology group.

CONTRIBUTORS

JEFFREY S. ABRAMS, M.D., Assistant Professor of Medicine and Oncology, University of Maryland Cancer Center, Baltimore, Maryland

JOSEPH AISNER, M.D., F.A.C.P., Professor of Medicine, Oncology, Pharmacology, and Experimental Therapeutics; Director, University of Maryland Cancer Center, Baltimore, Maryland

JEROME APPELBAUM, M.D., Clinical Assistant Professor of Medicine, Cornell University Medical College, North Shore University Hospital-Cornell University Medical College, Manhasset, New York

GLAISTER AYR, M.SC., Senior Physicist, State University of New York Health Science Center at Brooklyn, Brooklyn, New York

HASSAN AZIZ, M.D., Assistant Professor of Radiation Oncology, State University of New York Health Science Center at Brooklyn, Brooklyn, New York

VLADIMIR BENISOVICH, M.D., Assistant Professor, Department of Neoplastic Diseases, The Mount Sinai Medical Center, Medical Oncology, Department of Medicine, Mount Sinai Services, City Hospital Center at Elmhurst, Elmhurst, New York

ALBERT S. BRAVERMAN, M.D., F.A.C.P., Clinical Associate Professor of Medicine, State University of New York Health Science Center at Brooklyn, Brooklyn, New York

HOWARD BRUCKNER, M.D., Professor of Neoplastic Diseases, Mount Sinai School of Medicine, Mount Sinai Medical Center, New York City, New York

NEIL I. BRODY, M.D., PH.D., Associate Professor of Dermatology, State University of New York Health Science Center at Brooklyn, Brooklyn, New York

DOROTHY L. BUCHHAGEN, PH.D., Naval Medical Oncology Branch, National Cancer Institute, and the Uniformed University of the Health Sciences, Bethesda, Maryland

HUGH CARROLL, M.D., Professor of Medicine, State University of New York Health Science Center at Brooklyn, Brooklyn, New York

ANNE C. CARTER, M.D., Professor of Medicine, New York Medical College, Valhalla, New York; Visiting Professor of Medicine, State University of New York Health Science Center at Brooklyn, Brooklyn, New York

ABRAHAM CHACHOUA, M.D., Assistant Professor of Medicine, New York University School of Medicine, New York City, New York

ENGRACIO P. CORTES, M.D., Associate Clinical Professor of Medicine, Albert Einstein College of Medicine, New York City, New York; staff, Long Island Jewish Medical Center, New Hyde Park, Long Island, New York

JANET CUTTNER, M.D., Professor of Clinical Medicine and Neoplastic Diseases, Mount Sinai School of Medicine, Mount Sinai Medical Center, New York City, New York

HOSOON P. DINCSOY, M.D., Attending Pathologist, Northshore University Hospital, Long Island, New York

HARVEY DOSIK, M.D., F.A.C.P., Director of Medicine, Interfaith Medical Center; Professor of Medicine and Clinical Associate Dean, State University of New York Health Science Center at Brooklyn, Brooklyn, New York

JOSEPH FELDMAN, PH.D., Professor of Preventive Medicine, State University of New York Health Science Center at Brooklyn, Brooklyn, New York

THOMAS J. FORLENZA, M.D., F.A.C.P., Director of Oncology, St. Vincent's Medical Center of Richmond, Staten Island, New York; Clinical Assistant Professor of Medicine, New York University School of Medicine, New York City, New York

SIDNEY GLANZ, M.D., Professor and Co-director of Cardiovascular and Interventional Radiology, State University of New York Health Science Center at Brooklyn, Brooklyn, New York

DAVID H. GORDON, M.D., Professor of Radiology and Director of Body Computed Tomography and Magnetic Resonance Imaging, State University of New York Health Science Center at Brooklyn, Brooklyn, New York

MICHAEL GREEN, M.D., F.A.C.P., F.R.A.C.P., Deputy Director, Department of Clinical Haematology and Medical Oncology, The Royal Melbourne Hospital, Victoria, Australia

MARK HOROWITZ, M.D., Clinical Instructor, State University of New York Health Science Center at Brooklyn, Brooklyn, New York

GWENDOLYN HOTSON, M.D., Assistant Professor and Director of Neuro Computed Tomography and Magnetic Resonance Imaging, State University of New York Health Science Center at Brooklyn, Brooklyn, New York

MUTHUSWAMY KRISHNAMURTHY, M.D., F.A.C.P., Chief of Hematology, Interfaith Medical Center; Associate Professor of Clinical Medicine, State University of New York Health Science Center at Brooklyn, Brooklyn, New York

GOBIND LAUNGANI, M.D., Associate Professor of Urology, State University of New York Health Science Center at Brooklyn, Brooklyn, New York

RICHARD J. MACCHIA, M.D., Professor and Chairman, Department of Urology, State University of New York Health Science Center at Brooklyn, Brooklyn, New York

JOSE R. MARTI, M.D., Associate Professor of Surgery, State University of New York Health Science Center at Brooklyn; Chairman, Department of Surgery, Brooklyn Hospital Center, Brooklyn, New York

LARRY NORTON, M.D., Chief, Breast and Gynecological Cancer Medicine Service, Memorial Sloan-Kettering Cancer Center, New York City, New York.

RUTH ORATZ, M.D., Assistant Professor of Medicine, New York University School of Medicine, New York City, New York

SREEDHAR P. RAO, M.D., Associate Professor of Clinical Pediatrics, State University of New York Health Science Center at Brooklyn, Brooklyn, New York

JEAN CLAUDE REMY, M.D., Clinical Associate Professor of Obstetrics/Gynecology, State University of New York Health Science Center at Brooklyn, Brooklyn, New York

SEYMOUR RITTER, M.D., Assistant Professor of Medicine, State University of New York Health Science Center at Brooklyn, Brooklyn, New York

C. JULIAN ROSENTHAL, M.D., Professor of Medicine and Oncology, State University of New York Health Science Center at Brooklyn, Brooklyn, New York

ALEXANDER SEDLIS, M.D., Professor of Obstetrics/Gynecology, State University of New York Health Science Center at Brooklyn, Brooklyn, New York

ASHOK SHAHA, M.D., Associate Professor of Surgery, State University of New York Health Science Center at Brooklyn, Brooklyn, New York

ROBERT SILBER, M.D., Professor of Medicine and Director, Division of Hematology, New York University Medical Center, New York City, New York

WILLIAM B. SOLOMON, M.D., Assistant Professor of Medicine, State University of New York Health Science Center at Brooklyn, Brooklyn, New York

ROBERT L. STAHL, M.D., Assistant Professor of Medicine, Division of Hematology and Medical Oncology, Emory University School of Medicine, Atlanta, Georgia

RICHARD S. STARK, Director of Hematology/Oncology, Interfaith Medical Center, Brooklyn, New York

DAVID J. STRAUS, M.D., Associate Attending Physician, Memorial Sloan-Kettering Cancer Center, New York City, New York

N. SIMON TCHEKMEDYIAN, M.D., F.A.C.P., Newport Beach, California

WILLIAM L. THELMO, M.D., Chief of Surgical Pathology and Cytology, Kings County Hospital Center; Associate Professor of Clinical Pathology, State University of New York Health Science Center at Brooklyn, Brooklyn, New York

KEVIN M. TROY, M.D., Assistant Professor of Medicine, Mount Sinai School of Medicine, Mount Sinai Medical Center, New York City, New York

JACK TWERSKY, M.D., Associate Professor, State University of New York Health Science Center at Brooklyn, Brooklyn, New York

JAIME URIBARRI, M.D., Assistant Professor of Medicine, Mount Sinai School of Medicine, Mount Sinai Hospital, New York City, New York

GEORGE A. VAS, M.D., Associate Professor of Neurology, State University of New York Health Science Center at Brooklyn, Brooklyn, New York

RAM S. VERMA, PH.D., M.R.C. PATH., Chief, Division of Genetics, Long Island College Hospital; Professor of Medicine, Anatomy, and Cell Biology, State University of New York Health Science Center at Brooklyn, Brooklyn, New York

RAMASWAMY VISWANATHAN, M.D., D.SC., Associate Professor of Clinical Psychiatry, State University of New York Health Science Center at Brooklyn, Brooklyn, New York

CAROLINE A. WEBBER, M.D., Attending Pathologist, Kings County Hospital Center; Clinical Assistant Professor of Pathology, State University of New York Health Science Center at Brooklyn, Brooklyn, New York

1

EPIDEMIOLOGY OF CANCER

Joseph Feldman, Ph.D.

IN 1990, CANCER WAS the second leading cause of mortality in the United States and was responsible for an estimated 510,000 deaths or approximately 23% of total mortality.[1] Table 1-1 shows the number of deaths and new cases by site of cancer for males and females in 1990.

In males, cancer of the lung, colon-rectum, and prostate accounted for an estimated 55% of new cases and 57% of deaths. In females, cancers of the breast, lung, and colon-rectum were responsible for an estimated 54% of the new cases and 52% of deaths.

Table 1-1. Number of Cases and Expected Deaths at the Most Common Cancer Sites in the United States: 1990 Estimates

Site	Incidence		Deaths	
	Female	Male	Female	Male
Breast	150,000	—	44,000	
Prostate		106,000	—	30,000
Lung	55,000	102,000	50,000	92,000
Colon and Rectum	79,000	76,000	30,900	30,000
Uterus	46,500	—	10,000	—
Ovary	20,500	—	12,400	—
Bladder	13,000	36,000	4,200	6,500
Pancreas	14,500	13,600	12,900	12,100
Stomach	13,000	13,900	5,400	8,300
Lymphomas	20,200	22,800	9,300	10,500
Leukemias	12,100	15,700	8,300	9,800

Source: American Cancer Society (ref 1)

Trends

Mortality. Relatively little increase has been seen over time in overall cancer mortality after adjusting for the increased number of the aged in the population. About 85% of the increase in cancer mortality from 1930–80 can be explained by aging of the population.[2] The remaining 15% increase is at least partly due to better diagnosis and death certification. An analysis of age-adjusted cancer mortality in the United States between 1962 and 1985 showed an average annual increase of 0.4%/yr.[3,4]

Incidence. Patterns of cancer incidence also show little change over time. Data from 2 national surveys of cancer incidence conducted between 1947 and 1970 show that cancer incidence declined by 5% over this period.[4] Among males, the overall rate increased by 8%, but among females the rate declined by 13%. Data from 1973–85 from the SEER program (Surveillance, Epidemiology

Table 1-2. Average Annual Age-Adjusted (1950) Standard Cancer Incidence Rates, White Males, 1937, 1947, 1969–71, 1973–77, and Percentage Change, 1973–85

	1937	1947	1969–71	1973–77	Average change, 1973–85 (%)
Stomach	41.8	32.4	12.1	10.7	−2.0
Colon	20.7	25.1	29.8	30.9	−1.0
Rectum	17.8	20.7	16.0	16.5	−0.2
Pancreas	6.7	8.9	10.7	10.2	−1.1
Lung	13.7	29.5	68.0	68.2	−1.0
Prostate	32.0	37.4	45.2	52.7	+2.2
Bladder	14.1	17.2	21.3	23.0	+0.9

Sources: Young JL, Pollack, ES. The incidence of cancer in the United States. In: Schottenfeld D, Fraumeni J, eds. Cancer epidemiology and prevention. Philadelphia: Saunders, 1982; U.S. Department of Health & Human Services (ref 4)

Table 1-3. Average Annual Age-Adjusted (1950) Standard Cancer Incidence Rates, White Females, 1937, 1947, 1969–71, 1973–77, and Percentage Change 1973–85

	1937	1947	1969–71	1973–77	Average change, 1973–85 (%)
Stomach	25.4	17.8	5.8	4.7	−2.1
Colon	20.7	25.1	29.8	30.9	+0.4
Rectum	11.2	13.9	9.6	10.0	+0.2
Pancreas	5.0	5.6	6.5	6.6	+0.8
Lung	4.1	6.7	4.9	20.4	+5.4
Breast	67.1	73.6	73.3	81.8	+1.1
Cervix uteri	NA	38.3	15.1	11.3	−4.3
Corpus uteri	NA	22.9	23.2	29.0	−3.0
Bladder	6.6	7.1	5.6	6.1	+1.0

Source: see table 1-1

Table 1-4. Percent Five-Year Relative Survival, White Male, 1960–85

	1960–63	1970–73	1973–80	1980–85
Lung and bronchus	7	9	10	12
Prostate	50	63	68	73
Colon	42	47	48	54
Rectum	36	43	46	50
Bladder	53	61	73	78

Source: Biometry Branch, National Cancer Institute (Data from National End Results and SEER programs)

Table 1-5. Percent Five-Year Relative Survival, White Female, 1960–85

	1960–63	1970–73	1973–80	1980–85
Breast	63	68	74	76
Colon	44	50	52	55
Rectum	41	48	51	53
Cervix uteri	58	64	68	67
Corpus uteri	73	81	88	83
Lung and bronchus	11	14	15	16

Source: see table 1–4

and End Results), a series of population-based tumor registries encompassing 25 million people, indicated an increase in cancer occurrence of 1% per year.[4,5] However, substantial changes have taken place in cancer occurrence over time for specific sites. Tables 1-2 and 1-3 show substantial increases in lung cancer for both males and females since 1937. There is a possibility that the incidence of lung cancer has begun to level off in males. Cancer of the prostate has increased consistently, whereas stomach and cervical cancer have declined consistently.

5-Year Survival. Cancer survival rates have changed little for the more common sites over the 20-yr period 1960–85. Tables 1-4 and 1-5 show 5-yr relative survival rates for white males and females. The relative survival rate adjusts for deaths from causes other than cancer and equals the ratio of cancer patients who survive 5 yr to the number expected in the general population of comparable age, sex, and race. For males, little change has occurred in the prognosis for lung and colorectal cancer. For bladder and prostate cancer, improvements in survival have been seen. Among females, substantially increased survival is seen for cancer of the breast and modestly increased survival for colorectal and uterine cancer; little improvement is seen for lung cancer. It has been suggested that some of the improvement in 5-yr survival rates may be artifactual, resulting from misdiagnosis of noninvasive tumors, lead time bias, and staging bias.[4,6] Because trends in mortality, occurrence, and survival have been relatively stable, it has been argued that more resources should be devoted to prevention of cancer and less to treatment.[3,7]

Genetics

Oncogenes—genes capable of inducing neoplastic change in cells—were first described in retroviral induced animal cancer.[8] In their normal state, these genes are referred to as proto-oncogenes and are present in all human and animal cells. Although they are diverse in function, proto-oncogenes are alike in exerting essential control over cellular replication and differential. The similarity between the DNA sequences of a number of human proto-oncogenes and those in low vertebrates suggest a fundamental role in cell growth.[9] The transformation of a proto-oncogene into an oncogene can occur either through deregulation of the gene or modification of the transcribed segment of the gene.[10] Deregulation implies that the gene is overexpressed, whereas modification implies that the protein product of the gene is changed. Chromosomal translocation and gene amplification are the most common mechanisms by which proto-oncogenes become oncogenes. In translocation, the proto-oncogene is moved from its normal location to another location where it may come under the influence of a promoter of other genes. With gene amplification, the increased number of copies may result in evasion of normal cellular control.[11]

Table 1-6. Range of Incidence Rates for Common Cancers Among Males and Females Around 1976

Site	High incidence	Males Rate per 100,000*	Low incidence	Rate per 100,000	Ratio
	AREA		AREA		
Colon	U.S. (Connecticut)	32.3	India (Poona)	3.1	10.4
Rectum	Canada	22.6	Israel, non-Jews	3.1	7.3
Pancreas	U.S. (Bay Area) black	18.3	India (Bombay)	2.0	9.2
Lung	U.S. (New Orleans) black	107.2	U.S. (New Mexico) American Indian	8.1	13.2
Prostate	U.S. (Alameda) black	100.2	Shanghai	0.8	125.3
Bladder	Switzerland (Geneva)	30.2	India (Poona)	2.4	12.6
		Females			
Colon	U.S. (Bay Area) Japanese	27.4	India (Poona)	2.8	9.8
Rectum	Switzerland (Neuchatel)	13.4	Israel, non-Jews	1.5	8.9
Cervix uteri	Colombia (Cali)	52.9	Israel, non-Jews	2.1	25.2
Corpus uteri	U.S. (Alameda) white	38.5	Japan (Fukuoka)	1.0	38.5
Breast	U.S. (Hawaii) Hawaiian	87.5	Japan (Osaka)	8.9	9.8
Pancreas	U.S. (New Mexico) American Indian	10.4	India (Bombay)	0.9	11.6
Lung	New Zealand, Maori	48.8	Spain (Navarra)	2.6	18.8
Bladder	U.S. (New Orleans) white	6.5	Hungary (Szabolcs)	0.5	13.0

*Age-standardized to standard world population
Source: Waterhouse J, Muir C, Powell J, eds. Cancer incidence in five continents, vol. 4 IARC Scientific Pub no. 42. Lyon, France: Int Agency for Research on Cancer, 1982

Table 1-7. Proportions of Cancer Deaths Attributed to Various Factors

| | Percent of all cancer deaths | |
Factor or class of factors	Best estimate	Range of acceptable estimates
Tobacco	30	25–40
Alcohol	3	2–4
Diet	35	10–70
Food additives	<1	5–2
Reproductive & sexual behaviour	7	1–13
Occupation	4	2–8
Pollution	2	<1–5
Industrial products	<1	<1–2
Medicines & medical procedures	1	0.5–3
Geophysical factors	3	2–4
Infection	10?	1–?
Unknown	?	?

Source: Doll R, Peto R. The causes of cancer: quantitative estimates of avoidable risks of cancer in the United States today. JNCI 1981; 66:1256.

Another type of oncogene appears to exert its influence by suppressing growth, and risk may be elevated if the gene is deleted or deactivated.[12]

Oncogenes can be activated by chemicals, viruses, or point mutations and may interact with environmental factors such as diet.[11] Evidence suggests that oncogene activation is but one step of a multistage process and that environmental factors play an important role in that process.[13] The wide variation in cancer occurrence throughout the world as described below is consistent with a multistep model.

Environmental Factors

The potential for prevention of cancer is illustrated in table 1-6, which shows the range of international variation in incidence for the more common sites. The range, never less than 7-fold and as high as 125-fold, immediately indicates an important environmental component. Some of this variation is genetic, but the similarity of cancer occurrence in migrant groups to that in the host population indicates that much cancer is environmentally determined. In this discussion, the meaning of the term *environment* is broadened to include culture and life-styles as well as the physical environment. The environmental factors and the percentage of cancers caused by each as estimated by Doll and Peto are shown in table 1-7.[7]

A brief discussion of each of the factors shown in table 1-7 follows.

Tobacco is the single most important scientifically documented cause of cancer. Tobacco has been estimated to cause 43% of male cancer deaths and 15% of female cancer deaths.[14] Although the relationship of tobacco is strongest for lung cancer, several other sites such as the oral cavity, larynx, esophagus, bladder, and pancreas are associated with tobacco use. The more tobacco used, the higher the risk for most sites. The use of filtered low-tar cigarettes is associated with a reduction in risk, but the risk remains many times greater than that for a nonsmoker.[15]

The use of pipes, cigars, chewing tobacco, and snuff increases risks of cancer of the oral cavity and throat. The number of epidemiology studies that have implicated smoking and various cancer sites is in the many thousands, leaving little doubt that tobacco is the premier cause of cancer. Analytic chemistry studies have shown that tobacco smoke contains almost 4,000 compounds, many of them either initiators, promoters, or co-carcinogens.[16]

Alcohol use is associated with an increased occurrence of cancers of the oral cavity, pharynx, larynx, and esophagus. It has been difficult to isolate the role of drinking in increasing risks of cancer because ethanol by itself doesn't produce cancer in animals. However, there is no doubt that individuals who are heavy drinkers and who smoke have a risk 15–20 times greater than that of nonsmokers and nondrinkers of developing cancer in the above sites.[17] Furthermore, age of diagnosis is considerably younger in patients who both smoke and drink heavily.[18]

Diet is believed to play a very large role in cancer causation, but the scientific evidence is less clear-cut than for tobacco, and the range of acceptable estimate is much larger.[19] In spite of the uncertainty, several authorities, including the American Cancer Society, National Cancer Institute, and the National Research Council of the National Academy of Sciences, have issued dietary guidelines or recommendations to reduce the risk of cancer.[20,21] These guidelines, which reflect prudent judgments based on current, though incomplete, scientific evidence, are summarized below.

- *Avoid obesity.* Animal studies have shown that incidence of cancer is reduced and life span lengthened by providing nutritionally adequate diets that maintained animals at ideal weight. In humans, obesity has been associated with cancers of the uterus, gallbladder, colon, and breast.
- *Reduce total fat intake.* Evidence from both epidemiological and laboratory studies suggests that excessive fat intake increases the risk of developing cancers of the breast, colon, and prostate. Excessive intake of both saturated and unsaturated fats—whether from plant or animal sources—has been reported to increase risk of cancer. It has been recommended that Americans reduce their total calories derived from fat from 40% to 30%.
- *Eat high fiber foods.* These foods include whole grain cereals, fruits, and vegetables. Fiber refers to food components that are not readily digested in the intestinal tract. Some studies have shown that fiber reduces risk of colon cancer, possibly by speeding transit time of fecal matter, thus decreasing the concentration of carcinogens, or by changing the intestinal flora.
- *Eat food rich in vitamins A and C.* These foods include dark-green and deep-yellow vegetables and certain fruits containing carotene, which is a precursor of vitamin A. Preformed vitamin A, or retinol, is found in whole milk, cheese, butter, egg yolks, and liver. In many studies, inverse associations have been found between dietary vitamin A, or carotenoids, and the risk of developing cancers of the lung, oral cavity, pharynx,

esophagus, and stomach. A recent review has concluded that carotenoids rather than retinoids are responsible for the lower risk.[22]

Vitamin C has been associated with a lesser risk of developing gastric cancer. Animal studies have shown that even small amounts of vitamin C can inhibit the formation of nitrosomines, which are potent carcinogens.

* *Reduce consumption of salt-cured smoked and nitrate-cured foods.* Studies in various parts of the world have found an association between these foods and the risk of gastric cancer. It has been suggested that widespread refrigeration in the United States is responsible for the decline in stomach cancer because of the reduced need to cure foods and the wider availability of fruits and vegetables.

Other aspects of diet, such as food additives, artificial sweeteners, coffee, trace elements, and vitamin E, have been implicated in increasing or decreasing cancer risk, but the relationships are less well documented and more controversial than those noted above.

Reproductive and sexual behavior. The most obvious association is between sexual intercourse and cancer of the cervix uteri. This disease is most common in the sexually active and those who have started intercourse at an early age.[16] The disease is very rare in nuns and uncommon in women with a single marital sexual partner. Pregnancy and childbirth influence the risks of cancers of the breast, endometrium, and ovary. In each, the disease is less common in women with more children and in those who bear children early.

Occupation. Most occupational carcinogens were detected because of clustering of rare cancer cases. However, on occasions in which the site was more common, the risk has been overlooked. Occupational carcinogens are believed to account for a small proportion of all cancers because of the relatively limited exposure of people to them. Asbestos represents an occupational carcinogen that has been released into the general environment with the potential to affect many people. At present, occupational carcinogens are believed to be responsible for < 10% of all cancers.[14]

Air pollution can be linked to the etiology of cancer only indirectly. Little evidence has been gathered to date showing that carcinogens in the air pose a serious cancer hazard.[16] In the workplace, exposures to coal gas, tar pitch, and coke oven emissions are many times greater than the levels in circulating air around us, but even the occupational levels have not been found to increase cancer risk. Passive cigarette smoking represents another form of indoor pollution that may carry risks.[23] Exposure to radioactive emissions from radon in uranium mines has been found to increase risks of lung cancer in miners. Radon can enter the home from soil, water, or building materials. The extent of risks from both passive smoking and radon is currently uncertain. Drinking water can contain known and suspected carcinogens, including asbestos, metals, radioactive substances, and industrial chemicals, but the levels are so small that there is probably little risk. Trihalomethanes, which can be formed when the chlorine that is used to purify water reacts with organic chemicals, are associated with an increased risk of G.I. cancers.[24]

Many *industrial products,* including detergents, hair dyes, certain cosmetics, plastics, paints, dyes, polishes, solvents, fabrics, and printer's ink, show carcinogenic potential in animals, but their effect in man in unknown. Current trends in cancer incidence give no reason for alarm, but many of these substances have been only recently introduced.[14]

Among *therapeutic and diagnostic agents,* about 20 substances are suspected carcinogens. The current view is that these agents are responsible for few cases of cancer and that the only reason their effect has been apparent to clinicians is the unusual microscopic appearance of the tumor or the site of occurrence.[25] An example is the epidemic of clear-cell adenocarcinoma of the vagina due to prenatal administration of diethylstilbestrol.[26] Ionizing radiation is believed to have caused 5–10% of the childhood malignancies in the 1950s and 1960s.[25] The wide use of postmenopausal estrogens may have accounted for an increase in the incidence of endometrial cancer in middle-aged women in the early 1970s. The impact of oral contraceptives on cancer risk is still not fully known. Most studies have found no increased risk of cancer among women who use oral contraceptives, and for some sites such as the ovary and endometrium, the risk is reduced.[27,28] Some recent studies have found an increased risk of cervical cancer among these women even after adjusting for sexual activity.[16]

Geophysical factors include natural ionizing radiation and ultraviolet (UV) light, both of which have been found to be carcinogens. The average exposure to an individual from natural radiation is 0.1–0.2 rems/yr, or about 50% of total exposure.[29] Based on a background dose of 20 million rems/yr, it is estimated that natural radiation produces 5,500 cancer deaths in this country annually—about 1.4% of all deaths from cancer.[14] UV light is the principal cause of basal cell carcinoma; it also causes a large number of squamous cell skin cancers. The incidence of melanoma in white-skinned populations is highly correlated with exposure to UV light. Overall, up to 2% of all cancers may be due to UV light.[14]

Infectious agents only rarely have been found to be a direct cause of neoplastic disease; cancer is not an infectious disease in the sense of other communicable diseases. Reports of clusters of cases, often leukemias or lymphomas, have failed to point to a common etiologic factor and are likely chance occurrences. Certain viruses have been associated with particular cancer sites in both animals and humans. The linkage between the hepatitis B virus and liver cancer initially was based on epidemiological and geographic observations. This association has been strengthened by results of studies of integration of viral DNA with the DNA of the host gene. It has been shown that carriers of the hepatitis B surface antigen have 100 times greater risk of developing liver cancer than noncarriers.[30]

Extensive evidence has been accumulated showing that Burkitt's lymphoma and cancer of the nasopharynx are associated with the Epstein-Barr virus. In high-risk areas, these cancers occur nearly always in individuals infected by the Epstein-Barr virus, and the viral DNA seems to be present in all the tumor cells.[25] Other viruses associated with cancer include herpes simplex type 2 and/or human papillomavirus (cervical cancer) and the human T cell leukemia lymphoma virus.

The total percentage reduction in cancer that is achievable is complicated by the fact that some cancers may have multiple causes, and elimination of one cause may not produce the expected decline. Based on current information, it is possible to reduce cancer mortality by 40%, with most of the reductionresulting from avoidance of tobacco. However, it has been difficult to convince smokers to give up the habit, even though substantial progress has been made.

In the future, opportunities for cancer prevention should increase as new information is gathered and existing information is modified and expanded for the factors described above, especially in the area of nutrition.

References

1. American Cancer Society. Cancer facts and figures, 1990. Atlanta: the society.
2. Devesa S, Schneiderman M. Increase in the number of cancer deaths in the United States. Am J Epidemiol 1977; 106:1–5.
3. Bailar J, Smith E. Progress against cancer? N Engl J Med 1986; 314-1226–32.
4. Dept. Health Human Services. NIH NCI annual cancer statistics review including cancer trends, 1950–85. US Govt Printing Office, 1988; 201-7788:61215.
5. Devesa S, Silverman DT. Cancer incidence and mortality trends in the United States 1935–1974. JNCI 1978; 60:545–71.
6. Enstrom J, Austin D. Interpreting cancer survival rates. Science. 1977; 195:847–51.
7. Cairns J. The treatment of diseases and the war against cancer. Sci Am 1985; 253:51–59.
8. Bishop JM. Viral oncogenes. Cell 1985; 42:23–28.
9. Slamon DJ, Boore TC, Murdock DC, et al. Studies of the human c-myb gene and its product in human acute leukemics. Science 1986; 233:347–51.
10. Hayward WS. Viral and cellular oncogenes in cancer etiology: In: Chagenti RSK, German J, eds. Genetics in clinical oncology. New York: Oxford University Press, 1985; 22–38.
11. Taylor JA. Oncogenes and their applications in epidemiologic studies. Am J Epidemiol 1989; 130:6–13.
12. Cavenee WK, Hansen MF. Molecular genetics of human familial cancer. Cold Spring Harbor Symp Ovont Biol 1986; 51:829–35.
13. Lard H, Paradu LF, Weinberg RA. Tumorigenic conversion of primary embryo fibroblasts requires at least two cooperating oncogenes. Nature 1983; 304:596–602.
14. Doll R, Peto R. The causes of cancer: quantitative estimates of avoidable risks of cancer in the United States today. JNCI 1981; 66:1191–1308.
15. Lee P, Garfinkel L. Mortality and type of cigarette smoked. J Epidemiol Commun Health 1981; 35:16–22.
16. Page H, Asire A. Cancer rates and risks. 3rd ed. U.S. Dept Health Human Services. NIH Pub. no. 85-691, 1985.
17. Tuyns AJ. Alcohol. In: Schottenfeld D, Fraumeni JF, Jr, eds. Cancer epidemiology and prevention. Philadelphia: Saunders, 1982; 293–303.
18. Feldman J, Boxer P. Relationship of drinking to head and neck cancer. Prev Med 1979; 8:507–19.
19. Willett W, MacMahon B. Diet and cancer—an overview (2 pts). N Engl J Med 1984; 310:633–38, 697–703.
20. ACS. Nutrition and cancer: cause and prevention. CA 1984; 34:121–26.
21. Committee on Diet, Nutrition and Cancer, National Research Council. Diet, nutrition and cancer. Washington, D.C.: National Academy Press, 1982.
22. Freudenheim JL, Graham S. Toward a dietary prevention of cancer. Am J Epidemiol 1989; 11:229–35.
23. Spengler J, Sexton K. Indoor air pollution: a public health perspective. Science 1983; 221:9–16.
24. Crump K, Guess H. Drinking water and cancer: review of recent epidemiological findings and assessment of risks. Annu Rev Pub Health 1982; 3:339–57.
25. Doll R. Strategy for detection of cancer hazards to man. Nature 1982; 265:589–96.

26. Herbst A, Ulfelder H, Poskanzer D. Adenocarcinoma of the vagina: association of maternal stilbestrol therapy with tumor appearance in young women. N Engl J Med 1971; 284:878–81.
27. Centers For Disease Control. Oral contraceptive use and the risk of ovarian cancer. JAMA 1983; 249:1600–04.
28. Centers for Disease Control. Oral contraceptive use and the risk of endometrial cancer. JAMA 1983; 249:1600–04.
29. Boice J, Land C. Ionizing radiation. In: Schottenfeld D, Fraumeni J Jr, eds. Cancer epidemiology and prevention. Philadelphia: Saunders, 1982; 231–76.
30. Beasley R. Hepatitis B virus as the etiologic agent in cellular carcinoma: epidemiologic considerations. Hepatology 1982; 2:215–65.

2

VIRAL CARCINOGENESIS

Dorothy L. Buchhagen, Ph.D.

IT IS WELL ESTABLISHED that viruses are responsible for a wide variety of tumors that appear in frogs, cats, mice, monkeys, and other animals.[1,2] The causative agents include viruses that have DNA as well as those that have RNA as their genetic material. Virus involvement in human cancers, which has been more difficult to assess, frequently arises as a result of "guilt by association," i.e., a virus infection is found to precede the appearance of a tumor, or a virus is isolated from a human tumor. The ethical prohibition to fulfilling Koch's postulates in humans precludes the direct induction of a tumor by inoculation of purified virus. In spite of this prohibition, evidence continues to accumulate implicating a viral etiology for a number of human cancers, including Burkitt's lymphoma, nasopharyngeal carcinoma, hepatoma, prostatic adenocarcinoma, Kaposi's sarcoma, cervical carcinoma, and T cell lymphoma.

Approaches that have been used to assign a viral etiology to human cancers represent indirect applications of Koch's postulates.* Evidence of viral infection prior to the appearance of the tumor includes the following:

- Presence of serum antiviral antibodies, characteristic viral-induced benign lesions, or epidemiology of the disease suggesting the involvement of a transmissible agent
- Detection of viral structural components, such as DNA, RNA, or protein molecules in the pretumor or tumor tissues
- Isolation of infectious virus from target or tumor tissue

---

*A statement of the kind of experimental evidence required to establish the etiologic relationship of a given microorganism to a given disease.

- The susceptibility of in vitro cultured human cells to infection and transformation by the suspected viral agent
- The ability to induce the cancer by purposely inoculating primates or by accidentally inoculating humans.

The DNA-containing viruses associated with human cancers include Epstein-Barr virus, hepatitis B virus, papillomavirus, cytomegalovirus, and herpes simplex virus type 2. The RNA-containing viruses belong to the HTLV class of retroviruses.

Epstein-Barr Virus

Early epidemiological studies on Burkitt's lymphoma (BL) in central Africa showed a clustering of the disease that suggested the involvement of a transmissible agent.[3] Subsequently, the Epstein-Barr virus (EBV), a virus of the herpes group with DNA as its genetic material, was isolated from cell lines established from BL tissues[4] and was shown to confer immortality to human B lymphocytes.[5] EBV is one of the most widespread of human viruses. The age at which infection occurs is determined by the level of hygiene: Adolescents are infected in affluent countries, whereas individuals in poorly developed countries are infected before the age of 3.[6] The 3 main diseases now associated with EBV infection vary in geographic distribution and with living standards. Infectious mononucleosis (IM), a self-limiting lymphoproliferative disorder, appears in affluent countries; BL, a poorly differentiated lymphocytic lymphoma most frequently located in the jaw, is endemic in central parts of Africa and New Guinea; and nasopharyngeal carcinoma (NPC), an undifferentiated or poorly differentiated carcinoma of the nasopharynx, appears in Southeast Asia. The absence of significant viral strain differences among EBVs in these 3 categories suggests that other factors, such as environment, diet, or genetics, might play a role in the development of EBV-associated cancers in 2 different cell types—lymphocytes and epithelium. EBV also has been implicated in the etiology of cervical and testicular carcinomas and may be sexually transmitted.[44-46,50] Most cases of BL develop in EBV-infected individuals living in tropical regions of Equatorial Africa where there is a high incidence of malaria.

EBV is a large virus containing 33 proteins and a linear double-stranded DNA genome of about 112 kilobase pairs (kbp). After infection of B lymphocytes in vitro, up to 40 newly synthesized viral proteins can be detected. Several of these proteins, both structural and nonstructural, serve as markers for EBV infection. Serological studies demonstrate that 97% of all BL patients carry antibodies to the EBV capsid antigen (VCA) as well as to a viral early antigen (EA).[7] Viral-specific antibodies can be detected in 5-mo-old infants, whereas the peak incidence of BL occurs between ages 6 and 8. The EBV nuclear antigen (EBNA) can be detected by immunofluorescence in BL tumors. Neutralizing antibodies in human sera are directed against EBV membrane antigen (MA). In an attempt to interfere in the pattern of infant infection, the MA glycoprotein is being purified and incorporated into liposomes for use as a vaccine.[8] Monkeys inoculated with a recombinant vaccinia virus expressing the EBV membrane glycoprotein gp340 do not succumb to EBV-induced lymphomas.[51] The preferred treatment for symptomatic BL is a single dose of cyclophosphamide.[9] Only some explanted BL tumor tissues and biopsy specimens express virus. Nearly all, however, contain EBV DNA as a supercoiled episome, a double-stranded linear molecule, or integrated into the chromosomal DNA. BL cells have an activated c-myc oncogene resulting from a translocation of the c-myc proto-oncogene on chromosome 8 to chromosome 14, 2, or 22, where it is placed under control of immunoglobulin promoters and enhancers.[10] Two other oncogenes, N-ras and C-myc, have been found to be activated in BLs and in cell lines established from them.[12] It is possible that EBV might act to promote continued proliferation of B lymphocytes and induce genetic recombinations, thus predisposing these cells to neoplastic transformation. BL is viewed as a model for multistep carcinogenesis where (1) EBV-induced B cell proliferation is aggravated by (2) malarial infection, thereby increasing the population of cells at risk for (3) chromosomal translocations of c-myc that result in unregulated growth.[42]

B cell lymphomas carrying EBV DNA and proteins have been detected in immunodeficient individuals suffering from x-linked lymphoproliferative syndrome, Chediak-Higashi syndrome, ataxia telangiectasia, and severe combined immunodeficiency, including immunosuppressed AIDS patients.[41,48,49]

The evidence linking EBV and NPC is largely seroepidemiological. NPC patients develop high IgG and IgA antibody titers against the VCA and several components of the EA complex.[47] The peak incidence of NPC is seen in Southeast Asian males aged 45–50 yr, and other factors such as exposure to nitrosamines and plant toxins as well as genetic constitution are thought to increase the risk of NPC. NPC cells contain multiple genomes of EBV DNA per cell. Intact virus or viral proteins are detected in cultured specimens or tumor cells passaged in nude mice,[6] and the latent membrane protein is expressed in 65% of fresh NPC tumors analyzed.[43]

Hepatitis B Virus

Primary hepatocellular carcinoma (PHC) is one of the most common cancers in Africa and Southeast Asia. Epidemiological studies show a strong correlation between the occurrence of this hepatoma and persistent infection by hepatitis B virus (HBV) as determined by the presence of high levels of a viral surface antigen (HBsAg or Australia antigen) in the circulating blood of PHC patients.[14,59] The initial HBV infection occurs in an immunologically immature or impaired individual who is unable to provide antibodies to eliminate the infecting virus. The route of infection is thought to be from infected mothers to their young children; subtypes of HBV within a family remain the same.

HBV is a small enveloped virus having a diameter of 45 nM (Dane particle) and containing a circular, partially double-stranded DNA genome of 3.2 kbp within an inner core particle.[15] These particles are found in sera from patients along with a preponderance (1,000-fold greater) of pleiomorphic spherical 22 n*M* particles and some tubular forms. The last 2 forms contain virion proteins, including the HBsAg, but lack viral DNA.

An HBV carrier state is established in an immune-compromised individual when the HBV DNA replicates in infected liver cells. It is estimated that there are 200 million carriers of this virus, and that one out of 250 of them will develop PHC, frequently preceded by chronic hepatitis and cirrhosis.[16,60] Both the low incidence of PHC among carriers and the lack of success in inducing this cancer in HBV-injected laboratory animals have prompted the suggestion that other cofactors are involved in the neoplastic process. Cofactors proposed are age at initial HBV infection, virus dose, and chemicals, such as nitrosamines. PHC tumors usually develop about 35 yr after the carrier state is established. However, 6 cases of childhood primary PHC have been confirmed.[61] Although both males and females are equally susceptible to virus infection and establishment of the carrier state, the incidence of PHC cases is 6-fold higher in males.

The association between persistent HBV infection and PHC is strengthened by the finding that the HBsAg can be identified histologically in normal hepatocytes from the livers of 94% of PHC patients, compared with 3% of non-PHC patients.[17] Hepatoma cells in HBsAg-positive patients cease to express HBsAg. Both episomal and integrated HBV DNA has been detected in cultured PHC cell lines, in PHC tumor and adjacent healthy liver tissue, and in liver tissues from chronic HBV carriers without PHC.[18,60] It is not known what role, if any, viral DNA integration plays in tumor development. The integration appears to be random with regard to the cellular genome as well as the viral genome. No known oncogenes have been implicated, although loss of a putative anti-oncogene on the long arm of chromosome 4 has been proposed.[62]

Prevention of carrier states in up to 85% of treated infants can be effected by administration of an HBV vaccine, although carrier states already established at the time of vaccination are not altered.[19] The HB vaccine is prepared from inactivated HBsAg purified from the 22 n*M* particles present in sera of carriers. Antigenic peptides of HBsAg DNA have been synthesized using sequence information obtained from molecularly cloned HBV DNA, and their effectiveness as vaccines are being tested.

Papilloma Virus

Human papillomavirus (HPV) is best characterized as the agent responsible for the induction of benign squamous epithelial lesions with hyperplasia of the papillae. The epidermis and mucosa of the larynx and the genital area are the most common sites of these lesions, although HPV proteins have been detected in 97% of cases of invasive carcinoma of the colon.[53] Basal layer cells are persistently infected with the episomal form of the virus but do not produce virion components; particle production is noted only in the superficial keratinized portions of papillomas in which the viral genome is integrated into the cellular chromosomes.[41]

Thirty distinct HPV isolates have been described. All contain about 8 kbp of double-stranded DNA in a protein capsid, but only a few of these isolates are associated with malignant transformation. HPV-6 and HPV-11 are associated with laryngeal papillomas that contain HPV particles and viral DNA.[20] Most cases of malignant conversion of these papillomas appear after a course of radiation therapy. HPV-6 and HPV-11 are associated also with anogential warts (condyloma acuminata), and their DNAs have been detected in 40% of cases of cervical dysplasia (CINII or CINIII). There is a low incidence of conversion of condyloma acuminata to a malignant carcinoma of vulva or penis, which can occur about 30 yr after initial detection.

HPV-16 and HPV-18 have been isolated from cervical cancers, and the viral DNAs have been detected in up to 90% of these tumors.[21,22,54] Up to 20% of cases of cervical dysplasia (CINII or CINIII) demonstrate HPV-16- and HPV-18-related DNA sequences. Overall, about 90% of all cervical cancers hybridize to papillomavirus sequences of a variety of subgroups. The presence of HPV-6, HPV-10, and HPV-11 DNAs indicate a low risk for development of cervical cancer, whereas the presence of HPV-16 and HPV-18 DNAs represent a high risk. Both heavy cigarette smoking and herpes simplex virus type 2 infection are considered cofactors for cervical cancer development.[23,52]

Cytomegalovirus

Human cytomegalovirus (HCMV) is a member of the herpes group of viruses. HCMV is ubiquitous in humans, is able to cause persistent latent infections, and can be reactivated in individuals who are immunosuppressed as a result of malignant disease or chemotherapy.[24] The ability of HCMV to transform human fibroblasts in vitro at low efficiencies suggests that this virus might play a role in human malignancies.[25] Various strains of this virus have been isolated from human saliva, urine, blood, milk, cervical secretions, feces, and semen, as well as from a prostate cell line. The HCMV genome consists of about 160 kbp of double-stranded DNA. A portion of the DNA is homologous to sequences of a human pseudogene of the myc oncogene. Two defined fragments, distinct from the myc-related sequences, are able to transform mammalian cells in vitro.[26]

One of the most prevalent tumors of males is adenocarcinoma of the prostate, frequently preceded by benign hypertrophy of the prostate (BHP). Serum antibodies to HCMV and immune lymphocytes cytotoxic to cells bearing CMV-specific membrane antigens are found in nearly 84% of patients with prostate tumors.[27] Analyses of HCMV DNA, messenger RNA, and nuclear and cytoplasmic proteins in normal, BHP, and adenocarcinoma prostate tissues indicate an increased presence of HCMV with increasing abnormality of the tissues. At least 60% of prostatic tumors also show existence of herpes simplex virus macromolecules, raising the possibility that HSV might act as a cofactor with HCMV to induce prostatic malignancies.[28,46]

Kaposi's sarcoma (KS) is a unique and complex tumor found in different forms among Equatorial African blacks, older males from the southern parts of Europe, and in male homosexuals worldwide. HCMV antibodies and virus titers were found in almost all of the European and North American KS cases studied,[29] although exposure to CMV was no higher than that seen in controls.[63] HCMV DNA and antigens are detected in most KS biopsies and established cell lines studied. HCMV has been detected in cervical and vaginal discharges and in cervical biopsy specimens, although serological data do not indicate involvement of this virus with cervical neoplasms. It is possible that HCMV might be adventitiously present in cervical tumors or that it might act as a cofactor in tumor development.[46]

Herpes Simplex Virus Type 2

It has been demonstrated that epithelial abnormalities of the cervical epithelium, atypia or dysplasia, progress to carcinoma *in situ* (CIS) or invasive cancer in 40% of untreated cases. Analyses of women with no evidence of cervical changes and those with preneoplastic or cancerous lesions indicate that both early and frequent sexual activity and hormonal factors are implicated in the progression to invasive carcinoma. The possible involvement of a sexually transmitted infectious agent responsible for the cervical lesions was suggested by the significantly higher levels of antibodies to herpes simplex virus type 2 (HSV-2) proteins in women with cervical cancer than among controls.[30,55,58] HSV-2 RNA and proteins can be detected in > 30% of cervical carcinoma tissues examined.[31,56] Whereas 90% of the seroepidemiological studies suggest an association between HSV-2 and cervical cancer,[32] recent studies have shown no direct correlation between the presence of HSV-2 viral information and development of cervical cancer.[33,57] It has been proposed that the role of HSV-2 in these cancers might be as a cofactor to a carcinogenic agent such as human papillomavirus or cytomegalovirus.[46]

Human T Cell Lymphotropic Virus (HTLV)

Retroviruses, a group of viruses having single-stranded RNA of about 8 kb as their genetic material, induce many types of tumors in animals.[2] These enveloped viruses possess an enzyme, reverse transcriptase, which transcribes the virion RNA into a complementary DNA that is made double-stranded using the DNA polymerase of the infected cell. This double-stranded DNA becomes integrated into the host chromosomes at random sites in a specific orientation with regard to the viral genome.

Epidemiological studies have shown that a rare form of adult T cell lymphoma (ATL) was predominant on 2 islands—Shikoku and Kyushu—in southwestern Japan.[34] Serological analyses demonstrated that patients had high titers of antibodies to components in their tumor cells. These components were later identified as structural proteins of a new human retrovirus that was isolated in the United States from T cell lymphomas in vitro.[35] Isolates of other human T cell lymphotropic viruses (HTLVs) were subsequently made from individuals in widely scattered areas worldwide. Analyses of patients and individuals in endemic areas of the Caribbean, South America, and Japan show that $\leq 5\%$ of the healthy population and 100% of patients with ATL have antibodies against these viruses.[36,64-66] Infection is thought to to occur in childhood by close contact with an infected individual and between adults through sexual activity.[65,66,68] In one study, >25% of the ATL patients were from families with histories of ATL, lymphoma, or other hematopoietic malignancies.[67]

HTLV is able to infect fresh human leukocytes of the OKT-4 phenotype in culture and readily transforms them. The transformed cells become independent of exogenous T cell growth factor (TCGF), express high levels of TCGF receptors on their cell surfaces, grow rapidly, and undergo such morphological alterations as the development of lobulated nuclei and multinucleated giant cells.[37]

Analyses of high-molecular-weight cellular DNAs from tumor cells demonstrate the presence of integrated HTLV provirus. This provirus is not detected in nontumor cells from the same patient or from healthy individuals. In a comparison of virus isolates and proviral DNAs from a variety of sources, no major strain differences were detected, although minor differences in restriction enzyme sites were seen.[38]

The overall genome organization of HTLV is similar to those seen for other retroviruses, consisting of 3 genes encoding the virion structural proteins and reverse transcriptase. However, the HTLV genome has an additional region containing 3 open-reading frames following the env gene, one of which is believed to encode a polypeptide of 42,000 daltons.[39] This polypeptide has been shown to be responsible for transactivation or transcription of the provirus in T lymphocytes and is thought to be responsible for the ability of this virus to successfully replicate in (and transform) T cells.[40]

References

1. Viruses in naturally occurring cancers (Books A & B). In: Cold Spring Harbor Laboratory Conferences on Cell Proliferation. Essex M, Todaro G, zur Hausen H, eds. New York: Cold Spring Harbor Laboratory, 1980.
2. Weiss R, Teich N, Varmus H, Coffin J, eds. RNA tumor viruses (vol 1&2). 2nd ed. New York: Cold Spring Harbor Laboratory, 1984, 1985.
3. Burkitt D. A children's cancer dependent on climatic factors. Nature 1962; 194:232–34.
4. Epstein MA, Achong BG, Barr YM. Virus particles in cultured lymphoblasts from Burkitt's lymphoma. Lancet 1964; i:702–703.
5. Henle W, Diehl V, Kohn G, zur Hausen H, Henle G. Herpes-type radiated Burkitt cells. Science 1967; 157:1064–65.
6. Henle W, Henle G. Epstein-Barr virus and human malignancies. In: G. Klein, ed. Viruses as the causative agents of naturally occurring tumors. Advances in viral oncology, vol 5. New York: Raven Press, 1985; 201–38.
7. Henle G, Henle W, Klein G, et al. Antibodies to early Epstein-Barr virus induced antigens in Burkitt's lymphoma. J Natl Cancer Inst 1971; 46:861–71.

8. Epstein MA, Morgan AJ. Prevention of endemic Burkitt's lymphoma in Africa. In: Lenoir GM, O'Conor GT, Olivery CLM, eds. Burkitt's lymphoma: A human cancer model. France: IARC Scientific Publications no. 60, 1985; 293–302.

9. Oliveny CLM, Nkruma FK. Treatment of Burkitt's lymphoma: the African experience. In: Lenoir GM, O'Conor GT, Olivery CLM, eds. Burkitt's lymphoma: A human cancer model. France: IARC Scientific Publications no. 60, 1985; 375–82.

10. Leder P. Translocations among antibody genes in human cancer. In: Lenoir GM, O'Conor GT, Oliveny CLM, eds. Burkitt's lymphoma: A human cancer model. France: IARC Scientific Publications No. 60, 1985; 341–57.

12. Murray M, Cunningham J, Parada L, Dautry F, Lebowitz P, Weinberg RA. The HL60 transforming sequence: a ras oncogene coexisting with altered myc genes in hematopoietic tumors. Cell 1983; 33:749–57.

13. Henle W, Ho HC, Henle G, Kwan HC. Antibodies to Epstein-Barr virus-related antigens in nasopharyngeal carcinoma. Comparison of active cases with long term survivors. J Natl Cancer Inst 1973; 51:361–69.

14. Melnick JL. Approaching the control of primary liver cancer by means of a virus vaccine. In: Melnick JL, Ochoa S, Oro J, eds. Viruses, oncogenes, and cancer. Basel: Karger, 1985; 22–38.

15. Melnick JL. Hepatitis B virus and liver cancer. In: Phillips LA, ed. Viruses associated with human cancer. New York: Marcel Dekker, 1983; 337–67.

16. Nishioka K. Hepatitis B virus and hepatocellular carcinoma: postulates for an etiological relationship. In: Klein G, ed. Viruses as the causative agents of naturally occurring tumors. Advances in viral oncology, vol 5. New York: Raven Press, 1985; 173–99.

17. Nayak NC, Schdeva R. Localization of hepatitis B surface antigen in conventional paraffin sections of the liver. Am J Pathol 1975; 81:479–92.

18. Miller RH, Lee SC, Liaw YF, Robinson WS. Hepatitis B viral DNA in infected human liver and in hepatocellular carcinoma. J Infect Dis 1985; 151:1081–92.

19. World Health Organization report. Prevention of hepatocellular carcinoma by immunization. WHO bull 61, 1983; 731–44.

20. Gissmann L, Wolnick L, Ikenberg H, et al. Human papillomavirus type 6 and 11 DNA sequences in genital and laryngeal papillomas and some clinical cancers. Proc Natl Acad Sci USA 1983; 80:560–63.

21. Durst MI, Gissmann L, Ikenberg H, zur Hausen H. A papilloma-virus DNA from a cervical carcinoma and its prevalence in cancer biopsy samples from different geographic regions. Proc Natl Acad Sci USA 1983; 80:3812–15.

22. Boshart M, Gissmann L, Ikenberg H, Kleinheim Z, Scheurlen W, zur Hausen H. A new type of papillomavirus DNA, its presence in genital cancer biopsies and in cell lines derived from cervical cancer. EMBO J 1984; 3:1151–57.

23. Zur Hausen H. Human genital cancer: synergism between two virus infections or synergism between a virus infection and initiating event. Lancet 1982; ii:1370–72.

24. Stagno S, Reynolds DW, Huang ES, Thames SD, Smith RJ, Alford Jr CA. Congenital cytomegalovirus infection: occurrence in an immune population. N Engl J Med 1977; 296:1254–58.

25. Geder L, Lausch R, O'Neill F, Rapp F. Oncogenic transformation of human embryo lung cells by human cytomegalovirus. Science 1976; 192:1134–37.

26. Spector DH, Spector SA. The oncogenic potential of human cytomegalovirus. In: Melnick JL, ed. Progress in medical virology, vol 29. Basel: Karger, 1984; 45–89.

27. Dagen JE, Sanford EJ, Rohner TJ, Geder L, Rapp F. Recognition of virally transformed cells by lymphocytes from patients with prostatic cancer. Urology 1978; 12:532–36.

28. Huang ES, Boldogh I, Mar EC. Human cytomegaloviruses: evidence for possible association with human cancer. In: Phillips LA, ed. Viruses associated with human cancer. New York: Marcel Dekker, 1983; 161–94.

29. Giraldo G, Beth E, Henle W, et al. Antibody patterns to herpes viruses in Kaposi's sarcoma. II. Serological association of American Kaposi's sarcoma with cytomegalovirus. Int J Cancer 1978; 22:126–31.

30. Gillman SC, Docherty JJ, Clarke A, Rawls WE. Reaction pattern of herpes simplex virus type 1 and type 2 proteins with sera of patients with uterine cervical carcinoma and matched controls. Cancer Res 1980; 40:4640–47.

31. McDougall JK, Crum CP, Fenoglio CM, Goldstein LC, Galloway DA. Herpres virus-specific RNA and protein in carcinoma of the uterine cervix. Proc Natl Acad Sci USA 1982; 79:3853–57.

32. Rapp R. The challenge of herpes viruses. Cancer Res 1984; 44:1309–15.

33. Vonka V, Kanka J, Hirsch I, et al. Prospective study on the relationship between cervical neoplasia and herpes simplex type 2. II. Herpes simplex type 2 antibody presence in sera taken at enrollment. Int J Cancer 1984; 33:61–66.

34. Takatsuki K, Uchijama T, Sagawa K, Yodoi J. Adult T cell leukemia in Japan. In: Seno S, Takaku F, Irino S, eds. Topics in hematology. Amsterdam: Excerpta Medica, 1984; 73–77.

35. Poiesz, BJ, Ruscetti FW, Gazdar AF, Bunn PA, Minna JD, Gallo RC. Detection and isolation of type C retrovirus particles from fresh and cultured lymphocytes of a patient with cutaneous T cell lymphoma. Proc Natl Acad Sci USA 1980; 77:7415–19.

36. Salahuddin SZ, Markham PD, Wong-Staal F, Gallo RC. The human T-cell leukemia-lymphoma virus family. In: Viruses, Oncogenes, and Cancer. Melnick JL, Ochoa S, Oro J, eds. Viruses, oncogenes, and cancer. Progress in medical virology, vol 32. Basel: Karger, 1985; 195–211.

37. Popovic M, Gunhild, LW, Sarin PS, Mann D, Gallo RC. Transformation of human umbilical cord blood T cells by human T-cell leukemia/lymphoma virus. Proc Natl Acad Sci USA 1983; 80:5402–06.

38. Wong-Staal F, Hahn B, Magasi V, et al. A survey of human leukemias for sequences of a human retrovirus, HTLV. Nature 1983; 302:626–28.

39. Seiki M, Hattoari S, Hirayama Y, Yoshida M. Human adult T cell leukemia virus: complete nucleotide sequence of the provirus genome integrated in leukemia cell DNA. Proc Natl Acad Sci USA 1983; 80:3618–22.

40. Sodroski JG, Rosen CA, Haseltine WA. Trans-acting transcriptional activation of the long terminal repeat of human T-lymphotropic viruses in infected cells. Science 1984; 225:381–85.

41. Raab-Traub N. The human DNA tumor viruses: human papilloma virus and Epstein-Barr virus. Cancer Treat Res 1989; 47:285–302.

42. Goldstein JA, Bernstein RL. Burkitt's lymphoma and the role of Epstein-Barr virus. J Trop Pediatr 1990; 36:114–20.

43. Fahraeus R, Fu HL, Ernberg I, et al. Expression of Epstein-Barr virus-encoded proteins in nasopharyngeal carcinoma. Int J Cancer 1988; 42:329–38.

44. Turner MJ, White JO, Soutter WP. Human seminal plasma inhibits the lymphocyte response to infection with Epstein-Barr virus. Gynecol Oncol 1990; 37:60–65.

45. Singh P, Ilancheran A, Ratnam SS, Kim LT, O'Reilly AP. Cervical adenocarcinoma in women with nasopharyngeal carcinoma (NPC). Cancer 1989; 64:1152–55.

46. Schmauz R, Okong P, deVilliers EM, et al. Multiple infections in cases of cervical cancer from a high-incidence area in tropical Africa. Int J Cancer 1989; 43:805–09.

47. Cevenini R, Donati M, Moroni A, et al. Specific Epstein-Barr virus serological response in patients with nasopharyngeal carcinoma detected by immunoblotting. Eur J Epidemiol 1988; 4:301–05.

48. Kersey, JH, Shapiro, RS, Filipovitch, AH. Relationship of immunodeficiency to lymphoid malignancy. Pediatr Infect Dis J 1988; 7 (suppl):S10–12.

49. Harrington DS, Weisenburger DD, Purtilo DT. Epstein-Barr virus-associated lymphoproliferative lesions. Clin Lab Med 1988: 8:97–118.

50. Algood CB, Newell GR, Johnson DE. Viral etiology of testicular tumors. J Urol 1988; 139:308–10.

51. Morgan AJ, Mackett M, Finerty S, et al. Recombinant vaccinia virus expressing Epstein-Barr virus glycoprotein gp340 protects cottontop tamarins against EB virus-induced malignant lymphomas. J Med Virol 1988; 35:189–95.

52. Bosch FX, Cardis E. Cancer incidence correlations: genital, urinary and some tobacco-related cancers. Int J Cancer 1990; 46:178–84.

53. Kirgan D, Manalo P, McGregor B. Immunohistochemical demonstration of human colon neoplasms. J Surg Res 1990; 48:397–402.

54. Van den Brule AJ, Claas EC, du Maine M, et al. Use of anticontamination primers in the polymerase chain reaction for the detection of human papilloma virus genotypes in cervical scrapes and biopsies. J Med Virol 1989; 29:20–27.

55. Corbino N, Guglielmino S, Petrina M, et al. The role of anti-herpes specific serum IgA levels as a marker in cervical oncogenesis. Eur J Gynaecol Oncol 1989; 10:103–08.

56. Gupta MM, Sharma BK, Singh V, Luthra UK. Immunocytological demonstration of HSV-II antigen on exfoliated cells from precancerous and cancerous lesions of the uterine cervix. Diagn Cytopathol 1988; 4:48–49.

57. Matiland, NJ. The aitiological relationship between herpes simplex virus type 2 and carcinoma of the cervix: an unanswered or unanswerable question? Cancer Surv 1988; 7:457–67.

58. Kjaer SK, de Villiers EM, Haugaard BJ, et al. Human papillomavirus, herpes simples virus and cervical cancer incidence in Greenland and Denmark. A population-based cross-sectional study. Int J Cancer 1988; 41:518–24.

59. Lu SN, Lin TM, Chen CJ, et al. A case-control study of primary hepatocellular carcinoma in Taiwan. Cancer 1988; 62:2051–55.

60. Wogan GN. Dietary risk factors for primary hepatocellular carcinoma. Cancer Detect Prev. 1989; 14:209–13.

61. Cheah PL, Looi LM, Lin HP, Yap SF. Childhood primary hepatocellular carcinoma and hepatitis B virus infection. Cancer 1990; 65:174–76.

62. Buetow KH, Murray JC, Israel JL, et al. Loss of heterozygosity suggests tumor suppressor gene responsible for primary hepatocellular carcinoma. Proc Natl Acad Sci USA 1989; 86:8852–56.

63. Bendsoe N, Dictor M, Blomberg J, Agren S, Merk K. Increased incidence of Kaposi sarcoma in Sweden before the AIDS epidemic. Eur J Cancer 1990; 26:699–702.

64. Andrada-Serpa MJ, Tosswill J, Schor D, et al. Seroepidemiologic survey for antibodies to human retroviruses in human and non-human primates in Brazil. Int J Cancer 1989; 44:389–93.

65. Tajima K. Malignant lymphomas in Japan: epidemiological analysis of adult T-cell leukemia/lyphoma (ATL). Cancer Metastasis Rev 1988; 7:223–41.

66. Reeves WC, Saxinger C, Brenes MM, et al. Human T-cell lymphotropic virus type I (HTLV-I) seroepidemiology and risk factors in metropolitan Panama. Am J Epidemiol 1988; 127:532–39.

67. Tajima K. The 4th nation-wide study of adult T-cell leukemia/lymphoma (ATL) in Japan: estimates of risk of ATL and its geographical and clinical features. Int J Cancer 1990; 45:237–43.

68. Kondo T, Kono H, Miyamoto N, et al. Age- and sex-specific cumulative rate and risk of ATL for HTLV-1 carriers. Int J Cancer 1989: 43:1061–1064.

3

DOMINANT AND RECESSIVE ONCOGENES: CLINICAL APPLICATIONS IN MALIGNANCY

Dorothy L. Buchhagen, Ph.D.

ANALYSES OF THE GENETIC changes that occur during the progression of a cell from normal to neoplastic serve as the basis for molecular oncology. The observation from human pedigrees of an inherited familial predisposition to certain forms of cancer helped form the notion of "cancer genes."[1] The isolation and identification of cancer genes, or oncogenes, by several experimental approaches established a genetic basis for cancer.

Dominant Oncogenes

An oncogene is a gene that is capable of transforming a normal cell to a neoplastic phenotype; oncogenes act in a dominant fashion. Genetic sequences that can initiate and maintain neoplastic transformation were identified in the early 1970s in avian retroviruses (tumor viruses having RNA as their genetic material). As an example, Rous sarcoma virus induces sarcomas in chickens; the oncogene carried by this virus is called src.[2] To date, 27 different oncogenes have been discovered in retroviruses isolated from chickens and other birds, mice, rats, cats, monkeys, and humans. They cause carcinomas, sarcomas, leukemias, and lymphomas. These retroviral oncogenes, the species of animals the retroviruses were isolated from, and the diseases they induce are listed in table 3-1.

In 1976, it was discovered that the src gene is not a viral gene. Rather, it is a normal cellular chicken gene (proto-oncogene) that had been picked up, or transduced, by a retrovirus and had become activated during the process.[3] Further investigations have shown that all retroviral oncogenes have cellular

Table 3-1. Retroviral Oncogenes

Oncogene	Species of origin	Tumorigenicity
src	Chicken	Sarcoma
fps/fes	Chicken/cat	Sarcoma
yes	Chicken	Sarcoma
ski	Chicken	Sarcoma
myc	Chicken	Carcinoma, sarcoma, myelocytoma
crk	Chicken	Sarcoma
jun	Chicken	Sarcoma
erb A	Chicken	Erythroleukemia, sarcoma
erb B	Chicken	Erythroblastosis, myeloblastosis
ets	Chicken	Erythroid/myeloid leukemia
myb	Chicken	Myeloblastic leukemia
mil/raf	Chicken/mouse	Sarcoma
rel	Turkey	Lymphatic leukemia
ros	Turkey	Sarcoma
mos	Mouse	Sarcoma
abl	Mouse/cat	B-cell lymphoma
fos	Mouse	Sarcoma
Ha-ras/bas	Rat/mouse	Sarcoma, erythroleukemia
Ki-ras	Rat	Sarcoma, erythroleukemia
fms	Cat	Sarcoma
fgr	Cat	Rhabdomyosarcoma
kit	Cat	Sarcoma
sis	Monkey	Sarcoma
tax-1	Human	Adult T cell lymphoma

counterparts.[4,31-33] However, oncogenes, or activated proto-oncogenes, not associated with retroviruses were isolated from human and animal tumors in experiments done in several laboratories in the late 1970s and early 1980s.[5-7] These oncogenes were detected by adding DNAs extracted from tumors to NIH3T3 cells, an established line of mouse fibroblasts, in tissue culture.

In these gene-transfer experiments, the added DNA is taken up by the cells and stably incorporated in the chromosomes. Foci of transformed cells appear in the monolayers, indicating that an active oncogene has been introduced into the cells. Many of the oncogenes detected by this approach belong to the ras family, which consists of oncogenes acquired from the rat genome by rat and mouse sarcoma viruses. Also included in the ras family are oncogenes that have a high degree of nucleic acid homology to the retrovirally transduced ras oncogenes. Three members of this ras group are found to be activated in several specific human cancers. Harvey ras (Ha-ras) is activated in bladder, lung, and mammary carcinomas; Kirsten ras (Ki-ras) is activated in colon, lung, bladder, and pancreatic carcinomas and in sarcomas; N-ras is activated in neuroblastomas, melanomas, lung and colon carcinomas, and sarcomas.[8,32,34-36] Although a few new oncogenes have been isolated using the DNA transfection assay, most oncogenes detected are the same as, or closely related to, those found in retroviruses. Several new oncogenes have been identified by hybridization of genome DNA or cDNA with known oncogene probes and by activation following integration of a retrovirus proviral DNA near by.[31-33]

Several lines of evidence indicate that the number of proto-oncogenes resident in the human genome is limited. First, the same (or closely related) oncogenes have been detected in several independent isolates of retroviruses and in independent gene transfer experiments from the same animal species. Second, the same or closely related oncogenes are found in retroviruses and in DNA transfer experiments from different animal species. Third, some retroviruses contain 2 oncogenes, 1 or both found individually in retroviruses. These repeated transductions and isolations of the same or related oncogenes suggest that the number of proto-oncogenes is small, perhaps <50 per genome. To date, nearly 40 oncogenes have been isolated by all methods.

Analyses of DNAs from a diverse selection of organisms show that proto-oncogenes are present and expressed as messenger RNA and proteins in yeast, slime molds, and fruit flies, as well as in fish, amphibians, reptiles, birds, and mammals, including humans.[9,33] Such a high degree of conservation over a period of >600 million yr indicates that the protein products of the proto-oncogenes must be vital to the functioning of normal cells.

Two of the most pressing questions relating to the molecular biology of the cancer problem are how proto-oncogenes are activated to become oncogenes and how oncogenes cause tumors.

Activation of Proto-Oncogenes

Activation of proto-oncogenes can be induced by four mechanisms: insertional mutagenesis, gene mutation, chromosomal translocation, and gene amplification.

Insertional Mutagenesis

Not all retroviruses carry oncogenes, yet those lacking oncogenes are able to induce tumors. Retroviruses are converted to double-stranded DNA copies of the RNA genome shortly after infecting a cell. These DNA copies (proviruses) are inserted randomly into the chromosomes. One possible consequence of this random insertion, or integration, could be the placement of proviral regulatory sequences near cellular genes, thereby influencing the expression of those genes. This phenomenon has been documented in chicken bursal lymphomas, where many avian leukemia viruses have integrated into the DNA near the proto-oncogene myc, enhancing its expression.[10] The DNAs of retroviruses that induce mammary carcinomas and leukemias in mice integrate into defined regions of DNA and activate specific unidentified cellular genes.[11,12] It is believed that these activated cellular genes contribute to cellular transformation.

Gene Mutation

A gene is a linear array of bases (deoxynucleoside triphosphates) dictating the amino acid content of a protein. A mutation in 1 or more of the bases might result in an altered protein. A change in an important functional domain of the protein could have a profound impact on the ability of that protein to perform its normal role. Mutations can be introduced by a variety of environmental hazards (X rays, chemical carcinogens, ultraviolet light) as well as by mistakes that can occur during the normal enzymatic replication of the DNA. Using the technique of DNA sequence analysis of molecularly cloned oncogenes, several laboratories have determined that Ki-ras oncogenes isolated from a variety of human tumors have an alteration in the codon for amino acid 13, 59, or 61 when compared with the normal proto-oncogene. The human Ha-ras and N-ras oncogenes are also mutated in 1 of the same 3 codons in tumor DNAs.[32,34-36]

Chromosomal Translocations

This activation of proto-oncogenes most likely results from removing the proto-oncogene from normal control elements that regulate its function or from placing it under the control of a strong transcriptional promoter. It has been observed experimentally that several molecularly-cloned proto-oncogenes are transforming when placed under the control of retroviral promoters present in the long terminal repeats.[13,14] In addition, chromosomal translocations have been observed in a variety of human tumors, and it is now known that proto-oncogenes map to the break points for many of these translocations.[37,38] This correlation was first noted for the myc oncogene, which is located on human chromosome 8 and is translocated to chromosome 14 in Burkitt's lymphoma cells.[15] In its new location on chromosome 14, the myc oncogene comes under the control of a transcriptional element within the immunoglobulin heavy chain locus; myc expression increases dramatically. Other translocations found in human tumors and the proto-oncogenes mapped to them are listed in table 3-2.

Table 3-2. Some Translocations of Human Tumors and Proto-Oncogenes Mapped to Them

Proto-oncogene	Human tumor	Translocation
myc	Burkitt's lymphoma	t (8:14)
	Acute lymphoblastic leukemia	t (2:8)
	Acute myeloblastic leukemia	t (8:15)
	Renal cell carcinoma	t (3:8)
mos	Acute nonlymphocytic leukemia	t (8:21)
	Acute myeloblastic leukemia	t (8:21)
abl	Chronic myelogenous leukemia	t (9:22)
fes	Acute promyelocytic leukemia	t (15:17)
sis	Chronic myelogenous leukemia	t (9:22)
	Burkitt's lymphoma	t (8:22)
myb	Ovarian carcinoma	t (6:14)

Activation of these proto-oncogenes can occur if they are moved adjacent to transcriptional control sequences or if they are dissociated from sequences that repress their expression.

Gene Amplification

In addition to insertional activation, mutation, and translocation, proto-oncogenes can transform cells when their protein products are present in dosages higher than normal. Many tumor cells contain amplified proto-oncogenes in the form of extremely small pieces of chromosomes called double minutes or homogenously staining regions on chromosomes. The abl and myc oncogenes have been shown to be amplified and expressed in human chronic myelogenous leukemias and neuroblastomas, respectively.[16,17] Amplified proto-oncogene expression may be related to development of a more malignant phenotype, as has been observed in certain lung tumors. The variant type of small-cell carcinoma of the lung can have 20–75 times as much myc DNA as normal lung cells.[18]

Proto-Oncogene Proteins

Because all known oncogenes are derived from proto-oncogenes that are expressed at some time in normal cells, it should be possible to approach an understanding of neoplasia by elucidating the roles of the proto-oncogene proteins. The proto-oncogenes can be organized into 4 groups on the basis of the functions and cellular localizations of their protein products. In some instances, specific biochemical differences between the normal and oncogenic forms of the proteins have been determined.

Nonreceptor Tyrosine Kinases

Tyrosine kinases are tyrosine-specific phosphokinases that are located in the cytoplasm or in cytoplasmic membranes; they include the src, yes, fgr, abl, fps/fes, lyn, lck, fyn, hck, tkl, crk and ros proteins. Phosphorylation of tyrosine residues is rare in normal cells but is increased >10-fold in transformed cells, with some specific proteins demonstrating >20-fold increase. It is unknown how tyrosine phosphorylation effects cellular transformation, but it may be through the ability of 1 kinase to alter numerous substrates, thereby controlling cell growth and division. Among the known specific targets of this tyrosine phosphorylation are vinculin, a protein that anchors actin filaments in adhesion plaques, 3 enzymes in the glycolytic pathway (enolase, phosphoglycerate mutase, and lactate dehydrogenase), and a 36,000-dalton plasma membrane-associated protein (p36).[19] The function of each of these proteins is altered following phosphorylation.

Growth Factor Receptor-Tyrosine and Serine/Threonine Kinases and Growth Factors

Members of this category of proto-oncogenes possess DNA sequence homology to nonreceptor tyrosine kinases, yet their products may or may not exhibit the tyrosine kinase activity. This class includes erb-A, erb-B, fms, mil/raf, rel, sis, neu, met, kit, trk, and mos, whose products are located in the cytoplasm or in cytoplasmic membranes. The erb-B protein is a truncated form of the receptor for epidermal growth factor (EGF), and the fms protein appears to encode an altered cell surface receptor for colony-stimulating factor-1 (CSF-1) that is responsible for macrophage proliferation.[20,21] The proto-oncogene product, sis, is 1 subunit of the platelet-derived growth factor.[22] The growth factor connection of 3 oncogene products provides clues as to how transformed cells may be able to grow uncontrollably. The erb-B protein lacks the EGF-binding domain and can function independently of an EGF signal. Therefore, its growth-stimulating activity is unregulated. The fms protein also may be able to act independently of bound CSF-1. The sis protein is secreted from transformed cells and is thus present at higher than normal levels to provide a continuous proliferation signal. Some members of this group, such as mos, mil/raf, and rel, are serine/threonine kinases.

GTP-Binding Proteins

The ras proto-oncogene family comprises group 3, the members being Ha-ras/bas, Ki-ras, and N-ras. The products of all 3 proto-oncogenes are 21,000-dalton guanosine triphosphate (GTP)-splitting proteins (p21s) that are located on the inner surface of the plasma membrane.[23,25] They are thought to activate adenylate cyclase, the enzyme that catalyzes the formation of cyclic adenosine monophosphate (AMP) from adenosine triphosphate (ATP) when hormones or neurotransmitters bind to specific cell surface receptors. It is unclear how the ras proteins activate adenylate cyclase. It has been observed that the oncogenic ras p21 proteins have lost the ability to split GTP to guanosine diphosphate (GDP) and p_i and retain GTP much longer than normal p21 proteins.[39] This retention of the reaction product might result in the continuous transmission of a proliferation signal that contributes to cellular transformation.

Nuclear Proteins

Proto-oncogenes whose products are found in the nucleus are assigned to group 4 and include fos, myc, myb, ski, jun, rel, ets, and tax-1. The most intensively studied of these is the myc protein. The myc proto-oncogene product is induced in normal cells by treatment with growth factors; it appears before the onset of DNA replication and binds to DNA.[24] Increased synthesis of myc protein in transformed cells may serve to immortalize the cell by forcing the DNA to undergo continuous rounds of replication. Table 3-3 presents a summary of the classification of the oncogenes.

Table 3-3. Summary of Oncogene Classifications

Group	Proto-oncogene	Product	Localization
1	src, yes, fgr, abl, fps/fes, ros, lck, fyn, hck, tkl, crk	Nonreceptor tyrosine kinase	Cytoplasm
2	erb-B, mil/raf, sis, fms, mos, erb-A, neu, rel, met, kit, trk	Growth factor receptor tyrosine and serine/threonine kinases	Cytoplasm, cytoplasmic membrane
	sis	Growth factor	Cytoplasmic membrane
3	Ha-ras/bas, Ki-ras, N-ras	GTP-binding protein	Plasma membrane (inner surface)
4	fos, myc, myb, jun, rel, ski, ets, tax-1	DNA-binding protein	Nucleus

Recessive Oncogenes

During the past several years, a new class of genes involved in tumorigenesis has been described.[40-43] Since 1 normal copy of these genes protects cells against malignant transformation, members of this class of genes are referred to as recessive oncogenes, tumor suppressors, or antioncogenes.[42,44] Predisposition to cancer results from the recessive nature of these genes and represents the inheritance of 1 defective copy of such a gene followed by mutation or loss of the normal copy. The existence of these genes was postulated to explain the appearance of childhood retinoblastoma,[45] and the retinoblastoma (RB1) gene at human chromosome 13q14 was the first tumor suppressor gene identified.[46,47]

The RB1 gene product is a DNA-binding protein of about 110 kd (pRB) located in the nucleus. It is expressed in all cell types and is phosphorylated at multiple sites prior to cell division at the transition from G-1 to S.[48,49] Transforming proteins of several DNA viruses can complex with the pRB to inactivate it, resulting in uncontrolled growth of the cell. These transforming proteins are SV40 virus large T antigen,[49] adenovirus E1a protein,[50] and papillomavirus E7 protein.[51]

Other Candidate-Recessive Oncogenes

Since the identification and characterization of the pRB, several other putative recessive oncogenes have been defined. The wild type p53 recessive oncogene, encoded by a gene at human chromosome 17p13, is a tumor suppressor, whereas mutants of p53 act as dominant oncogenes.[52] Wild type p53 is a nuclear protein active during the G-0 to G-1 phase of cell division. It is inactivated by binding to SV40 large T Ag,[53] to adenovirus E1b protein,[53] to papillomavirus E6,[64] and to mutated p53, with which it forms heterodimers.[54] Recent identifications of 2 additional human recessive oncogenes include the Wilms' tumor gene at 11p14[55,56] and the DCC gene, first detected as a frequent deletion in colon carcinoma at chromosome 8q22.[57]

Chromosomal Locations of Proposed Recessive Oncogenes

Cytogenetic analyses of human tumor cell lines and loss of heterozygosity studies on DNAs from tumors and tumor cell lines have delineated a number of other chromosomal regions thought to harbor recessive oncogenes. Among these regions are: 3p in lung,[58] uterine cervical,[59] and renal cell[60] carcinomas; 9p in various leukemias;[61] 5q21-q22 in familial adenomatous polyposis;[62] and 1p in multiple endocrine neoplasia (MEN2).[63]

Dominant and Recessive Oncogenes: Roles in Carcinogenesis (General View)

Cells become transformed when normal cellular genes (proto-oncogenes) are mutated to have altered functions or are rearranged so that they escape their usual regulatory mechanisms. Cells can also be transformed if both copies of a recessive oncogene, or tumor suppressor gene, are inactivated. Continued growth and division of a transformed call results in a clone of identical cells, which form a tumor. Numerous investigators have hypothesized that cancer is a multistep process in which a cell progresses from premalignant to malignant *in situ* to metastatic.[26,27] Results from recent oncogene research support the hypothesis that both tumor genesis and tumor progression involve multiple genetic alterations in both dominant and recessive oncogenes. It is important to note that DNA tumor viruses (adenovirus, papillomavirus) implicated as etiologic agents in some human cancers encode transforming proteins that inactivate known tumor suppressor genes.[31-33]

An analysis of a large number of human tumors for messenger RNA expression of proto-oncogenes showed that more than 1 oncogene was expressed in 52/54 tumors analyzed, with some tumors expressing 7/9 oncogenes studied.[28] This expression was amplified in the malignant tissue in comparison to the normal tissue. These results indicate that the cancer process is more complex than overexpression or alteration of 1 or 2 oncogenes. Because this study focused on developed tumors, no information regarding an ordered sequence of expression of the oncogenes was obtained.

Two groups of researchers have demonstrated that single oncogenes are unable to transform cells cultured immediately after being taken from animals.[29,30] However, certain pairs of oncogenes such as myc and ras can cooperate to transform such cells. Other "transforming" proteins fall into complementation groups based on their ability to interact with either myc or ras to transform these cells. It is postulated that the myc gene product, a DNA-binding protein, functions to immortalize the cell, whereas the ras protein, which is localized to the plasma membrane, provides a transforming function.

Recently, a human DNA gene, Nm 23, which maps to human chromosone 17q and whose expression is inversely correlated with metastatic capabilities, was isolated.[26] The interpretation of the data is that the protein product of this gene, which has amino acid sequence homology with a Drosophila gene that regulates development, may be involved in preventing an early step of metastasis, such as malignant invasion.[65] Other DNA sequences may be involved in later steps in the metastatic process.

Future Prospects

The picture that is emerging from oncogene research is that cancer is the result of aberrations in normal cell processes. The aberrations that have been documented are intracellular events ranging from catastrophic alterations such as chromosomal translocations to seemingly trivial single-base changes in the DNA. Yet the effects on the cells in which these changes occur are dramatic; they lose their contact inhibition of movement and division, growing to much higher saturation densities at a faster rate than their normal neighbors. They gain the ability to grow in reduced nutrients and at lower CO_2 tensions. They begin to grow independently of a solid substrate and eventually metastasize to distant sites. Each of these properties may reflect one or more distinct genetic changes. The fact that cell transformation results from normal processes run amok gives the basic scientist a convenient tool for understanding how a normal cell functions. By deciphering how dominant oncogenes transform cells and how recessive oncogenes protect cells against transformation, we may be able to understand how cancer from all causes arises and how it can be prevented.

References

1. Li RF, Fraumeni JR Jr. Soft-tissue sarcomas, breast cancer, and other neoplasms: a familial syndrome? Ann Intern Med 1969; 71:747–52.
2. Wang L-H, Duesberg P, Beemon K, Vogt PK. Mapping RNAse T resistant oligonucleotides of avian tumor viruses RNAs: Sarcoma-specific oligonucleotides are near the poly (A) end and oligonucleotides common to sarcoma and transformation-defective viruses are at the poly (A) end. J Virol 1975; 16:1051–70.
3. Stehelin D, Varmus HE, Bishop JM, Vogt PK. DNA related to the transforming gene(s) of avian sarcoma viruses is present in normal avian DNA. Nature 1976; 260:170–73.
4. Weiss R, Teich N, Varmus HE, Coffin J, eds. RNA tumor viruses. Cold Spring Harbor (NY): Cold Spring Harbor Press, 1982.
5. Shih C, Shilo B-Z, Goldfarb MP, Dannenberg A, Weinberg RA. Passage of phenotypes of chemically transformed cells via transfection of DNA and chromatin. Proc Natl Acad Sci USA 1979; 76:5714–18.
6. Goldfarb M, Shimizu K, Perucho M, Wigler M. Isolation and preliminary characterization of a human transforming gene from T24 bladder carcinoma cells. Nature 1982; 296:404–9.
7. Pulciani S, Santos E, Lauver AV, Long LK, Robbins KC, Barbacid M. Oncogenes in human tumor cell lines: Molecular cloning of a transforming gene from human bladder carcinoma cells. Proc Natl Acad Sci USA 1982; 79:2845–49.

8. Varmus HE. The molecular genetics of cellular oncogenes. Annu Rev Genet 1984; 18:553–612.
9. Weiss R, Teich N, Varmus HE, Coffin J, eds. RNA tumor viruses: supplement. Cold Spring Harbor (NY): Cold Spring Harbor Press, 1985.
10. Hayward WS, Neel BG, Astrin SM. Activation of a cellular oncogene by promotor insertion in ALV-induced lymphoid leukosis. Nature 1981; 290:475–79.
11. Nusse R, Varmus HE. Many tumors induced by the mouse mammary tumor virus contain a provirus integrated in the same region of the host genome. Cell 1982; 31:99–109.
12. Cuypers HT, Selten G, Quint W, et al. Murine leukemia virus-induced T-cell lymphomagenesis: integration of proviruses in a distinct chromosomal region. Cell 1984; 37:141–50.
13. Blair DG, Oskarsson M, Wood TG, McClements WL, Fischinger PJ, VanderWoude GG. Activation of the transforming potential of a normal cell sequence: a molecular model for oncogenesis. Science 1981; 212:941–43.
14. DeFeo D, Gonda MA, Young HA, et al. Analysis of two divergent rat genomic clones homologous to the transforming gene of Harvey murine sarcoma virus. Proc Natl Acad Sci USA 1981; 78:3328–32.
15. Dalla-Favera R, Bregni M, Erickson J, Patterson D, Gallo RC, Croce CM. Human c-myc oncogene is located on the region of chromosome 8 that is translocated in Burkitt lymphoma cells. Proc Natl Acad Sci USA 1982; 79:7824–27.
16. Collins S, Groudine M. Rearrangement and amplification of c-abl sequences in the human chronic myelogenous leukemia cell line K-562. Proc Natl Acad Sci USA 1983; 80:4813–17.
17. Kohl NE, Kanda N, Schreck RR, et al. Transposition and amplification of oncogene-related sequences in human neuroblastomas. Cell 1984; 35:359–67.
18. Little CD, Nau MM, Carney DN, Gazdar AF, Minna JD. Amplification and expression of the c-myc oncogene in human lung cancer cell lines. Nature 1983; 306:194–96.
19. Cooper JA, Hunter T. Regulation of cell growth and transformation by tyrosine-specific protein kinases: the search for important cellular substrate proteins. Curr Top Microbiol Immunol 1983; 107:125–161.
20. Downward J, Yarden Y, Mayes E, et al. Close similarity of epidermal growth factor receptor and v-erb-B oncogene protein sequences. Nature 1984; 307:521–27.
21. Sherr CJ, Rettenmeier CW, Sacca R, et al. The c-fms proto-oncogene product is related to the receptor for the mononuclear phagocyte growth factor, CSF-1. Cell 1985; 41:665–76.
22. Doolittle RF, Hunkapiller MW, Hood LE, Devare LG, Robbins KC, et al. Simian sarcoma virus oncogene is derived from the gene (or genes) encoding a platelet-derived growth factor. Science 1983; 221:275–76.
23. Papageorge A, Lowy D, Scolnick EM. Comparative biochemical properties of p21 ras molecules coded for by viral and cellular ras genes. J Virol 1982; 44:509–19.
24. Kelly K, Cochran BH, Stiles CD, Leder P. Cell-specific regulation of the c-myc gene by lymphocyte mitogens and platelet-derived growth factor. Cell 1983; 35:603–10.
25. Grand RJA, Smith KJ, Gallimore PH. Purification and characterization of the protein encoded by the activated human N-ras gene and its membrane localisation. Oncogene 1987; 1:305–07.
26. Steeg PS, Bevilacqua G, Kopper L, et al. Evidence for a novel gene associated with low tumor metastatic potential. JNCI 1988: 80:200–04.
27. Farber E, Cameron B. The sequential analysis of cancer development. Adv Cancer Res 1980; 31:124–226.
28. Slamon DJ, deKernion JB, Verma IM, Cline MJ. Expression of cellular oncogenes in human malignancies. Science 1984; 224:256–62.
29. Land H, Parada LF, Weinberg RA. Tumorigenic conversion of primary embryo fibroblasts requires at least two cooperating oncogenes. Nature 1983; 304:596–602.
30. Ruley HE. Adenovirus early region 1A enables viral and cellular transforming genes to transform primary cells in culture. Nature 1983; 304:602–6.
31. Weinberg RA. Oncogenes and the molecular origins of cancer. Cold Spring Harbor, N.Y.: Cold Spring Harbor Press, 1989.
32. Cooper GM. Oncogenes. Boston: Jones and Bartlett, 1990.

33. Pimentel E. Oncogenes. 2nd ed. Boca Raton, Fla.: CRC Press, 1989.
34. Reddy EP, Reynolds RK, Santos E, Barbacid M. A point mutation is responsible for the acquisition of transforming properties by the T24 human bladder oncogene. Nature (London) 1982; 300:149–152.
35. Capon DJ, Chen, EJ, Levinson AD, Seeburg PH, Goeddel DV. Complete nucleotide sequences of the T24 human bladder carcinoma oncogene and its normal homologue. Nature (London) 1982; 302:33–37.
36. Pulciani S, Santos E, Lauver AV, Long LK, Aaronson SA, Barbacid M. Oncogenes in solid human tumors. Nature 1982; 300:149–52.
37. Nowell PC, Croce CM. Chromosomal approaches to oncogenes and oncogenesis. FASEB J 1988; 2: 3054–60.
38. Sandberg AA. The chromosomes in human cancer and leukemia. 2nd ed. New York: Elsevier, 1990.
39. Gibbs JB, Sigal IS, Poe M, Scolnick EM. Intrinsic GTPase activity distinguishes normal and oncogenic ras p21 molecules. Proc Natl Acad Sci USA 1984; 81:5704–08.
40. Klein G. The approaching era of the tumor suppressor genes. Science 1987; 238:1539–45.
41. Hansen MF, Cavanee WK. Genetics of cancer predisposition. Cancer Res 1987; 47:6174–79.
42. Knudson AG. Hereditary cancer, oncogenes, and anti-oncogenes. Cancer Res 1985; 45:1437–43.
43. Ponder B. Gene losses in human tumors. Nature 1988; 335:400–02.
44. Green AR, Wyke JA. Anti-oncogenes: a subset of regulatory genes involved in carcinogenesis? Lancet 1985; ii:475–77.
45. Knudson AG. Mutation and cancer: statistical study of retinoblastoma. Proc Natl Acad Sci USA 1971; 68:820–23.
46. Friend SH, Bernards R, Rogely S, et al. A human DNA segment with properties of the gene that predisposes to retinoblastoma and osteosarcoma. Nature (London) 1986; 323:643–46.
47. Lee W-H, Bookstein R, Hong F, et al. Human retinoblastoma susceptibility gene: cloning, identification and sequence. Science 1987: 235:1394–99.
48. Buchkovich K, Duffy L, Harlow E. The retinoblastoma protein is phosphorylated during specific phases of the cell cycle. Cell 1989: 58:1097–1105.
49. DeCaprio JA, Ludlow JW, Lynch D, et al. The product of the retinoblastoma susceptibility gene has properties of a cell cycle regulatory element. Cell 1989; 58:1085–95.
50. Whyte P, Buchkovich KJ, Horowitz JM, et al. Association between an oncogene and an anti-oncogene: the adenovirus E1A proteins bind to the retinoblastoma gene product. Nature 1988; 334: 124–29.
51. Dyson N, Howley PM, Munger K, Harlow E. The human papillomavirus-16 E7 oncoprotein is able to bind to the retinoblastoma gene product. Science 1989; 243:934–37.
52. Lane DP, Benchimol S. p53: oncogene or antioncogene? Genes & Development 1990; 4:1–8.
53. Sarnow P, Ho YS, Williams J, Levine AJ. Adenovirus E1b-58 kd tumor antigen and SV40 large tumor antigen are physically associated with the same 54 kd cellular protein in transformed cells. Cell 1982; 28:387–94.
54. Eliyahu D, Goldfinger N, Pinhasi-Kimhi O, et al. Meth A fibrosarcoma cells express two transforming mutant p53 species. Oncogene 1988; 3:313–21.
55. Rose EA, Glaser T, Jones C, et al. Complete physical map of the WAGR region of 11p13 localizes a candidate Wilms' tumor gene. Cell 1990; 60:509–520.
56. Call KM, Glaser T, Ito CY, et al. Isolation and characterization of a zinc finger polypeptide gene at the human chromosome 11 Wilms' tumor locus. Cell 1990; 60:509–20.
57. Fearon ER, Cho KR, Nigro JM, et al. Identification of a chromosome 18q gene that is altered in colorectal cancers. Science 1990; 247:49–56.
58. Whang-Peng J, Kao-Shan CS, Lee EC, et al. Specific chromosome defect associated with human small-cell lung cancer: Deletion 3p (14–23). Science 1982; 215:181–82.
59. Yokota J, Tsukada Y, Nakajima T, et al. Loss of heterozygosity on the short arm of chromosome 3 in carcinoma of the uterine cervix. Cancer Res 1989; 49:3598–3601.
60. Cohen AJ, Li FP, Berg S, et al. Hereditary renal cell carcinoma associated with a chromosomal translocation. N Engl J Med 1979; 301:592–95.

61. Chilcote RR, Brown E, Rowley JD. Lymphoblastic leukemia with lymphomatous features associated with abnormalities of the short arm of chromosome 9. N Engl J Med 1985; 313:286–91.
62. Leppert M, Dobbs M, Scambler P, et al. The gene for familial polyposis coli maps to the long arm of chromosome 5. Science 1987; 238:1411–13.
63. Matthew CGP, Smith BA, Thorpe K, et al. Depletion of genes on chromosome 1 in endocrine neoplasia. Nature (London) 1987; 328:524–26.
64. Werness BA, Levine AJ, Howley PM. Association of human papillomavirus types 16 and 18 E6 proteins with p53. Science 1990; 248:76–79.
65. Rosengard AM, Krutzsch HC, Shearn A, et al. Reduced Nm23/Awd protein in tumor metastasis and aberrant Drosophila development. Nature 1989; 342:177–80.

4

BIOCHEMISTRY OF INTRACELLULAR SIGNAL TRANSMISSION IN NORMAL AND NEOPLASTIC CELLS

Jerome Appelbaum, M.D.

THE PATHWAY USED BY a cell in response to a peripheral signal is similar to the one it employs in response to other signals that elicit a variety of responses such as those induced by hormones and lymphokines. A number of substances (e.g., growth factors, antigens, lymphokines, oncogenes, mitogenes and lectins) are capable of inducing a proliferative response. After mitosis, a cell enters the G-1 phase, in which a decision is made either to continue cycling and enter the proliferative S phase or to stop proliferating and enter the G-0 phase, during which it differentiates to perform a specific function. Whereas some cells (e.g., muscle and nerve cells) terminally differentiate and remain in G-0 permanently, other cells retain their capacity to reenter the cell cycle and proliferate in response to a proliferative signal. The neoplastic phenotype can be characterized as an uncoupling of these 2 coupled events. The cell, no longer subject to normal constraints, continuously divides. The events that make up the intracellular signal transmission pathway are shared by the differentiation and proliferating signals. A variety of proliferating signals thus share a common metabolic pathway for the transmission of their signals into the interior of the cell, where DNA synthesis results. In order to understand how the malignant transformation occurs, one must also understand how the proliferative signal acts to stimulate DNA synthesis.

Proliferation in Response to an External Signal

The early events initiating proliferation in response to an external signal are mediated intracellularly by 2 pathways. One pathway involves the generation of cyclic adenosine monophosphate (CAMP) as a second messenger, whereas the other activates phosphatidylinosital (PI) turnover, releasing 2 second messengers, 1,2 diacylgycerol (DAG) and inositol 1,4,5, trisphosphate (IP_3).[1] These pathways have features in common. A wide variety of substances such as growth factors, antigens, lymphokines, and polypeptide hormones act as external signals and are capable of eliciting a proliferative response via 1 of these pathways. Binding of an external signal (first messanger) to its specific cell surface receptor induces a conformational change in the receptor. The latter in turn induces a conformational change in a membrane protein called the G protein because it binds guanosine diphosphate (GDP). This results in the exchange of GDP for guanosine triphosphate (GTP), thereby inducing a second conformational change in the G protein. This in turn activates an enzyme within the membrane. The activated enzyme acts on a precursor molecule, converting it to a second messenger. Activation of the membrane-bound enzyme phosphatidylinositol-4,5-bisphosphate (PIP_2) by phospholipase C results in the breakdown of PIP_2 to generate the 2 second messengers, DAG and IP_3.

The external signal is transduced through the cell membrane via the G protein. The signal is then amplified by the enzyme within the membrane via the formation of an increase in the amount of second messenger(s) from the precursor molecule. Second messengers such as CAMP, DAG, IP_3, and calcium ions all have been implicated in the control of cell growth through conveying their signals to the interior of the cell, which results in the induction of the synthesis of DNA preparatory to mitosis.[2] PI turnover recently has emerged as the central event in the transmission of the proliferative signal intracellularly. The steps in the breakdown and resynthesis of PI constitutes points of entry into the PI cycle for a variety of proliferating signals as well as representing a common converging pathway through which the different proliferation signals elicit their common response, i.e., the synthesis of DNA.

Intracellular Changes

The binding of an external signal (first messenger) to its specific membrane receptor activates the membrane-bound G protein, which in turn activates PIP_2 phosphodiesterase (phospholipase C). The latter enzyme hydrolyzes a minor lipoprotein within the membrane PIP_2 to DAG and IP_3. These 2 products are the 2 second messengers. DAG remains within the cell membrane and transduces the proliferative signal within the plane of the membrane to activate the enzyme protein kinase-C (PK-C). PK-C is also activated by the phorbol esters, which are potent tumor promoters. In fact, PK-C is the receptor for both DAG and the phorbol esters, which compete with each other for their common binding site.[3]

The role of an increased intracellular pH is (1) as a signal for proliferating and (2) as a mediator of the transition of the cell from the resting to the dividing stage and vice versa.[4] The activation of the Na+-H+ exchange activates the Na+-H+ ATPase (sodium pump), where hydrogen ions are exchanged for potassium ions. The intracellular level of postassium ions arrests the cell at a point after the initiation of the cell cycle and before the G-1/S boundary. The Na+ -K+ -ATPase exchange is latent in quiescent cells in G-0, but is rapidly activated (e.g., by growth factors and phorbol esters).

PK-C is not an integral membrane protein but is found in the cytoplasm. It migrates to the cell membrane. Interleukin (IL-2) induces the subcellular distribution of the PK-C receptor from the cytosol to the membrane. IL-2 also induces the activation of the PK-C receptor. PK-C has emerged as a pivotal regulation element in signal transmission, cell regulation, tumor promoters, and (perhaps) oncogenes. PK-C may also be the link enabling the 2 transmembrane signaling systems to interact. Phorbol-ester treated cells have an increased adenylate cyclase activity. This may be the result of PK-C phosphorylating the catalytic subunit of adenylate cyclase.[5]

The other signal pathway resulting from the hydrolysis of the PIP_2 involves the second messenger, IP_3. IP_3 mobilizes calcium ions from their intracellular stores localized within the endoplasmic reticulum. Calcium ions are also second messengers that have been implicated in the regulation of proliferation by many different cell types. In vitro, each limb of the hydrolysis of the PIP_2 can be activated separately. The calcium ionophore A23187 can increase intracellular calcium levels directly from the endoplasmic reticulum stores, thus bypassing IP_3. The phorbol esters can also activate PK-C directly by binding to it as a ligand. The calcium ionophore A23187 and the phorbol esters thus mimic the action of second messengers IP_3 and DAG, respectively. The calcium ionophore and phorbol esters are used to study each item of PIP_2 turnover separately. They have been used together on platelets where their simultaneous use elicited the maximum secretion of serotonin. However, when used individually, there was no effect.

The signal for proliferation and differentiation is regulated by PIP_2 turnover. Proliferation is characterized by an increase in PIP_2 turnover and differentiation is characterized by a decrease in PIP_2 turnover. PIP_2 turnover governs the ionic events that have been implicated in the regulation of some but not all proliferative signals. Growth factors such as epidermal growth factor (EGF) and insulin do not act via PIP_2 turnover. The increase in intracellular calcium following the binding of EGF to its receptor is from extracellular sources and is not by the mobilization from intracellular stores. Insulin does not stimulate PIP_2 turnover.

Functions of Oncogene Products

The gene products encoded by oncogenes may function in the signal pathway. Platelet-derived growth factor (PDGF) is the product encoded by the sis-oncogene and is an activator of PIP_2 hydrolysis. The binding of PDGF to its membrane receptor activates phospholipase-C. The latter in turn hydrolyzes PIP_2 to DAG and IP_3. The activation of DAG via the binding of PDGF to its receptor activates PK-C, inducing an increase in the the level of c-myc expression.[6] As stated above, not all growth factors act via the turnover of PIP_2. EGF, for example, upon binding to its receptor bypasses PK-C because it does not elicit an increase in the turnover of PIP_2 but activates the expression of c-myc independent of PK-C. PDGF also has been found to act independently of PIP_2 turnover, inducing an increase in the level of c-myc expression independent of PK-C (similar to EGF).

PDGF induces the expression of the c-fos oncogen. The proteins encoded by both c-myc and c-fos are localized in the nucleus and may function to control DNA synthesis.[7] PDGF may induce DNA replication directly, perhaps through the activation of its tyrosine kinase activity by autophosphorylation.

Another oncogene product implicated in the signal pathway is the p21 c-ras protein encoded by the ras oncogene. P21 c-ras may be a member of the G proteins, thus functioning as a transducer of the proliferation signal. Evidence for this are studies showing the p21 c-ras (1) couples receptor to the enzyme phosphodiesterase, (2) its binding to GTP, and (3) its location within the cell membrane, properties it shares with the other members of the G protein family. The function of p21 c-ras may then be similar to the G proteins, i.e., the coupling of the receptor-ligand complex to the amplifier enzyme phosphodiesterase, which hydrolyzes PIP_2 to DAG and IP_3.

Cells transformed by the Rous sarcoma virus (RSV) have an increased PIP_2 turnover. The RSV encodes the phosphorylated protein pp60 v-src, which is localized in the cell membrane and has a protein kinase activity (i.e., it transfers phosphorus groups from ATP to proteins). Pp60 v-src can also decrease the level of DAG by adding phosphorus groups to DAG and converting it to phosphotidic acid, thus making DAG unavailable for binding to PK-C. By reducing the level of DAG, pp60 v-src indirectly controls the activation of PK-C, activating the Na+/H+ exchange and the level of intracellular pH, which regulates the competence of the cell to synthesize DNA, go into S phase, and go on into proliferation.

P68 v-ros is the gene product of the avian sarcoma virus UR2. It is also a kinase that is localized in the cell membrane. P68 v-ros, like pp60 v-src, controls the level of DAG by phosphorolyating PI_2 to IP_4 and IP_4 to PIP_2. The increase in PIP_2 when activated generates DAG that in turn controls the ionic events involved in the Na+/H+ exchange, raising the intracellular pH that produces the proliferative signal.

Summary

In summary, the products of oncogenes may regulate self-proliferation at different stages, leading to the synthesis of PIP_2 or during its hydrolysis as follows: The src and ros oncogene products are kinases that phosphorylate PI_2 and PIP_2. P21 c-ras acts like a transducer G protein to couple the receptor corresponding to the first messenger as a ligand to the amplifying enzyme (PDE). PDGF, encoded by the c-sis-oncogene after binding its receptor, activates the enzyme phosopolipase-C, which in turn hydrolyzes PIP_2 to DAG and IP_3.

The end result of mitogen stimulation of the lymphocyte in proliferation is characterized by an increase in the DNA content of the lymphocyte. This synthesis is detectable only 48–72 hr after stimulation of the lymphocyte. The synthesis of DNA is dependent on an increase in the intracellular calcium concentration. Within 3 min of stimulation there is an 18-fold increase in the turnover of PIP_2. Thus, PIP_2 turnover is an early event in lymphocytic activation and occurs prior to DNA synthesis and precedes the prerequisite increase in the intracellular calcium ion level. Recent experimental work suggests that the phosphorylation of IP_3 to inositol 1,3,4,5-tetrakiphosphate produces another second messenger that regulates the entry of calcium from extracellular stores.[8]

The role of the second messenger cAMP, generated through the adenyl cyclase pathway in the proliferation response, is controversial and will not be reviewed here.

The biochemistry of intracellular signal transmission, insofar as it involves the PI cycle and the turnover of PIP_2, represents a mechanism through which some of the different types of proliferation signals are delivered to the interior of the cell. It also turns out that a particular proliferation signal, e.g, PDGF, can adapt more than 1 pathway by which to elicit a cellular response. The processing of the proliferation signal at the level of the cell membrane to the interior of the cell remains a stimulating area for future research into the insight of the process of neoplastic transformation.

It has recently been suggested that the human gamma interferon (IFN) transmits its effect intracellularly by using the transmembrane signaling pathway. Human gamma IFN stimulates an early and transient increase in the concentration of DAG and IP_3.[9] The action of human IFN may thus involve the activation of the same metabolic pathways employed by other peripheral signals.

References

1. Berridge MJ, Irvine RF. Nature 1984; 312:315–21.
2. Hokin LE, Rana RS. Physiol Rev 1990; 70:115–64.
3. Bell MR. Cell 1986; 45:631–32.
4. Berridge, MJ. Biochim Biophys Acta 1987; 907:33–45.
5. Yoshimasa T, Sibley DR, Bouvier M. Nature 1987; 327:67–70.
6. Macara IG. Am J Physiol (Cell Physiol 17) 1985; 248:C3–C11.
7. Curran T, Franza RB. Cell 1988; 55:395–97.
8. Gupta S. Mol Cell Biochem. 1989; 91(1–2):45–50.
9. Yap WH, Teo TS, Tan YH. Science 1986; 234:355–57.

5

CHROMOSOMAL ABNORMALITIES IN NEOPLASTIC DISEASES

Ram S. Verma, Ph.D., M.R.C. Path.

THE ROLE OF CHROMOSOMES in the transformation of a normal cell to a neoplastic one was first postulated more than 75 yr ago by the German zoologist Theodor Boveri.[1] However, it has been over only the past 2 decades that great strides have been made toward understanding the chromosomal basis of human neoplasias by the application of various banding techniques.[2] This has resulted in the discovery of more than 100 human neoplasms associated with specific cancer, thus implicating the involvement of certain regions in the process of malignant transformation.[3] An overview of the evidence regarding particular patterns of chromosomal changes in various human neoplasms is given in this review. Much of the detailed information about relevant chromosomal rearrangements has been described in a number of recent reviews.[4-8] Although a detailed discussion of recent discoveries in the field of molecular genetics is beyond the scope of this chapter, an introductory explanation of the events that occur at the DNA level in these chromosomal regions is appropriate here.

Consistent Chromosomal Abnormalities

It is an accepted fact that chromosomal abnormalities are characteristics of malignant cells. The acquired abnormalities are consistent and shared by multiple cells, suggesting clonal origins. These findings have greatly stimulated interest in the cytogenetic aspects of cancer and have established a definite correlation between specific chromosomal abnormalities and proliferative anomalies (table 5-1). To elucidate some principles of chromosomal changes in

Table 5-1. Neoplasms with a Known Consistent Chromosomal Defect

Disease	Chromosomal defect
Chronic myelogenous leukemia	t(9;22)(q34.1;q11.21)
Acute nonlymphocytic leukemia	
M1,M2	inv(3)(q21q25–27)
M1,M2,M4,M5,M6	− 5 or del(5)(q13q31) +
M1,M2	t(6;9)(p22.2;q34)
M1,M2,M4,M5,M6	− 7 or del(7)(q31.2q36) +
M1,M2,M4,M5,M6	+ 8
M2	t(8;21)(q22.1;q22.3)
M2,M4,M5a	t(9;11)(p22;q23) +
M1,M2	t(9;22)(q34.1;q11.21)
M3	t(15;17)(q22;q11.2?)
M2,M4,M5b	inv(16)(p13.1q22.1)
Myelodysplasia-preleukemia	
RA,RAEB-CMML	t(1;3)(p36;q21)
RA,RA-S,RAEB	t(2;11)(p11;q23)
RA	del(5)(q13q31) +
RA,RA-S,RAEB,RAEB-T,CMML	− 7 or del(7)(q31q36) +
RAEB	del(7)(p11.2p22)
RA,RAEB	+ 8
RAEB,RAEB-T	del(9)(q13q22)
RA-S,RAEB	del(20)(q12q13)
Chronic lymphocytic leukemia	
B cell	t(11;14)(q13;q32.3)
B cell	+ 12
T cell	inv(14)(q11.2q32.3) or
	t(14;14)(q11.2;q32.3)
Acute lymphocytic leukemia	
L1,L2, pre-B cell	t(1;19)(q21-23;p13?)
L1,L2, null	t(4;11)(q21;q23)
L2, null	del(6)(q21q25) +
L3, B cell	t(8;14)(q24.1;q32.3)
L1,L2, null	t(9;22)(q34.1;q11.21)
L1,L2, T cell	t(11;14)(p13-
	14.1;q11.2-13)
Non-Hodgkin's lymphoma	
Diffuse large noncleaved cell	del(6)(q21q25) +
Burkitt, non-Burkitt	t(8;14)(q24.1;q32.3)
Small-cell, immunoblastic	
Small lymphocytic, B cell	del(11)(q14.2q23.3)
Small lymphocytic, B cell	t(11;14)(q13;q32.3)
Small lymphocytic, B cell	+ 12
Diffuse mixed small and large T cell	t(12;14)(q13;q32.3)
Small lymphocytic T cell	inv(14)(q11.2q32.3) or
Sézary syndrome, mycosis fungoides	t(14;14)(q11.2;q32.3)
Follicular small cleaved follicular cell and	t(14;18)(q32.3;q21.3)
follicular mixed small and large cell	

Table 5–1 (cont.). Neoplasms with a Known Consistent Chromosomal Defect

Disease	Chromosomal defect
Carcinoma	
Melanoma	del(1)(p21–22p36) +
Neuroblastoma	del(1)(p31.2p36)
Small-cell lung carcinoma	del(3)(p14p23) +
Renal cell carcinoma, familial	t(3;8)(p14.2;q24.1)
Renal cell carcinoma	t(5;14)(q13;q22)del (14)(q22q32)
Ovarian papillary cystadenocarcinoma	t(6;14)(q21;q24)
Carcinoma of prostate	del(10)(q23–24q36)
Ewing's sarcoma, neuroepithelioma, Askin's tumor	t(11;22)(q23;q11.23)
Constitutional Wilms' tumor, Wilms' tumor	del(11)(p13)
Seminoma, teratoma	i(12p)
Constitutional retinoblastoma, retinoblastoma, osteosarcoma	del(13)(q14.1)
Multiple endocrine carcinoma	del(20)(p12.2)
Benign solid tumor	
Mixed parotid gland tumor	t(3;8)(p21;q12)
Meningioma	– 22

Source: adapted from Yunis (ref 5)

neoplastic disorders, a few examples were chosen, answering fundamental questions such as whether specific chromosomal aberrations are related to etiologic factor(s) or to the type of target cell(s) in human neoplasia.

Prior to the advent of banding techniques, only numerical and structural rearrangements were classified. The most intriguing discovery was the presence of a small deleted chromosome in patients with chronic myelogenous leukemia (CML).[9] The abnormality, while formerly thought to involve a deletion of the long arm of chromosome 22, has now been shown to involve a balanced translocation between the long arms of chromosomes 9 and 22.[10] This finding greatly stimulated interest in exploring chromosomal abnormalities in other neoplasias.[11]

Remarkable discoveries have resulted from the application of new banding techniques that have permitted precise information not only on the involvement of a band but also that of a sub-band.[12] The recent application of high-resolution chromosome analysis[13] of synchronized cells has proved to be a more refined level of analysis, one that has permitted the visualization of defects that previously went undetected.[14-16] Despite the tremendous strides that have been made, some neoplasias have point mutation that is not detectable as chromosomal aberration.

More than 70 human neoplasias are known to have 1 of the more than 40 specific recurrent chromosomal abnormalities. These abnormalities could be either translocations, deletions, duplications, inversions, or trisomies.[17-20] Translocations are seen in leukemias and non-Hodgkin's lymphomas, whereas deletions are found more frequently in myelodysplasia and solid tumors. Consistent chromosomal defects are an important parameter used in the prognosis of a specific neoplasia; however, some chromosomal abnormalities are shared among related disorders (table 5-2). One of the most common chromosomal abnormalities is the translocation t (9;22), found primarily in patients with CML but also seen in acute lymphocytic leukemia (ALL) and acute nonlymphocytic leukemia (ANLL). The recent review on this subject is well covered by Yunis,[5] thus only a brief and comprehensive tabulation is provided here.

Chromosomal Basis of Childhood Cancer

In recent years, it has become more and more evident that many genetic factors play an important role in the etiology of pediatric malignancies. Although it is beyond the scope of this discussion to review the myriad recent discoveries that have been made in pediatric neoplasias,[21] for present purposes childhood cancer can be grouped into 2 classes, hereditary and nonhereditary. Among hereditary malignancies, retinoblastoma and Wilms' tumor are well-investigated diseases. Nonhereditary pediatric malignancies include chronic myelogenous leukemia (CML), acute nonlymphocytic leukemia (ANLL), and acute lymphoblastic leukemia (ALL). The following paragraphs attempt to shed some light on these neoplasias.

Retinoblastoma is a malignant congenital tumor that characteristically arises multicentrically in one (unilateral) or both (bilateral) retinas.[22] The most reliable estimates of incidence range from 1/15,000 to 1/28,000 population, with a trend toward a higher incidence than presently found.[23] Retinoblastoma cases occur unilaterally in about 65% of cases and bilaterally in the remaining

Table 5-2. Neoplasias with a Shared Single Recurrent Chromosomal Defect

Chromosomal defect	Disease
del 1p	Neuroblastoma Melanoma
t(1;3)(p36;q21)	Myelodysplasia Acute nonlymphocytic leukemia,M4
inv(3)(q21q27)	Myelodysplasia Acute nonlymphocytic leukemia,M1,M2
t(4;11)(q21;q23)	Acute lymphocytic leukemia,L1,L2 Acute myelomonocytic leukemia
del(5)(q13q31)	Myelodysplasia Acute nonlymphocytic leukemia,M1,M2,M4,M5,M6
del(6)(q21q25)	Diffuse large-cell lymphoma Acute lymphocytic leukemia,L2
t(6;9)(p21.2;q34)	Acute nonlymphocytic leukemia,M1,M2

Table 5-2 (cont.). Neoplasias with a Shared Single Recurrent Chromosomal Defect

Chromsomal defect	Disease
del(7)(q31.2q36)	Myelodysplasia Acute nonlymphocytic leukemia,M1,M2,M4,M5,M6
+8	Myelodysplasia Acute nonlymphocytic leukemia,M1,M2,M4,M5,M6
t(8;14)(q24.1q32.3)	Burkitt's lymphoma Acute lymphocytic leukemia,L3 Small noncleaved non-Burkitt's lymphoma Immunoblastic lymphoma,B cell
t(8;21)(q22.1;q22.3)	Acute myelogenous leukemia,M2,M4
t(9;11)(p22;q23.3)	Acute monocytic leukemia,M5 Acute myelomonocytic leukemia,M4 Acute nonlymphocytic leukemia,M2
t(9;22)(q34.1;q11.21)	Chronic myelogenous leukemia Acute myelogenous leukemia,M1,M2 Acute lymphocytic leukemia,L1,L2
t(11;14)(q13.3;q32.3)	Chronic lymphocytic leukemia, B cell Small-cell lymphocytic lymphoma, B cell Diffuse large-cell lymphoma, B cell
t(11;22)(q23;q11.2)	Ewing's sarcoma Neuropithelioma Askin's tumor
+12	Chronic lymphocytic leukemia, B cell Small-cell lymphocytic lymphoma, B cell
iso12p	Seminoma Teratoma
del 13(q14)	Retinoblastoma Constitutional retinoblastoma Osteosarcoma
inv(14q11.2q32.3) or t(14;14)(q11.2;q32.3)	Chronic lymphocytic leukemia, T cell Small lymphocytic lymphoma, T cell Sézary syndrome Mycosis fungoides
t(14;18)(q32.3;q21.3)	Follicular small cleaved cell lymphoma Follicular mixed cell lymphoma Follicular large-cell lymphoma
inv(16)(p13.1q22.1)	Acute monocytic leukemia,M5b Acute myelomonocytic leukemia,M4 Acute nonlymphocytic leukemia,M2

Source: adapted from Yunis (ref 5)

35%. Retinoblastoma is one of the known cancers in humans inherited through a dominant autosomal gene, with penetrance of about 90%.[24] The hereditary tendency is governed by a locus (or loci) mapped on the long arm of chromosome 13 bands 13q13.1–q14.5.[25] Although the inheritance pattern is an autosomal dominance, molecular studies clearly suggest that the retinoblastoma locus is recessive, and both alleles must undergo mutation before the tumor is expressed.[26] This author's in-depth review on this subject was published in 1985.[27]

Nephroblastoma, commonly known as Wilms' tumor (WT), is a malignant embryonal neoplasm of the kidney that is very similar to retinoblastoma. The incidence of Wilms' tumor in the general population is 7.8 per million in the United States; it comprises 6.2% of all neoplasias in Caucasians and 7.9% of all malignancies in black children. Wilms' tumor occurs in both hereditary (40%) and nonhereditary forms. The cytogenetic findings revealed that the distal half of band 11p13 is deleted.[28,29] Besides the involvement of band 11p13 in a deletion or mutation, other chromosomal defects have been reported.[30-32]

CML, ANLL, and ALL are nonhereditary types of childhood cancers. Significant strides have been made in understanding these acquired malignancies in children. Most, if not all, malignant neoplasms have chromosomal abnormalities. Chromosomal abnormalities of pediatric cancers are thoroughly reviewed by Arthur.[21]

Neoplasms of Chromosome Breakage Syndromes

Certain individuals who are predisposed to develop neoplasia are referred to as cancer prone. The terms *chromosome breakage* or *instability syndrome* also have been used to describe these individuals.[33,34] Fanconi's anemia, ataxia-telangiectasia, and Bloom syndrome are the most common disorders, but xeroderma pigmentosum, Werner's syndrome, Kostmann's agranulocytosis, and anemia also can be included in this group.

Fanconi's anemia (FA) is an autosomal recessive disorder that was first described in 1964.[35] The chromosome breakage was manifested in 10 to 100 of cultured lymphocytes. All kinds of aberrant chromosomal constitutions were seen in individuals with the disorder, including chromosome and chromatid breaks, fragments, rings, translocations, triradials, quadriradials, and various kind of markers involving many chromosomes. These abnormalities were observed in fibroblasts as well as in lymphocytes. These individuals are very sensitive to certain clastogenic agents and show a high rate of sister chromatid exchange (SCE).[36] A faulty DNA repair mechanism has been postulated in these patients,[37] and an increased rate of acute leukemia also has been reported.[38] It cannot be concluded that FA disposes to leukemia, however, because chromosomal instability in FA is not understood.

Bloom syndrome (BS) is another autosomal recessive disorder with an increased frequency of symmetrical quadriradials in lymphocyte metaphases. An increased rate of SCE is also observed,[39] and there is nonrandom involvement of chromosomal abnormalities in this neoplasia.[40] BS, with its greatly increased incidence of malignancies, constitutes a prime example of gene defect predisposing to malignancy.[41]

Ataxia-telangiectasia (AT), also an autosomal recessive disorder in addition to being an immune deficiency disorder, is associated with an abnormally increased frequency of lymphoid malignant proliferation. A significantly high rate of spontaneous chromosome breakage is found when lymphocytes are exposed to X rays. This approach has helped in detecting heterozygotes of AT. The SCE frequency is normal, but the tandem translocation involving both chromosomes 14 with breakpoints in band q11–12 is demonstrated.[42] In addition, translocations affecting chromosomes 7 and 14 are found much more often in AT T lymphocytes. The role of chromosome instability of AT in the cancer prone is unknown, but the fact that an individual with AT is at such an impressively greater than normal risk of malignant neoplasia conceivably indicates that multifactorial events are responsible in persons with homozygous status for these rare genes. However, genetic instability and a defective immune system may be the leading factors in chromosomal abnormalities in AT.

A report by Cleaver in 1968 demonstrated that ultraviolet-irradiated cells of patients with xeroderma pigmentosum (XP) undergo an abnormally small amount of "repair replication" of damaged DNA.[43] Only the *induced* rate of chromosomal breakage is abnormally high,[44] a syndrome German has referred to as "conditional chromosome breakage."[121] XP is inherited as an autosomal recessive trait, the clinical features of which have been reviewed elsewhere.[45] Based on several facts, one might expect to see an increased susceptibility of individuals with XP to tumors, but no such susceptibility has been found because of early death of most XP patients and lack of autopsy records.[46]

The first report of neoplasia in a person with Werner's syndrome (WS) appeared in 1939.[47] Unusual chromosomal changes in WS patients are seen in both fibroblasts and lymphocytes. Predominantly stable translocations that were clonal in nature were the most common abnormalities.[48,49] The distribution of chromosomes involved in these translocations appeared to be nearly random, although chromosomes 2,3,10, and X were most commonly seen. An increase in chromosomal breakage has been noted in these patients,[50] who have a markedly reduced life span and a high frequency of sarcomas.

The Chromosomal 'Fragile Site' in Cancer

Although the mechanisms that trigger translocations in cancer are still unknown, several attempts are being made to understand the chromosomal as well as molecular basis of human neoplasias. A research area that has drawn considerable interest is the so-called "fragile site" in cancer, i.e., when cultures are grown in a medium deprived of folic acid and thymidine, certain chromosomes have a tendency to break at certain sites.[51] Several investigators have observed a remarkable association between the location of oncogenes and these fragile sites.[52] At least 33 constitutive fragile sites (c-frg) have been mapped close to the breakpoints found in 38 of the 41 specific structural chromosomal defects known thus far in cancer.[53] In addition to c-frg, 16 heritable chromosomal fragile sites (h-frg) have been identified.[54] The precise mechanism(s) of fragile site formation and their biological significance remain unknown. However, at the Seventh Human Gene Mapping workshop,[55] a statistically significant association between 21 fragile sites and 50 cancer-specific breakpoints was established.[56] Indeed, the function and identity of genes located at fragile sites remain an enigma, but inherited (f-frg) fragile sites are related to genetic predisposition and the development of neoplastic tissues. The occurrence of fragile sites in somatic cells may also be an indication of fragile sites in germ cells, something that may further uncover the mysteries of heritable cancer.

Chromosomal Basis of Oncogenesis

Astonishing progress has been made in recent years toward understanding the chromosomal basis of oncogenesis. The status of chromosomal localization of the cellular homology of the retroviral oncogene (c-onc) has recently been reviewed.[57] It is emphasized that the breakpoints of many of the consistent rearrangements that characterize individual cancers involve the specific bands to which various c-onc genes have been assigned (table 5-3). The role of oncogenes in chromosomal aberrations has been the major factor in their localization. Thus, it has been stated, "Chromosomes in a cell of the immune system sometimes 'trade' segments of DNA. This process can activate cancer-causing genes by placing them near genetic sequences that enhance activity."[58] The voluminous literature on the subject bears witness that there has been no dearth of theories and postulates on the causation of neoplasia in humans. The following few paragraphs focus on the primary role of chromosomal changes with respect to oncogenes and cancer.

Table 5-3. Localization of Proto-Oncogenes in the Human Genome

Chromo-somes	Band location	Oncogene	Chromo-somes	Band location	Oncogene
1	p12→cen & p22	N-ras	9	q34.1	ab1
	p32	L-myc & B-			
		lym-1	11	p13	tcl-2
	p32→p35	1ck		p15.5	H-ras-1
	p34→p36	fgr		q13	bcl-1,int-2,sea
	p36	src		q23→q24	est-1
	q22→q24	ski			
	q24→q25	arg	12	p12.1	K-ras-2
	q32	trk		q12→q13	int-1
				q13→q14.3	gli
2	p13→cen	rel		q24.2	K-ras-2
	p23.2→q24	N-myc			
	q21→q31	fos	13	q12	flt

Table 5-3 (cont.). Localization of Proto-Oncogenes in the Human Genome

Chromo-somes	Band location	Oncogne	Chromo-somes	Band location	Oncogene
3	p21→pter or p17	A-erb-2	14	q21→q31	fos
	p25	raf-1,mil,mht		q32	akt-1
				q32.3	tcl-1
4	q11→q22	kit			
	?	raf-2	15	q26.1	fes or fps
5	p13→p14	M-1vi-2	16	?	fos
	q33→q34	csf-1r			
	q34	fms	17	p13	p53
				q11→q21.3	A-erb-1
6	p21	pim-1		q21→q22	ng1
	p23→q12	K-ras-1		?	neu
	q12→p11	P-kas-1			
	q21	syr	18	q21.3	yes-1 &bcl-2
	q22	ros			
	q22→q23	myb	19	p13.2→q13.2	me1
	?	yes-2		?	R-ras
7	p12→p13	egf-R	20	q11→q12	hck
	p12→p14	B-erb-1		q13.1	src-1
	p14→q21	A-raf-2			
	p15→p22	ra1	21	q22.3	est-2
	pter→q22	pks-2			
	q21→q31	met	22	q12.3→q13.1	sis & P-dgf-B
	q35	tcl			
			X	p21→q11	A-raf-1
8	q13→qter	lyn		pter→q22	pks-1
	q22.1→q22.3	mos		pter→q28	H-ras-2
	q24	pvt-1		q27	mcf-2
	q24.1	C-myc			

Source: adapted from Verma (ref 100)

Highly significant data pertaining to translocations and activation of oncogenes are rapidly accumulating.[59] A number of these consistent translocations (described above) have demonstrated the nature of activation. For example, in patients with CML, 95% have 9q;22q translocation. The oncogene c-abl, located on the terminal band of the long arm of chromosome 9 at band 9q34, has been demonstrated to be translocated to the Ph chromosome (22q−).[60] If the breakpoints in chromosome 22q are at the light chain gene, then c-abl may be activated by the immunoglobulin gene promoters. However, in 5–8% of cases, in which c-abl gene is not involved in translocation, an oncogene other than c-abl has been shown to be activated.[61] Another oncogene known as c-sis has been localized to band 22q11→qter, which is involved in this disease.[62] Recently, the consistent presence of c-abl RNA transcript in CML with t(9;22) suggests that it is a consequence of c-abl translocation, which plays a role in development of this leukemia.[63]

Perhaps the second most interesting correlation between oncogenes and chromosomal translocation is found in Burkitt's lymphoma, where chromosome 8 is most commonly involved in a reciprocal translocation with chromosome 2, 14, or 22, of which 8;14 translocation is by far the most frequent.[64] The c-myc proto-oncogene has been localized on chromosome 8 band 8q24, and chromosomes 2, 14, and 22 each are known to code for immunoglobulin chains, again in the region of the translocation. As a result of the t(8;14) in Burkitt's lymphoma cells, c-myc transcription may increase $\leq$ 20 times over the normal level. The mechanisms by which the chromosomal rearrangement triggers malignant growth are intriguing. However, rearranged immunoglobulin genes that then associate with oncogenes may be an attractive hypothesis.[66,67] Again, it is intriguing to note that the long arm of chromosome 8 (q22) also contains an oncogene known as c-mos,[68] and the long arm of chromosome 15 band q22 contains another oncogene known as c-fes.[69,70] The oncogene c-fes has been correlated with the 6(15;17) that occurs in ANLL-M3. Furthermore, the oncogene c-myb is located on 6q23 and translocated to chromosome 14 in ovarian carcinoma.[71] These are some of the examples that strongly support the model of translocation-mediated oncogene activation in the origin of neoplastic transformation.[72,73] In many—if not all—cancers, both tumorigenesis and tumor progression is a multifactorial event. This can be further documented by using chromosomal deletions such as retinoblastoma, neuroblastoma, and Wilms' tumor.[74-80]

There is good reason for excitement as conflicting evidence for specific genes in the causation of tumors continues to unfold. The chromosomal events seen in these tumors may not be limited. Clearly, these observations indicate the widespread importance of these events in oncogenesis; the lack of an adequate mechanistic explanation for their developmental processes and their derangement does not justify ignoring them.

Individuals with congenital anomalies are well correlated with chromosomal defects.[81] In addition, these individuals are at higher risk than those who are chromosomally normal. For example, those with Down syndrome have an 11-fold increased risk of leukemia as compared to the normal population.[82] Patients with aneuploidy for sex chromosomes are again at higher risk than the general population. Neoplasms are occasionally reported in patients with structural and numerical mosaicism.[83] Retrospectively, patients with skin cancer have been found to have a significantly increased rate of chromosomal aberrations.

Conclusion

To date, > 100 neoplasms with a specific chromosomal defects have been documented since Boveri first proposed the association between mitotic errors and the origin of neoplasia. The consistent chromosomal abnormalities that are closely associated with particular neoplasms provide convincing evidence for the fundamental role in the transformation of a normal cell to a malignant cell. Over the past few years, with the advent of high-resolution banding techniques, it has become more and more apparent that every patient with a specific neoplasm has abnormal chromosomes. It has become possible to identify the specific breakpoint in localizing the function of DNA sequences that are important in carcinogenesis.

Cancer cytogenetics stand on the threshold of a molecular revolution. Recent developments in the recognition and characterization of human oncogenes are providing a better understanding of neoplastic development. Although the evidence implicating oncogenes as causes of human cancers is still circumstantial, it is accumulating rapidly. More than 50 such oncogenes have been localized, and it has been suggested that chromosomal rearrangements occur near proto-oncogenes. Understanding the organization of these oncogenes will be one of the next landmarks in the exploration of the molecular and cellular biology of carcinogenesis. Recent technical advances have revealed the inadequacy of many past efforts in this highly specialized area, and application of new techniques will clearly provide researchers with greater understanding of the chromosomal as well as the molecular basis of human cancer.[85-100]

References

1. Boveri T. Zur frag de enstehung maligner tumoren. Jena: Fischer, 1914; 1–6.
2. Yunis JJ. The chromosomal basis of human neoplasia. Science 1983; 221:227–36.
3. Mitelman F. Catalogue of chromosome aberrations in cancer. Cytogenet Cell Genet 1983; 36:1–458.
4. LeBeau MM, Rowley JD. Chromosomal abnormalities in leukemia and lymphoma: clinical and biological significance. In: Advances in human genetics. vol 15. New York: Plenum Publishing, 1986; 1–54.
5. Yunis JJ. Chromosomal rearrangements, genes, and fragile sites in cancer: clinical and biological implications. In: DeVita VT, Hellman S, Rosenberg SA, eds. Important advances in oncology. Philadelphia: JB Lippincott, 1986; 93–128.
6. Sandberg AA. The chromosomes in human leukemia. Semin Hematol 1986; 23:201–17.
7. Croce CM, Klein G. Chromosome translocations and human cancer. Sci Am 1985; 252:54–60.
8. Rowley JD, Testa JR. Chromosome abnormalities in malignant hematologic disease. Adv Cancer Res 1983; 36:103–48.
9. Nowell PC, Hungerford DA. A minute chromosome in human chronic granulocytic leukemia. Science 1960; 132:1497.
10. Rowley JD. A new consistent chromosomal abnormality in chronic myelogenous leukemia identified by quinacrine flourescence and Giemsa staining. Nature 1973; 243:290–93.
11. Gilbert F. Chromosomal abnormalities, gene amplification and tumor progression. In: Evans AE, D'Angio GJ, Seeger RC, cds. Advances in neuroblastoma research. New York: Alan R. Liss, 1985; 151–59.
12. Verma RS, Dosik H. Recent advances in detecting human chromosomal abnormalities by various banding techniques. Pathol Annu 1982; 17 (pt 2):261–86.
13. ISCN. An international system for human cytogenetic nomeclature. Birth defects: original article series vol 21:1. New York: March of Dimes Birth Defects Foundation, 1985.
14. Yunis JJ, Bloomfield CD, Ensrud K. All patients with acute nonlymphocytic leukemia may have a chromosomal defect. N Engl J Med 1981; 305:135–39.
15. Rowley JD. Do all leukemic cells have an abnormal karyotype? N Engl J Med 1981; 305:154–66.
16. Yunis JJ. New chromosome techniques in the study of human neoplasia. J Hum Pathol 1981; 12:540–49.
17. Yunis JJ, Oken MM, Theologides A, Howe RB, Kaplan ME. Recurrent chromosomal defects are found in most patients with non-Hodgkin's lymphoma. Cancer Genet Cytogenet 1984; 13:17–28.

18. Sandberg AA. The chromosomes in human cancer and leukemia. New York: Elsevier, 1980.
19. German J. Chromosome mutation and neoplasia. New York: Alan R. Liss, 1983.
20. Mitelman F. Catalogue of chromosome aberrations in cancer. Cytogenet Cell Genet 1983; 36:1–458.
21. Arthur DC. Genetics and cytogenetics of pediatric cancers. Cancer 1986; 58:534–40.
22. Ellsworth RM. Retinoblastoma. Clin Ophthal 1983; 3:1–18.
23. Vogel F. Genetics of retinoblastoma. Hum Genet 1979; 52:1–54.
24. Sparks RS. The genetics of retinoblastoma. Biochemica Biophy Acta 1985; 780:95–118.
25. Yunis JJ. Retinoblastoma and sub-band deletion of chromosome 13. Am J Dis Child 1978; 132:161–165.
26. Cavenee WK, Murphre AL, Shull MM, et al. Prediction of familial predisposition of retinoblastoma. N Engl J Med 1986; 314:1201–07.
27. Verma RS, Kopelowitz N. Oncogenesis of retinoblastoma. Ann Opthalmol 1985; 17:701–04.
28. Franke U, Holmes LB, Atkins L, Riccardi VM. Aniridia-Wilms' tumor association: evidence for specific deletion of 11p13. Cytogenet Cell Genet 1979; 24:185–192.
29. Slater RM, de Kraker J. Chromosome 11 and Wilms' tumor. Cancer Genet Cytogent 1982; 5:237–245.
30. Kondo K, Chilcote RR, Maurer HS, Rowley JD. Chromosomal abnormalities in tumor cells from patients with sporadic Wilms' tumor. Cancer Res 1984; 44:5376–81.
31. Douglas EC. Wilimas JA, Green AA, Look AT. Abnormalities of chromosomes 1 and 11 in Wilms' tumor. Cancer Genet Cytogenet 1985; 14:331–38.
32. Reeve AE, Housiaux PJ, Gardner RJM, Chevings WE, Grindley RM, Millow LJ. Loss of Harvey ras allelle in sporadic Wilms' tumor. Nature 1984; 309:174–76.
33. German JL. Chromosome breakage syndromes. New York: The National Foundation, 1969. Birth defects. Original article series 5:117–131.
34. Hecht F, McCaw BK. Chromosome instability syndromes. In: Mulvihill JJ, Miller RW, Fraumeni JF, eds. Genetics of human cancer. New York: Raven Press, 1977; 105–23.
35. Schroeder TM, Anschutz F, Knopp A. Sponfane chromosomenaberratuinnen bei bei familiarer panmyelopathie. Humangenetic 1964; 1:194–96.
36. Ray JH, German J. The cytogenetics of the "chromosome-breakage syndrome" In: German J, ed. Chromosome mutation and neoplasia. New York: Alan R. Liss, 1983; 97–134.
37. Polani PE. DNA repair defects and chromosome instability disorders. In: Human genetics: possibilities and realities (Ciba Foundation series 66). Amsterdam: Exerpta Medica, Elsevier, 1979; 81–117.
38. Berger R, Bernheim A, Le Coniat M, Vecchione D, Schaison G. Chromosomal studies of leukemic and preleukemic fanconi anemia patients. Examples of acquired "chromosomal amplication". Hum Genet 1980; 56:59–68.
39. Ved Brat S. Sister chromatid exchange and cell cycle in fibroblasts of Bloom's syndrome. Hum Genet 1979; 48:73–79.
40. Ved Brat S, Verma RS, Dosik H. Chromosome fragility in Bloom's syndrome cell line GM 1492. Cancer Genet Cytogenet 1984; 12:267–74.
41. Schonberg S, German J. Sister chromatid exchange in cells metabolically coupled to Bloom's syndrome cells. Nature 1980; 284:72–74.
42. McCaw BK, Hecht F, Harnden DG, Teplitz RI. Somatic rearrangement of chromosome 14 in human lymphocytes. Proc Natl Acad Sci 1975; 72:2071–75.
43. Cleaver JE. Defective repair replication of DNA in xeroderma pigmentosum. Nature 1968; 218:652–56.
44. Sasaki MS, Tonomura A, Matsubara S. Chromosomal constitution and its bearing on chromosomal radiosensitivity in man. Mutat Res 1970; 10:617–33.
45. Bootsma D. Xeroderma pigmentosum. In: Hanawalt PC, Friedberg EC, Fox CF, eds. DNA repair mechanisms. New York: Academic Press, 1978; 589–601.
46. Cairns J. The origin of human cancer. Nature 1981; 289:353–57.
47. Agatston SA, Gartner S. Precocious cataracts and scleroderma (Rothmund's syndrome; Werner's syndrome). Arch Ophthalmol 1939; 21:492–96.

48. Hoehn H, Bryant EM, Au K, Norwood TH, Boman H, Martin GM. Variegated translocation mosaicism in human skin fibroblasts cultures. Cytogenet Cell Genet 1975; 15:282–98.

49. Salk D, Au K, Hoehn H, Martin GM. Cytogenetics of Werner syndrome cultured skin fibroblasts: variegated translocation mosaicism. Cytogenet Cell Genet 1981; 30:92–107.

50. Nordenson I. Chromosome breaks in Werner's syndrome and their prevention in vitro by radical scavenging enzyme. Hereditas 1977; 87:151–54.

51. Yoder FE, Vincent RA, Morgan SK, Grush OC. Chromosome fragile sites. Cancer Genet Cytogent 1985; 14:369–70.

52. LeBeau MM, Rowley JD. Heritable fragile sites in cancer. Nature 1984; 308:607–09.

53. Yunis JJ, Soreng AL. Constitutive fragile sites and cancer. Science 1984; 226:1199–1204.

54. Yunis JJ. Fragile sites and predisposition to leukemia and lymphoma. Cancer Genet Cytogenet 1984; 12:85–88.

55. Human gene mapping: seventh international workshop on human gene mapping. Cytogenet Cell Genet 1984; 37:274.

56. LeBeau MM. Chromosomal fragile sites and cancer-specific rearrangements. Blood 1986; 67:849–58.

57. Rowley JD. Human oncogene locations and chromosomal aberrations. Nature 1983; 301:290–91.

58. Croce CM, Klein G. Chromosome translocations and human cancer. Sci Am 1985; 252:54–60.

59. Sandberg AA. A chromosomal hypothesis of oncogenesis. Cancer Genet Cytogenet 1983; 8:277–85.

60. Heisterkamp N, Stephenson, et al: Localization of the c-abl oncogene adjacent to a translocation breakpoint in chronic myelogenous leukemia. Nature 1982; 306:239–42.

61. Groffen J, Heisterkamp N, et al. *C-sis* translocated from chromosome 22 to chromosome 9 in chronic myelogenous leukemia. J Exp Med 1983; 158:9–15.

62. Dalla-Favera R, Gallo RC, Giallongo A, Croce CM. Chromosomal localization of the human humolog (c-sis) of simian sarcoma virus *onc* gene. Science 1982; 218:686–88.

63. Gale RP, Canaai E. An 8-kilobase *abl* RNA transcript in chronic myelogenous leukemia. Proc Natl Acad Sci 1984; 81:5648–52.

64. Sandberg AA, Wake N. Chromosomal changes in primary and metastatic tumors and in lymphoma: Their nonrandomness and significance. In: Arrighi FE, Rao PN, Stubblefield E, eds. Genes, chromosomes and neoplasia. New York: Raven Press, 1981; 297.

65. Rappold GA, Hameister H, Cremer T, et al. *C-myc* and immunoglobulin light chain constant genes are on the 8q+ chromosome of three Burkitt's lymphoma lines with t(2;8) translocation. EMBO J 1984; 3:2951–55.

66. Land H, Parada LF, Weinberg RA. Cellular oncogenes and multistep carcinogenesis. Science 1983; 222:771–78.

67. Lenoir GM, Preud'homme JL, Bernheim A, Berger R. Correlation between immunoglobulin light chain expression and variant translocation in Burkitt's lymphoma. Nature 1982; 298:474–76.

68. Neel BG, Jhanwar SC, Chaganti RSK, Hayward WS. Two human c-onc genes are located on the long arm of chromosome 8. Proc Natl Acad Sci 1982; 79:7842–46.

69. Harper ME, Franchini G, Love J, Simon MI, Gallo RC, Wong-Staal F. Chromosomal sublocalization of human *c myb* and c-fes cellular *onc* genes. Nature 1983; 304:169–71.

70. Heisterkamp N, Groffen J, Stephenson JR, et al. Chromosomal localization of human cellular homologues of two viral oncogenes. Nature 1982; 299:747–49.

71. Wake N, Hershchyshyn MM, Piver SM, et al. Specific cytogenetic changes in ovarian cancer involving chromosomes 6 and 14. Cancer Res 1980; 40:4512–18.

72. Klein G. The role of gene dosage and genetic transposition in carcinogenesis. Nature 1981; 294:313.

73. Robinson HL. Retroviruses and cancer. Rev Infect Dis 1982; 4:1015–25.

74. Horwich A. Oncogenes and human cancer. Br J Hosp Med 1984; 32:262–66.

75. Willecke K, Schafer R. Human oncogenes. Hum Genet 1984; 66:132–42.

76. Gallie BL, Phillips RA. Retinoblastoma: a model of oncogenesis. Opthalmology 1984; 91:666–72.

77. Phillips RA, Gallie BL. Retinoblastoma: importance of recessive mutations in tumorigenesis. J Cell Phys (suppl) 1984; 3:79–85.

78. Fearson ER, Vogelstein B, Feinberg AP. Somatic deletion and duplication of genes on chromosome 11 in Wilms' tumors. Nature 1984; 309:174–79.

79. Reeve AE, Housiaux PJ, Gardner RJH, et al. Loss of a Harvey *ras* allele in sporadic Wilms' tumors. Nature 1984; 309:174–79.

80. Orkin SH, Goldman DS, Sallan SE. Development of homozygosity for chromosome 11p markers in Wilms' tumors. Nature 1984; 309:172–74.

81. Gericke GS, Hesseling PB, Brink S, Becker WB. Leukaemogenesis in Down's syndrome. S African Med J 1977; 51:158–63.

82. Harnden DG, Longlands AO, McLean N. Carcinoma of the breast and Klinefelter's syndrome. J Med Genet 1971; 8:460–70.

83. Nordenson I, Beckman L, Liden S, Stjernberg N. Chromosomal aberration and cancer risk. Hum Heredity 1984; 34:76–81.

84. Verma RS. Oncogenetics: a new emerging field of cancer. Mol Gen Genet 205:385–89.

85. Sager R. Genetic suppression of tumor formation: a new frontier in cancer research. Cancer Res 1986; 46:1573–80.

86. Sandberg AA. The chromosomes in human leukemia. Semin Hematol 1986; 23:201–17.

87. Varmus H. Retroviruses. Science 1988; 240:1427–35.

88. Verma RS. Chromosomal and molecular basis of human neoplasia. In Vivo 1988; 2:257–70.

89. Schwab M. Genetic principles of tumor supression. Biochem Biophys Acta 1989; 989:49–64.

90. Spandidos DA, Anderson MLM. Oncogenes and onco-suppressor genes: their involvement in cancer. J Pathol 1989; 157:1–10.

91. Botti AC, Verma RS. The molecular biology of acute lymphoblastic leukemia. Anticancer Res 1990; 10:519–26.

92. Barbacid M. *Ras* oncogenes: their role in neoplasia. Eur J Clin Invest 1990; 20:225–35.

93. Arnheim N. The possible role of Z DNA in chromosomal translocation. Cancer Cell 1990; 2:121–22.

94. Sager R. Tumor suppressor genes: the puzzle and the promise. Science 1989; 246:1406–12.

95. Lane DP, Benchimol S. p^{53}: oncogene or antioncogene?— Genes Dev 1990; 4:1–8.

96. Wood RD, Lindahl T. A gene for tumour prevention. Nature 1990; 348:13–14.

97. Witkowski JA. The inherited character of cancer—an historical survey. Cancer Cells 1990; 2:229–57.

98. Hollingsworth RE, Lee W-H. Tumor suppressor genes: new prospects for cancer research. JNCI 1991; 83:91–96.

99. Stanbridge EJ. Human tumor suppressor genes. Annu Rev Genet 1990; 24:615–57.

100. Verma RS. Genomeic diversity in neoplasia and the retroviral genome. In: Verma RS, ed. The genome. New York: VCH Publishers, 1990; 237–87.

6

TUMOR GROWTH KINETICS

Larry Norton, M.D.

MODERN CANCER THERAPY IS founded on the study of the biology of neoplasia and the chemistry of various therapeutic modalities. If current treatments will seem primitive in a few years—a fervent hope—this will reflect as much on the dramatic rate of advance of these sciences as on our present imperfect knowledge. We have every reason to expect that the modern explosion of information regarding the molecular and cellular biology of cancer and the immune system will prove to be of concrete diagnostic and therapeutic value. In our enthusiasm for the future, however, we must not forget that currently available concepts and data are far from limited and have already generated effective, even curative treatments for a significant number of neoplastic diseases.

Many of these valuable concepts concern the metabolism of mitosis. If cancer cells did not divide, they would not be cancerous. Invasion, metastasis, and immunologic idiosyncrasy are important aspects of neoplasia and in the future may be critical targets for anticancer therapy. At present, however, the most vulnerable aspect of a malignant tumor mass is the division of its individual cells. Mitosis creates cancer, and chemotherapy kills mitotic cells.

This chapter will briefly review mitosis, using this central biological event to classify subpopulations of tumor cells. The relationships of these subpopulations over time and their changes in absolute and relative numbers defines the growth of the cancer. These changes will be described by means of basic mathematical concepts, and the association of such growth with the clinical behavior of the cancer will be illustrated. The relationship between tumor growth and the development of cellular heterogeneity in such important characteristics as metastatic potential and biochemical drug resistance will be examined. The influence of therapy on the pattern of growth will be discussed in relation to the concepts of sensitivity and curability and to the variability of growth and regression that is a consequence of biological heterogeneity. These concepts have specific implications for the design and (especially) analysis of anticancer therapeutics.

Mitosis and Mitotic Compartments

All somatic cells, normal as well as neoplastic, divide by mitosis: Genetic material in the nucleus is duplicated, chromosomes are formed, an apparatus for the separation of paired chromosomes is synthesized and assembled, the chromosomes are segregated, and the nuclear material and cytoplasmic envelopes are divided. Errors in DNA synthesis and chromosome formation and separation occur in normal cells, and are frequently fatal. Such errors, including chromosome translocations, deletions, and amplification or mutation of genetic information, occur more commonly in the division of cancer cells, where they may not be fatal. Hence, cancer cells contain many errors in chromosome number, morphology, and the construction and instruction of genes.

Some cell mutations underlie fundamental aspects of tumor biology. These errors occur with a certain probability per cell division. Populations with more mitoses per unit of time therefore would be correctly assumed to have a higher error and mutation rate. For this reason, the number of mitoses that occur in the life history of a tumor (or of any growing body of cells) is directly related to the probability of emergence of genetic variability in that population.

There are 3 major determinants of the number of mitoses in the life history of a population. The first is the fraction of cells actually involved in mitosis. The other 2, to be considered below, are the time required for mitosis and the rate of cell loss. Regarding the fraction of cells in mitosis, in certain experimental tumors (mouse leukemia) and a few clinical cancers (Burkitt's lymphoma in children), up to 90% of the cells at any point in time are in some phase of their dividing process.[1,2] This fraction is termed the *growth fraction*.[3] Most human cancers, in contrast, have much smaller growth fractions, closer to 10% or 5% or less. Cells in the growth fraction progress through an orderly sequence of events (figure 6-1). Immediately after dividing, the cell enters a G-1 phase of active protein synthesis and active lipid and polysaccharide metabolism, but a period of relative inactivity in DNA synthesis. The G-1 phase can vary widely in duration; in fact, G-1 is the most variable phase of the mitotic process. It ends when the rate of DNA duplication increases to the point that it can be measured by enzyme activity, other markers, or—most classically—the incorporation of radioactive precursors into DNA. The initiation of this new phase, marked by DNA synthesis, ends the G-1 phase and starts the S phase. Several hours before active DNA synthesis, specific biochemical events take place in the cell (events that can be inhibited by arresting protein synthesis) preparing the cell to end G-1 and enter S phase.[4] The transition from G-1 to S phase also involves changes in cell geometry related to ionic fluxes between the intracellular and extracellular spaces.[5]

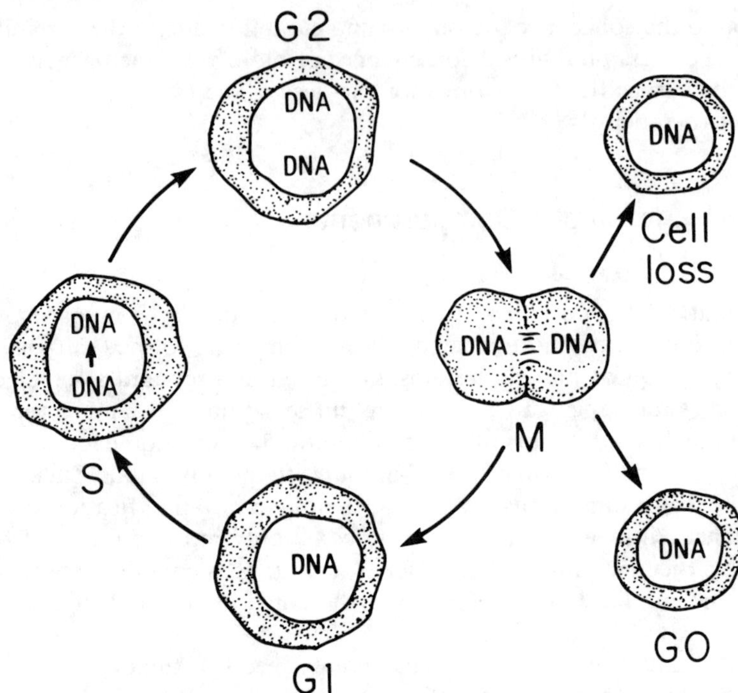

Figure 6-1. Phases of the cell cycle. Cells in G_0 and G_1 contain a diploid content of DNA (termed 2N), during the S phase, the DNA content increases from 2N to 4N, and G_2 cells are tetraploid with 4N DNA. At mitosis (M phase) there are 3 possible fates of a cell: more mitosis (the proliferative P compartment), rest (the G_0 state or the quiescent Q compartment), or death (the cell loss compartment). G_0 and G_1 cannot be distinguished cytokinetically. The tritiated thymidine labeling index measures the S phase. Flow cytometry graphs DNA content, which gives the relative proportions of G_0/G_1, G_2/M, and, by mathematical calculation, S.

The S phase is of special interest to the chemotherapist because most of the agents used in the treatment of cancer are thought to exert their major influence against the process of DNA production.[6] Antimetabolites, for example, may rob cells of essential nucleotide constituents. As part of their activity, anthracyclines, along with alkylating agents and bleomycin, may structurally destroy DNA. Steroids and procarbazine may adversely affect the process of DNA-directed protein synthesis. Such drugs as vincristine and vinblastine may interfere with the production of metaphase-spindle protein that occurs during S phase. It is clear, therefore, that S phase cells are particular targets of chemotherapy agents, even when these drugs are not "specific" for S phase, and are also active in other phases of the mitotic process. In addition, the interface of G-1 and S is a critical target for many agents. Steroid hormones and antihormones, for example, cause a G-1:S arrest. Antimetabolites can have a similar effect by delaying or preventing fruitful DNA synthesis.

Another aspect of the S phase that underscores its importance to the chemotherapist is that errors in DNA replication, including important gene mutations, occur and are propagated during this part of the mitotic process. If a cell's S phase is prolonged, the probability of mutation during that mitosis may be increased.[7] Some of these mutations may result in increased metastatic potential, whereas others may cause true biochemical drug resistance.[8] In general, most behaviors associated with neoplastic virulence, such as invasiveness, destructiveness, and immunological and biochemical variability—all features of tumor heterogeneity—in fact develop in large measure by random gene alteration. Therefore, the strong tendency of cancers to evidence increasingly malignant behavior over time, a phenomenon known as *tumor progression,* is closely related to kinetic, mitotic events.[9]

Biochemical Drug Resistance

Progression toward biochemical drug resistance is of particular concern to the sytemic therapist. Cells that are resistant by any mechanism to all of the drugs used in a chemotherapeutic program are, by definition, incurable with that program. Resistance to more than 1 agent might occur by random independent events or by a type of collateral resistance; that is, mutation toward impaired ability to transport a specific drug across the cell membrane may carry with it reduced ability to transport additional (otherwise unrelated) drugs. Panresistance to a wide variety of agents might be associated with a specific cellular protein.[10] Fortunately, however, most cells are not resistant to all chemotherapy drugs, even if they are resistant to 1 or some. Hence, in theory, by applying multiple agents simultaneously, all of the cells in a tumor might be subject to toxic damage by 1 or more components of the program. This is the conceptual basis for the observed superiority of combinations of agents, as opposed to single drugs, in the treatment of human malignancy.[11]

Once the DNA in the cell is replicated, the rate of synthesis drops. This marks the end of the S phase and the beginning of the G-2 phase. Some cells may remain in G-2 for long periods, but usually there is a timely passage into the actual division of the cell in the M phase. The cell "rounds up," chromosomes form discrete units and are separated in characteristic metaphase plate (associated temporally with disruption of the nuclear envelope), and the cell membrane pinches itself centrally, dividing into spheres containing complementary genetic material. The time from the very beginning of G-1 to the successful completion of M is the *cell cycle time.* This is the second major determinant of the rate of mitosis over time, the first being the actual number of cells engaged in the process. Given a uniform growth fraction, a short cell-cycle time implies more mitoses per unit of time and hence more opportunities for mutation.

Each of the 2 daughter cells produced by the division of the parent cell can meet only 1 of 3 possible fates: (1) It can progress through a new G-1 to S and thereby, ultimately, to another division; (2) it can stay in early G-1 for a long period; or (3) it can die, either immediately or after entry into any phase of the mitotic process. A cell that goes on to divide is regarded as belonging to the growth fraction; it is known as a *proliferative,* or P, cell. Because some cells progress through G-1, S, G-2, and M and then reenter G-1, etc., repeatedly, the mitotic process is sometimes thought of as a cycle. In fact, it is only the terms used to label the phases of the mitotic process that actually cycle, not individual cells.

The many techniques available for assessing cell cycle variables have given rise to several measures now used to describe the kinetic state of a tumor.[12] Three of these are in sufficiently common use to merit attention by clinicians. The *labeling index* is the percent of cells that pick up a radioactive precursor of DNA. Because only S phase cells are actively making DNA, these are the cells that label by this technique. The *mitotic index* is the percent of cells visibly in (or close to) M phase. Both of these measures are commonly—but erroneously—used to signify growth rate. In fact, they do convey information regarding the potential growth rate of a tumor but, as pointed out below, other factors may modify their influence.

Use of Flow Cytometry

Currently, a great deal of interest among clinicians has been focused upon the use of flow cytometry for assessing the kinetic state of a tumor. Unlike tritiated thymidine labeling, flow cytometry can readily be performed rapidly enough to aid in making therapeutic decisions.[12] This method uses dissociated tumor cells from fresh or—less optimally—paraffin-embedded specimens, sorting them by their degree of uptake of a fluorescent marker. If a dye that binds stoichiometrically to DNA is used, the cells can be sorted and counted by their DNA content. Hence, the percentage of cells with diploid content (termed 2N) can be measured, as also can the percentages of cells with other amounts of DNA. Cells in the G-1 and G-0 phases of the cell cycle should have 2N DNA. Cells in G-2 and M phases should have 4N DNA. Cells in S phase should have a DNA content between 2N and 4N. The percentage of cells in S (S phase fraction or SPF) is generally calculated by the use of computer programs for curve-fitting and area-measuring. In expert hands, the correlation is excellent between S phase estimates by flow cytometry and the classical tritiated thymidine labeling method.[13] If a population of cells contains <2N DNA (hypodiploid) or >4N DNA (hypertetraploid), or if there is a clear G-0/G-1 peak other than at 2N, that population is considered aneuploid, usually representing chromosomal aberrations of a significant degree. Ploidy (DNA content) can now be measured in >90% of solid tumors and SPF in about 80% of specimens.

The presence of aneuploidy in a biopsy usually signifies malignancy (rather than benignity), and, in conjunction with SPF, has been shown to have prognostic implications in a variety of tumors. In breast adenocarcinomas, for example, aneuploidy and high SPF usually correlate positively with such poor prognostic factors as estrogen/progesterone receptor negativity, premenopausal status, axillary lymph node involvement, and poorly differentiated histology.[14] About three-quarters of ovarian carcinomas are aneuploid, a finding that may correlate positively with stage and seemingly predicts shorter survival.[15] In diploid ovarian carcinomas, the finding of high SPF may convey negative prognostic information.[16] Aneuploidy also is found in prostate adenocarcinomas, but results linking this finding to prognosis are conflicting.[17,18] In colon cancer, both aneuploidy[19] and high SPF[20] point to a poor prognosis. Flow cytometry has been used to screen for transitional cell carcinoma using urinary bladder washings, but results are somewhat equivocal. Nevertheless, the presence of aneuploidy in biopsy specimens is a poor prognostic sign.[21] The flow cytometric approach to the kinetic analysis of clinical specimens has most recently been applied to other solid cancers, including those of the adrenal gland, endometrium, lung, skin (melanoma), thyroid, and testes. In neuroblastoma, in contrast to the general findings in other solid tumors, the discovery of aneuploidy seems to convey a positive prognostic influence,[22,23] which may be related to an association of N-myc amplification and the absence of aneuploidy.[24] In acute lymphoblastic leukemias, the prognostic significance of aneuploidy must be regarded as secondary to the more detailed analyses of chromosome composition/function afforded by the techniques of immunophenotyping, gene rearrangement studies, and cytogenetic classification.[25]

The Unique Abilities of Stem Cells

The vast majority of P cells in all organisms have finite capacities for S phase, and can progress through just so many S phases before they stop dividing or die; therefore, their life span is limited. Some special P cells, however, have greater capacity for repeated S phases than other cells and can divide without limit during the entire life span of the organ, tumor, or organism. These *stem cells* may have cell-cycle phase durations that differ significantly from those of more ordinary P cells. A mature tumor cell is doomed to die from its inception, so that its death by chemotherapy or any other treatment is merely accelerating the inevitable. On the other hand, a stem cell, by continuing to divide indefinitely, is a constant source of mature tumor cells and disease. For this reason, it is the death or arrest of tumor stem cells that is the real goal of cancer treatment.

In some human cancers—leukemias and lymphomas in particular—a high percentage of the cells produced at each mitosis rejoin the growth fraction. The relationship between the number of cells joining the growth fraction per mitosis and the size of the growth fraction is mathematically specifiable: The larger the percent allocation to the growth fraction at mitosis, the larger the absolute growth fraction.[26] In other cases, especially in the so-called "solid tumors," or cytomas, relatively few cells recycle after each mitosis, so the growth fraction is commensurately smaller. Some of these cells enter prolonged G-1 phases, never in the life of the host entering the late G-1 period in preparation for renewed DNA synthesis. These cells are physiologically in G-1 but are termed G-0 cells to identify the retrospective view that they are permanently nonmitotic. It is understood, however, that under certain circumstances, viable G-0 cells can be induced to reenter G-1 and progress to S, G-1, and M. This process is known as *recruitment*. The importance of recruitment is clear when we remember that S phase is important for maximum chemotherapeutic impact, and that if a large bulk of the tumor is in G-0–G-1, the tumor will be *kinetically refractory* to drug-induced regression. This type of drug resistance is as important as biochemical drug resistance, for both can preclude cure with conventional drugs, doses, and schedules.

Cells in G-0 are termed *quiescent,* or Q, cells. The growth fraction is the ratio of P over P + Q numbers. It is important to recognize that growth fraction is not equivalent to labeling index, which is the number of cells in S phase divided by the sum of the P + Q numbers. Because labeling index can be influenced by the relative duration of S phase in the cell cycle time, full knowledge of the durations of cell cycle phases is necessary to relate labeling index to growth fraction. Such knowledge is usually gained by a radioactive-DNA-precursor/autoradiographic technique known as the *percent of labeled mitoses,* or *PLM curve.* The mitotic index is also strongly related to cell cycle parameters. A long cycle time may yield a slow growth rate even if a high percentage of cells appear to be in M phase at any given point, especially if the duration of M phase is prolonged.

The Importance of Cell Loss

The P and Q compartments are 2 of the 3 possible fates of a cell leaving M phase. The third fate is cell death or cell loss, which is far from a trivial consequence.[27] A cell can be lost to the tumor by myriad mechanisms: necrosis, exfoliation, surgical extirpation, drug toxicity, death by ionizing radiation, and terminal differentiation, to name a few. A cell that enters the cell-loss fraction is no longer considered a part of the tumor, but this event is of critical importance in cancer biology.

Along with growth fraction and cell-cycle time, cell loss is a major determinant of tumor growth rate. High growth fraction and short cycle time cannot lead to a rapid growth rate if most of the cells produced by mitosis are lost. Even if the mitotic index is high, a high rate of cell loss could lead to a slow growth rate. An example of this phenomenon is basal cell epithelioma. On the other hand—and this is as important a role as in the determination of growth rate—the cell-loss fraction is quantitatively related to the emergence of gene alterations. This is because the 3 factors of cell loss, growth fraction, and cell-cycle time all determine the rate of accumulation of mitoses over time. A tumor with a high cell-loss rate must have an even higher cell production rate to sustain positive growth. A tumor with a high growth fraction and reasonably short cycle time that nevertheless grows slowly may be doing so in spite of a large number of mitoses over time because some of these products of mitosis are being lost. For every cell lost, another, its mitotic twin, must remain. If both products of mitosis are lost, a rarity in an actively growing mass, the mitotic twin of the parent cell (or its progeny) may remain. The remaining mitotic twin counts as a product of mitosis and adds to the cumulative number of mitoses in the life history of the tumor. Because mutation incidence is related to this accumulated number of mitoses, high-cell-loss tumors would be expected to exhibit marked heterogeneity. Examples are breast and colorectal adenocarcinomas. In contrast, tumors with lower cell loss rates, such as the acute leukemias and some lymphomas, may have had fewer mitoses to reach a clinically apparent tumor size; therefore, they may be more homogeneous than the adenocarcinomas. This concept applies as well to states associated with iatrogenetic chronic cell loss, such as maintenance chemotherapy of tumors in complete or low-volume partial remission (*vide infra*). Chemotherapy given as maintenance increases cell loss in the residual tumor and in host tissues affected by the chemotherapy. This could lead to heterogeneity not only in the tumor (drug resistance) but in the host tissues, such as oncogenesis in leukocyte precursor cells, leading to "second malignancies" in treated cancer patients.[28]

Growth Curves

The combination of growth fraction, cell-cycle time, and cell-loss fraction determines not only the growth rate of the tumor and its rate of mutation but also its pattern of growth. Assume, for the sake of illustration, that the growth fraction is 100%, the cycle time is 1 day, and the cell-loss factor is zero. After 1 day, a single cell has become 2 cells. After 2 days, each of these 2 cells has divided so that the tumor now measures 4 cells. At the end of the first week, the single cell has doubled 7 times to yield 128 cells. This pattern of growth is called "simple" exponential. The tumor doubles in size each cell-cycle time, in this case 1 day. Some primitive organisms and very young embryos divide by this pattern, but cancer growth is almost always more complicated. An example is a tumor with a growth fraction of 50%. After 1 day, the 2 cells now constitute a tumor mass, of which 1 cell is a Q cell and 1 a P cell. Only the P cell divides, so that at the end of 2 days there are 3 cells. Of these 3 cells, only 1 or 2 divide, so that at the end of the third day there will be 4 or 5 cells. At the end of 1 wk there will be 19–27 cells—considerably less than the 128 produced with a growth fraction of 100%. The third factor, cell loss, also exerts a growth-inhibitory influence. Using a starting point of 100 cells, without cell loss and at a growth fraction of 50% and a cycle time of 1 day, there will be 150 cells after 1 day, about 225 after 2 days, and slightly more than 1,700 cells at the end of the first week. The tumor doubles in size each 1.7 days. If 10% of cells are lost with each cycle, however, at the end of 1 day there will be 140 cells instead of 150. After 2 days there will be 196 instead of 225, and after 1 wk only slightly more than 1,050 instead of 1,700. The tumor now doubles about every 2 days. In this example, the potential doubling time is 2 days. It is clear that the ratio of potential to actual doubling times measures the cell loss fraction, and is frequently used for this purpose.

The combination of a growth fraction of 50% and a cell-loss fraction of 10% is equivalent to a growth fraction of 40% in terms of the overall growth rate of the tumor. However, a growth fraction of 50% and a cell-loss fraction of 10% requires more mitoses to produce 1,050 cells than a tumor with a growth fraction of 40% and no cell loss; therefore, there will be more opportunities for mutation in the growth pattern that includes cell loss, and thereby more heterogeneity.

As long as the 3 kinetic factors remain constant, the pattern of growth will be exponential, even if it is no longer simple. In all clinical and most laboratory examples, the numbers of cells involved are greater than those used in the illustrations above. As a shorthand, therefore, we express tumor cell numbers in exponential (to the base 10) notation. By this method, 100 cells are 2 logs of cells and 10 million cells are 7 logs of cells. A tumor must double about 3⅓ times to increase by 1 log. As illustrated above, the time required for the tumor to double—the doubling time—is always constant in exponential growth. Because the doubling time is constant, the time required for 3⅓ doublings is constant, so the time required for increase by 1 log is constant. As a consequence, when exponential growth is drawn on a semilogarithmic plot, with time on a regular arithmetic scale and volume on a logarithmic scale, the pattern has the appearance of a straight line (lower graph of figure 6-2).

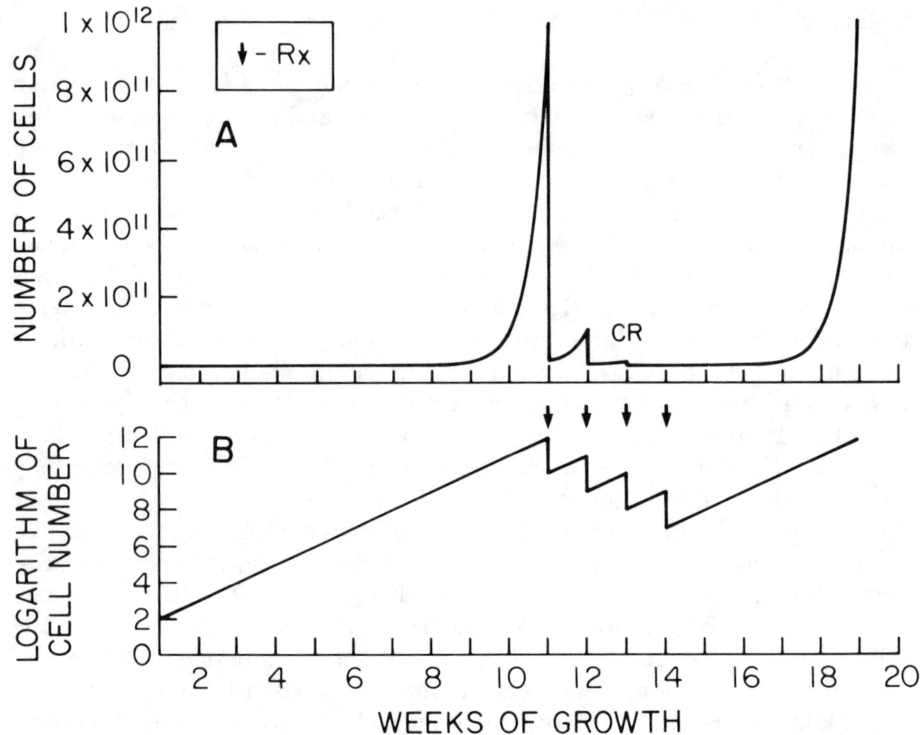

Figure 6-2. Exponential growth. The arithmetic scale (as the clinician would view the tumor) is shown in the upper graph (A), and the same tumor growth is shown on a logarithmic scale of tumor size in the lower graph (B). Therapy causing a 2-log (99%) reduction in tumor size is indicated by the arrows. Silent growth prior to clinical appreciation is apparent. Complete remission is shown to leave a considerable burden of tumor cells, leading to relapse (see text for details).

Figure 6-2 illustrates several characteristics of exponential growth of major importance in clinical oncology. The first is *silent growth*. With reference to the arithmetic scale (top graph), the 2-log tumor at the end the first week is invisible to the unaided eye of the clinician. It is only one-tenth of one-millionth of a cubic centimeter in size (assuming that the tumor cells are the size of small lymphocytes and are closely packed). The tumor illustrated in this figure has the same kinetics as described above: a growth fraction of 50% and a cell-loss fraction of 10%, which, for a cell cycle time of 1 day, results in a doubling time of about 2 days. The lower graph presents the same data as the arithmetic plot above it, but uses a semilogarithmic scale. After 3⅓ doubling times, or just less than 1 wk, the tumor grows from 2 to 3 logs. It is still invisible, as it is just one-millionth of a cubic centimeter. But another week brings the tumor to 4 logs, still microscopic, and so on, until, about the eighth week, the tumor measures about 9 logs, which is just 1 cc in size. The tumor would just reach the clinical limits of detection, then, between weeks 7 and 8. The entire growth period from 100 (2 logs) cells to 1 billion (9 logs) cells is truly invisible and therefore silent. Yet almost 1⅓ *billion* mitoses have taken place prior to the eighth week, each mitosis carrying a finite risk of mutation. It would be no surprise to find at least 1 cell in such a mass that had already mutated toward biochemical resistance to any particular chemotherapeutic drug. Indeed, this is more likely to be the rule rather than the exception. Additionally, mutations toward metastatic behavior and other characteristics of a virulent tumor would also be likely to have occurred. Even though the growth of the tumor is silent to the clinician, it may be very important to the biology of the tumor and may eventually have important clinical ramifications.

From wk 8 to wk 9, the tumor, still with a 50% growth fraction and a 10% cell loss per 1-day cycle time, grows from 1 cc to 10 logs, or 10 cc. In another week it reaches 11 logs, or 100 cc. By wk 11 it has reached 1 L in size. Hence, this same tumor, following unchanged kinetics, takes 8 wk to grow from 100 cells to clinical detectability, but only 3 wk to grow from 1 cc to a full liter in size.

The "explosive" nature of exponential growth can be particularly compelling when the tumor grows as a sheet rather than as a nodule. For example, a sheet of lymphangitic pulmonary metastasis 1 cell thick can be invisible radiographically and insignificant clinically. However, 3 or 4 doublings can result in thickness sufficient to cause a compromise in gaseous exchange and a dramatic alteration in chest x-ray appearance. Here, prolonged growth is needed to create the silent unicellular layer, whereas a short subsequent period leads to severe disease.

To an untutored eye, the 3 wk of clinically measurable tumor growth in figure 6-2 might represent a change in tumor kinetics in favor of more aggressive behavior. Although changes toward more aggressive growth can happen (especially as a consequence of mutation or of hormonal changes), most cases of explosive growth can be explained by basic exponential kinetics. It is clear, then, that the silent period and the explosive period of exponential growth are really part of a continuum, that constant doubling time leads to constant log-growth periods (in this case 1 wk), which gives the illusion of a change in kinetics once significant size is achieved.

Models of Tumor Response to Therapy

One of the major conceptual and experimental advances in modern oncology occurred with the development of a theory relating the growth of an exponential tumor to its pattern of response to effective therapy.[29] This theory, the *log-kill model,* was important partially because it allowed for the analysis and screening of chemotherapeutic drugs in a murine leukemia model. The model was important in equal part because the experimental work it permitted led directly to influential concepts of drug use.

The observation that is fundamental to the log-kill concept is illustrated in figure 6-2. At wk 11, a certain dose of chemotherapy is given as a bolus. The tumor regresses rapidly from 12 logs (1 trillion cells) to 10 logs (10 billion cells). This is a change of 2 logs, or a log-kill of 2. The tumor regrows over 1 wk by 1 log to 11 logs (100 billion cells, 100 cc). In actual practice, the tumor would not be observed to change volume as rapidly as seen in this graph, because of

(1) delayed cell death; (2) slow removal of dead cells from the mass; and (3) edema, fibrosis, and other nonmalignant components of tumor bulk. Nevertheless, the tumor should shrink by the end of 1 wk of therapy toward 100 cc, or one-tenth of the original tumor mass. If at 11 wk the tumor is spherical in shape, its diameter should be 12.4 cc. The usual clinical method of recording tumor size is the product of 2 mutually perpendicular diameters; therefore, the mass would be measured at 12.4 by 12.4 cc, or 154 sq cm. At the end of the first week of therapy—at 11 logs or 100 cc—the mass should measure 5.76 by 5.76 cc, or 33.18 sq cm. Since 33.18 is < ½ of 154, the tumor at 1 wk would be in partial remission.

The characteristic log-kill effect is seen at wk 12 when a second dose of the same agent at the same dose level is applied. Here the tumor size changes from 11 logs to 9 logs, or 1 billion cells. This mass is at the limits of clinical detection. The change from 11 logs to 9 logs is also a log-kill of 2: According to the log-kill model, the fractional change induced by an agent (disregarding drug resistance) is always the same, in this case a change of 2 logs. This tumor also regrows over the next week, so that at wk 13 it measures 10 logs or 10 cc in volume (2.67 by 2.67 cm in product of diameters). It should be noted that at the end of the first week of therapy, the tumor at 100 cc was one-tenth of its pretreatment size of 1 L; now, at the end of the second week of therapy, the tumor at 10 cc is one-tenth of the size that it was at the end of the first week.

Implications of Log-Kill Concept

The implications of the log-kill concept are broad. In the example above, the drug has reduced the tumor to one one-hundredth of its pretreatment volume with just 2 doses. A third dose is given at wk 13, which also causes a log-kill of 2. The cell number is reduced from 10 logs to 8 logs. Even with a 1-log growth over the next week, the tumor has in effect disappeared from clinical view. This complete remission (CR) is achieved in just 2 wk of treatment. The tumor appears to be quite sensitive. A last dose of therapy is given at wk 14. In the absence of a kinetic analysis (i.e., just inspecting the upper graph of figure 6-2 without attempting a mathematical analysis) it may seem that a fourth dose at wk 14 should be able to eradicate the residual tumor. Such fallacious reasoning would cite the observation that 1 L of tumor cells were "eliminated" from clinical view rapidly, hence the tumor cell population should be homogeneously sensitive to the drug. In fact, however, the fourth dose is limited to causing but another log-kill of 2. Nine logs of cells are reduced to 7 logs, a small volume (one one-hundredth of 1 cc), but at 10 million cells, still far from disease eradication. The tumor regrows not because of biochemically resistant cells but because of the kinetic "resistance" inherent in the log-kill model. There is a discrepancy between the sensitivity of the tumor in terms of rate of attainment of a CR and curability in terms of likelihood of disease ablation.

It is important to note that the regrowth of this tumor would not be immediately apparent to the clinical observer. From the tumor nadir of 7 logs at wk 14 it takes 2 wk for the tumor to reach the smallest discernible size of 9 logs at wk 16. The appearance of explosive growth is only detectable after wk 17. Because a CR is achieved at wk 13, the duration of the CR (3–4 wk) is longer than the 2 wk used to obtain it. Beyond 17 wk, the tumor demonstrates progressive disease. This example illustrates that many clinically relevant terms are merely descriptions of kinetic growth curves. Many widely held beliefs about optimal cancer chemotherapy are derived directly from the log-kill model.[30] Giving drugs in pulses of equal intensity and equally spaced over time is 1 such concept. Using more than 1 drug simultaneously (in an effort to sum their log-kills) is also supported by the model. The need to treat beyond CR is based on the kinetic resistance illustrated above. These ideas have had a major influence on the development of modern cancer medicine.

The exponential pattern depends upon a constancy of the 3 determinants of growth. Some animal cancers do indeed demonstrate such constancy, and a few human tumors (primarily lung nodules) have been observed to follow exponential kinetics for short periods of observation.[31] However, the vast majority of animal tumors, and most clinical cancers as well, do not follow strict exponential growth. The average cell cycle time remains fairly constant, and cell loss seems to remain a constant proportion of the total cell number; the growth fraction, on the other hand, declines over time.[32] The result is that when the tumor is small, its growth appears to be almost exponential, but as it becomes larger, the growth rate of the cancer becomes progressively slower than would be expected for an exponential tumor. If the growth fraction

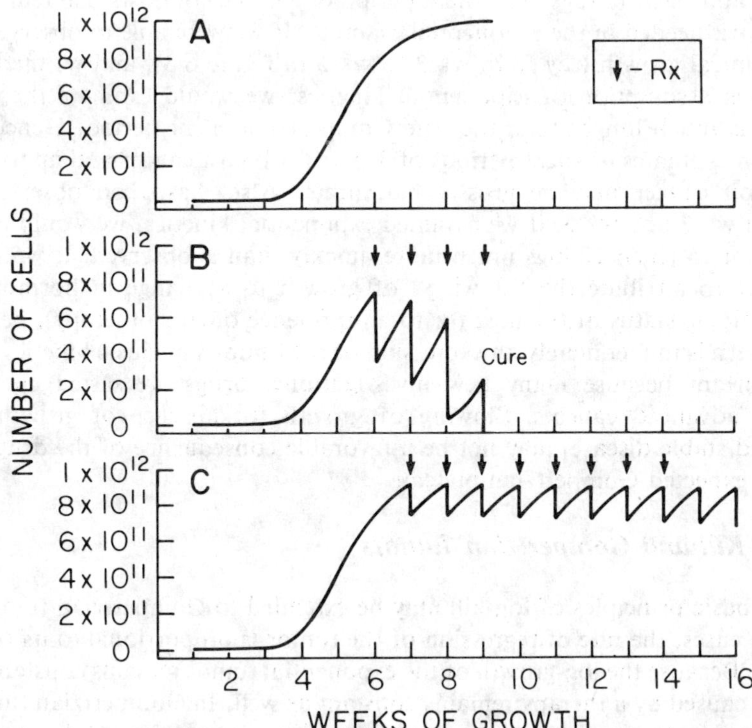

Figure 6-3. Gompertzian growth on an arithmetic scale of tumor size. Untreated (A), therapy started during the rapid growth phase (B), and therapy started at advanced tumor size close to the plateau phase (C) (see text for details).

declines according to a certain pattern, the tumor growth curve has a particular "S" shape or *Gompertzian* sigmoid form (figure 6-3, upper graph).[33]

A few clinical cancers have been documented as following Gompertzian kinetics.[34,35] In addition, the appropriateness of the sigmoid pattern is intuitive: Many tumors (breast and colon adenocarcinoma, nodular lymphomas, some hypernephromas) may spontaneously enter a phase of slow growth after an earlier period of more rapid growth. For example, in figure 6-3 the tumor "explodes" from its silent period between wk 3 and 4. By wk 7 or 8, a cell number of close to 12 logs is achieved. Most of this growth occurs between wk 4 and wk 6, with slow growth thereafter. After wk 8, the tumor is clearly in *plateau phase,* with little significant further growth. Benign tumors, or premalignant neoplasms, may reach a Gompertzian plateau at a small size. This does not mean that there is little mitotic activity, however; if the cell loss fraction is large, the tumor may require a great number of mitoses to replace the cells lost. Each of these mitoses carries a risk of mutation, so tumor heterogeneity may develop even during the plateau phase of a Gompertzian tumor. This may be a mechanism by which especially virulent clones of leukemia cells arise by mutation out of a plateau phase of chronic leukemia. Breast cancer may arise from premalignant lesions by a similar process.[36]

The upper graph of figure 6-3 illustrates another important feature of Gompertzian growth. Here the tumor, starting at 2 logs of cells, requires just 7 wk to approach 12 logs. The silent period of 3–4 wk contrasts markedly with the 7–8 wk needed in the exponential example. If we were able to observe only early clinical growth (say from wk 3 to wk 5 in figure 6-3), and we made the erroneous assumption of exponential kinetics, we would estimate the silent period as much longer than the true Gompertzian silent period. Hence, the common estimates of silent periods of 3–5 yr for breast cancer and up to 20 yr for colon cancer may be grossly inaccurate. Also, based on observations between wk 3 and wk 5, if we assumed exponential kinetics, we would expect the tumor to reach 12 logs much more quickly than is observed. It would be incorrect to attribute the "slowing" of growth to a change in hormone or immunologic status of the host (or to an influence of some therapy), because the pattern is in fact merely an expression of the tumor's intrinsic kinetics. This is important because many new investigational drugs are tested clinically against advanced cancers. Slowing of growth (or absence of growth, the so-called stable disease) may not be a favorable consequence of the drug, but just an expected Gompertzian plateau.

Log-Kill and Gompertzian Tumors

The basic principles of log-kill may be extended to Gompertzian tumors.[37] In both cases, the rate of regression of the tumor is proportional to its rate of growth. Because the log-growth of the exponential tumor remains constant, the log-kill caused by a therapy remains constant as well. In Gompertzian tumors, however, growth is not constant. This leads to important points of dissimilarity with the log-kill of exponential kinetics. In the middle graph of figure 6-3, the first dose of therapy at wk 6 reduces the tumor by 400 billion cells, from 700 billion cells to 300 billion residual cells. It would take this tumor 8 days to regrow from 300 billion to 700 billion, but our therapeutic plan does not allow this recovery. Instead, we treat again only 7 days later (at wk 7) with the same dose level of the same drug and kill even more cells than with the first treatment. The reason for this increased cell-kill is that although there are fewer cells at wk 7 compared to wk 6, more cells are engaged in mitosis; that is, the product of the increased growth fraction and the smaller number of cells is actually a larger number of cells in division. More cells in mitosis means more cells at risk for chemotherapeutic damage. The cells left after therapy at wk 7 would enable the tumor to regrow to its pretreatment size in 8 days, but we prevent this from happening by re-treating 7 days later and again accomplishing a significant cell-kill.

In exponential kinetics, a given dose of drug kills a constant number of logs of tumor volume. By contrast, in Gompertzian kinetics a given dose of drug kills a variable fraction of cells, but always kills enough cells so that it would take a constant period of time for the tumor to recover if left undisturbed. In this example, the constant period is 8 days. If therapy can be given more often than this constant recovery period, tumor regression and eventual eradication can be accomplished.

The bottom graph in figure 6-3 simulates the influence of the same dose and schedule as in the middle graph, but starts therapy at wk 7 instead of wk 6. Here the treatment also results in an 8-day displacement, i.e., it would take this tumor 8 days to recover from the cell-kill caused at wk 7. Because the tumor volume here is higher than at the first treatment in the middle graph, however, the impact of the drug in terms of the number of cells killed is quite different. For this larger volume tumor, closer to its plateau size, less growth takes place over 8 days—only 160 billion cells compared with 400 billion in the previous example. Over 7 days, the tumor comes closer to replenishing these lost cells, so that the impact of therapy at wk 8 is only slightly more substantial. Weekly therapies thereafter do cause a rate of tumor volume regression, but because this rate is insufficient to even approach a cure volume, treatment is very unrewarding. In addition, the significant regrowth between cycles of therapy adds many mitoses to the cumulative number in the life history of the tumor, which increases the chances of mutation to biochemical drug resistance.

The lower graph in figure 6-3 illustrates one of the cardinal features of Gompertzian kinetics. Starting therapy at too large a tumor size can result in a poor rate of tumor regression—not because of biochemical drug resistance but because of kinetic factors. Slow-growing tumors regress slowly in response to therapy; if a tumor is close to its plateau phase, the relatively large number of Q cells may resist antimitotic therapy. This distinguishes Gompertzian growth from the exponential pattern in which the largest tumors (as in figure 6-2) respond the most briskly to treatment. This is because the constant log-kill in the exponential case (here 2 logs, or 99%) represents the largest number of cells (99% of a large number of cells is a large number and a sizable cell-kill).

Even if therapy is started at a more moderate tumor size, however, cure can sometimes be elusive on a kinetic basis. The concept of kinetic resistance for subclinical tumors, illustrated in figure 6-2 for the exponential case, is operative here as well. Rapid regression of the tumor during the rapidly growing portion of the Gompertzian curve may lull the clinician into a false sense of confidence, so that after the attainment of CR, insufficient therapy is applied to maximize the chances of cure. Sensitivity—the rate of macroscopic regression—may not correlate with curability. This reason for treatment failure may be quite common in practice. As just 1 example, patients with advanced Hodgkin's disease who achieve CRs with combination chemotherapy sometimes relapse after going off treatment, some of the relapses occurring a year or more after therapy is terminated. Such patients have a 50% chance of reentering complete remission by the reapplication of the same drugs used to attain the initial CR.[38] If the relapse was due to biochemical drug resistance, the induction of a second remission with the same agents would be impossible.

Kinetics and Treatment Design

It is clear, then, that factors other than biochemical drug resistance may hamper our ability to eradicate a given neoplasm. This is especially valid when we consider the heterogeneity of most clinical cancers. The mutations arising from the mitoses during the silent period of growth can give rise to various subclones with different kinetics as well as metastatic behavior. Some of these subclones may be biochemically resistant to treatment, whereas others, because of long cycle time, short S phase, or small growth fraction, may be kinetically resistant. From the above discussion, it is clear that aggressive therapy during CR may be needed to eradicate such cells. If these same cells are also biochemically resistant, the aggressive therapy would best be composed of agents not used to induce the original remission. This plan of *crossover intensification* has met with some success in clinical trials in breast cancer,[39] Hodgkin's disease,[40] ovarian carcinoma,[41] and other diseases.[42] Marrow-ablative chemotherapy with bone marrow transplantation as rescue is a late-intensification concept of present investigational interest.[43]

A view alternative to the crossover plan is that it would be best to alternate different combinations in an effort to eliminate multiple clones simultaneously.[44] This plan is also intended to reduce the size of all subpopulations as quickly as possible in order to minimize the risk of further mutations toward biochemical drug resistance. The theory underlying this hypothesis depends strongly on subpopulations of equal size, each with the same growth rates and the same degrees of sensitivity to their respective therapies. Such rigid biological conditions may be difficult to find in clinical practice. However, an alternating chemotherapy trial in advanced Hodgkin's disease has resulted in a longer CR duration than a conventional plan using a single drug combination in equally spaced cycles.[45] Many other programs have applied alternating cycles without apparent benefit. While no concrete therapeutic recommendations should be made at this time, this is an active area of kinetic research that should be watched for direct clinical applicability.

Also of current interest and potential importance are studies of the kinetic relationship between tumor subpopulations. Evidence suggests that the elimination of 1 subline may release others from a type of growth inhibition, with the result that the growth fraction of the residual populations may increase.[46]

If the cycle time and cell loss fraction remain constant, the increase in growth fraction can have 2 consequences: (1) the larger number of dividing cells are a bigger target for chemotherapy and (2) the increased number of mitoses can increase the chances for mutation. For this reason, giving chemotherapy immediately after the inhibition release would be essential for maximum therapeutic response. This is clinically relevant for debulking surgery, which suddenly eliminates large numbers of tumor cells. Perioperative chemotherapy, or even the "neoadjuvant" approach in which chemotherapy is given before surgery, may be indicated by this reasoning.[12] Clinical trials in this regard should be watched carefully, not only for their particular therapeutic effects, but also for the kinetic lessons they convey.

Tumor kinetics forms the vocabulary unique to cancer medicine. Topics as diverse and as important as tumor heterogeneity, drug resistance, and the impact of dose scheduling are dependent on kinetic reasoning. These comprise an essential part of the foundation for modern cancer therapy. An understanding of the relationship between mitosis and cancer growth illuminates many clinically relevant principles of today and may provide the basis for therapeutic advances in the future.

References

1. Simpson-Herren L, Lloyd HH. Kinetic parameters and growth curves for experimental tumor systems. Cancer Chemother Rep 1970; 54:143–74.
2. Norton L. Cell kinetics in normal tissues and in tumors of the young. In: Levine AS, ed. Cancer in the young. New York: Masson, 1982; 53–82.
3. Mendelsohn ML. The growth fraction: a new concept applied to tumors. Science 1960; 132:1496.
4. Pardee AB, Campisi J, Gray HE, et al. Cellular oncogenes, growth factors, and cellular growth control. In: Ford RJ, Maizel AL, eds. Mediators in growth control and differentiation. New York: Raven, 1985; 21–29.
5. Folkman J, Moscona A. Role of cell shape in growth control. Nature 1978; 273:345–49.
6. Valeriote F, van Putten L. Proliferation-dependent cytotoxicity of anticancer agents: a review. Cancer Res 1975; 35:2619–30.
7. Novick A, Szilard L. Experiments with the chemostat on spontaneous mutations of bacteria. Proc Natl Acad Sci USA 1950; 36:708–19.
8. Poste G, Fidler IJ. The pathogenesis of cancer metastases. Nature (London) 1980; 283:139–46.
9. Nowell PC. The clonal evolution of tumor cell populations. Science 1976; 194:23–28.
10. Deuchars KL, Ling V. P-glycoprotein and multi-drug resistance in cancer chemotherapy. Semin Oncol 1989; 16:156.
11. DeVita VT. The influence of information on drug resistance on protocol design. Ann Oncol (in press).
12. DeVita VT. Primary chemotherapy can avoid mastectomy, but is there more to it than that? (edit) JNCI 1990; 82:1522–52.
13. McDivitt RW, Stone KR, Meyer JS. A method for dissociation of viable human breast cancer cells that produces flow cytometric kinetic information similar to that obtained by thymidine labeling. Cancer Res 1984; 44:2628–33.
14. Dressler LG, Seamer L, Owens MA, et al. DNA flow cymetry and prognostic factors in 1331 frozen breast cancer specimens. Cancer 1988; 61:420–27.
15. Friedlander ML, Hedley DW, Taylor IW, et al. Influence of cellular DNA content on survival in advanced ovarian cancer. Cancer Res 1984; 44:397–400.

16. Kallioneiemi OP, Punnonen R, Mattila J, et al. Prognostic significance of DNA index, multiploidy, and S-phase fraction in ovarian cancer. Cancer 1988; 61:334–39.

17. Fordham MVP, Burdge AH, Matthews J, et al. Prostatic carcinoma cell DNA content measured by flow cytometry and its relation to clinical outcome. Br J Surg 1986; 73:400–03.

18. DeVere White R, Tesluk H, Deitch A. The paradox of aneuploidy in the benign and malignant prostate (abstract). Cytometry 1987; 1:3.

19. Wolley RC, Schreiber K, Koss LG, et al. DNA distribution in human colon carcinomas and its relationship to clinical behavior. J Natl Cancer Inst 1982; 69:15–22.

20. Bauer KD, Lincoln ST, Vera-Roman JM, et al. Prognostic implications of proliferative activity and DNA aneuploidy in colonic adenocarcinomas. Lab Invest 1987; 57:329–35.

21. Murphy WM, Chandler RW, Trafford RM. Flow cytometry of deparaffinized nuclei compared to histological grading from the pathological evaluation of transitional cell carcinomas. 1986; J Urol 135:694–97.

22. Oppedal BR, Storm-Mathisen I, Lie SO, Brandtzaeg P. Prognostic factors in neuroblastoma: clinical, histopathologic and immunohistochemical features and DNA ploidy in relation to prognosis. Cancer 1988; 62:772–780.

23. Taylor SR, Blatt J, Costantino JP, Roederer M, Murphy FF. Flow cytometric DNA analysis of neuroblastoma and ganglioneuroma: A 10-year retrospective study. Cancer 1988; 62:749–54.

24. Dominici C, Negroni A, Romeo A, et al. Association of near-diploid DNA content and N-myc amplification in neuroblastomas. Clin Exp Metastasis 1989; 7:201–211.

25. Sobol RE, Bloomfield CD, Royston I. Immunophenotyping in the diagnosis and classification of acute lymphoblastic leukemia. Clin Lab Med 1988; 8:151–62.

26. Norton L. Implications of kinetic heterogeneity in clinical oncology. Semin Oncol 1985; 12:231–49.

27. Steel GG. Cell loss as a factor in the growth of human tumors. Eur J Cancer 1967; 3:381–87.

28. Glicksman AS, Pajak TF, Gottlieb A, Nissen N, Stutzman L, Cooper, MR. Second malignant neoplasms in patients successfully treated for Hodgkin's disease. Cancer Treat Rep 1982; 66:1035–45.

29. Skipper HE. Laboratory models: the historical perspective. Cancer Treat Rep 1986; 70:3–7.

30. DeVita VT Jr, Simon RM, Hubbard S, et al. Curability of advanced Hodgkin's disease with chemotherapy. Ann Intern Med 1980; 92:587–95.

31. Collins VP, Loeffler RR, Tivey H. Observations on growth rate of human tumors. Am J Radiol 1956; 76:988–1000.

32. Laird AR. Dynamics of growth in tumors and normal tissues. Monographs Natl Cancer Inst 30, 1969.

33. Winsor CP. The Gompertz curve as a growth curve. Proc Natl Acad Sci USA 1932; 18:1–8.

34. Sullivan PW, Salmon SE. Kinetics of tumor growth and regression in IgG multiple myeloma. J Clin Invest 1972; 51:1697–1708.

35. Demicheli R. Growth of testicular neoplasm lung metastases: tumor-specific relation between two Gompertzian parameters. Eur J Cancer 1980; 16:1603–09.

36. Norton L. A Gompertzian model of human breast cancer growth. Cancer Res 1988; 48:7067–71.

37. Norton L. Implications of kinetic heterogeneity in clinical oncology. Semin Oncol 1985; 12:231–49.

38. Fisher RI, DeVita VT Jr, Hubbard SP, et al. Prolonged disease-free survival in Hodgkin's disease with MOPP reinduction after first relapse. Ann Intern Med 1979; 90:761–63.

39. Buzzoni R, Bonadonna G, Valagussa P, Zambetti M. Sequential vs. alternating chemotherapy in the adjuvant treatment of breast cancer with more than three positive axillary nodes. Proc Am Soc Clin Oncol 1990; 9:67.

40. Glick J, Tsiatis A, Prosnitz L, et al. Improved survival with sequential Bleo-MOPP followed by ABVD for advanced Hodgkin's disease. Proc Am Soc Clin Oncol 1984; 20:926.

41. Coleman M, Pasmantier MW, Silver RT. HAC-Cytoxan chemotherapy for ovarian carcinoma: alternating chemotherapy with intensification. Cancer 1985; 55:2342–47.

42. Livingston RB, Greenstreet ML. Reinduction prolongs survival in complete responders with small-cell lung cancer. Proc Am Soc Clin Oncol 1982; 1:151.

43. Peters, WP, Davis R, Shpall EJ, et al. Adjuvant chemotherapy involving high dose combination cyclophosphamide, cisplatin and carmustine and autologous bone marrow support for stage II/III

breast cancer involving ten or more lymph nodes (CALGB 8782): a preliminary report. Proc Am Soc Clin Oncol 1990; 9:80.

44. Goldie JH. Scientific basis for adjuvant and primary (neoadjuvant) chemotherapy. Semin Oncol 1987; 14:1-7.

45. Valagussa P, Santoro A, Boracchi P, Viviani S, Bonadonna G. 9-year results of two randomized studies with MOPP and ABVD in Hodgkin's disease: multiple regression analysis. Proc Am Soc Clin Oncol 1989; 8:976.

46. Canellos GP, Propent K, Cooper R, et al. MOPP vs. ABVD vs. MOPP alternating with ABVD in advanced Hodgkin's disease: a prospective randomized CALGB trial (abstr). Proc Am Soc Clin Oncol 1988; 7:888.

47. Fisher B, Gunduz N, Saffer EA. Influence of the interval between primary tumor removal and chemotherapy on the kinetics and growth of metastases. Cancer Res 1983; 43:1488-92.

7

CANCER METASTASES AND PRINCIPLES OF STAGING

Albert S. Braverman, M.D., F.A.C.P.

Pathogenesis of Metastasis

EXCEPT FOR CERTAIN BRAIN and lung tumors, death from malignancy is always the result of metastases, for the reason that modern surgical and radiotherapeutic techniques usually can completely control primary tumors. Tumors fulfilling the morphologic criteria of malignancy are almost always able to metastasize. The more anaplastic the primary tumor and the higher its growth fraction—i.e., proportion of cells in cycle, as determined by mitotic index or S phase level—the more likely it is to have metastasized, the greater number of metastatic sites, and the earlier the metastases are likely to become apparent. (This correlation does not seem to hold for B immunocyte neoplasms because the well-differentiated, slowly proliferating follicular forms are typically widely disseminated at presentation; however, this may not be a true metastatic phenomenon). Flow cytometry techniques, which can determine the percentage of tumor cells in cycle, are now routinely applied to clinical specimens, sometimes yielding significant prognostic data.[1]

Multiple malignant tumors of similar histology are usually, but not invariably, evidence of metastasis. Exceptions are Kaposi's sarcoma, low-grade transitional cell bladder carcinomas, familial medullary thyroid carcinomas, retinoblastomas. In these cases, because of a preneoplastic, sometimes inherited mutation affecting all cells in the involved field, multiple primary malignancies occur, which, unlike primary tumors and their metastases, are *polyclonal.*

Studies of metastasis in animal models, in which tumor cells are transplanted into hosts genetically identical (syngeneic) to the animals in which they arose, have greatly increased our understanding of metastatic mechanisms.[2-4] These studies have led to the following conclusions:

1. Although almost always *monoclonal* (the progeny of a single cell), and therefore initially genetically identical, tumor cells rapidly acquire a variety of mutations.

2. The ability to metastasize depends on mutations acquired by only a small proportion of the cells in any tumor.

3. Subsets of these cells are genetically endowed with the ability to metastasize to particular organs. Lines can be obtained which preferentially colonize lung, brain, etc.

4. The ability of such a tumor line to colonize a particular organ does not depend primarily on its ability to grow within it but rather on its ability to become fixed to the organ parenchymal or vascular endothelial cells or to invade the organ.[5]

The precise mechanisms of metastasis are now under active investigation.[6] They may include the following:

- Production of angiogenesis factors to elicit new blood vessel growth[7]
- Production of enzymes necessary to penetrate the basement membrane, in order to leave the primary tumor and invade the host organ; these include collagenases and cathepsins[6,8]
- Ability to become attached to host organ-specific adhesion molecules on vascular endothelial or basement membrane or parenchymal cells[5,6]
- Ability to evade host immune defenses insofar as they may be directed against tumor antigens[9]
- Ability to proliferate in the host organ in response to specific local growth factors.[6]

Patterns of Human Metastasis

From the clinical (in vivo) behavior of tumors, 3 determinants of the distribution of metastases can be deduced: (1) vascular pathways, (2) organ receptivity, and (3) intracellular attributes.

The first capillary bed that cells liberated from the primary tumor encounter is a favored metastatic site. This probably accounts for the tendency of tumors arising from organs whose venous drainage is the portal circulation (e.g., G.I. tract above the rectum; pancreas) to form hepatic metastases. The same principle presumably accounts for the high frequency of pulmonary metastases from most other tumors and perhaps for the tendency of bronchogenic carcinomas to spread to the brain.

Lymphatic vessels are also important conduits for metastases. If they have metastasized at all, carcinomas typically involve local draining nodes; sarcomas often bypass them. In some cases, such as squamous tumors arising in the head and neck region, there is a sequential spread, first to nodes, and then to distant sites. In others, such as breast cancer, lymphatic and hematogenous spread appear to occur simultaneously.[31] Breast tumors also employ lymphatic vessels for spread to more distant sites, such as pleura (90% of malignant effusions are homolateral in breast cancer[10]) and to lung.[11]

Certain organs, such as spleen, kidney, and skeletal muscle, appear constitutively resistant to metastasis, though the spleen is characteristally receptive to lymphomas and myeloproliferative cells; splenomegaly should always suggest these latter neoplasms rather than carcinoma.

When tumors do spread to bone, they most commonly involve the axial skeleton, especially the vertebrae. The slow flow of blood in Batson's venous plexus, which drains these bones, may facilitate the fixation of tumor cells.[12]

The ability to colonize certain organs is an intrinsic attribute of certain types of tumor cells. In 80% of prostate and differentiated thyroid carcinoma patients and in 50% of breast cancer cases, bones are the exclusive site of metastases. In these tumors, osseous metastases are uniquely *blastic,* indicating that perhaps because of the relatively indolent character of the metastasis, some new bone formation occurs in response to tumor cell osteolysis—though never enough to prevent a net loss of bone. Radiologic evidence of areas of increased bone density, in addition to lytic regions and intense radionuclide scan positively, are typical.

Kaposi's sarcoma has a unique predilection for spread to the G.I. tract. T cell lymphomas, high-grade B immunocyte neoplasms, and acute lymphoblastic leukemia commonly spread diffusely to the meninges (although not to CNS parenchyma; metastatic CNS mass lesions are very uncommon in hematologic neoplasms, occurring only in primary brain lymphoma).

Principles of Tumor Staging

Following are the objectives of tumor staging:
- To determine the local and local nodal extent of a primary tumor, in order to decide whether adjuvant systemic therapy and/or radiation are appropriate
- To establish the presense of distant metastases in order to avoid unnecessary surgery on the primary tumor
- To define the extent of Hodgkin's disease in order to determine whether it is potentially curable by radiation (XRT) alone
- To establish the presence of dangerous CNS metastases (brain and epidural masses), which may be effectively palliated in incurable patients.

Nomenclature

A standard staging system exists for each tumor type.[13] In each case, the specific attributes of the primary tumor (T), its draining nodes (N), and distant metastases (M) are defined, and grouped, by roman numerals, into successive prognostic categories. As an example, the system for breast cancer is shown in table 7-1. These are prognostic groups. Stages 0 and I are usually cured by surgery alone; most IIb patients relapse if they do not receive systemic therapy; surgery is never sufficient local treatment for III; and stage IV patients are all ultimately incurable with any therapy.

History and Physical Examinations

The medical history is among the most sensitive staging procedures. For example, radionuclide bone scanning is routinely performed in stage II breast cancer patients prior to surgery because of its great sensitivity. Yet this procedure detects metastases in bone (the most common metastatic site in this disease) in <5% of patients without complaint of pain.[14-16] Conversely, the physician should investigate complaints of pain the patient ascribes to long-standing, preexisting causes such as lumbar disc disease. Cancer patients often subconsciously reassure themselves by attributing new symptoms to old, familiar, and unthreatening diseases. In general, the first principle of staging is that clinical leads should be elucidated before gratuitous screening studies are obtained. Bone metastases are far more common than brain metastases in breast cancer patients, but a CT head scan should be the first diagnostic procedure in a breast patient who complains of hemiparesis or seizures or is inexplicably demented.

The physical examination is probably less sensitive than the history, but decidedly more specific. Very firm or hard nodes, even when not >1 cm in size, may be diagnostic. Homolateral supraclavicular adenopathy is common in bronchogenic and breast cancer (particularly at the sterno-clavicular junction in the latter); Virchow's node (on the left) is often detected in gastric, pancreatic, and advanced bladder carcinoma. This examination is best performed with the patient in a sitting position. Although the inguinal regions are usually palpated, the femoral triangles—where adenopathy is more specific— are often ignored. Organomegaly and abdominal masses are often missed because of the patient's position, which should be completely recumbent (on a flat bed). Bone tenderness is highly specific; sternal or vertebral tenderness is a reliable sign of infiltrative metastatic disease or hematologic neoplasm, such as myeloma or acute leukemia. Tenderness is not a sensitive finding, however.

Table 7-1. TNM Staging System for Breast Cancer

Primary tumor (T)

T0	Carcinoma *in situ*
T1	<2 cm
T2	2–5 cm
T3	>5 cm
T4	Any size, fixed to skin or chest wall

Regional lymph nodes (N)

N0	Local nodes
N1	1 or more + nodes
N2	Nodes fixed

Distant metastases (M)

M0	No distant metastases
M1	Distant metastases

Stage grouping

Stage 0	T0
Stage I	T2, N0, M0
Stage IIa	T2, N0, M0
Stage IIb	T2, N1, M0; or T3, N0, M0
Stage IIIa	T3, N1, M0
Stage IIIb	T4, N1 or N2, M0
Stage IV	Any T, any N, M1

Painful vertebrae are often nontender because of the distance of the involved vertebral bodies from the percussing fist.

Blood Studies

Routine laboratory studies provide fairly sensitive (though nonspecific) data. The serum alkaline phosphatase (AP) is usually elevated in patients with blastic bone metastases; this may be the earliest evidence of neoplastic hepatic infiltration. The serum lactic dehydrogenase (LDH) level correlates with rapid tumor proliferation and is a strong negative prognosticator. Serum calcium, although insensitive, is fairly specific. Although an elevated reading occasionally can be the result of hyperparathyroidism, in tumor patients it is strong evidence of either lytic bone metastases or the production of a parathormone-like substance by the tumor, which has an almost equally bad prognosis.

Despite the vast amount of literature on the subject and the diversity of clinically available assays, very few specific markers are known. Prostatic acid phosphatase (PAP) and a specific antigen (PSA) play an important role in diagnosis and staging. PAP is highly specific, but sensitive only to osseous metastases, being positive in 75–90% of cases. PSA is much more sensitive to localized prostatic carcinoma than PAP but less specific because it may also be elevated in benign prostatic hypertrophy (adenoma).[33] Very high levels of PSA, however, are diagnostic of malignancy. These markers are useful in following the response of prostatic carcinoma to therapy—a particularly difficult problem in tumors whose metastases are limited to bone.

Serum levels of the beta subunit of human chorionic gonadotrophin (BHCG) and alpha-fetoprotein (AFP) play a major role in the staging and therapeutic evaluation of testicular germ cell tumors, being significantly elevated in at least two-thirds of metastatic cases. BHCG is also elevated in male and female choriocarcinoma. Both markers may be elevated in occasional patients whose histological diagnosis is seminoma; their elevation in such cases implies the need for chemotherapy in addition to (or instead of) the usual XRT. AFP or BHCG elevations play an important role in the diagnosis of extragonadal germ cell tumors, often arising in midline structures of older adults.[32] AFP is markedly elevated in two-thirds of hepatoma cases, often providing conclusive evidence for this diagnosis.

When elevation of the total serum globulin is associated with a sharply defined (Gaussian) peak on the standard serum protein electrophoresis (S-PEP), a monoclonal gammopathy is diagnosed. This diagnosis, which can be made only by visual inspection of the pattern, is evidence of a B immunocyte neoplasm—usually myeloma. Identification of the subclass of immunoproteins to which the monoclonal species belongs (usually IgG or IgA in myeloma) by immunoelectrophoretic or diffusion techniques, is helpful, but not essential.

Histo- and Cytopathologic Confirmation of Metastases

In recently diagnosed tumor patients, the results of imaging are often quite specific and do not necessarily require pathologic confirmation. But when long intervals have elapsed since primary tumor diagnosis, or when imaging results are ambiguous, such confirmation may be necessary.

Guided fine-needle aspiration procedures have been a major advance in tumor diagnosis and staging.[17-23] Directed by CT scanning or sonography, such needles may be inserted into tumor masses at a number of inaccessible sites, such as pancreatic masses, retroperitoneal nodes, adrenals, deep breast masses, the hepatic dome or left lobe, or pulmonary masses not diagnosed by bronchoscopic procedures. The risk is very low, but experienced invasive radiologists and pathologists familiar with evaluating such specimens are essential for these procedures. It is desirable that the cytopathologist be available for immediate reading of specimens so that needle position can be altered when the results are negative. The specimen obtained is usually an aspirate, yielding cytology only, but this is often sufficient for confirmation of metastases. In lymphoma diagnosis, the ability to determine whether the aspirated cells are monoclonal, by immunofluorescent staining for sIg kappa or lambda, or DNA analysis to demonstrate Ig or T receptor gene rearrangement, may greatly increase the value of such studies.[24]

A common error in institutions in which these aspiration techniques are available is an assumption that they have supplanted traditional core biopsy procedures, such as liver or node biopsy, or mediastinoscopy. These procedures, unlike fine-needle aspiration, provide histology rather than cytology. They are much more helpful in the primary diagnosis of less common tumors, such as lymphomas, sarcomas, and germ cell neoplasms, and are also capable of establishing the presence of nonneoplastic pathology. Accessible nodes and hepatic masses should not be aspirated, but rather resected or biopsied.

Detection of Metastases at Specific Sites

Nodes

Physical examination, when practical, is quite specific, although rather insensitive. When large (>2 cm), firm nodes are palpated, they contain tumor in 90% of cases, but the false-negative rate is at least 30%, even in accessible nodes, as in breast cancer. CT scanning is also specific when marked adenopathy is reported, but relatively insensitive to small nodal metastases.

The false-positive rate of lymphangiography is the lowest of any imaging procedure, and it can detect metastases in minimally enlarged nodes as filling defects. But it opacifies parailiac and aortic nodes only below the coeliac axis, is relatively invasive, painful, and is associated with some pulmonary complications. It has some value in the staging of certain Hodgkin's lymphoma patients, but cannot reliably rule out local node involvement in uterine, prostatic, or testicular tumor patients. Surgical resection of draining nodes is often essential for adequate staging if a significant therapeutic decision is to be made.

Liver and Spleen

The demonstration by imaging procedures of discrete, hypodense regions in the liver is diagnostic of carcinomatous or sarcomatous infiltration. However, solitary hypodense areas, especially in women, may be the result of hemangiomas (hemartomas), so that confirmation by aspiration may be necessary.

Although radionuclide hepatic scanning remains useful, contrast CT and MRI scanning are more sensitive, and MRI can distinguish a hemangioma from a metastasis.

Neither Hodgkin's lymphoma nor other lymphomas commonly produce discrete hepatic abnormalities when they involve the liver. Rather, they produce mostly diffuse changes that no imaging procedure can distinguish from inflammatory processes. Imaging procedures also have little role in the elucidation of splenomegaly, and the physical examination is sufficient to demonstrate (though not rule out) enlargement.

Bone

Routine radiologic evaluation of the axial skeleton and upper femurs remains a useful procedure. Although the procedure is not very sensitive, it is highly specific; the discovery of discrete lytic and/or blastic abnormalities is diagnostic. Typical lytic bone lesions are diagnostic of myeloma, but they are not the most common radiologic change in this disease, which is diffuse osteopenia (permeative bone involvement). This condition is often indistinguishable from osteoporosis, except in the context of the patient's age, sex, and general health. Conversely, in patients from such endemic areas as the Caribbean, multiple lytic skull lesions may be the result of HTLV I leukemia-lymphoma.

Radiologic study is the primary procedure of choice for localized bone pain. Bone scanning with technitium pyrophosphate is the procedure of choice for global screening for bone metastases. It is far more sensitive than routine radiologic study (although much less specific); at least 20% of scan-positive patients lack radiologic evidence of metastasis. Scan-positive areas are studied radiologically either to confirm the presence of metastases by more specific findings or to establish nonmalignant pathology such as osteoarthritis, Paget's disease, or osteoporotic fractures.

A scan-positive, radiologically negative area must be presumed to contain tumor metastases. When the scan reveals multiple, discrete, intense areas of increased uptake, it may be considered diagnostic. But when only a few asymptomatic, scan-positive, radiologically negative areas are found, the results are ambiguous.

MRI may help to elucidate such cases. It can detect the presence of marrow infiltration without cortical disruption (which is often painless) and is particularly useful in myeloma, where radionuclide scanning has little value.[25] MRI may replace radionuclide scanning for global bone staging in the next decade. CT scanning is especially useful for symptomatic areas in which other studies are ambiguous because it is more sensitive than MRI to the cortical disruption, which is often a cause of pain. Although radionuclide scanning is most sensitive in tumors that produce blastic metastases (e.g., breast and prostate), it is usually positive in the lytic metastases of other tumors such as lung and hypernephroma.

Central Nervous System

Postcontrast CT scanning can rule out mass brain metastases as a source of clinical symptoms and can detect asymptomatic metastasis in many cases.

When contrast cannot be used, or when posterior fossa involvement is suspected, MRI is the procedure of choice; it can be the primary staging procedure when convenient.

A major goal of staging is to establish the presence of epidural masses above L-1 before neurologic deficits occur, because cord compression and paraplegia can be prevented by timely radiotherapeutic or surgical intervention in almost all such cases.[26,27] When pain, especially in radicular distribution (i.e., girdling chest pain) is associated with any cervical or thoracic spine metastasis, epidural mass lesions must be ruled out. MRI has largely replaced contrast myelography for this purpose[28] because it is noninvasive. CT scanning is generally not helpful for ruling out epidural masses.

Imaging procedures do not detect lymphomatous, leukemic, or carcinomatous meningitis; lumbar puncture is the procedure of choice here. When the clinical index of suspicion is high (e.g., mononeuritis multiplex syndrome in a high-grade lymphoma patient) a second lumbar puncture, performed a few days after the first, will often be diagnostic when the first was not.

Chest

Routine chest film remains a sensitive and specific procedure for detecting nodular or lymphatic spread to the lungs. However, CT scanning can demonstrate pulmonary metastases in 10% of high-grade sarcoma patients in whom the chest film is negative; its value for the detection of pulmonary parenchymal metastases in other neoplasms has not been established. CT scanning is also the procedure of choice in establishing the presence of mediastinal or hilar adenopathy in bronchogenic carcinoma and lymphoma patients. The false-negative rate, however, is significant.

Staging of Specific Tumors

Many staging procedures cause serious anxiety in already badly frightened patients, further disrupt their lives, raise false hopes (because physicians and patients habitually overestimate the sensitivity of these procedures), and consume limited medical resources. These are often the only accomplishments of staging. Below are listed the staging procedures actually indicated in patients in whom a primary malignant diagnosis has been made and whose initial medical history, physical examination, and routine blood studies are negative except for problems attributable to the primary tumor itself.

Breast. None, in clinically node-negative patients.[16] Bone scanning and chest films are indicated in patients who are node +, or whose tumors are >5 cm, or involve skin.

Bronchogenic. Chest and head postcontrast CT scanning or MRI.[29] (Chest CT scanning will demonstrate the adrenal metastases that commonly occur in squamous cell tumors.)

Colorectal, gastric. Abdominopelvic contrast CT scanning, which includes liver.

Hodgkin's lymphoma. In the usual presentation of supradiaphragmatic disease without subdiaphragmatic physical findings, total body CT scanning is the primary procedure. Splenic or abdominal nodal involvement cannot be ruled out without staging laparotomy, which is indicated in many younger patients without B symptoms (fever and weight loss). It should always be preceded by bone marrow biopsy. Older patients with B symptoms are usually presumed to have disseminated disease; they rarely require laparotomy.[38] Lymphangiography should be performed when the results can determine whether or not laparotomy is indicated. The precise evaluation of the size of large mediastinal masses by CT scanning is most important, because masses whose horizontal diameter is more than one-third that of the chest imply the need for bimodality therapy, thus reducing the potential significance of subdiaphragmatic staging.[37]

Hypernephroma. Abdominal CT scanning; chest film.

Non-Hodgkins lymphoma. Staging laparotomy is almost never indicated. In patients with overtly disseminated nodal disease, staging procedures, such as bone marrow biopsy, are not helpful.[30] CT scanning and bone marrow biopsy are important in localized disease, especially at extranodal sites such as stomach or thyroid. A positive bone marrow biopsy, which is obtained in 30–50% of non-Hodgkin's lymphoma patients, may obviate the need for laparotomy in patients with a purely visceral presentation (retroperitoneal or mediastinal adenopathy; splenomegaly; pleural effusions). Lumbar puncture is indicated in all high-grade (Burkitt's, immunoblastic, T cell) lymphoma patients.

Myeloma. Radiologic bone survey of axial skeleton, skull, and femurs.

Pancreas. Abdominal CT scanning. Pancreatic and bile duct imaging (ERCP) is not indicated when a definite pancreatic mass is demonstrated by CT scan.

Prostate. Radionuclide bone scanning in locally advanced (>stage I or a) or marker-positive patients. The value of imaging procedures (transrectal sonography; MRI) for local staging is under investigation.[34]

Sarcoma. Local staging by MRI in limb sarcomas, CT in trunk. Chest CT in all high-grade sarcomas.

Testicular. Postorchiectomy beta-HCG, alpha-fetoprotein or LDH if positive prior to surgery. Abdominal CT scanning may help to establish adenopathy at renal vessel level, but laparotomy is usually necessary to rule it out and for therapeutic resection of residual nodal metastases.

Uterine body and cervix. Abdominal and pelvic CT scanning.

Evaluation of Response of Metastases to Therapy

In general, a >50% decrease in the product of the 2 greatest diameters of a metastatic mass, such as a node or pulmonary nodule, is considered objective evidence of response. Certain results are false-negative, however. Cytopathologic evidence of chemotherapy-induced tumor cell damage or death, or actual tumor necrosis, may precede shrinkage of the mass by weeks or months.[39] CT scanning of masses may reveal necrosis liquifaction before the size of the mass has changed. This may be particularly striking in the case of hepatic metastases.

In nodular sclerosing Hodgkin's lymphoma, residual fibrosis may lead to incomplete regression of nodal masses, especially in the mediastinum and retroperitoneum, in which all tumor has actually been destroyed.[36] The persistance of pulmonary nodules after chemotherapy in germ cell tumor patients is sometimes the result (as demonstrated by surgical resection) of differentiation to benign teratoma.[35]

Evaluating the response of bone metastasis to therapy remains a major problem, especially in such tumors as prostate, in which bone is the only metastatic site. Radiologic evidence of blastic changes is permanent, and at least 3 mo must elapse before sclerosis of lytic lesions is radiologically apparent. The radionuclide bone scan has been of very limited value. During the healing phase of responding metastases, isotope uptake may actually increase; in the case of relatively old traumatic fractures, areas of increased isotope uptake may persist for months or years. The serum AP level is equally unreliable, although the LDH may be useful if it was significantly elevated initially. Specific markers such as the PAP or PSA or monoclonal proteins (in myeloma patients) may be quite useful in such situations. The obvious difficulty with employing the amelioration of bone pain as an indication of response to therapy is the pronounced placebo effect of treatment. However, if the improvement is associated with durable elimination of the need for narcotic analgesics and if a previously bedridden patient becomes fully ambulatory, pain control may be considered valid evidence of therapeutic control of bone metastasis. MRI may have the ability to demonstrate objectively the regression of marrow infiltration, but this remains to be demonstrated.

References

1. Clark GM, et al. Prediction of relapse or survival in patients with node-negative breast cancer by DNA flow cytometry. N Engl J Med 1989; 320:627–33.
2. Fidler IJ, Kripke ML. Metastasis results from pre-existing variant cells within a malignant tumor. Science 1977; 197:893–95.
3. Nicolson GL. Cancer metastasis. Sci Am 1979; 240:66–76.
4. Nicolson GL, Custead SE. Tumor metastasis is not due to adaptation of cells to a new organ environment. Science 1982; 215:176–78.
5. Netland PA, Zetter BR. Organ-specific adhesion of metastatic tumor cells *in vitro.* Science 1984; 224:1113–15.
6. Zetter BR. The cellular basis of site-specific tumor metastasis. N Engl J Med 1990; 322:605–12.
7. Folkman J, Klagsbrun M. Angiogenic factors. Science 1987; 235:442–47.
8. Sloane BF, Dunn JR, Honn KV. Lysosomal cathepsin B: correlation with metastatic potential. Science 1981; 212:1151–53.
9. Feldman M, Eisenbach L. What makes a tumor cell metastatic? Sci Am 1988; 259:60–85.
10. Raju RN, Kardinal CG. Pleural effusion in breast carcinoma. Cancer 1981; 4:2524–27.
11. Thomas JM, Redding WH, Sloane JP. The spread of breast cancer: importance of the intrathoracic thoracic route. Br J Cancer 1979; 40:540–47.
12. Batson OV. The role of the vertebral veins in the metastatic process. Ann Intern Med 1942; 16:38–45.
13. American Joint Cancer Committee. Manual for staging of cancer. 3rd ed. Philadelphia: Lippincott, 1988.

14. Lee T-TN. Bone scanning in patients with early breast carcinoma: should it be a routine staging procedure? Cancer 1981; 47:486–95.
15. Pedrazzini A, et al. First repeated bone scan in the observation of patients with operable breast cancer. J Clin Oncol 1986; 4:389–84.
16. Ciatto S et al. Preoperative staging of primary breast cancer. Cancer 1988; 61:1038–40.
17. Tao LC et al. Percutaneous find needle aspiration biopsy. Cancer 1980; 45:1480–85.
18. Ho CS et al. Guided fine-needle aspiration biopsy of the liver. Cancer 1981; 47:1781–85.
19. Friedman M et al. Second malignant tumors detected by needle aspiration cytology. Cancer 1983; 52:699–706.
20. Berkman WA et al. The computer tomography-guided adrenal biopsy. Cancer 1984; 53:2098–2103.
21. Crosby JH, Hager B, Hoeg K. Transthoracic fine needle aspiration. Cancer 1985; 56:2504–07.
22. Bootles K et al. Fine needle aspiration biopsy. Am J Med 1986; 81:525–31.
23. Remvikos Y et al. DNA flow cytometry applied to fine needle sampling of human breast cancer. Cancer 1988; 61:1629–34.
24. Hu E et al. Diagnosis of B cell lymphoma by analysis of immunogene rearrangements in biopsy specimens obtained by fine needle aspiration. J Clin Oncol 1986; 4:278–83.
25. Ludwig H et al. Magnetic resonance imaging of the spine in multiple myeloma. Lancet 1987; 364–66.
26. Rodichek LD et al. Early diagnosis of spinal epidural mets. Am J Med 1981; 70:1181–88.
27. Ruff RL, Lanska DJ. Epidural mets in prospectively evaluated veterans with cancer and back pain. Cancer 1989; 63:2234–41.
28. Hagenau C et al. Comparison of spinal MRI and myelography in cancer patients. J Clin Oncol 1987; 5:1663–69.
29. Sorenson JB et al. Brain mets in adenocarcinoma of the lung. J Clin Oncol 1988; 6:1474–80.
30. Bennett JM et al. The significance of bone marrow involvement in non-Hodgkin's lymphoma. J Clin Oncol 1986; 4:1462–69.
31. Fisher B, Fisher ER. The interrelationship of hematogenous and lymphatic tumor dissemination. Surg Gyne Obstet 1966; 122:791–99.
32. Richardson RL et al. The unrecognized extra-gonadal germ cell tumor syndrome. Ann Intern Med 1981; 94:181–86.
33. Stamey TA et al. Prostatic specific antigen as a serum marker for prostatic adenocarcinoma. N Engl J Med 1987; 317:909–16.
34. Rifkin MD et al. Comparison of MRI and ultrasonography in staging early prostate carcinoma. N Engl J Med 1990; 323:621–26.
35. Hong WK et al. The evolution of mature teratoma from malignant testicular tumors. Cancer 1977; 40:2987–92.
36. Canellos GP. Residual mass in lymphoma may not be residual disease. J Clin Oncol 1988; 6:931–3.
37. Willett CG et al. Stage IA to IIB mediastinal Hodgkin's disease: three dimensional volumetric assessment of response to treatment. J Clin Oncol 1988: 6:819–24.
38. Rosenberg SA. Exploratory laparotomy and splenectomy for Hodgkin's disease: a commentary. J Clin Oncol 1988; 6:574–75.
39. Morrow M et al. Multimodality therapy for locally advanced breast cancer. Arch Surg 1986; 121:1291–96.

8

BIOLOGIC RESPONSE MODIFICATION IN CANCER

C. Julian Rosenthal, M.D., F.A.C.P.

IN A BROAD SENSE, biologic response modifiers (BRMs) include a variety of agents, viable cell concentrates, and cell products that are capable of altering interactions between tumors and host toward a therapeutic advantage. Available BRMs can act through 3 mechanisms: modification of the host response to tumors, regulation of tumor growth and differentiation, and direct cytotoxic effect on tumor cells.

In the past, BRMs were generally discussed under the term *immunotherapy* as used in its broad meaning. Passive nonspecific immunotherapy has proved significantly disappointing because of initial claims of therapeutic success that could not be later confirmed. Nevertheless, it is now evident that some type of immunotherapy can be effective under conditions present in any one patient only at certain stages of the evolution of tumor/host interactions. The rapid progress registered during the past few years in obtaining large amounts of biologicals in a pure form through modern DNA recombinant biotechnology made them suitable for a precise definition of their therapeutic benefits. Thus, these biologicals are becoming members in good standing of a human pharmacopeia that includes agents with well-defined chemical structure. They differ from the initial immunotherapy agents, which were complex products of living cells with an unknown chemical composition.

The action of most BRMs has several common denominators.[1] Most BRMs act through a specific receptor or binding structure on the surface of cells directly affected by the agent. Exceptions are found among some immunomodulating chemicals and among bacterial products; these can have selective action on the intracellular metabolism of target host cells not requiring an agent-specific surface receptor moiety.

Most of the natural BRMs have a primary cellular action that affects neither the synthesis nor the function of DNA, the major cellular site of action of the cytotoxic chemotherapeutic antineoplastic agents. Nevertheless, with the exception of differentiation agents, BRMs ultimately cause tumor cell elimination either through a cascade of events resulting in increased antitumor action of host defenses or through direct cytotoxic action on tumor cells.

Based on their cellular action, BRMs can be divided somewhat dogmatically into 2 categories:

- Antigen-dependent, which includes interferons and other lymphokines, certain anti-T cell monoclonal antibodies, thymic factors, adaptively transferred T cytotoxic cells and lymphokine-activated killer cells, and antitumor monoclonal antibodies
- Antigen-independent, including primarily those BRMs inducing activation of macrophages and natural killers, of which muramyl dipeptide derivatives are ready for clinical trials.

With the help of monoclonal antibodies, tumor-associated antigens (TAAs) have been demonstrated in acute leukemia cells, in melanomas, renal cell carcinomas, and astrocytomas, but in many other solid tumors TAAs have not yet been detected. In some cases of melanomas, it was found that TAAs were immunogenic in the patient of origin through the demonstration of circulating antibodies to the melanoma cells. In most other tumors, such antibodies are not found, probably because of the tumor escape phenomenon.

Because BRMs, acting through the augmentation of host immune defense, may have maximum antineoplastic effect at a dosage lower than the maximally tolerated dose (MTD), a new term, *optimal immunomodulatory point* (OIP), was introduced to define maximal antineoplastic effect through immune augmentation.[2] This is the dose and schedule producing maximum enhancement of the effector cell function of interest without compromise of other immunologic responses. Consequently, it is helpful to determine both doses—the MTD and OIP—for most BRMs.

In the following brief discussion of the most important BRMs, they are subdivided in 3 groups: (1) those causing modifications of the host response, (2) those promoting differentiation of malignant cells, and (3) those representing an adoptive immune transfer.

BRMs Causing Modifications of Host Response to Malignant Cells

This category, which includes most of the available BRMs, can be divideded into major subgroups as follows:

Immunomodulating Noncellular Agents

This group includes a variety of compounds that during the past 3 decades were thought to be able to favorably alter the host response to malignant cells (the immune network). The group comprises 3 classes: (1) microorganisms of microbial and fungal products, (2) synthetic compounds, and (3) cytotoxic anticancer drugs.

Initial clinical trials in immunotherapy were all performed with natural microbial and fungal products (bacille Calmette-Guerin [BCG] and Corynebacterium parvum have been the most widely tested among them). These trials yielded little progress after initially published biased results suggested efficacy in patients with small tumor masses. In a few trials, BCG was found to induce measurable responses primarily when administered regionally and intralesionally. Ninety percent of the melanoma lesions injected with $0.5-1 \times 10^8$ viable BCG organisms/ml showed significant local regression without evidence of systemic effect.[4,5] BCG instilled into the pleural cavity after surgical excision of lung cancer was found to prolong survival in a randomized study that was not subsequently confirmed. Consistent results were reported only after the intravesical administration of BCG following fulguration of recurrent superficial transitional cell carcinoma of the bladder.[5,6]

Several other extracts of microbial natural products are currently being tested, primarily in Japan, and have already shown modest clinical efficacy. These substances include a protein-bound polysaccharide, which is mostly a macrophage activator; a streptococcal preparation, OK432, which is a natural killer cell stimulator; nocardia rubra cell wall skeleton, also a macrophage activator; and lentinan, a T cell stimulator. Each of these agents is composed of many chemical elements and can also affect other immune function. For this reason, clinical trials on natural products should be postponed until their active moiety can be prepared synthetically or by genetic engineering procedures.

Among synthetic immunomodulating compounds, 3 of the tested agents, levamisole, bestatin, and polyA-polyU, showed statistically significant antitumor activity. Even so, this activity did not translate therapeutically into significant prolongation of patient survival.

Levamisole, an orally active synthetic phenylimidazole, was found to be a potent inhibitor of tumor tissue alkaline phosphatases and to alter T lymphocyte and macrophage function in vitro. In experimental animals, greater antitumor effect for levamisole was noted when it was used in conjunction with chemotherapy, especially with nitrosoureas and alkylating agents. In clinical trials, levamisole as a single agent adjunct to surgery was not found effective after excision of bronchogenic carcinomas, melanomas, and breast carcinoma.[7] However, it was found to be effective in prolonging survival as compared with control groups in combination with other cytotoxic agents in:

- Patients with Duke B_3 and C colorectal carcinoma in conjunction with 5-fluorouracil (5-FU 10 mg/kg/day I.V. $\times$ 5 every 6 wk; levamisole 2.5 mg/kg p.o. $\times$ 2 days every week between 5-FU cycles)
- Patients with acute lymphoblastic leukemia with low risk for recurrence (WBC 50,000/μl), who received levamisole 100 mg/m^2/day $\times$ 2 each week in conjunction with maintenance chemotherapy
- Patients with multiple myeloma in partial (PR) or complete remission (CR) who received 100 mg/m^2/day $\times$ 2 every week between the 3-wk chemotherapy cycles with alkeran, cyclophosphamide (CTX), prednisone, and vincristine (VCR).

PolyA-PolyU (polyadenylic-polyuridylic) acid is a double-stranded complex of synthetic polyribonucleotides found to be an interferon inducer through the increase in the 2–5A synthetase and protein kinases. To date, it has been found to significantly prolong survival at 7 yr in patients with stage I and II infiltrating ductal carcinoma of the breast after surgery and/or regional radiotherapy. In one trial, response was exceptionally good in patients with positive lymph nodes when 30 mg PolyA-PolyU was administered weekly for 6 wk a month after surgery (at 7 yr, 60% of the treated group were alive compared with only 19% of the control group).[8] Other synthetic compounds, including Azimexon, Tufstin, and Isoprimosine were found ineffective.

Muramyl dipeptide derivatives, with primary macrophage activating action in animals, are currently being tested in clinical trials. Certain cytotoxic anticancer drugs have also been found to have immunomodulating activity in experimental systems and in preliminary studies in humans. CTX was found to enhance antibody production and to delay cutaneous hypersensitivity when administered at a relatively low dose (100 mg/kg in mice, 300 mg/m^2 in humans) at least 1 day (but preferably 3 days) before the administration of the antigen due to specific inhibition of T suppressor lymphocytes, an activity more discriminatory than that of the available anti-T cell monoclonal antibodies. This activity facilitated the development of cytotoxic T lymphocytes.[9,10] Adoptive transfer of normal T lymphocytes abrogated immunopotentiation by CTX.

Adriamycin (ADR) selectively induces maturation of macrophages and eliminates an adherent T down-regulator cell in mice, at the same time stimulating lymphokine production. Together with mitomycin-C, methotrexate, VCR, and 5-FU, ADR can also augment the delayed cutaneous hypersensitivity response to an antigen administered 3–4 days later.[10]

Cytokines

In a broad sense, cytokines are cell products with biological activity on another cell or on themselves that are produced in response to a variety of endogenous or exogenous stimuli. In terms of their cellular origin and primarily to their function, cytokines that enhance the host response to malignant cells can be subdivided into the following classes:
- *Interferons.* Cytokines made by polymorphonucleated leukocytes, fibroblasts or lymphocytes in response to viral infections or to other inducers
- *Lymphokines.* Cytokines made by lymphocytes and monocyte-macrophages that regulate the interactions between various cellular components of the immune system
- *Lymphotoxins.* Cytokines produced by activated lymphocytes, which have a direct suppressive effect on foreign organisms or cells (including malignant cells) when they invade the eukaryotic organisms; capable of inducing tumor cell killing, but poorly characterized and available only as cellular extracts of very low purity
- *Cytotoxic factors* produced by macrophages: tumor necrosis factor
- *Growth factors* with immune stimulating activity: colony stimulating factors.

The most important of the cytokines are briefly described below.

INTERFERONS

Interferons (INF) are a group of proteins and glycoproteins discovered in connection with viral stimulation of various cells; they were subdivided according to differences in antigenic, biologic, and chemical properties.[11] The 3 distinct antigenic types of INFs are designated as α, β and γ; the last one is inactivated at pH 2 or lower and is exclusively produced by T lymphocytes after stimulation by antigens or mitogens. INF α and β can be induced in cells of diverse origin, although those used in clinical trials have been induced respectively in leukocytes or lymphoblastoid cell lines and fibroblasts by viruses or synthetic polyribonucleotides. The production of human INF β and γ was found to be under the control of single genes, whereas a dozen different genes are coding for INF α subtypes, which were found to have somewhat different biological activity. However, all classes of INFs possess antiviral immunomodulatory and antiproliferative activities that may play a part in tumor control. These activities are usually expressed after the activation of 2 intracellular enzymatic systems (of the 2–5A synthetase and of a phosphoril-protein kinase) that ultimately suppress protein synthesis. In addition to this, INFs can also promote differentiation through direct modulation of the production of certain cell surface antigens by mechanisms that are still unknown.

Numerous clinical trials have tested the potential use of INFs in the treatment of malignant tumors. The INF α initially prepared from human leukocytes and INF β prepared from the supernatant of cultured foreskin fibroblasts induced by synthetic polyribonucleotides had a low-grade purity (½–1%) and an activity of 10^6 U per mg of protein for INF α and 10^7 U/mg protein for INF β. The application of molecular cloning and DNA recombinant technology has permitted large-scale production of several highly purified single molecular species of INF α as well as INFs β and γ. The 2 most intensively studied recombinant INF α preparations—the INF α 2a produced by Schering-Plough and INF α 2b produced by Hoffman-LaRoche Co.—have been refined to 98% purity and have specific activity of at least 2×10^8 U/mg protein. INF α 2a and 2b are also equally pure, but unlike their counterparts they can be induced in eukarytic human cells; they are not glycosilated. Still, in clinical trials they showed biological effects in vitro similar to those of the native glycosilated products.

Phase 1 studies have established the MTDs of recombinant INFs α, β, and γ as well as their most common side effects, including chills, fever, myalgias, anorexia, weight loss, fatigue, decreased alertness, thrombocytopenia, and occasional neutropenia and elevation of transaminases. The last 2 side effects are usually dose-limiting.[11] Phase 2 studies continue to be conducted in a variety of tumors. The results of completed trials are available for recombinant α INF in most but not all human malignancies.

Research results so far indicate that α INFs appear to be clearly active in hairy cell leukemia, non-Hodgkin's lymphomas having favorable histology, chronic myelogenous leukemia, Kaposi's sarcoma, and renal cell carcinoma. Their activity in other malignancies such as mycosis fungoides, non-Hodgkin's lymphomas with unfavorable histology, nasopharyngeal carcinoma, malignant gliomas, and superficial bladder carcinoma remains to be confirmed. On the other hand, α INFs are clearly inactive as single agents in bronchogenic carcinoma, colorectal carcinoma, and osteosarcomas. In other human malignancies, equivocal or conflicting results were reported on the effectiveness of recombinant α INFs. A dose-related effectiveness of α INFs was noted in patients with Kaposi's sarcoma and renal cell carcinoma. It was less apparent for the other tumors in which INFs were active; in these cases, determining the OIP appears to be more important.

In all active cases, partial and (rarely) complete remissions (defined by the usual criteria of a decrease in maximal tumor diameter of >50% for PR and disappearance of measurable lesions for CR) were seen. The duration of these remissions was limited, varying between 6 and 14 mo.

To date, α INFs are prescribed as first-line treatment (3 mil U/m^2 every other day up to 1 yr) in hairy cell leukemia patients;* they are recommended as second-line therapy for the other tumors in which they were found active. INF β and especially INF γ are expected to have an even broader range of indications due to the uniqueness of their genetic control. In view of the fact that many mammalian fluids contain mixtures of various interferons and some eukaryotic cells can produce all or most of them, it is likely that best clinical results can be obtained when various INFs are used in combination and in conjunction with lymphokines.

LYMPHOKINES

Lymphokines are peptide molecules secreted by lymphocytes or macrophages that affect the interaction between various cellular elements—predominently lymphocytes—of the immune defense through differentiation, amplification, or inhibition of cell functions.

Of the lymphokines, 2 compounds—interleukin-2 (IL-2) and interleukin-1 (IL-1)—were purified, then genetically engineered through DNA recombinant techniques and produced on a large scale, making extensive clinical trials possible.

IL-2 originally was known as T cell growth factor because it stimulates in vitro the differentiation and replication of T lymphocytes. IL-2 was found to bind to a receptor site on the T cell surface, whose molecular nature was discovered. This IL-2 receptor molecule turned out to be a useful reagent for the identification of histocompatibility gene products. IL-2 was shown to be able to (1) boost the generation of antigen-specific T cells, (2) augment NK (natural killer) cell activity, (3) reverse immune suppression caused by glucocorticosteroids, (4) enhance antibody secretion in vitro by B lymphocytes through predominant stimulation of the T helper cell replication, and (5) potentiate the therapeutic effect of a special subgroup of killer cells, the LAK (lymphokine-activated killers).[12]

In preliminary clinical trials, IL-2 alone appears capable of inducing PRs and CRs in patients with lymphomas and renal cell carcinoma.[19] Other preliminary clinical trials have suggested that IL-2 could be more effective in combination

---

*They are suggested as first-line treatment (5 mil U/m^2/day up to 6 mo) in patients with CML who were found to achieve hematologic remission in 65% of cases and to return a normal kariotype devoid of Philadelphia chromosome in 10% of cases.[18]

with other biologicals and as a potentiator of killer cell activity (see Adoptive Immunotherapy, page 88).

IL-1 is a protein compound produced by macrophages; it was found capable of a variety of activities including: (1) thymocyte and T lymphocyte proliferation, (2) inducing fever (endogenous pyrogen), (3) inducing proliferation of fibroblasts (which explains its wound-healing capability), (4) promoting bone resorption and cartilage degradation through the release of collagenase and prostaglandins from synovial cells, and (5) initiating a series of reactions leading to acute phase protein synthesis and release from liver cells.[12]

It was discovered that 2 distinct genes are capable of coding for protein products with IL-1 activities. Molecular cloning was used to produce 2 molecules in *Escherichia coli* plasmids. IL-1 and IL-1B have in common only 25 amino acids at their C terminal. Nonetheless, they share the same receptor site on the cell surface and can equally express some IL-1 activities while differing for others: IL-1 primarily promotes fibroblast proliferation, whereas IL-1B is primarily an inducer of bone resorption. The clinical potential of IL-1 is currently being explored in phase 1 trials and appears significant.

TUMOR NECROSIS FACTOR

Tumor necrosis factor (TNF) is a glycoprotein produced by macrophages conditioned by BCG, some reactive proteins, and possibly viral agents; it is triggered by endotoxin but does not contain endotoxin.[1] In contrast to endotoxin, TNF is toxic in vitro for murine and human tumor cells but not for normal cells. Recently, TNF polypeptide was obtained by DNA recombinant techniques in a pure form, with well-defined molecular structure and with biological effects identical with natural TNF. It was found that specific receptors exist on sensitive tumor target cells and that the tumor sensitivity to TNF is related to the number of such receptors. TNF is cytotoxic only if it penetrates the cell lysosome after binding to its receptor. Injection of TNF directly in the cytoplasm or the disruption of lysosomes (enzymatic treatment) eliminates TNF cytotoxic activity.

Recent data have suggested that the TNF molecule is almost identical with cachetin, another polypeptide produced by macrophages responsible in part for the cytotoxic effect of lipopolysaccharide endotoxin. This and other biological effects of cachetin are different from those of TNF. The latter was also found to have 30% structural identity with recently characterized lymphotoxin produced by T lymphocytes. Ongoing phase 1 clinical trials will define the therapeutic role of this biological, which has shown significant antineoplastic effect in experimental studies.

Growth Factors

Among the growth factors that have been described to date, most were found useful in antineoplastic therapy through the promotion of malignant cell differentiation to benign cells. One of them, the granulocyte-macrophage colony-stimulating factor (GM-CSP), in addition to promoting differentiation of leukemic cells, has an important role in enhancing host response to neoplastic proliferation through (1) promotion of bone marrow engraftment after transplantation, (2) boosting the release in circulation of white cells following autoreductive therapy, and (3) activating macrophages, which in a number of experimental models (A375 melanoma cell line, etc.) became capable of killing human tumor cells.[12]

GM-CSF also was found to activate macrophages in experiments in which they were able to kill parasites (e.g., trypanosoma cruzi) and bacteria. GM-CSF was recently produced in pure form using DNA recombinant technology and is currently administered to patients in phase 1 trials. Preliminary data suggest that GM-CSF could be especially effective in combination with interleukins.

Adoptive Immunotherapy

The possible transfer of lymphocytes selectively immunized against tumor cells to syngeneic animals has been demonstrated for more than a decade. The results were, however, erratic and limited by the inability to easily generate large numbers of syngeneic lymphoid cells.

In 1980, Rosenberg described the LAK cell phenomenon.[13] Incubation of human peripheral blood lymphocytes or of normal murine splenocytes with the lymphokine interleukin-2 resulted in the generation of lymphoid cells with the ability to lyse fresh noncultured natural killer-resistant cancer cells in short-term chromium release assays. They were not lytic to fresh normal lymphocytes nor to liver or lung cells. The administration of very high doses of IL-2 alone to mice was capable of generating LAK cells in vivo and also mediated antitumor effects.[14] Extensive studies in experimental animals have shown that optimal therapeutic effects against established pulmonary and hepatic metastases are obtained when a combination of LAK cells and IL-2 is given.

When recombinant IL-2 became available in large quantities, a clinical trial was initiated at the National Institutes of Health in 1984; when initial preliminary results proved favorable, the trial was continued in 5 other centers. Patients first received IL-2 q. 8 hr for 5 days; 2 days later, a 5-day program of daily leukapheresis from the patients was performed. Cells so obtained were cultured, and after 3–4 days they were harvested and infused autologously along with the administration of IL-2 q. 8 hr for another 5 days, starting with the last day of leukapheresis. At this writing, close to 200 patients have been entered in these phase 1 studies. The results appear to be consistent, confirming the initial Rosenberg observations. CRs have been seen in 30–60% of cases of renal cell carcinoma and in 1 case of melanoma. PRs have been attained in >30% of cases; they were seen in patients with renal cell carcinoma, malignant melanoma, and colorectal carcinoma. However, significant side effects occurred in >50% of cases, including hypotension (requiring vasopressors), diarrhea, nausea and vomiting, fever, dyspnea, water retention, anemia (requiring blood transfusions), transient renal insufficiency, and hepatic dysfunction. For this reason, adoptive therapy with LAK cells requires significant improvement before it is acceptable for widespread clinical application. This may become possible when LAK cells specific to the respective tumor can be selected, treated with IL-2 in vivo, then infused autologously. It is likely that most of the side effects that are due to lack of specificity of the currently administered LAKs will no longer occur.

BRMs Capable of Promoting Tumor Cell Differentiation

This class of BRMs represents a new area of active investigation in cancer therapy but one in which clinical application is still limited. The idea of treating cancer by promoting differentiation came from experimental data indicating that malignant cells represent a blockade in the physiologic maturation of their cell of origin—a blockade that may not be irreversible. Instances were reported of infants with neuroblastoma that was transformed into a benign ganglioneurofibroma by the time the infants were 1–2 yr old.

Most experimental studies focusing on differentiation agents were conducted either by studying myeloid cell differentiation in mice or by studying the effect of these agents on differentiation of murine and human leukemic cell lines K562 (human early myeloblast and erythroblast), KG-1 (myeloblast), and HL-60 (promyelocyte). The inducers of myeloid cell differentiation are divided into 5 categories: chemotherapeutic agents, polar compounds, vitamin analogues, phorbal diesters, and cytokines. Their effect is quantitated by the plating efficiency 2 (PE-2) index—the amount of decrease in self-renewal potential of clonogenic cells differentiation.

Chemotherapeutic Agents

Among chemotherapeutic agents, ADR, daunomycin, bleomycin, methotrexate, hydroxyurea, 5-FU, prednisone or dexamethasone, and especially 5 azacytidine and cytosine arabinoside (ara-C) were found capable of inducing either direct leukemic cell differentiation or potentiating the differentiation effect of a protein serum factor when used in low doses alone or in combination; these doses do not induce direct cytotoxicity.

Ara-C was investigated in extensive experimental studies and in preliminary clinical trials for its ability to promote leukemic cell differentiation when used at low doses; this is probably due to the induction of DNA hypermetilation causing inhibition of genes required for neoplastic cell differentiation. In larger doses, ara-C is one of the most effective cytotoxic antileukemic agents because of its ability to inhibit DNA replication.

Preliminary results in clinical trials using low-dose ara-C (5 mg/m^2/day subcutaneously) in patients with myelodysplastic syndromes and acute non-lymphocytic leukemia have been contradictory despite the fact that, in vitro, low-dose ara-C consistently reduces the number of blasts and increases the number of mature granulocytes and macrophages in two-thirds of leukemic marrow cultures studied.

Polar Compounds

Among the polar-planar compounds, dimethyl-sulfoxide (DMSO) and hexamethylene bisacetemide (HMBA), 2 low-molecular-weight substances with a polar hydrophilic moiety and a planar hydrophobic portion, were found to be capable of triggering differentiation of cell lines derived from a number of neoplasms, including neuroblastoma, glioblastoma multiforme, teratocarcinoma, melanoma, and promyelocytic leukemia. Because it binds with glutathione, HMBA penetrates slowly in the neoplastic cells, usually manifesting its action on differentiation 18 hr later. For this reason, in an ongoing clinical trial, HMBA is administered by continuous infusion at a dose ranging from 4.8 to 42.3 g/m^2/day.[15]

Vitamin Analogues

Among the vitamin analogues, retinoic acid, a metabolite of vitamin A, is known to play an important physiologic role in the maturation of epithelial cells and normal hematopoietic cells. One of its analogues, 13-cis-retinoic acid, at concentrations of 10 M/L was found to induce differentiation of leukemic cell lines. Also, in preliminary clinical studies it was found to lead to a therapeutic benefit in patients with promyelocytic leukemia but not in patients with chronic myelogenous leukemia or myelodysplastic syndromes.[15]

Vitamin D analogues (especially 1,25 dihydroxyvitamin D), besides being major regulators of calcium transport, were found to induce in vitro maturation of normal myeloid cells and of leukemic cell lines; they are currently being studied in patients with myelodysplastic syndrome. It was recently found that 1,25 (OH)$_2$D$_3$ induces a reduction in the c-myc mRNA levels within 4 hr of HL-60 cell exposure; this reduction precedes by 8 hr the onset of other phenotype changes.

Phorbol Esters and Cytokines

Phorbol esters are another group of differentiation agents that have been found to induce macrophage differentiation on leukemic cell lines, probably because of their binding to the protein kinase C. Phorbol myristate acetate currently is under investigation in patients with myelodysplastic syndrome.

Among cytokines, as previously mentioned, GM-CSF (granulocyte monocyte colony-stimulation factor) and gamma interferon appear to be effective differentiation agents; the latter compound promotes differentiation of immature myeloid lines along the monocyte pathway through the increased expression of class 2 HLA antigens. Recently, it was found that T cell lymphocytes also can produce a differentiation factor for the HL-60 promyelocytic leukemic cell line.

BRMs with Direct Cytotoxic Antineoplastic Activity

The major compounds of this class of biologic modifiers have been identified with some of the *monoclonal antibodies* (m.abs) to malignant cells. Monoclonal antibodies resulted from application of the hybridoma technology introduced by Kohler and Milstein.[16] Briefly, mice are immunized with a source of antigen, i.e., neoplastic cells. Splenocytes from the immunized animals, which include a rich suply of immune B lymphocytes, are fused with an established myeloma cell line that preferably is producing but not secreting a monoclonal immunoglobulin. Under selective conditions, hybrid cells grow that are capable of killing nonhybridized mouse myeloma cells and splenocytes. Hybrid cells combine 2 critical phenotypes from the original starting cell populations: the ability to produce a specific antibody (from the immune B splenocyte) and the property of immortality (from the myeloma cell). Immortalized hybrid cells of interest can be isolated by cell-cloning procedures that allow identification of hybrid clones that secrete individual antibodies of required specificity.

With the monoclonal antibodies so generated, an intensive search for tumor-specific antigens has been performed over the past 5 yr. Although it has been difficult to develop m.abs with absolute specificity for cancer cells, it has been possible to produce antibodies that identify antigens with higher expression on malignant cells when compared to their normal cell counterpart. Monoclonal antibodies have been produced and extensively studied for use in the early diagnosis and therapy of human malignant tumors. The potential therapeutic use of m.abs was explored in 3 areas of investigation, resulting in the following data:

1. Monoclonal antibodies were found able to mediate destruction of tumor target cells through an immune mechanism that included—

- Activation of complement; this can produce lysis of tumor target cells. It can be produced only by IgM, IgG_3, IgG_{2a}, and IG_{2b} immunoglobulin subclasses. It was reported in nude mice carrying human breast tumor implants and in patients with metastatic malignant melanoma with a complement fixing IgG_3 antibody to G_{D3} ganglioside. The complement mediated lysis of melanoma cells was more effective when 2 m.abs directed against distinct determinants of melanoma cells were administered.
- Activation of antibody-directed effector cells, including macrophages, natural killer (NK) lymphocytes, neutrophils, and (occasionally) platelets causing tumor cell lysis, a phenomenon known as antibody-dependent cell-mediated cytotoxicity (ADCC). Only m.abs of the subclasses IgG_2 and IgG_3 were found to be effective in the nude mouse ADCC assays in inhibiting the growth of a variety of human tumor implants (e.g., melanoma, renal cell carcinoma, colon carcinoma, breast carcinoma).
- Production of anti-idiotypic antibodies resulting after the binding of antibodies to antigen (the idiotypic determinant of the antibody). Some experimental evidence suggests that anti-idiotypes can elicit delayed hypersensitivity and protection against tumors and microorganisms.

2. Monoclonal antibodies to autocrine growth factors were found able to inhibit tumor growth by blocking the production of growth factors by malignant cells that self-stimulate the growth of malignant cells secreting these factors. In animal models, squamous cell carcinoma tumors were inhibited after the administration of a m.ab to the receptor for epidermal growth factor, which is the product of oncogene V-erb-B. Small-cell carcinomas were inhibited after treatment with m.abs directed against bombesin, one of the major autocrine growth factors of small-cell carcinoma of the lung.

3. One of the most attractive uses of m.abs to tumor cell antigens (which when given alone generally are not directly cytotoxic) is to administer them after being conjugated to a radiolabeled or cytotoxic agent or to protein toxins.

To date, conjugation of m.abs to radiolabeled isotopes has led to successful antineoplastic agents used in experimental animals. The isotopes used have included particle emitters (^{131}iodine, ^{47}scandium, ^{90}yttrium), alpha emitters (^{212}bismuth and ^{211}astatine), auger electron emitters (^{125}iodine and ^{77}bromine, and ^{10}boron). M.abs were also conjugated to the protein toxins ricin and diphtheria, which have an extremely potent active A chain fragment. This requires a second peptide, the B chain, in order to bind to target cells. When the A chain is attached to a m.ab, it is inactive unless delivered to a tumor cell by the m.ab. Among the chemotherapeutic agents conjugated to m.ab that were successful in inhibiting tumor growth, vindesine, methotrexate, daunorubicin, ADR, ara-C, and 5-FU were found to be the most useful. Clinical application of the conjugated m.ab is not yet practical because of a number of technical problems in the stability, biological activity, and specificity of these conjugates.

References

1. Hersey P. Biological agents in the treatment of cancer. Aust NZ J Med 1990; 20:85–98.
2. Hawkins MJ, Hoth DF, Wittes RE. Clinical development of biological response modifiers: comparison with cytotoxic drugs. Semin Oncol 1986; 13:132–40.
3. Talmadge JE, Hartman D. Optimization of an immunotherapeutic protocol with poly (1,C). LCJ Biol Rep Modif 1985; 4:484–89.
4. Morton DL, Eilber FR, Malmgreen RA, et al. Immunological factors which influence response to immunotherapy in malignant melanoma. Surgery 1970; 68:158–64.
5. Pinsky CM. Local administration of immunomodulators. Semin Oncol 1986; 13:141–43.
6. Lamm DL, Thor DE, Winters WD, et al. BCG immunotherapy of bladder carcinoma: inhibition of tumor recurrence and associated immune responses. Cancer 1981; 48:82–88.
7. Borden EC, Hawkins MJ. Biologic response modifiers as adjuncts to other therapeutic modalities. Semin Oncol 1986; 13:144–52.
8. Lacour J, Lacour F, Sprio A, et al. Adjuvant treatment with polyadenylic-polyuridylic acid in operable breast cancer: updated results of a randomized trial. Br Med J 1984; 288:589–92.
9. Berk M, Mastrangelo MJ, Engstrom PF, et al. Augmentation of the human immune response by cyclophosphamide. Cancer Res 1982; 42:4862–66.
10. Mastrangelo MJ, Berd D, Maguire H Jr. Immune-augmenting effects of cancer chemotherapeutic agents. Semin Oncol 1986; 13:186–94.
11. Krown SE. Interferons and interferon inducers in cancer treatment. Semin Oncol 1986; 13:207–17.
12. Gillis S, Conlon PJ, Cosman D, et al. Lymphokines: from conjecture to the clinic. Semin Oncol 1986; 13:218–27.
13. Rosenberg SA. The adoptive immunotherapy of cancer: accomplishments and prospects. Cancer Treat Rep 1984; 68:233–55.
14. Rosenberg SA, Lotze MT, Meul LM, et al. Observations on the systemic administration of autologous lymphokine activated Killer cells and recombinant interleukin-2 to patients with metastatic cancer. N Engl J Med 1985; 313:228–33.
15. Gabrilove JL. Differentiation factors. Semin Oncol 1986; 13:228–33.
16. Kohler G, Milstein C. Continuous culture of fused cells secreting antibody of predefined specificity. Nature 1975; 256:495–96.

17. Houghton AN, Scheinberg DA. Monoclonal antibodies: potential applications to the treatment of cancer. Semin Oncol 1986; 13:165–79.
18. Ozer H. Biotherapy of chronic myelogous leukemia with interferon. Semin Oncol 1988; 15:14–20 (suppl 5).
19. Parkinson DR. Interleukin-2 in cancer therapy. Semin Oncol 1988; (suppl 6) 15:10–26.
20. Harris DT, Mastrangelo MJ. Serotherapy of cancer. Semin Oncol 1989; 15:180–98.

9

COMMON METABOLIC DISTURBANCES IN PATIENTS WITH CANCER

Jaime Uribarri, M.D., and Hugh Carroll, M.D.

DISTURBANCES IN WATER, ELECTROLYTE, and acid-base metabolism are very common in patients with cancer, and although none is unique to this disease state, some are frequent and some characteristic. This chapter will address the topic of these disturbances by first briefly describing the relevant pathophysiology, then discussing the clinical setting in which the metabolic disturbances develop, and finally offering suggestions on their recognition and management.

Edematous States

Edema can present either as interstitial edema or as fluid accumulation in the pleural, peritoneal, or other cavities. Under a variety of circumstances, some fluid extravasates from the capillaries and stays in the interstitium to form edema. At least 6 pathophysiologic mechanisms lead to edema.

1. *High hydrostatic pressure in capillaries.* This condition is seen in patients with venous obstruction (e.g., inferior or superior vena cava syndrome) or with congestive heart failure.

2. *Hypoalbuminemia with consequent decrease of oncotic pressure.* Observed in patients with malnutrition (cachexia) or in a case of replacement of liver parenchyma by tumor. It is also seen in patients with intestinal protein loss or urinary protein loss; in nephrotic syndrome[1] associated with Hodgkin's disease (minimal change disease); in multiple myeloma with renal amyloidosis; and in immune complex disease with tumor antigens (e.g., bronchogenic and colon carcinomas and melanoma).

94

3. *Increased capillary permeability to protein.* This disorder leads to a fall in serum albumin and a rise in the interstitial albumin; it is generally induced by mediators of the inflammatory process (e.g., kinins) and histamine that can cause leakage of protein and therefore water from the capillary at an increased rate. Increased permeability can be a local or general phenomenon.

4. *Loss of tissue hydrostatic pressure.* This event frequently is caused by a decrease in collagen formation. Collagen-rich connective tissue bands resist distention of the interstitial space. Cachexia and corticosteroids are 2 of the factors that can impair the formation of connective tissue protein and permit the accumulation of interstitial fluid.

5. *Obstruction of lymphatics by disease or therapy.* Pelvic tumors infiltrating or compressing lymphatics characteristically cause unilateral or asymmetric edema of the legs. Obstruction of the thoracic duct may contribute to ascites formation, including chylous ascites. Transection of lymphatics during radical axillary or groin resection is often (20% in radical mastectomy) followed by fibrosis and obstruction with accumulation of protein-rich edema. Poor operative technique, irradiation, and chronic low-grade infection are factors in the scar formation that prevents lymphatic revascularization. Management relies mainly on mechanical means of increasing interstitial pressure to force reentry of fluid into capillaries (e.g., fitted elastic garments).

6. *Severely malnourished patients, when refed with carbohydrates, may develop edema.*[2] The mechanism of this refeeding edema remains controverial.

Ascites, the accumulation of serous fluid in the abdominal cavity, is caused by increased formation and reduced drainage of coelomic lymph. Peritoneal metastases contribute to lymph formation because their capillaries are leaky to proteins and, if partially obstructed, are under increased hydrostatic pressure. It has been shown that lymphatic drainage is reduced in the presence of peritoneal implants. Obstruction of the porta hepatis or the portal vein increases pressure in the splanchnic vessels and favors increased formation of lymph, which transudes into the peritoneal cavity. Low serum albumin generally favors egress and inhibits the return of capillary water. In patients with hepatoma, the ascites may be due to underlying cirrhosis.

Treatment of edematous states includes specific treatment for the underlying cancer whenever possible, salt restriction, judicious use of diuretics, nutritional supplements to raise plasma protein concentration, and total parenteral nutrition as needed. In the case of intractable symptomatic ascites, peritoneovenous shunts (LeVeen) have been used despite the theoretical hazard of increased metastases. Small therapeutic paracentesis may be used when necessary, but it should be remembered that albumin is wasted by paracentesis. Intravenous albumin occasionally may be indicated. Edema and ascites often must be tolerated to a certain extent, inasmuch as removal of fluid may lead to decreased effective arterial volume with hypotension and azotemia.

Polyuria

Polyuria has 2 basic causes: excretion of increased amounts of solute (osmotic diuresis) and inability to form an osmotically concentrated urine (water diuresis). Osmotic diuresis may be seen with hyperglycemia of any cause, including total parenteral nutrition. Urea unloading may contribute to diuresis following relief of urinary tract obstruction. Water diuresis may be due to lack of antidiuretic hormone (ADH) or renal unresponsiveness to ADH (nephrogenic diabetes insipidus). Lack of ADH may be the result of: (1) primary or metastatic tumor involving the hypothalamus or pituitary, (2) removal of or injury to hypothalamic structures during operative therapy of brain lesions, and (3) drugs that diminish ADH release, such as diphenylhydantoin. Renal unresponsiveness to ADH may be the result of hypercalcemia, hypokalemia, amyloidosis, urinary tract obstruction (particularly after relief of obstruction), or drugs that diminish ADH action, such as lithium, demeclocycline, and amphothericin B.

Treatment of polyuria should first include discontinuation of the offending drug whenever possible. In the case of central diabetes insipidus, some residual release of ADH is usually present, and increasing the action of this ADH with drugs such as chlorpropamide (250 mg p.o. daily) is often useful.[3] However, injection or inhalation of ADH analogues may be necessary. Patients with nephrogenic diabetes insipidus are unresponsive to ADH. Therapy with salt restriction plus thiazide diuretics aims at mild volume depletion to reduce formation of dilute urine in the distal nephron.[4]

Disorders of Serum Sodium

Hyponatremia

The major concern in hyponatremic states is not the effect of a low concentration of sodium ions in the extracellular space but rather that low osmolality causes excessive cellular uptake of water. Hyponatremia not associated with low effective plasma osmolality may be observed in patients with hyperglycemia or during mannitol administration (because water is drawn osmotically from the cells and dilutes extracellular electrolytes) as well as in patients with hyperglobulinemia, a condition that may cause hyponatremia with normal osmolality because of positive charges in the protein substitute for sodium in the plasma.[5] Spurious hyponatremia may be found with hyperlipidemia and marked hyperglobulinemia.

Treatment of hyponatremic states depends upon their pathogenesis. Two major pathogenetic classes of patients can be differentiated by evaluation of the effective arterial volume and hemodynamics. The first class consists of hyponatremic patients with reduced effective arterial volume. It includes (1) patients who have lost sodium or sodium plus potassium from the body and therefore are depleted of salt and water; (2) patients who are actively forming edema (although patients with renal failure who receive excessive amounts of sodium-free water should be excluded because they are volume expanded); and (3) patients who accumulate fluid in a "third space" (e.g., intestinal fluid, ascites, or local edema behind severe venous thrombosis).

The second class comprises hyponatremic patients with normal or mildly expanded effective arterial volume. The syndrome of inappropriate secretion of ADH (SIADH) accounts for most patients in this category. The excess ADH causes fluid retention, volume expansion, and renal salt loss. The slight volume expansion is usually not evident on physical examination but may be detected by low BUN and serum creatinine and uric acid, indicators of increased renal perfusion. A wide variety of tumors may lead to SIADH, including oat cell carcinoma of lung, pancreatic cancer, and brain tumor.

A modest hyponatremia with serum sodium about 130 mEq/L can occur, due to resetting of the osmostat, in chronically debilitated patients with cancer.[6] An occasional patient with salt depletion may retain sufficient water to restore volume to normal, thus leading to hyponatremia. Various drugs may either enhance the release or the peripheral action of ADH, resulting in hyponatremia with manifestations indistinguishable from SIADH. These drugs include chlorpropamide, vincristine (VCR), cyclophosphamide (CTX), acetaminophen, morphine, and the barbiturates.

In all of the conditions listed above, the ADH levels are normal or high; therefore, the finding of hyponatremia with an osmotically concentrated urine is not a useful diagnostic feature of SIADH, an error widely promulgated.

Treatment of hyponatremia depends on its pathogenetic mechanism. Patients with volume depletion states due to salt loss are treated by salt and water replacement, given orally if possible, I.V. if necessary. Isotonic salt solutions suffice in patients without symptoms of hyposmolality. Patients with SIADH can be treated by water restriction and normal salt intake. For patients who cannot cooperate in water restriction, loop diuretics and salt replacement will usually be effective.[7] When hyponatremia is caused by drugs, the offending agent should be discontinued whenever possible.

In patients with symptomatic hyponatremia (altered consciousness or seizures) hypertonic NaCl is indicated. It is often advantageous to combine I.V. furosemide with hypertonic NaCl therapy because loop diuretics inhibit urinary concentration. The optimum rate of increase in serum sodium in symptomatic hyponatremia is uncertain, but a rise of 10 mEq/L in the first 4–6 hr of therapy, followed by a much slower subsequent return to normal, is a useful approach. The main risk of rapid correction of hyponatremia is the development of central pontine myelinolysis, a complex neurologic syndrome that may be manifested by pseudobulbar palsy and quadriplegia.

Hypernatremia

Hypernatremia is caused most frequently by water loss (e.g., diabetes insipidus) and less frequently by sodium retention without dehydration (e.g., treatment of lactic acidosis or cardiac arrest with hypertonic sodium bicarbonate). It is commonly the result of a combination of water loss and salt retention (as from diabetes insipidus), with reduced thirst and normal sodium intake. Continued hypernatremia results from inadequate water intake, loss of thirst mechanism, coma, lack of access to water, inability to drink water due to esophageal or oropharyngeal cancer, or continuous vomiting. Water loss can occur either because water intake is insufficient in the presence of normal insensible loss and normal renal water conservation, or because of excessive renal water loss (diabetes insipidus, osmotic diuresis) without commensurate increase in water intake.

Diagnosis of hypernatremia is based on the evaluation of urine and plasma osmolality. If urine osmolality exceeds 800 mOsm/L, hypernatremia is due to either insufficient water intake or extrarenal water loss. If urine osmolality is lower than plasma osmolality, the patient has central or nephrogenic diabetes insipidus. If urine osmolality is between the level of plasma osmolality and 800 mOsm/L, hypernatremia may be due to diabetes insipidus, osmotic diuresis, or renal failure. Central diabetes insipidus can be distinguished from nephrogenic diabetes insipidus by the rise in urine osmolality in response to pitressin— >15% in central and <10% in nephrogenic.

The immediate therapy of patients with hypernatremia is administration of water. The water requirement can be estimated as: total body water (liters) $\times (1 - \frac{\text{desired serum Na}}{\text{actual serum Na}})$.

In general, no more than half of the calculated deficit should be administered over the first 24 hr, with the remainder given over the next 2 days. When hypernatremia is accompanied by a degree of volume depletion that demands the rapid administration of large volumes of fluid for hemodynamic stabilization, therapy can begin with isotonic salt solutions to prevent too rapid a fall in osmolality. Long-term therapy will depend on the mechanism leading to hypernatremia; e.g., pitressin will be given for central diabetes insipidus.

Disorders of Potassium Metabolism

The body of an adult contains about 2,500–4,500 mEq of potassium. The concentration in intracellular fluid is 150 mEq/L; in extracellular fluid, concentration is generally in the range of 4–5 mEq/L. If serum potassium rises or falls, abnormal electrical events at cell membranes lead to abnormalities in cardiac impulse formation and conduction that can be lethal. Hypokalemia may lead to general muscle weakness, muscle necrosis, impaired insulin release, and nephrogenic diabetes insipidus. Hyperkalemia occasionally leads to peripheral muscle weakness.

The average American ingests about 50–100 mEq of potassium per day, of which 90% is excreted by the kidney and 10% by the intestine. Excessive potassium loss may take place by either route, but excessive retention can be blamed only on the kidney. Reduced or excessive intake seldom represents the sole cause of high or low serum potassium. Hypokalemia may be caused by potassium loss or by a shift of potassium into cells (acute alkalosis, insulin and epinephrine action).[8]

Disturbances in serum potassium are likely to be encountered in patients with cancer. Hypokalemia is encountered in patients with neoplasms in the following situations:

- During vomiting or gastric drainage. Potassium is lost in the urine because metabolic alkalosis due to loss of HCl leads to renal excretion of bicarbonate. Because bicarbonate cannot be effectively reabsorbed in the collecting duct, its negative charge pulls potassium into the urine.
- After glucocorticoid hormone administration. Also in patients with adrenal tumors or ACTH-producing tumors of nonendocrine origin (e.g., carcinoma of the lung). The glucocorticosteroid hormones contribute to

urinary potassium loss by increasing the filtration rate and hence the distal delivery of sodium to exchange with potassium.

- During the administration of certain drugs that lead to urinary potassium wasting. Such drugs include diuretics, amphotericin-B, and nonreabsorbable anions (e.g., penicillins).
- In patients with magnesium depletion, which leads to urinary potassium excretion by uncertain mechanism.
- In patients with leukemias, there are several potential mechanisms for hypokalemia, including (1) spurious results in patients with WBC count exceeding $1,000,000/\mu l^3$ (when left at room temperature, white cells extract potassium from plasma and lower the potassium level);[9] (2) rapid cell growth; (3) antibiotics (penicillins and aminoglycosides); and (4) chemotherapy (cisplatin). The presence of large amounts of urinary lysozyme is also associated with potassium wasting.
- In patients with diarrhea of whatever etiology.

Treatment of hypokalemia includes the removal of its cause whenever possible and supplements of potassium given orally or I.V. at a rate determined by the patient's needs. If I.V. replacement is used, a safe rate of administration is <20 mEq/hr; though faster rates can be used in case of emergency (e.g., arrythmias). Treatment may also include the use of potassium-sparing diuretics (e.g., spironolactone, triamterene), which can limit renal potassium loss.

Hyperkalemia can be spurious or true. Spurious (pseudohyperkalemia) occurs in vitro in tubes in which clotting of blood containing a large number of platelets or white cells may cause release of cell potassium and elevate serum potassium. In these cases, plasma potassium will accurately reflect extracellular potassium concentration. True hyperkalemia can result from:

- *Chemotherapy.* Although lysis of large numbers of cells during chemotherapy is unlikely to increase serum potassium significantly in the absence of renal failure, renal failure may result from chemotherapy if tubules are obstructed by uric acid aggregates and calcium phosphate complexes.
- *Acute metabolic acidosis* producing a shift of potassium from the cells, especially when renal function is compromised.
- *Heparin administration,* which interferes with aldosterone synthesis[11] and may cause increased serum potassium in a patient who already has some predisposition to hyperkalemia.

Treatment of hyperkalemia frequently starts with the oral or rectal administration of sodium polystyrene sulfonate (Kayexalate), a resin that removes potassium from the body. Administration of glucose and insulin causes potassium to enter cells rapidly. One can also antagonize the effects of hyperkalemia on the cardiac cell membrane with I.V. calcium. Finally, in the case of renal dysfunction or failure, potassium can be removed by dialysis.

Hypomagnesemia

Serum magnesium concentration of <1.7 mg/dl constitutes hypomagnesemia. Although this concentration does not necessarily reflect body magnesium stores, in a setting of predisposition to magnesium loss it can usually be used as an index of the need for magnesium replenishment. Hypomagnesemia can result (1) from poor intake of magnesium combined with G.I. loss as observed in patients with diarrhea and steatorrhea (e.g., radiation enteritis), or (2) from excessive renal loss after the administration of certain drugs, including aminoglycosides, cisplatin, and diuretics (furosemide and, less frequently, thiazides). Hypomagnesemia may also be seen in patients with other metabolic abnormalities, such as SIADH, hypercalcemia, and phosphate depletion.

Clinical manifestations of hypomagnesemia include paresthesias, tetany, carpopedal spasm, hyperreflexia, seizures, prolonged Q-T interval in the EKG, arrhythmias, increased sensitivity to digitalis toxicity, occasional urinary potassium wasting, and hypocalcemia with impaired parathyroid hormone release.

Treatment of hypomagnesemia is tailored to the severity of symptoms of magnesium depletion. In severe depletion with convulsions, 1 mEq of magnesium per kilogram of body weight of magnesium can be given I.V. over 4 hr and another 1 mEq/kg can be given over the rest of the first 24 hr. For less severe depletion, 0.25 mEq/kg can be given every 4 hr. One gram (1 cc) of 50% magnesium sulfate provides 8 mEq of elementary magnesium. The main limitation for oral magnesium supplementation is the frequent development of diarrhea.

Hypercalcemia

Primary hyperparathyroidism is the commonest cause of hypercalcemia, but in hospitalized patients the commonest cause is cancer.[12] Certain tumors, such as carcinoma of the breast, lung (squamous cell), multiple myeloma, and head and neck carcinomas, frequently lead to hypercalcemia, but the disorder is infrequent or rare in such tumors as oat cell tumor of the lung, and cervical and colon carcinoma.[13] Recently, a subset of T cell (HTLV-1) lymphomas has occurred in outbreaks in southern United States, West Indies, and Japan; this disease is almost universally associated with hypercalcemia.[14]

As is the case with other imbalances of electrolytes in the extracellular fluid, the nature and severity of symptoms of hypercalcemia, particularly those involving altered states of consciousness, depend on the rate of rise as well as the level of serum calcium reached. Renal effects of hypercalcemia include nephrogenic diabetes insipidus characterized by polyuria, polydipsia, thirst, and nocturia. These findings must be distinguished from those of central diabetes insipidus due to hypothalamic metastases. Anorexia, nausea and vomiting, abdominal pain, and constipation are frequent manifestations when serum calcium exceeds 13 mg/dl. The characteristic electrocardiographic manifestation of hypercalcemia is shortening of the Q-T interval. Lethargy, confusion, weakness, apathy, depression, drowsiness, altered personality, obtundation, and coma are neuromuscular findings of note. Pruritus, hypertension, band keratopathy, and nephrolithiasis are signs of hyperparathyroidism rather than malignancy-associated hypercalcemia, primarily because of the shorter life span in the latter case. Obviously, many of these signs and symptoms are identical to those attributable to cancer itself or to the effects of chemotherapy or radiotherapy.

The differential diagnosis of hypercalcemia includes the following disorders: (1) primary hyperparathyroidism, (2) malignancy, (3) granulomatous diseases (sarcoidosis, tuberculosis), (4) thiazide diuretics, (5) severe immobilization, (6) milk-alkali syndrome, (7) vitamin D intoxication, (8) vitamin A intoxication, (9) hyperthyroidism, (10) adrenal insufficiency, and (11) familial hypocalciuric hypercalcemia.

Most of these conditions are easily distinguishable on clinical evidence, and the principal problem in differential diagnosis is the distinction of cancer from primary hyperparathyroidism. The single most important laboratory test is measurement of the plasma level of parathyroid hormone (PTH). Although different antisera give variable results in immunoassays, most patients with primary hyperparathyroidism have clear elevation in immunoreactive PTH levels, whereas most tumor patients with the same degree of hypercalcemia have low or normal levels of immunoreactive PTH.[15]

Elevated urinary cyclic AMP, modulated by PTH, is characteristic of hyperparathyroidism, but it is also frequently elevated in hypercalcemic malignancy patients, reflecting the production of humoral substances with the ability to stimulate urinary cyclic AMP.[16] Hypercalcemia with hypophosphatemia suggests primary hyperparathyroidism, although many patients with cancer are also hypophosphatemic because of malnutrition, humoral substances that cause phosphaturia, or increase in urinary phosphate excretion as a direct effect

Table 9-1. Pathogenetic Classification of the Hypercalcemia of Cancer

Clinical group	Types of tumors	Bone histologic studies	Bone radiologic studies	Other features	Factors implicated	Local or systemic
Hematologic cancers	Myeloma, lymphosarcoma, Burkitt's lymphoma, adult T cell lymphoma	Increase in osteoclastic bone resorption adjacent to neoplastic cells	Mainly osteolytic lesions; occasionally diffuse osteopenia		Osteoclast activating factor: 1.25 dihydroxy-vitamin D	Local
Solid tumors with bone metastases	Breast, lung, pancreatic	Increase in local osteoclastic bone resorption; variable osteoblastic response	Discrete lytic lesions; variable sclerotic response		Prostaglandins: direct erosion by tumor cells	Local
Solid tumors without metastases	Lung, kidney, pancreatic, ovarian	Increased osteoclastic bone resorption: decreased bone formation	No abnormality	Increase in fractional excretion of phosphate: increase in nephrogenous cyclic: AMP; decrease in immunoreactive parathyroid hormone	I. Parathyroid hormone II. Prostaglandin III. Transforming growth factors IV. PTH-like peptide V. Colony-stimulating activity	Systemic

Source: Mundy GR, et al (ref 13)

of hypercalcemia.[17] Serum alkaline phosphatase levels are usually higher in malignancy than in primary hyperparathyroidism.[18]

Certain clinical features tend to distinguish cancer-associated hypercalcemia from primary hyperparathyroidism. In cancer, hypercalcemia worsens more rapidly, the degree of hypercalcemia tends to be greater, and renal stones are absent despite marked hypercalciuria.

The pathogenesis of hypercalcemia in cancer is related primarily to increased bone resorption, although serum calcium may occasionally rise because of increased intestinal absorption or because of reduced renal excretion, particularly with renal failure or dehydration. Resorption of bone is accompanied not only by hypercalcemia but also by the consequences of osteolytic bone loss, itself a severe problem. Calcium is released from bone through the activity of osteoclasts, which are stimulated by a variety of mechanisms (see table 9-1).

Increased levels of 1,25 dihydroxy vitamin D, probably of extrarenal origin, have been found in a few cases of malignant lymphoma, including T cell lymphoma associated with HTLV-1.[19] Chemotherapy and prednisone reduce the levels of both calcium and vitamin D; however, these are exceptional cases, and it is unlikely that vitamin D is a common humoral mediator of hypercalcemia. At the site of a metastasis, prostaglandins, which can stimulate osteoclastic activity, are produced by bone cells, tumor cells, monocytes, and macrophages.[20] The failure of nonsteroidal anti-inflammatory agents to lower serum calcium in patients with bone metastases suggests either that other factors are primarily responsible for hypercalcemia or that prostaglandin synthesis inhibitors are not effective in bone.[21] Circulating prostaglandins of tumor origin have been identified with certain tumors, but correlation with serum calcium is poor and response to prostaglandin synthesis inhibition very disappointing.[22]

Neoplasms of lymphoid origin, such as multiple myeloma, Burkitt's lymphoma and adult T cell lymphoma, produce a group of proteins—the osteoclast activating factors (OAFs)—that activate the osteoclasts.[23] Their structure is still uncertain, and their presence has been determined only by bioassay based on bone resorptive capacity. The humoral hypercalcemic factor in multiple myeloma is undoubtedly OAF, but such other factors as renal function may help to determine the final concentration of serum calcium. It is of interest that when myeloma cells are cultured with indomethacin the release of OAF is inhibited, but there is no clinical counterpart to this observation.[24]

The belief at one time was that ectopic secretion of PTH occurred commonly in hypercalcemic cancer patients, but now it seems that this ectopic PTH secretion is rare.[25] Recently, attention has been focused on a group of "PTH-like factors" produced by solid tumors.[26] These factors bind to PTH receptors and stimulate adenyl cyclase in renal membranes, increasing urinary cyclic AMP and decreasing renal tubular reabsorption of phosphate. They also increase the glucose-6-phosphate dehydrogenase content in renal tubular cells. Their effects on cellular systems in vitro are inhibited by synthetic PTH antagonists. However, unlike PTH, they do not increase renal tubular reabsorption of calcium, nor do they stimulate renal 1-alpha hydroxylase. Immunoassay for PTH usually has yielded negative results. The action of these substances on bone, studied histologically, reveals uncoupling of osteoclast/osteoblast activity, with exaggerated resorption and subnormal formation of bone. Extracts of tumors that produce PTH-like substances have only rarely been shown to synthesize the messenger RNA of PTH. Recently, a radioimmunoassay has been developed to measure this PTH-like peptide in cancer patients.[27]

Finally, transforming growth factors (TGFs) are a family of polypeptides with properties similar to those of epidermal growth factor and platelet-derived growth factor.[23] They stimulate cell growth and replication as well as osteoclast activity leading to increased bone resorption. Many tumors and normal tissues produce TGFs (e.g., experimental rat Leydig-cell tumor and human renal cell carcinoma). These factors are not related to PTH. The role of TGFs in hypercalcemia associated with cancer is still unsettled.

The treatment approach for hypercalcemia depends on whether the patient has experienced rapid elevation of serum calcium accompanied by deterioration of mental status or whether a chronic tendency to hypercalcemia is present. The emergency treatment of hypercalcemia includes the following stepped approach:

1. *I.V. NaCl solutions with or without furosemide.* Volume expansion with saline reduces reabsorption of sodium and calcium in the proximal tubule and delivers increased amounts of these ions to the ascending limb of Henle's loop. At this site, furosemide prevents reabsorption of both ions, and marked natriuresis and calciuresis occurs. Because patients are often dehydrated when treatment begins, 1–2 L of saline may be required merely to overcome dehydration. The subsequent rate of administration of saline containing K Cl at about 10 mEq/L ranges from 250 to 500 ml/hr, depending on the rapidity of diuresis and the cardiovascular state of the patient. Furosemide may be given I.V. 60–80 mg every 3–6 hr. Serum calcium, sodium, magnesium, and potassium should be measured 2–3 times/day and intake adjusted accordingly. In elderly and debilitated patients, volume expansion should be guided with measurement of central venous pressure.

2. If the above approach is contraindicated or ineffective, *calcitonin* at a dose of 4 MRC U/kg of body weight subcutaneously q. 12 hr can be used. Serum calcium begins to fall in 2 hr and remains at lower levels for up to 72 hr as calcitonin is continued. Tolerance to calcitonin may be due to down-regulation of receptors or immune response; addition of prednisone may prolong the action of calcitonin for periods up to several months.

3. *Mithramycin,* which suppresses RNA synthesis and bone resorptive activity of osteoclasts, takes 1–3 days for maximal hypocalcemic effect. The small quantity used avoids many toxic effects of this compound, but in patients with thrombocytopenia or hepatic or renal impairment, great caution must be employed. The use of mithramycin for long-term therapy is limited by its toxicity, but it can be tried if other measures fail. The dose is 15–25 μg/kg, given I.V. It can be repeated daily for 4–5 days.

4. *Hemodialysis or peritoneal dialysis* can lower calcium quickly but very transiently; dialysis may be needed in patients with heart failure or renal failure (e.g., myeloma kidney or acute uric acid nephropathy).

5. I.V. phosphate or chelating agents such as EDTA cannot be used because of excessive toxicity. Sodium sulfate is safer than phosphate or EDTA but is no more effective than normal saline.

6. The *diphosphonates* are a group of drugs that can be very effective in reducing hypercalcemia by inhibiting bone resorption. The I.V. form of

etidronate disodium (Didronel) is currently recommended for the treatment of hypercalcemia of malignancy; etidronate is infused at a dosage of 7.5 mg/kg/day × 3.

The long-term treatment of hypercalcemia includes such measures as liberal salt and water intake and avoidance of dehydration, immobilization, foods rich in calcium, and thiazides and other agents that promote hypercalcemia. Glucocorticoids have an unpredictable effect on serum calcium; only about a third of patients treated with prednisone 20–40 mg/day will respond. Myeloma and lymphomas are among the more responsive tumors. Oral phosphates work primarily by reducing reabsorption of calcium by the gut. The available preparations—Fleet Phospho soda, Neutra-Phos, and K-phos—cause diarrhea, but this may be treated with Lomotil. The usual dose is 1–3 g of elementary phosphorus per day in divided dosage. Phosphate is not used in patients with renal failure. Calcitonin and mithramycin can be used in the long-term control of hypercalcemia with the restrictions and caveats noted above.

Hypocalcemia is an infrequent problem in cancer patients. Rapid uptake of calcium by bone metastases in prostatic carcinoma, magnesium depletion, treatment with mithramycin, and hyperphosphatemia constitute most of the examples encountered. Neoplastic infiltration of the parathyroid glands is a rare cause of primary hypoparathyroidism. Tetany and Chvostek's and Trousseau's signs may be present, and the EKG may show a prolonged Q-T interval and arrhythmias. Symptomatic hypocalcemia is treated with I.V. infusion of calcium salts. The rate of calcium infusion should not exceed 50 mg/min, and a total dose of 1 g should not be exceeded without a repeat measurement of serum calcium.

Disorders of Phosphate Metabolism

Hyperphosphatemia

Serum phosphate may rise sharply with the release of phosphate that accompanies chemotherapy of certain tumors such as leukemias and Burkitt's lymphoma.[28] Renal failure, hypocalcemia, hyperuricemia, hyperkalemia, and extraskeletal calcifications are among the consequences. Treatment includes hydration and allopurinol before institution of chemotherapy. After the fact, glucose with insulin, alkaline diuresis, and oral phosphate binders are helpful. However, hemodialysis is often needed when renal failure supervenes.

Hypophosphatemia

Nonspecific causes such as malnutrition, diarrhea, and alkalosis (especially respiratory) may lower serum phosphate. Because total parenteral nutrition can cause acute hypophosphatemia, adequate phosphate supplements must be included in the formula. Tumor-associated mechanisms resulting in hypophosphatemia include (1) uptake of phosphate by rapidly growing tumor cells such as leukemias;[29] (2) Fanconi's syndrome, associated with multiple myeloma;[30] and (3) oncogenic osteomalacia associated with renal phosphate wasting.[31]

Treatment of hypophosphatemia should involve the oral route as much as possible. Preparations such as Neutra-Phos (liquid or tablets) may be given at a daily dose of 2–3 g of phosphate. In severe symptomatic hypophosphatemia, phosphate may be given I.V. as the sodium or sodium plus potassium salt at rates up to 10 mM of phosphate per hour; more rapid phosphate administration may lead to hypocalcemia.

Acid/Base Disturbances

Acid/base disturbances occur frequently in cancer patients, but very few are directly traceable to the presence of tumors. Rather, they tend to occur for the same reasons that are operative in any group of individuals suffering from severe illness and its treatment. An adequate approach to acid/base disturbances can be found in any standard acid/base textbook. Only lactic acidosis will be discussed here because this disorder may offer special features in cancer patients.

Lactic Acidosis

In cancer, lactic acidosis occurs for the following reasons:[32]
- Overproduction of lactic acid can be encountered in leukemia (cells may run on anaerobic metabolism like red blood cells when packed tightly in bone marrow);[33] in severe anemia, when oxygen supply to tissues is reduced; or in septic or hemorrhagic shock accompanied by decreased delivery of oxygen to both normal and neoplastic tissues.
- Reduced disposal of lactic acid, occurring primarily in patients with infiltration of the liver or reduced delivery of oxygen to liver secondary to hemorrhagic or septic shock.

The diagnosis of lactic acidosis is suspected in a patient with metabolic acidosis, high anion gap, and appropriate clinical setting, and is confirmed by measurement of serum lactate. One must be careful in evaluating the anion gap; if the patient has high serum chloride due to hypoalbuminemia, or low serum sodium due to accumulation of positively charged myeloma globulins, the baseline anion gap may be low and the development of lactic acidosis may only raise it to normal.

Treatment of lactic acidosis consists first of removing its cause through an increase in red cell mass, reduction in tumor burden, and reversal of sepsis and shock. Acidemia is treated with bicarbonate, using the smallest quantities possible to ensure continued survival under the circumstances. It has been repeatedly shown that treatment with bicarbonate increases lactic acid formation, presumably by raising cell pH.[34] Treatment of chronic lactic acidosis in anorectic, cachectic cancer patients poses a problem: Increased lactate formation leads to increased urinary lactate excretion. Because glucose cannot be made from fat, and because glycogen stores are depleted, gluconeogenesis from tissue protein is the ultimate mechanism to provide lactate precursors. The cost of therapy of chronic lactic acidosis with bicarbonate may be the rapid worsening of the cachectic state, as protein rapidly breaks down into carbon skeletons that are converted to lactate and wasted in the urine.

Uric Acid Metabolism Disorders

Hypouricemia

Hypouricemia, occasionally observed in cancer patients, can usually be attributed to increased renal clearance of uric acid (e.g., Fanconi's syndrome in myeloma; SIADH with hypouricemia in oat cell carcinoma of the lung).[35] Hypouricemia requires no treatment.

Hyperuricemia

The association between cancer (especially myeloproliferative disorders) and hyperuricemia is well known. This secondary hyperuricemia may give rise to the following clinical manifestations: acute gout, acute uric acid nephropathy, chronic urate nephropathy, and uric acid stones. Usually, only the first 2 manifestations are seen, as the latter 2 are associated with chronic hyperuricemia. Polycythemia vera is the disease most frequently associated with clinical gouty arthritis. Treatment includes that usually given for acute gout plus allopurinol to block uric acid synthesis.

Acute uric acid nephropathy is a well-recognized form of acute renal failure that occurs during treatment of leukemias and lymphomas.[36] The sudden lysis of tumor cells leads to increased production of uric acid, hyperuricosuria, and obstruction of renal tubules by precipitated uric acid. The diagnosis rests on finding hyperuricosuria (urine uric acid-to-creatinine ratio of >1) in the appropriate clinical setting. Early diagnosis is essential; prevention is preferable. Treatment includes maintenance of large urine volume, alkalization of the urine, and administration of allopurinol.

References

1. Alpers CE, Cotran RS. Neoplasia and glomerular injury. Kidney Int 1986; 30:465.
2. Wesner RL. Fasting—a review with emphasis on electrolytes. Am J Med 1971; 50:233.
3. Bode HH, Harley BM, Crawford JD. Restoration of normal drinking behavior by chlorpropamide in patients with hypodipsia and diabetes insipidus. Am J Med 1971; 51:304.
4. Earley LE, Orloff J. The mechanism of antidiuresis associated with the administration of hydrochlorothiazide to patients with vasopressin-resistant diabetes insipidus. J Clin Invest 1962; 41:1988.
5. Murray T, Long W, Narins RG. Multiple myeloma and the anion gap. N Engl J Med 1975; 292:574.
6. Flear CTG, Singh CM. Hyponatremia and sick cells. Br J Anaesth 1973; 45:976.
7. Decaux G. Treatment of the syndrome of inappropriate secretion of ADH by long loop diuretics. Nephron 1983; 35:82.
8. Uribarri J, Carroll HJ. Potassium metabolism and hypertension. J Clin Hypertens 1985; 4:283.
9. Adams PC, Woodhouse KW, Adela M, et al. Exaggerated hypokalemia in acute myeloid leukemia. Br Med J 1981; 282:1034.
10. Kerr DJ, McAlpine LG, Dagg JH. Pseudohyperkalemia. Br J Med 1985; 291:890.
11. Phelps KR, Oh MS, Carroll HJ. Heparin-induced hyperkalemia: report of a case. Nephron 1980; 25:254.
12. Fisken RA, Heath DA, Bold AM. Hypercalcemia: a hospital survey. Q J Med 1980; 196:405.

13. Mundy GR, Ibbotson KJ, Desouza SM, et al. The hypercalcemia of cancer. Clinical implications and pathogenetic mechanisms. N Engl J Med 1984; 310:1718.

14. Fukumoto S, Matsumoto T, Ikeda I, et al. Clinical evaluation of calcium metabolism in adult T cell leukemia/lymphoma. Arch Intern Med 1988; 148:921.

15. Habener JF, Segre GV. Parathyroid hormone radioimmunoassay. Ann Intern Med 1979; 91:782.

16. Rude RK, Sharp CF, Fredericks RS, et al. Urinary and nephrogenous adenosine 3, 5 - monophosphate in the hypercalcemia of malignancy. J Clin Endocrinol Metab 1981; 52:765.

17. Schussler GC, Verso MA, Nemoto T. Phosphaturia in hypercalcemic breast cancer patients. J Clin Endocrinol Metab 1972; 35:497.

18. Boyd JC, Ladenson JH. Value of laboratory tests in the differential diagnosis of hypercalcemia. Am J Med 1984; 77:863.

19. Breslau N, McGuire J, Zerwekh J, et al. Hypercalcemia associated with increased serum calcitriol levels in three patients with lymphoma. Ann Intern Med 1984; 100:1.

20. Atkins D, Ibbotson KJ, Hillier K, et al. Secretion of prostaglandins as bone-resorbing agents by renal cortical carcinoma in culture. Br J Cancer 1977; 36:601.

21. Caro JF, Besarab A, Flynn JT. Prostaglandin E and hypercalcemia in breast carcinoma: only a tumor marker? Am J Med 1979; 66:337.

22. Buckle RM, McMillan M, Mallinson C. Ectopic secretion of parathyroid hormone by a renal adenocarcinoma in a patient with hypercalcemia. Br Med J 1970; 4:724.

23. Mundy GR. Hypercalcemia of malignancy. J Clin Invest 1988; 82:1.

24. Josse RG, Murray TM, Mundy GR, et al. Observations on the mechanism of bone resorption induced by multiple myeloma marrow culture fluids and partially purified osteoclast-activating factor. J Clin Invest 1981; 67:1472.

25. Simpson, EL, Mundy GR, D'Souza SM, et al. Absence of parathyroid hormone messenger RNA in nonparathyroid tumors associated with hypercalcemia. N Engl J Med 1983; 309:325.

26. Stewart AF, Horst R, Reftos CJ, et al. Biochemical evaluation of patients with cancer-associated hypercalcemia—evidence for humoral and nonhumoral groups. N Engl J Med 1980; 303:1377.

27. Burtis WJ, Brady TG, et al. Immunochemical characterization of circulating parathyroid hormone-related protein in patients with humoral hypercalcemia of cancer. N Engl J Med 1990; 322:1106.

28. Matzner Y, Prococimer M, Polliack A, et al. Hypophosphatemia in a patient with lymphoma in leukemic phase. Arch Intern Med 1981; 141:805.

29. Maldanedo JE, Velosa JE, Kyle RA, et al. Fanconi syndrome in adults: a manifestation of a latent form of myeloma. Am J Med 1975; 58:354.

30. Drezner MK, Feinglos MN. Osteomalacia due to 1,25 dihydroxycholecalciferol deficiency; association with a giant cell tumor of bone. J Clin Invest 1977; 60:1046.

31. Gitelis S, Ryan WG, et al. Adult onset hypophosphatemic osteomalacia secondary to neoplasm. J Bone Joint Surg 1986; 68A:134.

32. Kreisberg RA. Pathogenesis and management of lactic acidosis. Annu Rev Med 1984; 35:181.

33. Waiver RA, Werink PH, Thompson WL. Metabolic and therapeutic studies of a patient with acute leukemia and severe lactic acidosis of prolonged duration. Am J Med 1973; 55:255.

34. Fraley DS, Alder S, Bruns FJ. Stimulation of lactate production by administration of bicarbonate in a patient with a solid neoplasm and lactic acidosis. N Engl J Med 1980; 303:1100.

35. Beck LH. Hypouricemia in the syndrome of inappropriate secretion of antidiuretic hormone. N Engl J Med 1979; 301:528.

36. Kjellstrand CM, Campbell DC, Van Hartitzch B, et al. Hyperuricemic acute renal failure. Arch Intern Med 1974; 133:349.

10

DIAGNOSTIC IMAGING IN NEOPLASTIC DISEASES

*David H. Gordon, M.D., Gwendolyn Hotson, M.D.,
Jack Twersky, M.D., and Sidney Glanz, M.D.*

Computerized Axial Tomography

THE ORIGIN OF THE specialty of diagnostic radiology can be traced to the discovery of X rays by Roentgen in 1895. Since 1972, X rays have been applied in clinical practice to a new field, that of computerized axial tomography, or CT scanning, a diagnostic technique based primarily on studies performed by 2 Nobel prize laureates, Alan McCormack and Godfrey Hounsfield. Their research suggested that computers and mathematics could be used to reconstruct an image from accurate x-ray measurements through the body from multiple angles. In 1968, employing a gamma source of radiation, the first computer-reconstructed image was produced; a period of 9 days was required to scan the object and 2½ hr to process a single image. With an x-ray tube as a source of photons, scan time was later reduced to 9 hr, leading to the production in 1972 of the first prototype clinical unit, which had a scan time of 4½ min. The initial results produced by this scanner were rapidly recognized as a major contribution to the field of neuroradiology. In 1975, a CT unit with an 18-sec scan time and no need for a water bag became available. The unit could also be used for imaging the chest and abdomen with satisfactory resolution, thereby introducing clinically useful body CT. Since 1975, rapid strides have been made in terms of scan time and image processing; the third and fourth generation scanners available today have scan times in the range of 2–10 sec with immediate reconstruction.[1-6] The Cine-CT scanner is capable of producing as many as 12 images per second for cardiac imaging procedures.

The production of a CT image can be described briefly as follows: Thinly collimated beams of X rays pass through the patient from many different angles. Some of the photons will be absorbed; the fraction that reaches a detector on the opposite side of the patient are measured. From the multiple simultaneous equations produced, the X ray attenuation coefficient of each tiny block of tissue in each known location can be calculated. These numbers can be converted to an image by the arbitrary assignment of a grey scale to all or part of this array of values. Because superimposition of different tissues is not relevant, CT produces tissue contrast differentiation markedly superior to that achieved by conventional radiography. The size of a structure or lesion that may be demonstrated by a state-of-the-art CT scanner may be as small as 5 mm, but this depends upon how different it is in its X ray attenuation coefficient from the tissue around it.

Software packages in combination with the basic hardware as described above enable measurement of tissue attenuation values in terms of "Hounsfield units" by placing a cursor over the tissue to be studied. By convention, water is placed at the center of the scale at 0 Hounsfield units, fat is in the -125 U range, air is in the -500 U range, soft tissue is in the $+30$ U range, and bone is in the $+500$ U range.

It is important to understand that the absolute CT numbers of tissues vary from machine to machine and even within the same machine from day to day. Machines must be calibrated daily, and excessive reliance on absolute CT numbers may be fraught with danger. However, by referencing the absolute CT number against an internal fluid reference such as the gallbladder, one may get a relative value scale that can be applied clinically.

The radiation exposure given to a patient receiving a CT scan is difficult to define precisely because the amount of exposure depends on the size of the field scanned. It is reasonable to state that CT examinations in general deliver no more radiation to the patient than conventional radiographic examinations, particularly if the radiation dose is assessed as an integral dose.

The reliability and clinical usefulness of the CT scanner has grown from a research tool in 1968 to a clinically vital area of the hospital, without which it is virtually impossible to practice satisfactory modern clinical medicine. It has interphased with and supplanted many other noninvasive clinical imaging modalities such as nuclear scanning and ultrasound. In addition, it has reduced or eliminated the need for angiography in many areas. It has had a major impact on both the diagnosis and treatment of cancer of all types.

The CT scan is often the initial screening modality performed when a patient enters the hospital with a suspicion of cancer or a clinically discovered mass. The CT scanner may be able to define the organ of origin, the extent of spread, and the nature of the tumor (solid, cystic, calcified); it has become an indispensable tool for the radiation therapist in terms of planning portals for radiation administration.

In addition to the purely diagnostic aspects of CT scanning, biopsies of masses and drainage of abscesses and fluid collections can be done with great precision using CT localization.

CT has become the major imaging modality in neuroradiology, with very high sensitivity and specificity in the detection and characterization of intracranial pathology.

Intracranial masses, whether primary or secondary, benign or malignant, are generally best seen on a contrast-enhanced CT scan. The normal brain does not enhance with I.V. contrast; the intact blood/brain barrier prevents the high-molecular-weight organic molecule from passing into the interstitium. Most pathological lesions enhance with contrast, either because of blood/brain barrier destruction or because the vessels of the lesion pool intravascular contrast, or both. The presence of enhancement increases the sensitivity of the examination; the pattern of enhancement increases its specificity. After the I.V. administration of iodine-containing contrast, the CT attenuation value of any structure perfused by vessels will be raised. This discriminates a solid structure containing blood vessels from a hollow organ or cyst. A noncontrast CT is required only if intracranial hemorrhage is a serious diagnostic possibility, if the detection of calcification in the lesion will alter its management, or if a medical contraindication to its use (e.g., renal failure, allergy) exists. Intrathecal contrast increases the spatial resolution of CT and helps detect and localize posterior fossa masses. CT-guided brain biopsies can be performed through a burr hole or craniotomy.

Angiography is less sensitive and less specific than CT in the evaluation of intracranial masses, but is occasionally still required preoperatively in masses that are poorly localized or intimately related to important vessels.

CT of the spine is sometimes important in evaluating bone lesions. It is more sensitive than a plain x-ray for bone destruction, although less sensitive than an isotope scan. It may be useful in planning reconstructive surgery, and is useful in planning a bone biopsy approach. It has not, however, replaced myelography in the evaluation of epidural tumor and cord compression nor in the detection of tumors within the cord or subarachnoid space. The small amount of epidural fat above the midlumbar region makes the differentiation of normal soft tissues around the cord from tumor difficult unless contrast has been injected into the subarachnoid space. In detecting abnormalities of the spine, the newest imaging technology of magnetic resonance has been found to be the most useful diagnostic technique.

Magnetic Resonance Imaging

Instead of X rays, magnetic resonance imaging (MRI) uses a high-strength external magnetic field and radio waves to discriminate among soft tissues on the basis of their hydrogen content and their biochemical surroundings. The signal intensity of a tissue depends upon proton density and 2 tissue relaxation times, T1 and T2. Changing imaging parameters (TR and TE) determines which of these 3 factors has the largest influence upon the brightness of the signal.

MRI has several advantages over CT in studying the brain. It is more sensitive in the detection of soft-tissue abnormalities, it is readily amenable to imaging in multiple planes, and it may not require the use of I.V. contrast. When necessary, gadolinium chelates may be used I.V. to detect blood/brain barrier breakdown, a property that is particularly useful in the discrimination of brain metastases from other destructive parenchymal lesions. Drawbacks of MRI include its nonspecificity, the long imaging times, and its unsuitability in very sick patients who require life support systems made of metal inadmissible to the magnet room.

In the CNS of cancer patients, MRI shows enormous usefulness in the evaluation of the spine. It is probably the most sensitive technique yet devised to detect bone marrow metastases and can readily demonstrate epidural spread of metastatic tumor. The spinal cord is directly displayed, so that cord compression is well shown; intramedullary metastases may show areas of prolonged T2 or enhancement with gadolinium DTPA. The ability to produce direct sagittal images makes MRI a more efficient imaging technique than CT.

Outside the CNS, the role of MRI has not been as well worked out as in the CNS. One main area of application of MRI relates to the signal void produced by flowing blood; this enables a form of MR angiography that may obviate the need for contrast-catheter angiography.

MRI has a strong ability to enable specific tissue characterization in terms of different signals produced by neoplasms and pathology within a solid organ. In general, most neoplasms have a prolonged T2 relaxation time on T2-weighted images. Coronal and sagittal sections, in combination with a more familiar axial section, make it possible to view the pathologic process in a 3-dimensional manner. Volume acquisitions enable very thin slices and multidimensional reconstruction from various angles. In vivo spectroscopy is another area that shows promise in characterizing specific tissues by means of a spectroscopic analysis in vivo. This is in an experimental stage at this time.

In terms of the specific applications of MRI to oncology, MRI has proven to be very useful in a number of areas and is in fact the procedure of choice in many instances. In the chest, although it is of little value for imaging the pulmonary parenchyma because of the respiratory motion of the lungs, MRI is excellent for imaging of the mediastinum and, because the flow void of the vessels of the hilum provide good contrast with any solid masses or nodes in apposition to the hilum, it is probably the procedure of choice for imaging the hilar structures.

The aorticopulmonary window, an area that is particularly difficult to evaluate on axial CT scans, can be well elucidated on coronal MRI scans. Axillary lymph nodes and the presence of mediastinal spread from a primary breast carcinoma are well delineated on MRI. The internal mammary node chain can also be well delineated. The application of MRI to delineation and characterization of primary breast tumors is of limited value because calcification, which is not imaged well on MRI, is a prime diagnostic consideration in the evaluation of breast carcinomas.

MRI is currently probably the study of choice in defining the presence of metastases or masses within the liver. At high field strength, heavily T2-weighted images compare favorably with the best CT scanning done. However, if colon carcinoma recurrence in the liver is suspected, a CT portogram should be done prior to resection of suspected metastases because this may be the most definitive imaging modality within the liver. On low-field-strength machines, heavily T1-weighted images are preferable to T2-weighted images in defining masses within the liver. MRI is useful in distinguishing between hemangiomas and malignant liver masses, especially when combined with gadolinium DTPA injection. MRI has not shown significant value in diagnosing carcinoma of the pancreas as compared to CT. This disease still appears to be beyond the currently available diagnostic modalities regarding the goal of arriving at an early diagnosis to make a surgical cure possible.

Characterizing and defining adrenal masses is another area in which MRI has shown promise. Nonfunctioning adenomas on T2-weighted imaging generally have a signal that is the same or less than that of the liver. Metastases and primary carcinomas have a higher signal than the liver, and pheochromocytomas, cysts, and hemangiomas of the adrenal have very high signal relative to the liver. However, there is significant (20–25%) overlap in these groups, so that when specific tissue characterization is needed to define a clinical algorithm (as in lung cancer) with an enlarged adrenal, a CT guided biopsy needs to be done. Gadolinium DTPA administration may improve diagnostic accuracy among adrenal masses.

MRI also shows promise as an aid in distinguishing between tumor recurrence and fibrosis, as in postradiation changes within the mediastinum in a patient with lymphoma, or in a patient's status postabdominal perineal resection, where there typically is a presacral fibrous plaque after the surgery. Imaging with MRI may be helpful in distinguishing between tumor recurrence, which would produce a bright signal on T2-weighted images, and fibrosis, which should give a dark signal on T2-weighted image because of the small number of available protons present in fibrous tissue. Again, this is not specific; if a clinical decision must be made on the basis of fibrosis versus recurrent tumor, a biopsy may ultimately be necessary.

MRI has established itself as the modality of choice in the assessment of bone marrow in diffuse processes such as multiple myeloma or metastatic disease. Although it is not as readily accomplished as bone scanning, it is more specific and in some instances may be more sensitive, as in myeloma or breast carcinoma, where bone scans can be negative in the presence of metastases. Metastatic disease to the marrow will produce a low signal that replaces the normal high signal of fatty marrow on T1-weighted images. These areas will then become bright on T2-weighted images, whereas the fat signal will go down on T2-weighted images. MRI is not valuable, however, in terms of defining cortical bone abnormalities, an area in which CT is the modality of choice. MRI has also established itself as the procedure of choice in the evaluation of bony and soft-tissue tumors for extent of tumor, degree of marrow invasion, and feasibility of a limb-sparing operation. The proximity of the neoplasm to the neurovascular bundle in the extremity can also be established, as can its relation to the joint space, utilizing its multiplanar capability and excellent tissue characterization.

In a patient who is allergic to I.V.-iodinated contrast, MRI may be of value in defining retroperitoneal adenopathy. However, MRI is currently limited by the fact that there is no good oral contrast available to opacify the bowel; this is a pitfall in imaging for retroperitoneal adenopathy.

MRI is of limited value in the kidneys because normal kidneys become extremely bright on T2 weighting, as do renal neoplasms, thereby providing little differentiation between the tumor and normal parenchyma. Results have been disappointing in staging bladder neoplasms as well. Nuclear scanning and sonography are more useful than MRI in evaluation of testicular masses.

MRI has been proven useful in the evaluation and follow-up of gynecologic malignancies. In cervical carcinoma, sagittal images can provide information on the degree of invasion outside the cervix, into the vaginal vault, and into the corpus uteri. Pelvic lymph nodes can also be well evaluated and the adnexa can be defined. In endometrial carcinoma, the depth of invasion can be established and lymph node enlargement can be defined. In follow-up of gynecologic malignancies after radiation or surgery, MRI is useful because of its multiplanar capacity and its tissue characterization abilities.

Although gadolinium has proven itself to be quite useful within the CNS, its application to the body outside the CNS is limited to the spine. In general, it has the effect of shortening T1 relaxation time. In instances in which this is of value, gadolinium may ultimately demonstrate itself to be useful particularly in conjunction with rapid imaging techniques such as gradient-recalled imaging and single-breath-hold scans. Much additional work remains to be done in assessing the ultimate role of MRI in the noninvasive imaging of neoplastic processes outside the CNS.

Sonography

Another imaging technique currently used less frequently in the diagnosis of cancer is that of sonography—the use of ultrasound to define tissue abnormalities. Ultrasound should be used whenever radiation dose is a major consideration, such as in women of child-bearing age and children. Ultrasound is preferable in thin patients and for the visualization of spaces filled with liquid material (cysts, biliary ducts, etc.), when contrast cannot be used in performing the CT scan. Because periorgan fat is the contrast material of CT scanning, the fatter the patient the better, in terms of producing a high-quality CT scan. The cost of the examination of the patient is similar in both modalities, as is the time needed to perform the studies. However, CT scanning in general is more reproducible, less operator-dependent, and gives a more panoramic view than ultrasound, which must be directed at a specific area. Also, CT scanning is the procedure of choice whenever air is in the region of the portion of the body to be scanned, such as in the chest, mediastinum and left upper quadrant. Air interferes markedly with the sound beam, whereas it has very little effect on CT scanning. Metal within the patient presents a problem for both ultrasound and CT scanning, producing streak artifacts in both.

Interventional Radiology

During the past 5 yr, interventional radiology interphased with CT scanning has become progressively involved in the definitive diagnosis and treatment of many neoplastic diseases. One such location in which interventional radiology can play an important role in defining the diagnosis is the retroperitonium.

CT scanning is the initial procedure of choice in the evaluation of the retroperitoneum. However, if the CT scan is negative or equivocal, a bipedal lymphangiogram may be performed. CT scanning will define only enlarged nodes; it will not depict partially replaced but normal-sized nodes. Because of its superior resolving power, a lymphangiogram is able to define partial replacement of nodes. In addition, if it is necessary to histologically define the cancerous nature of the nodes, a thin-needle biopsy under CT control can be performed. Thin-needle biopsies are cytologic aspiration biopsies rather than cutting biopsies because of the deep location of the retroperitoneum. However, this may be adequate to define the malignant nature of a process, and a small tissue core can often be obtained. When the diagnosis is lymphoma and tissue markers are needed for precise characterization, a surgical biopsy may be necessary to obtain more tissue.

Guided cytologic aspiration biopsy is a well-accepted and extremely useful procedure in the management of cancer patients. The procedure has the potential of making a laparotomy or thoracotomy for purely diagnostic purposes unnecessary, especially in patients with pancreatic tumors, extravisceral abdominal and pelvic masses, and peripheral lung masses difficult to reach by bronchoscopy. Illustrations of biopsies are given with the cases in the following section.

Palliation for the incurable cancer patient can also be achieved by application of other interventional radiologic techniques such as embolization. Therapeutic embolization of unresectable tumors may palliate necrotic bleeding tumors and reduce blood supply to tumors prior to surgical resection. In addition, there is some evidence that embolization and infarction of the primary tumor in widespread metastatic disease may prolong life by releasing tumor antigens into the circulation, producing an autologous antigen/antibody tumor reaction and thereby slowing the rate of tumor multiplication.

In the following pages, illustrations of some of the radiologic images helpful in the diagnosis of neoplastic disease will be presented. This presentation, although not comprehensive, has the primary aim of familiarizing the reader with some relatively common as well as some unusual diagnostic imaging problems encountered in patients with specific neoplastic diseases dealt with in other chapters of this book.

Case Examples

Case 1—Multifocal Hepatoma (Figures 10-1A & B, 10-2, 10-3)

Multifocal hepatoma cannot be readily distinguished from metastatic disease to the liver on CT.[7-11] Clinical correlation with underlying cirrhosis, elevated alpha-fetoprotein and clinical presentation may be helpful. The arteriographic pattern is suggestive but not pathognomonic of hepatoma. The presence of vena caval invasion interdicts operative resection. The presence of underlying liver disease usually means that the patient cannot undergo surgery in any event. Differential diagnosis includes multiple metastases, complex abscesses, regenerative nodules of cirhossis, and multiple liver adenomas.

Case 2—Metastatic Disease to the Liver from a Breast Primary (Figure 10-4)

Metastases to the liver occur frequently (30–45% of cases) in patients with advanced carcinoma of the breast. The liver is second only to bones among sites of metastatic dissemination of infiltrating ductal carcinoma of the breast.[12-14] Differential diagnosis includes multifocal hepatoma and multiple complex abscesses.

Case 3—Calcified Metastases to the Liver from a Primary Mucinous Adenocarcinoma of the Stomach, with Portal Vein Thrombosis (Figures 10-5A & B, 10-6)

Mucinous adenocarcinoma primary in the colon, stomach, or elsewhere may calcify when metastatic to the liver.[13-20] Ovarian carcinoma also may produce calcified metastatic lesions. When seen in the liver, a virtual histologic diagnosis of metastatic mucinous adenocarcinoma can be made.

Case 4—Cecal Adenocarcinoma with Peritoneal Implants (Figures 10-7, 10-8)

Metastatic tumor from multiple primary sources can produce this picture. G.I. neoplasms and ovarian and breast primaries are the most common. Aspiration of the ascites fluid may provide the diagnosis of malignant ascites.[21-23] CT or sonographically guided biopsy of these lesions (as was done in this case) is another way of providing a diagnosis without surgery or laparoscopy.

Case 5—Gallbladder Carcinoma (Figure 10-9A & B)

Gallbladder carcinoma is an occult disease that is being diagnosed with more frequency and at an earlier stage as a serendipitous finding on CT. Invariably, gallbladder carcinoma is associated with either stones within the gallbladder or a calcified (porcelain) gallbladder. The tumor may present as thickening of the gallbladder wall, as an endoluminal mass, or as an exophytic mass invading the liver.[24-26] Differential diagnosis includes lymphoma, metastatic disease, cholangiocarcinoma (Klatzkin's tumor), hepatoma, and pericholecystic abscess.

Case 6—Pancreatic Carcinoma Presenting as Obstructive Jaundice (Figures 10-10A,B,C,D, 10-11, 10-12)

Pancreatic carcinoma is the most common radiologic entity producing painless (obstructive) jaundice. The algorithm for evaluation includes a sonogram or a CT initially to define the presence of bile duct dilatation and the absence of stones.[27-30] The cross-sectional imaging modality may also be able to locate the obstructing mass. After the location of the obstruction is determined, a percutaneous transhepatic cholangiogram and drainage procedure should be performed in the same session. Alternatively, ERCP with cytologic sampling and slant placement may be performed. Aspiration of bile at the initial session may produce a positive cytologic diagnosis in ≤40% of patients. Percutaneous biopsy can establish the diagnosis in most of the remaining patients. Nonoperative management is usually desirable unless it can be clearly demonstrated that the patient is free of liver metastases and that no other contraindications to surgery (such as encasement of the major visceral vessels) are present. Differential diagnosis includes benign stricture of common bile duct, lymphoma, and metastatic disease to porta hepatis.

Case 7—Peripancreatic Lymphoma Producing Biliary Dilatation and Retroperitoneal Involvement and Encasement of the Left Renal Vein (Figure 10-13A & B)

The recognition on CT of a lymphoma that is producing obstructive jaundice is quite important because radiotherapy and/or chemotherapy of the lesion often produces a dramatic response with lysis of the obstructive jaundice picture.[31,32] The retroperitoneal involvement suggests lymphoma rather than metastatic disease from another primary. Differential diagnosis includes pancreatic carcinoma, metastatic disease, tuberculosis, and actinomycosis.

Case 8—Abdominal Non-Hodgkin's Lymphoma Producing Early Intestinal Obstruction (Figures 10-14, 10-15, 10-16, 10-17, 10-18)

Similarly to the previous case, the recognition on CT scan or a small-bowel series of a lymphoma that can produce intestinal obstruction is important, inasmuch as it can be treated by nonsurgical methods. The histologic diagnosis can be obtained by percutaneous fine-needle biopsy under CT scanning or sonographic guidance. However, occasionally, as in this case, intestinal obstruction due to intussusception caused by small bowel infiltration by lymphoma may occur as the first clinical manifestation of the disease that later spread below and above the diaphragm.[31-34]

Case 9—Primary Testicular Lymphoma Metastatic to the Retroperitoneum and Pelvic Nodes (Figure 10-19A & B)

The diagnosis of lymphoma was made on removal of the left testicle. The extensive metastatic spread mandates systemic chemotherapy. Differential diagnosis includes metastatic carcinoma, primary retroperitoneal lymphoma, tuberculosis, fungal disease, and retroperitoneal fibrosis. Frequently it can be made with the help of CT scanning and lymphangiography.[35-39]

Case 10—Retroperitoneal Liposarcoma (Figure 10-20)

The lesion in the figure is consistent with a primary retroperitoneal tumor, as in this case, or nodal metastases to the para-aortic or psoas region. Hemorrhagic complications from an aortic aneurysm may also simulate this appearance. Percutaneous biopsy is an easy way of defining the presence of a tumor.

Although lipomas can be diagnosed with near histologic certainty on CT if they have a uniformly fatty consistency,[40,41] liposarcomas may have a soft-tissue component that predominates. Any fatty tumor with a significant soft-tissue component must be considered liposarcoma until it is proven otherwise. Differential diagnosis: other primary retroperitoneal sarcomas, carcinomas, carcinosarcomas, retroperitoneal fibrosis, tuberculosis, and fungal disease.

Case 11—Metastatic Adenocarcinoma of the Prostate to the Retroperitoneum (Figure 10-21A & B)

Patients with prostatic carcinoma can present significant enlargement of the para-aortic and mesenteric nodes as illustrated in the figures. Differential diagnosis of this case includes lymphoma, leukemia, retroperitoneal fibrosis, metastatic disease from other primaries, tuberculosis, actinomycosis, and perianeurysmal fibrosis.[42-44]

Case 12—Carcinoma of the Cervix Stage 3B Metastatic to the Left Psoas Muscle Compartment (Figures 10-22, 10-23)

Although primary tumors of the psoas muscle in the retroperitoneum do occur, metastatic disease from gynecologic carcinomas may present as psoas and parapsoas masses.[45-54] There may be involvement of both the psoas compartment as well as periaortic adenopathy in these instances. A percutaneous aspiration biopsy may save the patient an exploratory laparotomy and enable further treatment without surgery.

Case 13—Metastatic Disease to the Left Adrenal Gland with Demonstration of Biopsy Technique in a Patient with Primary Carcinoma of the Lung (Figure 10-24A,B,C,D)

Routine scanning of the adrenal glands should be done in any patient with a primary potentially resectable carcinoma of the lung,[55-60] as there is an incidence of 15–25% of occult metastases to the adrenal that if discovered and biopsied will obviate an unnecessary lobectomy or pneumonectomy.[27]

That was the case in the patient shown in figure 10-24, who had no other evidence of metastatic disease. The right adrenal gland was normal.

Case 14—Adrenal and Retroperitoneal Metastases from Primary Carcinoma of the Bladder (Figure 10-25A & B)

Adrenal metastases from primary transitional cell carcinoma of the bladder have been reported in <10% of cases.[61-64]

Case 15—Necrotic Renal Cell Carcinoma Metastatic to the Left Iliac Bone with Angiographic Embolization of the Lesion Prior to Hip Replacement (Figures 10-26A & B, 10-27, 10-28, 10-29)

The figures illustrate the case of a 46-yr-old man with a large metastatic mass in his left iliac bone from a renal cell carcinoma primary tumor. After successful embolization, the patient went on to have an uneventful total hip replacement and was able to walk. At surgery there was minimal blood loss. Usually, replacement of the hip in the presence of hypervascular metastatic disease is associated with massive blood loss.

Palliative embolization of inoperable metastatic disease has been successfully performed[33] via a catheter inserted in the main arterial supply of a tumor that erodes the mucosa and causes bleeding (G.I. tract malignancies, bronchogenic carcinoma) or may have to be rendered ischemic before surgical resection if very vascular like renal cell carcinoma, hepatocellular carcinoma, or choriocarcinoma. Occasionally, bone neoplasms can be embolized via percutaneous injection of a tissue adhesive.[3,65-67]

Case 16—Chloromas of the Kidneys Secondary to Chronic Myelogenous Leukemic Invasion (Figure 10-30A & B)

Extracranial chloroma, although rare, can be well demonstrated by CT and response to therapy monitored by serial scans.[68-72] Differential diagnosis includes lymphoma, multiple abscesses, bilateral acute pyelonephritis, metastatic disease, tuberculosis.

Case 17—Carcinoma of the Colon in a Patient with Multiple G.I. Polyps (Familial Polyposis) (Figures 10-31, 10-32)

CT of malignant colonic lesions preoperatively may be helpful in defining the size of the mass, pericolonic fat invasion, and spread to nodes or the liver.[73-76] It is also useful in assessing postoperative recurrence.

Case 18—Carcinoma of the Stomach, Primary in the Antrum with a Large Node in the Gastrohepatic Ligament (Figures 10–33 and 10-34)

CT in gastric neoplasms may provide information regarding metastases to the gastrohepatic ligament and other extragastric sites including the liver.[77-79] The radiographic presentation of a gastric carcinoma has several distinguishing features such as its projection as a crater protruding inside the gastric lumen with irregular folds, the presence of filling defects, and (frequently) abnormalities of the mucosa surrounding the ulcer. These are better seen with the double contrast method with supplementary carbon dioxide or instilled air.

Case 19—Carcinoma of the Esophagus (Figure 10-35A & B)

Carcinoma of the esophagus is a highly lethal disease to which CT has contributed only minimally to this point. In several series, however, it has been reported that CT is able to define inoperability prior to surgery based on loss of the fat plane between the esophagus and aorta prior to surgery. In addition, the presence of mediastinal metastases and tracheoesophageal fistula can be demonstrated. Also, retrocrural and liver metastases may be defined on CT, thereby eliminating the possibility of curative resection.[80-84]

Case 20—Mediastinal Mass (Figure 10-36A & B)

Heavy smoker, 47, with complaint of periodic chest pain. Chest radiographs revealed mediastinal widening. Differential diagnosis includes bronchogenic carcinoma of mediastinal origin, lymphoma, malignant thymoma, and teratoma. A mediastinal thyroid mass is not included because the lesion was not contiguous with the thyroid gland. Biopsy of the mass revealed squamous cell carcinoma. Because of its axial plane of imaging and excellent contrast resolution, CT is the diagnostic study of choice in evaluating a widened mediastinum. CT examination determines if a mass is present, and if so, which mediastinal compartment it is in. It can also determine if a mass is cystic, vascular, or calcified.

Case 21—Bronchogenic Carcinoma (Figures 10-37, 10-38)

Differential diagnosis includes bronchogenic carcinoma, lymphoma, and (rarely) metastatic carcinoma and primary tuberculosis. Biopsy revealed small-cell carcinoma of the lung. CT clearly demonstrates which mediastinal nodal groups are involved with adenopathy. This determines the surgical indication for biopsy and possible radical surgery. Vascular obstruction and tracheal compression by tumor are also well demonstrated by cross-sectional imaging. CT also serves as the most sensitive test to determine tumor response following chemotherapy.

Case 22—Recurrent Bronchogenic Carcinoma After Surgery (Figures 10-39, 10-40)

In the postlobectomy or pneumonectomy patient, early recurrence of disease is difficult to detect. The ability of CT to distinguish between all the mediastinal structures makes it ideal for detecting a new or recurrent mass lesion.

Case 23—Pleural Mass (Figure 10-41)

Differential diagnosis includes lymphoma, localized mesothelioma, pleural metastases, and pleural scar from previous infection or trauma. Biopsy revealed histiocytic lymphoma. Pleural disease and its extent is best demonstrated by CT. CT clearly distinguishes between pleural masses and pleural effusions.[85-87]

Case 24—Soft-Tissue Mass of the Chest Wall (Figure 10-42)

A chest wall mass often has a clinically undetectable intrathoracic component. CT clearly outlines the extent of a chest wall mass and helps determine if the adjacent bone is destroyed.[90]

Case 25—Parosteal Chondrosarcoma (Figures 10-43, 10-44)

Differential diagnosis includes parosteal osteogenic sarcoma, parosteal chrondroma, parosteal chondrosarcoma, and parosteal hematoma from previous trauma. The type of calcification, however, is typical of a cartilaginous matrix. In this case, the pathologic diagnosis was parosteal chondrosarcoma. A plain radiograph of a bone tumor is the most valuable radiographic examination. CT is helpful in evaluating the exact location and extent of tumor[91,92] and sometimes in distinguishing benign from malignant disease.[93]

Case 26—Chondrosarcoma (Figure 10-45A & B)

Differential diagnosis includes metastatic carcinoma, and other rare malignancies of bone, such as hemangiosarcoma. In bony, anatomically complex areas such as the face and the pelvis, CT is helpful in detecting tumor and in delineating its extent.[94] Postoperatively, CT scanning is the radiographic method of choice for detection of recurrent disease.

Case 27—Ewing's Sarcoma (Figures 10-46, 10-47)

Girl, 10, with Ewing's sarcoma of the right femur. The characteristic features of these bone neoplasms of childhood are the onionskin pattern of periosteal new bone formation and the destruction of the bone cortex.

Case 28—Dermatofibrosarcoma (Figures 10-48A,B,C,D)

Differential diagnosis includes benign and malignant skin tumors and localized inflammatory lesions of the skin. CT often determines the extent of a soft-tissue mass of the extremities and its margination and possible involvement of adjacent structures.[95] A lipoma has a distinct, pathognomonic appearance on CT. However, masses of soft-tissue density cannot be histologically distinguished by CT.

Case 29—Metastasis in Soft Tissues (Figures 10-49, 10-50)

CT scanning is especially valuable in the diagnosis of soft-tissue masses and in resolving the differential diagnosis of leg swelling.

Case 30—Bone Metastasis (Figures 10-51A,B,C,D)

Bone metastases can be lytic, such as the one represented on the CT scan cuts of this case, or they can be blastic. Only a few primary tumors can present blastic lesions in the bones; they include adenocarcinoma of the prostate, ductal infiltrating carcinoma of the breast, folliculer or papillary carcinoma of the thyroid, and (occasionally) Hodgkin's lymphoma. With the exception of prostatic carcinoma, all of these tumors can also present metastatic lytic lesions in the bones. Differential diagnosis of a lytic expansile lesion of the bone includes bone metastasis from bladder, prostate, thyroid, breast, kidney, multiple myeloma, and a primary bone tumor. Pathologic diagnosis in this case was metastatic transitional cell carcinoma of the bladder.

Case 31—Histiocytosis X (Figure 10-52)

Girl, 2, with eosinophilic granuloma of bone. The most characteristic radiographic presentation of this disease is that of bones with multiple lytic lesions forming a "geographic pattern."

Case 32—Neuroblastoma (Figures 10-53, 10-54)

Neuroblastoma is a highly malignant tumor presenting in infants and young children with para-aortic and suprarenal masses (figure 10-53) and with a high incidence of marrow and bone metastases (figure 10-54).

Case 33—Wilms' Tumor (Figures 10-55, 10-56)

A poorly differentiated malignant neoplasm of the kidney encountered only in children.

Sequence 34—Metastatic Tumors of the Brain, Solitary (Figure 10-57A,B,C,D)

Metastases in the brain are single in about 30% of cases; they can present as a solid (figure 10-57B) or ring-enhancing (figure 10-57D) lesion surrounded by massive edema (figure 10-57A) identical with the presentation of primary astrocytoma or glioblastoma multiforma, or without perilesional edema (figure 10-57B). They are occasionally inherently hyperdense (figure 10-57C) but usually not. They usually show vivid enhancement (figure 10-57B) but occasionally little (figure 10-57D) or none after the administration of contrast material. The histology of a metastasis is not generally predictable from its CT appearance.

Sequence 35—Multiple Lesions of the Brain (Figure 10-58A,B,C,D)

Brain metastases are frequently multiple at the time of diagnosis (in 60–70% of cases). However, not all multiple brain lesions represent metastatic neoplasms; figure 10-58D demonstrates a case of primary glioblastoma multiforme with multiple ring lesions in 1 hemisphere at the time of diagnosis. Besides this, particularly in immunosuppressed patients, it must also be remembered that primary CNS lymphoma, toxoplasmosis, and other inflammatory lesions may present with multiple brain masses.

On the other side, glioblastoma multiforme (astrocytoma IV) is rarely multicentric at the time of diagnosis (in only 5–17% of cases).

Sequence 36—Ring Lesions of the Brain (Figure 10-59A,B,C,D)

A ring-enhancing nodule with surrounding edema is the most characteristic appearance of brain metastasis and a frequent appearance of primary astrocytoma; however, this radiographic appearance is seen as well in many other disorders: toxoplasmosis, fungal abscesses and other primary brain tumors, such as lymphomas, hemangioblastomas, and (occasionally) meningiomas.

Sequence 37—Solid Nodules of the Brain (Figure 10-60A,B,C,D)

A solid enhancing nodule in the brain is a common appearance of metastatic disease. CT scans of the head show nodular lesions of various size, but not all solid nodules are metastatic. Occasionally, a meningioma or lymphoma can present as solid nodules, and cerebral hemorrhages can also have a nodular presentation on CT scan; however, primary CNS hemorrhages are inherently hyperdense but do not enhance. Normal blood vessels as well as arterial and venous aneurysms are inherently hyperdense and do enhance.

Other disorders that can present as solid nodules include tuberculosis and histoplasmosis.

Sequence 38—Base of Skull Lesions (Figure 10-61A,B,C,D,E)

Metastases to the base of the skull can originate in any primary tumor, but are more frequently seen in patients with multiple myeloma, lymphomas, prostatic carcinoma, and squamous cell carcinoma of the head and neck. Local invasion by nasopharyngeal or sinus carcinoma is probably the most common cause of destruction of the skull base. Very aggressive sinus infections (e.g., mucomycosis) may also produce extensive basal destruction.

Sequence 39—Malignant Tumors of the Spine Detected by Myelography (Figure 10-62A,B,C)

Placement of iodinated contrast into the subarchnoid space enables the clinician to locate tumors in the following compartments: extradural, intradural-extramedullary, and intramedullary. The location helps determine the differential diagnosis.

Sequence 40—Malignant Tumors of the Spine Detected by CT Scan and MRI (Figure 10-63A & B)

CT scan of the spine is accurate in defining the contour of a mass but often cannot show the difference between normal and abnormal soft tissue within the canal. MRI, still in its early developmental phase, is likely the most precise imaging test for the detection of malignant tumors of the spine. It can detect the infiltration of the vertebral bone marrow not recognized by any of the other radiologic tests. Because of differences in signal may be able to differentiate malignant from benign tumors.

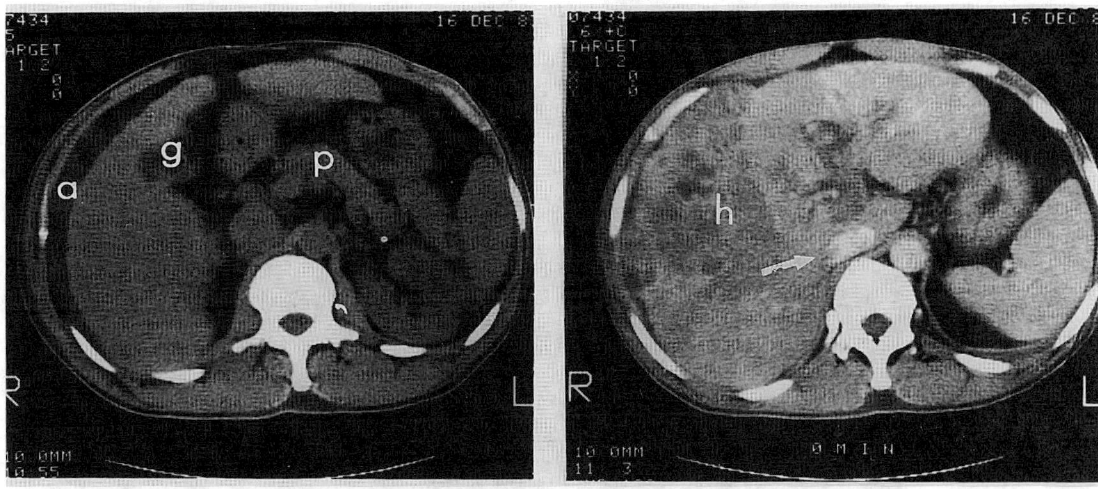

Figure 10-1A (left) & B (right). Axial sections mixed through the liver (A—pre- and
  B— postcontrast). Attenuation areas (h) are seen throughout the liver,
  predominantly in the right lobe; there is also evidence of ascites (a).
  Note extrinsic mass effect on the lateral aspect of the inferior vena cava
  (arrow) (g = gallbladder, p = pancreas).
Figure 10-2. Selective hepatic arteriogram demonstrates diffuse neovascularity
  throughout the liver consistent with mulifocal hepatoma.

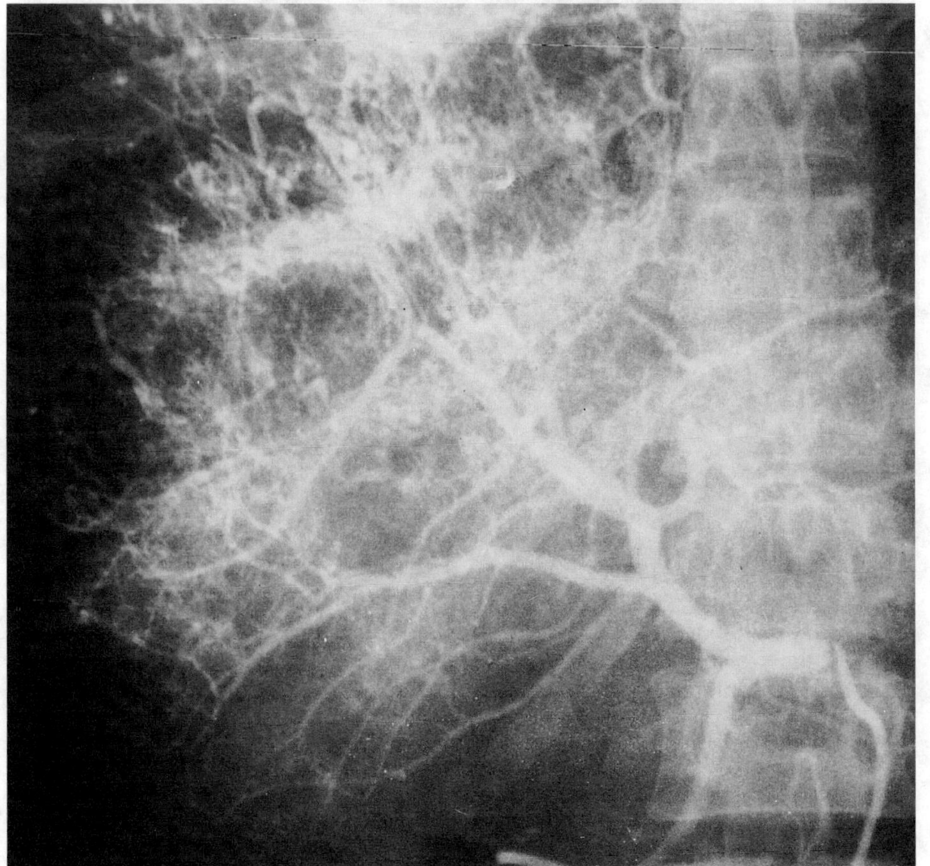

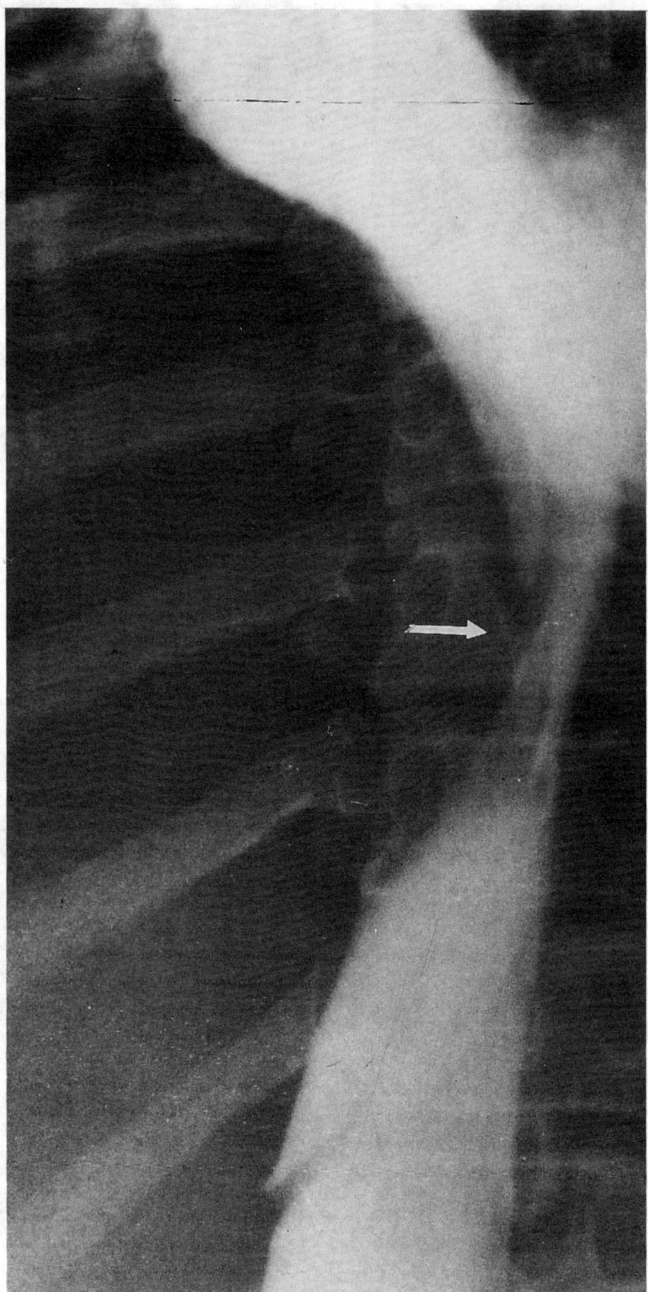

Figure 10-3. Inferior vena cavagram reveals extrinsic pressure corresponding to the previously noted CT defect (arrow). There is no intrinsic involvement of the inferior vena cava.

Figure 10-4. Representative section from an enhanced CT scan through the liver shows multiple low attenuation lesions throughout the liver with a hypo-dense center in the largest lesion indicating necrosis (N). This is typical of metastatic disease to the liver from any hypovascular primary (s = stomach; p = portal vein; a = aorta; i = inferior vena cava; v = vertebra; sp = spleen; k = kidney).

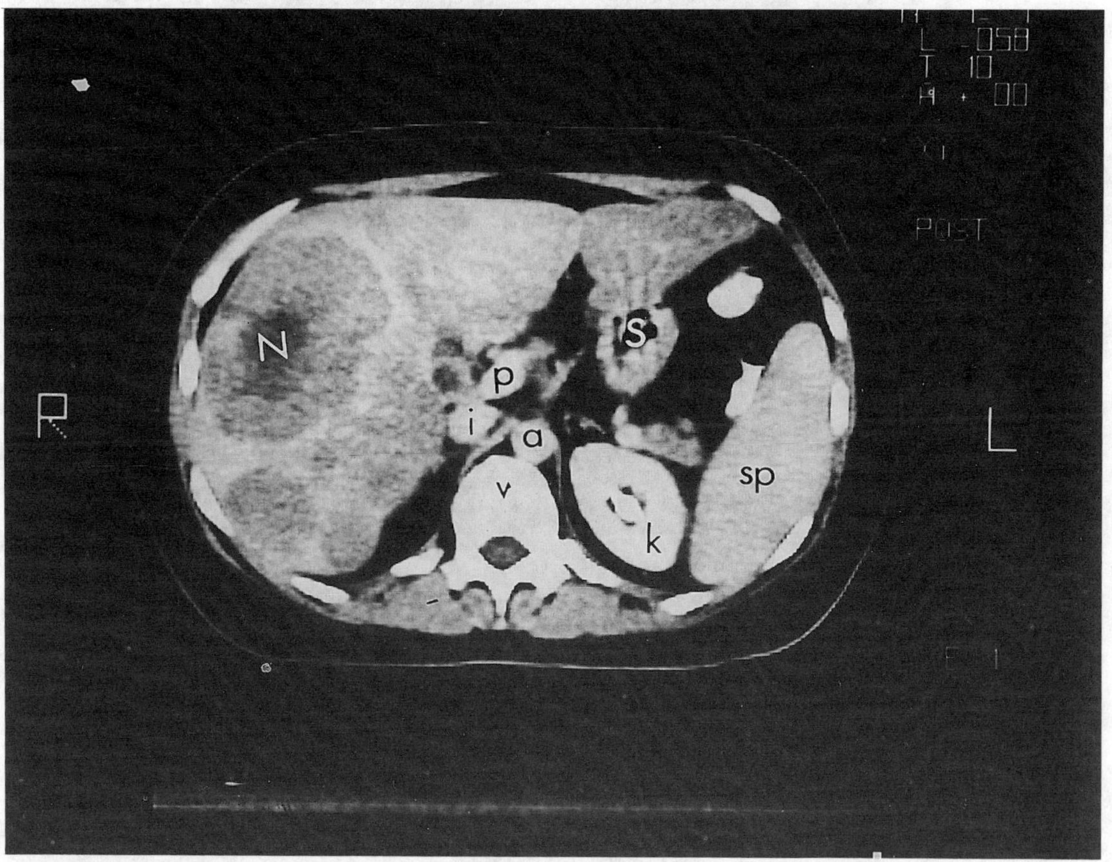

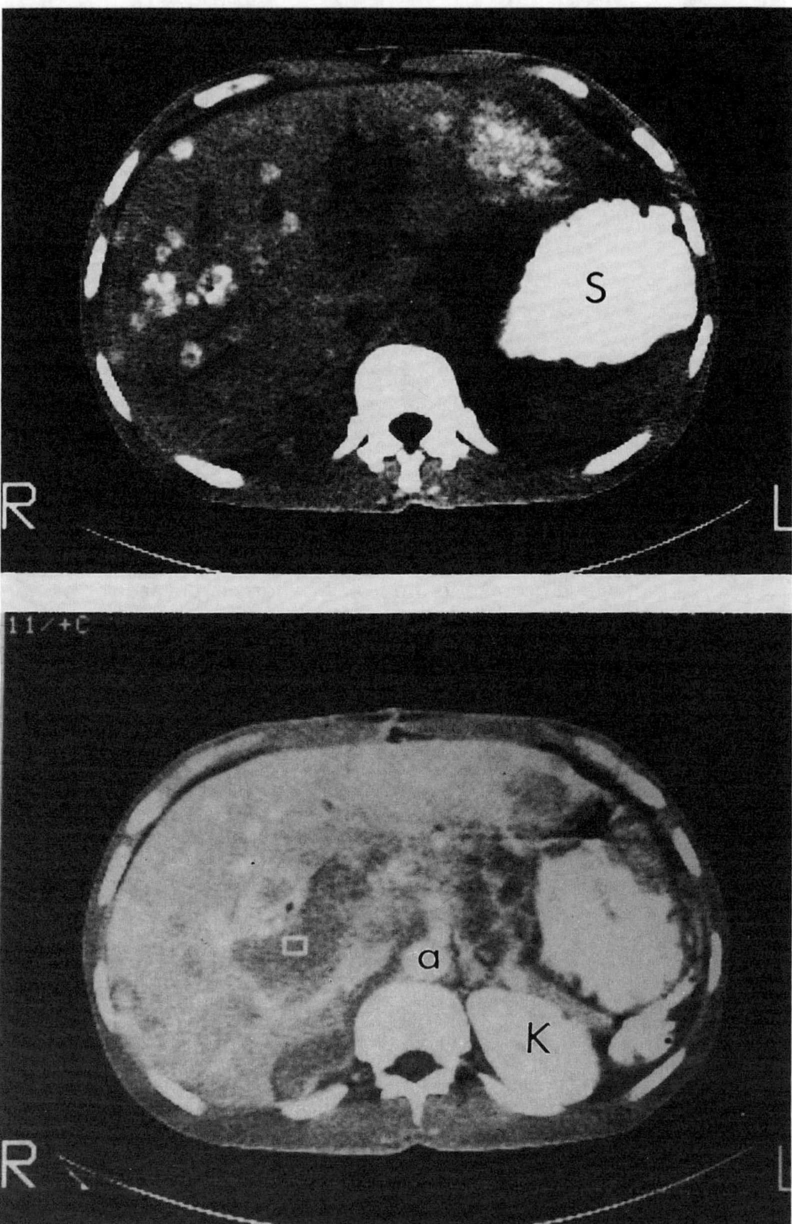

Figure 10-5. A nonenhanced CT of the liver in the top picture demonstrates multiple calcified metastatic lesions throughout the liver consistent with metastatic mucinous adenocarcinoma (s = stomach). After enhancement with I.V. contrast material, the enlarged region of the portal vein is seen on the bottom picture as a hypodense area in relation to the rest of the liver (9) indicating tumor thrombus within the portal vein (box). Note that the calcified metastases are seen much less well now as the rest of the liver parenchyma has enhanced to nearly the level of the calcified metastases (k = kidney; a = enhanced aorta).

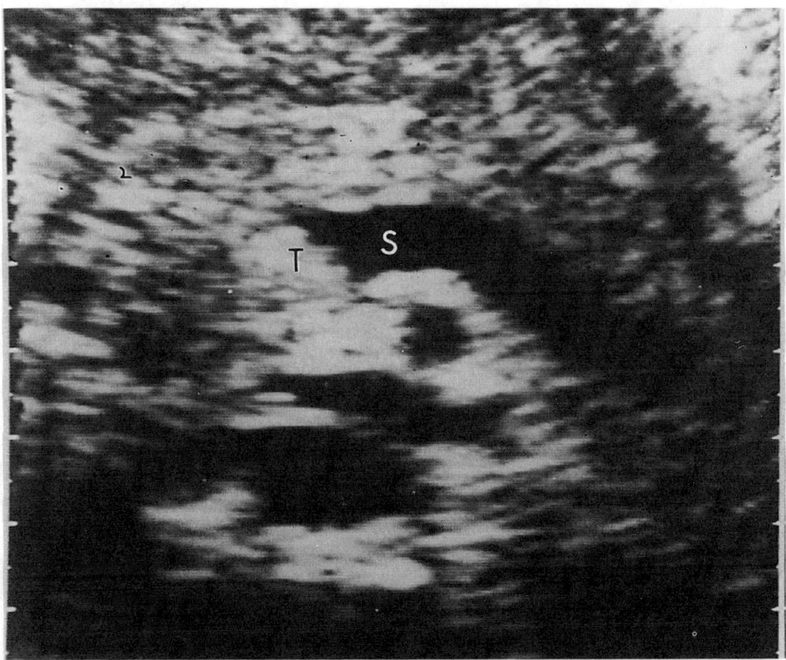

Figure 10-6. Sonography at the level of the junction of the splenic veins with the superior mesenteric vein shows a tumor thrombus (T) indenting the proximal splenic vein.

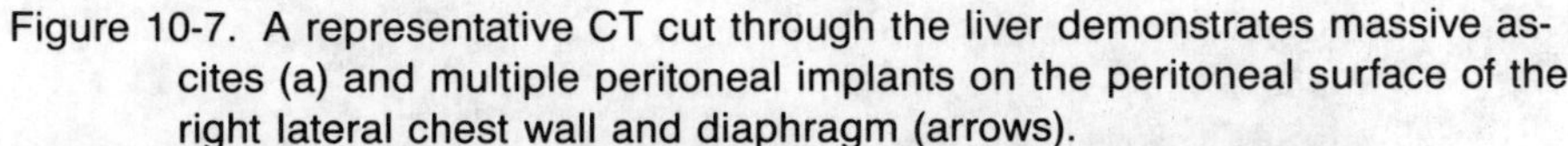

Figure 10-7. A representative CT cut through the liver demonstrates massive ascites (a) and multiple peritoneal implants on the peritoneal surface of the right lateral chest wall and diaphragm (arrows).

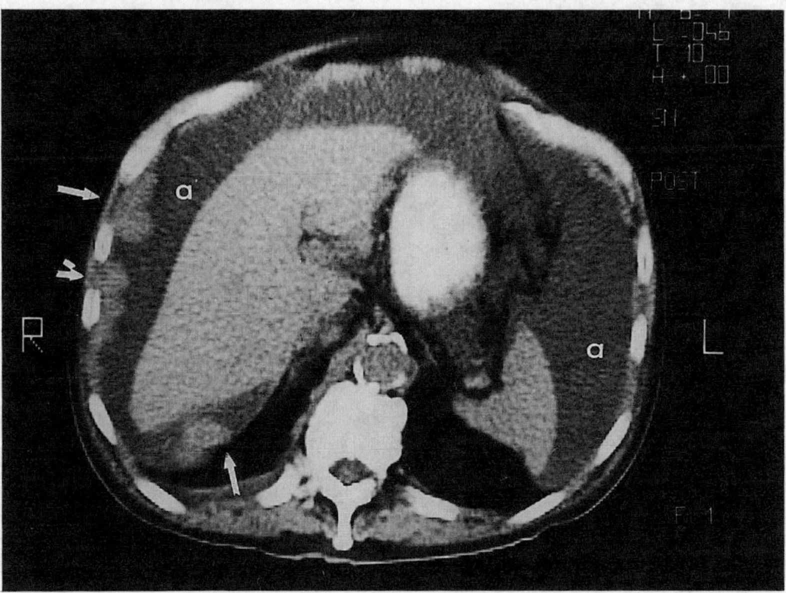

Figure 10-8. A sonographic sector scan of the same area again demonstrates the ascites (a) with the chest wall peritoneal implant (arrow).

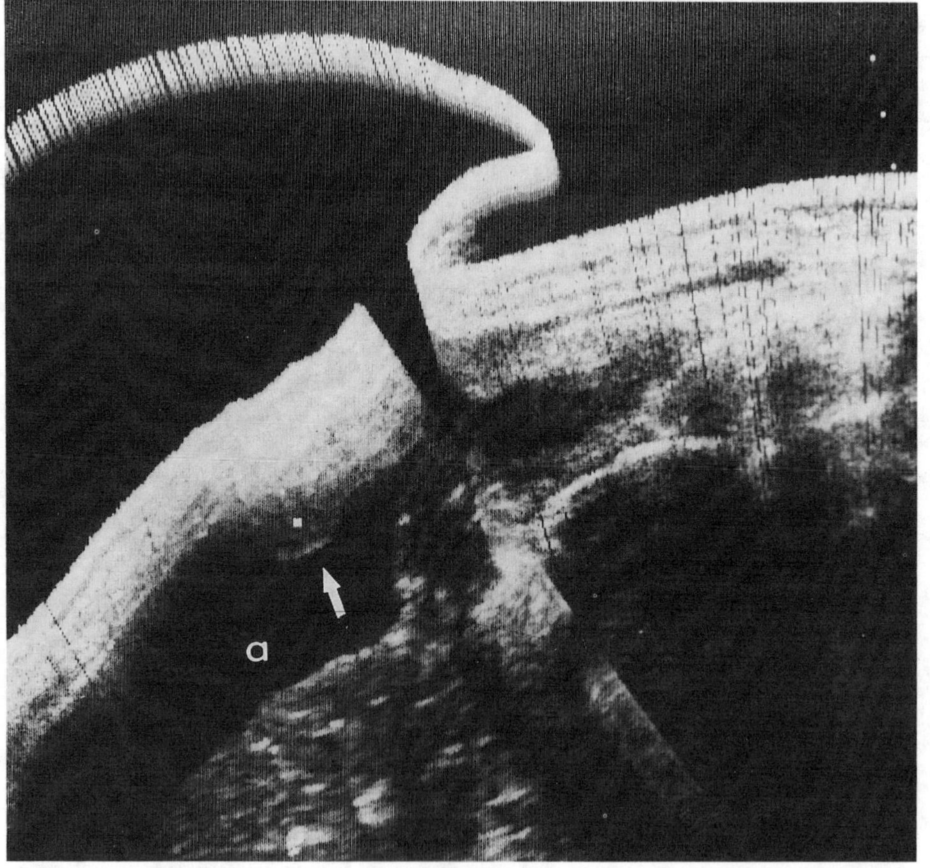

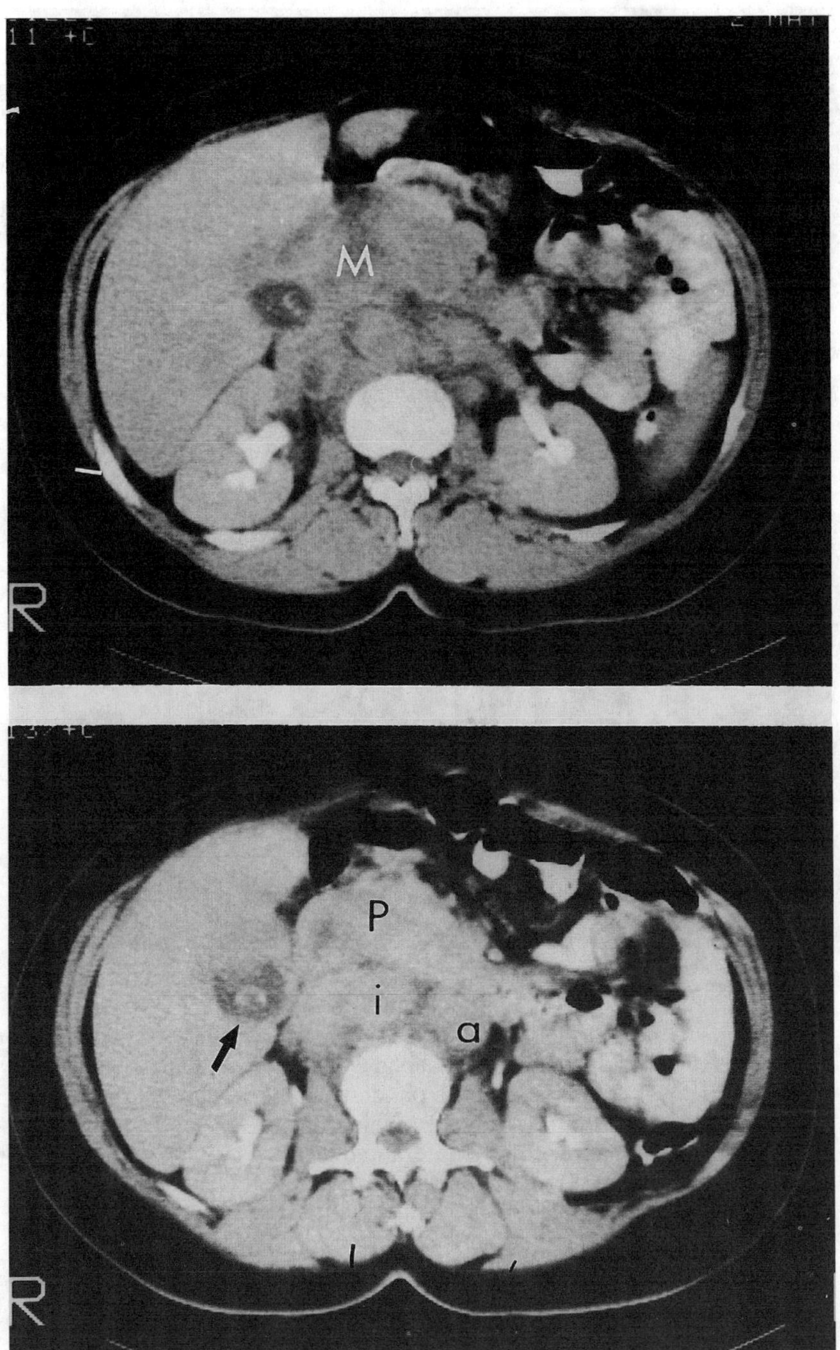

Figure 10-9. Two sections through the level of the gallbladder demonstrate a gall-
stone within the gallbladder (arrow in bottom view) and a large, poorly
defined low attenuation mass (M) that invades the region of the porta
hepatis and pancreatic head (p). Even though the porta hepatis nodes
are involved by contiguous spread of this tumor, there is no biliary dilatation. Note poor definition of aorta (a) and inferior vena cava (a) due to
retroperitoneal invasion.

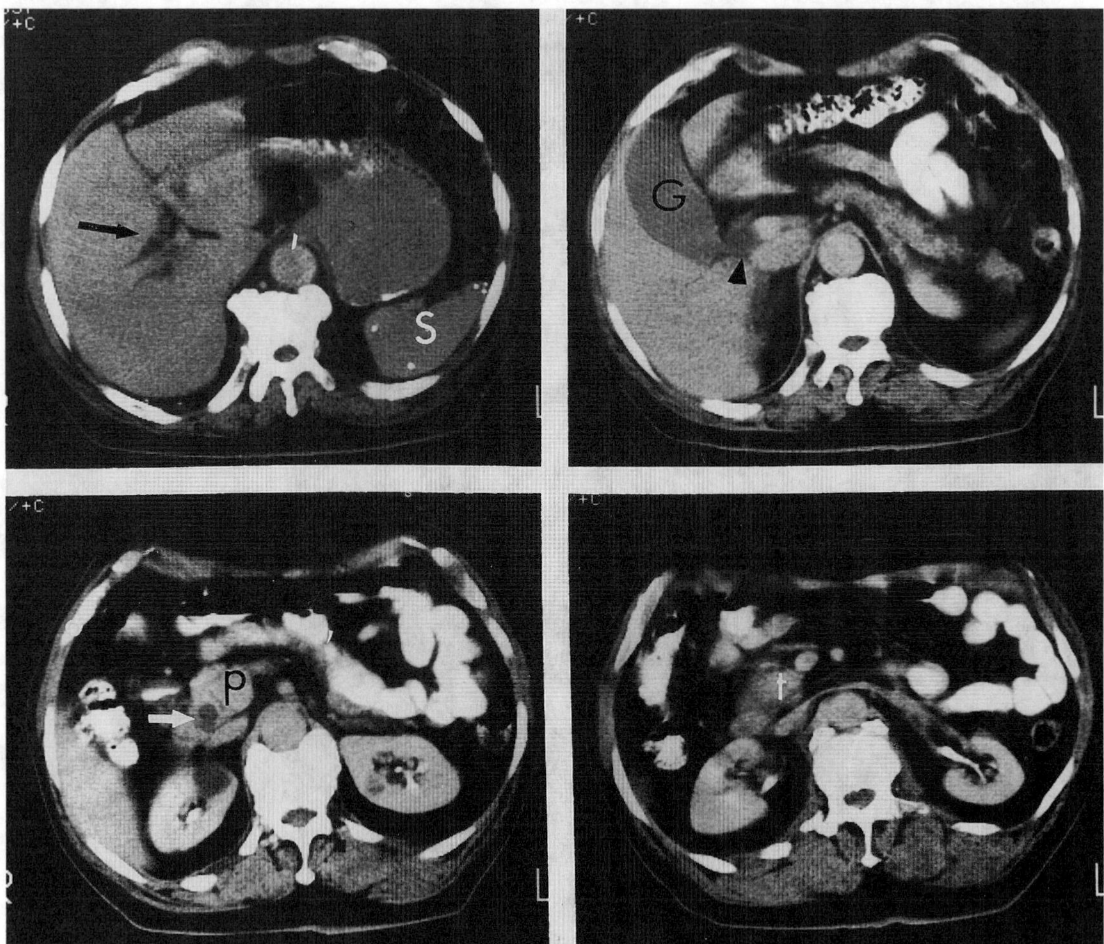

Figure 10-10A,B,C,D. Enhanced CT sections through the level of the porta hepatis and gallbladder (A&B, top left & right) reveal dilated intrahepatic bile ducts (arrow) and a dilated gallbladder (G) as well as a dilated common bile duct (arrowhead). Note calcifications within the spleen (S). Sections through the level of the head of the pancreas (C, lower left) shows the dilated common duct (arrow) located within the posterolateral aspect of a rounded prominent-appearing head of the pancreas (p). One centimeter lower (D, lower right), the bile duct is no longer seen, indicating that the tumor (t) is present at this level. By stacking these slices together, one can obtain a "CT cholangiogram."

Figure 10-11. A percutaneous transhepatic cholangiogram demonstrates the "rat tail" ending of the common bile duct (arrow) consistent with a carcinoma encasing it.

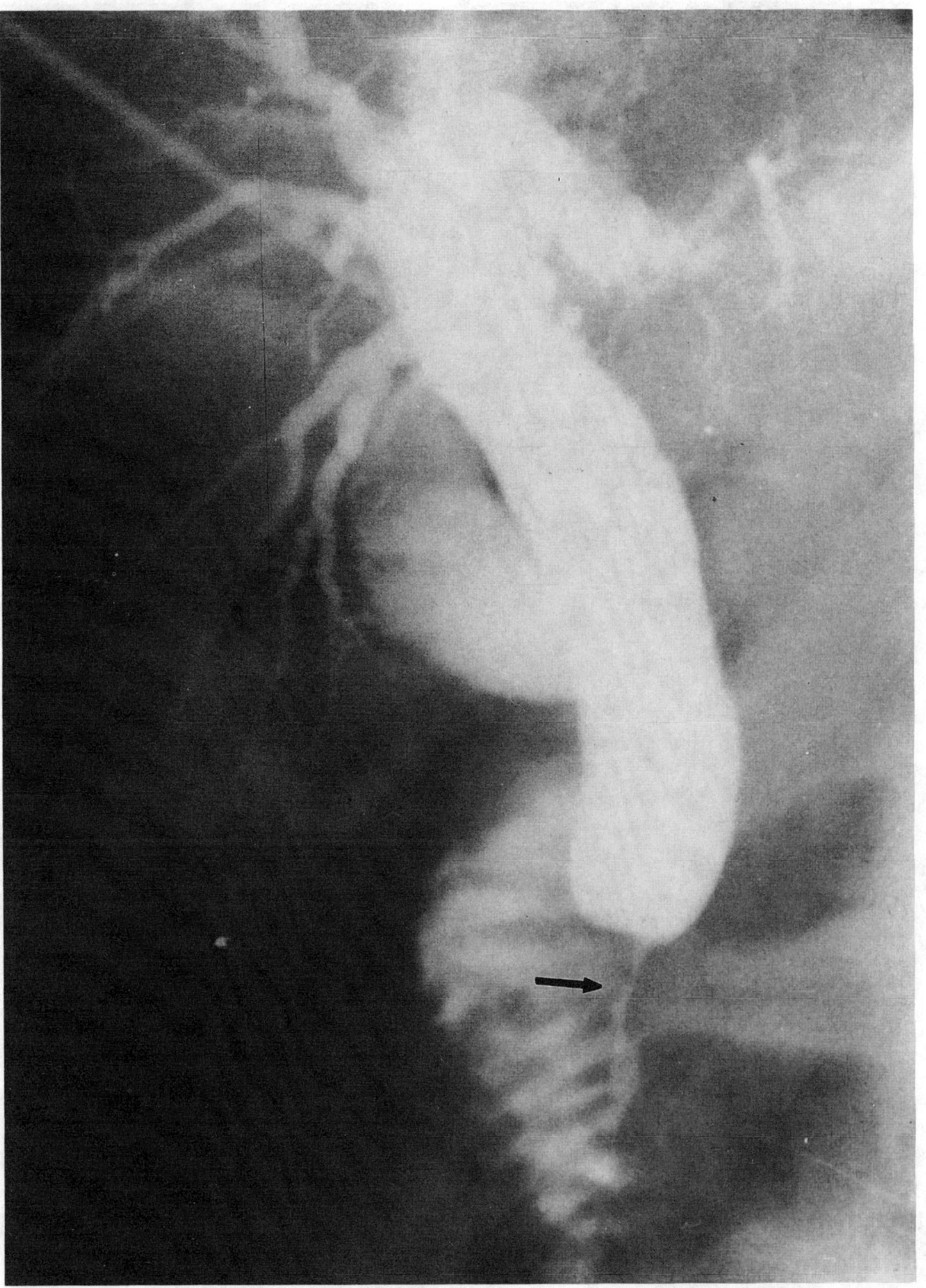

Figure 10-12. An internal/external drainage tube has been placed through the pancreatic tumor into the duodenum, with side holes above and below the lesion to provide drainage.

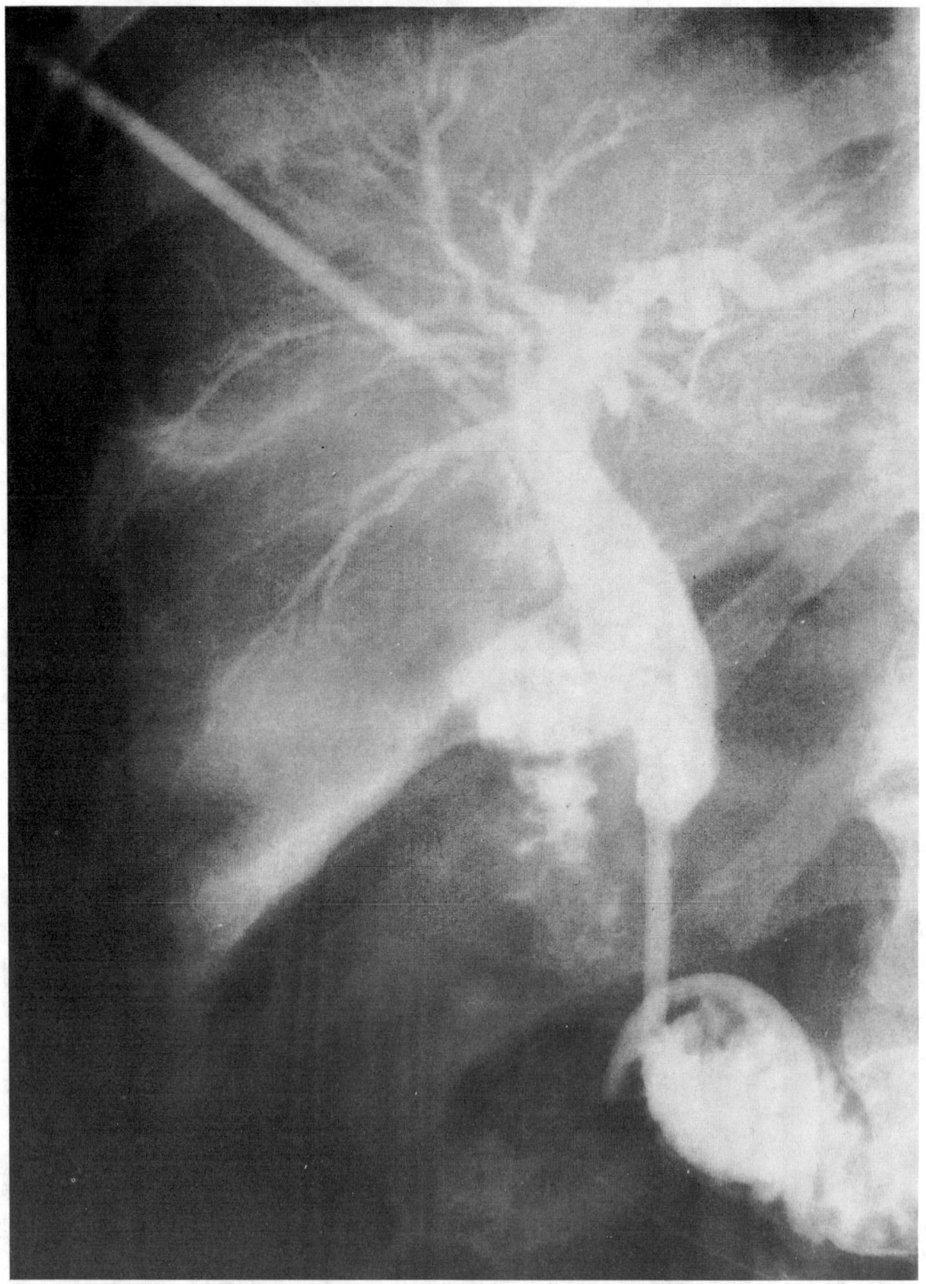

Figure 10-13. A section at the level of the crossing of the left renal vein anterior to the aorta (top photo) demonstrates the mass (M) encasing the renal vein (arrow) while invading the retroperitoneum and displacing the inferior vena cava (i) laterally. A CT scan through the level of the porta hepatis (bottom photo) demonstrates a large hypodense mass (m) involving the retroperitoneum and encroachment upon the superior aspect of the inferior vena cava (i) and bowing the portal vein (p) upward and producing massive dilatation of the biliary tree (b).

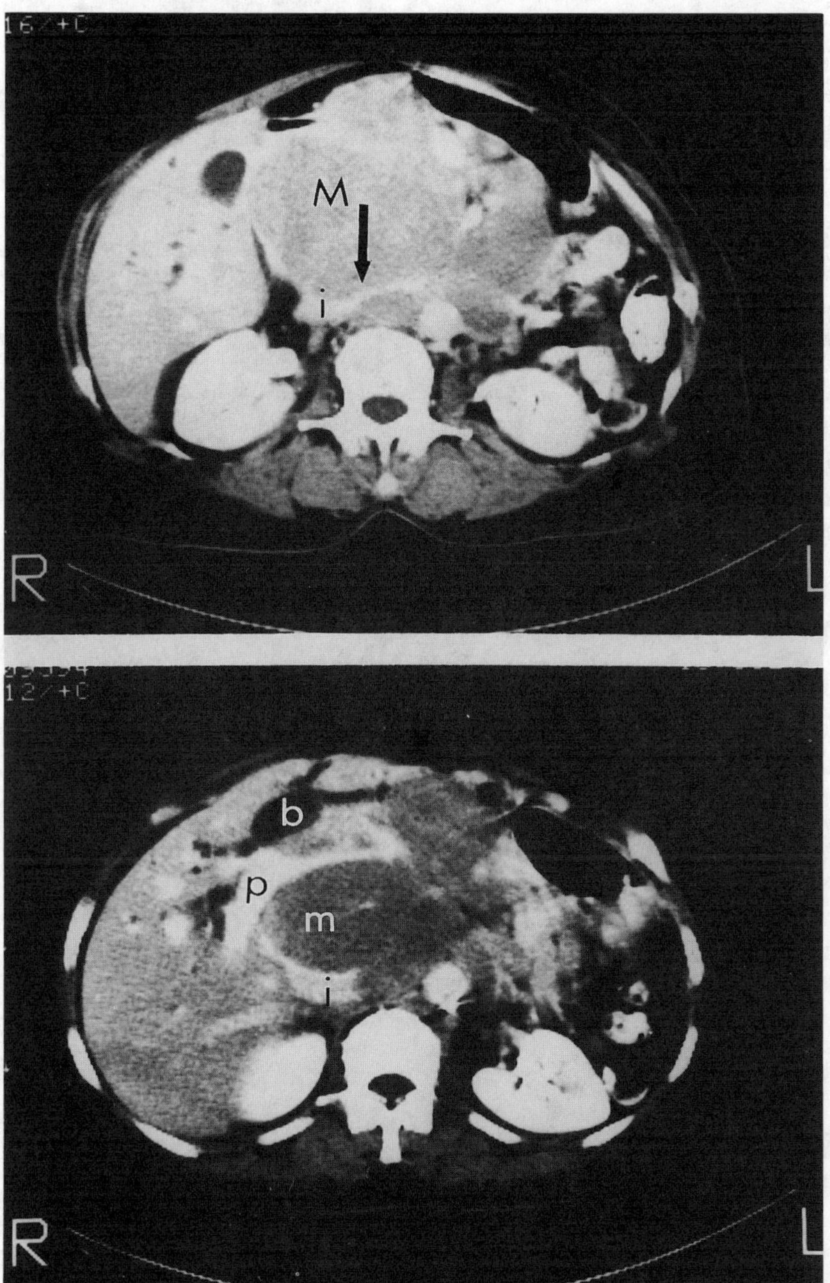

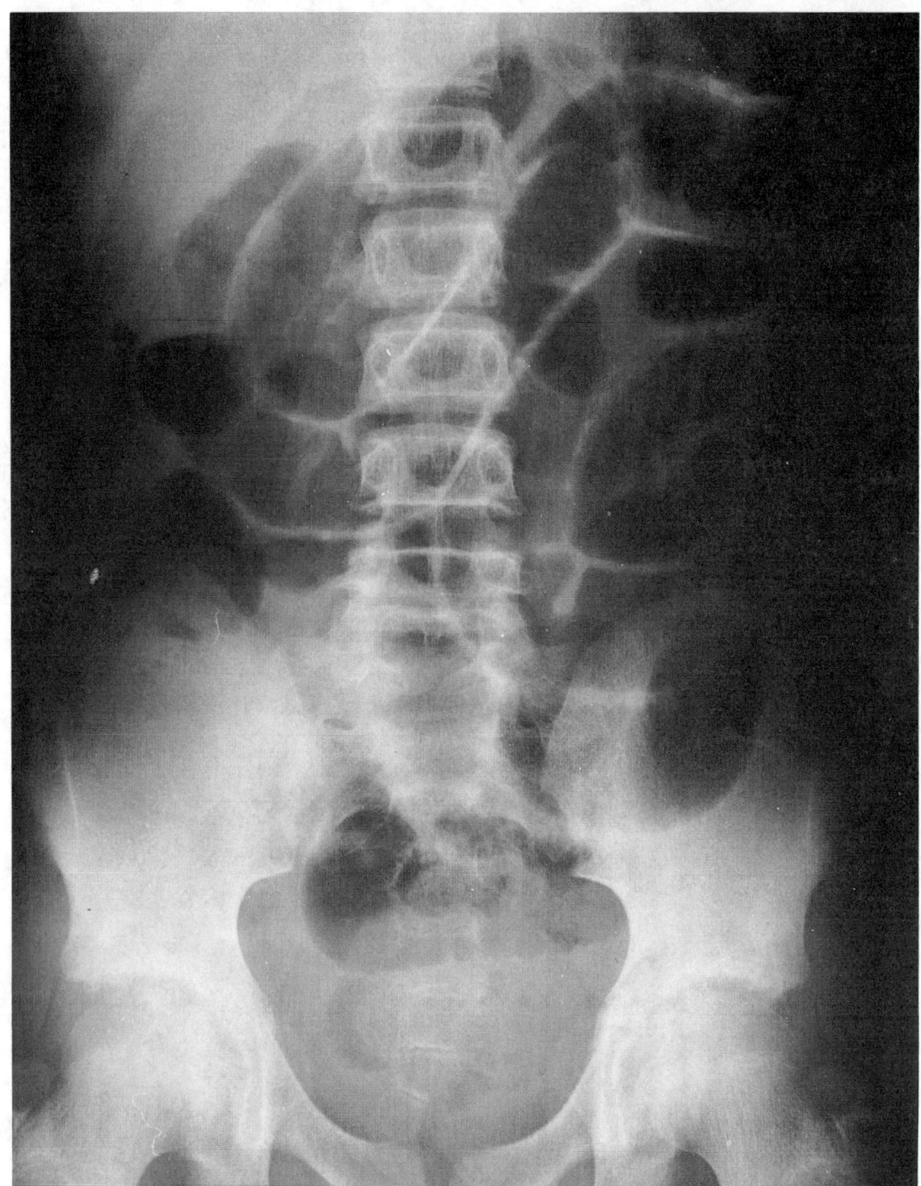

Figure 10-14. Initial examination shows typical small bowel obstruction. Exploratory laparotomy revealed ilio-colic intussusception. No tumor was identified. Subsequently, patient developed large abdominal and mediastinal masses.

Figure 10-15. Small bowel series shows large abdominal mass displacing small
bowel loops.

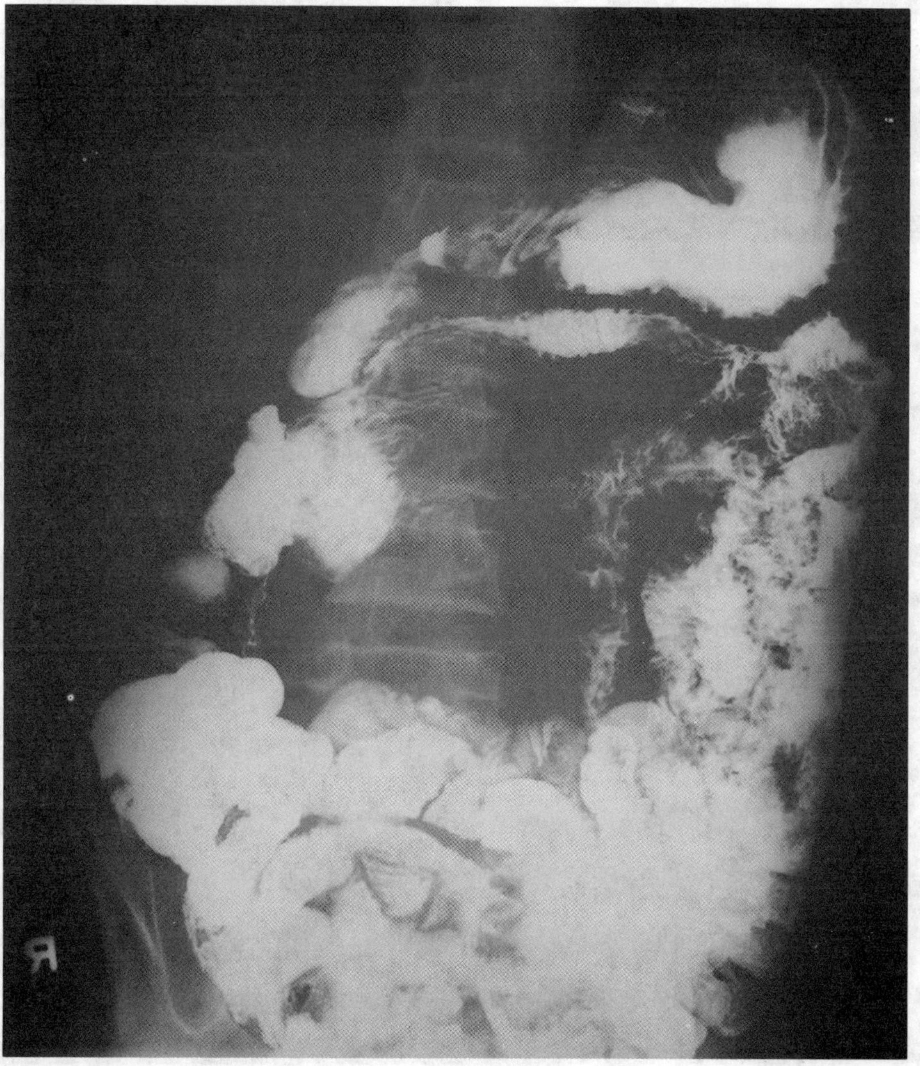

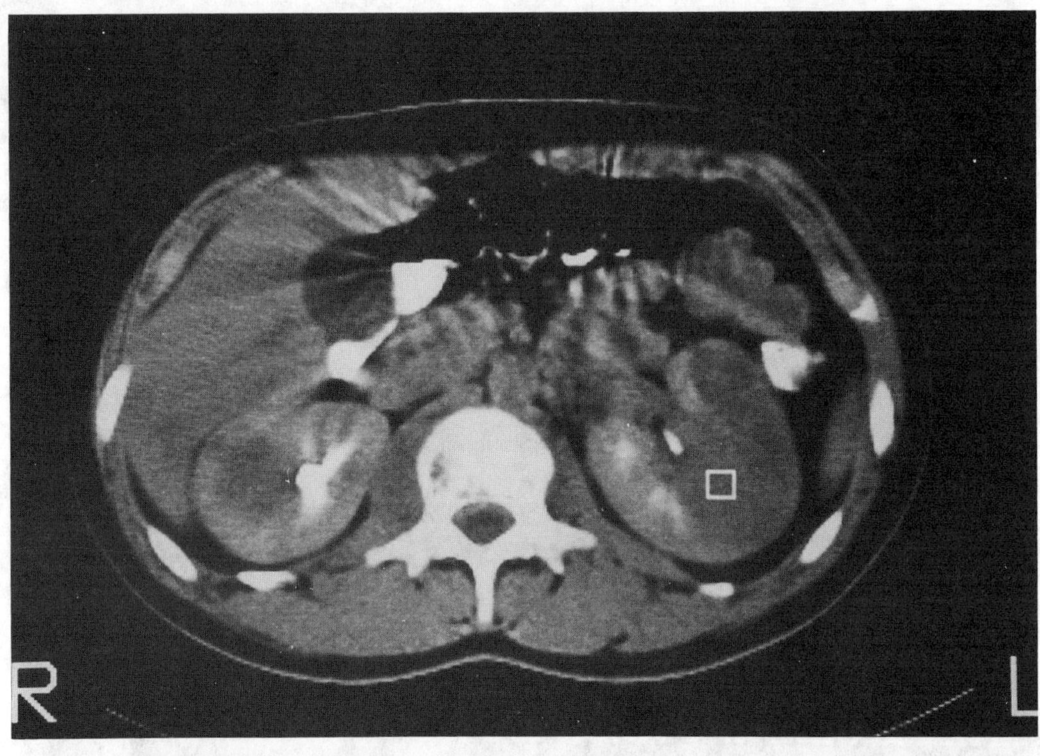

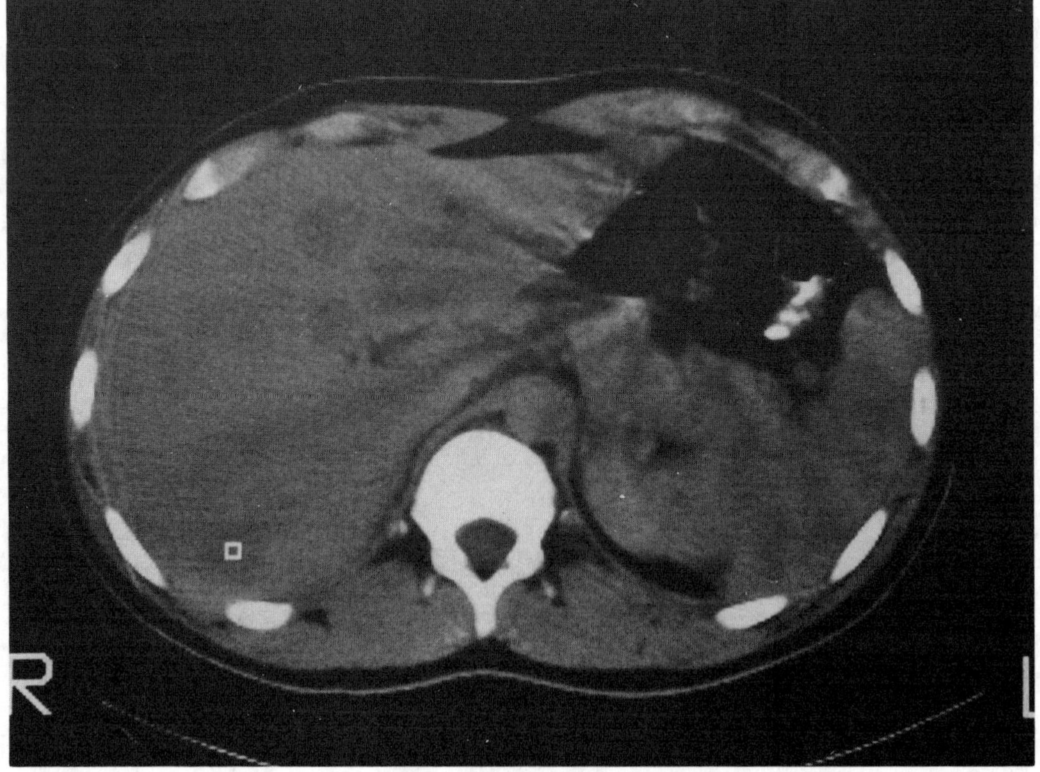

OPPOSITE PAGE, TOP

Figure 10-16. Enhanced CT scan through kidney showing low attenuation areas in both kidneys and paraspinal retroperitoneal adenopathy.

OPPOSITE PAGE, BOTTOM

Figure 10-17. Enhanced CT through liver showing numerous low attenuation areas within liver parenchyma. Note enlarged spleen.

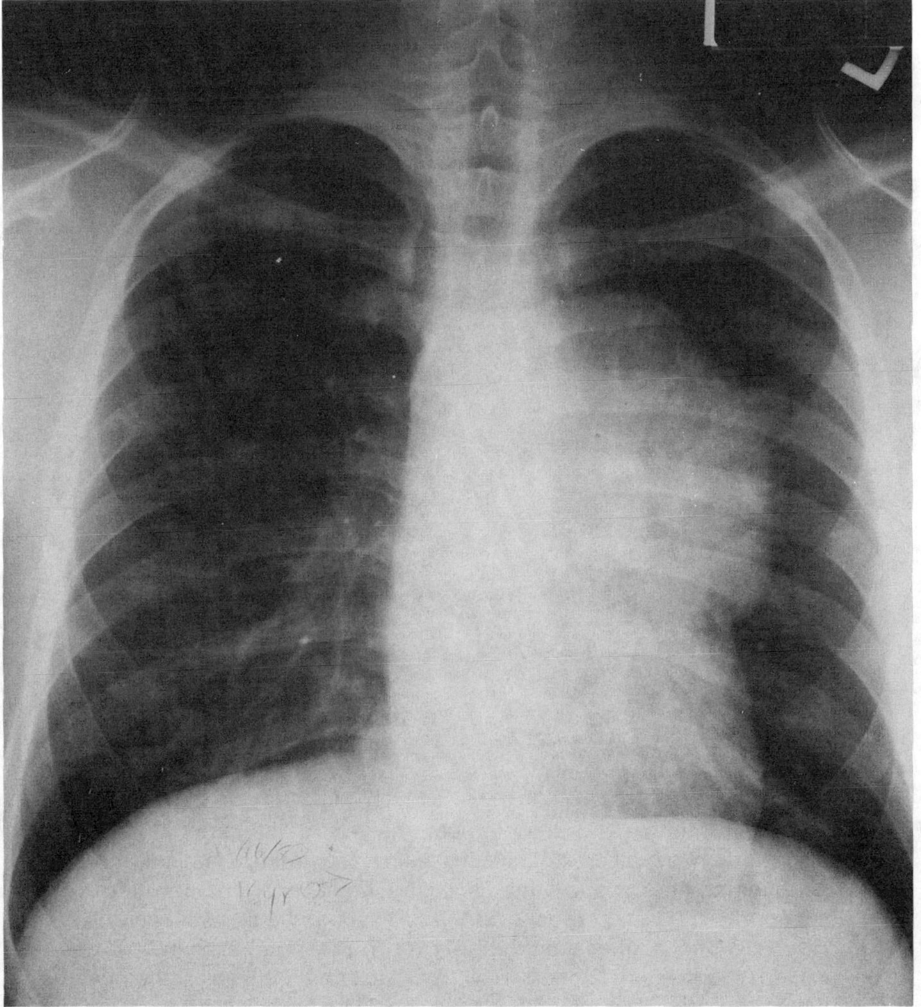

Figure 10-18. Posteroanterior view of the chest showing lobulated anterior mediastinal mass.

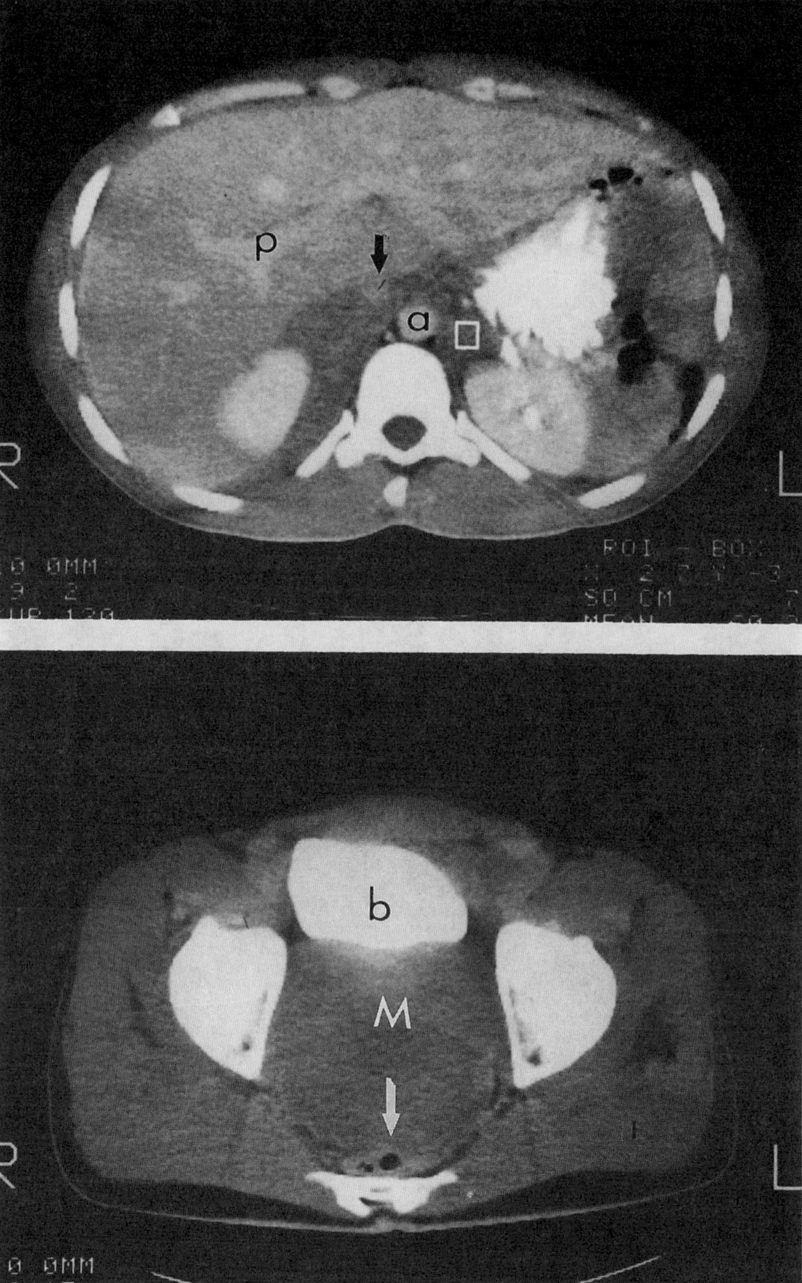

Figure 10-19. Postenhanced CT scan through the level of the upper kidneys (top picture) demonstrates extensive low attenuation retroperitoneal masses surrounding the aorta (a) and displacing the inferior vena cava (arrow) superiorly. The cursor (box) over the left para-aortic mass measures 60 Hounsfield units, indicating that this is soft tissue rather than fluid density. (p = portal vein). Bottom view: A CT scan at the level of the acetabulum in the pelvis demonstrates a huge pelvic soft-tissue mass (M) displacing the rectum posteriorly (arrow) and the bladder (b) anteriorly.

Figure 10-20. A single frame from an enhanced CT scan at the level of the renal hilar structures demonstrates a large variegated attenuation mass (M) displacing the left kidney (K) markedly anteriorly and invading and enlarging the left psoas muscle (P) (compare with right psoas).

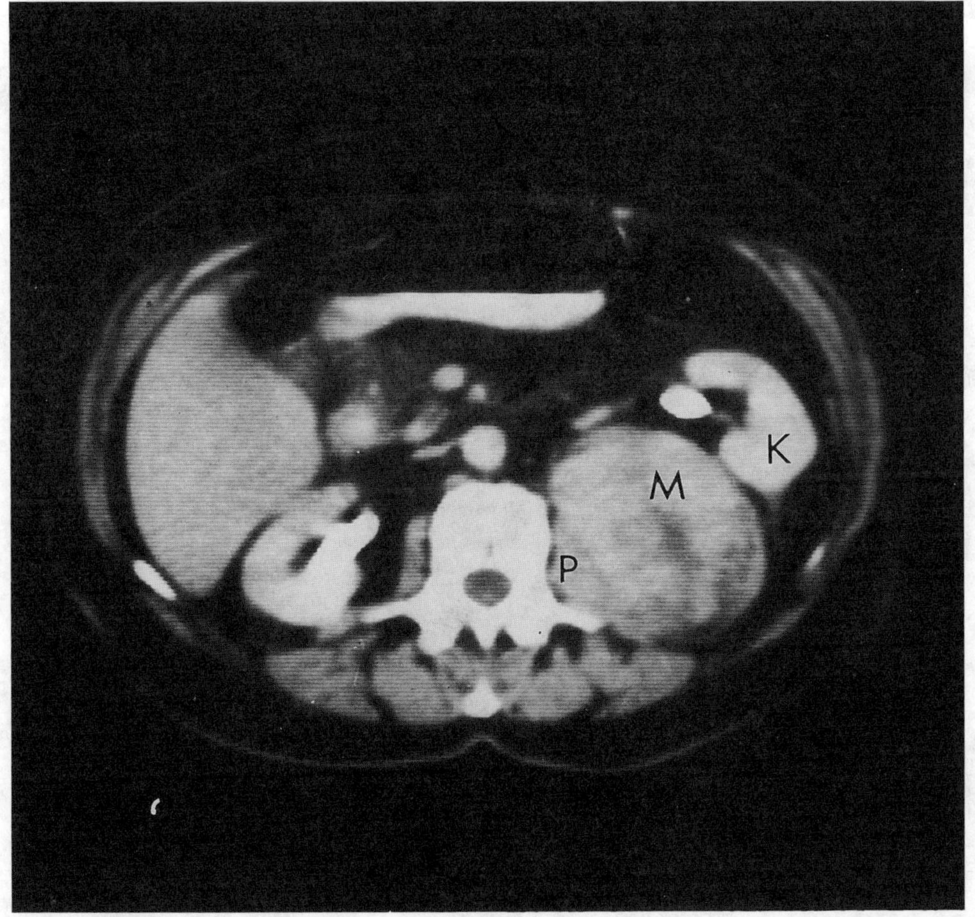

Figure 10-21. Postenhanced CT scan of the abdomen below the level of the kidneys (top view) demonstrates a huge mass of nodes (N) elevating the calcified aorta (a) anteriorly and obliterating the normal retroperitoneal landmarks. The mass (M) displaces the rectosigmoid (arrow) in the pelvis to the right (bottom view) and at this level consists of both prostate and metastatic adenopathy. Diagnosis was made by percutaneous aspiration biopsy.

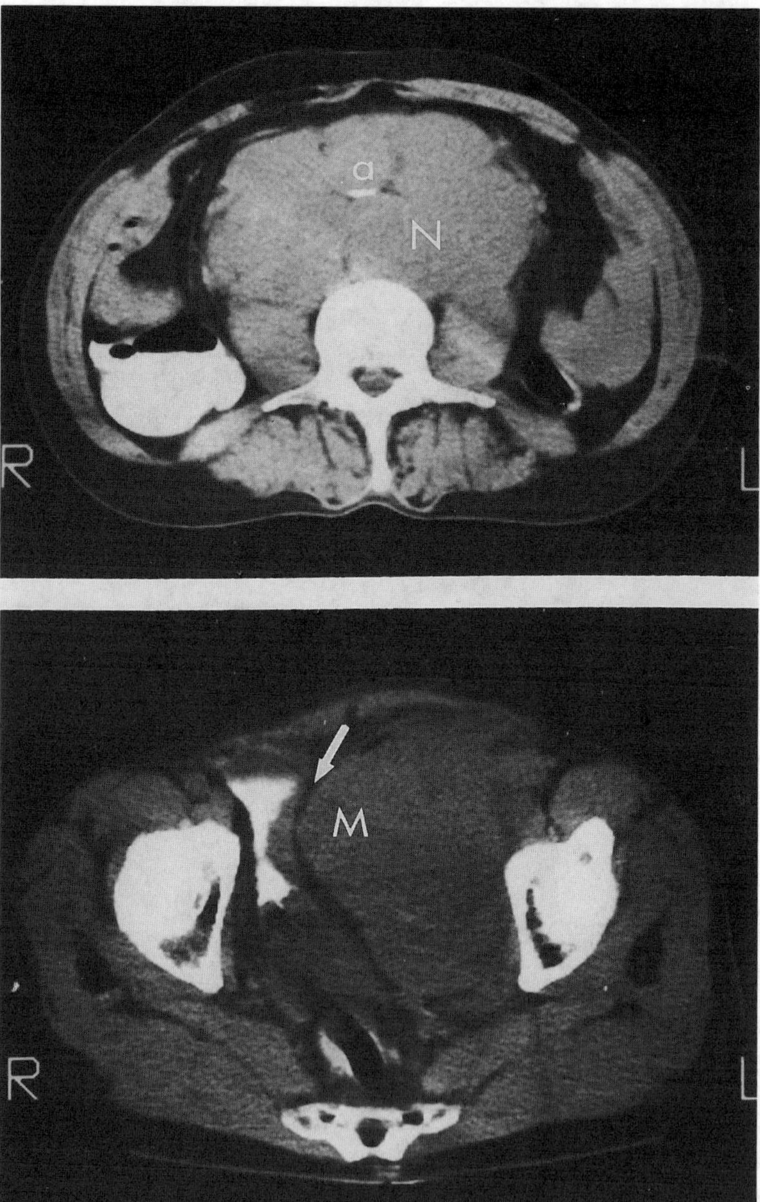

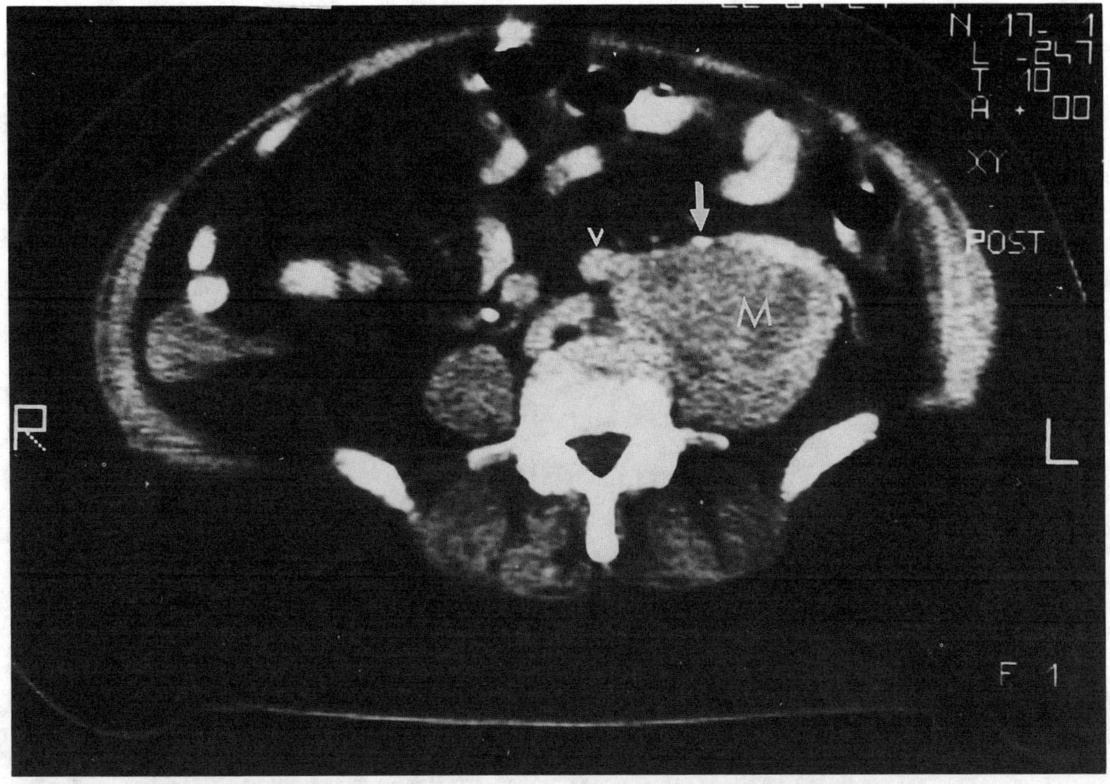

Figure 10-22. Enhanced CT scan below the level of the kidneys shows a large, low attenuation mass (M) with a necrotic center that displaces the left ureter anteriorly (arrow) and the left iliac vessels (v) to the right.

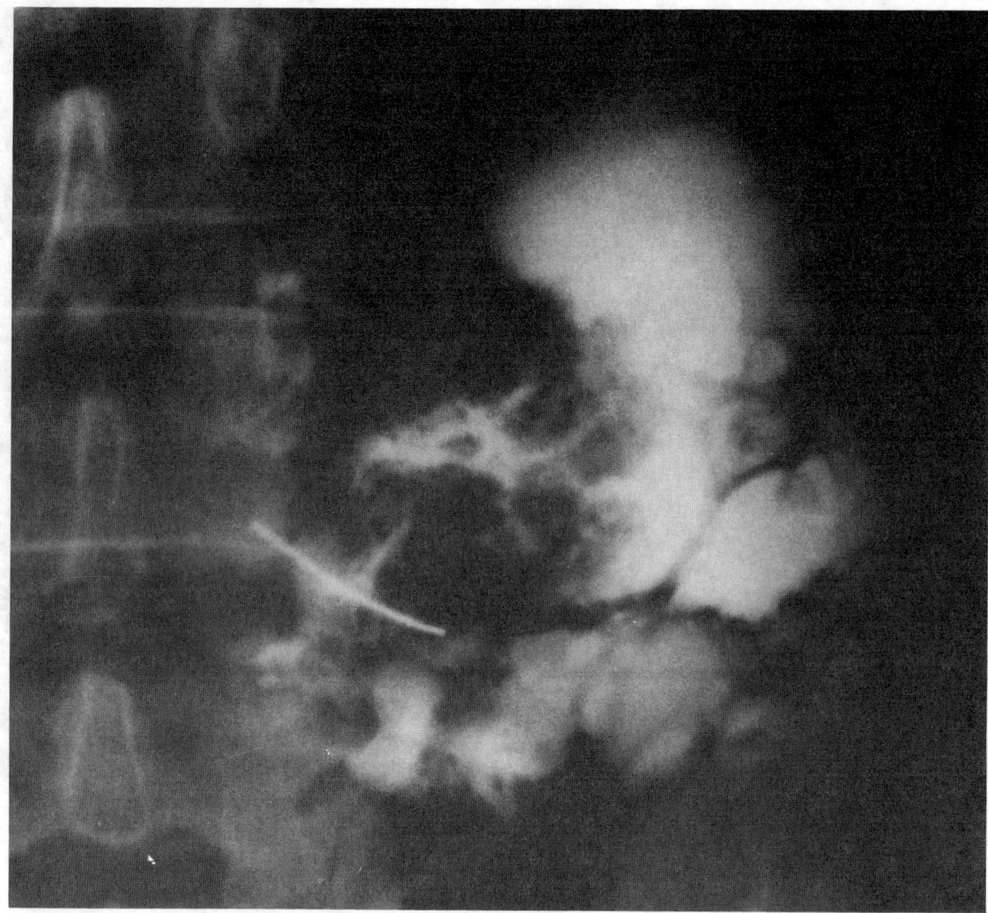

Figure 10-23. A plain x-ray film taken from a biopsy of this lesion after it was in-jected with contrast material shows the necrotic center and multilocu-lated character of this metastatic mass. The aspiration biopsy was posi-tive for metastatic cervical carcinoma.

Figure 10-24 A,B,C,D. CT scan at the level of the left adrenal gland (A, top left) demonstrates a prominent left gland with convex medial and lateral border (arrow). A computer line (l) drawn from the anterior abdominal wall defines the depth of the adrenal mass (B, top right). A needle (n) is positioned slightly lateral to the adrenal mass (C, lower left). The needle tip has been repositioned and is identified. Air has been injected to prove that the needle is passing through the adrenal gland (D, lower right). The biopsy was positive for epidermoid carcinoma identical to that of the lung primary (s = stomach, a = aorta, sp = spleen).

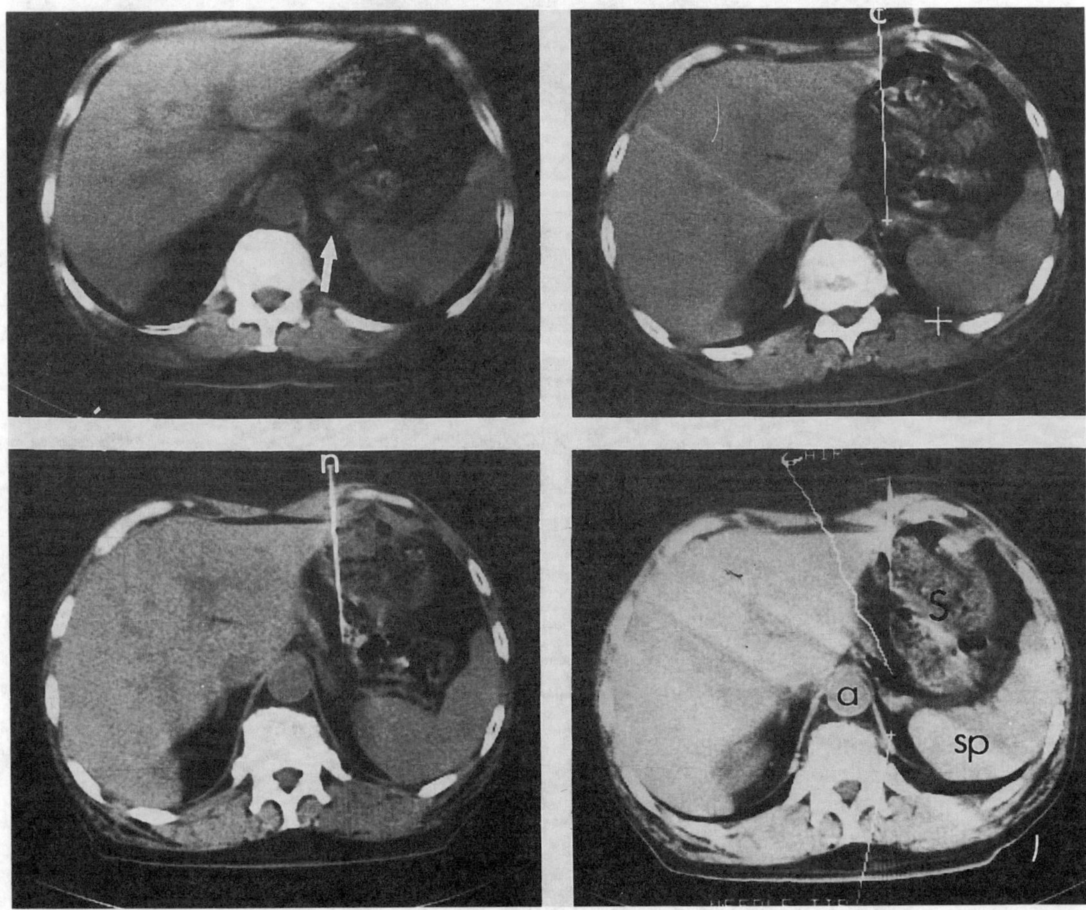

Figure 10-25. CT scan at the level of the adrenal glands (top view) demonstrates bilateral adrenal masses. The right adrenal is identified by the box cursor over it. The left adrenal (a) has biconvex borders and is markedly enlarged (A = aorta, I = inferior vena cava, p = pancreas, c = caudate lobe of liver, ca = celiac axis). Bottom view: Massive retroperitoneal adenopathy (n) elevates the heavily calcified aorta (A). Percutaneous biopsy of the retroperitoneal nodes demonstrated metastatic disease.

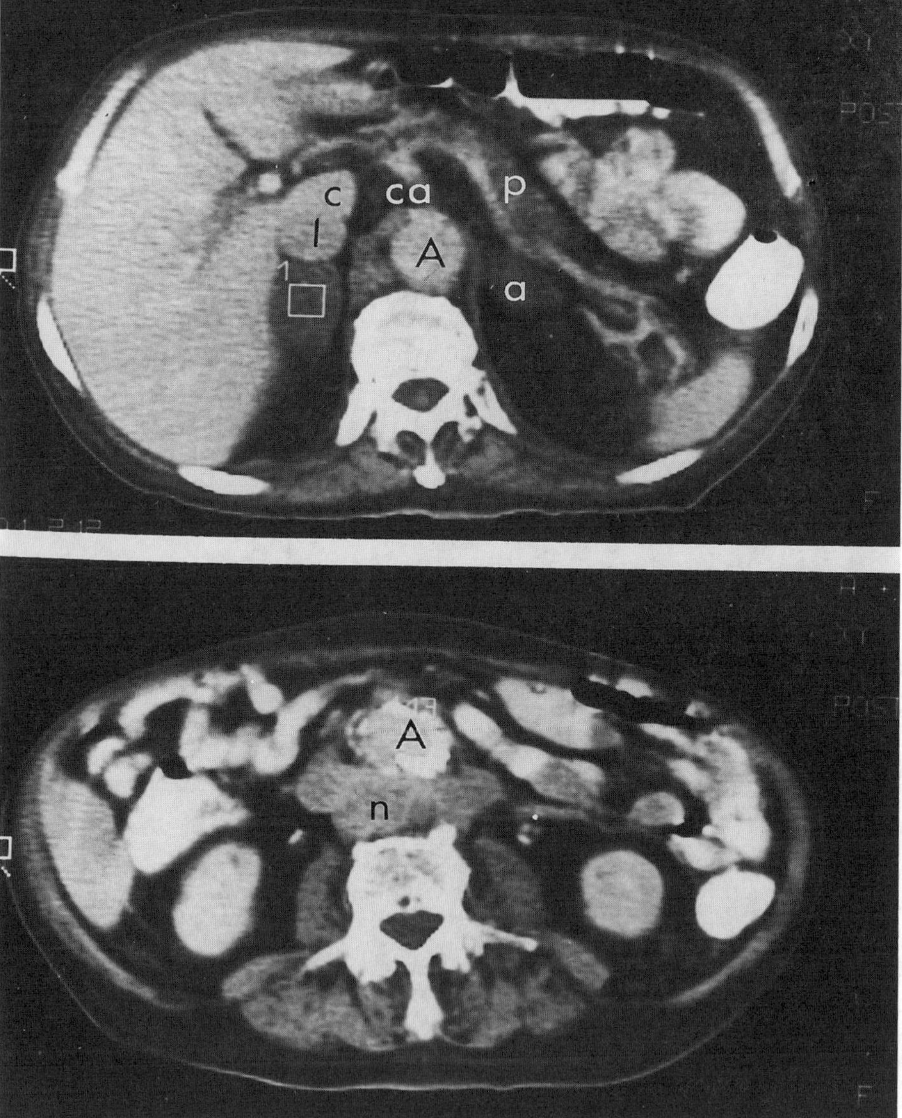

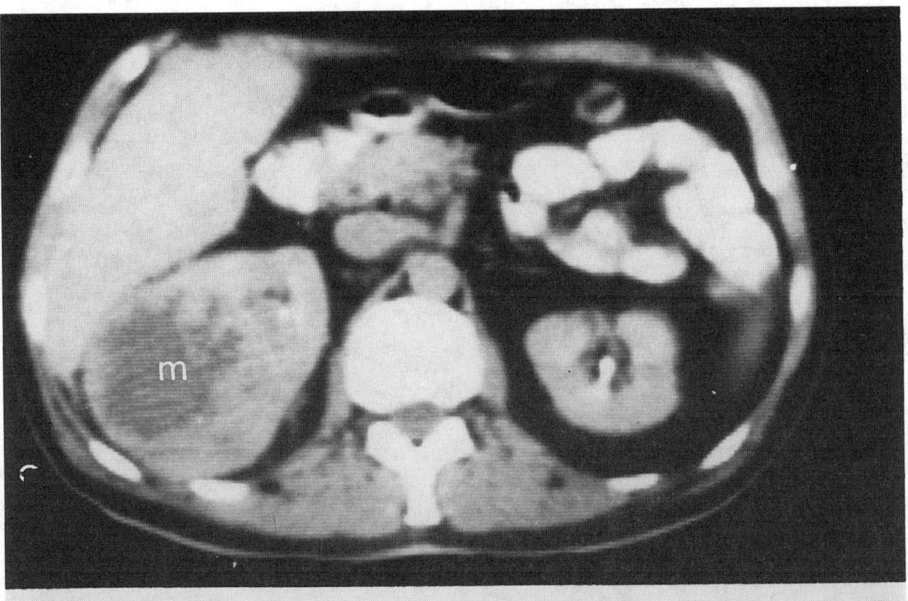

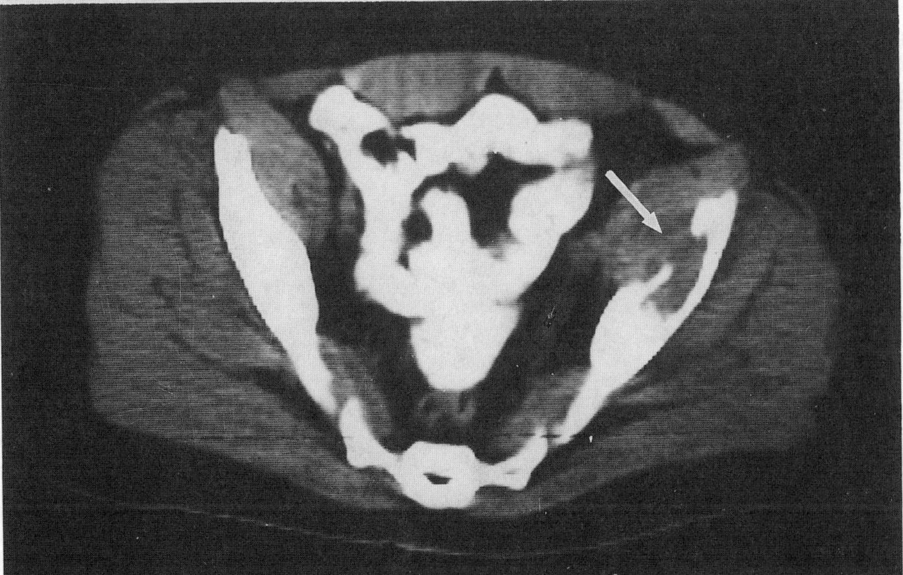

Figure 10-26. Enhanced CT section through the level of the right kidney (top view) demonstrates a large, necrotic low attenuation mass (m) in the right kidney. A section through the level of the iliac wing (bottom view) demonstrates destruction of the left iliac wing with a contiguous soft-tissue mass (arrow).

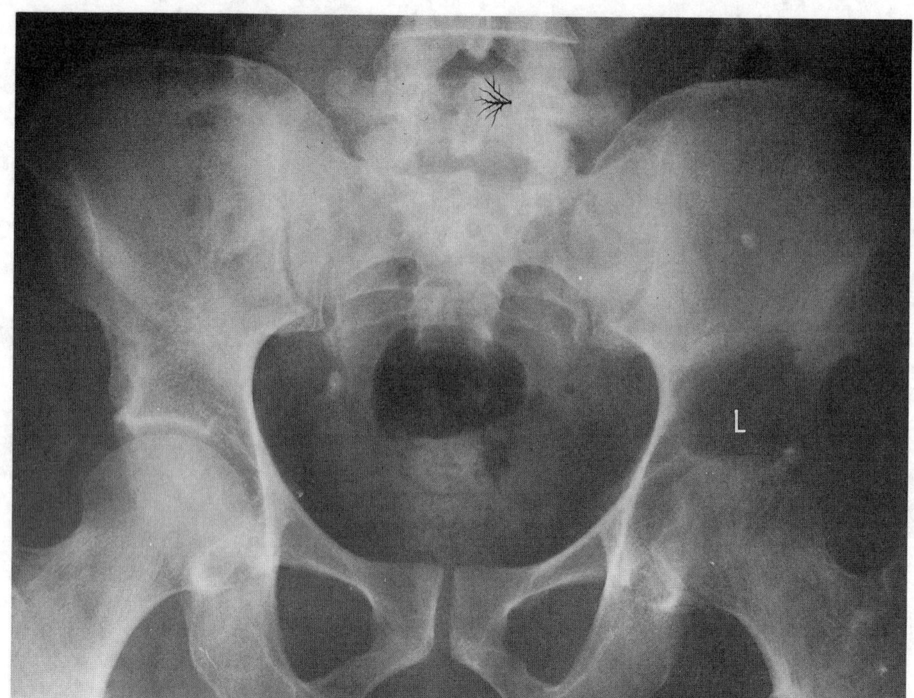

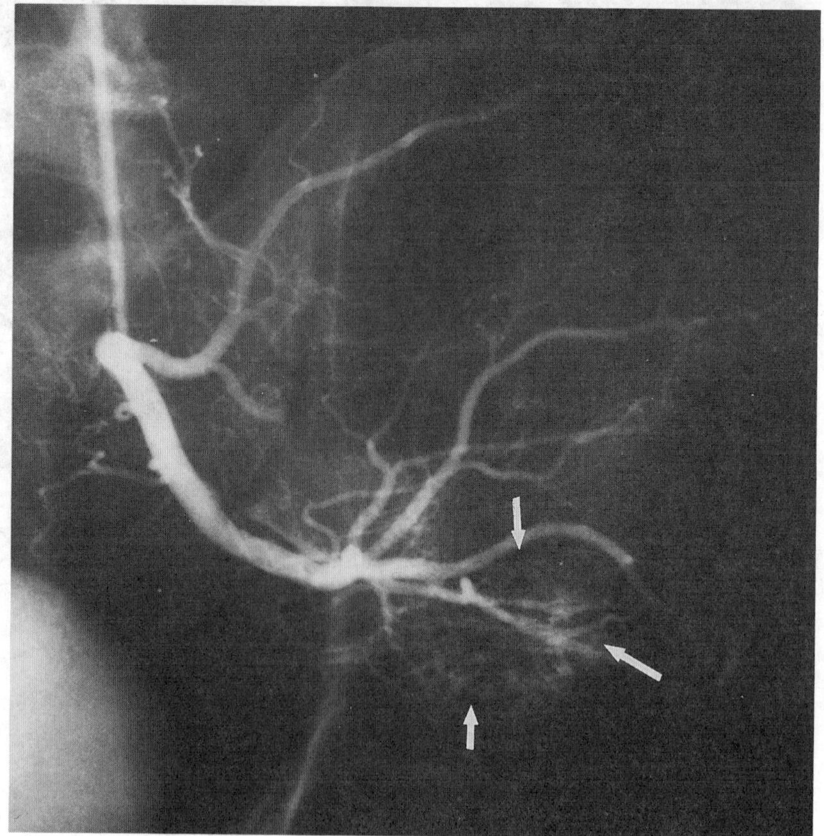

OPPOSITE PAGE, TOP

Figure 10-27. A plain x-ray of the pelvis also demonstrates the lytic lesion (L) and
its location at the roof of the left acetabulum.

OPPOSITE PAGE, BOTTOM

Figure 10-28. Preembolization films from a selective superior gluteal arteriogram
demonstrate the hypervascular nature of the lesion (arrows).

Figure 10-29. Postembolization film from a selective superior gluteral arteriogram
demonstrates that blood flow is stopped in the vessels after Gelfoam embolization. Note absence of neovascularity.

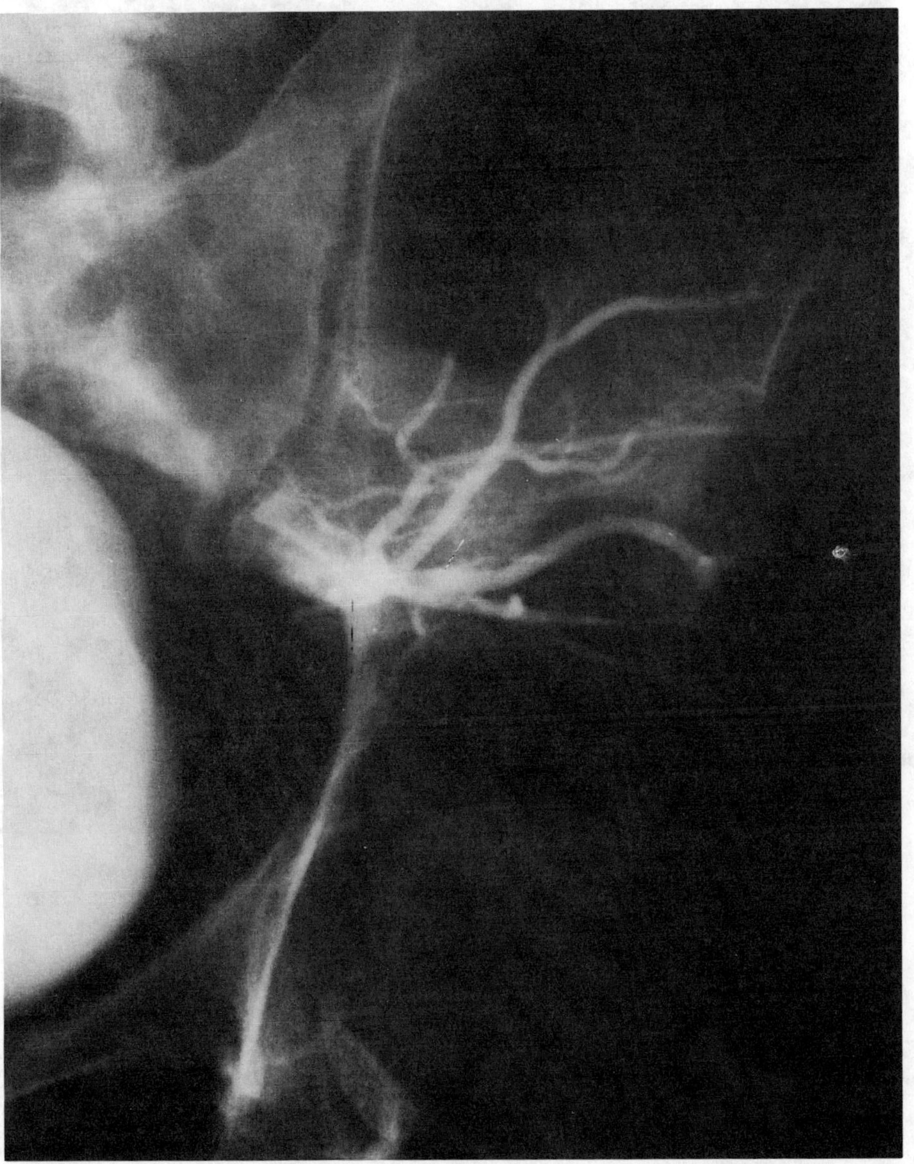

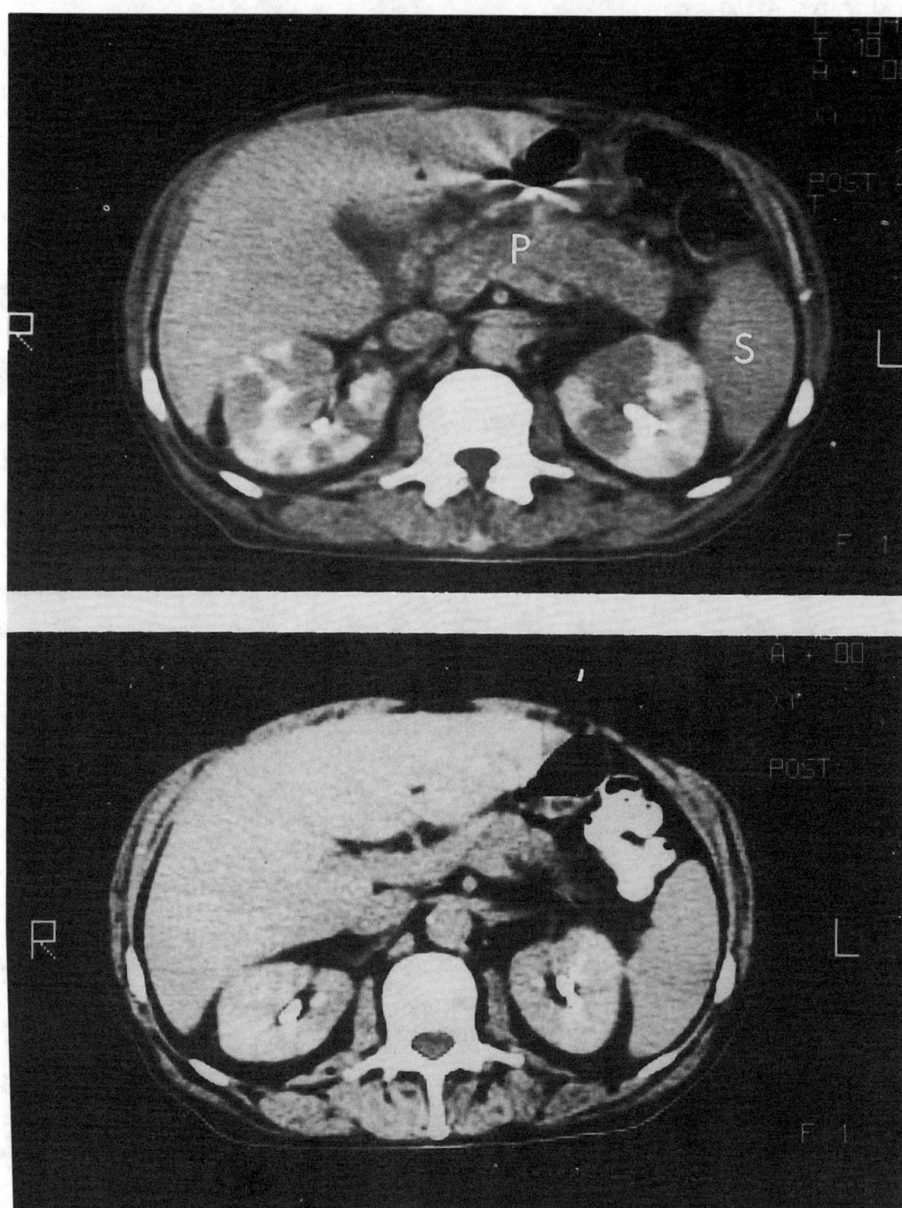

Figure 10-30. Top view: Initial CT scan after the administration of I.V. contrast demonstrates multiple low attenuation areas throughout enlarged kidneys bilaterally consistent with leukemic infiltrations of both kidneys (chloromas) (confirmed by percutaneous biopsy) (S = spleen, P = pancreas). Bottom view: Three weeks later, following radiation and chemotherapy, an enhanced CT at a comparable level demonstrates nearly complete resolution of the chloromas and marked reduction in size of the kidneys.

Figure 10-31. CT image through the level of the transverse colon demonstrates a large, mixed attenuation mass (m) associated within the transverse colon and effacing the lumen (white arrow). Also, note multiple low attenuation areas within the visualized small bowel representing other polyps in the small bowel (p and black arrows).

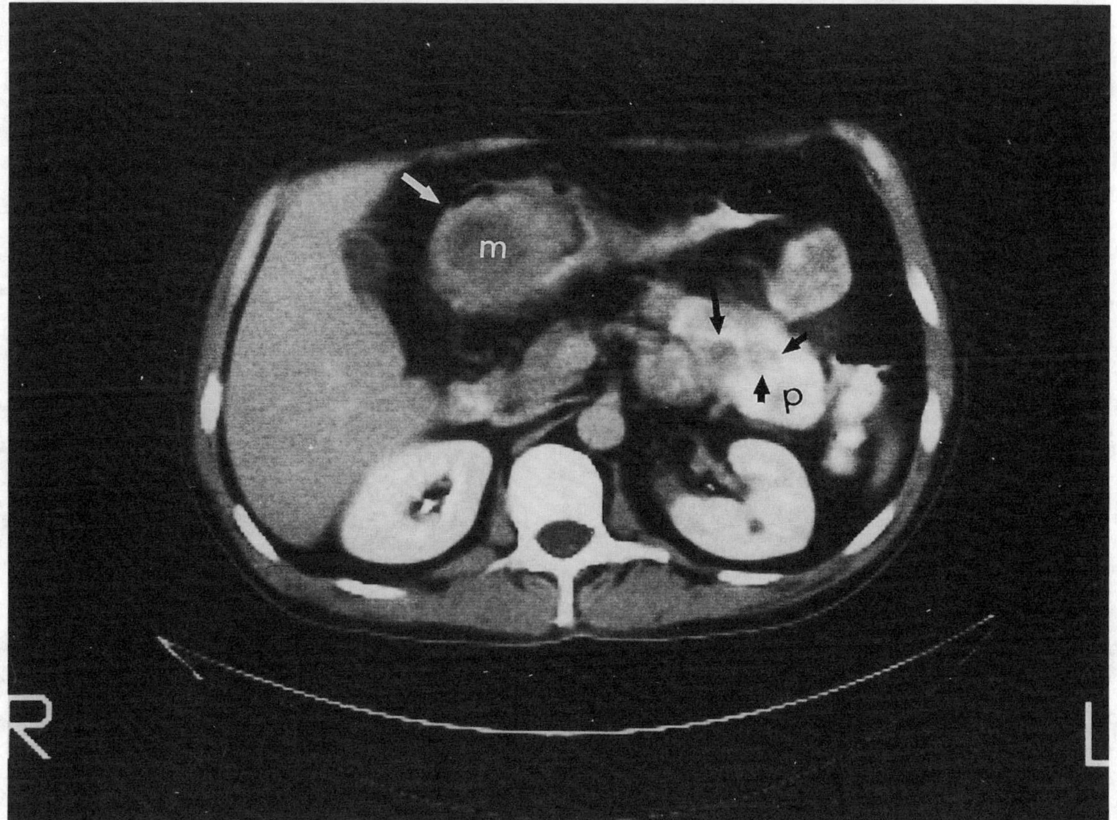

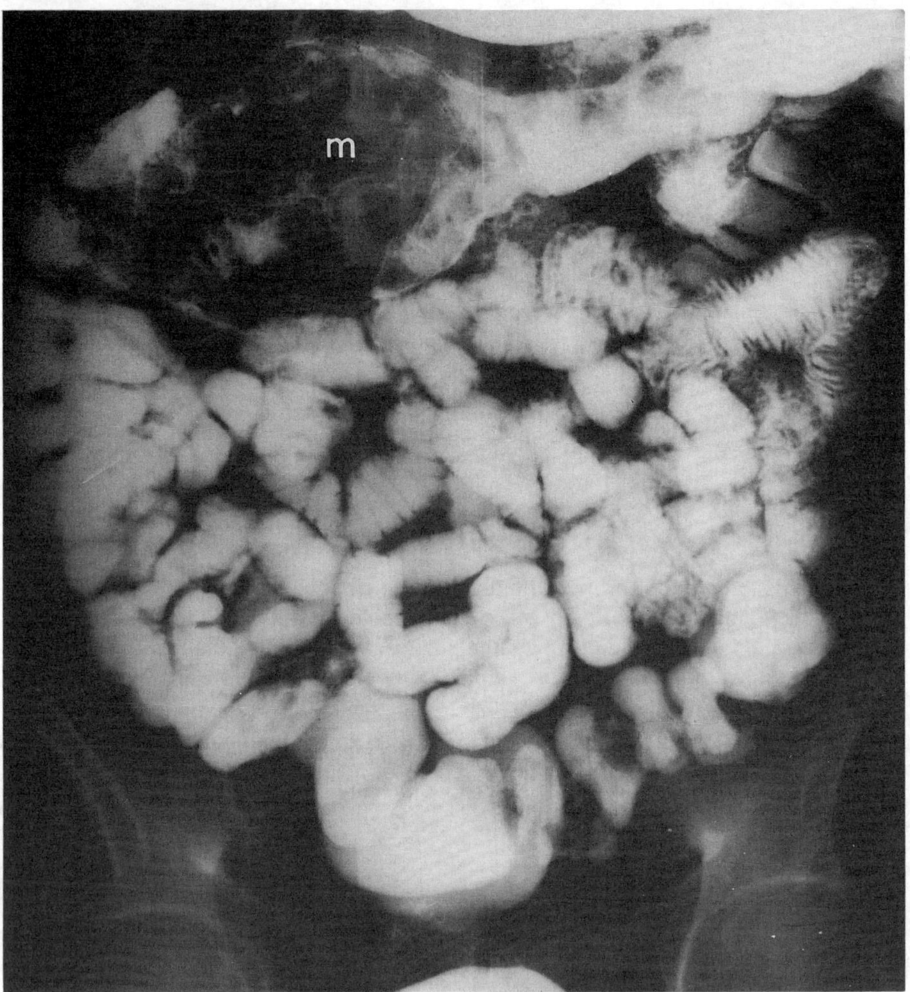

Figure 10-32. A film from an upper G.I. series and small bowel follow-through shows good clinical correlation of the ulcerated mass (m) within the transverse colon as well as visualizing multiple polyps within the small bowel.

Figure 10-33. Top: CT scan at the level of the gastric antrum (a) demonstrates tumor encasement of the gastric antrum with a suggestion of invasion of the head of the pancreas (p). Bottom: A section at a higher level demonstrates a large lymph node in the gastrohepatic ligament posterior to the body of the pancreas (P) (arrow). (C = caudate lobe of liver).

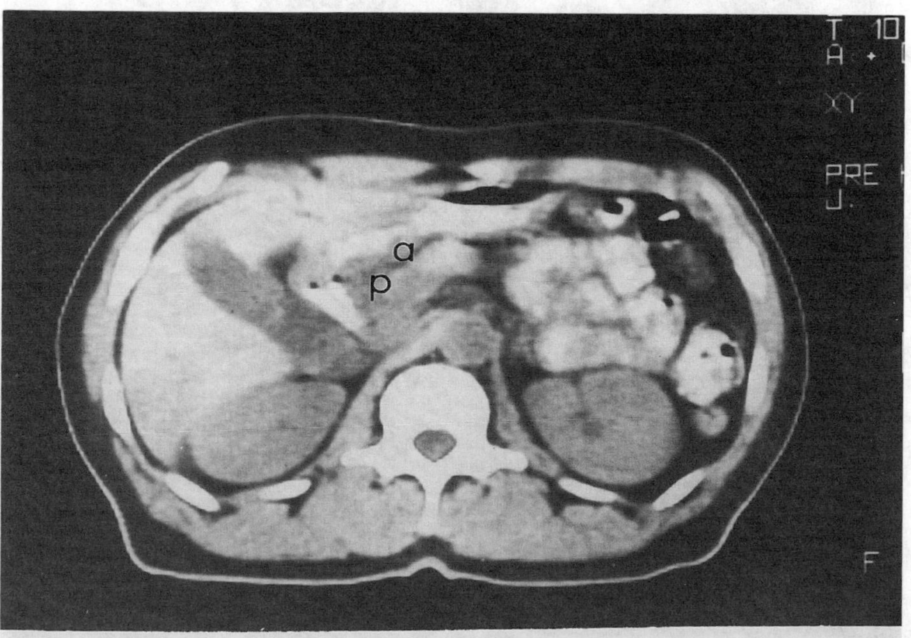

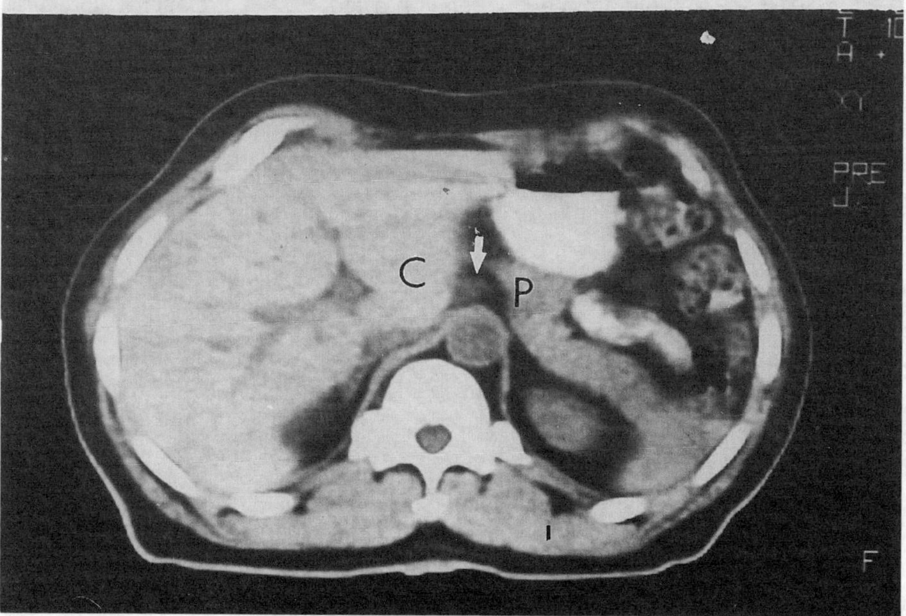

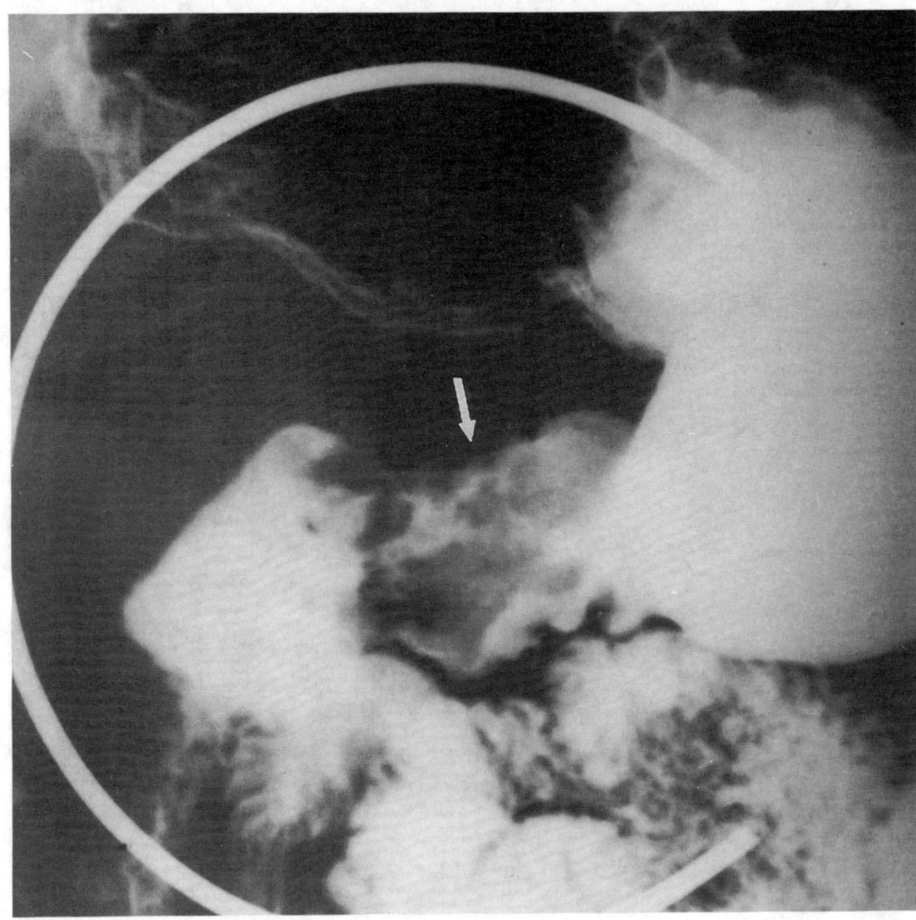

Figure 10-34. A spot film from a G.I. series provides x-ray correlation of the large ulcerated lesion in the gastric antrum (arrow). Lymphoma, primary carcinoma, metastatic disease from other primaries, tuberculosis, and actinomycosis, are in the differential diagnosis.

Figure 10-35. CT cuts at the level of the carina (top picture) demonstrates a stellate deformity of the esophagus (arrow) with invasion of the posterior mediastinum and obliteration of the fat plane between the esophagus and the aorta (A) indicating unresectability. Bottom picture: At a lower level, the extent of the mass (m) can be better appreciated encroaching upon the anterior aspect of the aorta (A) and the azygoesophageal recess (arrow) (P = main pulmonary artery, aa = ascending aorta, S = superior vena cava).

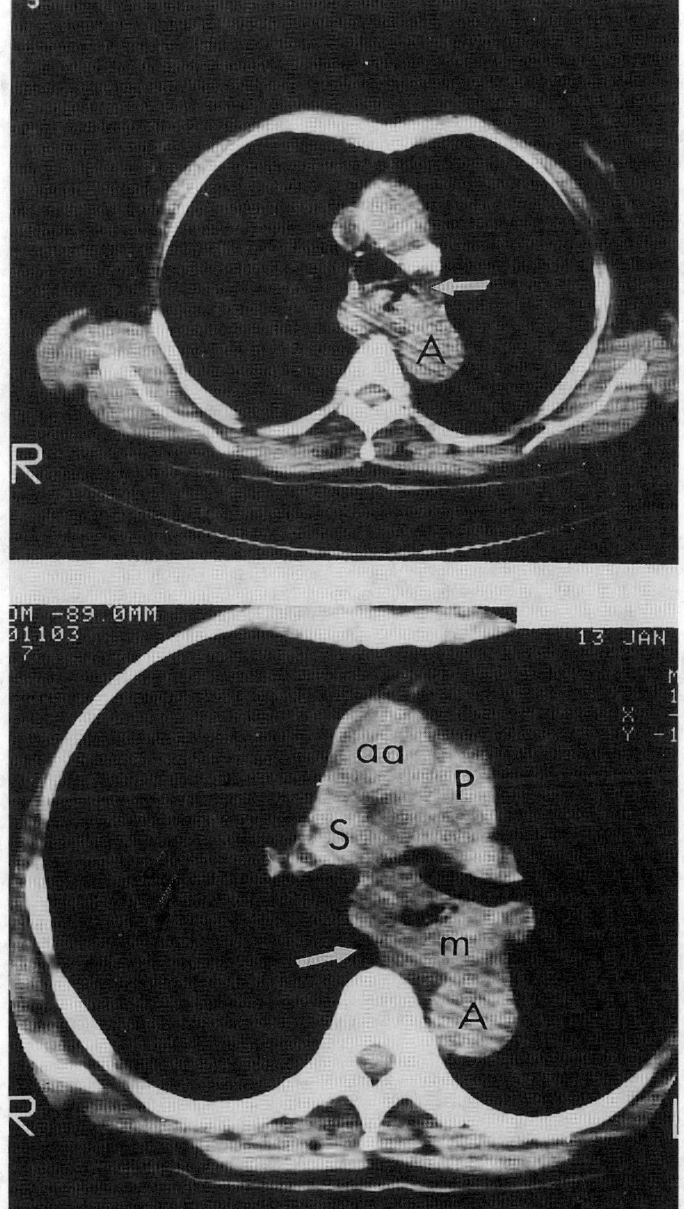

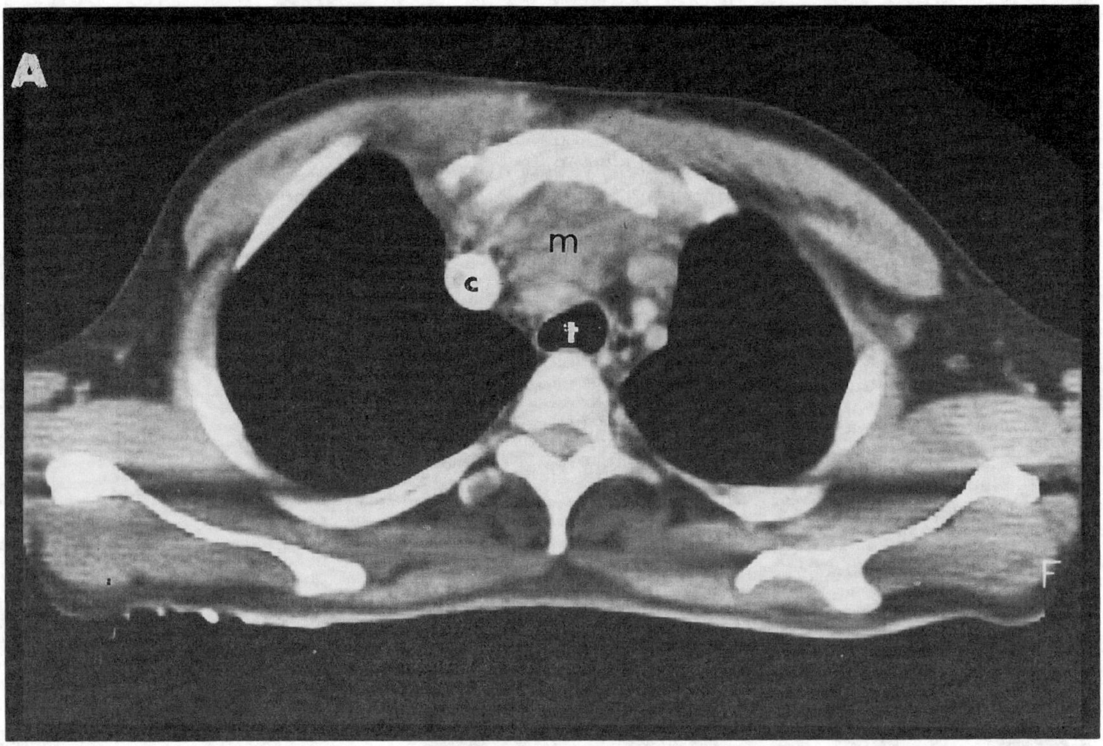

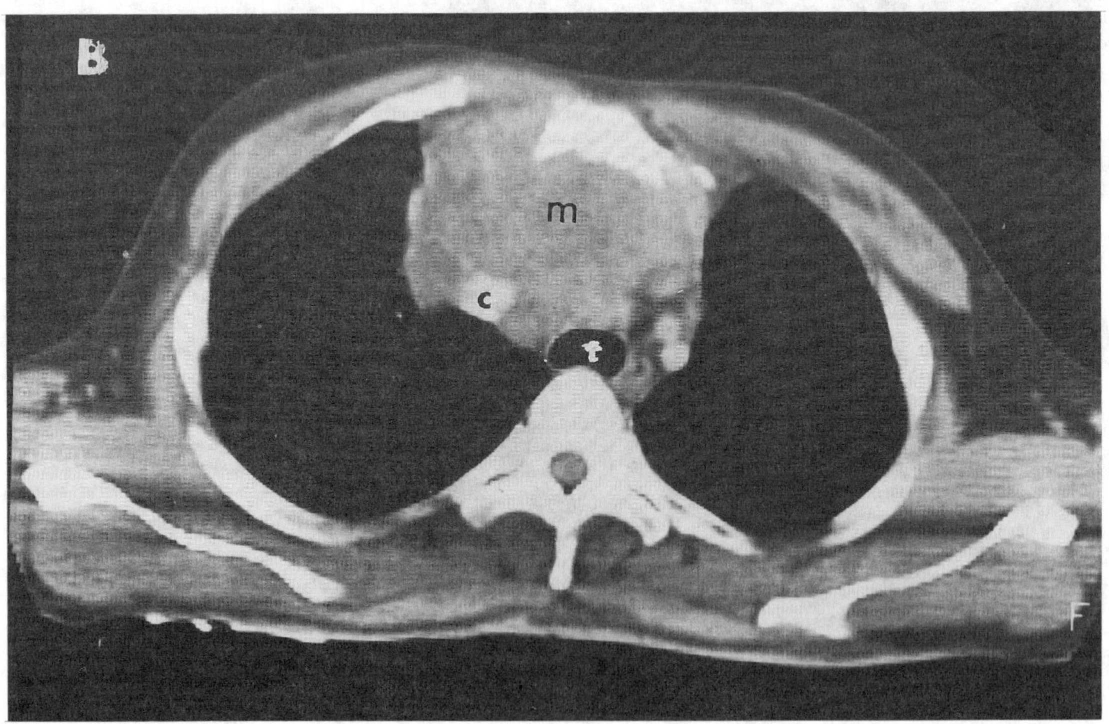

OPPOSITE PAGE

Figure 10-36 A & B. These pictures represent sequential axial sections of CT
          scan showing a large anterior mediastinal mass (m) with posterior dis-
          placement of the trachea (t) and blood vessels. Gradual narrowing of the
          SVC (c) is seen, indicating an impending SVC syndrome.

Figure 10-37. Posteroanterior view of the chest shows right middle lobe collapse
          and right pleural effusion.

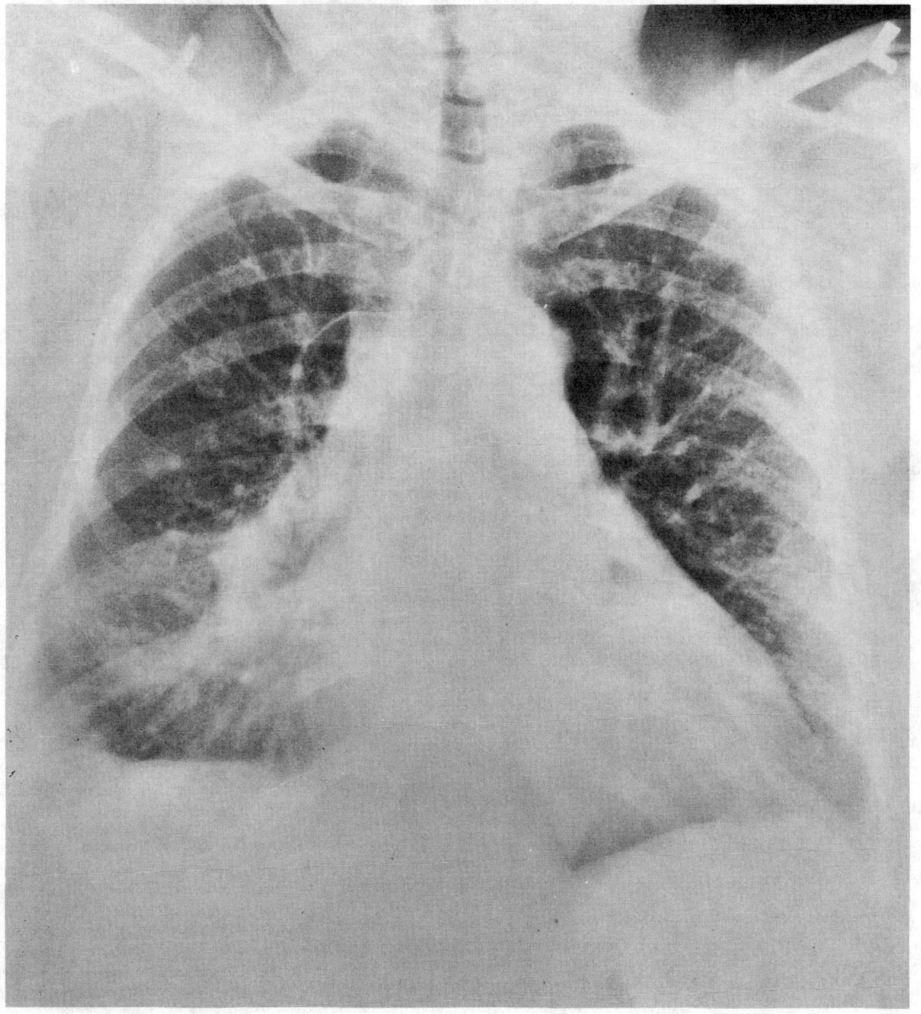

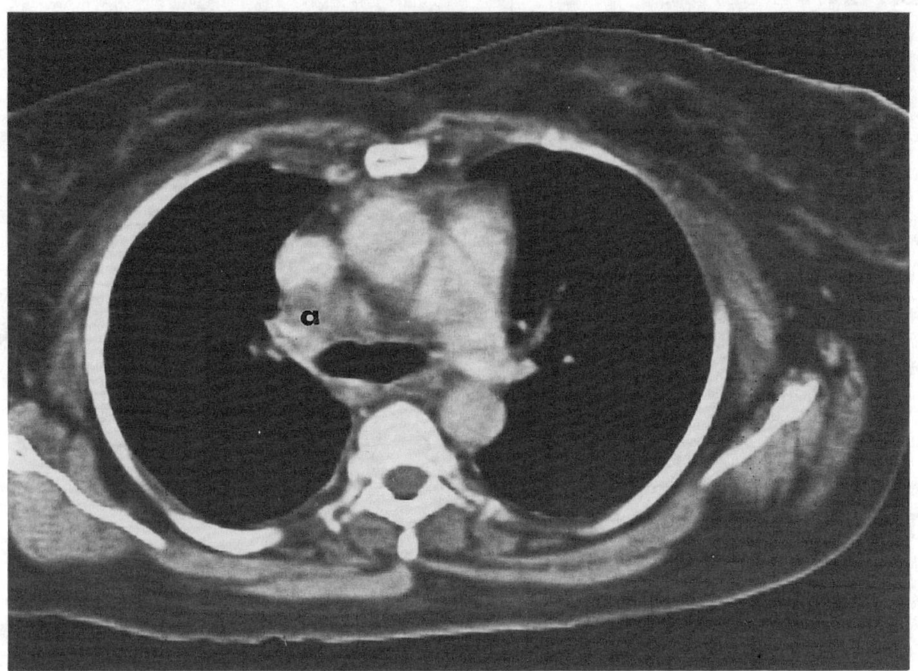

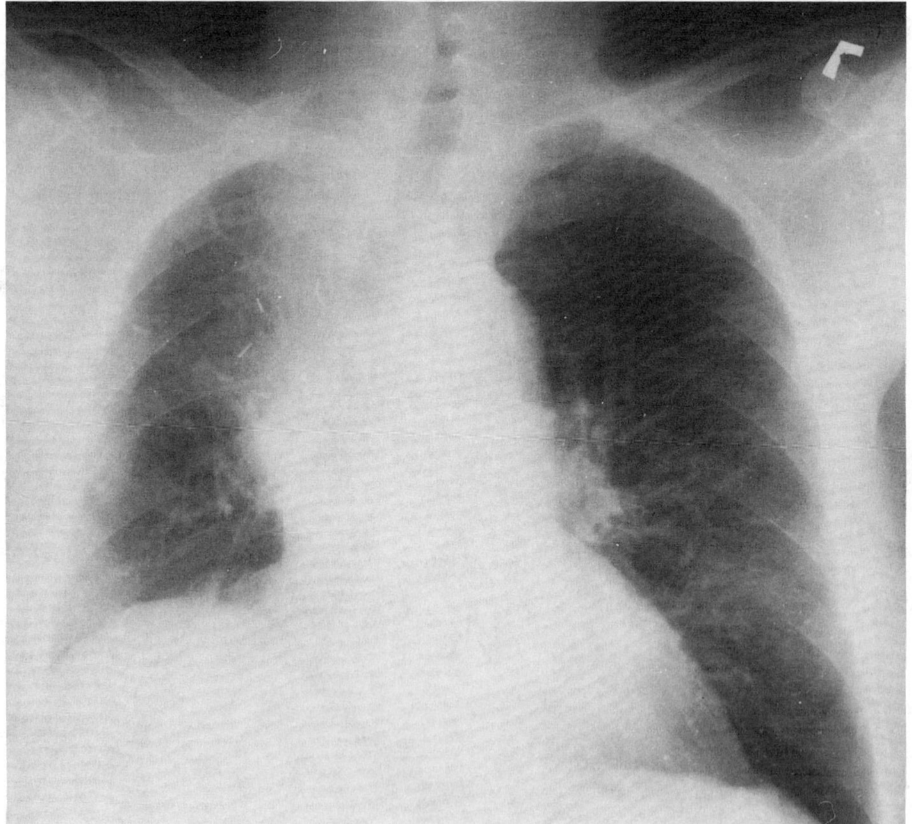

OPPOSITE PAGE, TOP

Figure 10-38. CT scan at the level of the carina. I.V. contrast material was injected to opacify the heart and major vessels. Extensive mediastinal and right hilar adenopathy (a) is present. This was the cause of the RML collapse.

OPPOSITE PAGE, BOTTOM

Figure 10-39. Posteroanterior view of the chest of a patient after right upper lobectomy for bronchogenic carcinoma. The radiograph reveals widening of the mediastinum, suggestive of tumor recurrence.

Figure 10-40. CT scan with I.V. contrast. Axial tomogram at the level of the aortic arch shows a mass of enlarged lymph nodes in the mediastinum surrounded by the aortic arch (a) on the left, the SVC (s) on the right and the trachea (t) posteriorly.

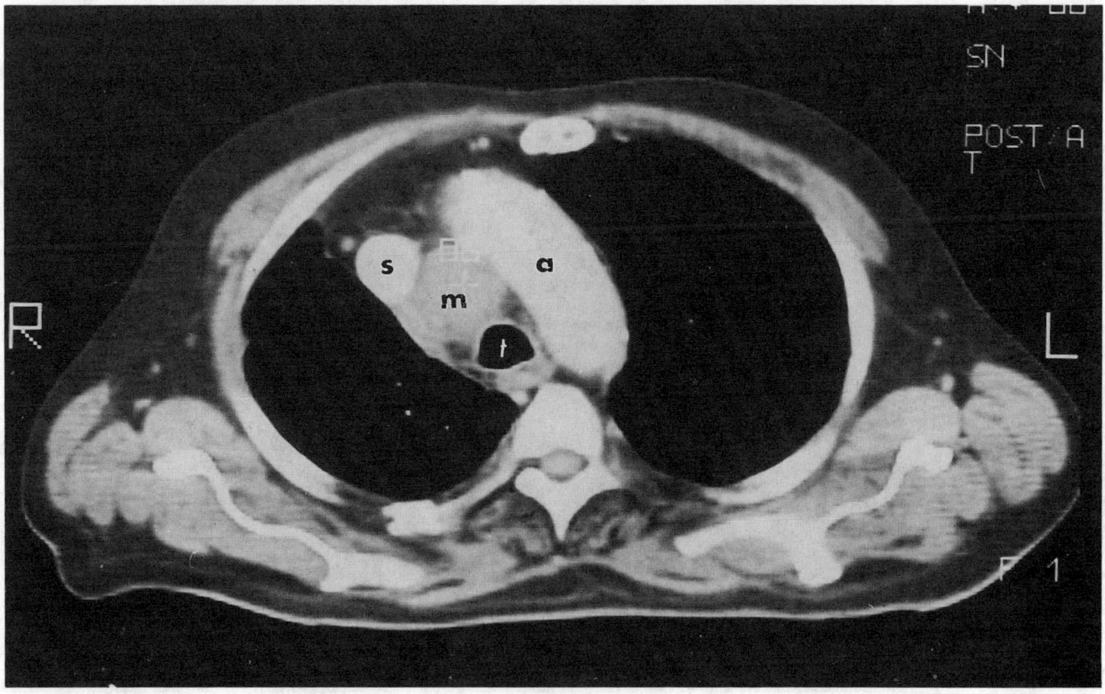

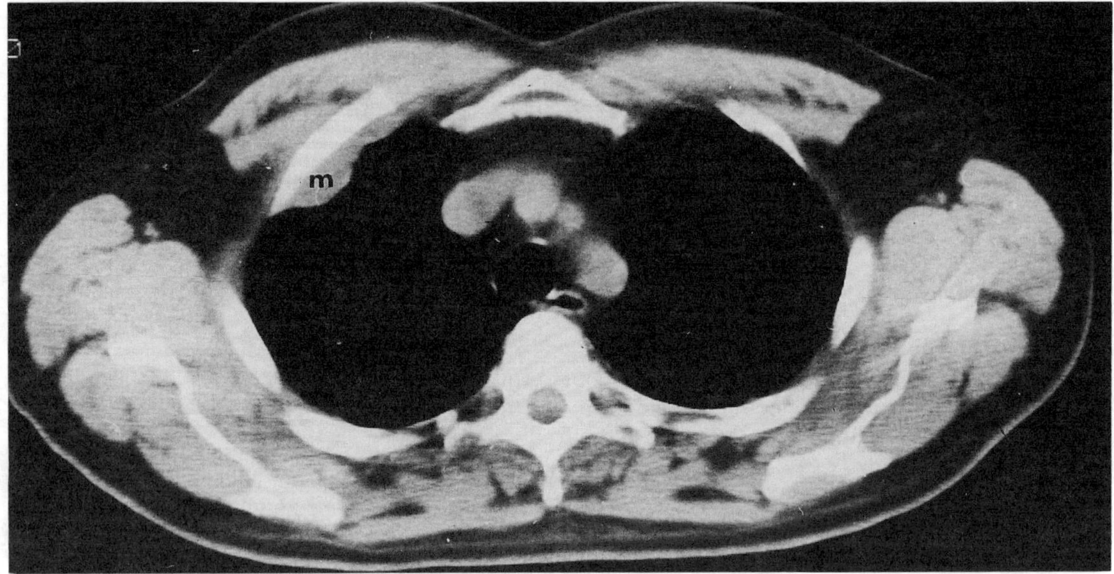

Figure 10-41. A localized lesion is present in the right pleural space (m) on CT scan.

Figure 10-42. The patient presented several years following mastectomy with a new soft-tissue mass in the right parasternal region. CT scan reveals a mass lesion (m) with bony destruction and an intrathoracic component. This recurrence of breast carcinoma may have originated in the internal mammary node. Also noted is an enlarged right axillary lymph node (n) and subcarinal lymphadenopathy (a).

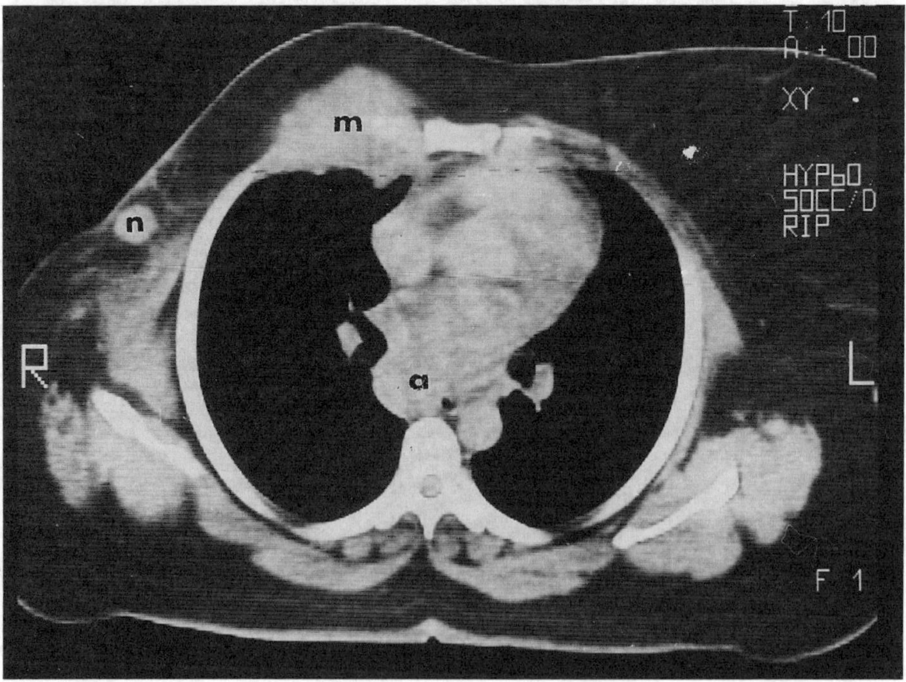

Figure 10-43. Anteroposterior x-ray view of the right shoulder: A localized calcifying tumor of the humerus is seen.

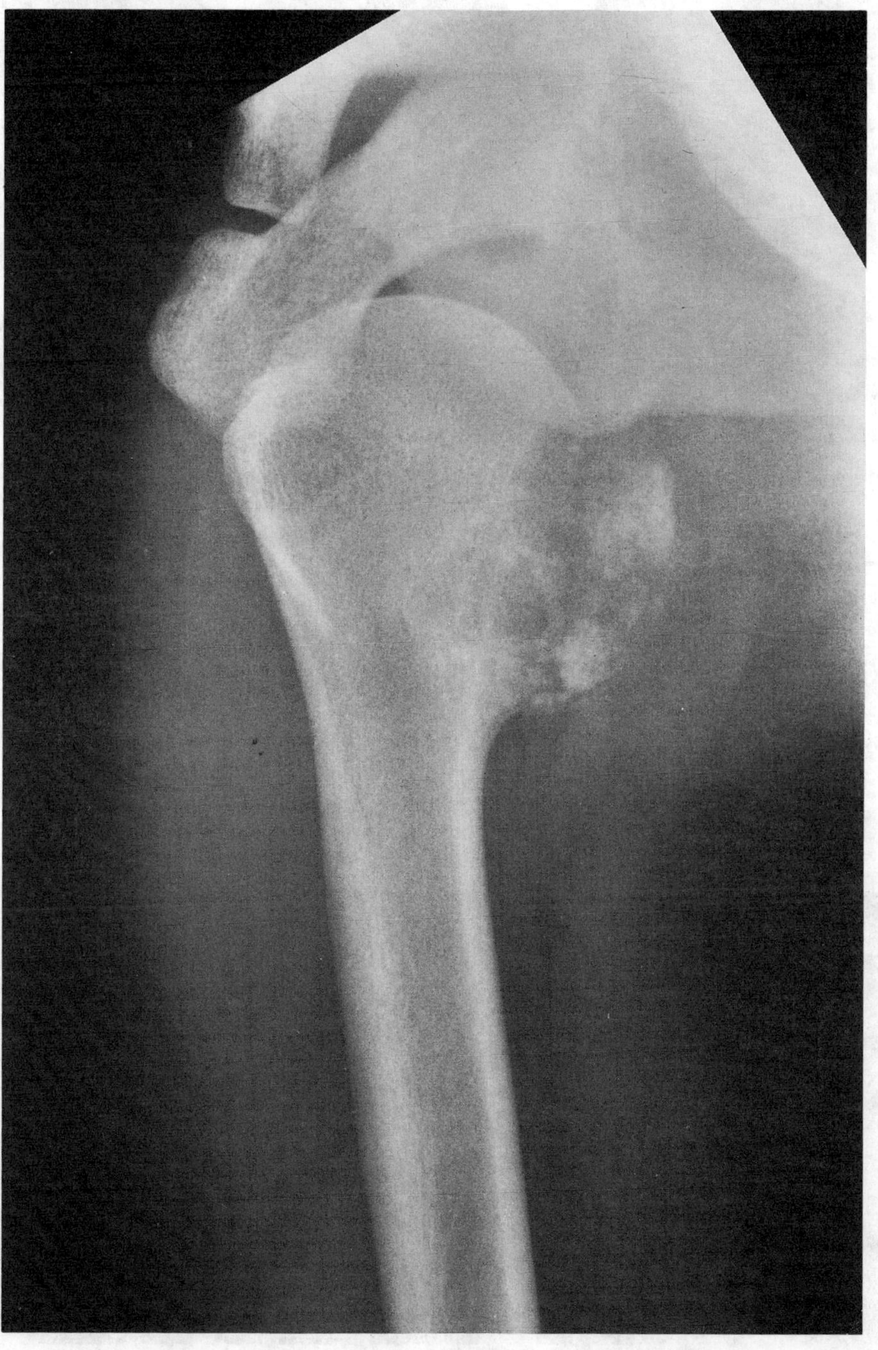

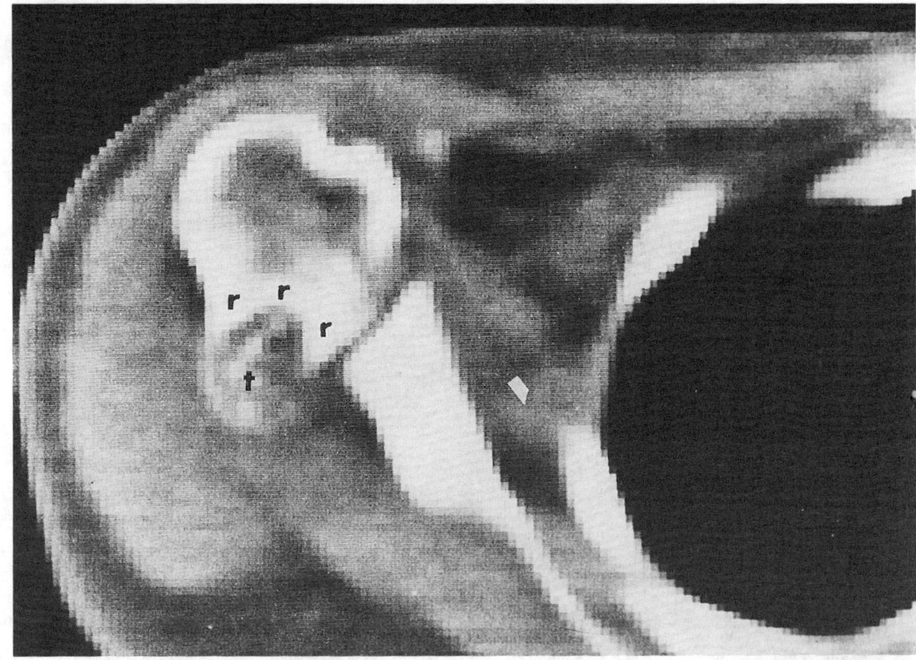

Figure 10-44. CT scan of the same shoulder shows that the tumor (t) involves the cortex and is demarcated from the humerus by a thick cortical rim (r). Therefore, it is a parosteal tumor.

Figure 10-45 A & B. A—CT scan reveals a permeative tumor (t) involving the left iliac bone (i) and the left side of the sacrum (s). B—Same scan seen with different scanning settings reveals wisps of calcification extending into the cystic components of the tumor anterior and posterior to the iliac bone. This appearance is typical of chondrosarcoma.

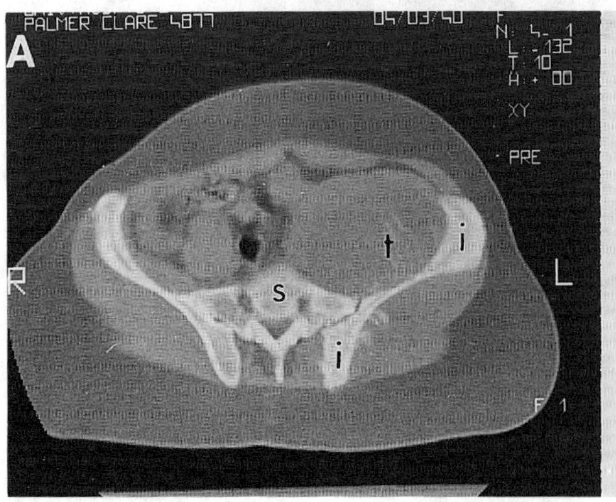

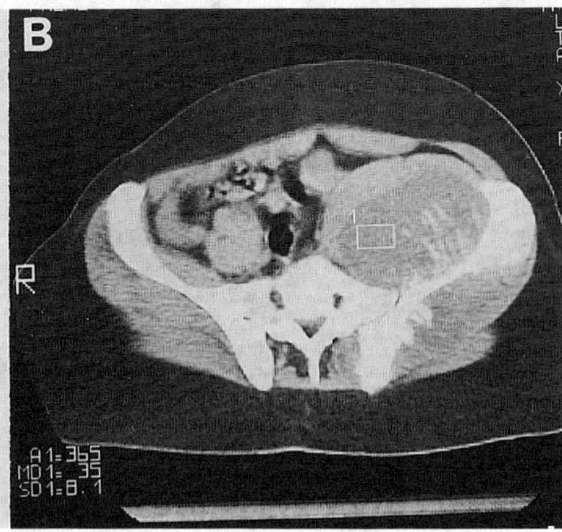

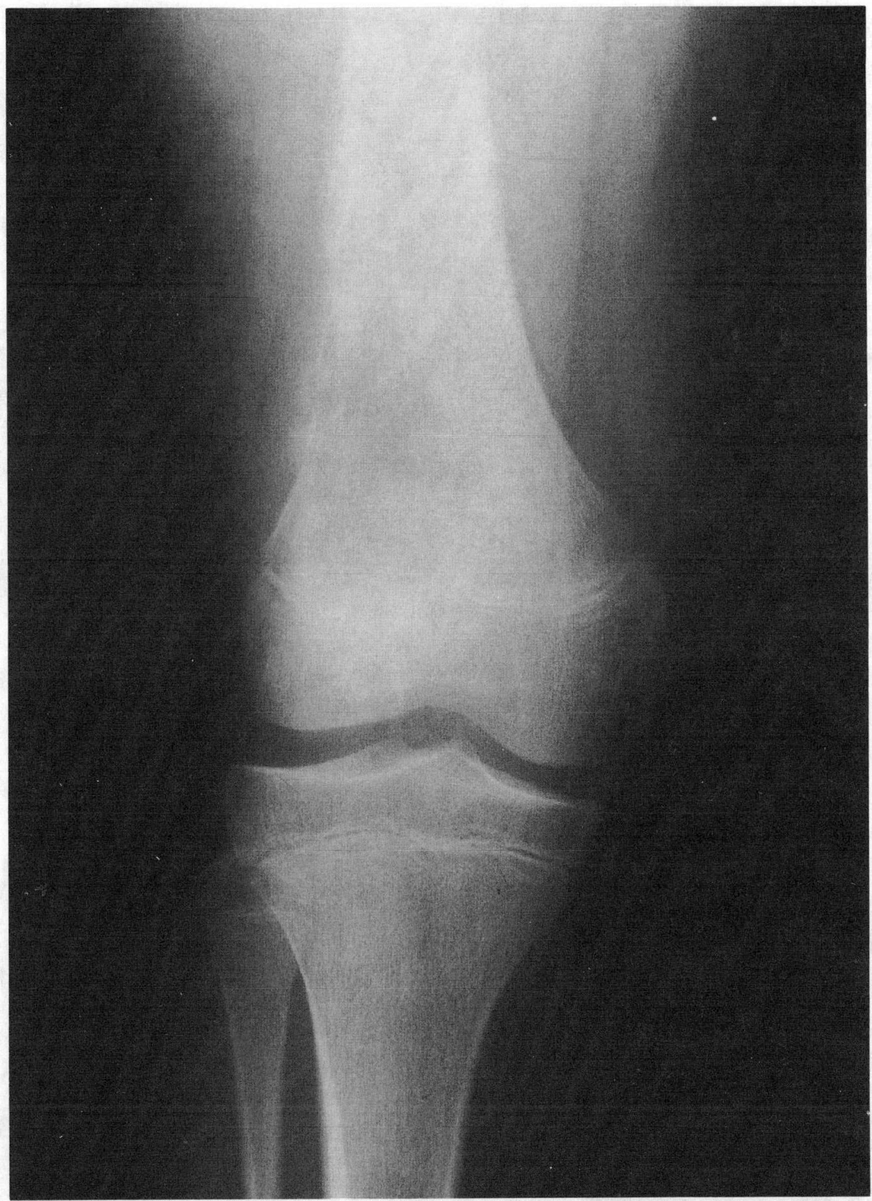

Figure 10-46. Frontal view of femur shows a lytic lesion of the distal femur involving both diaphysis and metaphysis. Note "onionskin" pattern of periosteal new bone and destruction of cortex.

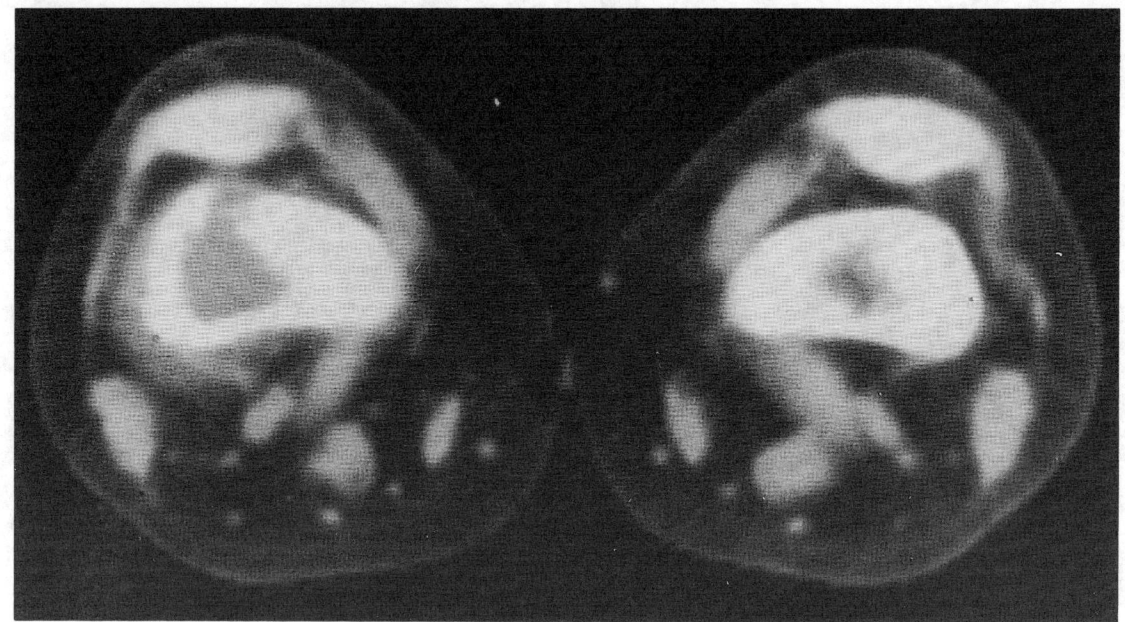

Figure 10-47. CT scan through distal femur at the upper part of patella of the patient in figure 10-46. It shows tumor in the medullary cavity, disruption of anterior cortex, and tumor in the soft tissue along the medial and posterior aspect.

Figure 10-48. Sequential CT scans of both thighs reveal a tumor of the skin (t) sharply demarcated from the underlying muscle. Pathologic diagnosis in this case was dermatofibrosarcoma protuberans.

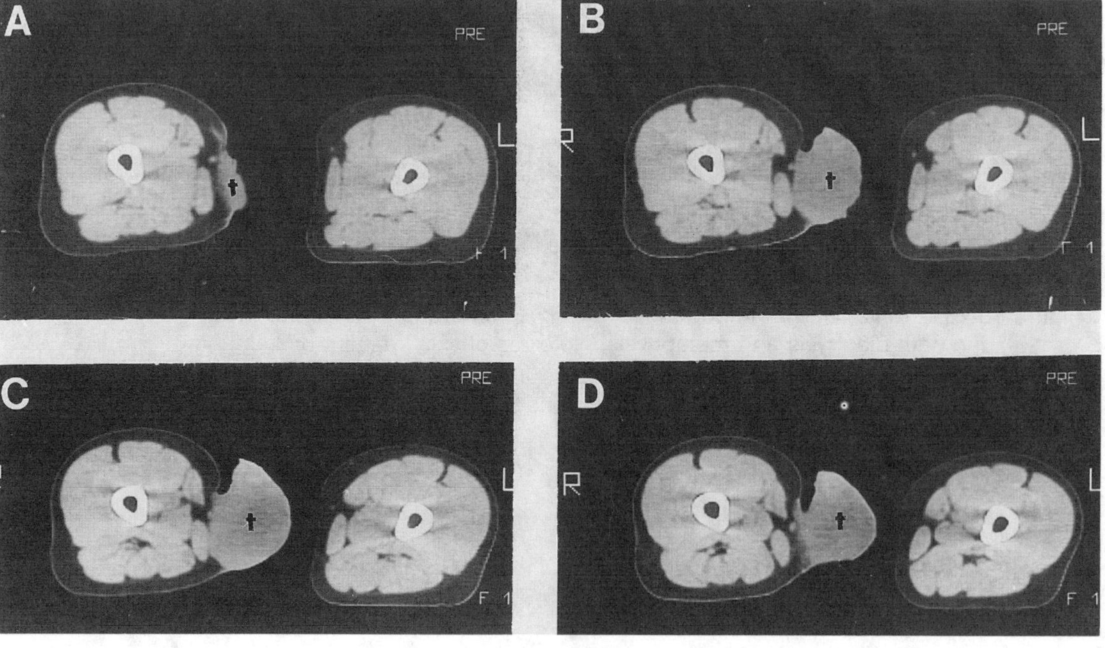

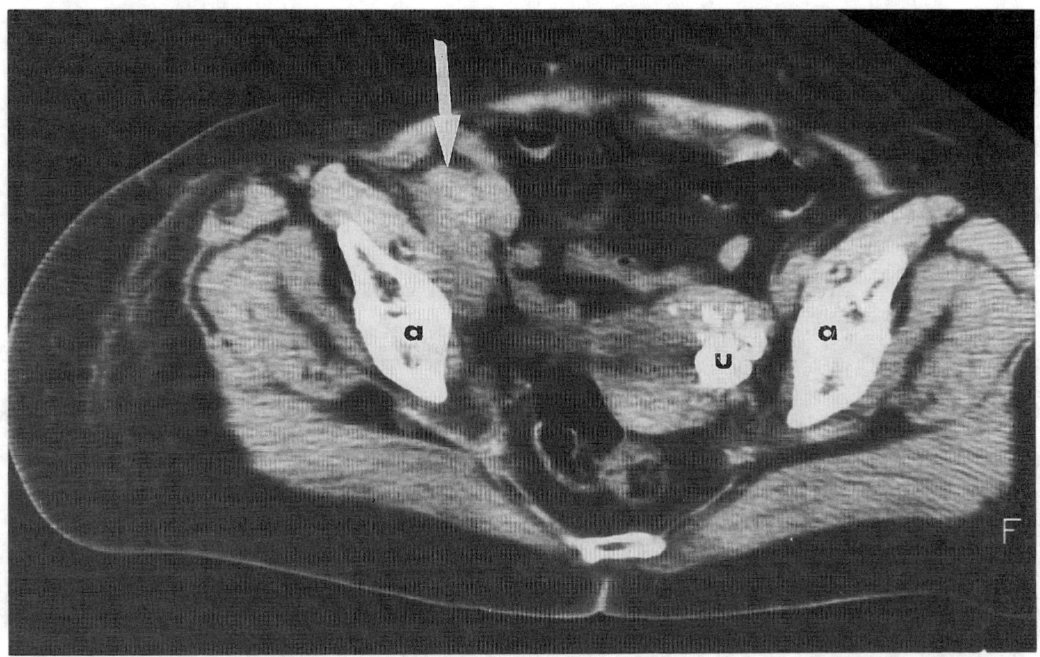

Figure 10-49. CT scan reveals an external iliac lymphanopathy (↓) (a = supra-acetabular bone, u = calcified uterine fibroid).

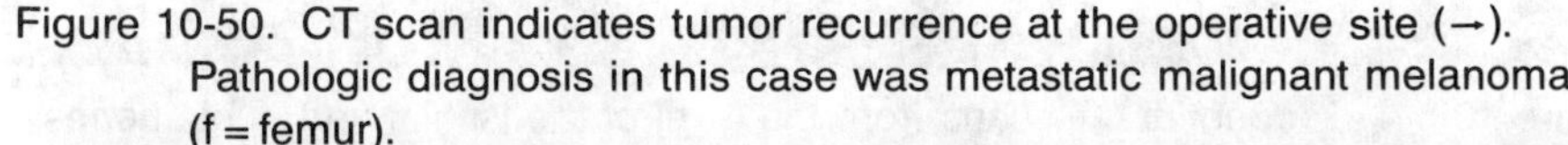

Figure 10-50. CT scan indicates tumor recurrence at the operative site (→). Pathologic diagnosis in this case was metastatic malignant melanoma (f = femur).

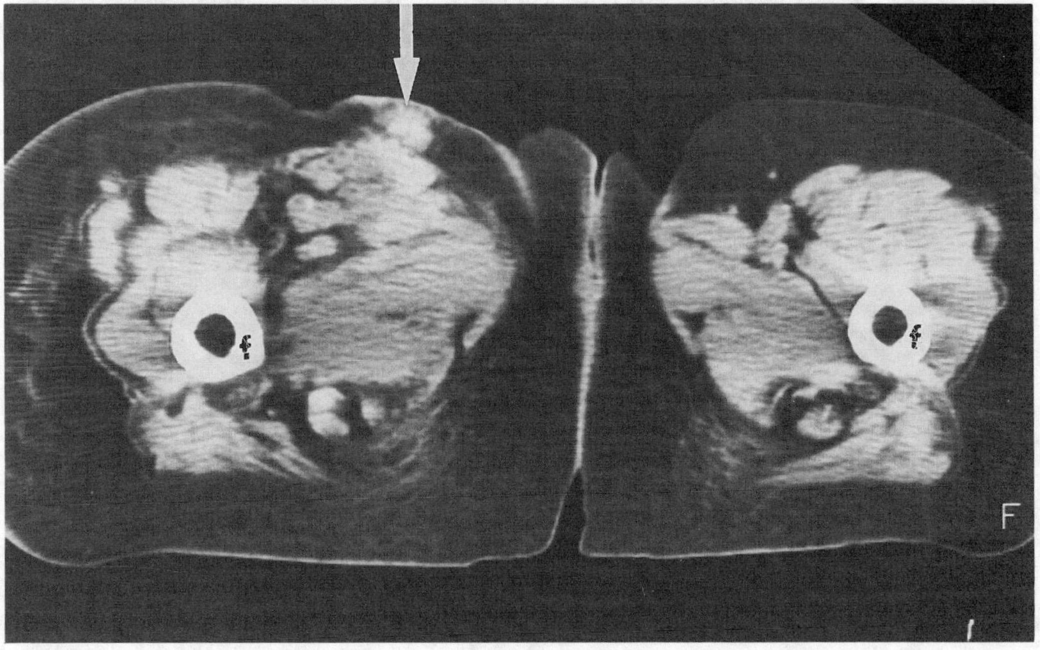

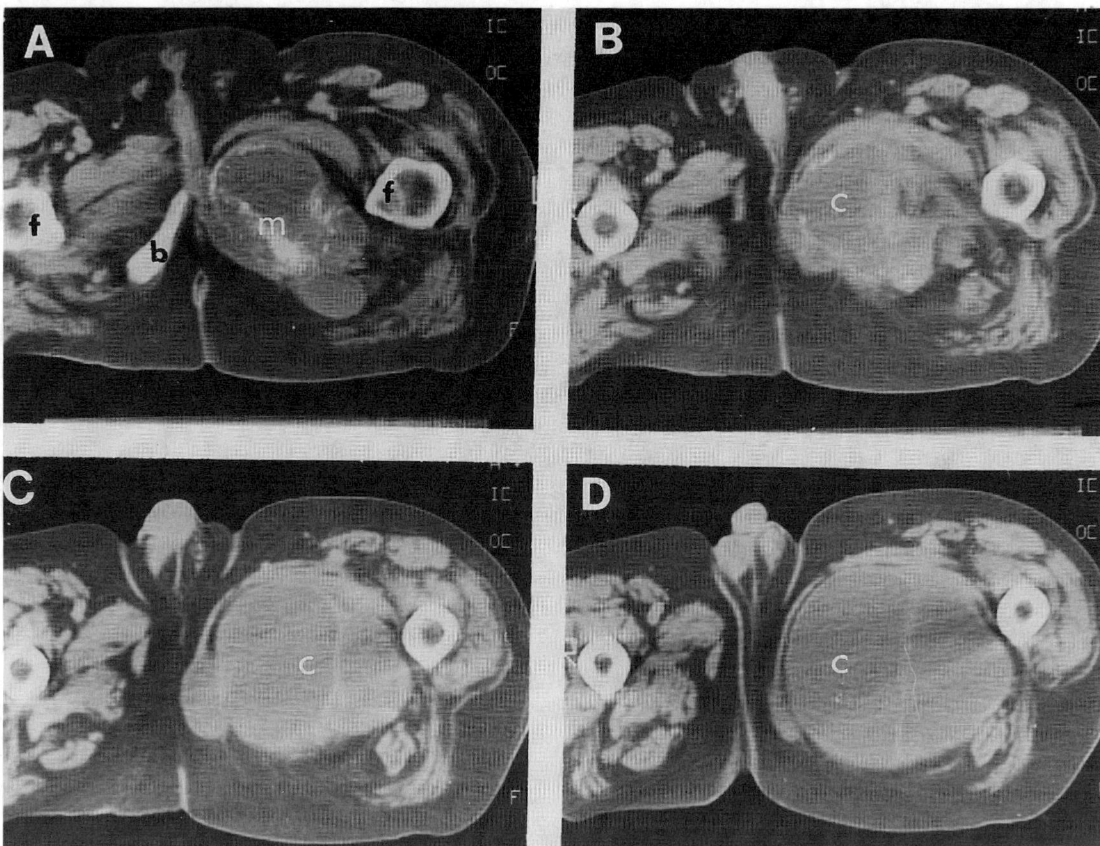

Figure 10-51. Sequential CT scans from the level of the ischial and pubic bones (A) going distantly by 1 cm intervals (B,C). The scans reveal an expansile metastasis (m) in the left pubic (b) and ischial bones. The large cystic component (c) of the bony metastasis extends into the thigh (m = metastasis, C = cystic component of the metastasis, b = parts of ischium and pubic bones, f = femur).

Figure 10-52. Lateral film of skull shows numerous lytic lesions with a "geographic pattern" of bone destruction.

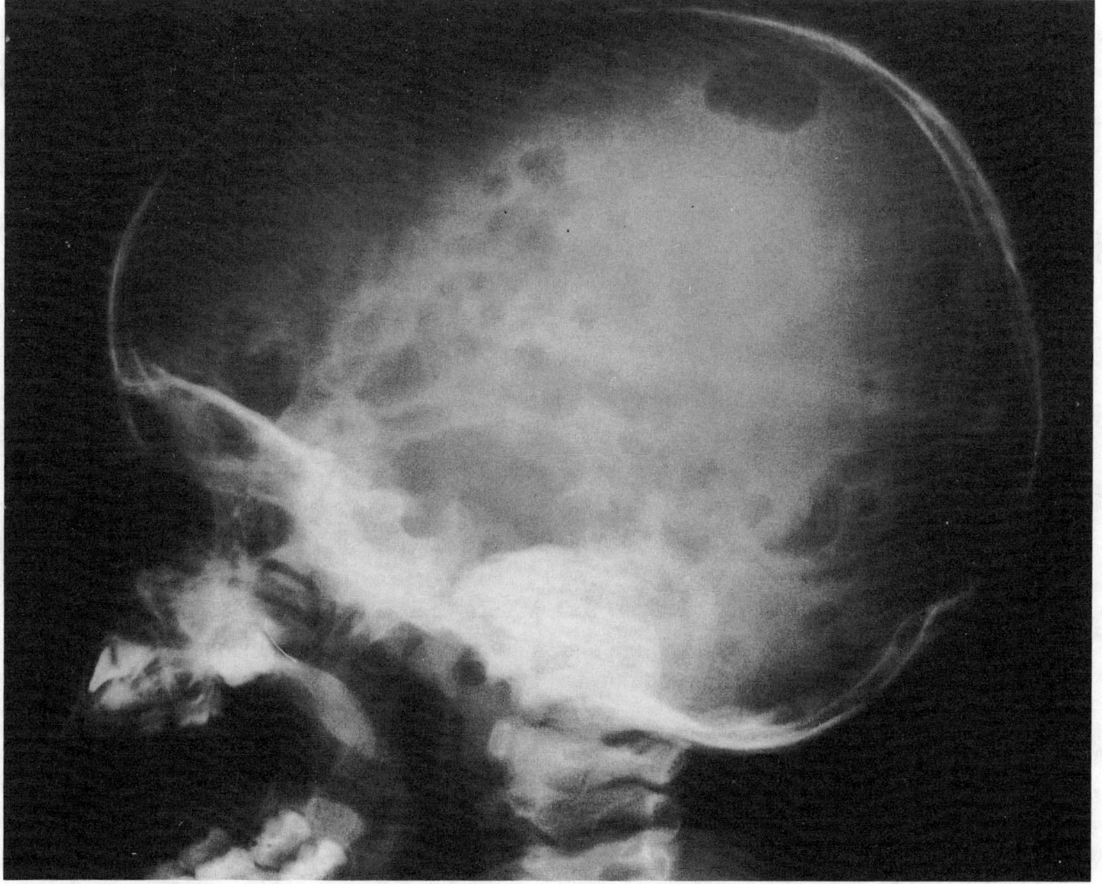

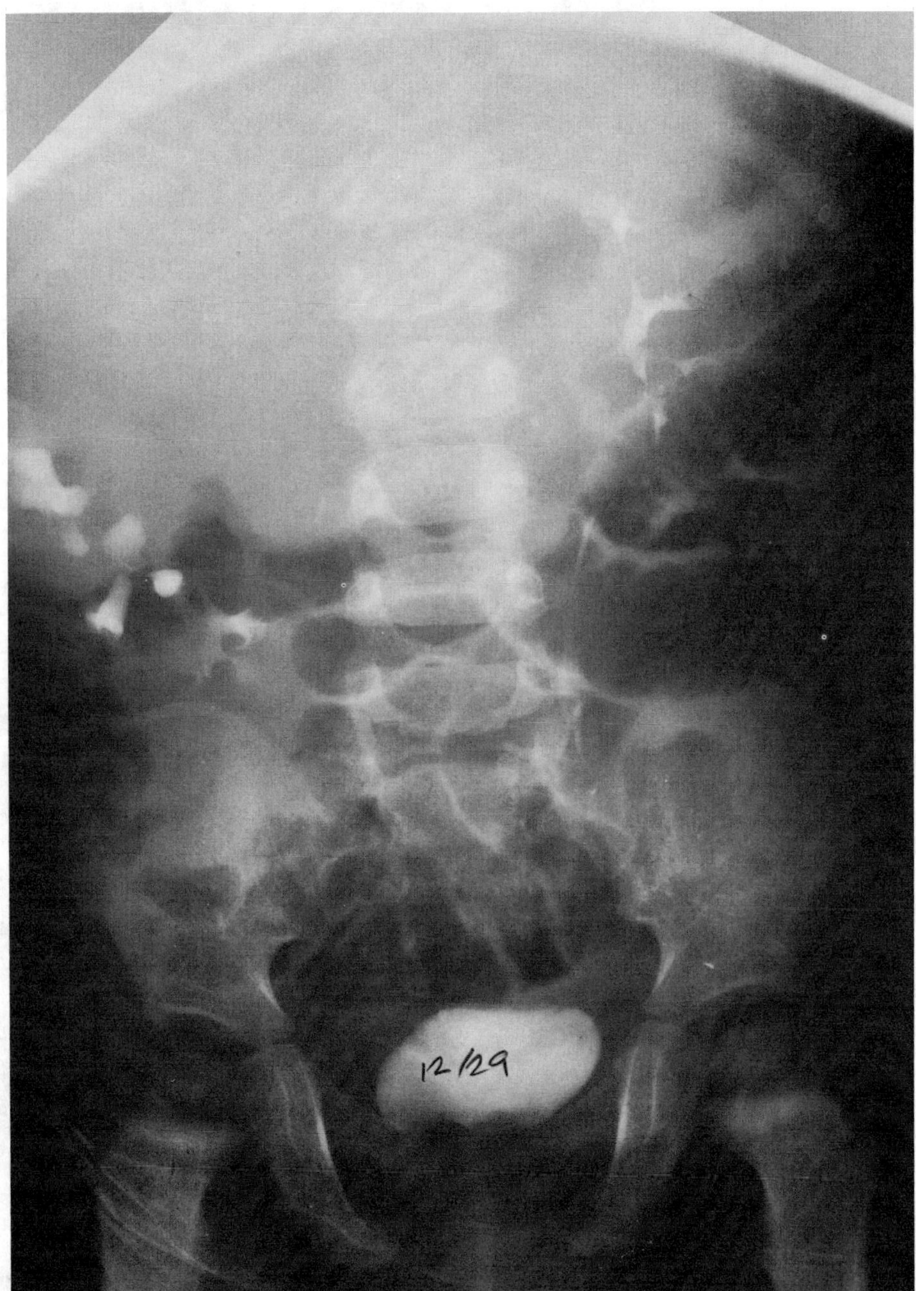

Figure 10-53. I.V. urogram shows normal left kidney. Right kidney is displaced downward and outward by a large suprarenal mass extending medial to the kidney.

Figure 10-54. Anteroposterior view of the knee of a child with metastatic neuroblastoma shows a poorly defined lytic lesion. Large soft-tissue mass extends medially, and there is a pathological fracture of femur. Note the
periosteal new bone formation. Also seen are destructive lesions in proximal tibia.

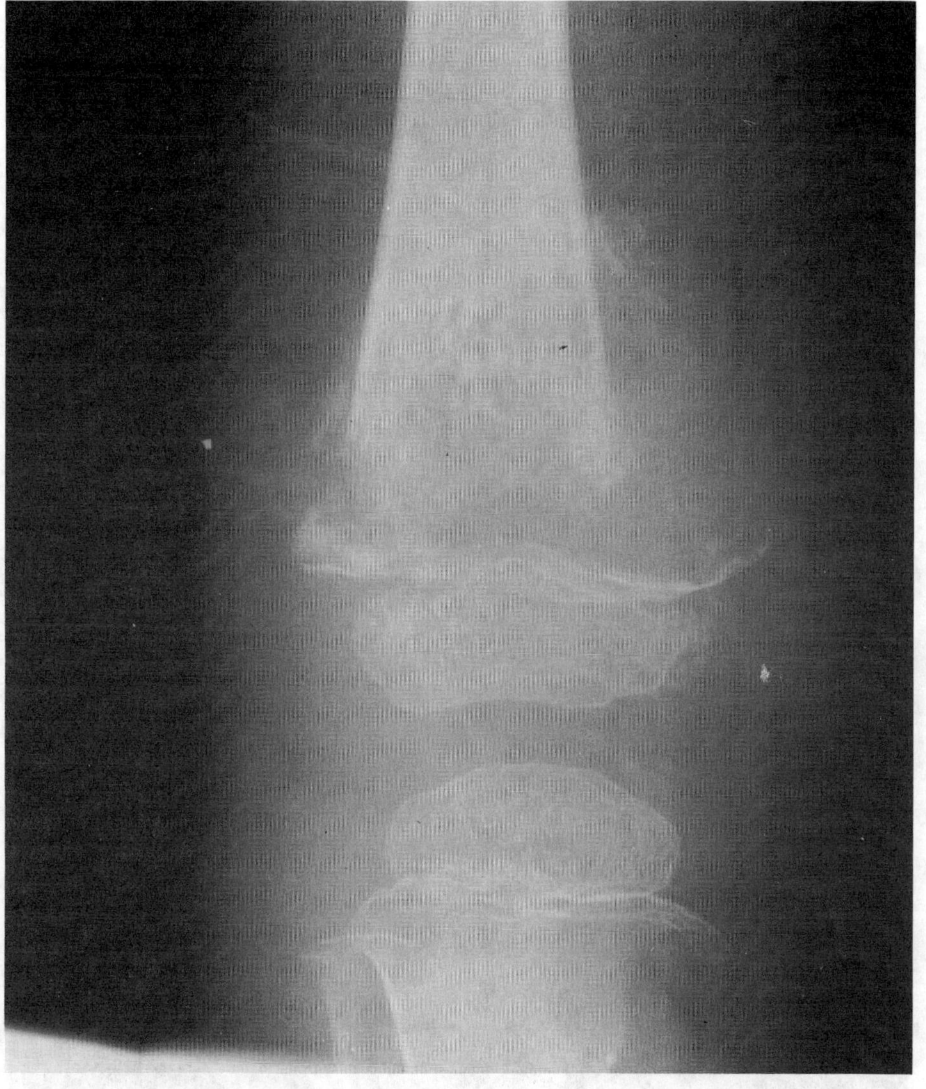

Figure 10-55. Oblique projection of I.V. urogram of a child with Wilms' tumor shows a large mass occupying the lower pole left kidney. The caliceal system is draped over the mass and the calyces are dilated.

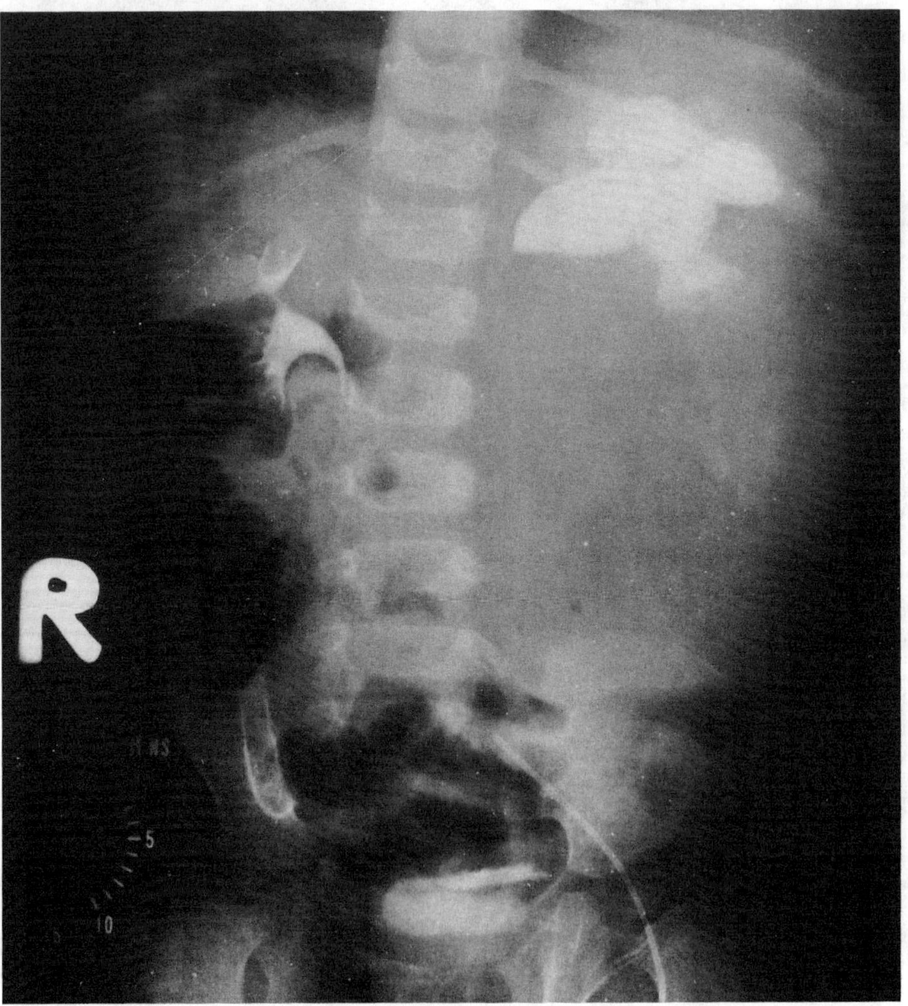

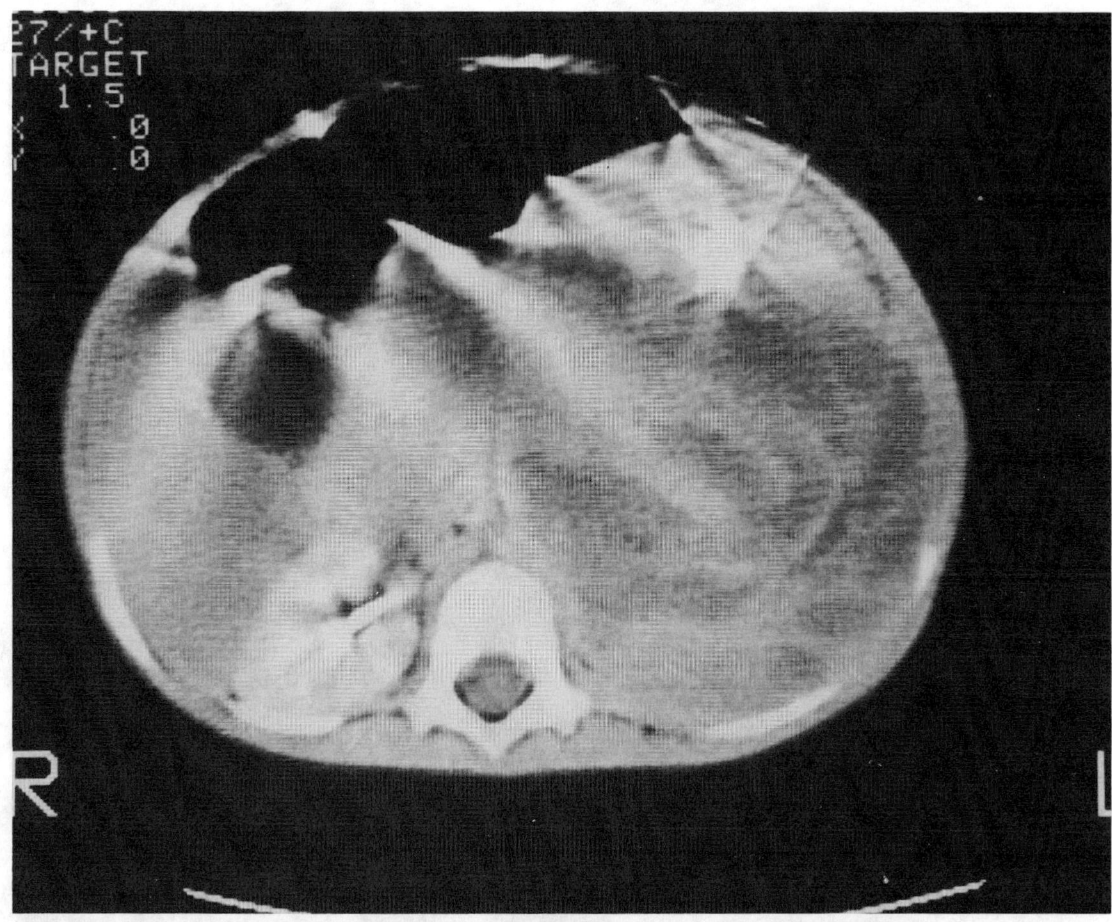

Figure 10-56. CT scan of the abdomen of a patient with Wilms' tumor shows a normal right kidney and markedly enlarged left kidney with areas of low attenuation within the tumor representing necrosis.

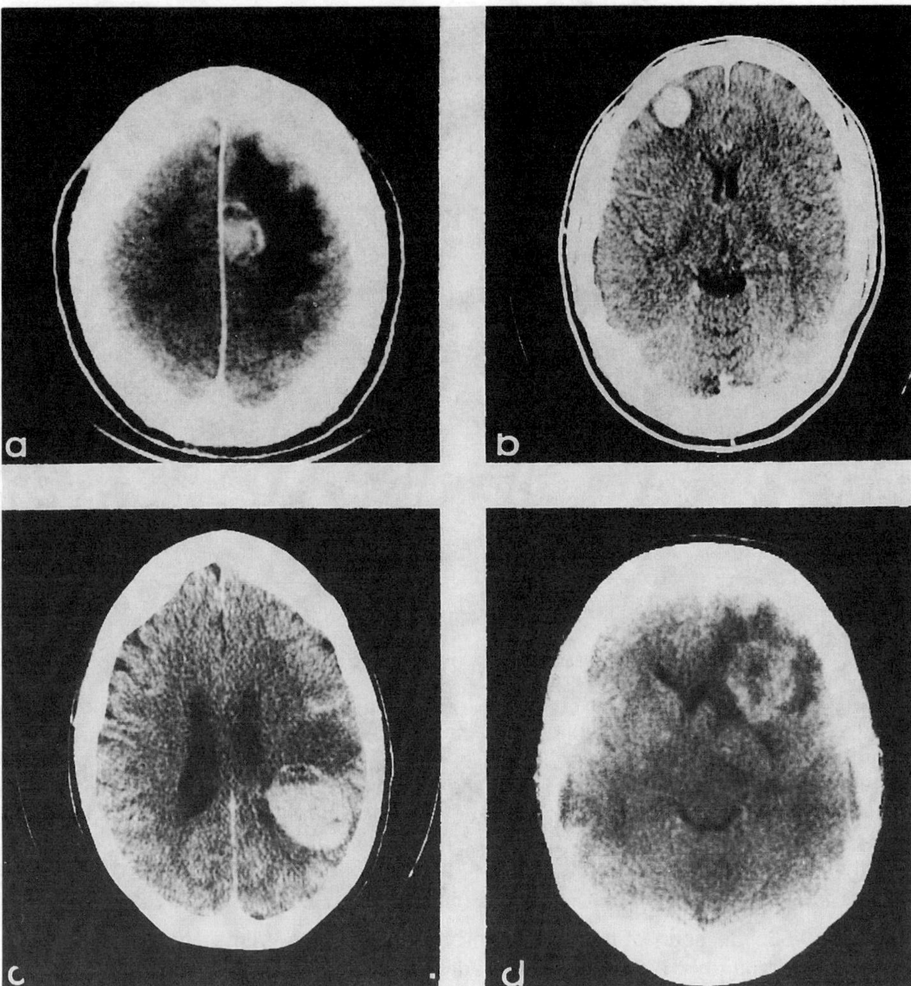

Figure 10-57. CT scans of the brain showing solitary metastases. A—Metastatic squamous cell carcinoma of the lung; B—metastatic terato carcinoma of the mediastinum; C—a hemorrhagic metastasis of malignant melanoma; D—metastatic rectal carcinoma.

Figure 10-58. CT scans of the brain showing multiple lesions. Scan A reveals multiple nodules, some solid, some ring-enhancing, with variable amounts of surrounding edema in a 29-yr-old female with metastatic adenocarcinoma of the lung. Scan B shows solid nodules, again with variable amounts of surrounding edema, this time caused by metastatic squamous cell carcinoma of the lung. Scan C shows many confluent solid enhancing nodules, all in the right hemisphere, with edema and mass effect in a 35-yr-old female with recurrent meningioma (the original tumor was intraventricular). Scan D reveals multiple ring lesions, all in the left hemisphere, with little edema or mass effect, proven to be "multicentric" glioblastoma multiforme in a 45-yr-old male.

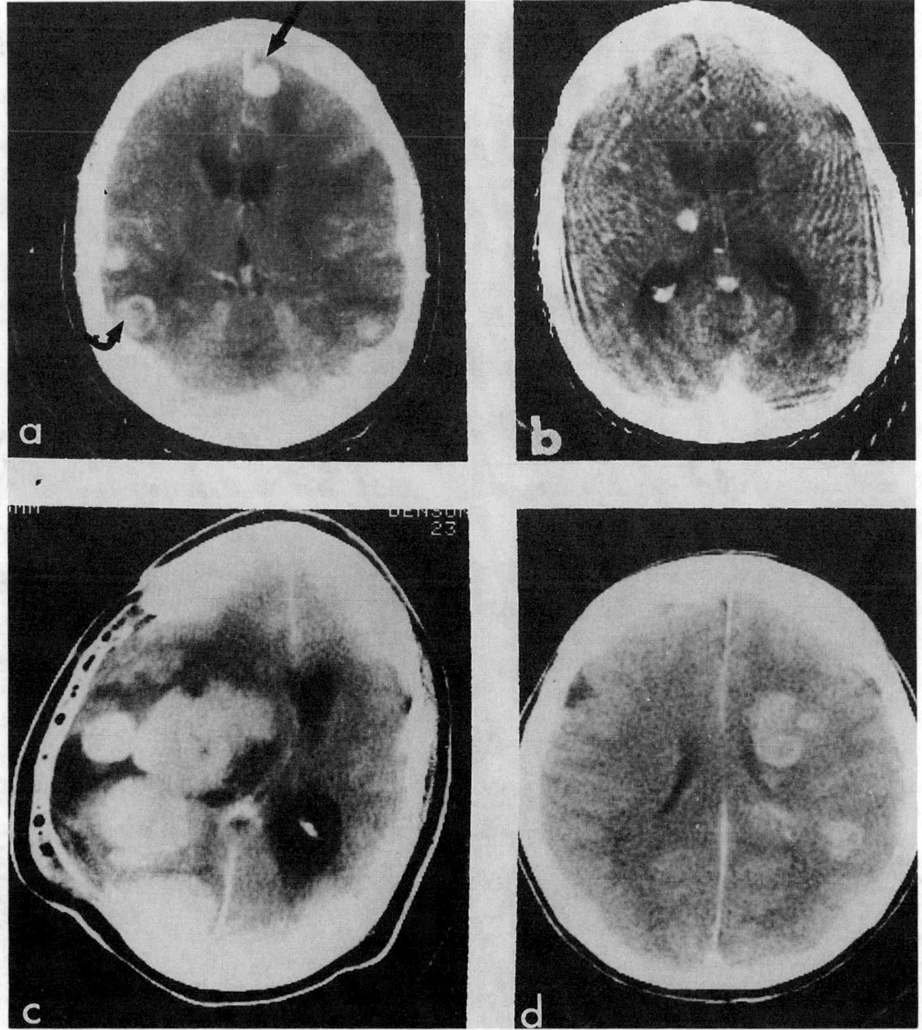

Figure 10-59. CT scans of the brain and skull with ring lesions in patients with various disorders. A—Metastatic leiomyosarcoma. B—Glioma. C—This scan offers a clue to the cerebellar abscess, namely sclerosis of the adjacent petrous bone and opacification of the mastoid air cells on the left. Scan D also shows 2 hyperdense nodules with peripheral ring enhancement in left frontal lobe, so-called "target" lesion, typical of resolving hemorrhage, in a patient 15 days after head trauma. Frequently, head trauma initially causes a solid single lesion that transforms into a target lesion 7 days after the traumatic event, when the hemorrhage starts resolving.

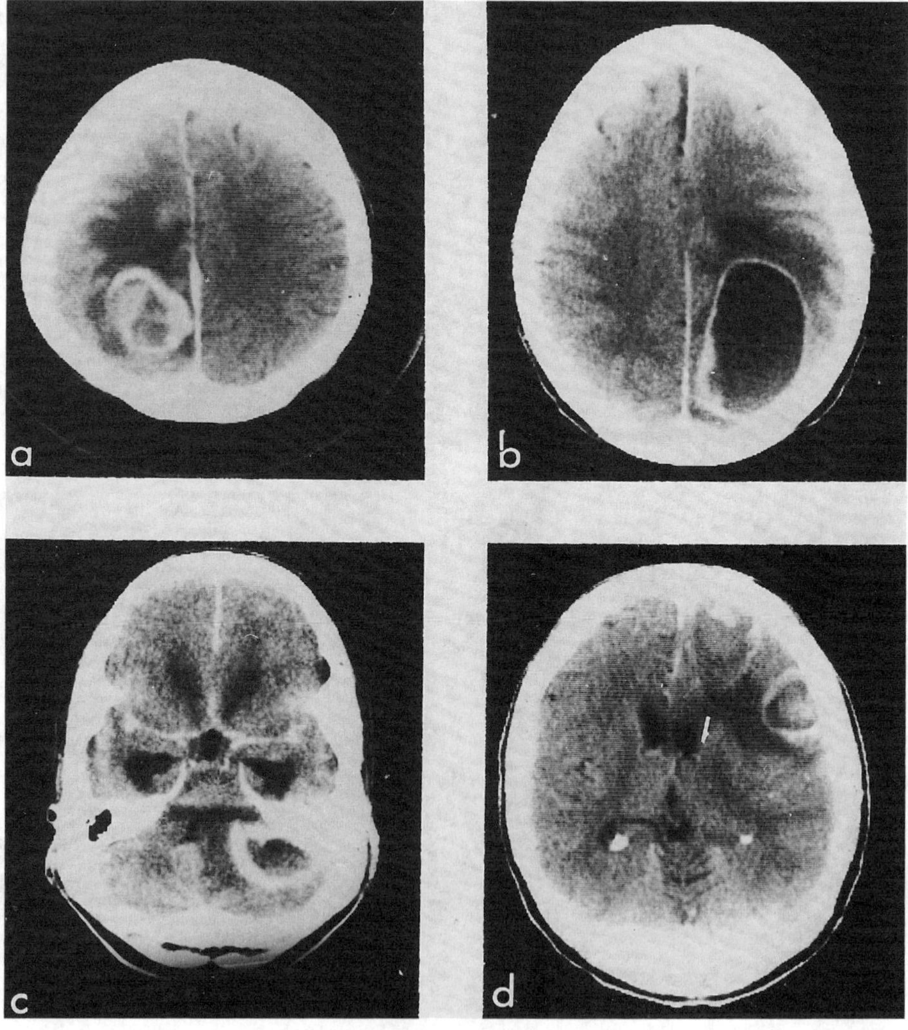

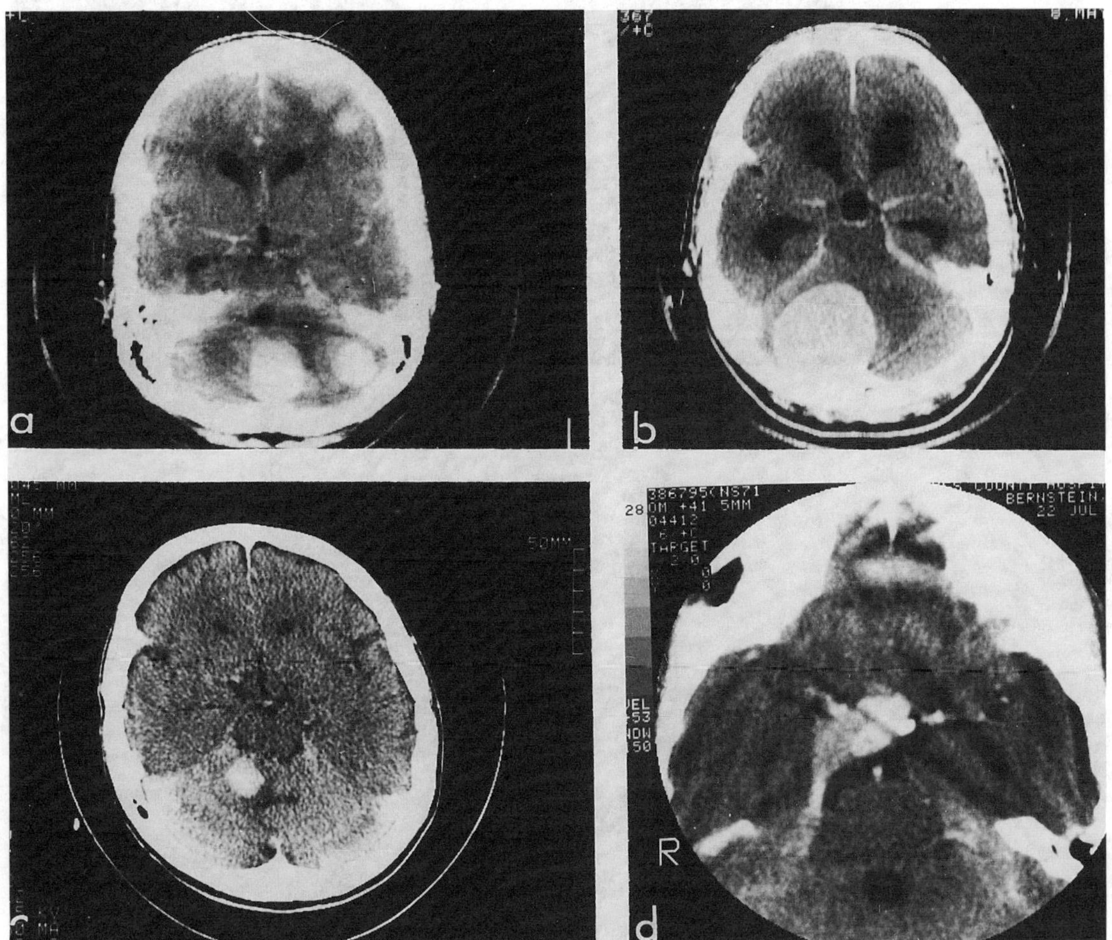

Figure 10-60. CT scans of the head showing nodular lesions of various sizes. Scan A shows 2 cerebellar and 1 left frontal nodule in a 29-yr-old female with metastatic lung cancer. The first 2 have surrounding edema and produce obstructive hydrocephalus; the last has almost no mass effect on the frontal horn. Not all solid nodules are metastatic, however. Scan B shows a large tentorial meningioma with little edema but obstructive hydrocephalus. Scan C is primary cerebellar hemangioblastoma, and scan D is a juxtasellar extra-axial primary lymphoma.

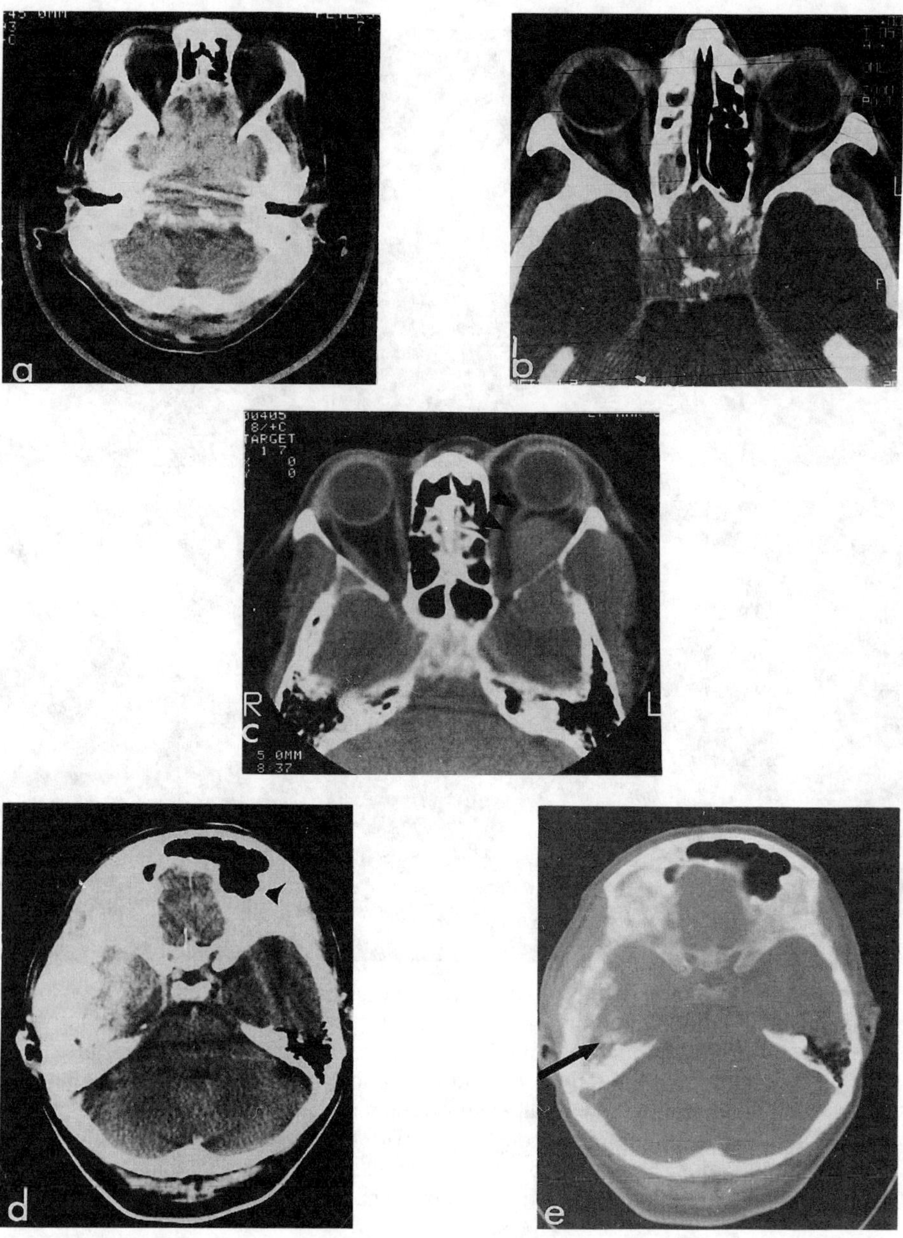

Figure 10-61. CT scans of the head showing various lesions of the base of the skull. Scans A & B show enlargement and destruction of the sella. The former is due to metastatic renal cell carcinoma, the latter to primary chordoma of the skull base. The soft tissue mass in scan C involves the orbit, the cheek, and middle cranial fossa, with destruction of the left sphenoid bone due to multiple myeloma. Severe stretching of the optic nerve (arrowheads) produced left blindness. Scan D shows a right middle cranial fossa mass (arrows), which on bone settings (scan E) is associated with flocculant calcification (arrow) and bone expansion. This appearance is frequent with meningioma, but this is a surgically proven metastasis to the dura from carcinoma of the prostate.

Figure 10-62. Malignant tumors of the spine as detected by contrast myelography. A—An expanded conus medullaris pushes the contrast away from itself in all directions. Although this appearance may be seen in any intramedullary mass, primary or secondary, this 12-yr-old child had ependymoma. B—A mass below the conus is capped by contrast in the subarachnoid space. Most intradural extramedullary masses are benign (neurofibroma, meningioma), but many CNS tumors seed the subarachnoid space, and systemic tumors may metastasize there. This 45-yr-old female has metastatic breast cancer. C—Circumferential "waisting" of the subarachnoid contrast by epidural disease. The pathological fracture of the superior end plate of L2 indicated bony metastasis with growth of tumor into the epidural space in this patient, who has squamous cell lung cancer. Primary epidural lymphoma could also produce these changes in the contrast column.

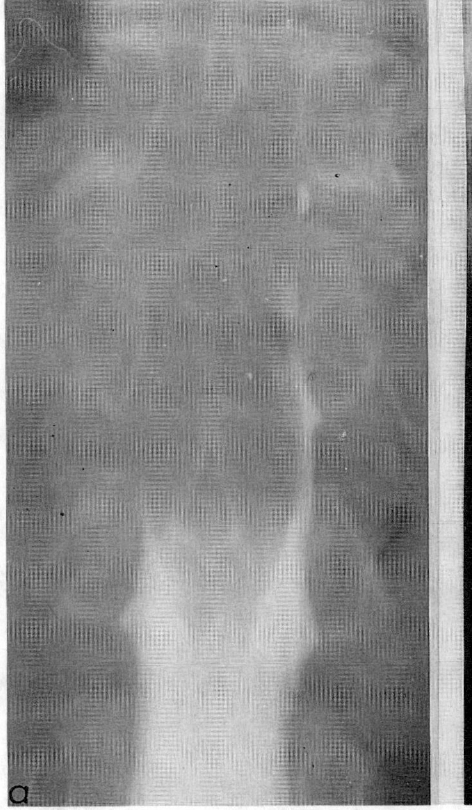
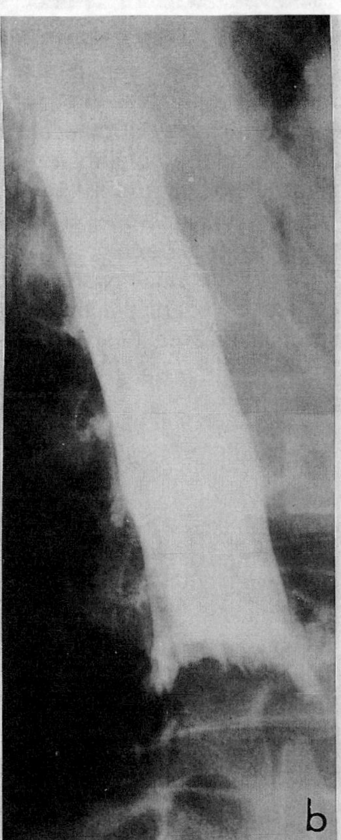
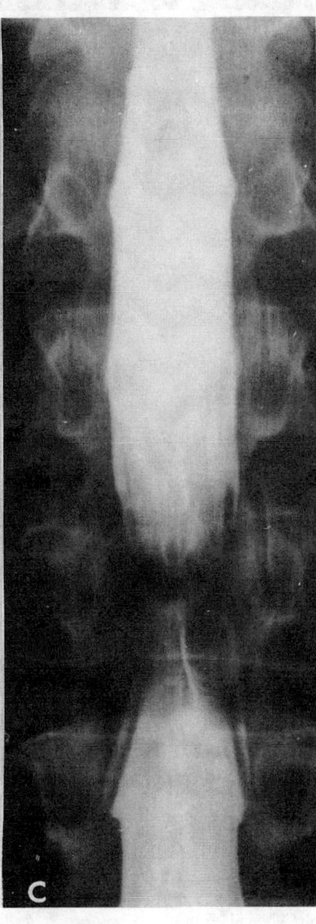

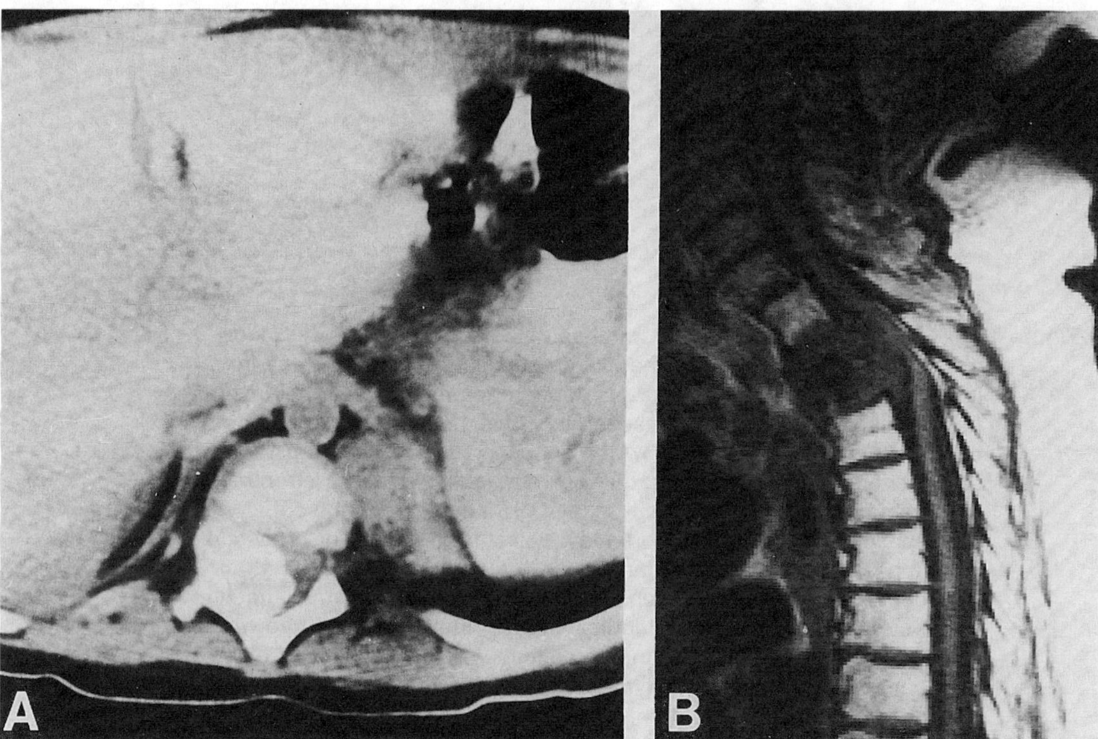

Figure 10-63. A sample of each of the 2 newest radiologic modalities used to diagnose malignant tumors of the spine—the CT scan and the magnetic
resonance image (MRI). A shows an axial CT scan of the spine at the
level of L2 vertebra; intrathecal contrast outlines the subarachnoid space
and shows the left epidural tumor as well as the left paraspinal neuroblastoma. B shows an MRI T1-weighted sagittal image of the cervicotho-
racic junction that reveals diminished signal intensity of the vertebral
bodies of T1 and T2 compatible with bone marrow replacement by tumor. This is associated with growth of tumor into the ventral epidural
space, and dorsal displacement of the thoracic spinal cord in a female
with metastatic breast cancer and leg weakness.

References

1. Lee JK, Sagel SS, Stanley RJ, eds. Computed body tomography. New York: Raven Press, 1983.
2. Naidich DP, Zerhouni EA, Siegelman SS. Computed tomography of the thorax. New York: Raven Press, 1984.
3. Ledley RS, Huang HK, Mazziota JC. Cross-sectional anatomy: an atlas in computerized tomography. Baltimore: Williams & Wilkins, 1977.
4. Kuhns LR, Seeger J. Atlas of computed tomography variants. Chicago: Year Book Medical Publishers, 1983.
5. Lee SH, Rao K. Cranial computed tomography. New York: McGraw-Hill, 1983.
6. Williams, Haughton, Victor. Cranial computed tomography. St. Louis: Mosby, 1985.
7. Takashima T et al. Diagnosis and screening of small hepatocellular carcinomas. Radiology 1982; 145:635–38.
8. Brandt DJ, Johnson CD, Stephens DH, Weiland LH. Imaging of fibrolamellar hepatocellular carcinoma. AJR 1988; 151:295–99.
9. Murayama S, Tsukamoto Y, Watanabe H, Nakata H. Computed tomography of residual hepatomas following transcatheter arterial embolization. J Comput Assist Tomogr 1986; 10(6):969–72.
10. Yoshikawa J, Matsui O, Takashima, et al. Fatty metamorphosis in hepatocellular carcinoma: radiologic features in 10 cases. AJR 1988; 151:717–20.
11. Case records of Massachusetts General Hospital: hepatocellular carcinoma. N Engl J Med, Aug 27, 1987; 556–64.
12. Knopf D et al. Liver lesions: comparative accuracy of scintigraphy and computed tomography. AJR 1982; 138:623–27.
13. Nelson RC, Chezmar JL, Sugarbaker PH, Barnardino ME. Hepatic tumors: comparison of CT during arterial portography, delayed CT, and MR imaging for preoperative evaluation. Radiology 1989; 172:27–34.
14. Sugarbaker, PH. Surgical decision making for large bowel cancer metastatic to the liver. Radiology 1990; 621–26.
15. Freeny PC. Portal vein tumor thrombus: demonstration by computed tomographic arteriography. J. Comput Assist Tomogr 1980; 4(2):263–64.
16. Araki T, Suda K, Sekikawa T, Ishii Y, Hihara T, Kachi K. Portal venous tumor thrombosis associated with gastric adenocarcinoma. Radiology 1990; 174:811–14.
17. Martin K, Balfe DM, Lee JKT. Computed tomography of portal vein thrombosis: unusual appearances and pitfalls in diagnosis. J. Comput Assist Tomogr 1989; 13(5):811–16.
18. Imaeda T, Yamawaki Y, Hirota K, Suzuki M, Seki M, Doi H. Tumor thrombus in the branches of the distal portal vein: CT demonstration. J Comput Assist Tomogr 1989; 13(2):262–68.
19. Scatarige JC et al. Computed tomography of calcified liver masses. J Comput Assist Tomogr 1983; 7(1):83–89.
20. Virgo M et al. CT demonstration of portal and superior mesenteric vein thrombosis in hepatocellular carcinoma. J Comput Assist Tomogr 1980; 4(5):627–29.
21. Jolles H et al. CT of ascites: differential diagnosis. AJR 1980; 135:315–22.
22. Walkey M, Friedman AC, Sohotra P, Radecki PD. CT manifestations of peritoneal carcinomatosis. AJR 1988; 150:1035–41.
23. Jeffrey RB Jr. CT demonstration of peritoneal implants. AJR 1980; 135:323–26.
24. Yeh C. Ultrasonography and computed tomography of carcinoma of the gallbladder. Radiology 1979; 133:167–73.
25. Lane J, Buck JL, Zeman RK. Primary carcinoma of the gallbladder: a pictorial essay. RadioGraphics 1989; 9(2):209.
26. So CB, Gibney RG, Scudamore CH. Carcinoma of the gallbladder: a risk associated with gallbladder-preserving treatments for cholelithiasis. Radiology 1990; 174:127–30.
27. Jafris Z et al. Comparison of CT and angiography in assessing resectability of pancreatic carcinoma. AJR 1984; 142:525–29.

28. Megibow A et al. Thickening of the celiac axis and/or superior mesenteric artery: a sign of pancreatic carcinoma on computed tomography. Radiology 1981; 141:449–51.

29. Freeny PC. Radiology of the pancreas: two decades of progress in imaging and intervention. AJR 1988; 150:975–81.

30. Friedman AC. Imaging pancreatic carcinoma. Appl Radiol Feb 1990; 21–28.

31. Ellert J. The role of computed tomography in the initial staging and subsequent management of lymphomas. J Comput Assist Tomogr 1980; 4(3):368–91.

32. Greco A, Jelliffe AM, Maher EJ, Leung WL. MR imaging of lymphomas: impact on therapy. J Comput Assist Tomogr 12(5):785–91.

33. Costello P, Duszlak EJ Jr, Kane RA, Lee RG, Clouse ME. Peripancreatic lymph node enlargement in Hodgkin's disease, non-Hodgkin's lymphoma, and pancreatic carcinoma. CT: J Comput Tomogr 1984; 8:1–11.

34. Cohan RH, Baker ME, Cooper C, Moore JO, Saeed M, Dunnick NR. Computed tomography of primary retroperitoneal malignancies. J Comput Assist Tomogr 1988;12(5):804–10.

35. Thomas J et al. Staging of testicular carcinoma: comparison of CT and lymphangiography. AJR 1981; 137:991–96.

36. Dunnick NR et al. Value of CT and lymphangiography: distinguishing retroperitoneal metastases from nonseminomatous testicular tumors. AJR 1981; 136:1093–99.

37. Stomper PC, Fung CY, Socinski MA, Jochelson MS, Garnick MB, Richie JP. Detection of retroperitoneal matastases in early-stage nonseminomatous testicular cancer: analysis of different CT criteria. AJR 1987; 149:1187–90.

38. Stomper PC, Socinski MA, Kaplan WD, Gasrnick MB. Failure patterns of nonseminomatous testicular germ cell tumors: radiographic analysis of 51 cases. Radiology 1988; 167:641–46.

39. Steinfeld AD. Testicular germ cell tumors: review of contemporary evaluation and management. Radiology 1990; 175:603–06.

40. Stephens DH et al. Diagnosis and evaluation of retroperitoneal tumors by computed tomography. AJR 1977; 129:395–402.

41. Lane RH, Stephens DH, Reiman HM. Primary retroperitoneal neoplasms: CT findings in 90 cases with clinical and pathologic correlation. AJR 1989; 152:83–89.

42. Levine MS et al. Detecting lymphatic metastases from prostatic carcinoma: superiority of CT. AJR 1981; 137:207–11.

43. Platt JF, Bree RL, Schwab RE. The accuracy of CT in the staging of carcinoma of the prostate. AJR 1987; 149:315–18.

44. Schnall MD, Bezzi M, Pollack HM, Kressel HY. Magnetic resonance imaging of the prostate. Magn Reson Quarterly 1990; 6(1):1–16.

45. Feldberg MA et al. Psoas compartment disease studied by computed tomographic analysis of 50 cases and subject review. Radiology 1983; 148:505–12.

46. Walsh et al. Recurrent carcinoma of the cervix: CT diagnosis. AJR 1981: 136:117–22.

47. Vick CW, Walsh JW, Wheelock JB, Brewer WH. Computed tomographic evaluation of parametrial extension from cervical cancer. Radiographics 1984; 4(5):787–99.

48. Ibid.

49. Jacques et al. CT assisted pelvic and abdominal aspiration biopsy in gynecologic malignancy. Radiology 1978; 128:651–55.

50. Eising EG, Reiser MF, Vassallo P, Peters PE. Cystic pelvic mass in a patient having recurrent carcinoma of the cervix. Invest Radiol 1990; 25:205–08.

51. Kim SH, Choi BI, Lee HP, et al. Uterine cervical carcinoma: comparison of CT and MR findings. Radiology 1990; 175:45–51.

52. Van Dyke JA, Holley HC, Anderson SD. Review of iliopsoas anatomy and pathology. RadioGraphics 1987; 7(1):53–84.

53. Toghashi KT, Nishimura K, Sagoh T, et al. Carcinoma of the cervix: staging with MR imaging. Radiology 1989; 171:245–51.

54. Gazelle GS, Haaga JR. Guided percutaneous biopsy of intraabdominal lesions. AJR 1989; 153:929–35.

55. Copeland P. The incidentally discovered adrenal mass. Ann Intern Med 1983; 88:94–95.

56. Sandler P et al. Computed tomographic evaluation of the adrenal gland in the preoperative assessment of bronchogenic carcinoma. Radiology 1982; 145:733–36.

57. Bernardino M et al. CT guided adrenal biopsy: accuracy, safety, and indications. AJR 1985; 144:67–69.

58. Francis IR, Smid A, Gross MD, Shapiro B, Naylor B, Glazer GM. Adrenal masses in oncologic patients: functional and morphologic evaluation. Radiology 1988; 166:353–56.

59. Cranston PE, Routh WD. Use of CT in metastatic adrenal gland tumor. Comput Med Imag Graph 1990; 14(2):143–46.

60. Falke THM, te Strake L, Sandler MP, et al. Magnetic resonance imaging of the adrenal glands. RadioGraphics 1987; 7(2):343.

61. Koss J et al. CT staging of bladder carcinoma. AJR 1981; 137:359–62.

62. Weyman P et al. Pelvic adenopathy from bladder and prostate carcinoma: detection by rapid sequential computer tomography. AJR 1983; 140:95–99.

63. Shirkhoda A, Dexeus FH, Logothetis CJ. Clinical and radiologic staging of locally advanced and inoperable bladder carcinoma. CT: J Comput Tomogr 1988:298–312.

64. Raghavan D, Shipley WU, Garnick MB, Russell PJ, Richie JP. Biology and management of bladder cancer. N Engl J Med 1990; 322(16):1129–38.

65. Keller F et al. Percutaneous embolization of bony pelvic neoplasms with tissue adhesive. Radiology 1983; 147:21–27.

66. Goldstein HM et al. Transcatheter arterial embolization in the management of bleeding in the cancer patient. Radiology 1975; 115:603–08.

67. Varma J, Huben RP, Wajsman Z, Pontes JE. Therapeutic embolization of pelvic metastases of renal cell carcinoma. J Urol 1984; 131:647.

68. Arki T et al. Leukemic involvement of kidneys in children: CT features. J Comput Assist Tomogr 1982; 6(6):781–84.

69. Dunnick NR et al. Computed tomography of extracranial chloroma. J Comput Assist Tomogr 1982; 6(1):83–85.

70. Breatnach E, Stanley RJ, Carpenter JT. Intrarenal chloroma causing obstructive nephropathy: CT characteristics. J Comput Assist Tomogr 1985; 9(4):822–24.

71. Olson M, Posniak H. CT characteristics of a hyperdense renal mass due to Richter syndrome. J Comput Assist Tomogr 1988; 12(4):669–70.

72. Pomeranz SJ, Hawkins HH, Towbin R, Lisberg WN, Clark RA. Granulocytic sarcoma (chloroma): CT manifestations. Radiology 1985; 155:167–70.

73. Ellert J et al. The value of CT in malignant colonic tumors. CT: J Comput Tomogr 1980; 4(3):225–40.

74. Fisher J. Abnormal colonic wall thickening on computer tomography. J Comput Assist Tomogr 1983; 7(1):90–97.

75. Balthazar EJ, Megibow AJ, Hulnick D, Naidich DP. Carcinoma of the colon: detection and preoperative staging by CT. AJR 1988; 150:301–06.

76. Freeny PC, Marks WM, Ryan JA, Bolen JW. Colorectal carcinoma evaluation with CT: preoperative staging and detection of postoperative recurrence. Radiology 1986; 158:347–51.

77. Balfe DM et al. Computer tomography of extracranial chloroma. J Comput Assist Tomogr 1982; 6(1):781–84.

78. Lee KR et al. Computer tomographic staging of malignant gastric neoplasms. Radiology 1979; 133:151–65.

79. Sussman SK, Halvorsen RA Jr, Illescas FF, et al. Gastric adenocarcinoma: CT versus surgical staging. Radiology 1988; 167:335–40.

80. Moss A et al. Esophageal carcinoma: pretherapy staging by computed tomography. AJR 1981; 136:1051–56.

81. Daffner R et al. CT of the esophagus: carcinoma. AJR 1979; 133:1051–55.

82. Recht MP, Coleman BG, Barbot DJ, et al. Recurrent esophageal carcinoma at thoracotomy incisions: diagnostic contributions of CT. J Comput Assist Tomogr 1989; 13(1):58–60.

83. Becker CD, Barbier PA, Terrier F, Porcellini B. Patterns of recurrence of esophageal carcinoma after transhiatal esophagectomy and gastric interposition. AJR 1987; 148:273–77.

84. Halvorsen RA Jr, Magruder-Habib K, Foster WL Jr, Roberts L Jr, Postlethwait RW, Thompson WM. Esophageal cancer staging by CT: long-term follow-up study. Radiology 1986; 161:147–51.
85. Press G, Glazer HS, Wasserman TH, et al. Thoracic wall involvement by Hodgkin's disease and non-Hodgkin's lymphoma: CT evaluation. Radiology 1985; 157:195–98.
86. Jafri SZ, Roberts JL, Bree RL, Tabor HD. Computed tomography of chest wall masses. RadioGraphics 1989; 9(1):51–68.
87. Mirvis S, Dutcher JP, Haney PS, et al. CT of malignant pleural mesothelioma. AJR 1983; 140:665–70.
88. Lynch DA, Gamsu G, Aberle DR. Conventional and high resolution computed tomography in the diagnosis of asbestos-related diseases. RadioGraphics 1989; 9(3):523–51.
89. Glazer HS, Aronberg DJ, Sagel SS, Emami B. Utility of CT in detecting post pneumonectomy carcinoma recurrence. AJR 1984; 142:487–94.
90. Meyer J, Munzenrider JE. Computed tomographic demonstration of internal mammary lymph node metastasis in patients with locally recurrent breast carcinoma. Radiology 1981; 139:661–63.
91. Lukens JA, McLeod RA, Sim PH. Computed tomographic evaluation of primary osseous malignana neoplasms. AJR 1982; 139:45–48.
92. Tehranzadeh J, Mnaymneh W, Ghavam C, Morillo G, Murphy B. Comparison on CT and MR imaging in musculoskeletal neoplasms. J Comput Assist Tomogr 1989; 13(3):466–72.

11

HISTOPATHOLOGY OF MALIGNANT TUMORS

William L. Thelmo, M.D., with contributions from Hosoon P. Dincsoy, M.D., Caroline A. Webber, M.D., and Janet Cuttner, M.D.

Introduction

This chapter, designed to serve as a quick reference for clinicians, consists of selected illustrations of the most common malignant and benign tumors of the different systems of the body. Illustrations are grouped according to body systems and corresponding organs, along with their respective diagnoses. Cytology and fine-needle aspirates are included whenever they are useful in establishing a more rapid and accurate diagnosis. Captions for the figures include stains employed and the degree of magnification used in producing the photomicrographs. (A list of the stains and their abbreviations appears in table 11-1.)

New advances in chemotherapy demand accurate diagnoses. The past 3 decades, which have seen the production of many commercially available monoclonal antibodies and the development of flow cytometry and DNA probes, have been called the era of immunohistochemistry. Techniques developed during the period have been applied in tumor studies, particularly those of lymphomas. However, the morphologic evaluation of malignant tumors by light microscopy remains the mainstay of surgical pathology examination. The newer techniques are best used whenever indicated as an adjunct to morphologic studies in order to improve diagnostic accuracy.

The working formulation for lymphoma is based primarily on H & E light microscopic preparation. This is not to undermine the importance of cell markers; in difficult cases, light microscopy has limitations. Cell markers and electron microscopy then play a major role in reaching an accurate diagnosis.

With its high diagnostic accuracy for neoplasms such as squamous cell carcinoma, adenocarcinoma, and large-cell anaplastic tumors, fine-needle aspiration has become a frequently used technique. Other tumors such as well-differentiated thyroid carcinomas have proven to be a challenge even with the use of core needle biopsy. Cell markers, electron microscopy, and DNA ploidy determinations may occasionally help reach a definitive diagnosis.

Table 11-1. Key to Abbreviations for Stains Used in Producing Photomicrographs

Stain	Abbreviation
Combined esterase	CE
Fontana	FT
Hematoxylin and eosin	H & E
Jenner-Giemsa	J-B
Myeloperoxidase	PX
Papanicolaou	Pap
Periodic acid Schiff	PAS
Prussian blue	Fe
Sudan Black B	SBB
Terminal deoxynucleotidyl transferase	TdT

Sometimes, only resection of the entire tumor, which may then reveal capsular and/or vascular invasion, will serve to distinguish atypical follicular adenoma from well-differentiated follicular carcinoma.

Distinguishing between malignant lymphoma and small-cell carcinoma of the lung—and occasionally large-cell carcinoma—can prove to be a very difficult if not impossible task, especially when only a small biopsy is available. The same is true with round-cell tumors of childhood and some soft-tissue sarcomas of adults, even with large resected specimens. It is in this context that cell markers and electron microscopy studies should be useful—indeed, they are sometimes indispensable—in arriving at an accurate diagnosis. Similarly, the accurate identification of various types and subtypes of acute leukemia cannot be made without special histochemical stains and/or use of specific cell markers.

In order to avoid redundancy, the histopathology of tumors of similar types will be illustrated in this chapter in only 1 or 2 systems in which occurrence is common. The same approach is taken for the cytopathology of fine-needle aspirates, malignant effusions, and cerebrospinal fluid.

Malignant Tumors of the Central Nervous System

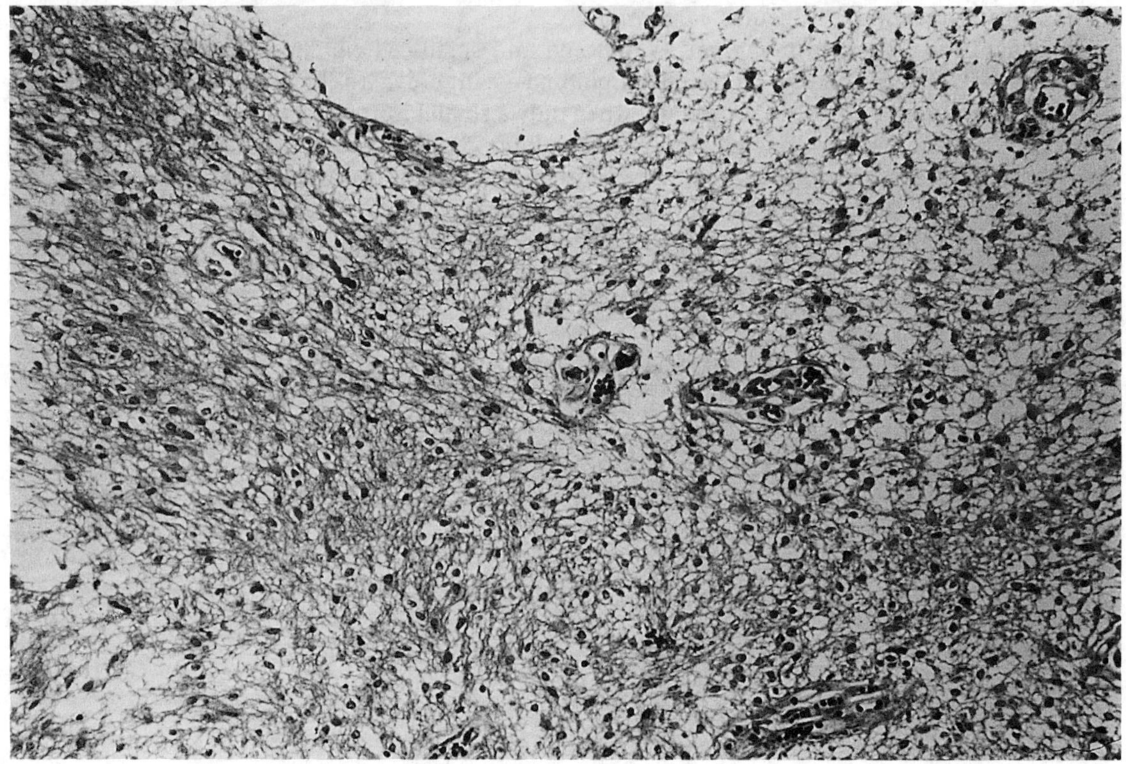

Figure 11-1. Astrocytoma of the brain. Tumor cells consist of small astrocytes somewhat larger than normal astrocytic cells, showing increased cellularity and pervading adjacent normal brain tissue without distinct tumor border. The cell types vary from fibrillary, pilocytic to gemistocytic. Depending upon the location, the tumor may exhibit more histologic uniformity as seen in cerebrum, whereas cerebellar astrocytoma shows more variation in cellular density and tendency to cyst formation. (H & E, X125)

Figure 11-2. Glioblastoma multiforme. Tumor cells vary from undifferentiated small pleomorphic cells with hyperchromatic nuclei and ill-defined processes to large, bizarre, plump giant cells with hyperchromatic to vesicular nuclei with coarse chromatin and prominent nucleoli in some. Necrosis with pseudopalisading arrangement by tumor cells is characteristic. Marked endothelial proliferation usually implies an aggressive glioma. The stromal background is fibrillar. (H & E, X125)

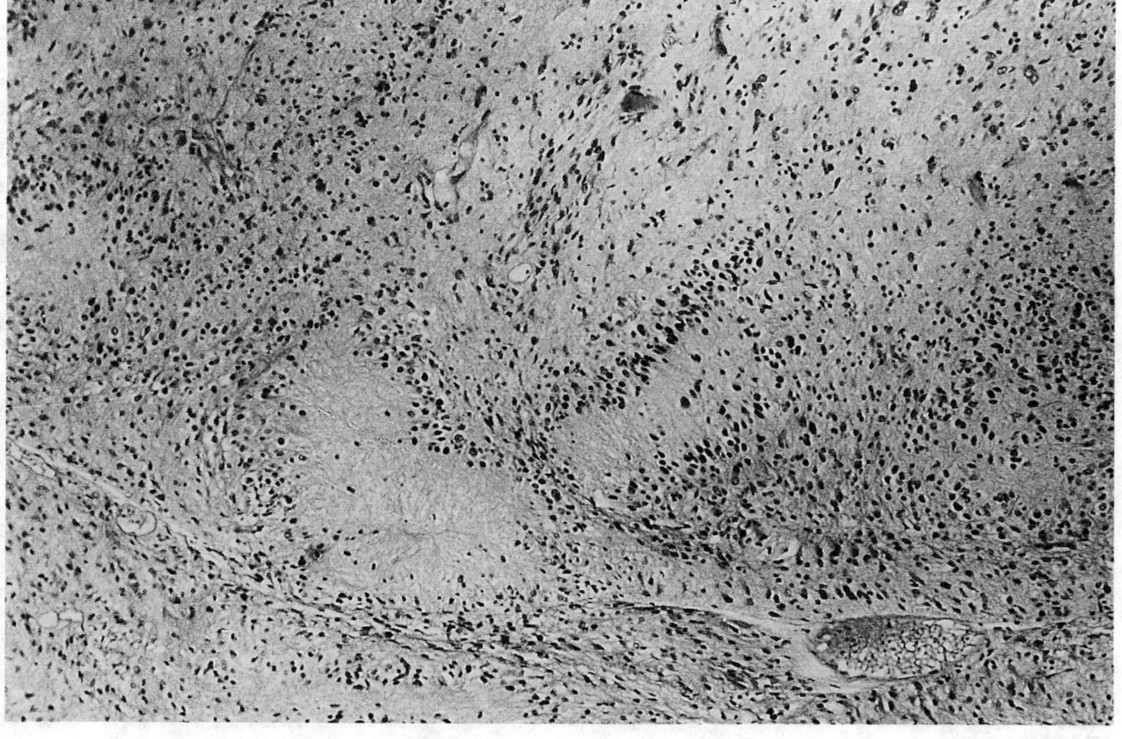

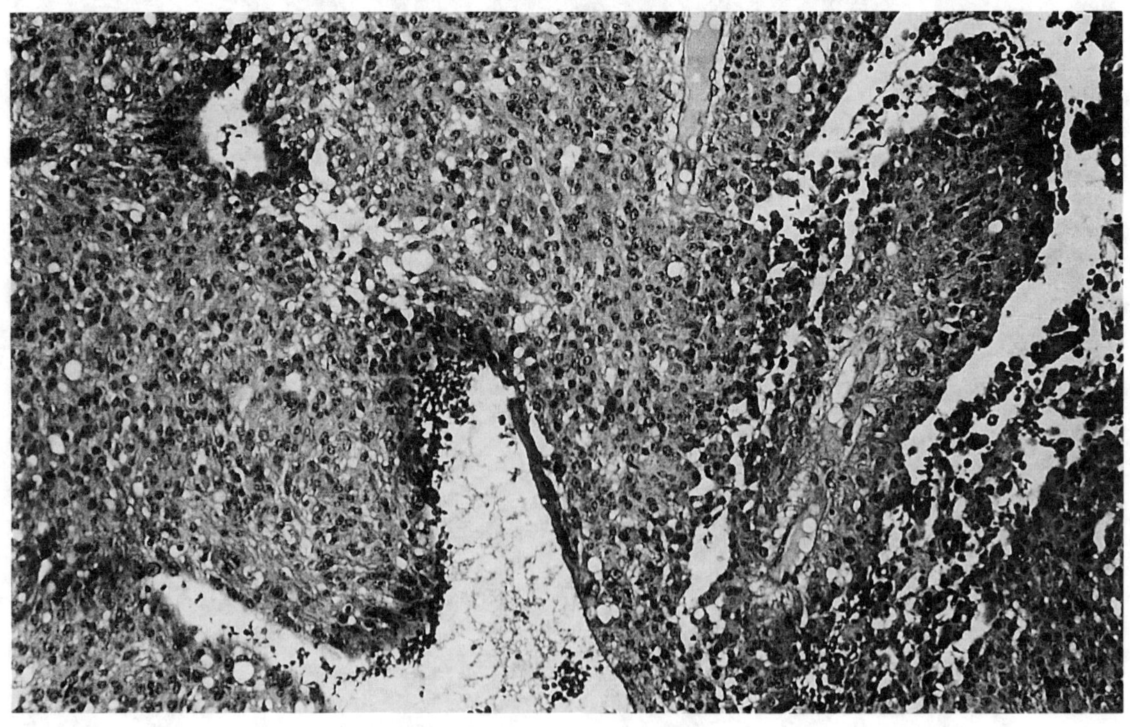

Figure 11-3. Ependymoma of the brain. Tumor cells vary from ovoid to fusiform cells with hyperchromatic nuclei having finely granular chromatin. Ependymal rosettes and perivascular pseudorosettes may be noted. The latter is more frequently seen. (H & E, X125)

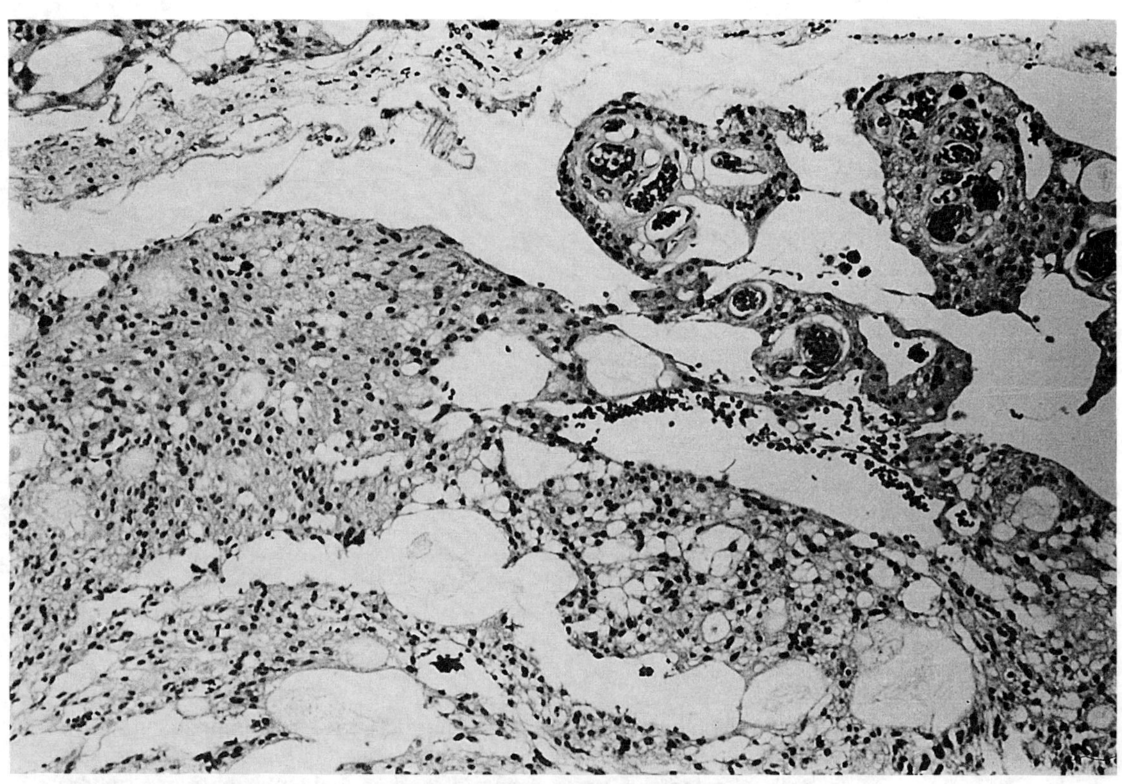

Figure 11-4. Myxopapillary ependymoma of the spinal cord. The tumor
comprises low columnar to cuboidal cells with clear cytoplasm arranged
around a core of fibrovascular tissue forming papillary pattern. Mucin
and PAS-positive material may be noted. The tumor is reminiscent of
filum terminale. (H & E, X125)

Figure 11-5. Medulloblastoma of the cerebellum. The tumor comprises small cells, round to ovoid to polar, with deeply hyperchromatic nuclei, scant or ill-defined cytoplasm proliferating in random fashion without any pattern except for occasional perivascular pseudorosette. Rosette formation is characteristic. (H & E, X125)

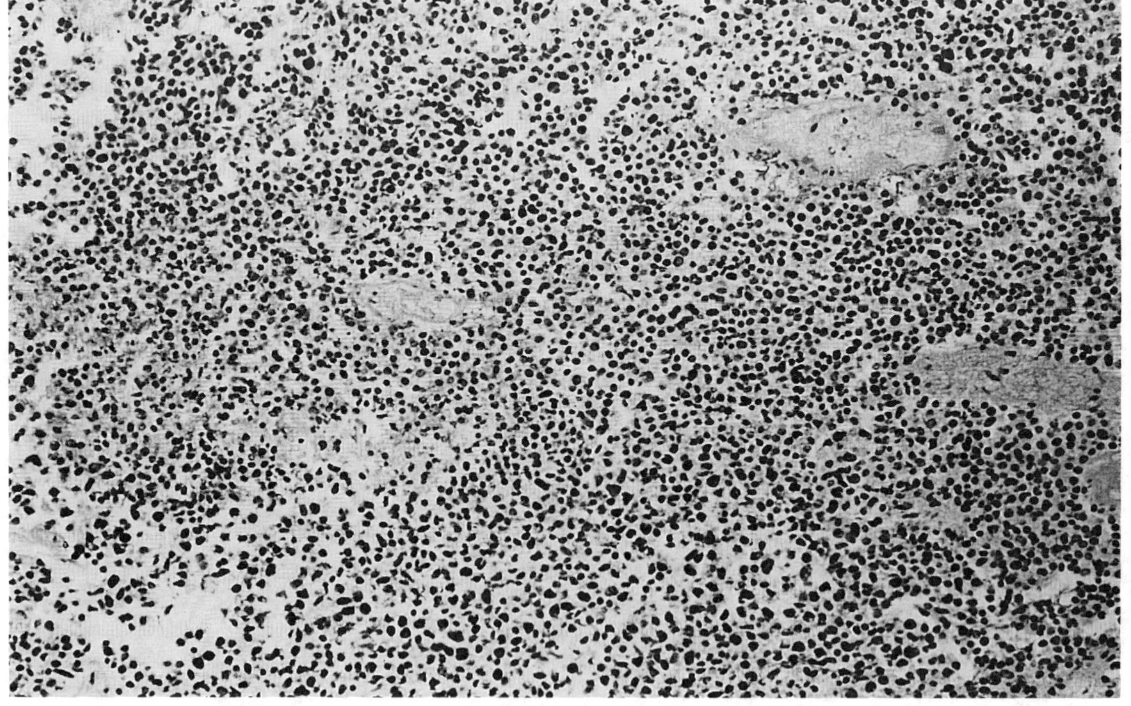

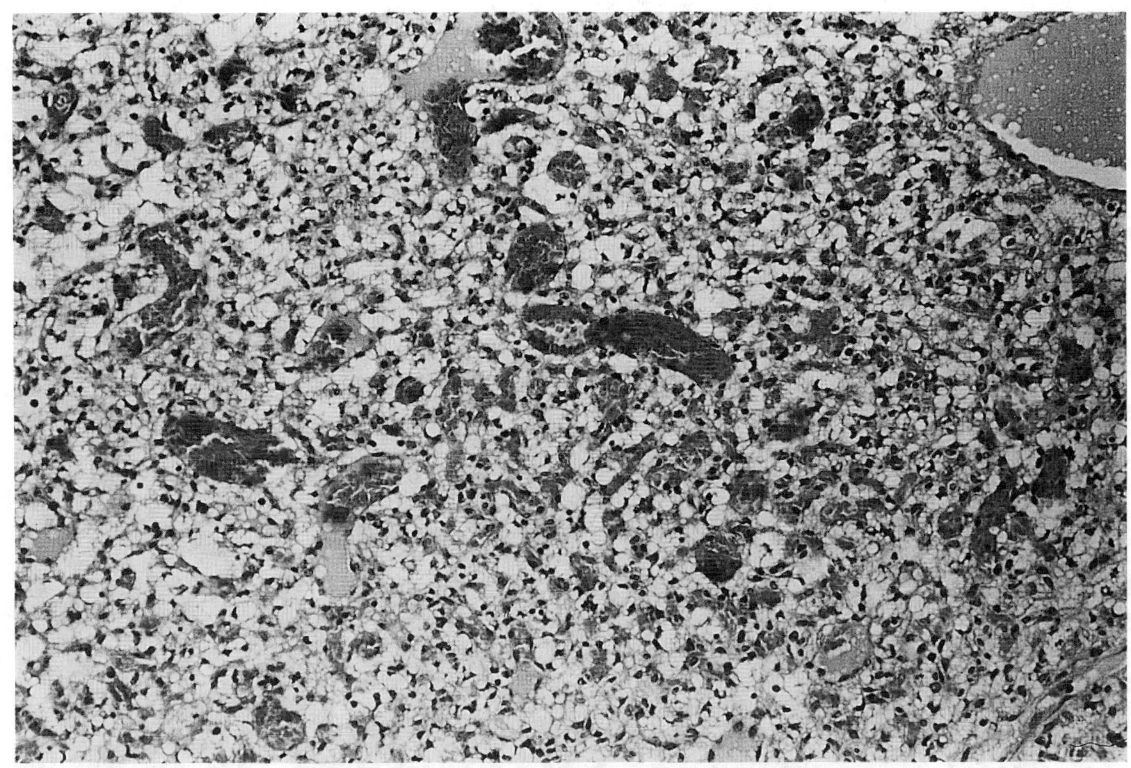

Figure 11-6. Cerebellar hemangioblastoma. The tumor comprises thin-walled blood vessels lined by plump endothelial cells and foamy cells noted between blood vessels. No mitosis is seen. The histology is reminiscent of renal cell carcinoma, from which it is not readily differentiated, particularly if the biopsy material is small. (H & E, X125)

Head and Neck Malignancies

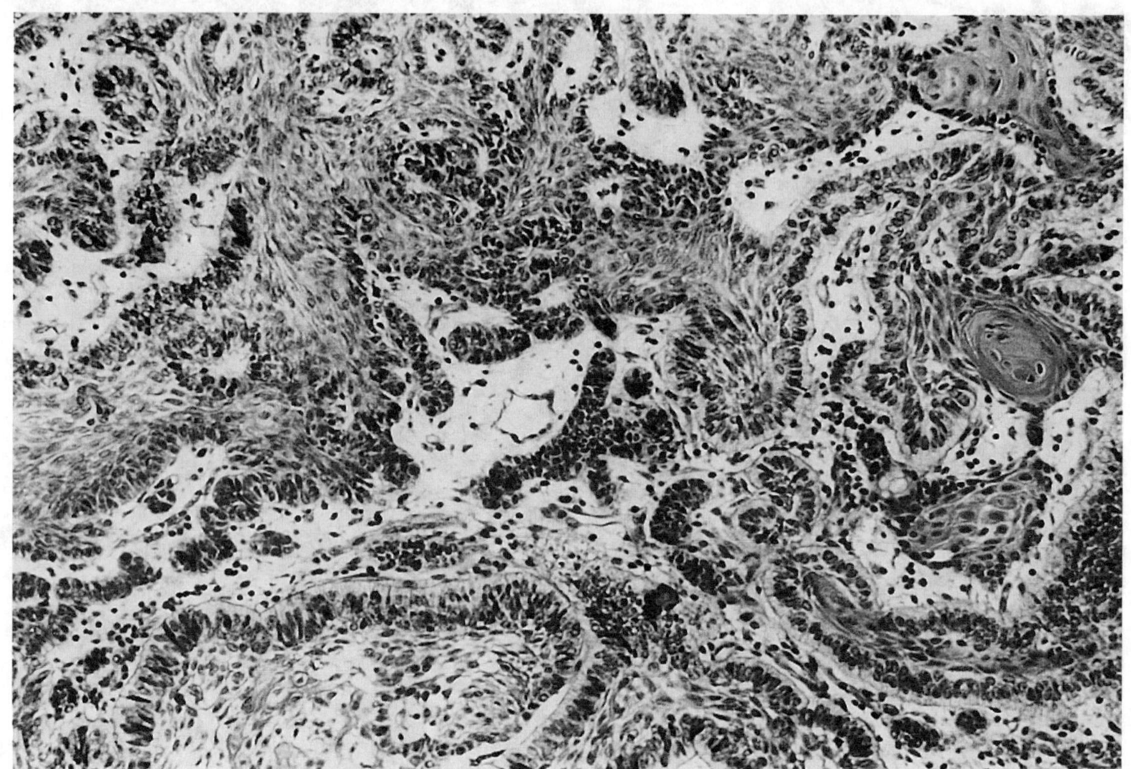

Figure 11-7. Dental lamina ameloblastoma. The tumor is locally invasive and has a high propensity to recur. Only rarely has it been reported to metastasize. The tumor consists of epithelial islands with a central portion made up of spindle cells or polyhedral cells resembling the stellate reticulum of a tooth bud. This is surrounded by a single layer of columnar cells with their nuclei polarized away from the basement membranes. The right side of the photo discloses a focal "acanthomatous" area. A well-differentiated squamous cell carcinoma must be ruled out as part of the differential diagnosis. (H & E, X125)

Figure 11-8. Salivary gland pleomorphic adenoma. A benign tumor, well encapsulated, that exhibits epithelial and mesenchymal elements. The cells
may exhibit tubular to cylindromatous pattern with squamous islands.
Mesenchymal elements are seen as myxoid, myxochondroid, chondroid,
and hyaline forms. It has a high rate of recurrence due to inadequate
excision. Malignant transformation usually exhibits squamous cell carcinoma predominantly with focal adenocarcinoma. (H & E, X125)

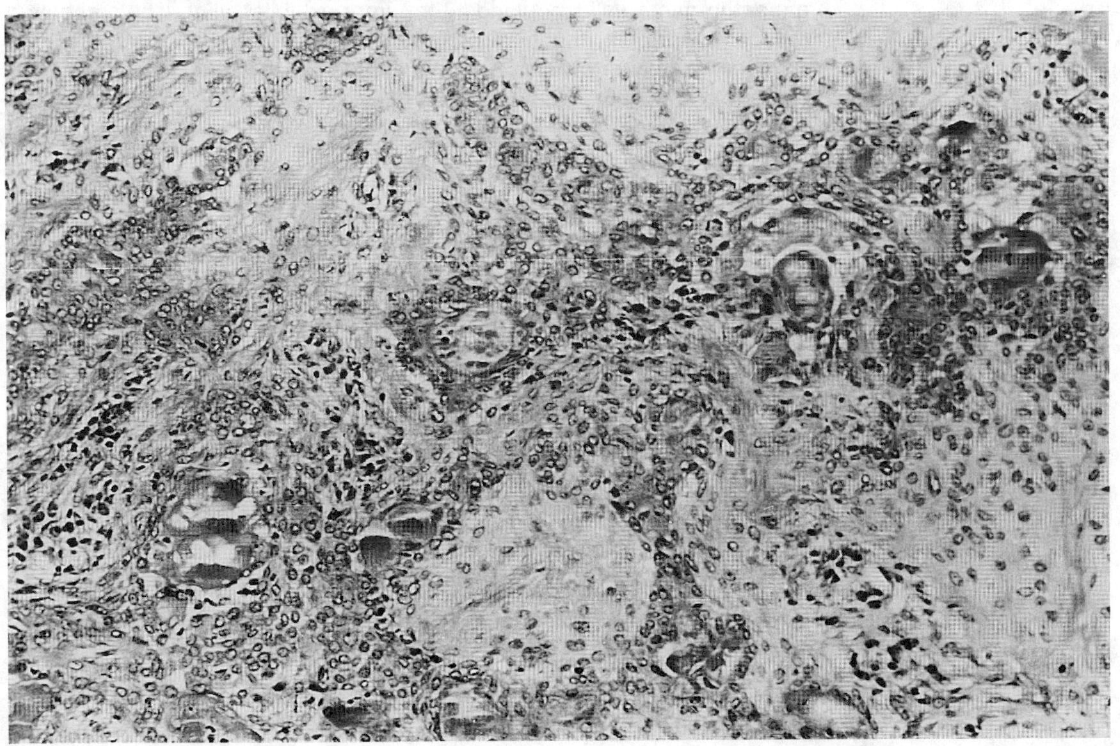

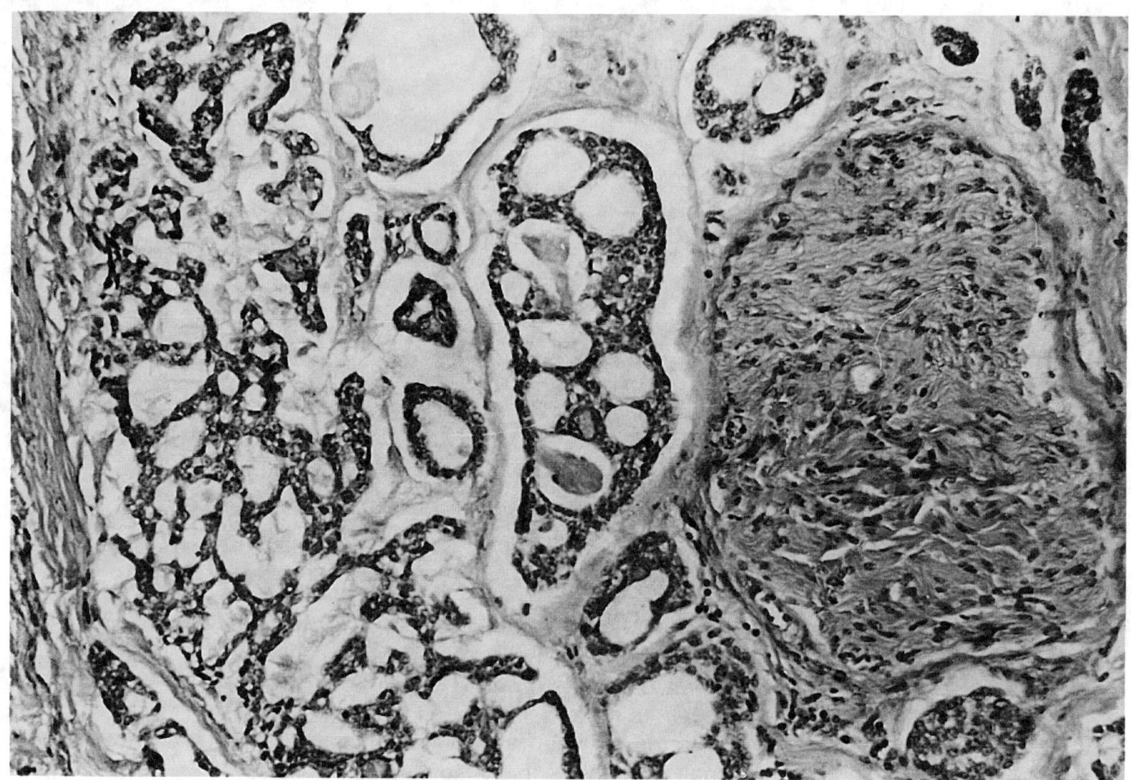

Figure 11-9. Salivary gland adenocystic carcinoma. Unencapsulated and more frequent in minor salivary glands, the tumor exhibits cylindrical to sheets and cords to cribriform pattern composed of hyperchromatic cells that may secrete mucin. Invasion of nerve bundles occurs early, as shown in photo. (H & E, X125)

Figure 11-10. Salivary gland mucoepidermoid carcinoma (low grade). Circumscribed tumor with cystic consistency composed of squamous cells and mucous-secreting cells arrayed in tubular cystic pattern. An intermediate cell is also present between the epidermoid and mucin-secreting cells. The low-grade tumor is composed primarily of well-defined squamous cells admixed with mucin-secreting cells and intermediate cells in random fashion. (H & E, X125)

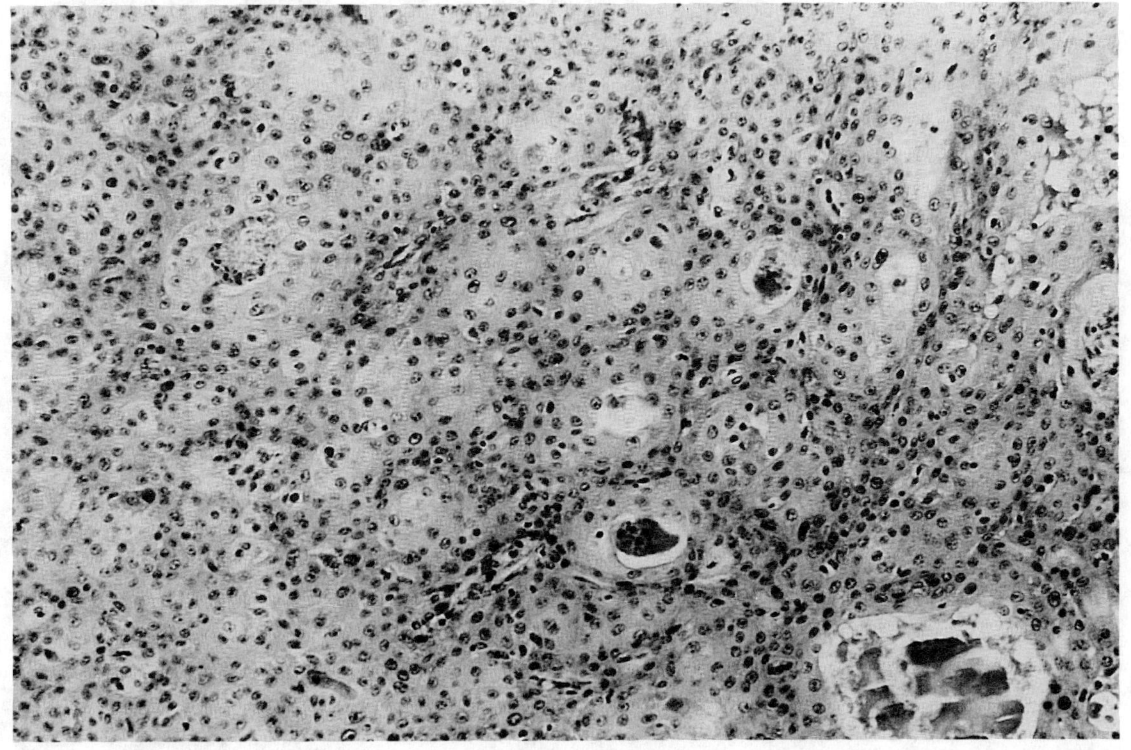

Figure 11-11. Salivary gland mucoepidermoid carcinoma (high grade). The high-grade malignancy consists of poorly differentiated pleomorphic epidermoid cells and less mucin-secreting and intermediate cells. Both will exhibit epithelial mucin, which is diastase fast PAS positive. This is the most common malignant salivary gland tumor in children. (H & E, X125)

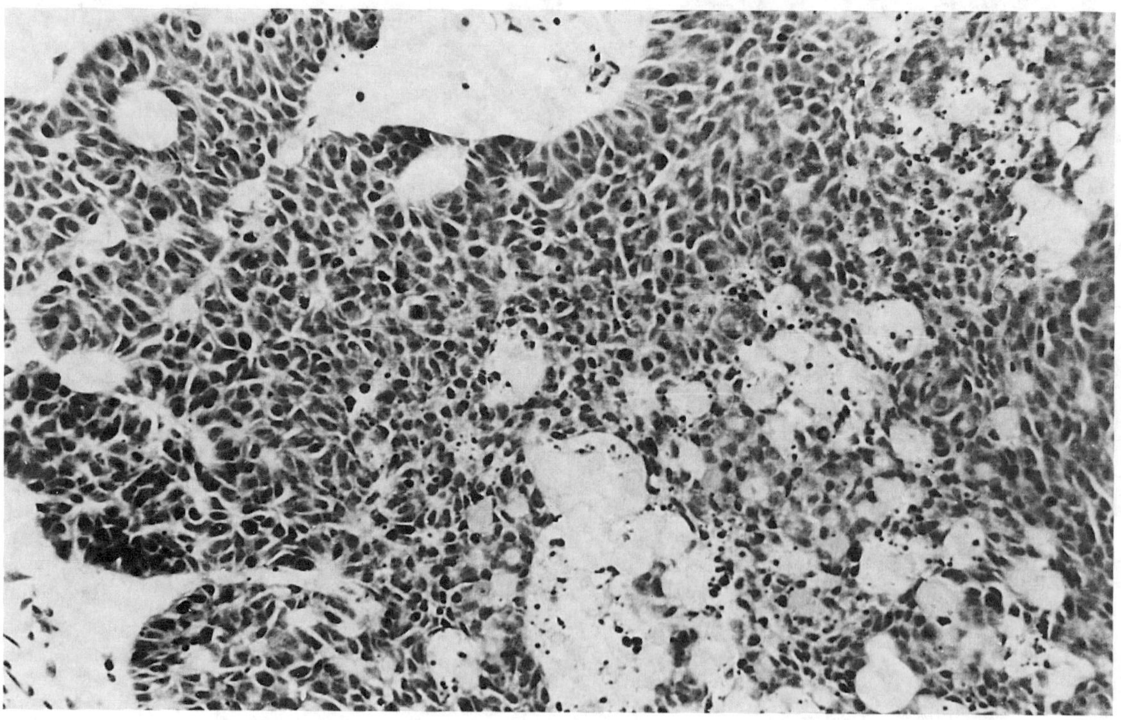

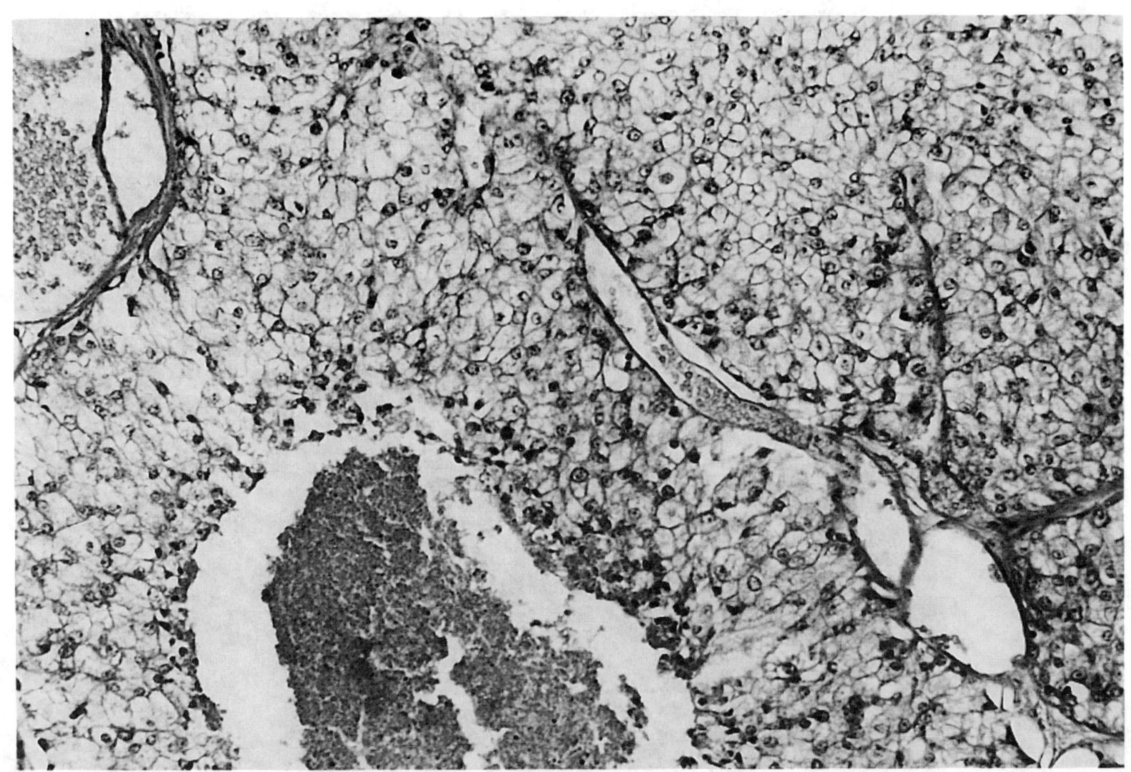

Figure 11-12. Salivary gland acinic cell adenocarcinoma. A well-encapsulated tumor composed of polygonal cells with a granular basophilic cytoplasm; some have clear, nongranular cytoplasm. Tumor may exhibit solid or trabecular or acinar pattern. (H & E, X125)

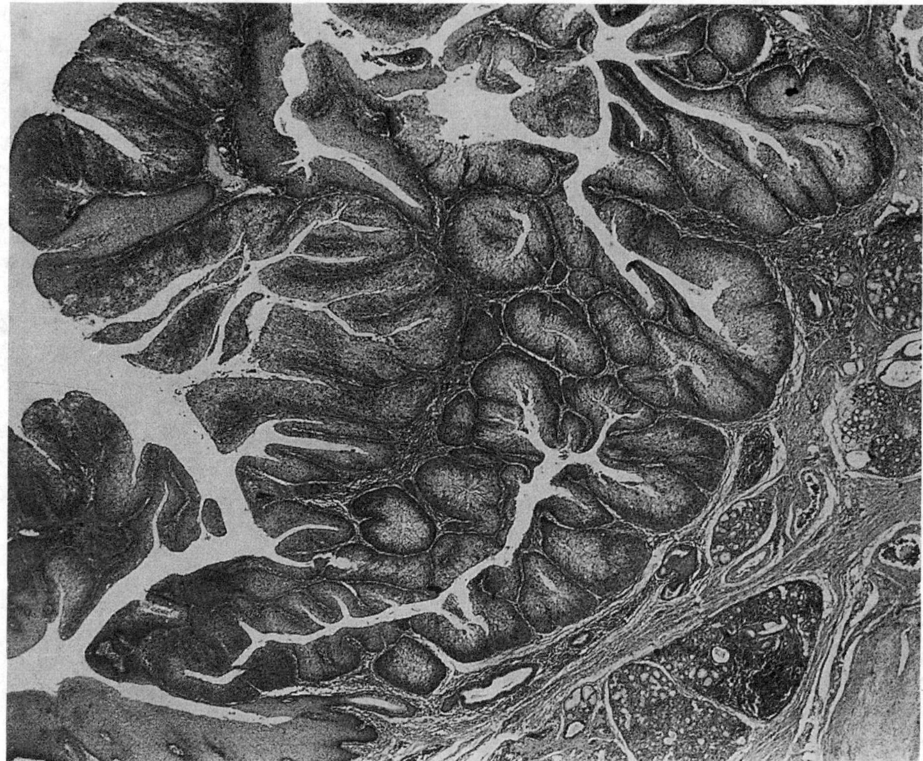

Figure 11-13A (above). Pharynx verrucous carcinoma. A variant of squamous carcinoma; consists of a well-differentiated squamous epithelium forming papillary fronds and their elongated bulbous rete ridges pushes adjacent connective tissue rather than infiltrate. Dysplastic changes are not conspicuous, so the lesion may be mistaken for condyloma or pseudoepitheliomatous hyperplasia. (H & E, X30)

Figure 11-13B (opposite page, top). Nasopharyngeal carcinoma. Two-thirds of malignant tumors in this region are made up of carcinomas and one-third are lymphomas. A fourth of the carcinomas are squamous, rarely adenocarcinomas, and a smaller number of cases are papillary transitional cell carcinomas (photo). The tumor has a tendency to retain basement membrane and histopathologically is similar to urothelial carcinoma. (H & E, X100)

Figure 11-13C (opposite page, bottom). Nasopharyngeal anaplastic carcinoma. About half of the nasopharyngeal carcinomas are anaplastic. The tumor has been called lymphoepithelioma due to intermingling of lymphocytes and histiocytes together with the syncitial-like anaplastic epithelial cells with ill-defined cell borders. Although highly radiosensitive early metastases to lymph nodes occur, this tumor may be misinterpreted as malignant lymphoma. The tumor has high prevalence in southern China and Malaysia, comprising 18% of all malignant tumors. Epstein-Barr viral genome has been shown in the malignant epithelial cells. T cell lymphocytes predominate the inflammatory infiltrate. (H & E, X100)

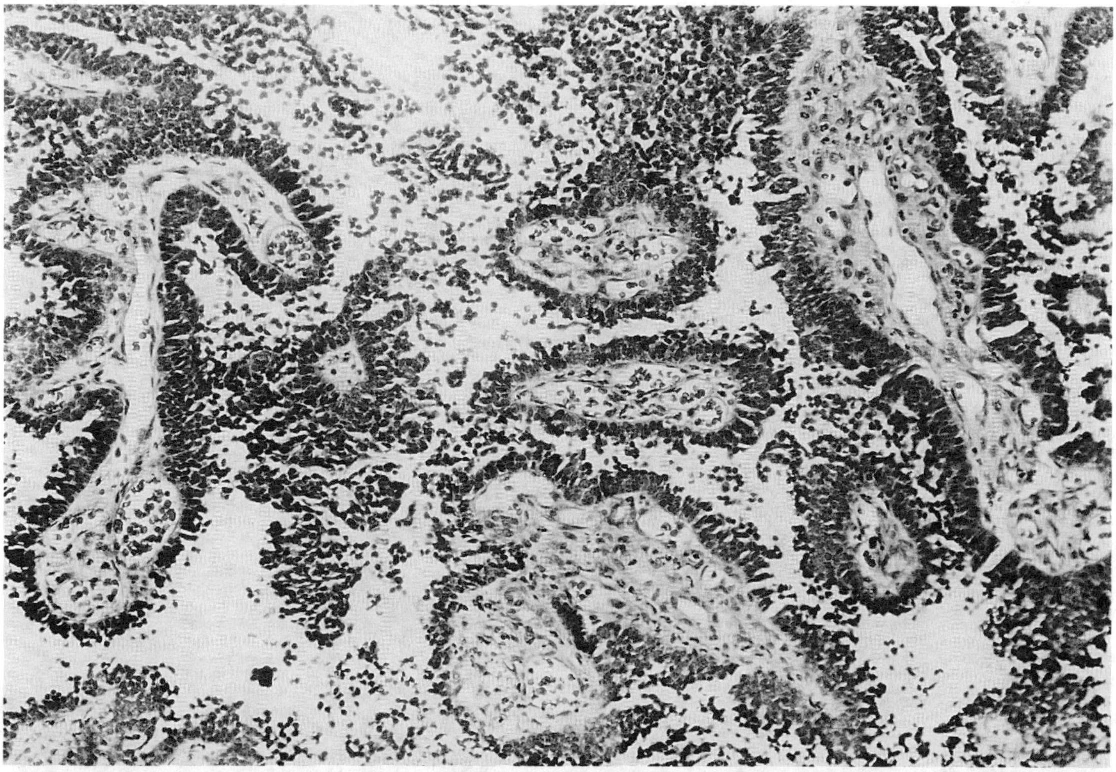

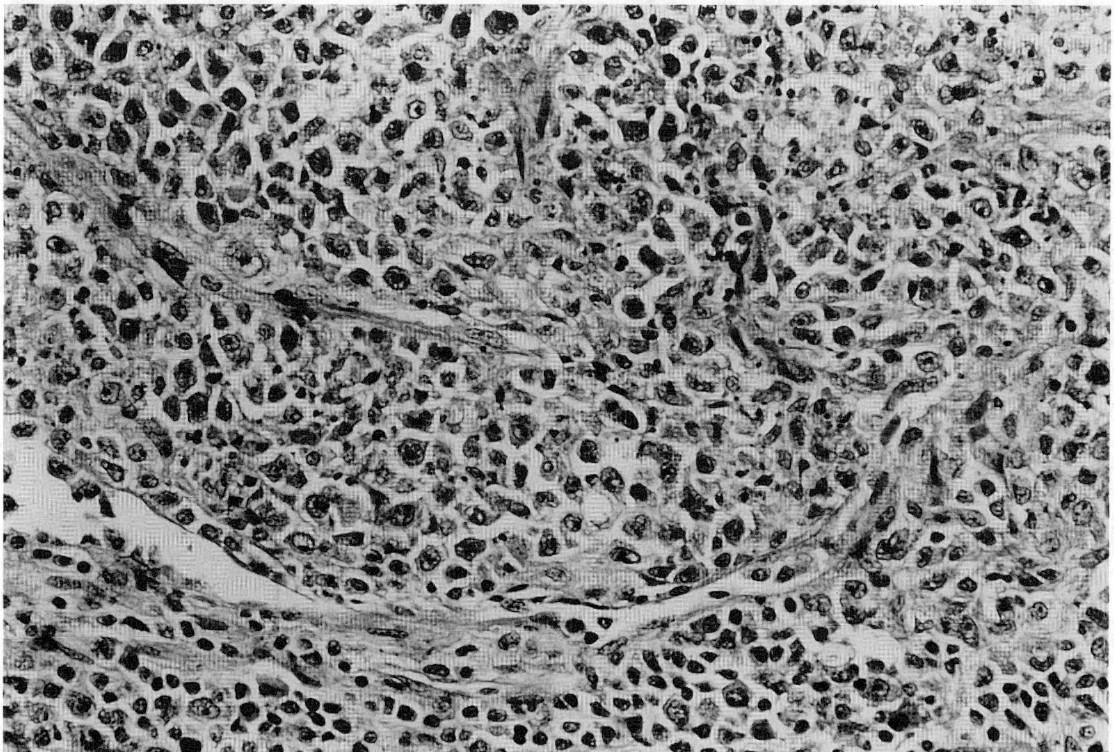

Malignancies of the Lower Respiratory System

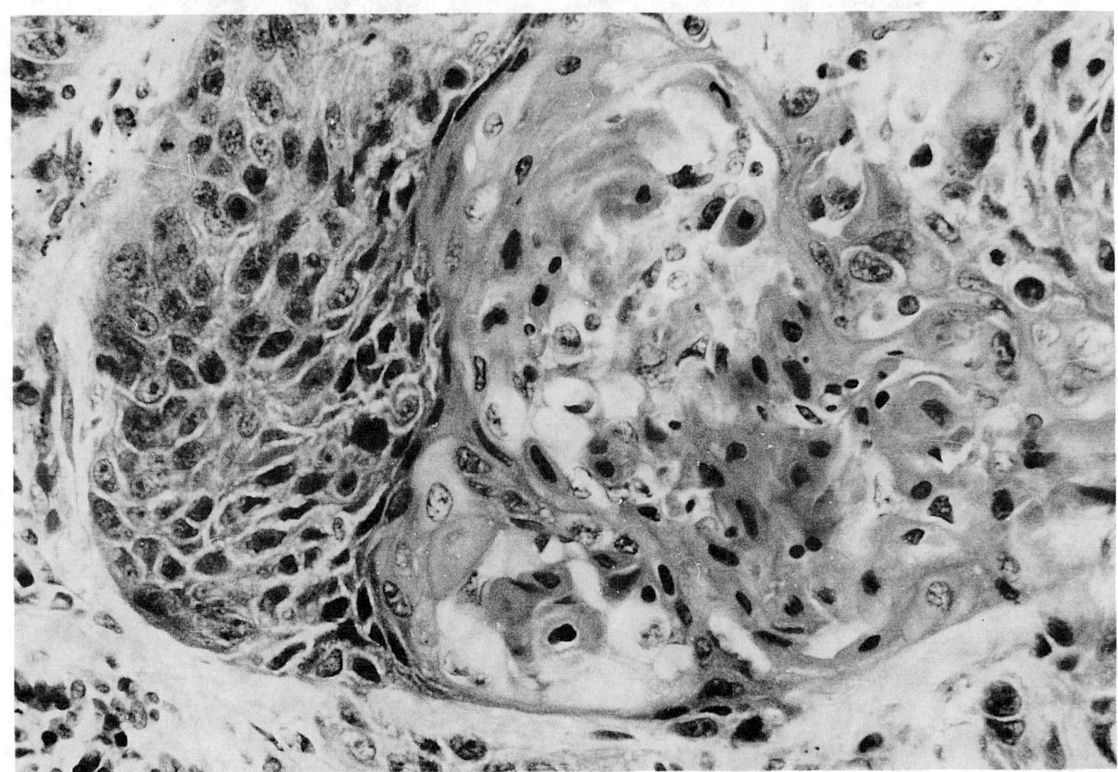

Figure 11-14. Squamous cell carcinoma of the lung. Sheet of tumor cells showing intercellular bridges and aborted pearl formation with keratinization.
Either intercellular bridges or keratinization should be present for such
classification. The poorly differentiated squamous cell carcinoma will
have only a few areas showing either feature or both, and the rest of the
tumor is largely undifferentiated. (H & E, X310)

Figure 11-15. Squamous cell carcinoma of the lung, cytology. Bronchial brushing with a loose sheet of spindle-shaped malignant cells with elongated, angulated flat hyperchromatic or pyknotic nuclei. Cytoplasm of these mature keratinized cells is bright orange, dense, opaque, homogenous and waxy, with a hard edge on Pap stain. Similarly shaped elongated keratinized squamous cells without nuclei are seen in the background, with an alveolar macrophage and erythrocytes. (Pap, X500)

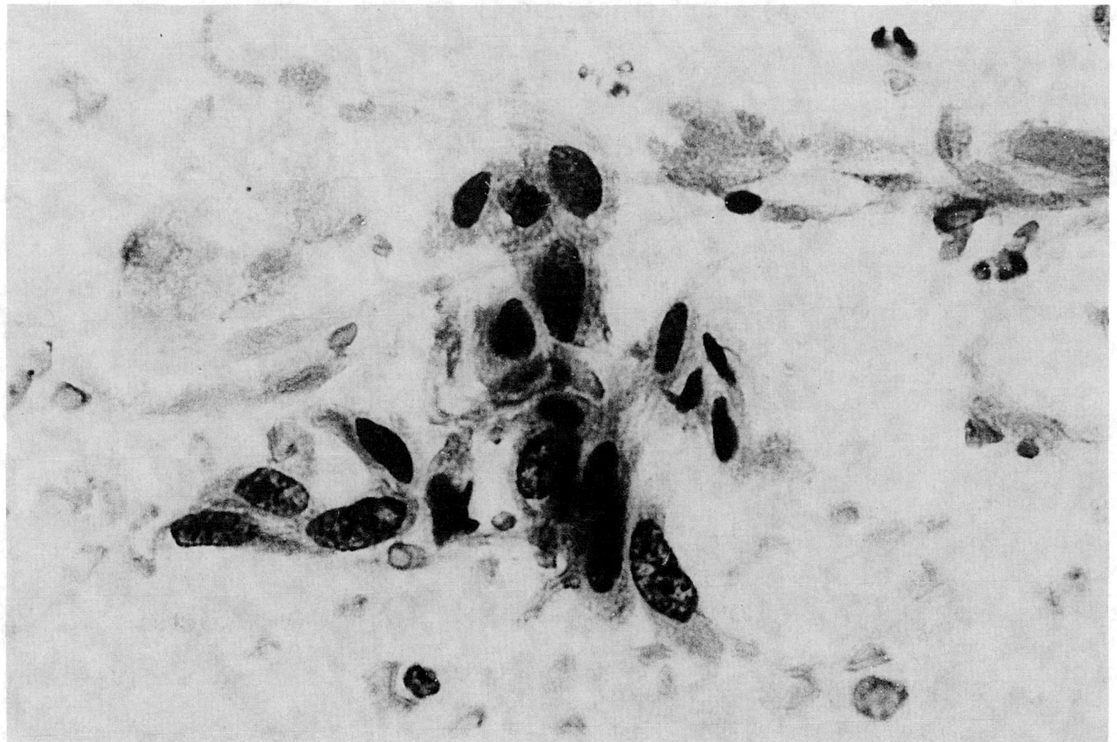

Figure 11-16A & B. Small-cell carcinoma of the lung. The tumor consists of cells larger than lymphocytes but having dense nuclear chromatin and inconspicuous nucleoli with hardly any cytoplasm. The cells may be uniformly ovoid, round, or fusiform. Tumor cells are usually similar in size but often exhibit nuclear pleomorphism, in shape and chromatin pattern with necrosis such as shown in photo A (below). When the tumor cells are homogenously round with uniform nuclear chromatin pattern, carcinoid tumor and malignant lymphoma must be ruled out. The tumor has a tendency to grow around blood vessels and palisade. Depending on the tangential cut, the cells may form a rosettelike pattern (photo B, opposite page). (H & E, 11-16A X310; 11-16B X125)

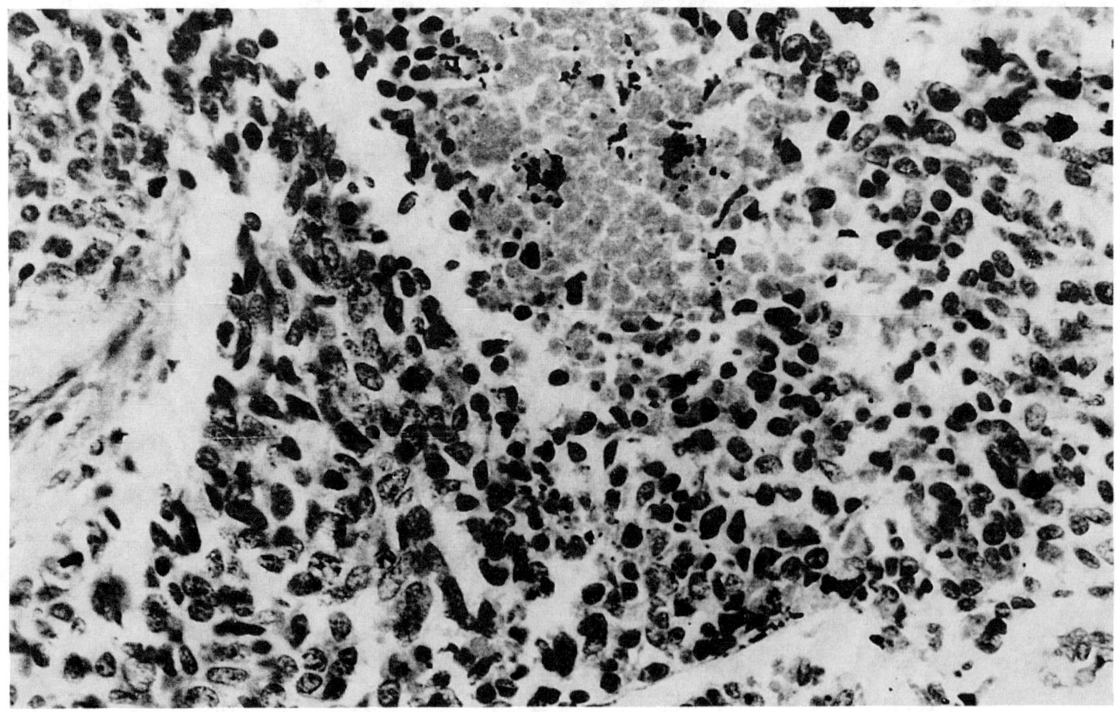

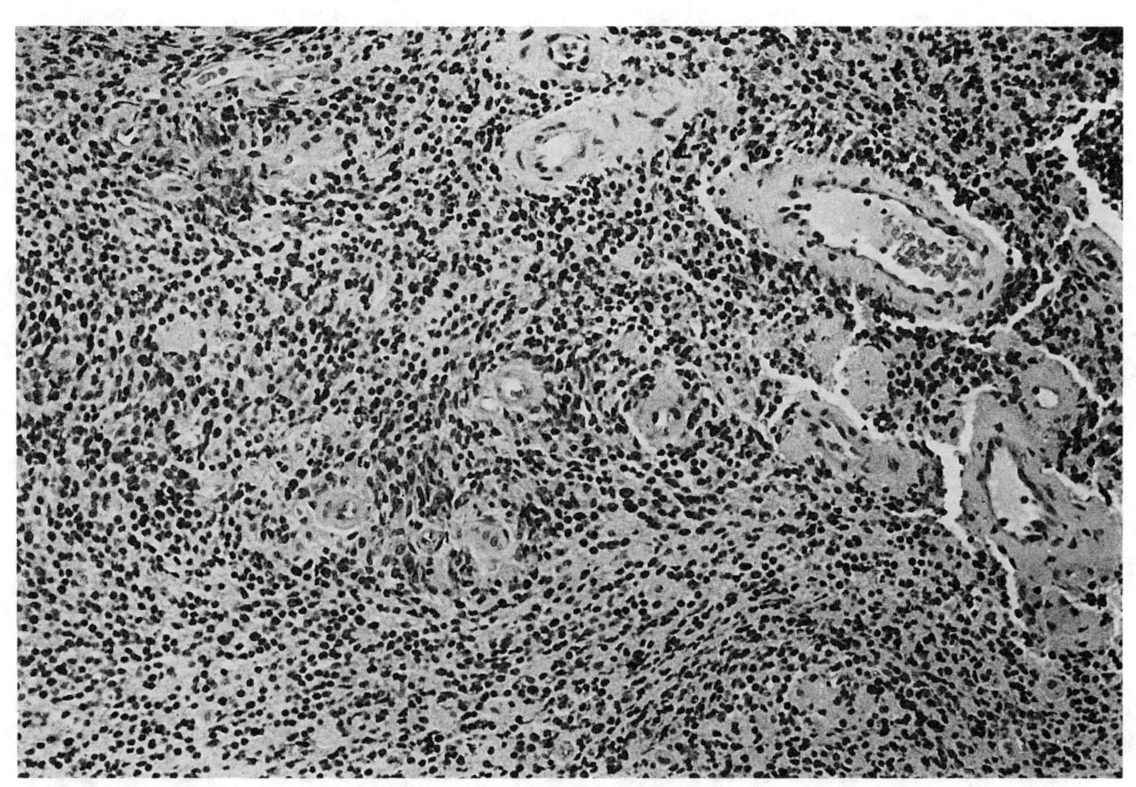

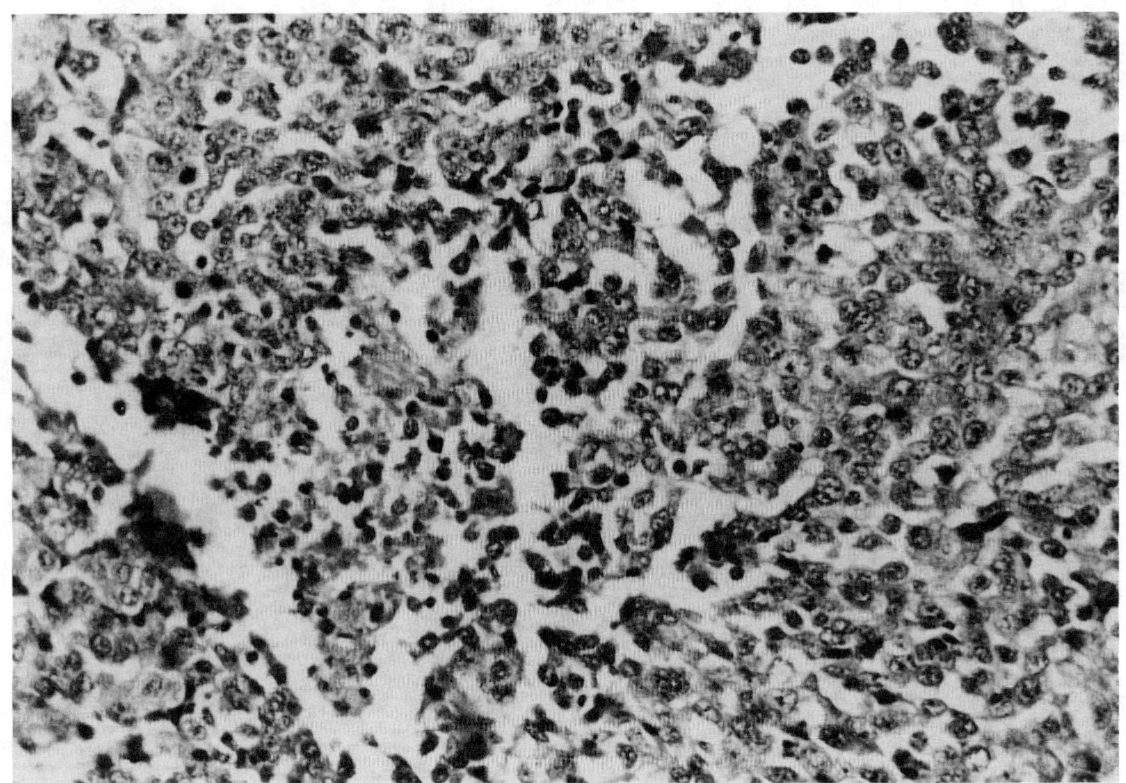

Figure 11-17. Small-cell carcinoma of the lung, intermediate type. The tumor is composed predominantly of small cells, with some cytoplasm. The cells are rather loose. Focal areas may disclose large-cell type also. (H & E, X310)

Figure 11-18. Small-cell anaplastic carcinoma of the lung—bronchial brushing
cytology. This loose cluster of small cells shows characteristic nuclear
molding. These flat cells have reversal of their nuclear cytoplasmic ratio.
Variation is seen in size and shape of the angular eccentric small nuclei,
which have dense chromatin and occasional discernible nucleoli. Nuclei
are larger than the degenerated small lymphocyte (at left edge of photograph), from which they must be distinguished. Cytoplasm is delicate
and extremely scanty. In addition to lymphocytes and other inflammatory
cells, small-cell carcinoma must also be distinguished from reserve cells
and groups of small, degenerated, darkly-staining bronchial cells. Nuclei
may vary in overall size from the small "lymphocyte-like" to the intermediate cell type. Cells from bronchial brushings (as these are) and from
needle aspirates are likely to be larger, better preserved, and exhibiting
better nuclear detail than cells from sputum and bronchial washings.
(Pap, X500)

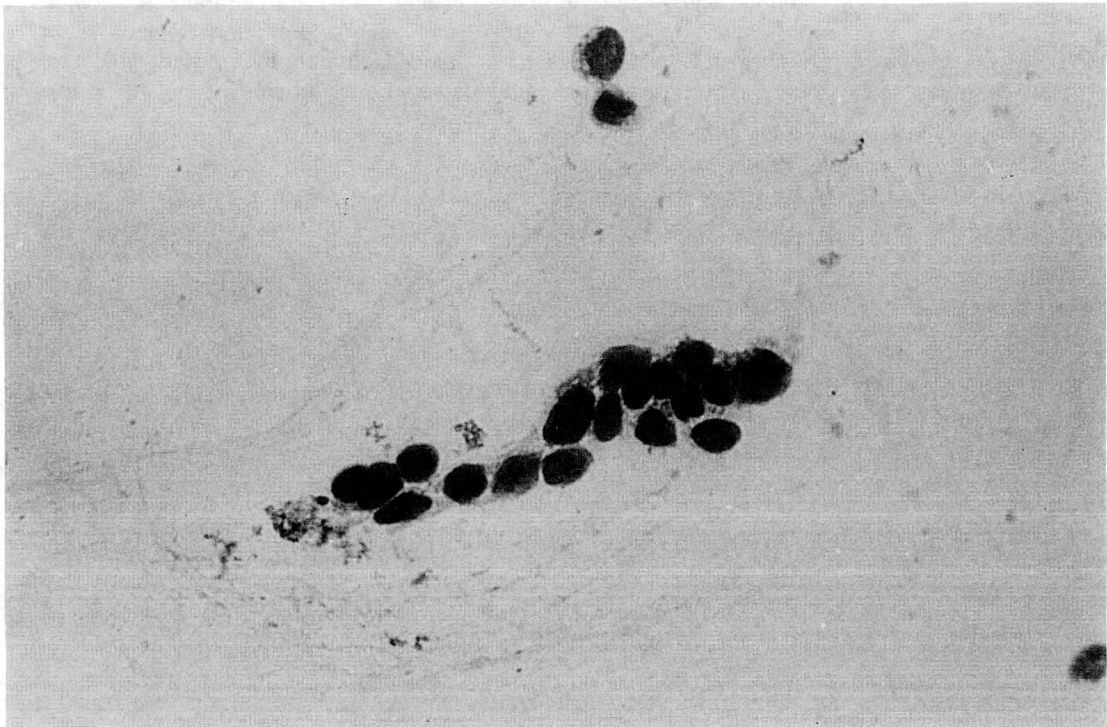

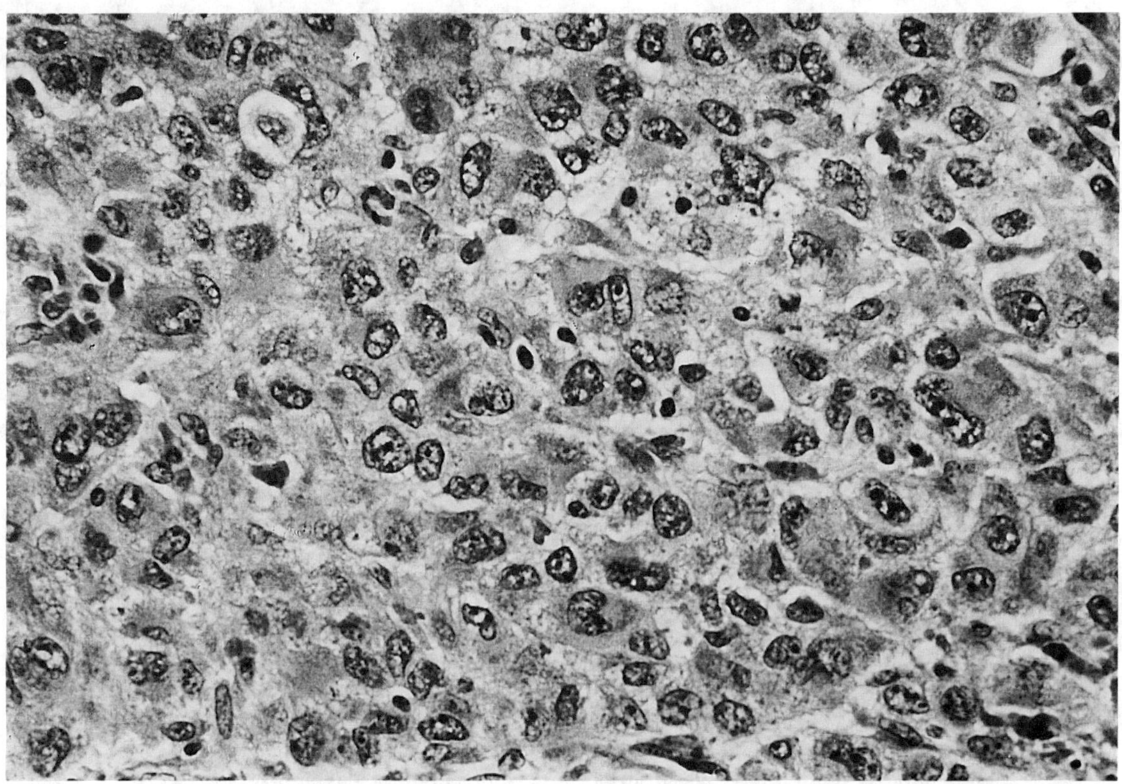

Figure 11-19A & B. Large-cell undifferentiated carcinoma of the lung. Tumor cells do not display any form or organization. They are generally large, with abundant cytoplasm, having large nuclei with prominent nucleoli (photo A, above). Some cases may exhibit predominant tumor giant cells and some extremely bizarre, multinucleated cells (photo B, opposite page) (H & E, 11-19A X310; 11-19B X200)

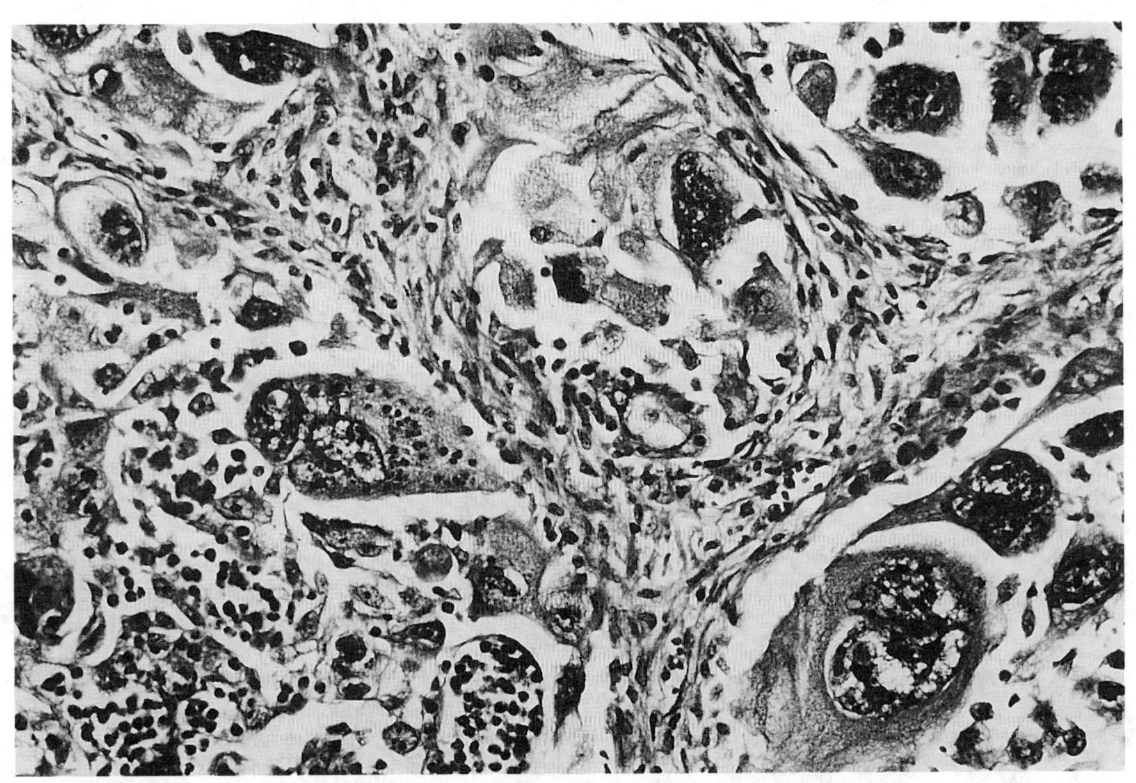

Figure 11-20. Large-cell undifferentiated carcinoma—bronchial brushing cytology. This cluster of malignant cells has extremely hyperchromatic round, oval, angulated, molded, or overlapped nuclei with lack of nuclear detail and scant, wispy cytoplasm without discernible cell borders. This field does not include the feature of granular background debris representative of a tumor diathesis. Nor does it show the considerable variation in nuclear size, the large nucleoli, and irregular nuclear margins that may be seen. Cells of poorly differentiated adenocarcinoma are likely to be diagnosed cytologically as large-cell undifferentiated carcinoma. Large-cell undifferentiated carcinoma is also to be distinguished from degenerated columnar cells. (Pap, X500)

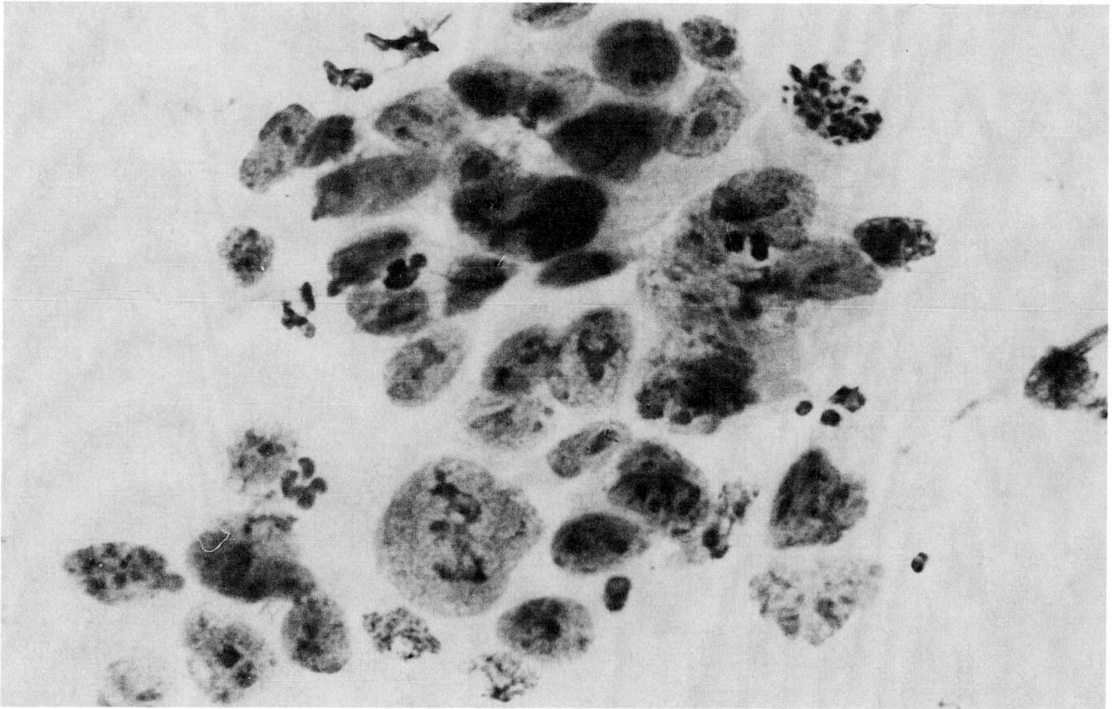

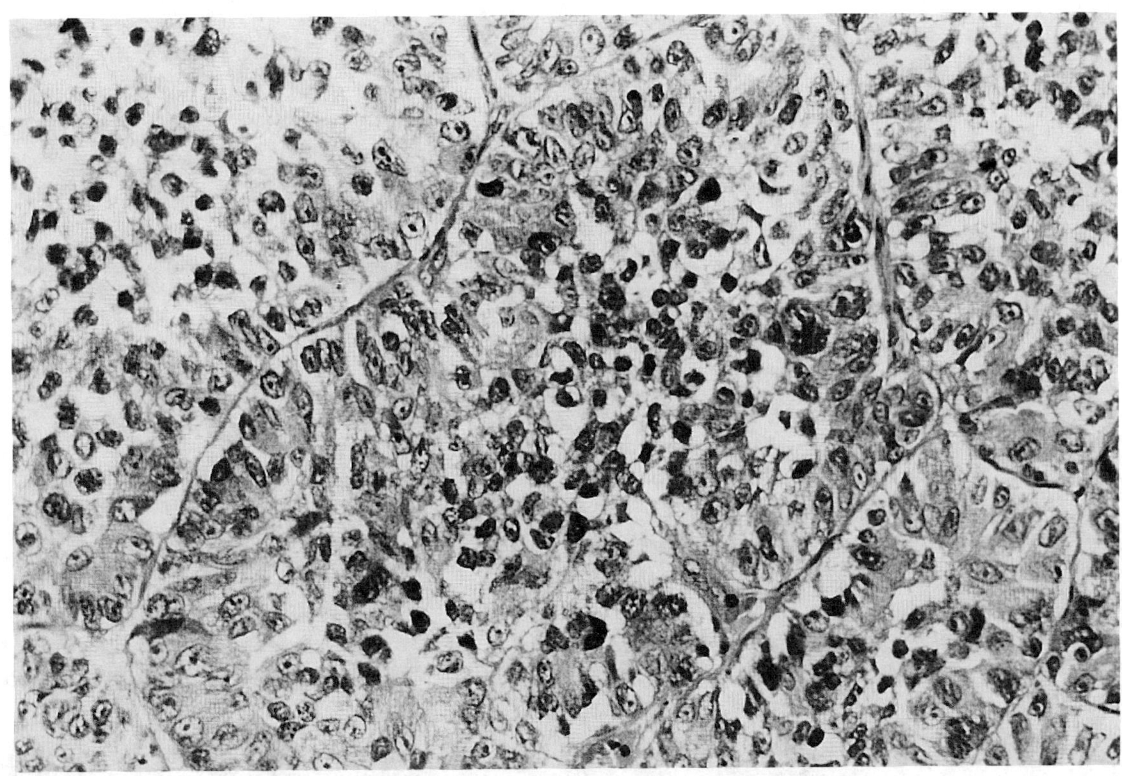

Figure 11-21. Adenocarcinoma of the lung. The tumor may exhibit acinar and tubular patterns admixed with solid areas. Cells are generally large with finely granular-to-foamy cytoplasm. The nuclei may be vesicular/or with coarse chromatin and prominent nucleoli. Moderate to poorly differentiated type cells make up most of this tumor. (H & E, X200)

Figure 11-22. Adenocarcinoma of the lung—sputum cytology. Note the variable size of round central or eccentric nuclei with well defined nuclear margins, central prominent nucleoli in every cell, distinct vacuoles, and granular cytoplasm with sharp cytoplasmic borders. (Pap, X640)

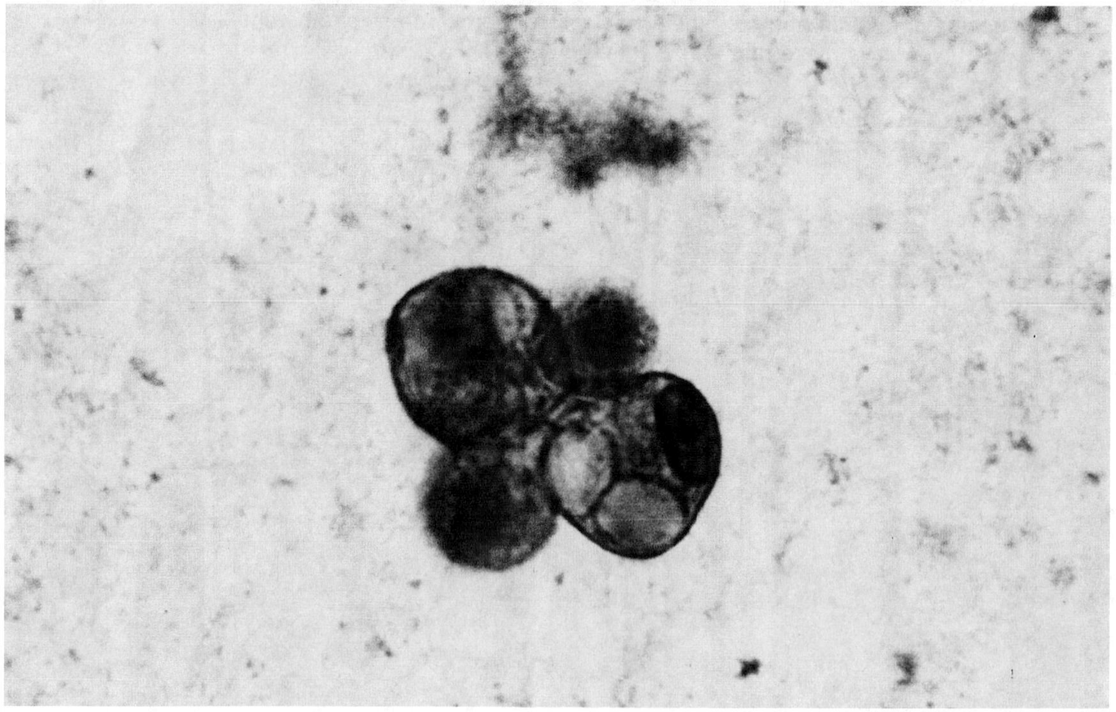

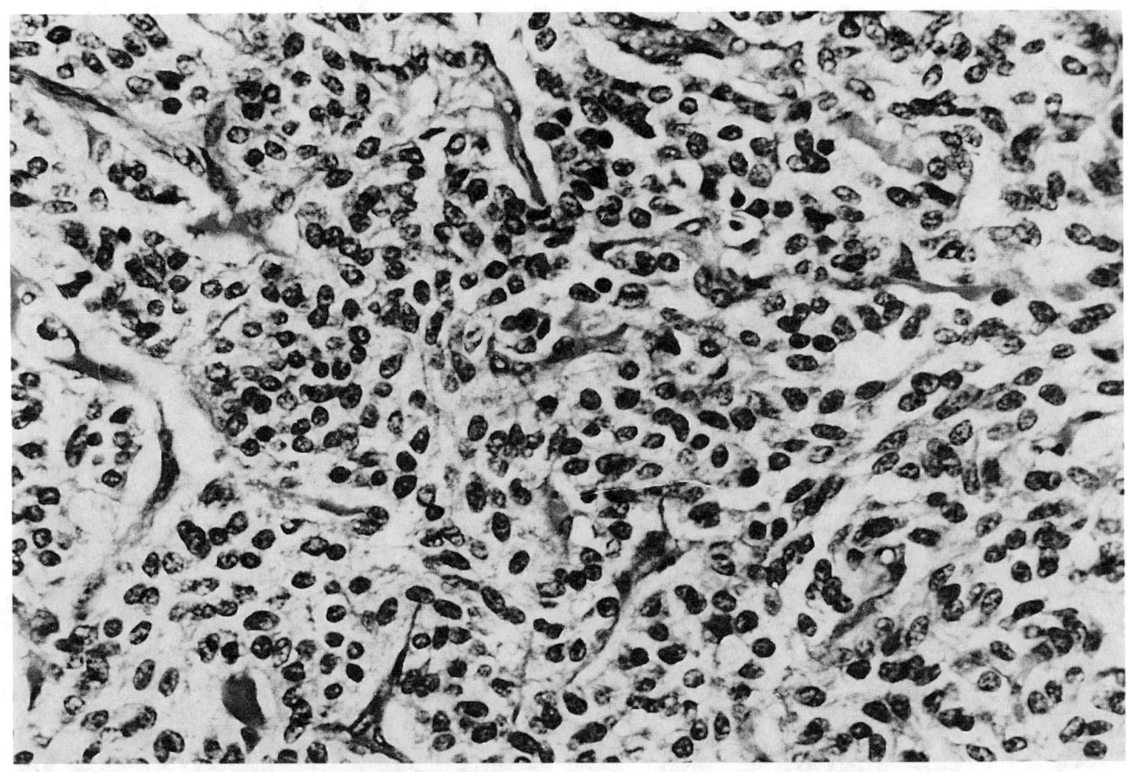

Figure 11-23. Carcinoid tumor of the lung. Tumor cells are relatively uniform in size, shape, and nuclear chromatin pattern. Islands of tumor cells are separated by thin fibrovascular stroma. This pattern is seen throughout the tumor without necrosis. (H & E, X310)

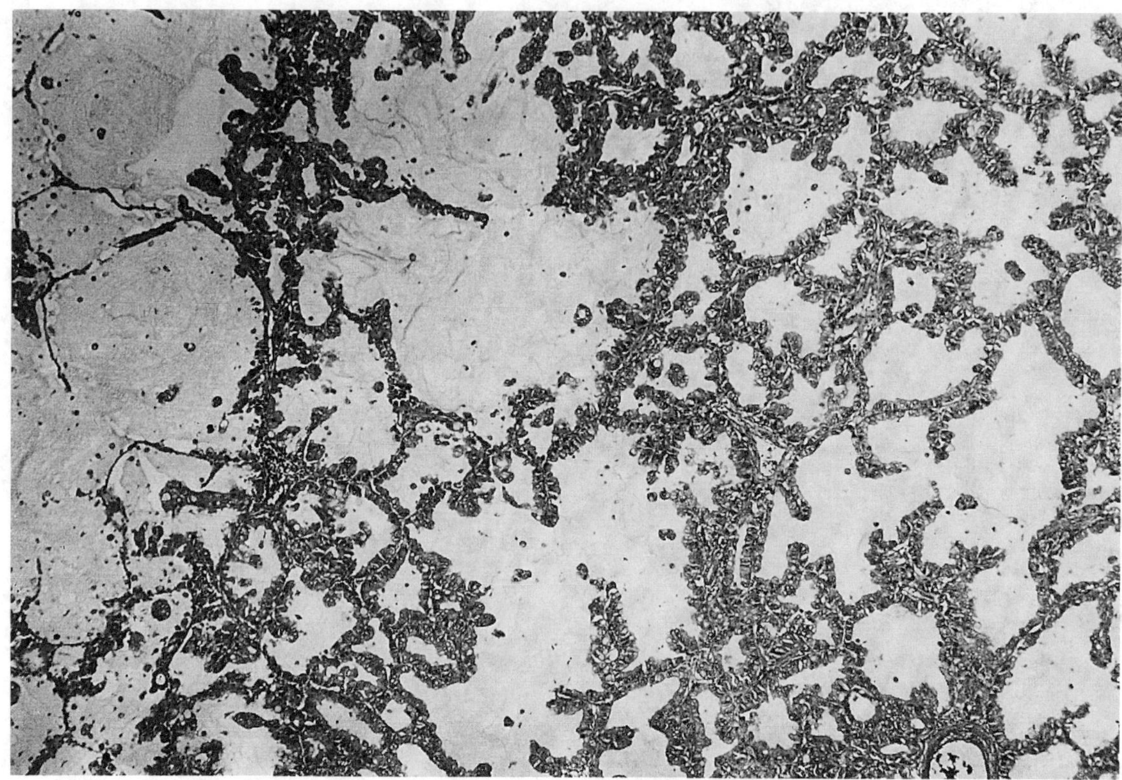

Figure 11-24A & B. Bronchiolo-alveolar carcinoma. A variant of adenocarcinoma composed of columnar cells that line up the alveolar wall structures and may form a papillary pattern (photo A, above). Tumor cells form a single layer and demonstrate intracytoplasmic and extracellular mucin without fibrosis (photo B, opposite page). (H & E, 11-24A X30; 11-24B X310)

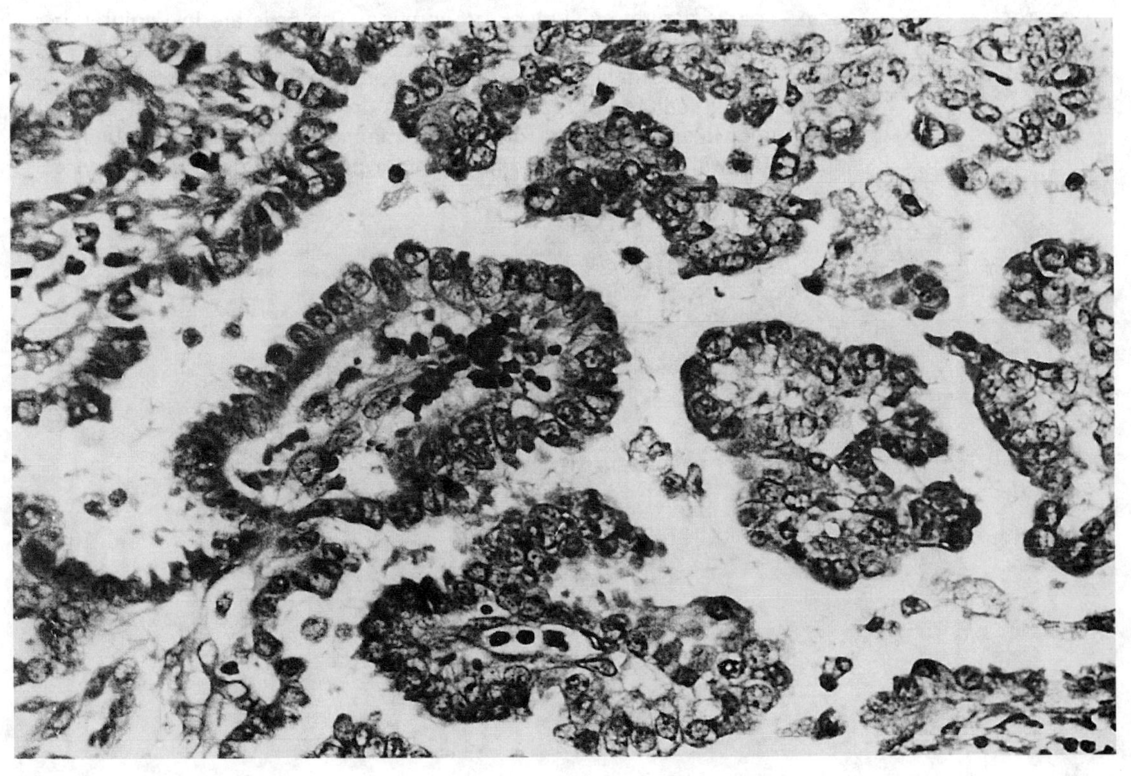

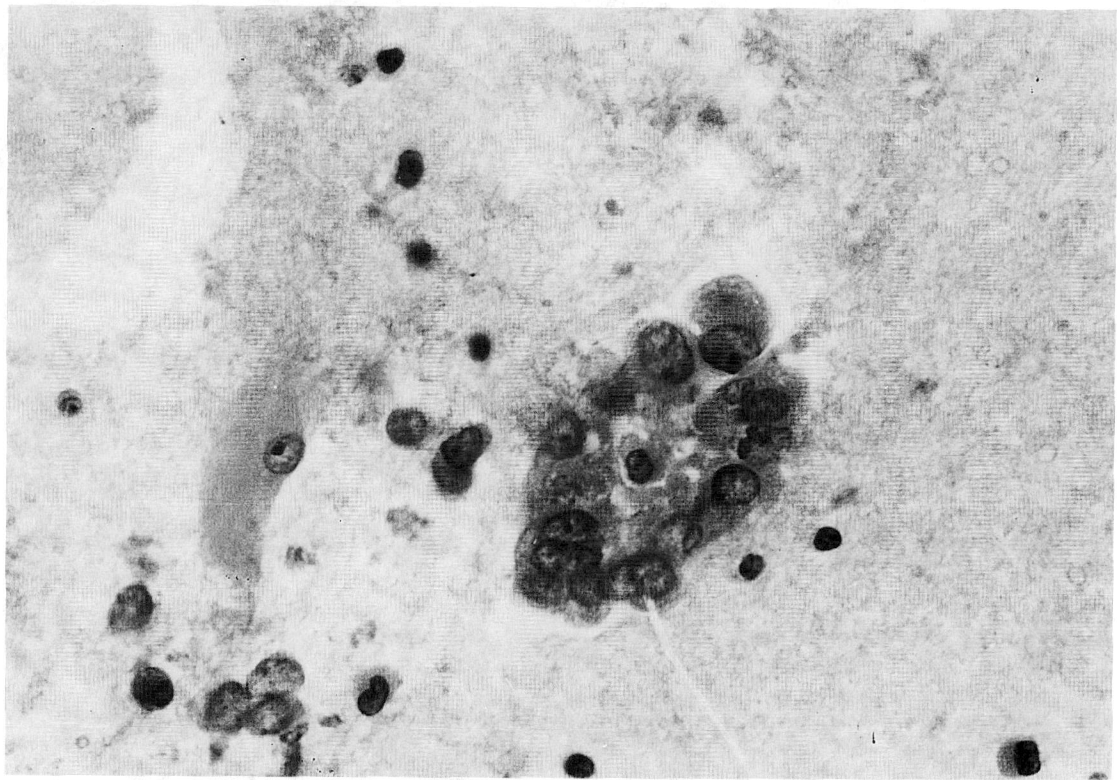

Figure 11-25. Terminal bronchiolo-alveolar cell carcinoma (cytology). This is a fine-needle aspirate cell block preparation. The cells are low columnar with vesicular nuclei having distinct nuclear membrane, small nucleoli, and coarse chromatin clumps. There is an abundant pale cytoplasm. The overall features of these tumor cells are not unlike reactive granular pneumocytes. One has to rule out an infarcted lung, which is usually associated with numerous reactive granular pneumocytes and histiocytes. (Pap, X500)

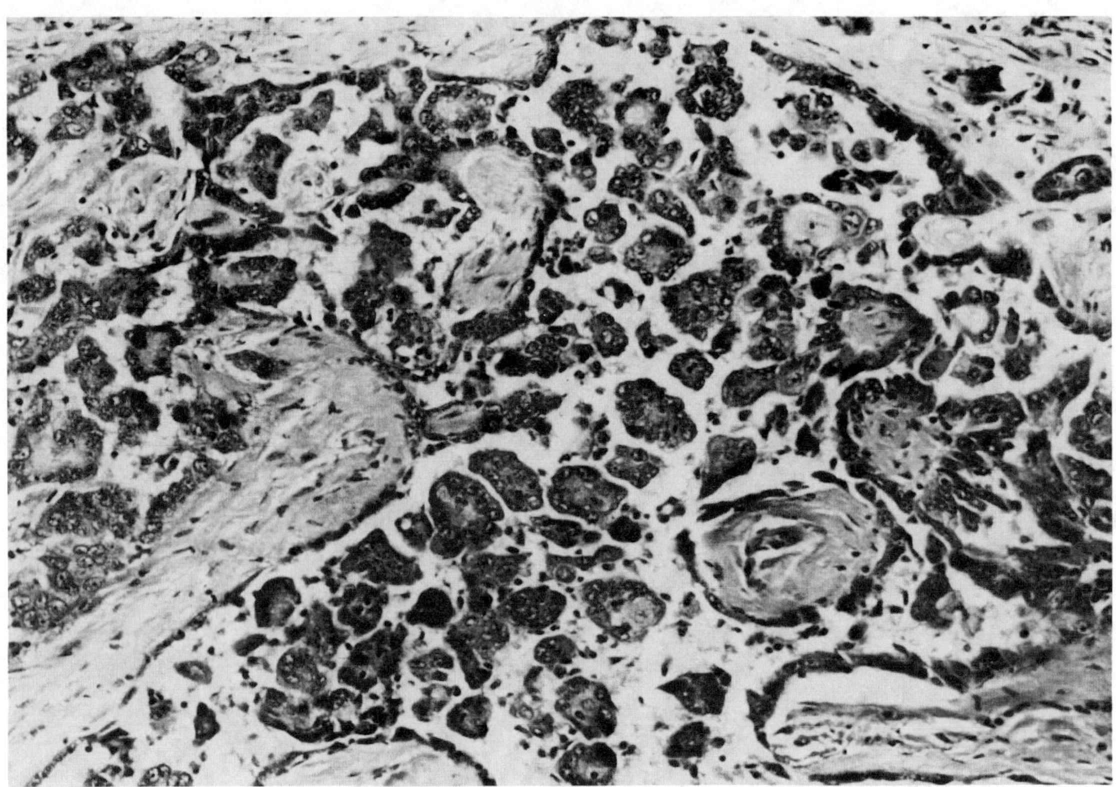

Figure 11-26A & B. Malignant mesothelioma. The tumor may show spindle cell sarcoma with spaces lined by low columnar cells that may form papillary patterns or sheets of tumor cells (photo A, above). When the tumor is predominantly epithelial (photo B, opposite page) differentiation from a peripheral adenocarcinoma of lung could be difficult on a biopsy specimen. Epithelial mucin can be distinguished from mesothelial acid mucin by a positive alcianophilic mucoid material removed by hyaluronidase in mesothelial tumor. A negative PAS-diastase, CEA, and Leu M1 immunoperoxidase stain also supports mesothelial cell type. Biopsy should be signed out as consistent with or probable mesothelioma. (H & E, 11-26A X125; 11-26B X310)

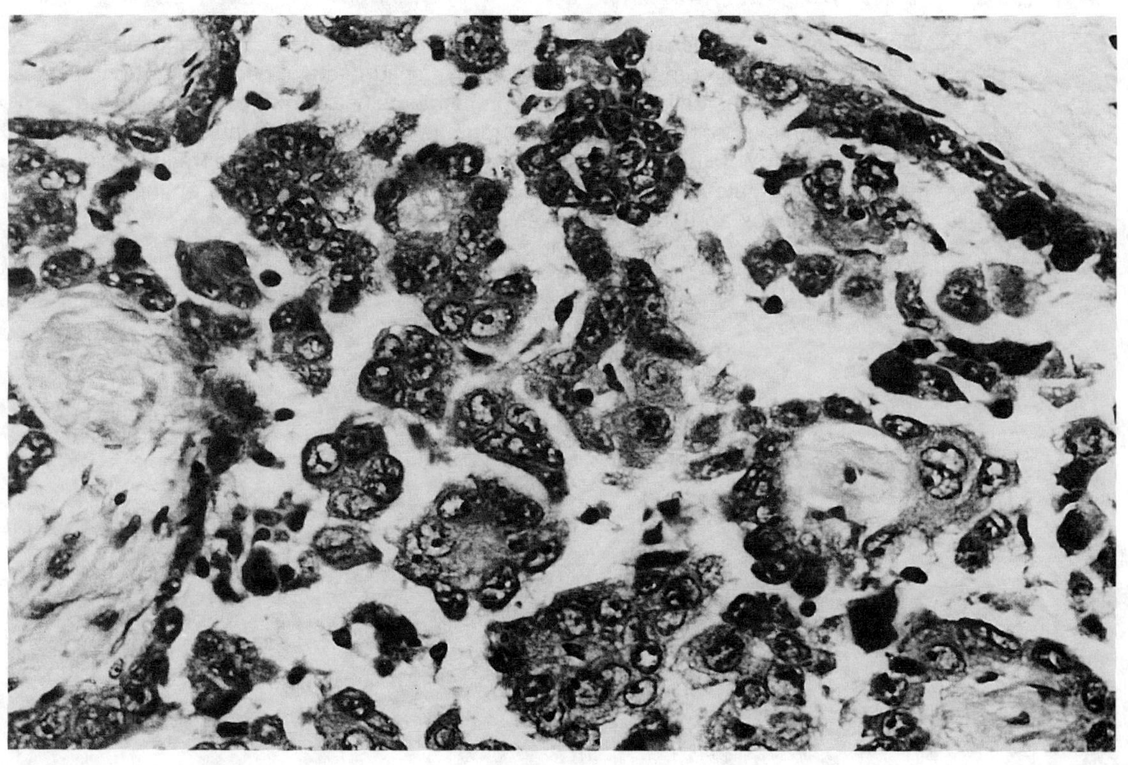

Malignant Tumors of the Digestive System

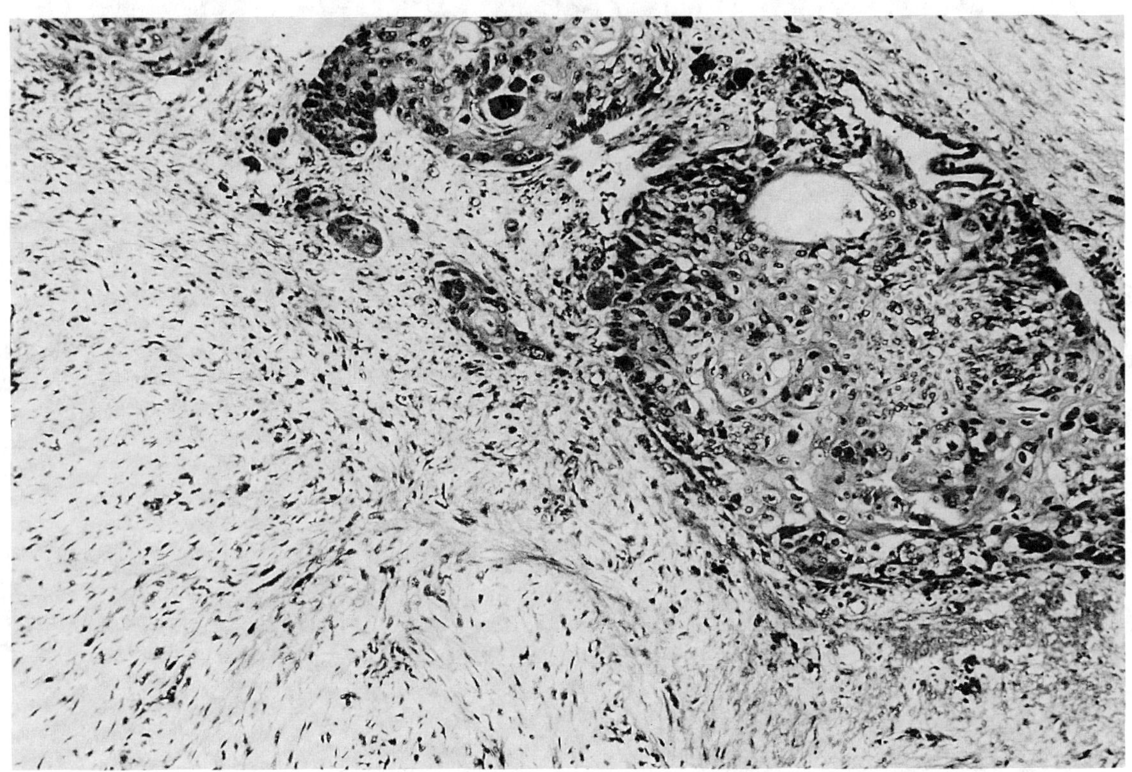

Figure 11-27. Carcinosarcoma of the esophagus. The tumor is composed of 2 malignant components consisting of solid nests of poorly differentiated squamous cell carcinoma and spindle cell sarcoma (pale area in the photo). Esophageal carcinosarcomas are usually polypoid or pedunculated. Whether the anaplastic spindle cell component represents truly sarcomatous or pseudosarcomatous element (squamous epithelial origin) remains an unresolved question. (H & E, X95)

Figure 11-28. Adenocarcinoma of the stomach, diffuse type (signet-ring cell carcinoma. The tumor cells are polyhedral or rounded, the cytoplasm is pale
and vacuolated, and the nuclei are hyperchromatic. These signet-ring
cells are produced by displacement of the nuclei to the periphery of tumor cells by intracytoplasmic accumulation of mucin. These tumor cells
are poorly cohesive and display a diffuse infiltrative growth pattern. Linitis plastica is the usual "gross appearance" of this tumor. A pure signet-
ring cell carcinoma has a much poorer prognosis than mixed pattern (adenocarcinoma with signet-ring cells) or pure adenocarcinoma. (H & E,
X200)

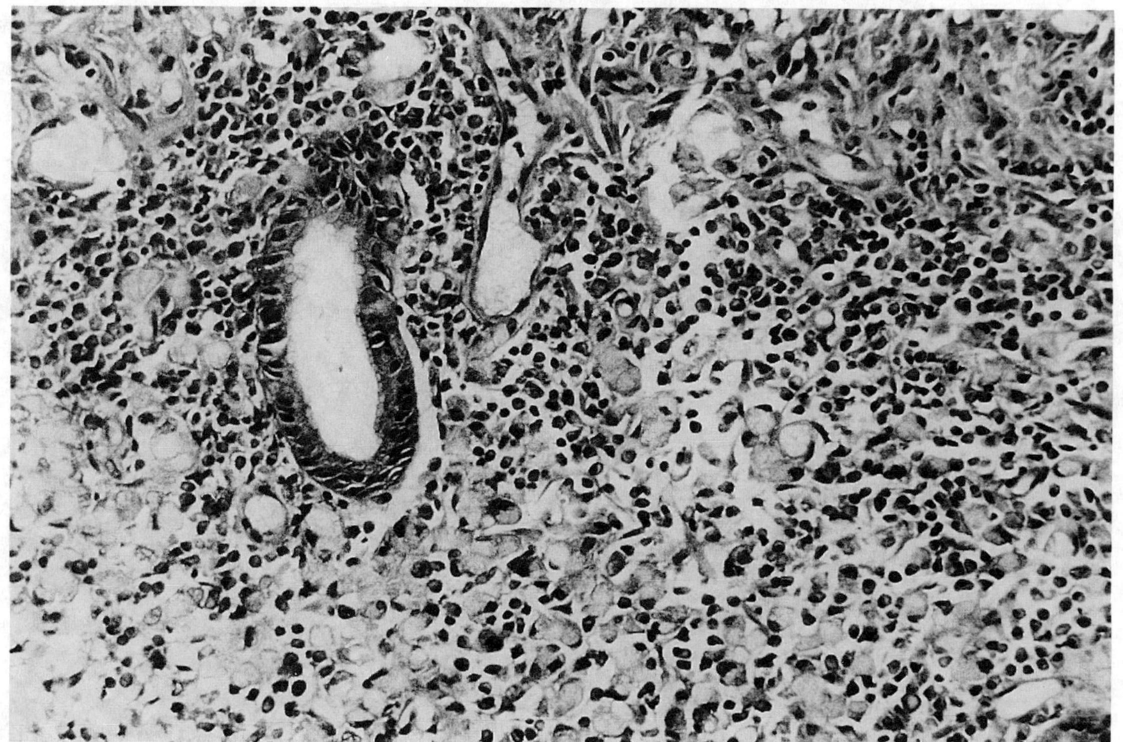

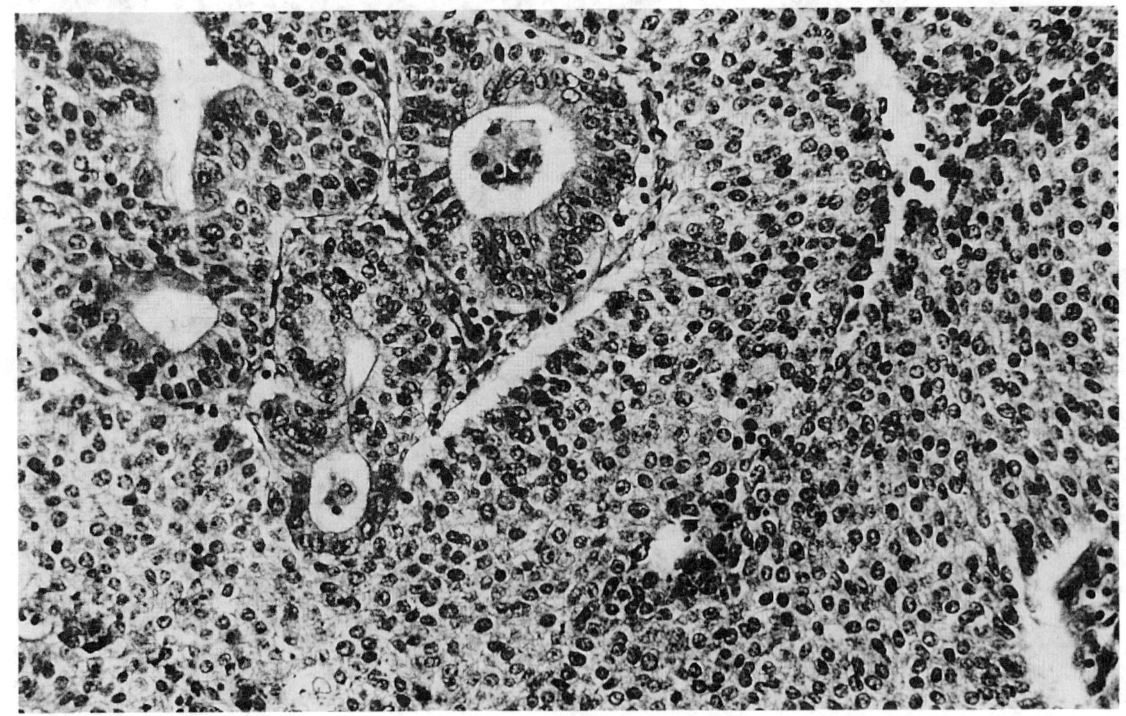

Figure 11-29. Adenocarcinoid of the stomach. This tumor is composed of 2 neoplastic components: One is an intestinal type of adenocarcinoma consisting of well-differentiated columnar cells forming glands; the other is formed of solid sheets of monomorphous round or polygonal cells with uniform, small, round nuclei representing a carcinoid tumor, in which cytoplasmic secretory granules can be demonstrated by means of an argyrophilic stain, i.e., Grimelius stain. (H & E, X200)

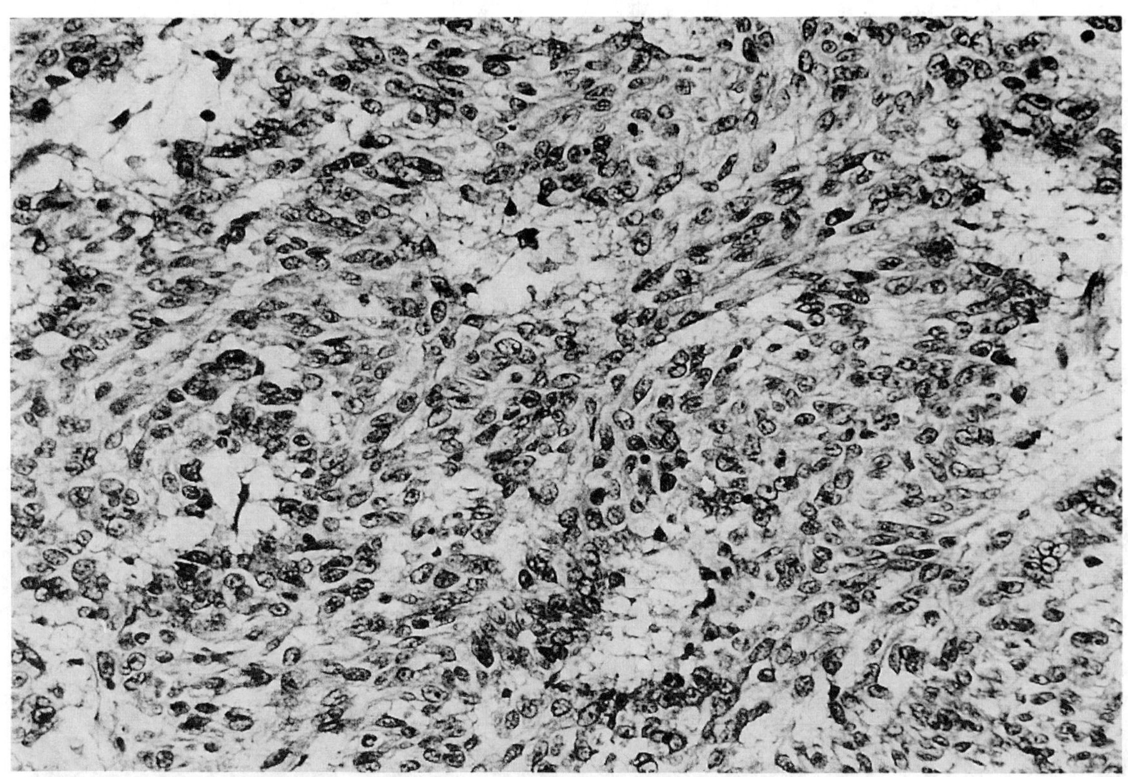

Figure 11-30. Leiomyoblastoma (epithelioid leiomyoma) of the stomach. The tumor is composed of plump polygonal or spindly cells having abundant acidophilic or clear cytoplasm with centrally placed round nuclei. This tumor is intermediate between leiomyoma and leiomyosarcoma in its biological behavior; tumors exhibiting 5 or more mitoses per 50 high-power fields metastasize. Endoscopic biopsy is insufficient to estimate the malignant potential. (H & E, X200)

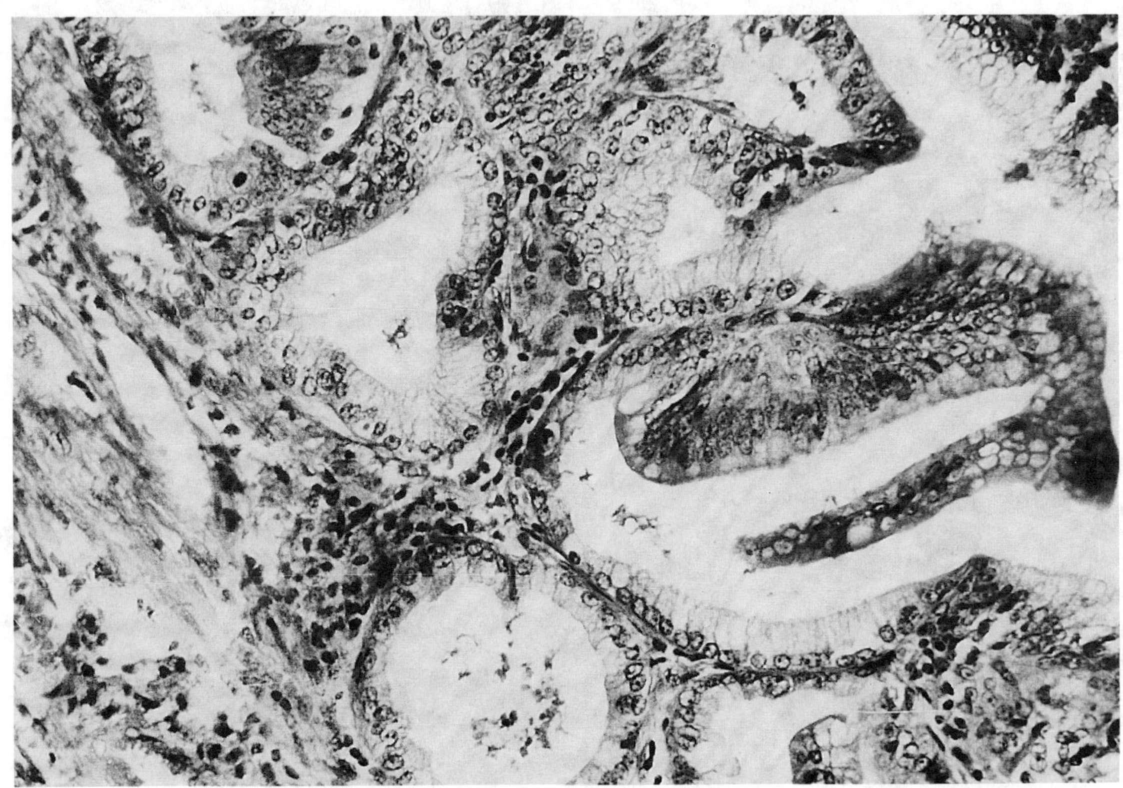

Figure 11-31. Ampullary adenocarcinoma. The tumor is composed of tall columnar cells with basal nuclei, forming glandular and papillary growth pattern. Histologic features are not distinguishable from those of duodenal or pancreatic adenocarcinoma. The ampullary carcinoma is usually well differentiated, and histologic diagnosis may be difficult if a biopsy sample is inadequate. (H & E, X200)

Figure 11-32. Carcinoid tumor of the ileum. The tumor is composed of large and small solid clusters of monomorphic cells. This tumor involves submucosa, but it may replace the mucosa or grow transmurally and extend into the serosa. (H & E, X75)

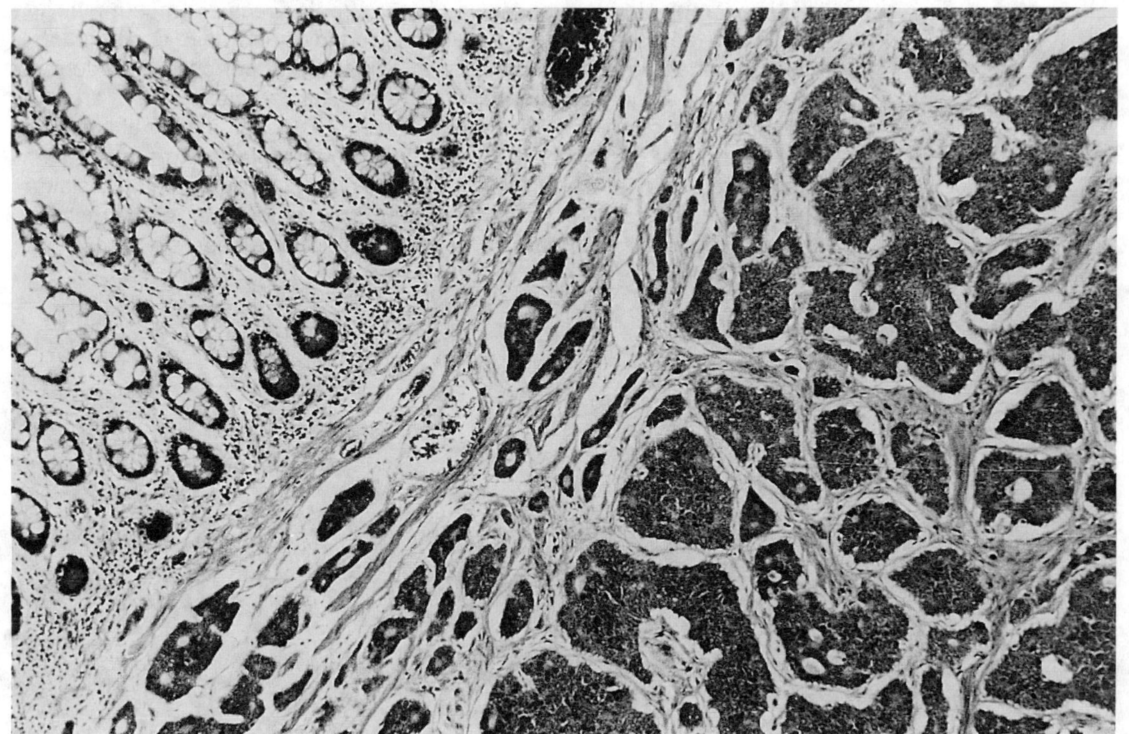

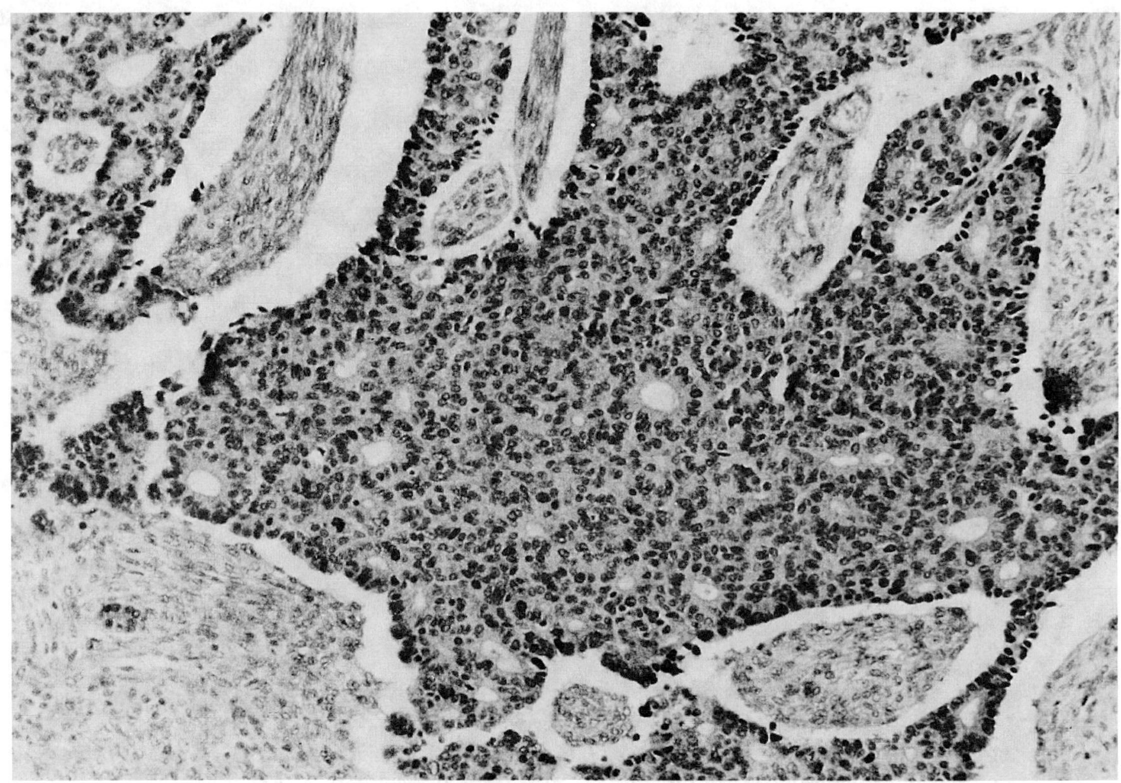

Figure 11-33A & B. Carcinoid tumor. Photo A, above, is a higher magnification of the tumor replacing the muscularis propria (pale areas of smooth muscle). Tumor cells are uniform, small, and rounded and have small, round nuclei. Scattered micrograndular arrangement of tumor cells is evident. Despite the benign appearance of the tumor, all carcinoid tumors are potentially malignant and may metastasize. Most small intestinal carcinoid tumors are functional (H & E, X125). Intracytoplasmic granules (black) are demonstrated in photo B, opposite page, by argentaffin stain. These granules correspond to the secretory granules seen ultrastructurally and is positive with chromogranin (immunoperoxidase stain). (FT, X600)

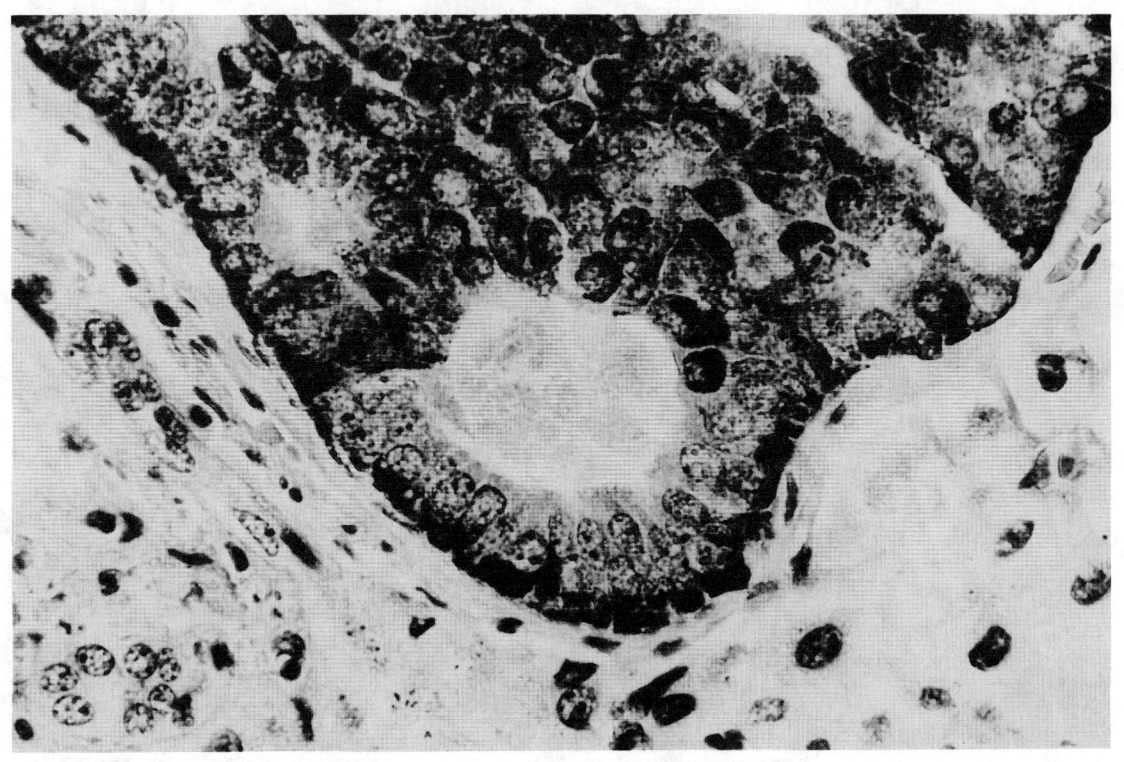

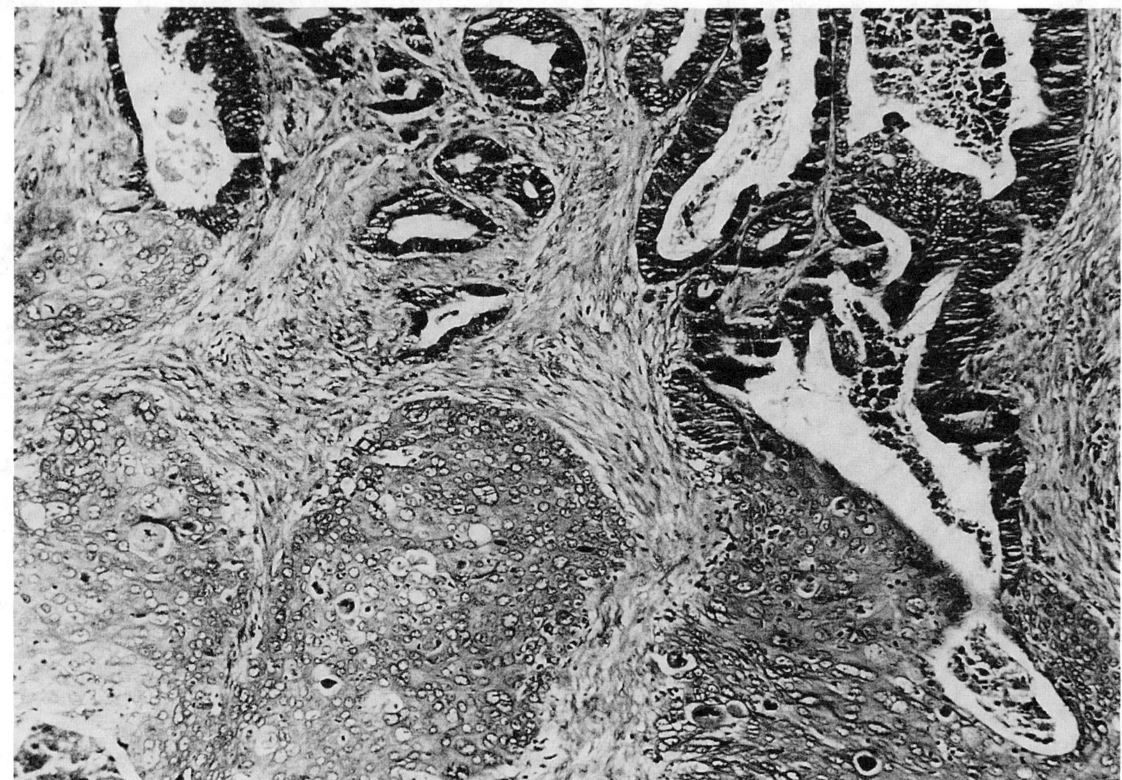

Figure 11-34. Colon adenosquamous cell carcinoma. The tumor comprises 2 components. One is a moderately differentiated adenocarcinoma composed of tall columnar cells forming a glandular pattern. The other is a moderately differentiated squamous cell carcinoma exhibiting islands of solid tumor cells with scattered keratin pearls (black, round structures). The transition between the adenocarcinoma and squamous cell carcinoma is clearly illustrated. When the squamous component is benign, the tumor is designated "adenoacanthoma." Pure squamous cell carcinoma of the colon has been reported. The predominant tumor of the colon is adenocarcinoma. (H & E, X75)

Figure 11-35. Hepatocellular carcinoma, trabecular pattern. The tumor is composed of well-differentiated cells resembling hepatocytes with
hyperchromatic nuclei and prominent nucleoli. Tumor cells are arranged
in irregular anastomosing trabeculae, and the intervening sinusoids are
lined by flattened endothelial cells. Most hepatocellular carcinomas are
well differentiated, despite the aggressive nature and poor prognosis. (H
& E, X150)

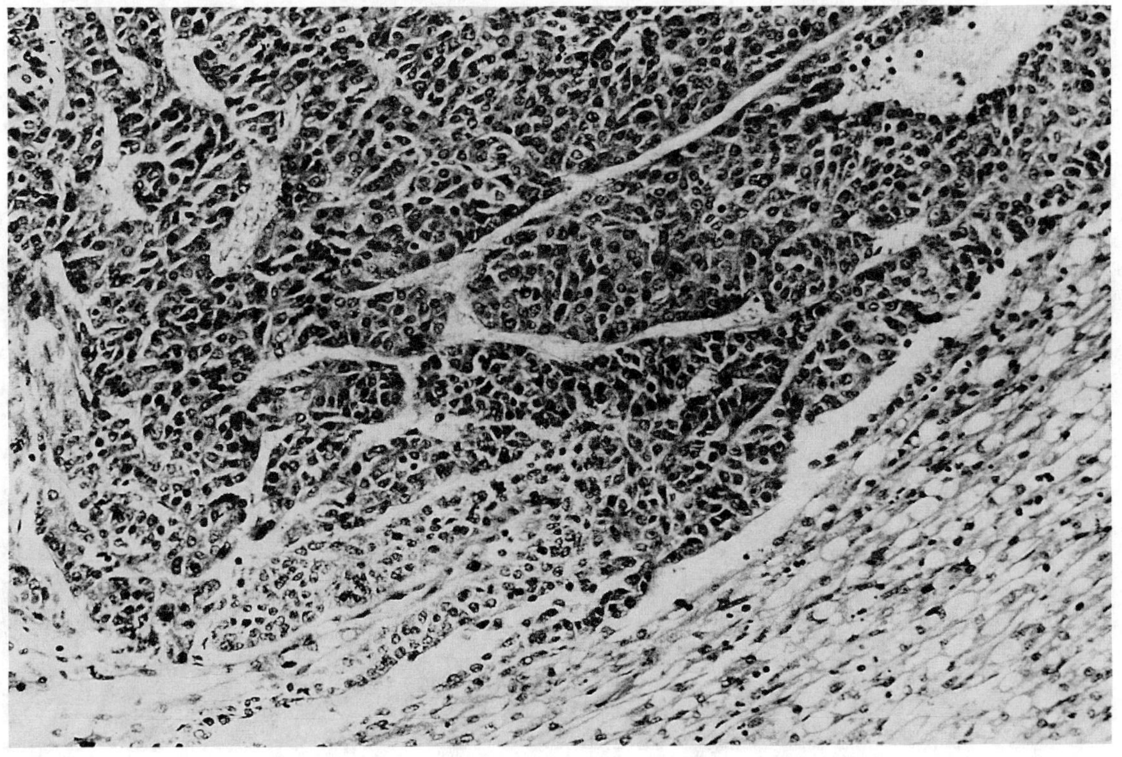

Figure 11-36. Hepatocellular carcinoma, acinar or pseudoglandular pattern. Tumor cells are arranged in small acini around a central lumen, which is formed by a bile canaliculus. These acinar lumens are distended and may contain bile or proteinaceous material. The trabecular pattern of tumor cells and flattened endothelial lining cells on the sinusoids are evident. This pattern is common in well-differentiated hepatocellular carcinoma and should not be confused with an adenocarcinoma. Alpha-1-antitrypsin, alpha-fetoprotein, and Mallory bodies may be present in the cytoplasm of the tumor cells and can be demonstrated by appropriate special methods. (H & E, X125)

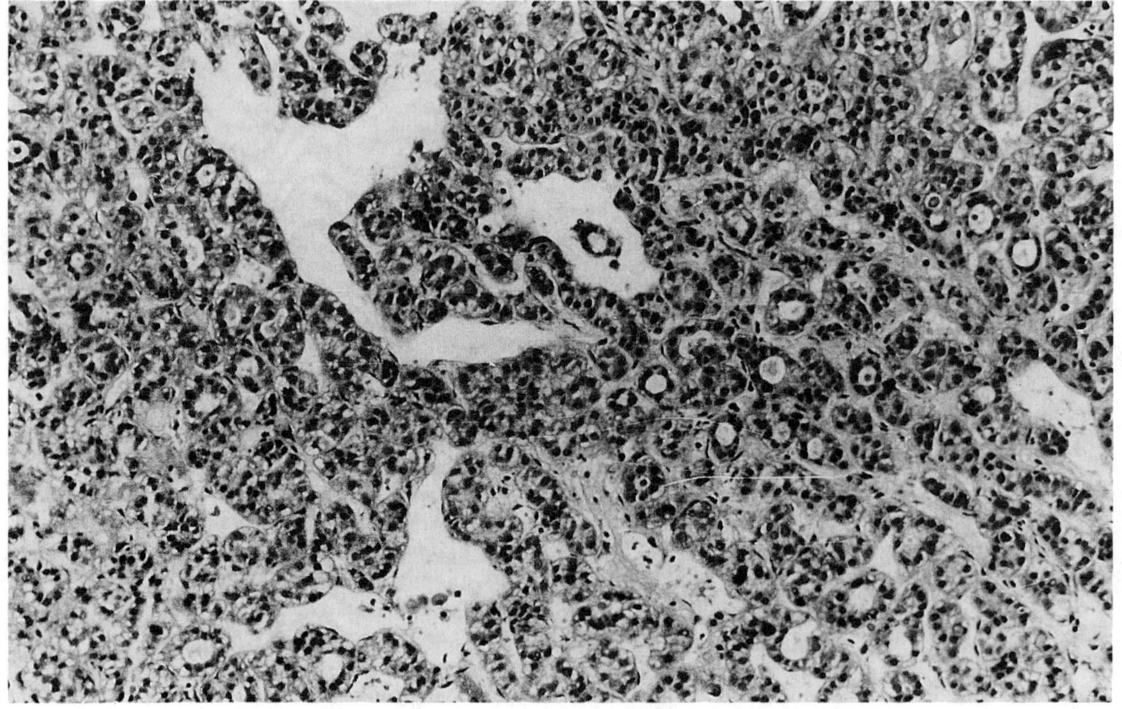

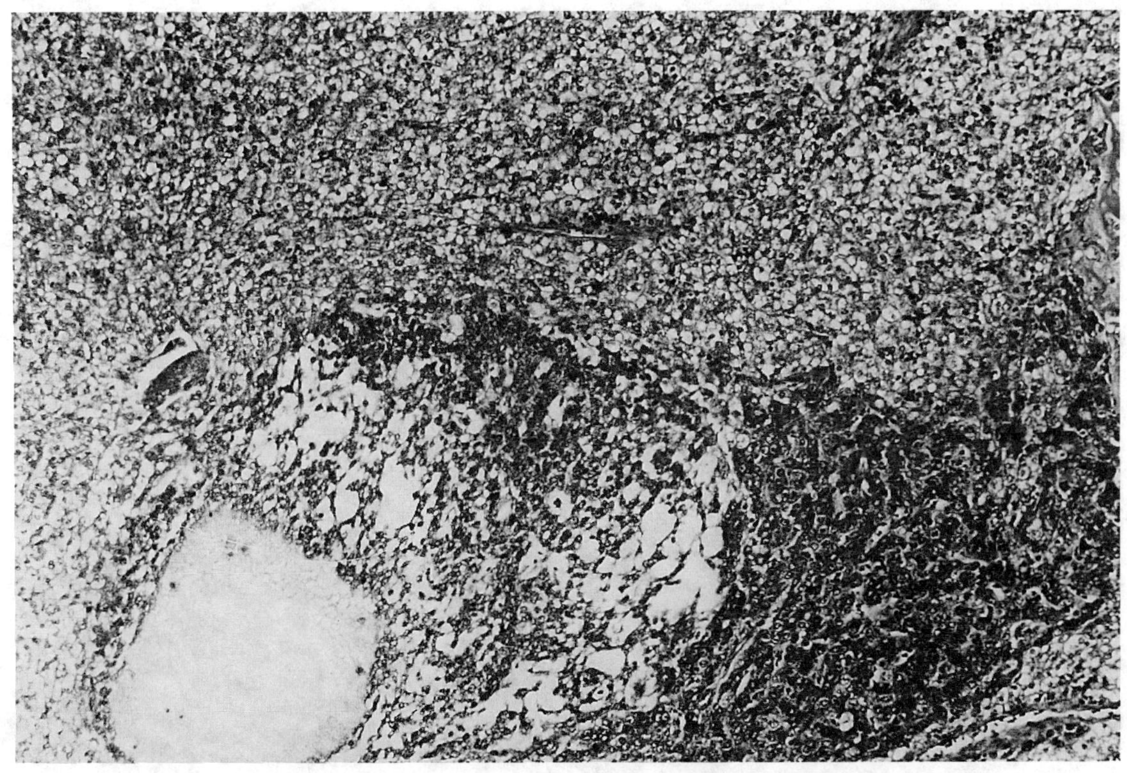

Figure 11-37. Hepatoblastoma, epithelial type. The tumor is composed of large
     solid sheets of the fetal type of small hepatocytes. A nodular area of em-
     bryonal type of hepatoblastoma and an island of trabecular hepatocellu-
     lar carcinoma are also present. Embryonal cells are more poorly differen-
     tiated than the fetal type of tumor cells. Hepatoblastoma is classified into
     an epithelial type and a mixed epithelial and mesenchymal type. In the
     mixed type, mesenchymal elements (not shown in this photo) consist of
     primitive spindle cells. Osteoid tissue is present in most mixed hepato-
     blastoma. (H & E, X75)

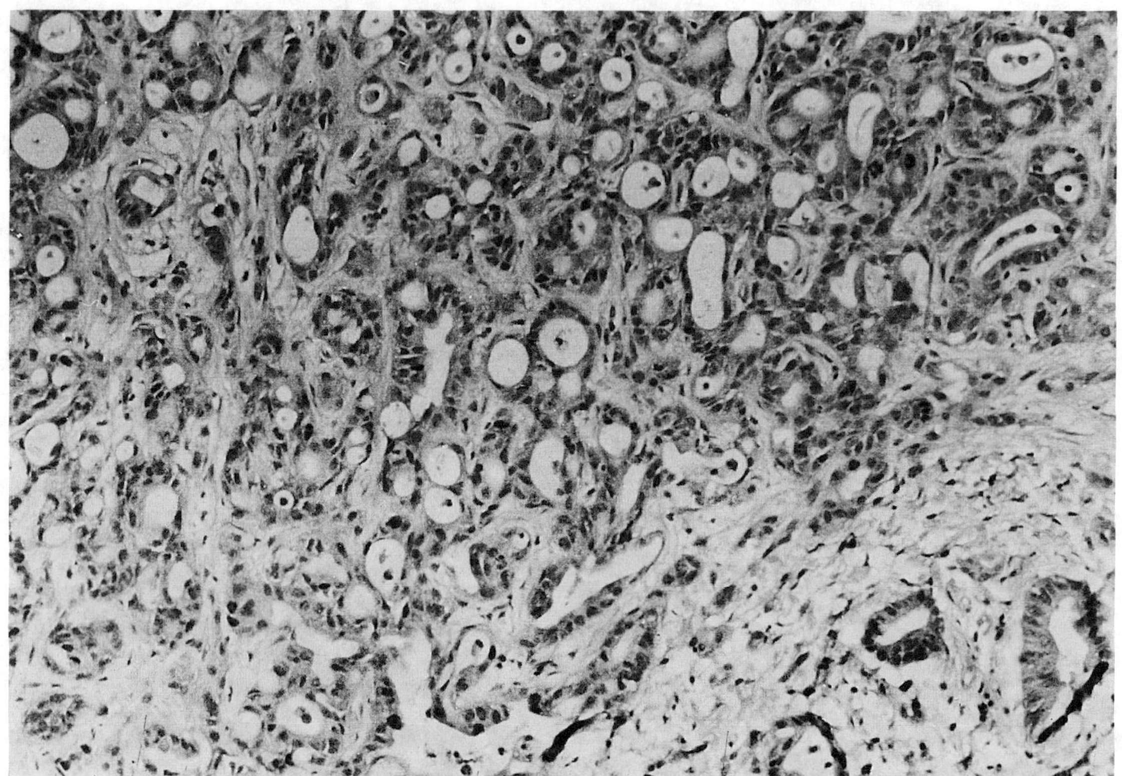

Figure 11-38. Cholangiocarcinoma. The tumor is composed of well-differentiated cuboidal cells forming a glandular pattern and accompanied by varying degrees of stromal desmoplasia. The glandular lumens are empty or may contain mucin. The cholangiocarcinoma is an adenocarcinoma and cannot be distinguished from metastatic adenocarcinoma originating from other primary sites. (H & E, X125)

Figure 11-39. Angiosarcoma of the liver. The hepatocytes are surrounded by malignant sinusoidal endothelial cells with ovoid hyperchromatic nuclei and scanty cytoplasm (sinusoidal pattern). The hepatocytes undergo atrophy as the tumor cells proliferate and replace the hepatocytes to form solid sarcomatous areas (sarcomatous pattern). Large blood-filled cystic spaces lined by malignant endothelial cells (not shown in this photo) are frequently encountered (cavernous pattern). Immunocytochemical stain may disclose the presence of factor VIII-related antigen in the tumor cells. (H & E, X95)

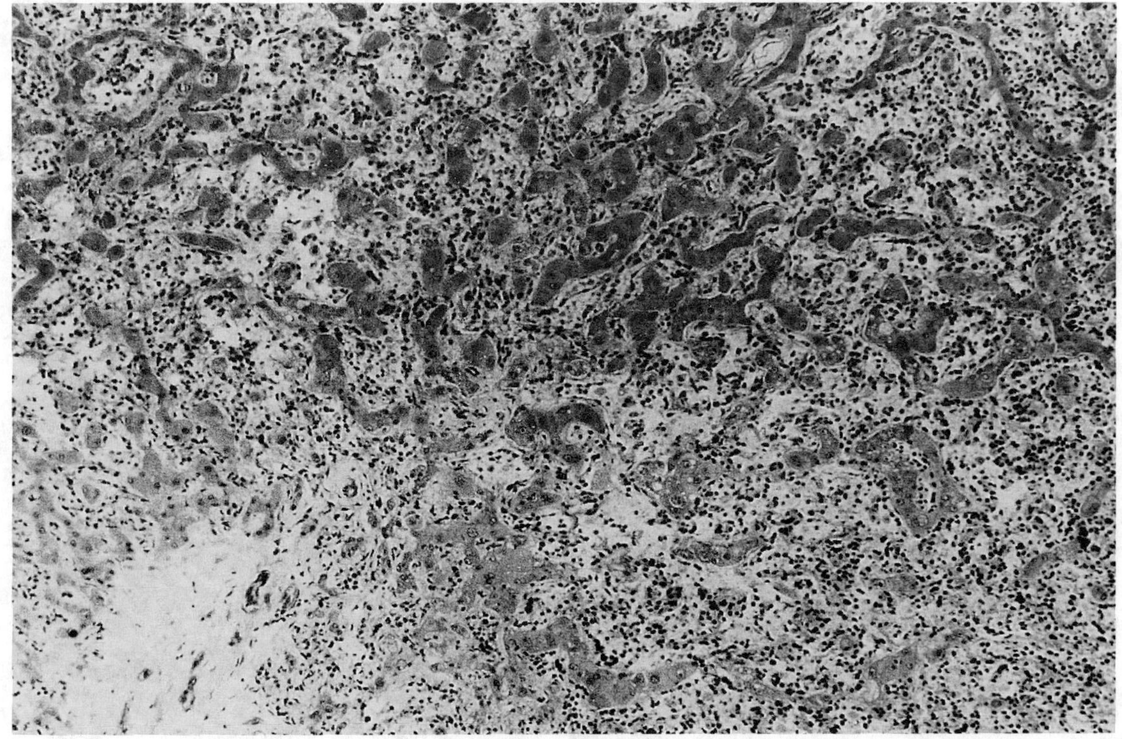

Figure 11-40. Anaplastic carcinoma of the gallbladder, signet-ring cell type.
Unlike the usual adenocarcinoma of the gallbladder, this tumor is composed of sheets of small cells, many of the tumor cells showing signet-
ring appearance due to intracytoplasmic mucin. The tumor cells diffusely
infiltrate the gallbladder wall, simulating the infiltrating carcinoma
(linitis plastica) of the stomach. (H & E, X200)

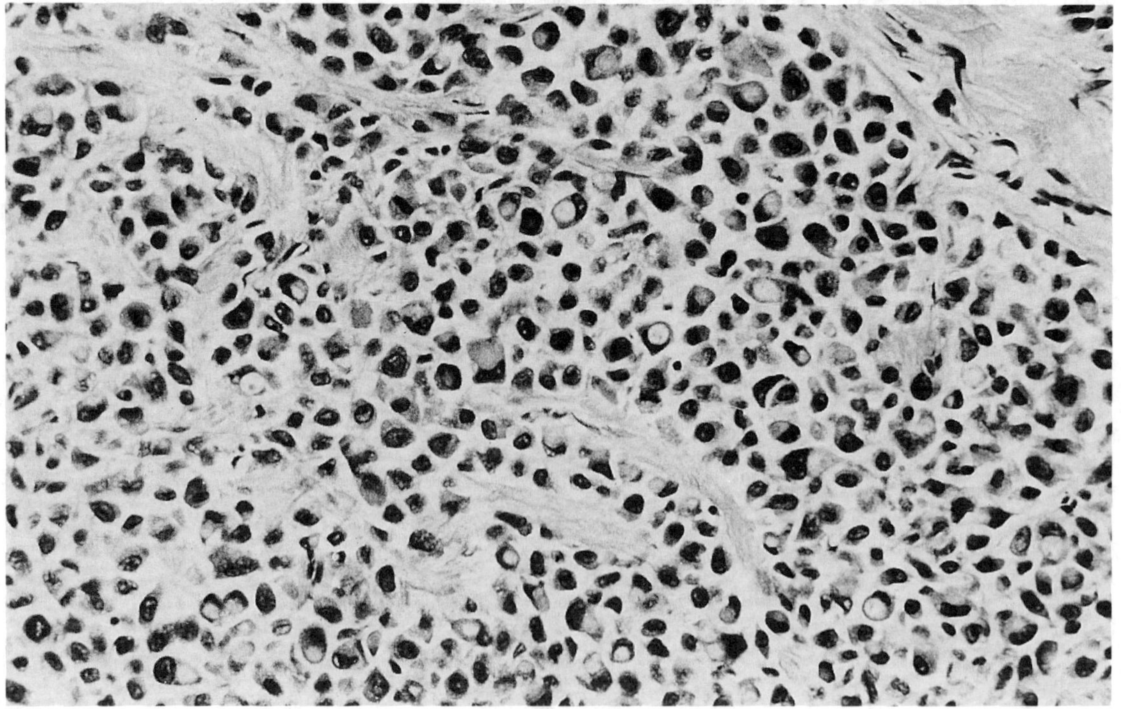

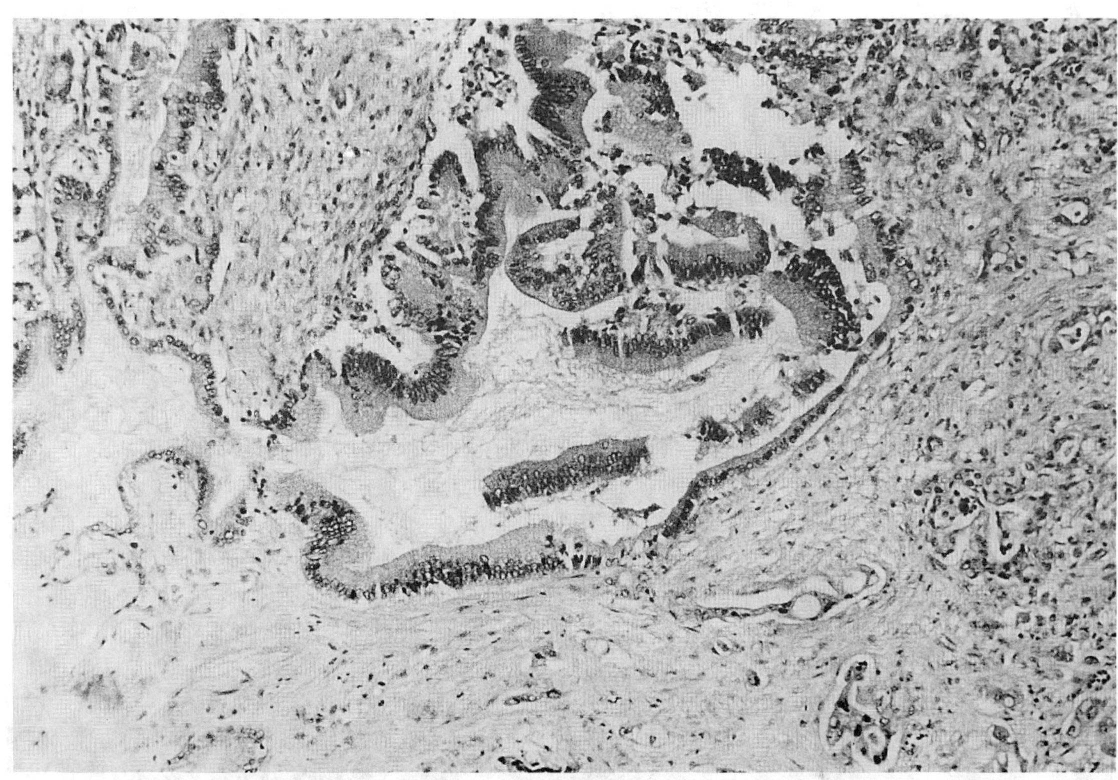

Figure 11-41. Pancreatic mucinous adenocarcinoma. The tumor exhibits 2 patterns. One is a cytadenocarcinoma showing a cystic space lined by well-differentiated tall columnar malignant cells with basal nuclei. The other is an adenocarcinoma invading the surrounding fibrous stroma. (H & E, X95)

Malignant Tumors of the Urinary System

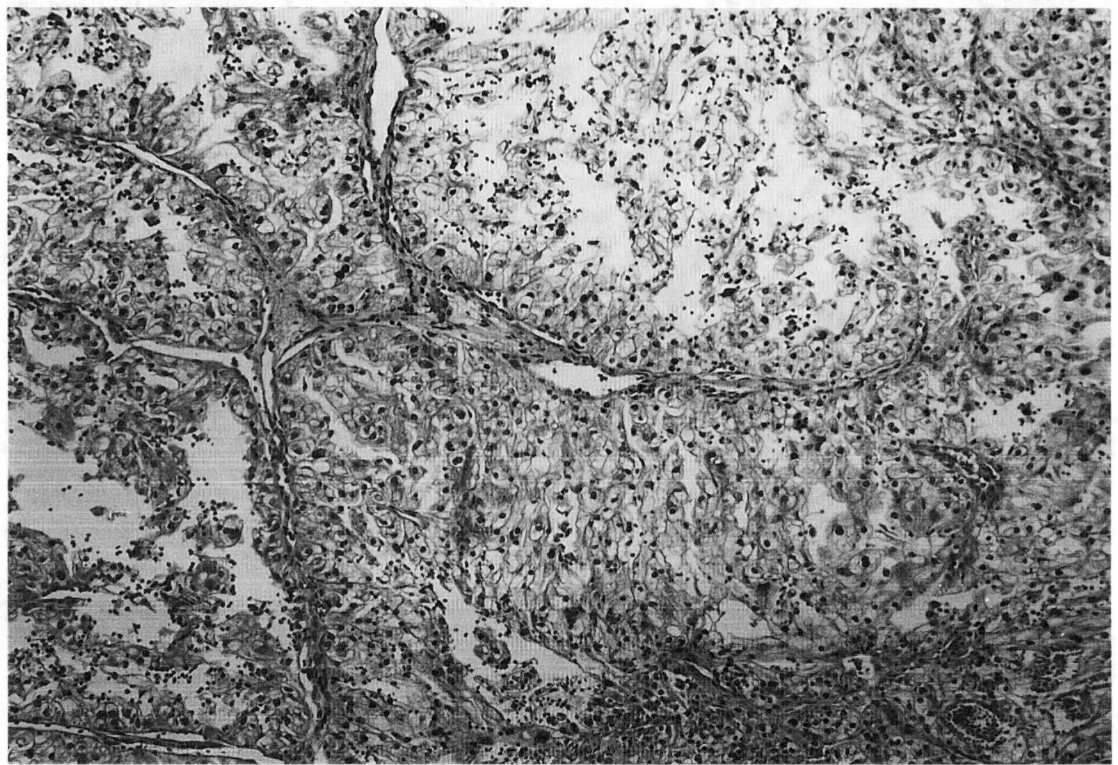

Figure 11-42A & B. Renal cell carcinoma (hypernephroma). The tumor cells may be either clear, granular, or spindle cells (sarcomatoid). Except for a few pure cases, the tumor often contains a mixture of cells. Nuclei of clear cells tend to be small, with abundant cytoplasm containing fat and glycogen. Granular cells have finely granular acidophil cytoplasm with irregular large nuclei (photo A, above). The spindle cells when prominent tend to be mistaken for sarcoma (photo B, opposite page). The tumor pattern may be solid sheets, papillary, or granular and may form cysts. Renal adenoma may show similar histology of clear to granular cells. Tumors of <3 cm are usually benign. Some authors consider these adenomas as potentially malignant. Renal pelvic tumors are commonly transitional cell carcinomas and a few are adenocarcinomas. (H & E, X75)

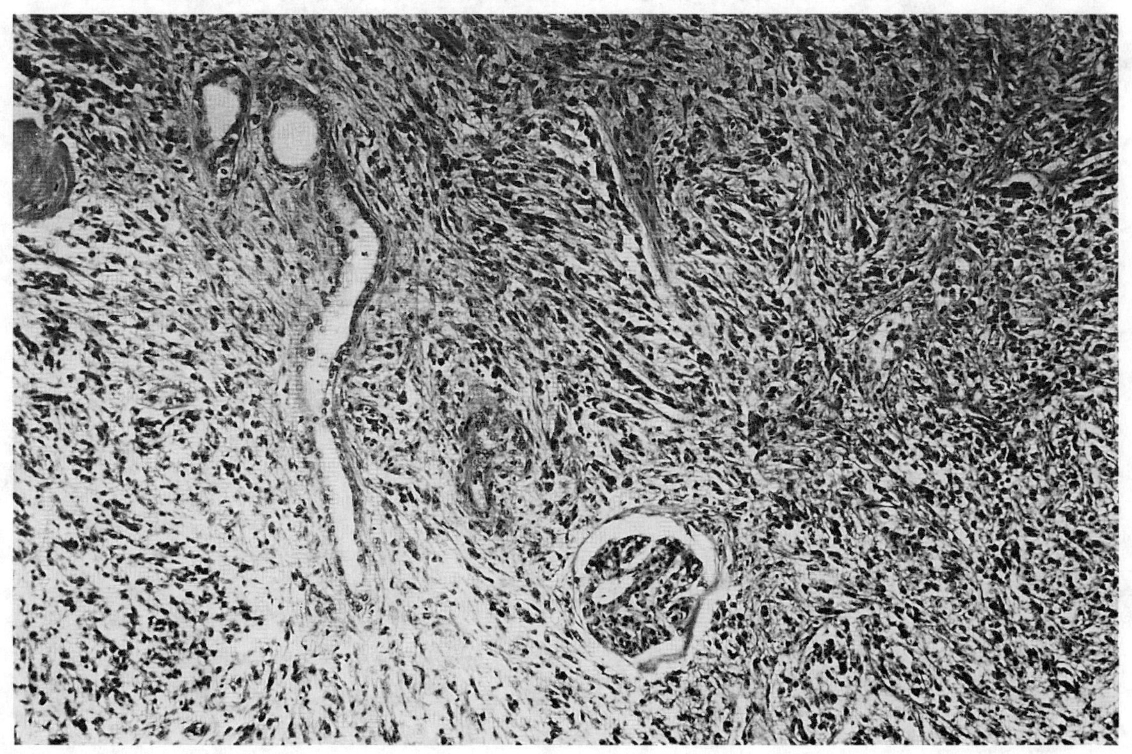

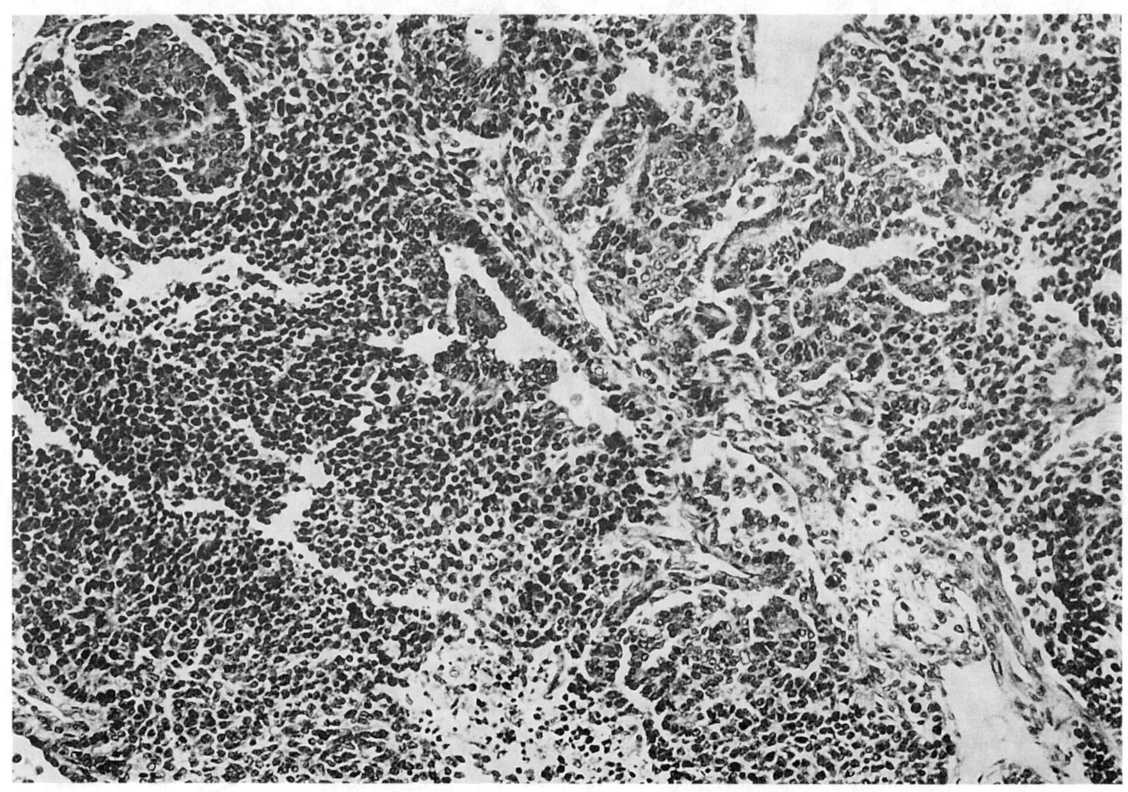

Figure 11-43. Wilms' tumor (nephroblastoma). The tumor is composed predominantly of undifferentiated round-to-ovoid hyperchromatic cells with tubules, glomeroid structures, and some minor components such as smooth and striated muscle, cartilage, bone, and fat tissue. Histologic types that preclude a more aggressive growth include the anaplastic and sarcomatous pattern. The sarcomatous pattern can present with rhabdomyosarcomatoid, clear-cell, and hyalinizing features. (H & E, X75)

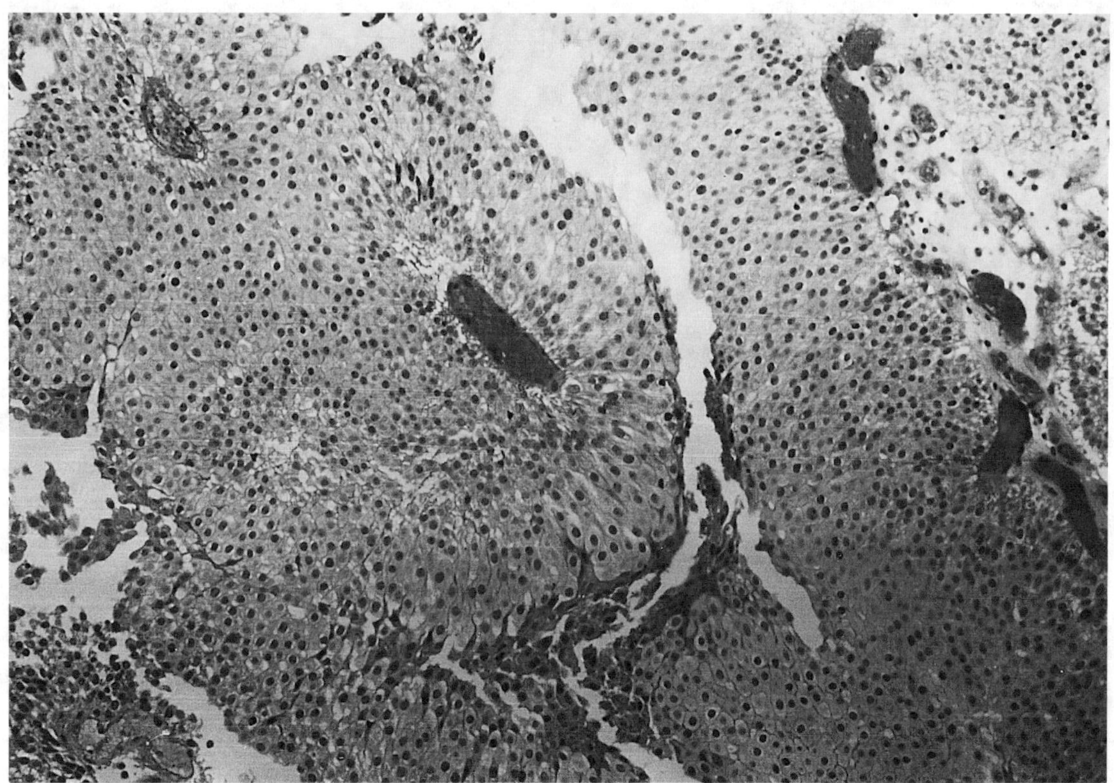

Figure 11-44A,B,C. Papillary transitional cell carcinoma of the bladder. Transitional cells lining a papillary structure indicates stratification, with cells showing slight nuclear pleomorphism and a few mitotic figures. This would be a grade I and may be classified by others as papilloma, particularly if the villi are delicate without fusion (photo A, above). Fifty percent of papillomas recur and <10% develop a higher grade of transitional cell carcinoma. Perhaps from a more practical viewpoint the papilloma would be included under grade I to ensure follow-up of patients. Grade III transitional cell carcinoma is less papillary due to fusion of villous processes. In grade III, epidermoid features are noted in focal or multiple areas with loss of stratification, conspicuous anaplasia, and frequent mitotic figures (photo C, opposite page, bottom). Grade II transitional cell carcinoma discloses papillary tumor showing moderate cellular pleomorphism and frequent mitoses (photo B, opposite page, top). Invasion of muscle layer should be noted for staging purposes. Transitional cell carcinoma involving other urothelial mucosa has the same histologic features. (H & E, X125)

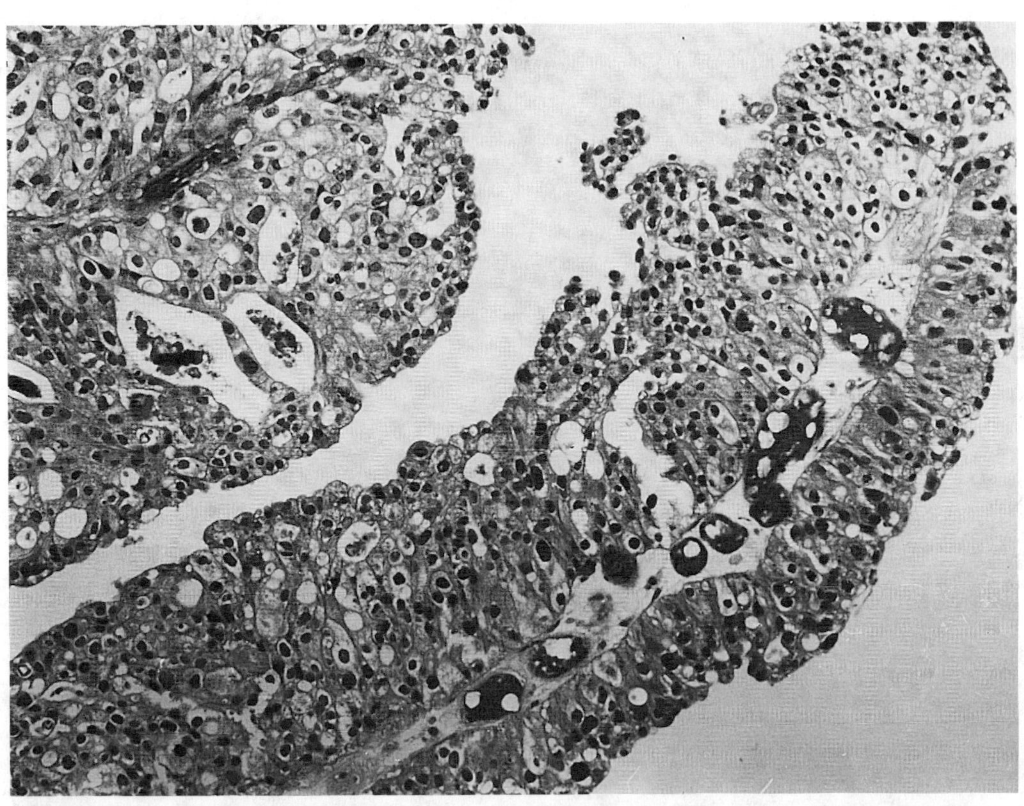

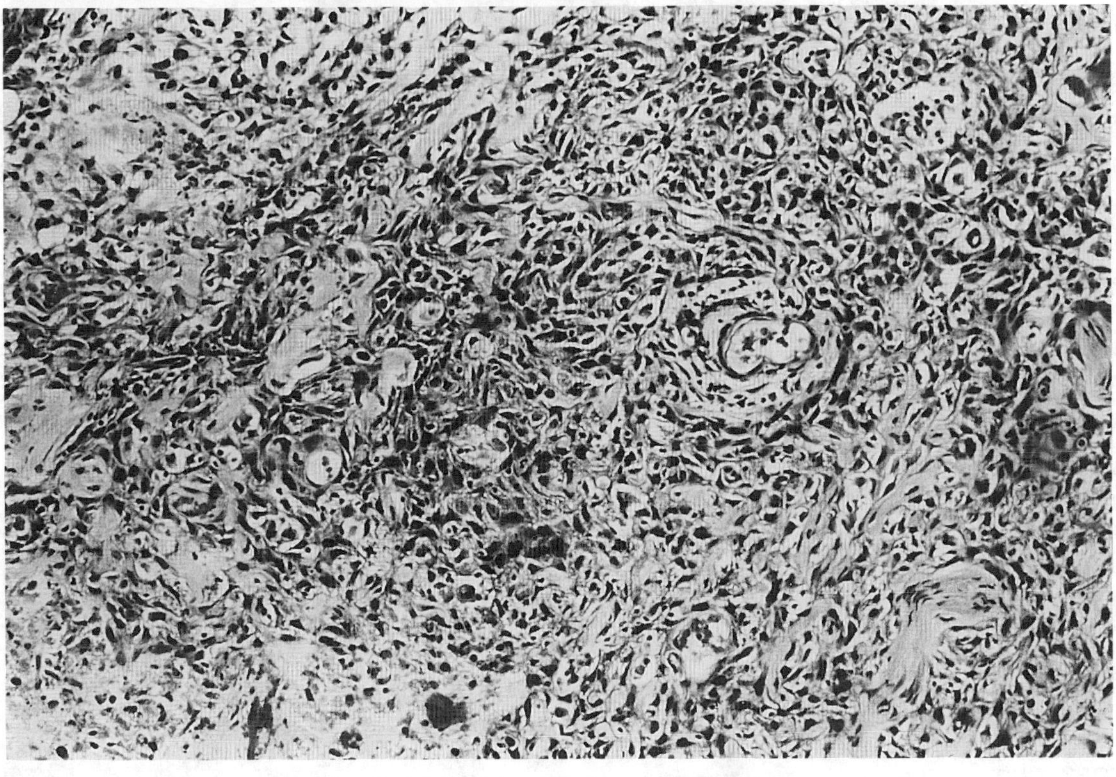

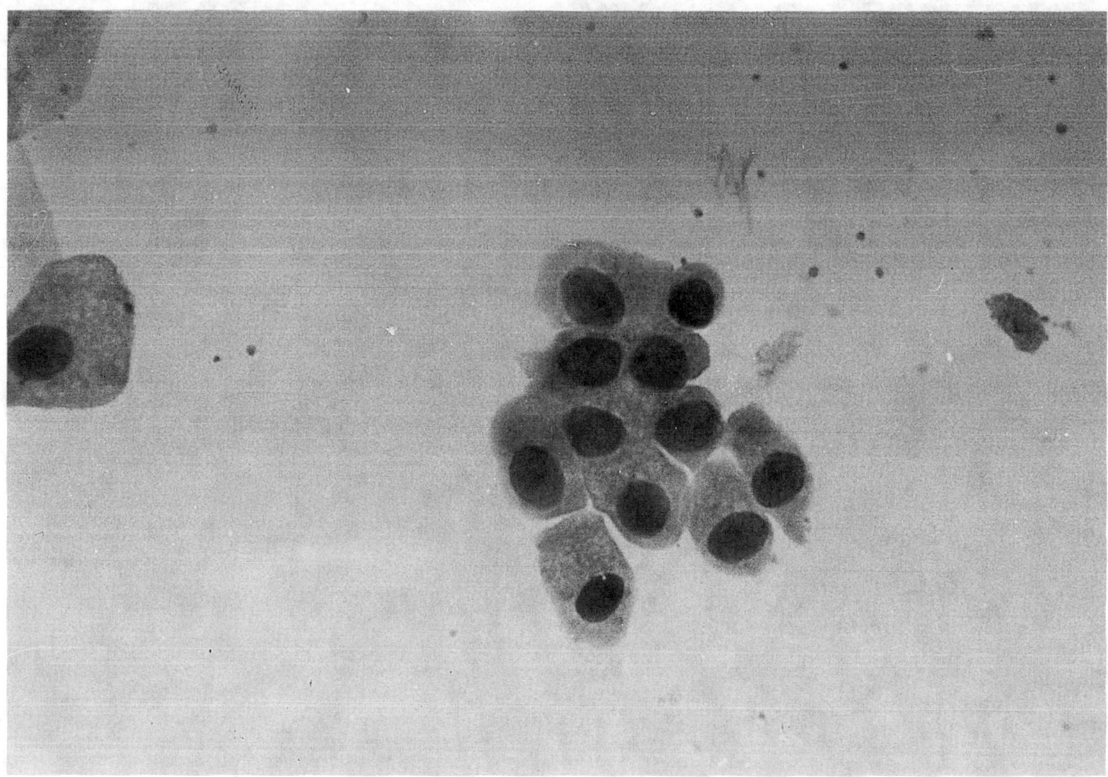

Figure 11-45A,B,C. Transitional cell carcinoma of the bladder (cytology). Exfoliated cells from a papilloma or a grade I transitional cell carcinoma are not distinguishable from normal urothelial cells (photo A, above). Tumor cells from grade III form clusters of polygonal to ovoid to irregularly shaped cells of varied sizes having dense hyperchromatic nuclei with irregular and angulated nuclear membrane. There is a scant to moderate amount of cytoplasm. Nucleoli may be prominent but are often obscured by dense, coarse nuclear chromatin. The nucleo/cytoplasmic ratio is decreased (photo C, opposite page, bottom). In grade II, the cells are less pleomorphic. The nuclear membrane is distinct, and most cells display smooth contours with less dense chromatin, so that nucleoli are often readily visible (photo B, opposite page, top). (Pap, X500)

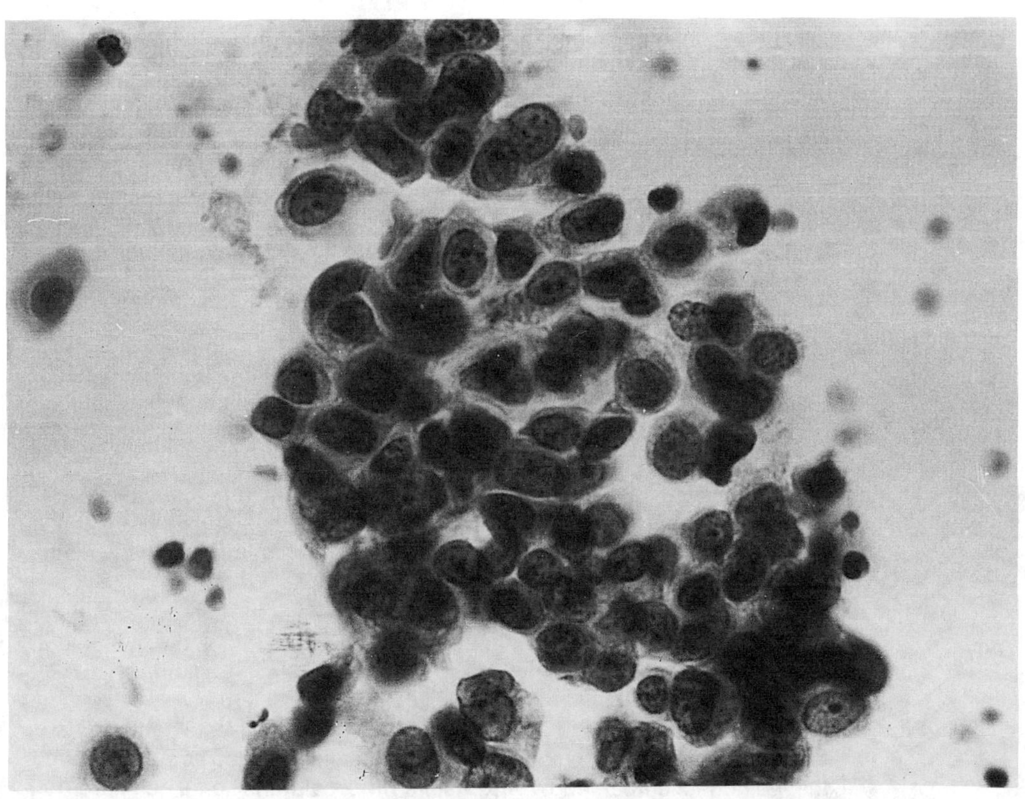

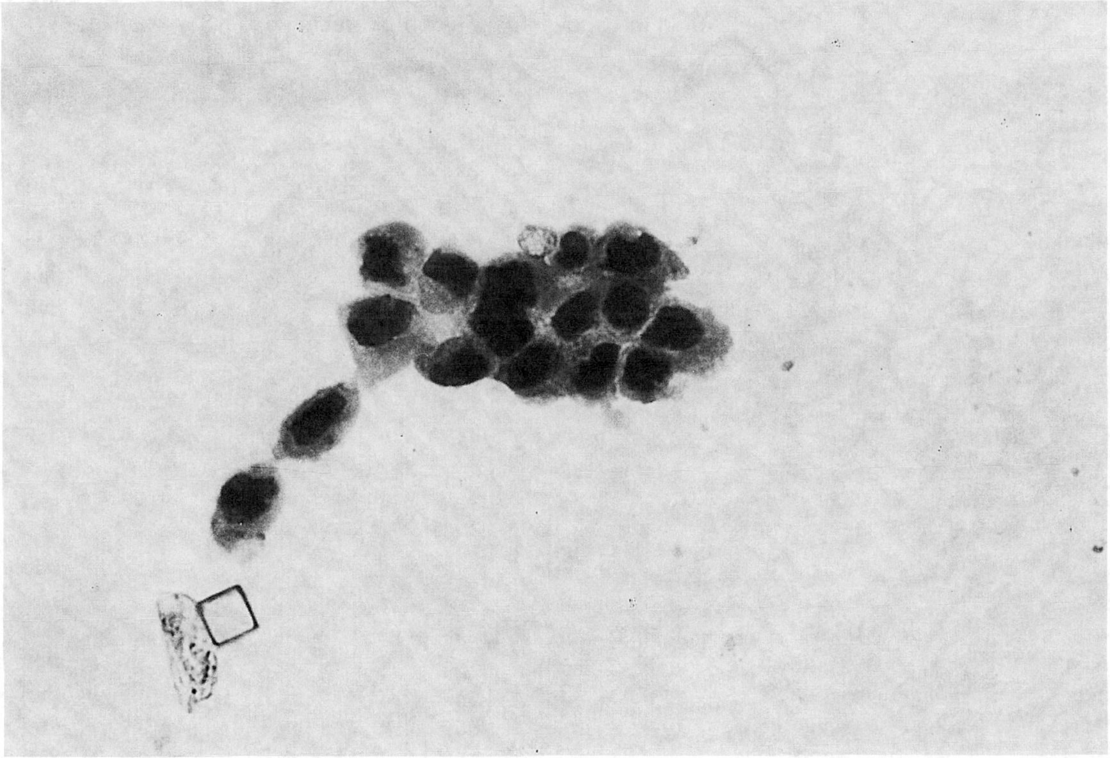

Figure 11-46. Adenocarcinoma of the bladder (linitis plastica-like). The tumor is composed of hyperchromatic cells with vacuolated cytoplasm infiltrating the wall unaccompanied by any visible mucosal transitional cell carcinoma. This is a rare type. Mucin-secreting adenocarcinoma occurs more frequently than the above and may be of urachal origin. (H & E, X125)

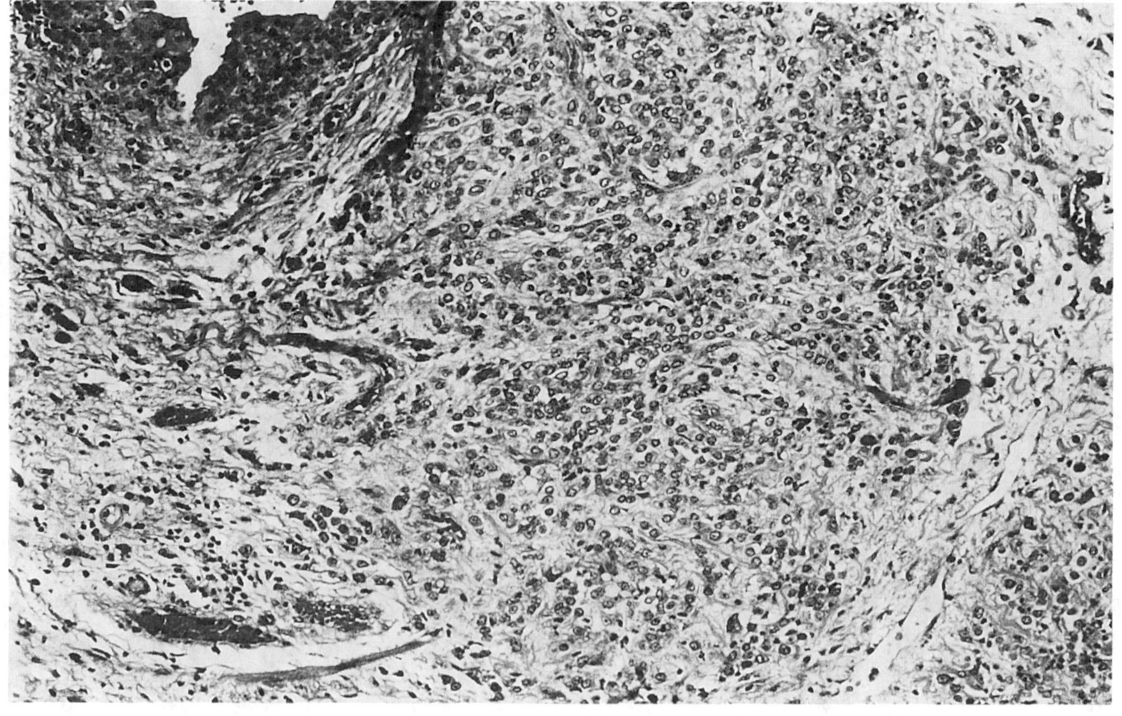

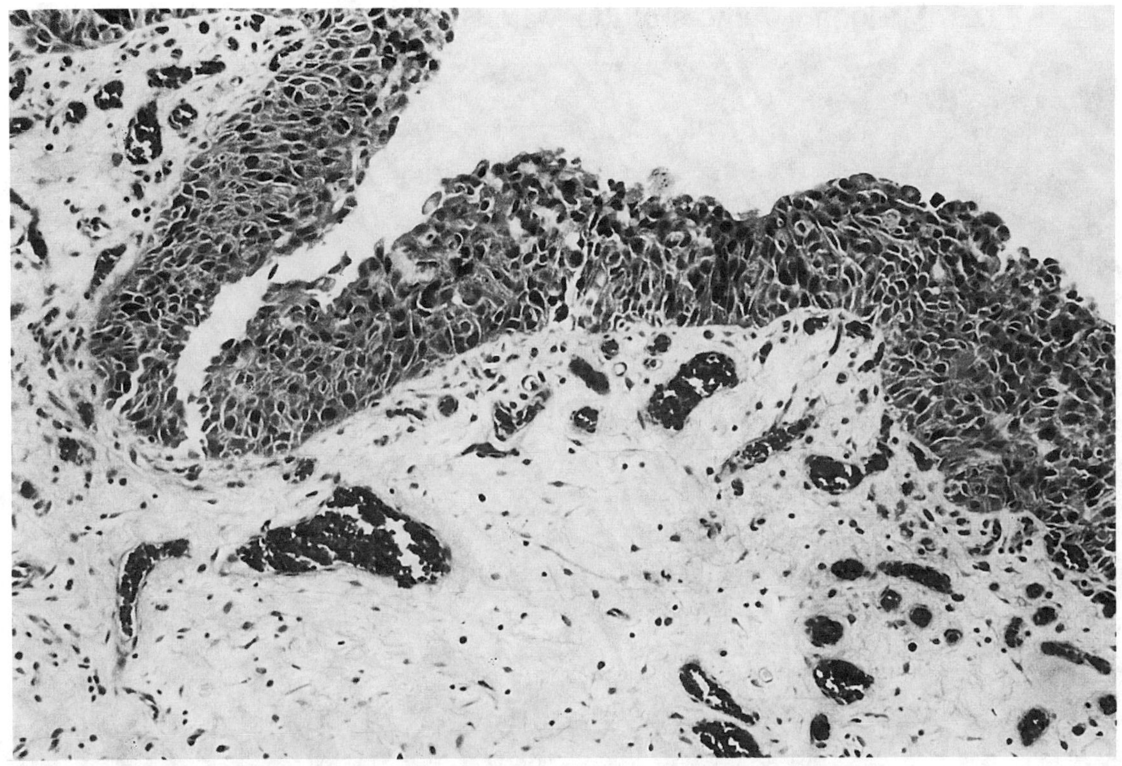

Figure 11-47. Bladder transitional cell carcinoma *in situ*. The lesion is characterized by dysplastic changes involving all layers of the urothelial mucosa. These may not be accompanied by any visible mucosal tumor and may occur in multiple areas if not throughout. (H & E, X125)

Malignant Tumors of the Male Reproductive System

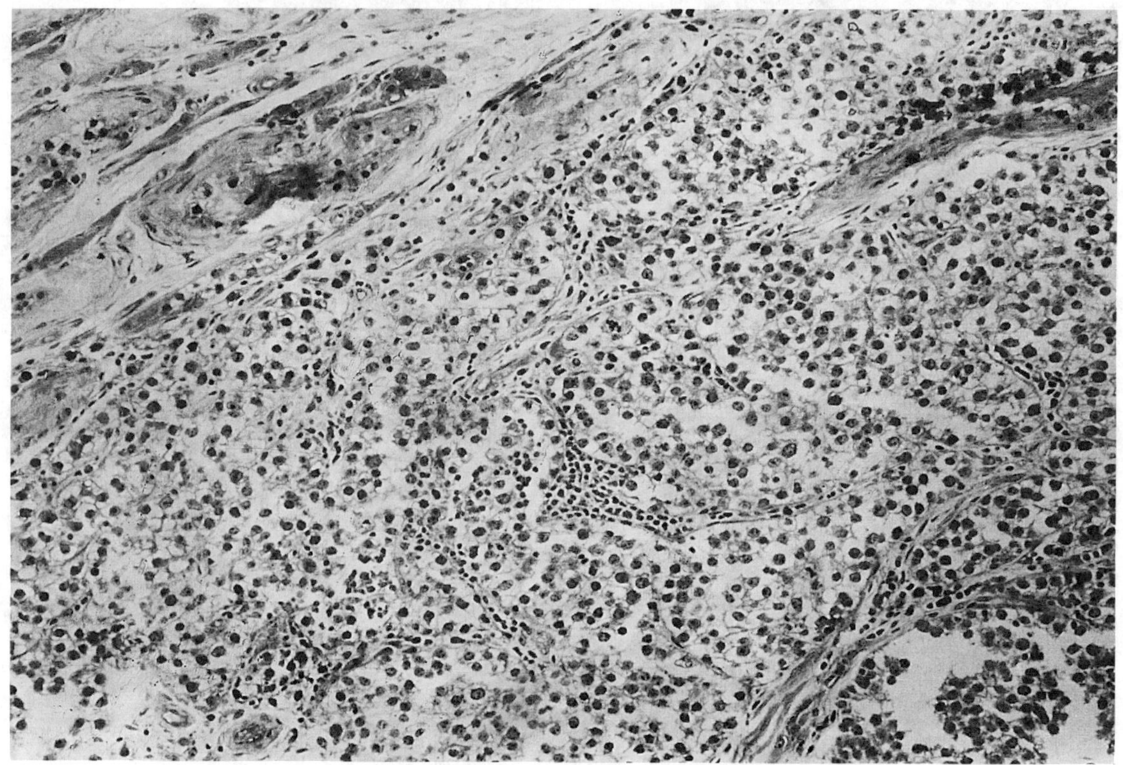

Figure 11-48. Testicular seminoma. It is composed of sheets of uniform round to polygonal cells with clear cytoplasm, centrally placed nuclei with prominent nucleoli, and distinct cell borders divided into lobules by thin fibrovascular stroma sprinkled with lymphocytes. Occasional syncytiotrophoblasts may be noted, but this does not necessarily imply the presence of choriocarcinoma. Anaplastic seminoma is categorized by the degree of cellular pleomorphism and the presence of 3 or more mitotic figures per high-power field. Rare in children. (H & E, X125)

Figure 11-49. Testicular embryonal carcinoma. Pleomorphic epithelial cells showing organoid pattern, papillary, tubular to solid sheets to an occasional
embryoid plates. Not reported in infants and children. (H & E, X125)

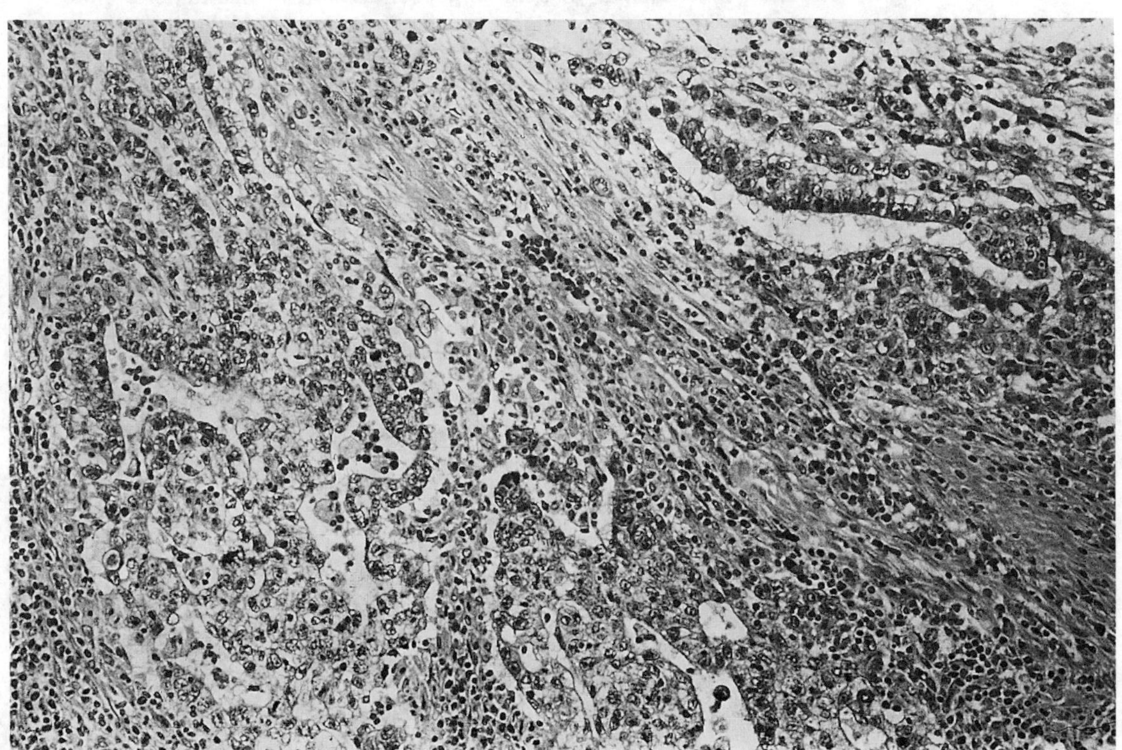

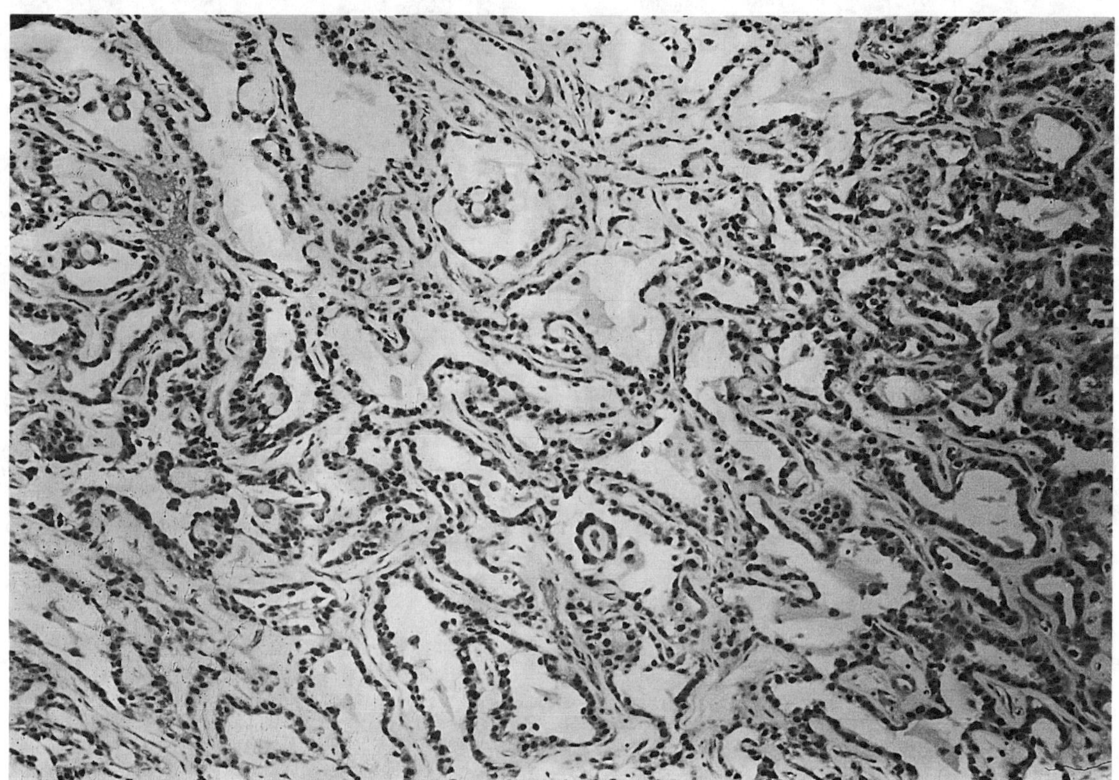

Figure 11-50A & B. Testicular yolk sac tumor (endodermal sinus tumor orchioblastoma). Tumor cells range from flattened endothelial-like cells to columnar or cuboidal type cells forming an irregular small and large acinar pattern. The nuclei are round to ovoid with 1 or 2 nucleoli having clear to acidophil cytoplasm containing PAS-diastase positive hyaline globules (photo A, above). Glomeruloid structure (Schiller-Duval body) may also be noted. It is a papillary structure with a central vessel covered by tumor cells projecting into a space lined by tumor cells simulating a glomerular structure (photo B, opposite page). This is the most common gonadal tumor in infants and children under 3½. This tumor also gives the strongest reaction with stains for alpha-fetoprotein, whereas embryonal carcinoma gives out a moderate intensity. Alpha 1-antitrypsin may also be positive. About 40% of nonseminomatous testicular tumors contain endodermal sinus tumor. (H & E, X125)

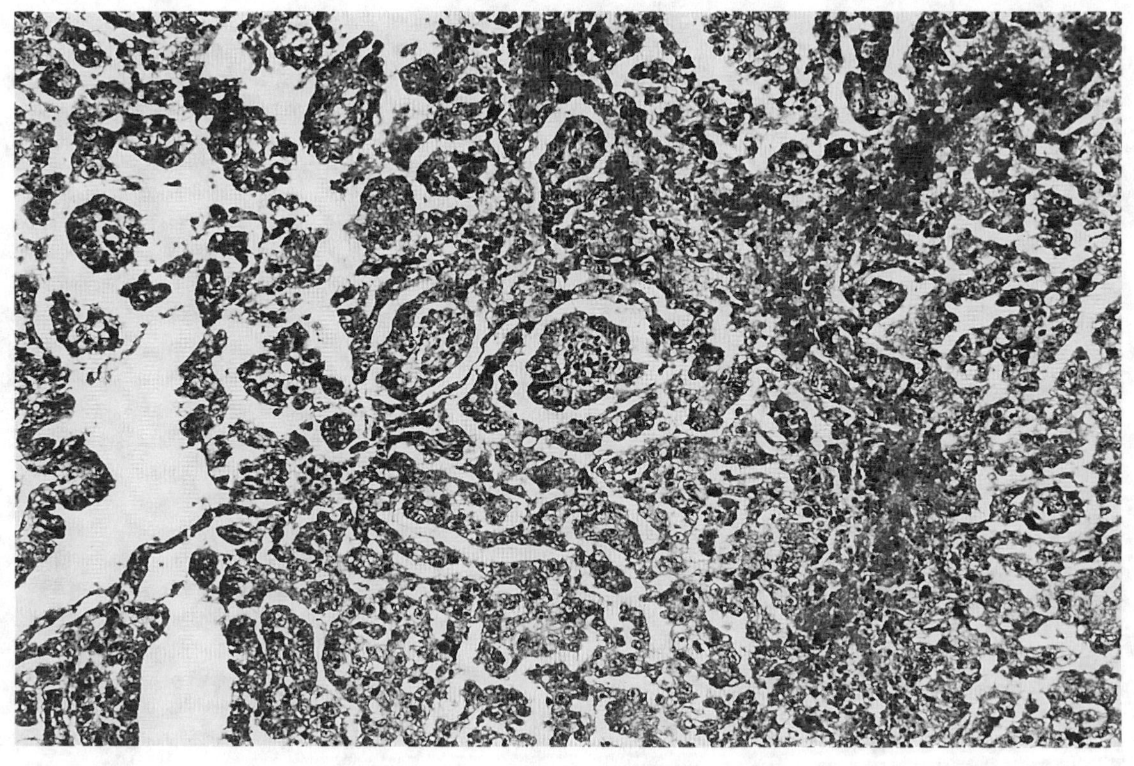

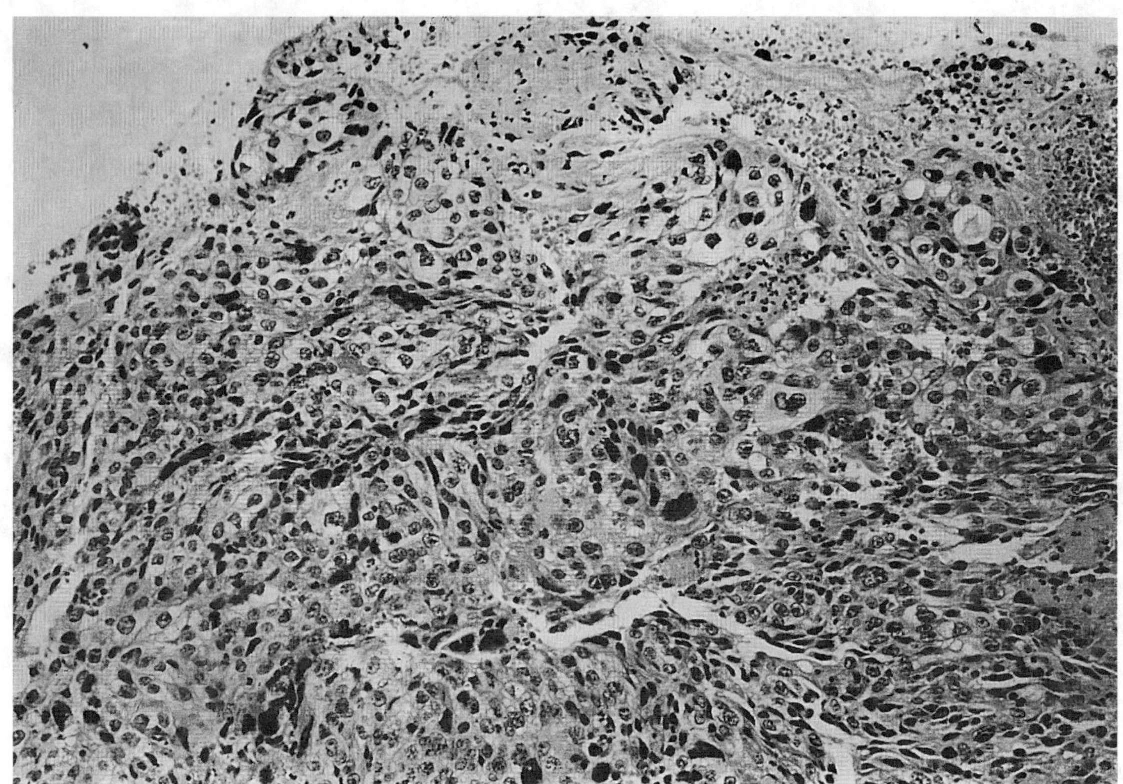

Figure 11-51. Testicular choriocarcinoma. The tumor consists of syncytiotropho-
blast and cytotrophoblast cells accompanied by necrosis and
hemorrhage. Syncytial cells alone are not sufficient for establishing the
diagnosis. Cytotrophoblasts are round-to-polygonal uniform-looking cells
arranged in sheets surrounded by multinucleated syncytial cells. Only
the syncytial cells will stain for HCG (human chorionic gonadotrophin).
Most of these tumors are mixed with other germ cell tumors. Pure choriocarcinoma is rare. (H & E, X125)

Figure 11-52. Testicular teratoma. The tumor may consist of mature to immature elements of more than 1 of the 3 primary germ layers (endoderm, ectoderm, and mesoderm). Mature and immature teratoma are capable of metastasizing in adults regardless of the absence of a malignant component. Forty percent of testicular tumors are mixed. Teratoma and embryonal carcinoma make up 24%, seminoma and embryonal carcinoma 5%. (H & E, X125)

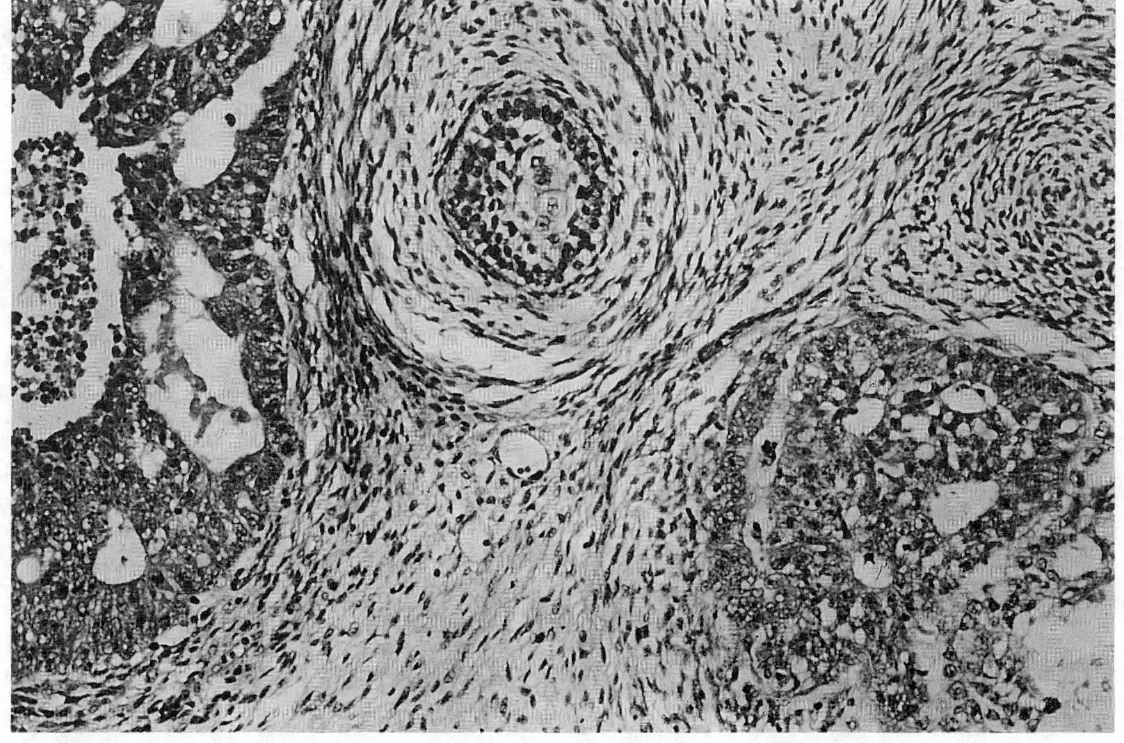

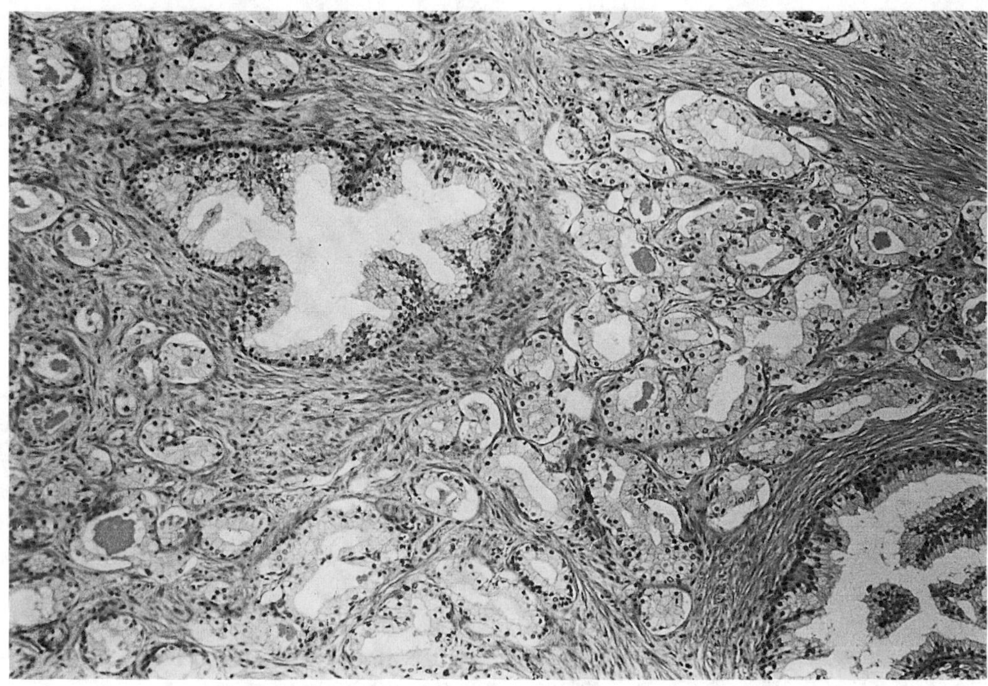

Figure 11-53A,B,C,D. Adenocarcinoma of the prostate. The tumor forms small acinar to cribriform patterns and solid forms or trabecular areas. The well-differentiated adenocarcinoma may simulate the normal-sized prostate gland except for its invasive features (photo A, above). The poorly differentiated adenocarcinoma forms solid tumor without discernible acinar pattern, readily recognized using scanning objective microscopy

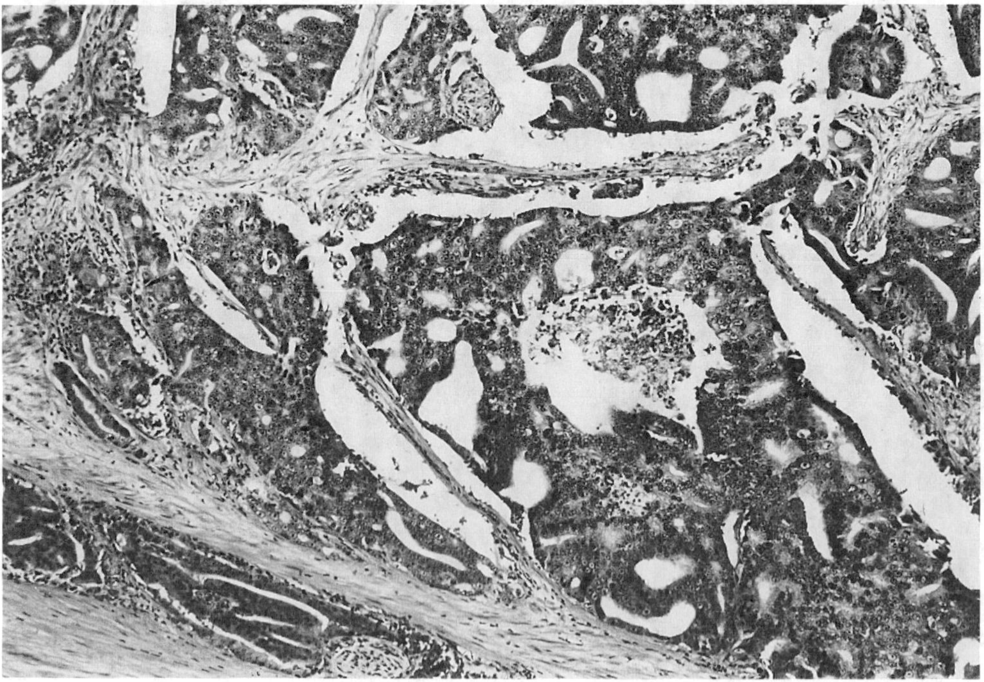

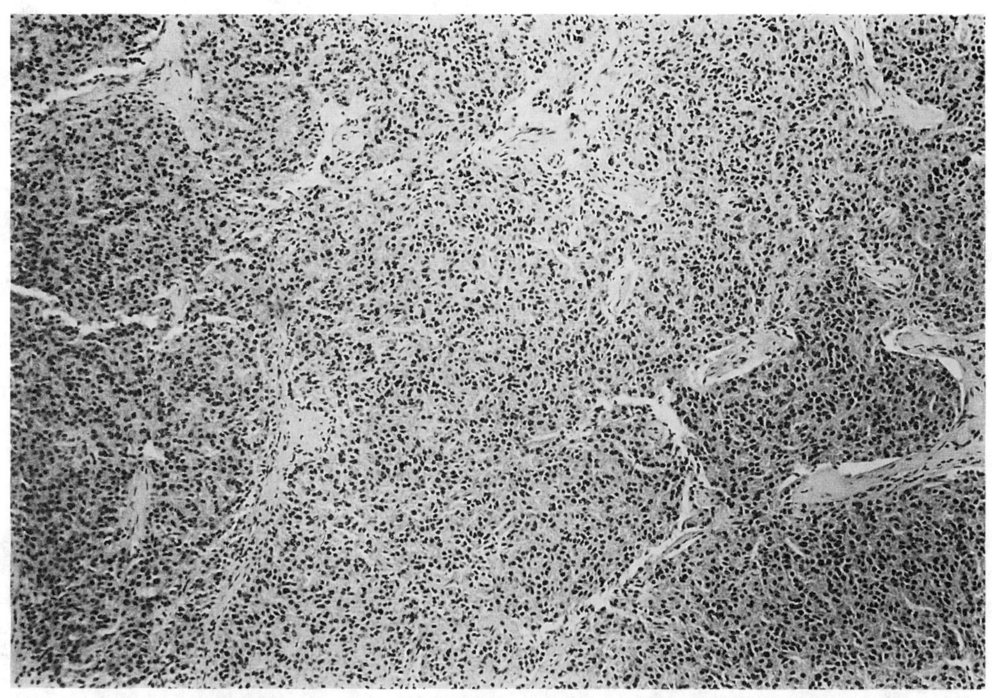

(photo C, above). Most cases, however, present as moderately differentiated tumors forming acinar and cribriform patterns (photo B, opposite page, below). Occasional undifferentiated adenocarcinoma may have clear cytoplasm remniscent of renal carcinoma (photo D, below). (H & E, X75)

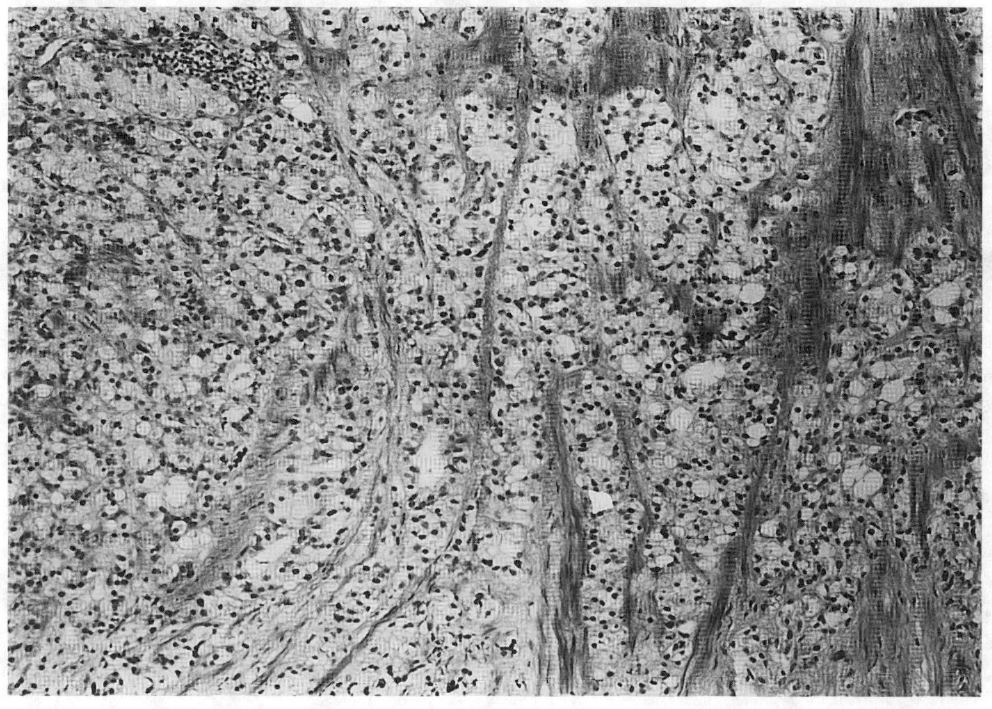

Figure 11-54. Adenocarcinoma of the prostate (cytology of fine-needle aspirate). The aspirate yields moderate cellularity made up of poorly cohesive cells that are round to ovoid, moderately pleomorphic, and have a decreased nucleo/cytoplasmic ratio. The nuclear membranes are distinct, with prominent nucleoli and coarse chromatin clumps. (Pap, X500)

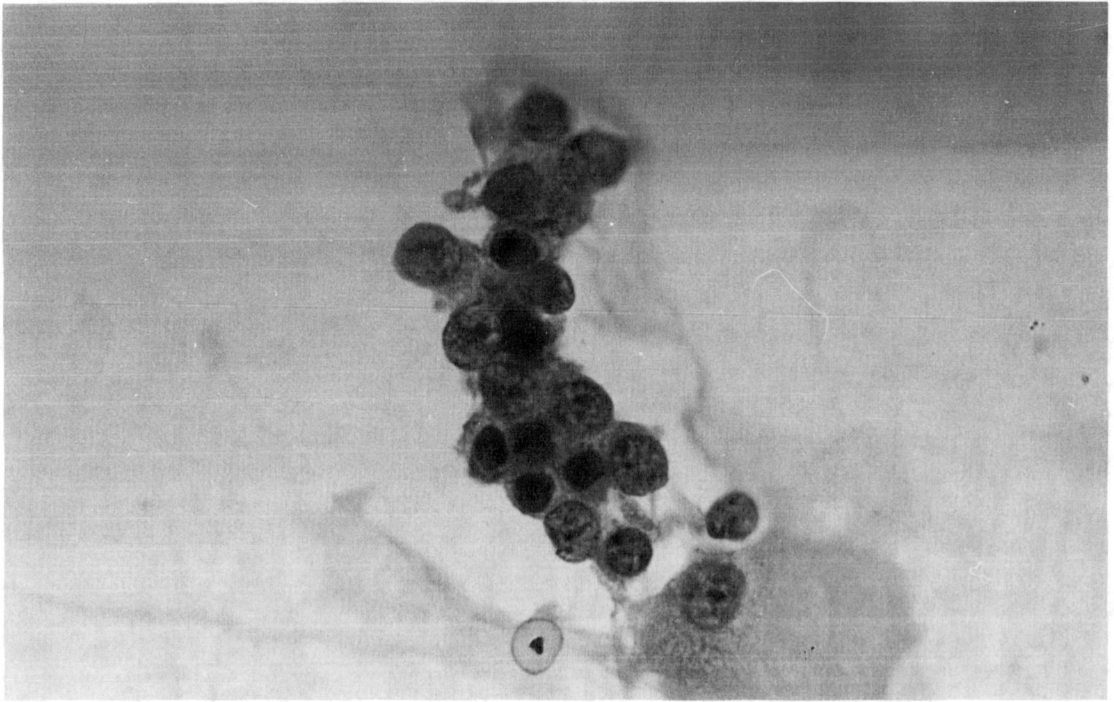

Malignant Tumors of the Female Reproductive System

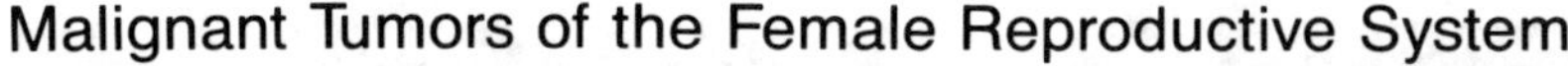

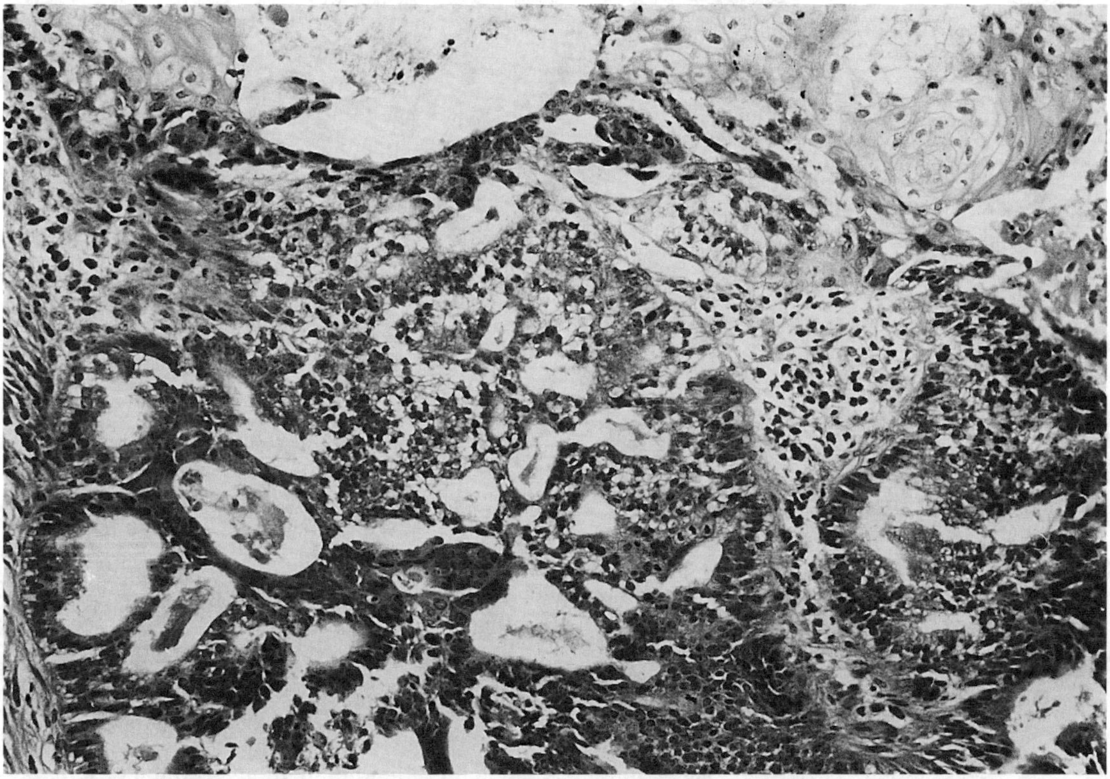

Figure 11-55. Endometrial adenocarcinoma. This tumor is composed of cells that are larger than the the normal cell of the endometrial glands, having acidophilic cytoplasm with hyperchromatic nuclei and prominent nucleoli. The tumor may vary from well-differentiated glandular patterns resembling atypical hyperplasia to poorly differentiated patterns forming very few or no glands. Typically, aberrant mitoses are present. Intraglandular epithelial bridges and disorganized piles of cells in the glands are the minimum criteria for malignancy, distinguishing well-differentiated adenocarcinoma from atypical hyperplasia. Intraglandular squamous metaplasia may be noted, usually only among well- to moderately differentiated adenocarcinoma. Histologically, tumors can be graded as follows: grade I for tumors forming purely glandular structures; grade II forming both glands and solid sheets of tumor; and grade III forming predominantly solid sheets of tumor. If it is a mixed squamous cell carcinoma, the tumor is called an adenosquamous carcinoma. Besides grading, depth of invasion and vascular infiltration are important to the patient's prognosis. The predominant tumor of the cervix is squamous cell carcionma. However, a good number of these will show mucin secretion and will be positive for CEA (carcino-embryonic antigen), classifying them as mucoepidermoid carcinoma, which has a higher incidence of lymph node involvement (33%) than pure squamous cell carcinoma.* (H & E, X125)

---

*Bostwick DG, et al. Ovarian epithelial tumors of borderline malignancy. A clinical and pathological study of 109 cases. Cancer 1986; 58:2052–65.

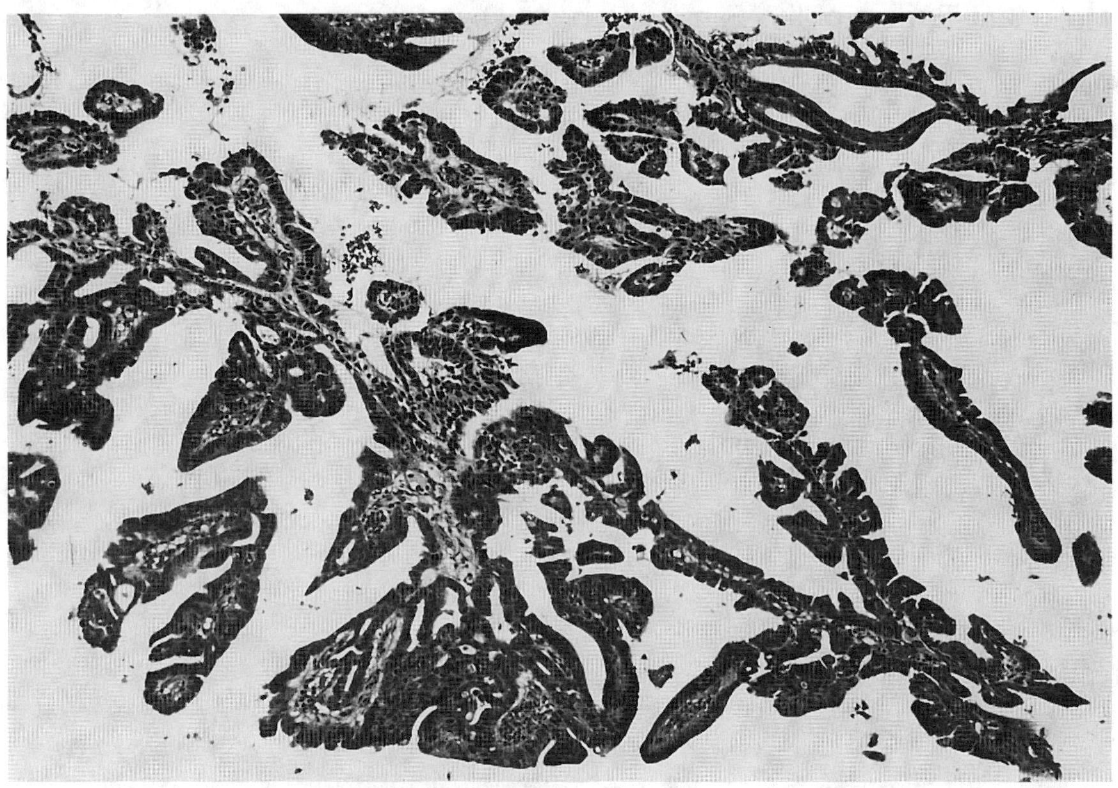

Figure 11-56A. Papillary serous carcinoma of the endometrium. The tumor forms distinct complex papillary structures with a broad fibrovascular core mantled by pleomorphic hyperchromatic epithelial cells with occasional large nucleoli and giant cells. Histologically it is indistinguishable from serous carcinoma of the ovary. Psammoma bodies may be noted. This is currently considered to be an aggressive tumor showing frequent lymphatic invasion; 40% of stage I cases have deep myometrial invasion. Very often, the uterus is not enlarged. (H & E, X75)

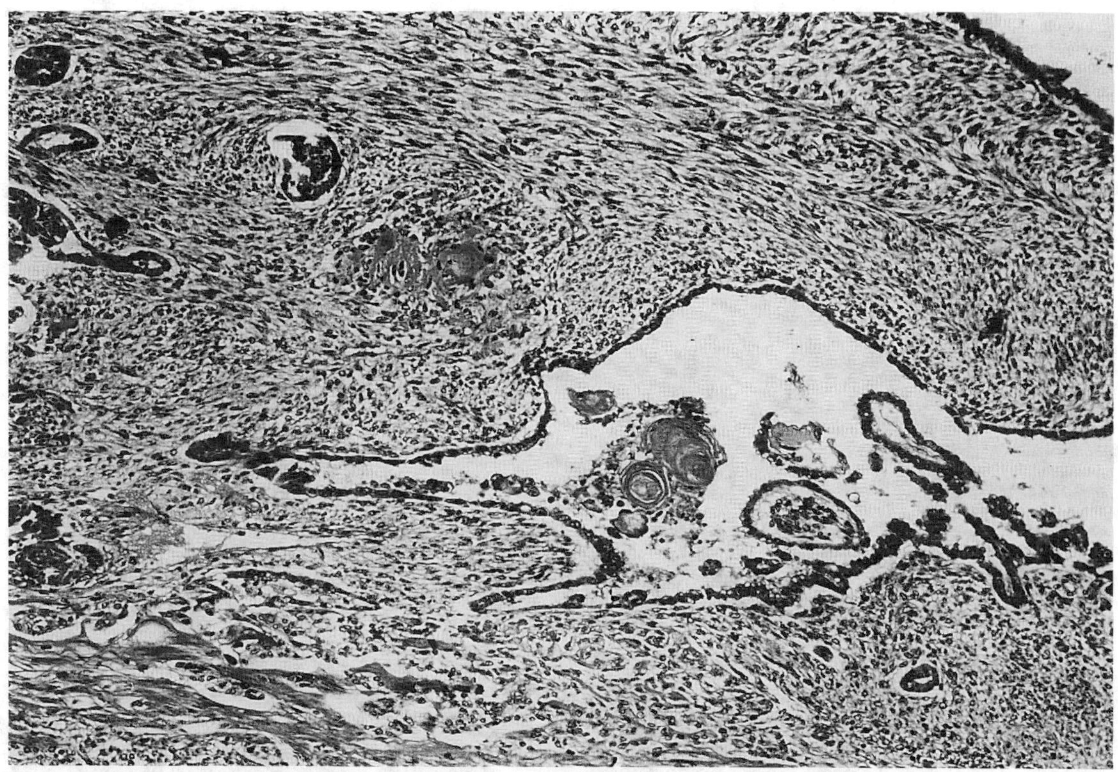

Figure 11-56B. Uterine malignant mixed mesodermal tumor. The tumor is composed of malignant epithelial adenocarcinoma, the most frequent epithelial element combined with any of the heterologous components (e.g., rhabdomyosarcoma, liposarcoma, or osteosarcoma). In the absence of any heterologous elements, the tumor is classified as carcinosarcoma. (H & E, X75)

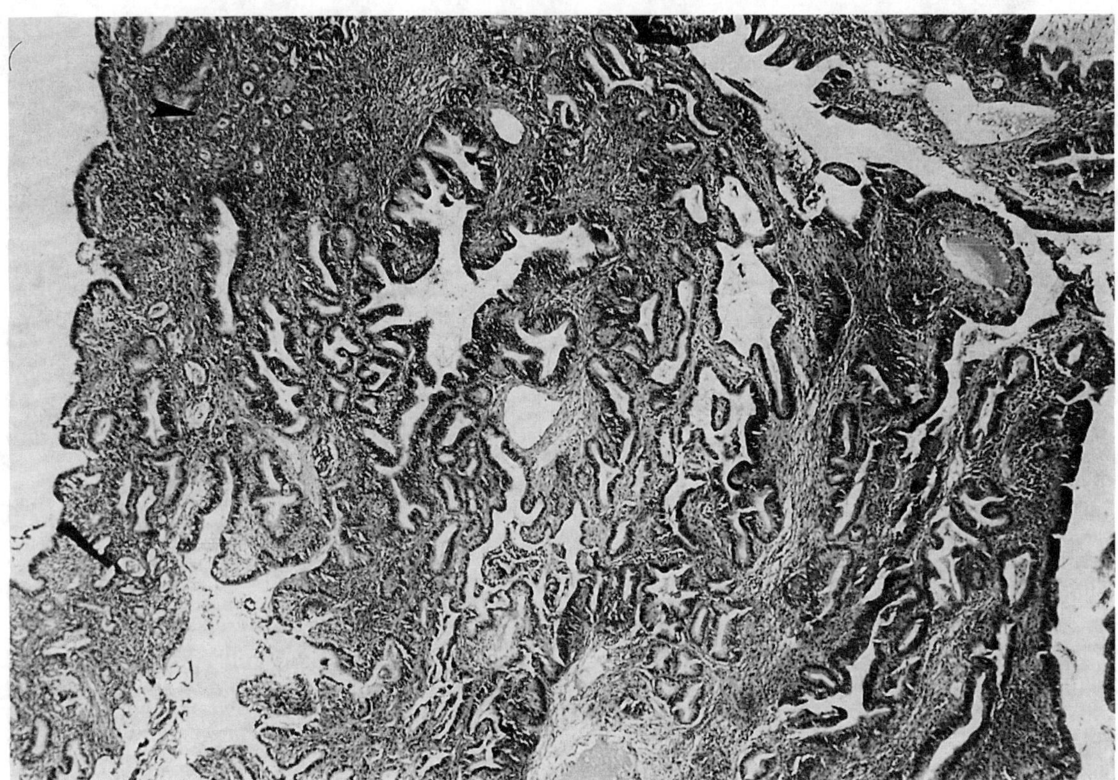

Figure 11-57. Well-differentiated adenocarcinoma of the cervix (adenoma malignum). The tumor cells display basal nuclear orientation with copious vacuolated to pale staining cytoplasm. The only clue as to its malignancy is the infiltrating architectural pattern with occasional dysplastic cells. (H & E, X30)

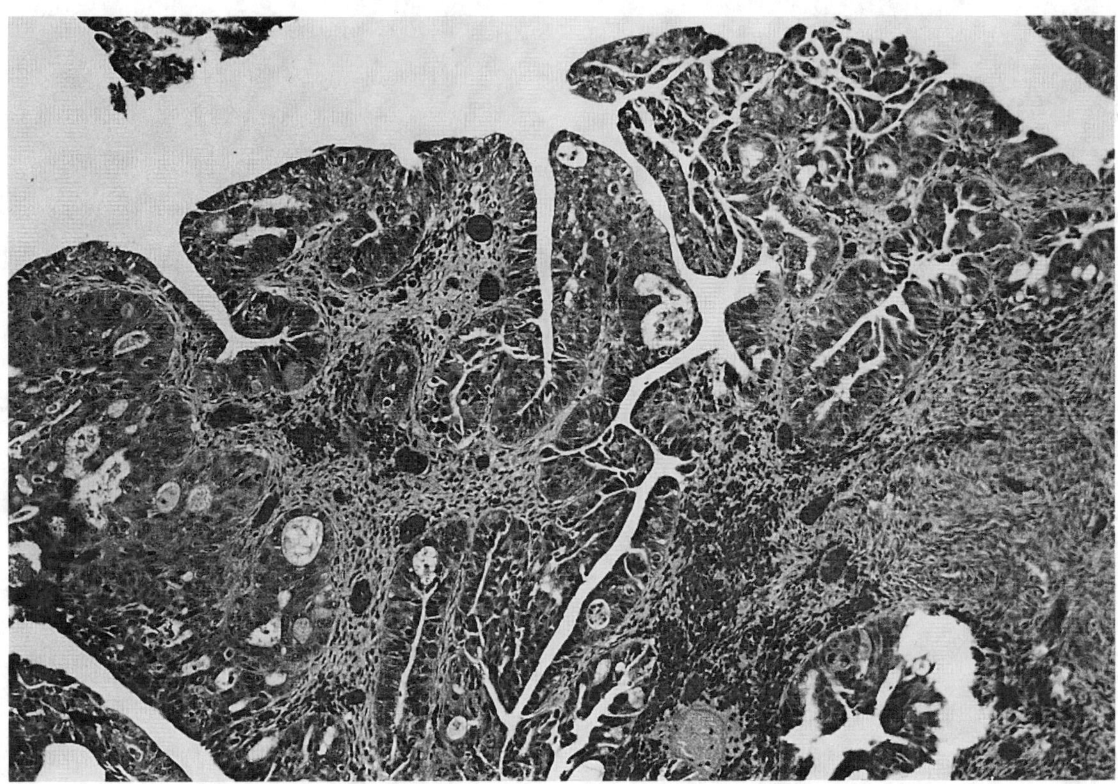

Figure 11-58A & B. Papillary serous cystadenocarcinoma of the ovary. The tumor cells are columnar with varying degrees of pleomorphism, some ciliated forming papillary structures. Histologic grading distinguishes well-formed papillary and glandular patterns as well-differentiated carcinoma from poorly differentiated tumors with solid patterns. Psammoma bodies and focal mucin secretion may also be noted (photo A, above). This is the commonest ovarian epithelial tumor; it is seen in about 40% of cases. Bilateral involvement of ovaries occurs in 50% of cases. Borderline malignancy* (photo B, opposite page)—carcinoma of low-grade malignant potential—histologically discloses atypical epithelial cellular stratification, microscopic papillary projection, and epithelial tufting besides mitoses. There is no stromal invasion. The distinction between borderline tumors (low malignant potential tumors) and fully malignant serous or mucinous carcinoma is important simply because the former has a 95% or more 5-yr survival rate in contrast to 20–45% for the latter (serous/mucinous carcinoma). (H & E, 11-58A X30; 11-58B X75)

---

*Thelmo WL et al. Mucoepirdermoid carcinoma of uterine cervix stage Ib. Int J. Gynecol Pathol 1990; 9:316–24.

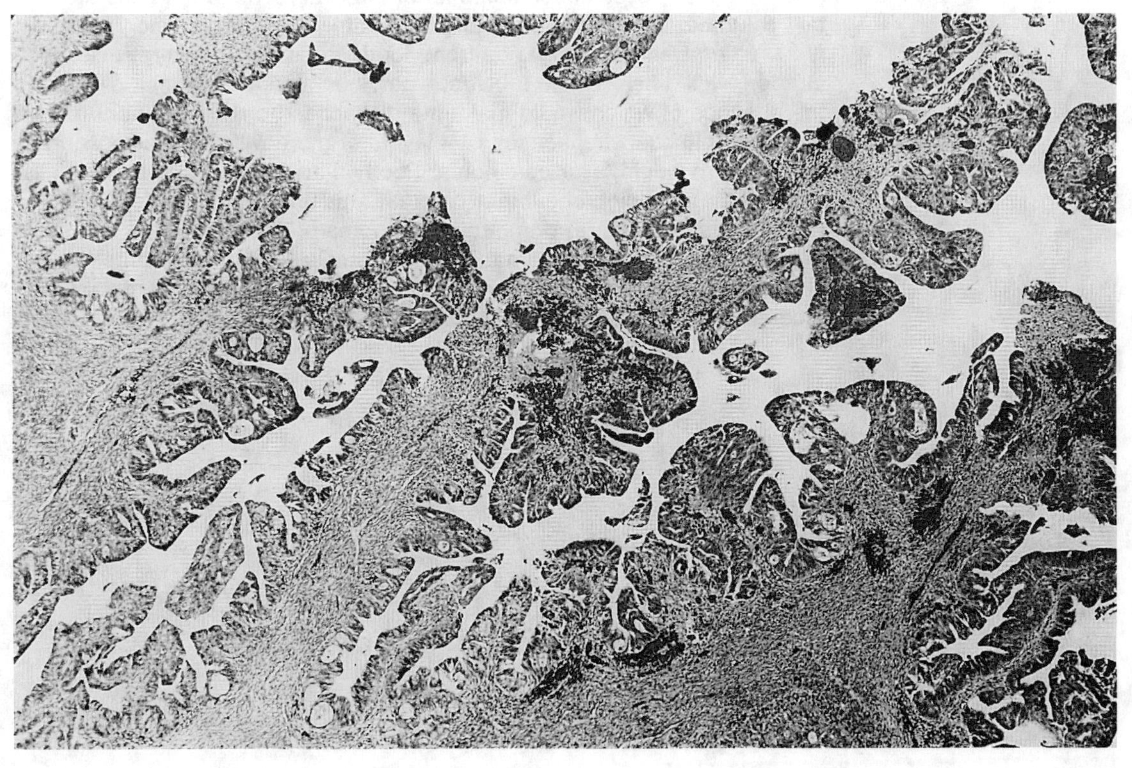

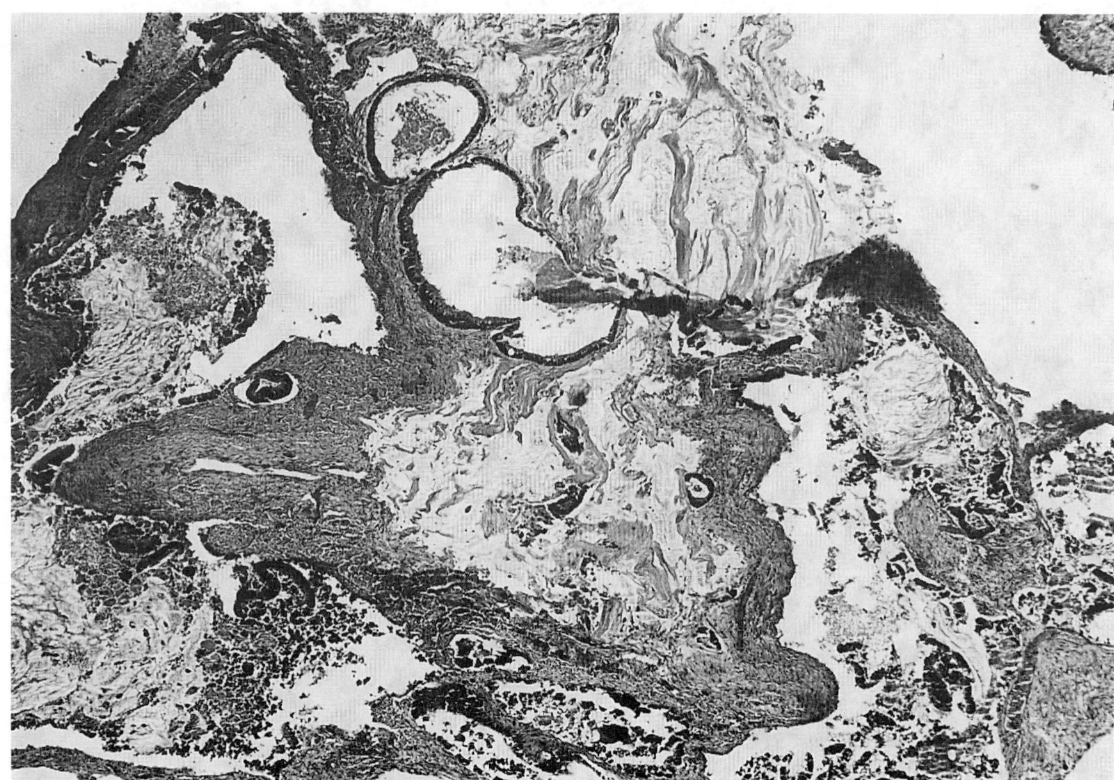

Figure 11-59. Mucinous cystadenocarcinoma of the ovary. The tumor cells are tall, columnar, and mucin-secreting, with a few mitoses. Histologic grade is based on well-formed glands from poorly formed glandular structures. Grade I, well-differentiated mucinous carcinoma shows stromal invasion, the absence of which would make the distinction from borderline tumors difficult. Epithelial stratification of 4 layers or more with or without cribriform pattern would favor carcinoma. Poorly differentiated cases present showing hardly any glandular structures. This tumor represents 3–10% of all ovarian tumors. Endometroid carcinoma of the ovary ranks second to serous cystadenocarcinoma. The histology is similar to endometrial adenocarcinoma, with half of cases showing some squamous metaplasia (acanthomatous areas). (H & E, X30)

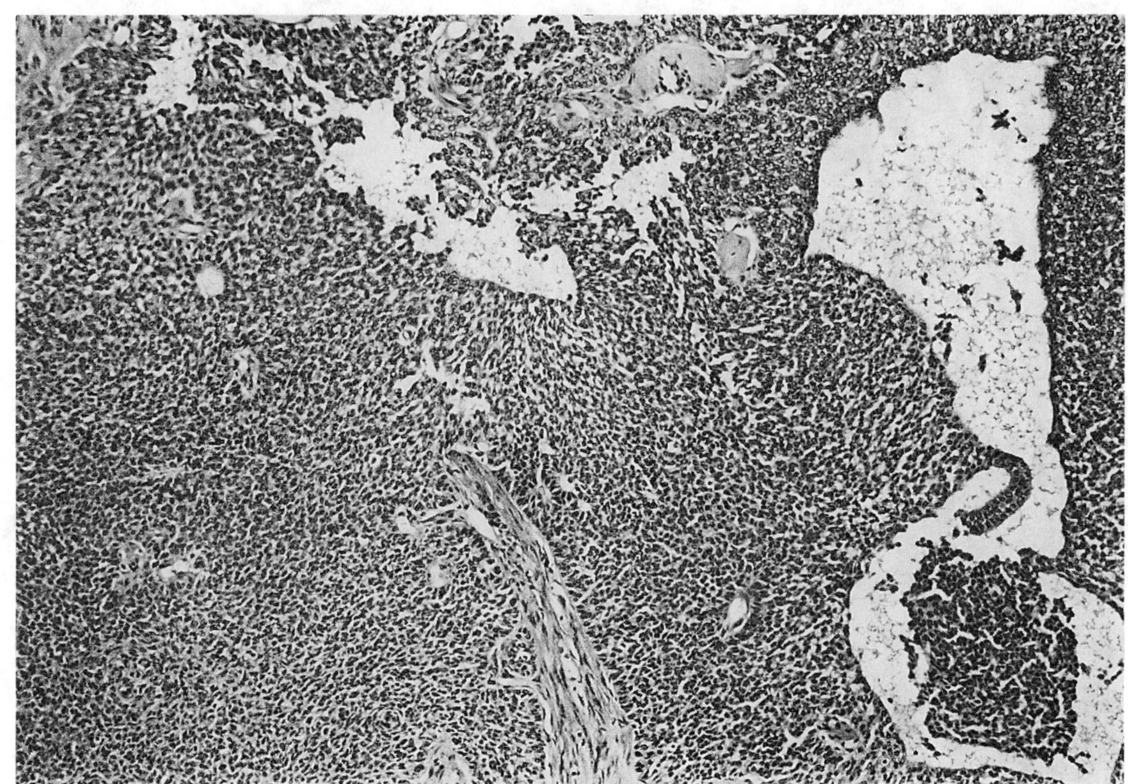

Figure 11-60A & B. Ovarian granulosa cell tumor. The tumor grows in a variety of patterns from micro to macrofollicular, from trabecular to a solid pattern (photo A, above). Cal-Exner bodies may be noted; they are characterized by small cavities filled with acidophilic fluid and a few degenerated nuclei surrounded by granulosa cells (photo B, opposite page). Theca cells are often seen in varying amounts. In a diffuse solid pattern, a reticulin stain sometimes will help outline the nest of granulosa cells noted as islands of cells without reticulin fibrils. The theca cells are surrounded individually by fibrils. (H & E, 11-60A X75; 11-60B X200)

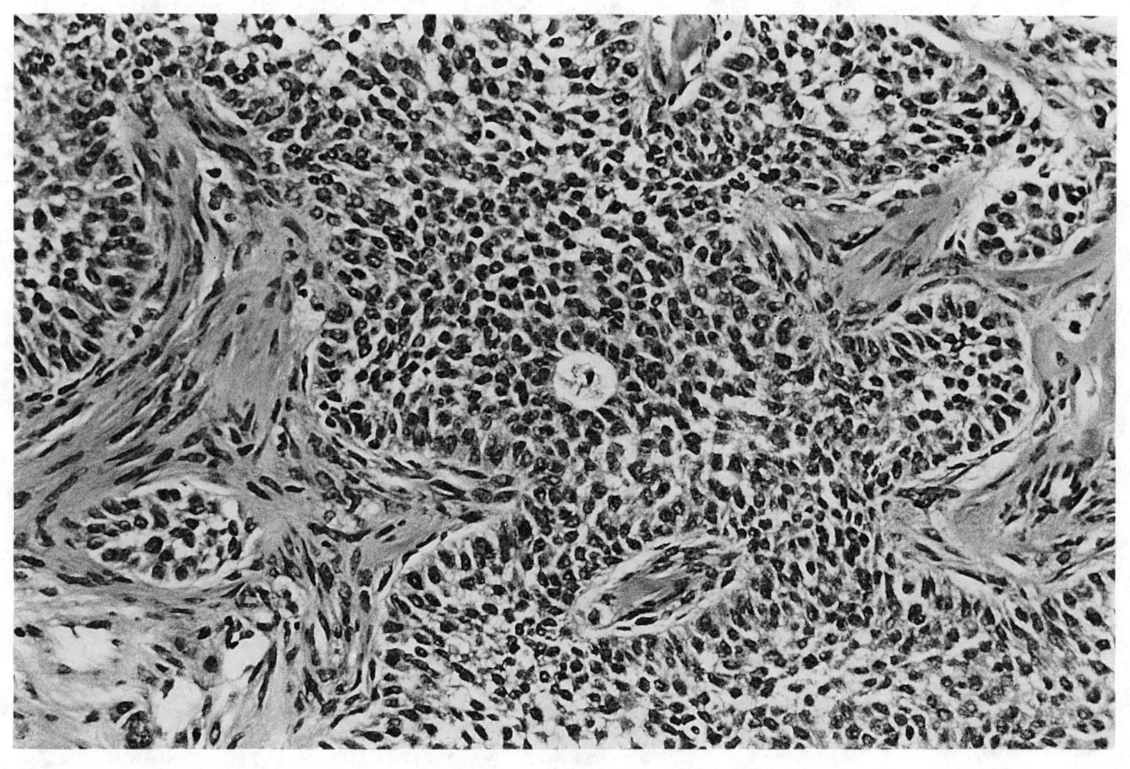

Soft-Tissue and Skeletal Malignant Tumors

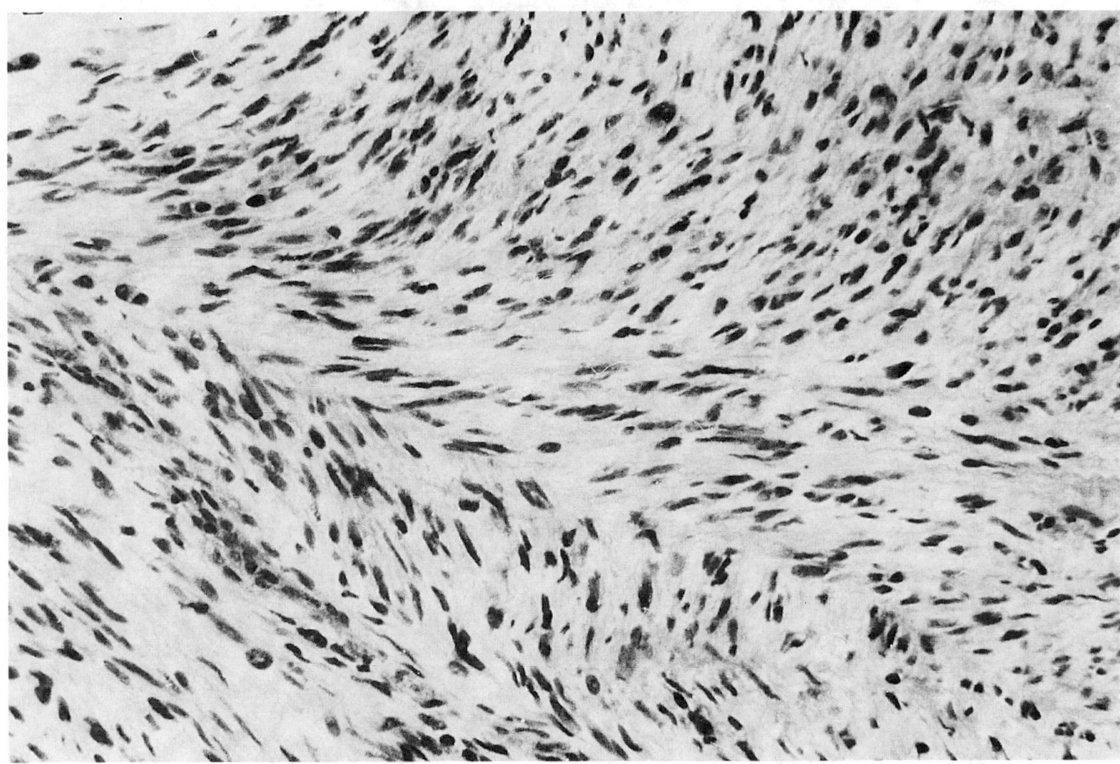

Figure 11-61. Fibrosarcoma. The tumor, removed from the thigh, is composed of spindle cells having tapered nuclear ends, scanty cytoplasm, and indistinct cell borders, with some collagen between spindle cells. The long fascicular (or herringbone) distribution seen throughout the tumor is a distinct feature of fibrosarcoma. Poorly differentiated fibrosarcoma may show some pleomorphism, with occasional giant cells, but the degree of pleomorphism is not as pronounced as that seen in malignant fibrous histiocytomas of the pleomorphic type. Nodular fasciitis may be mistaken for fibrosarcoma, but the size is often smaller, showing a disordered cellular pattern. The short fasicular pattern, with conspicuous myxoid background and chronic inflammatory infiltrate, also characterizes the fasciitis. Mitosis is not helpful except when it is aberrant, which may favor fibrosarcoma. (H & E, X200)

Figure 11-62. Malignant fibrous histiocytoma. It is characterized by the presence of plump spindle cells resembling fibroblasts, with a tendency to fasicular formation and cartwheel pattern (storiform pattern). Occasional giant cells and plump histiocytes with numerous typical and aberrant mitotic figures may be seen in a more aggressive tumor. The presence of a few scattered lymphocytes or plasma cells is also typical for this tumor. Depending upon predominant features, this tumor may be subclassified as giant cell, storiform-pleomorphic type, or myxoid type. Those tumors, which show diffuse neutrophilic leucocyte infiltration unaccompanied by necrosis, have been characterized by some as the inflammatory variant of malignant fibrous histiocytoma. This tumor apparently is more responsive to chemotherapy. Tumors with hemorrhagic cystic spaces simulating vascular spaces are known as the angiomatoid type. (H & E, X200)

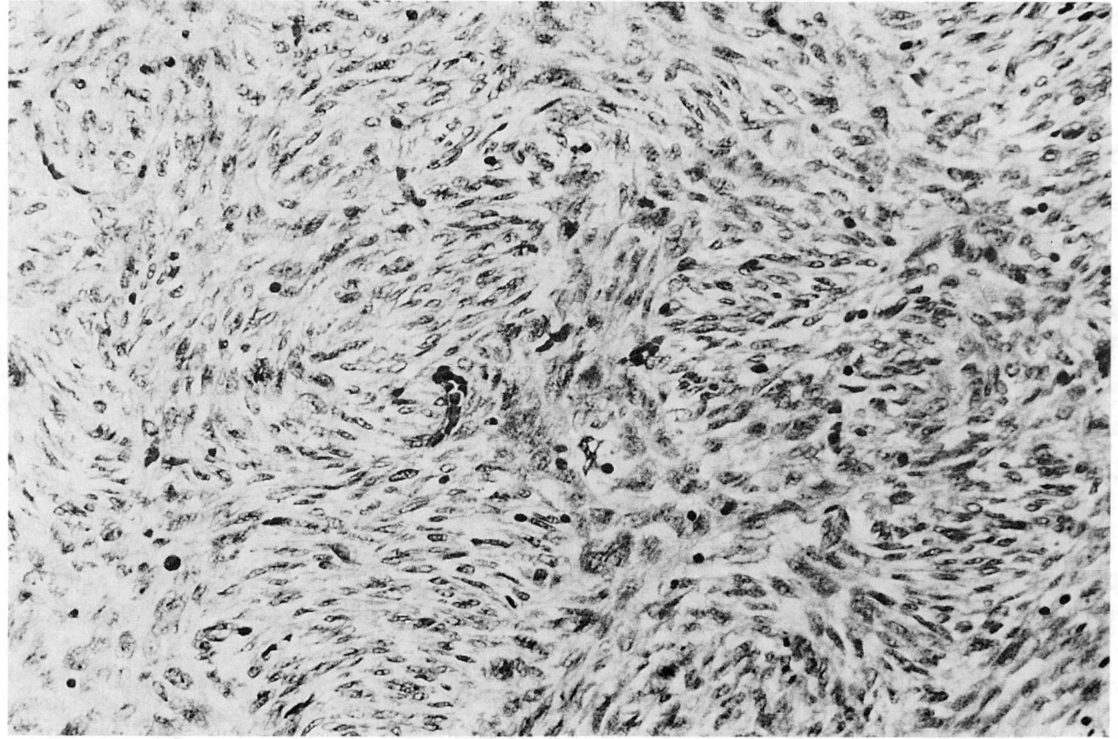

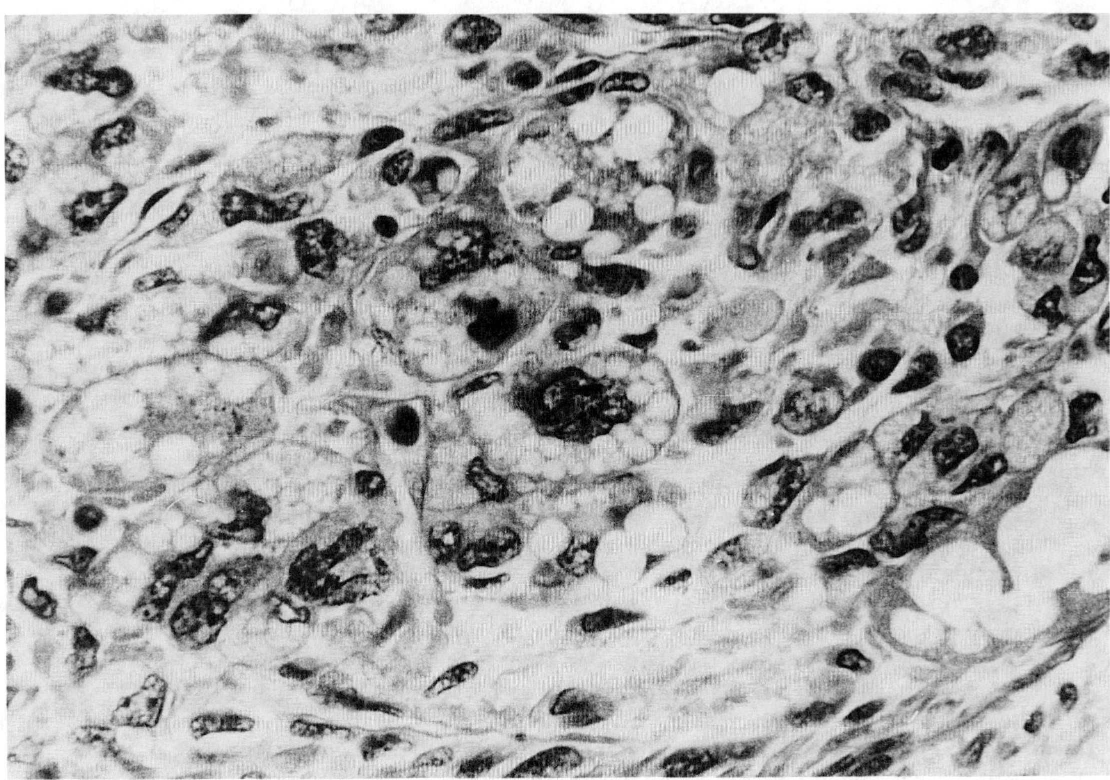

Figure 11-63A & B. Liposarcoma. The tumor, removed from the thigh, discloses a typical lipoblast with multiple intracytoplasmic lipid droplets with scalloped hyperchromatic nuclei (photo A, above). Other areas may show predominant spindle cells or a myxomatous pattern. Some of the small lipoblasts may mimic signet-ring cell carcinoma (photo B, opposite page). Myxoid liposarcoma is the commonest type, comprising about 40% of all liposarcomas. Well-differentiated and myxoid liposarcoma have been categorized as low grade, in that they virtually do not metastasize except in rare cases of myxoid liposarcoma. In contrast, the pleomorphic type, lipoblastic (round-cell) type, and the fibroblastic type are high grade, with 50% having distant metastases within 5 yr.* (H & E, 11-63A X500; 11-63B X200)

*Chang HR, Hajdu SI, et al. The prognostic value of histologic subtypes in primary extremity liposarcoma. Cancer 1989; 64:1514–20.

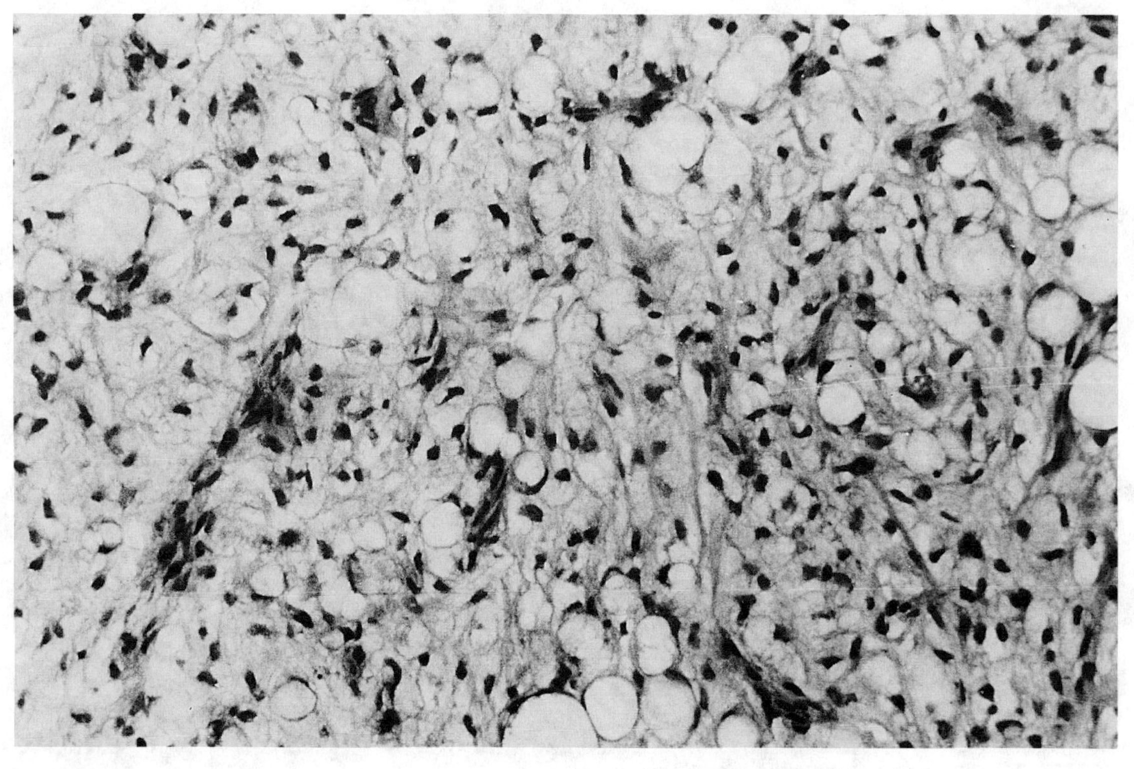

Figure 11-64. Leiomyosarcoma. The tumor consists of spindle cells with blunted nuclear ends, perinuclear vacuoles, dense acidophil cytoplasm, and display interlacing bundles with nuclear regimentation (palisading). The degree of aggressiveness is assessed on the basis of mitotic activity, pattern of growth on the adjacent tissue, and vascular invasion. Five to 10 mitotic figures per 10 high-power fields is considered low-grade sarcoma. However, one has to be wary of extra-uterine "leiomyomas"; even if mitotic figures average <5 per 10 high-power fields, this should be considered potentially malignant. (H & E, X200)

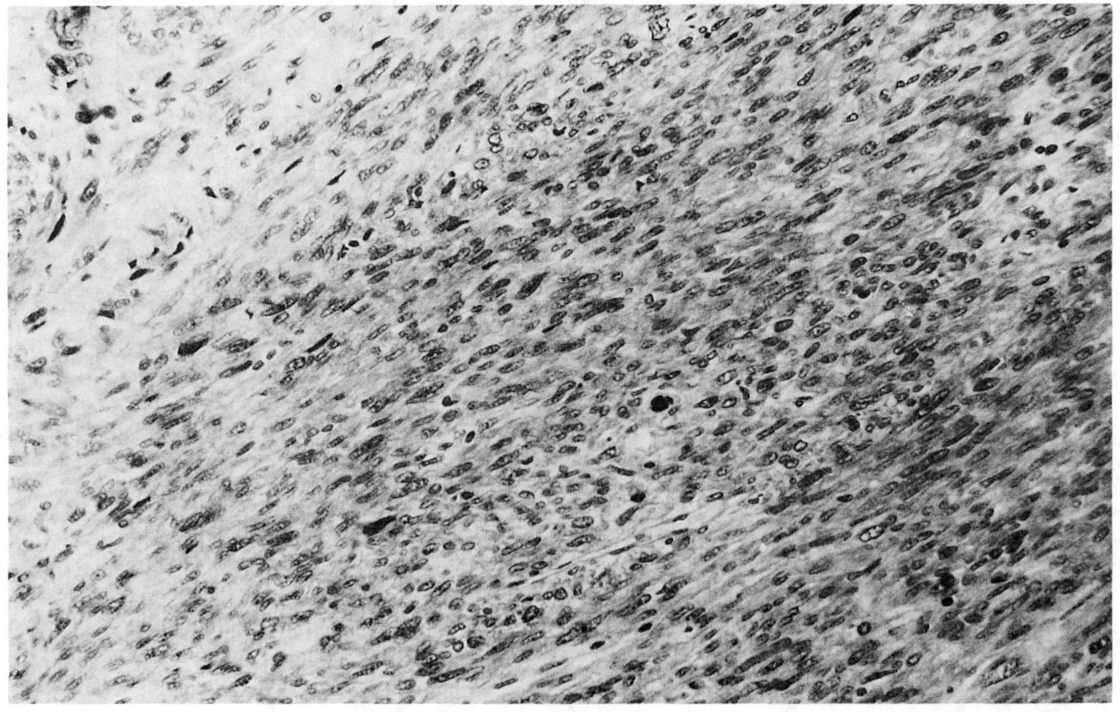

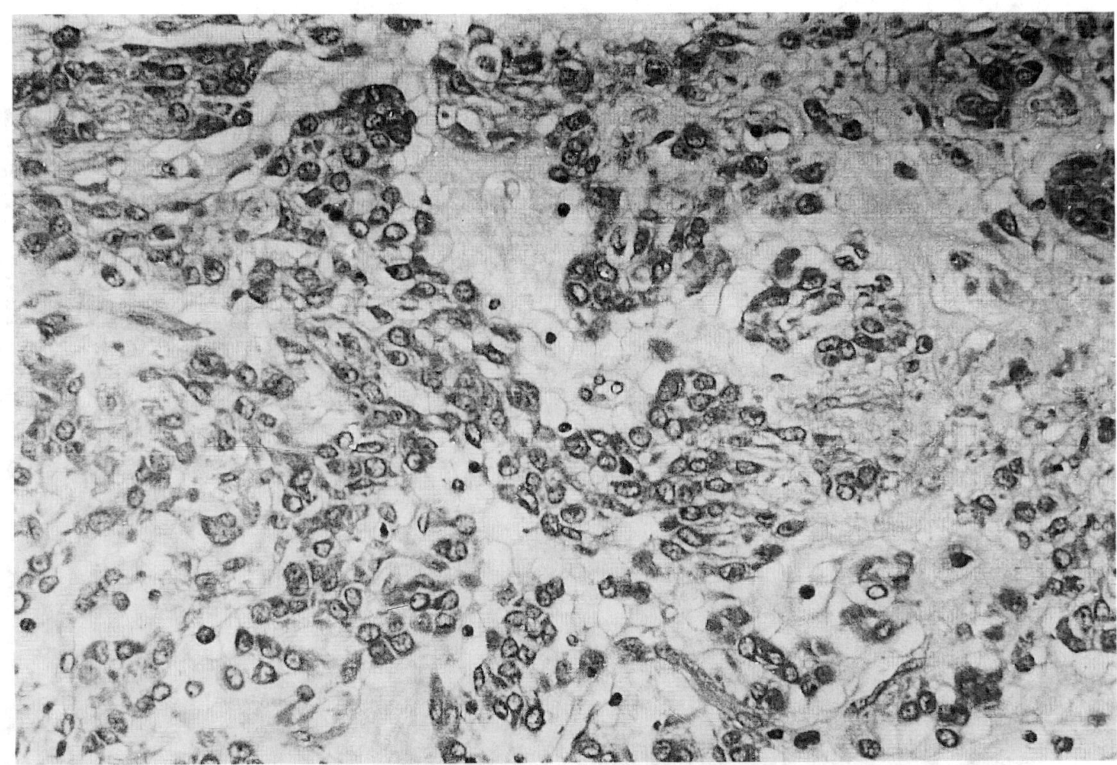

Figure 11-65. Leiomyoblastoma (epitheloid smooth muscle tumor). The tumor is composed of clusters of polygonal cells and short spindle stout cells with copious amphophilic or acidophilic cytoplasm and an eccentric nucleus suggesting signet-ring cell carcinoma or liposarcoma. The growth pattern mimics epithelial tumors. The malignant counterpart, malignant leiomyoblastoma (epitheloid leiomyosarcoma), discloses frequent mitotic figures and is usually larger in size. More than 5 mitotic figures per 50 high-power fields is considered malignant; however, there are cases with <5 mitoses per 50 high-power fields reported to have metastasized. Tumors >6 cm in diameter are considered malignant. For practical purposes, leiomyoblastoma should be considered potentially malignant. The majority arise in the stomach. (H & E, X200)

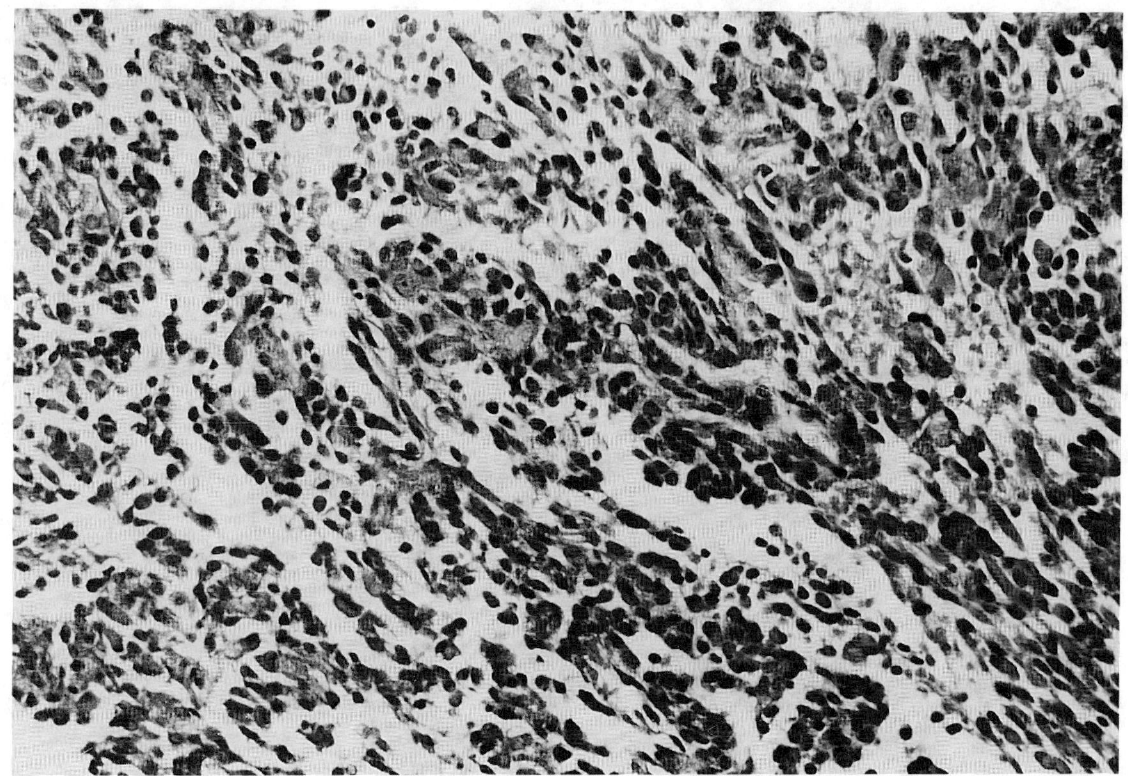

Figure 11-66A & B. Rhabdomyosarcoma. This tumor, removed from the thigh, consists of round to ovoid to spindle cells with a moderate amount of acidophil cytoplasm. Some areas may display unipolar, bipolar to tadpole-like cells (photo A, above). Striations may or may not be seen. The embryonal type makes up 90% of rhabdomyosarcomas. It is not unusual to find mixed histologic pattern in some cases (photo B, opposite page). The pleomorphic type discloses more differentiation into myocytes and is seen mostly in adults. The embryonal type is seen mostly in children. (H & E, 11-66A X200; 11-66B X500)

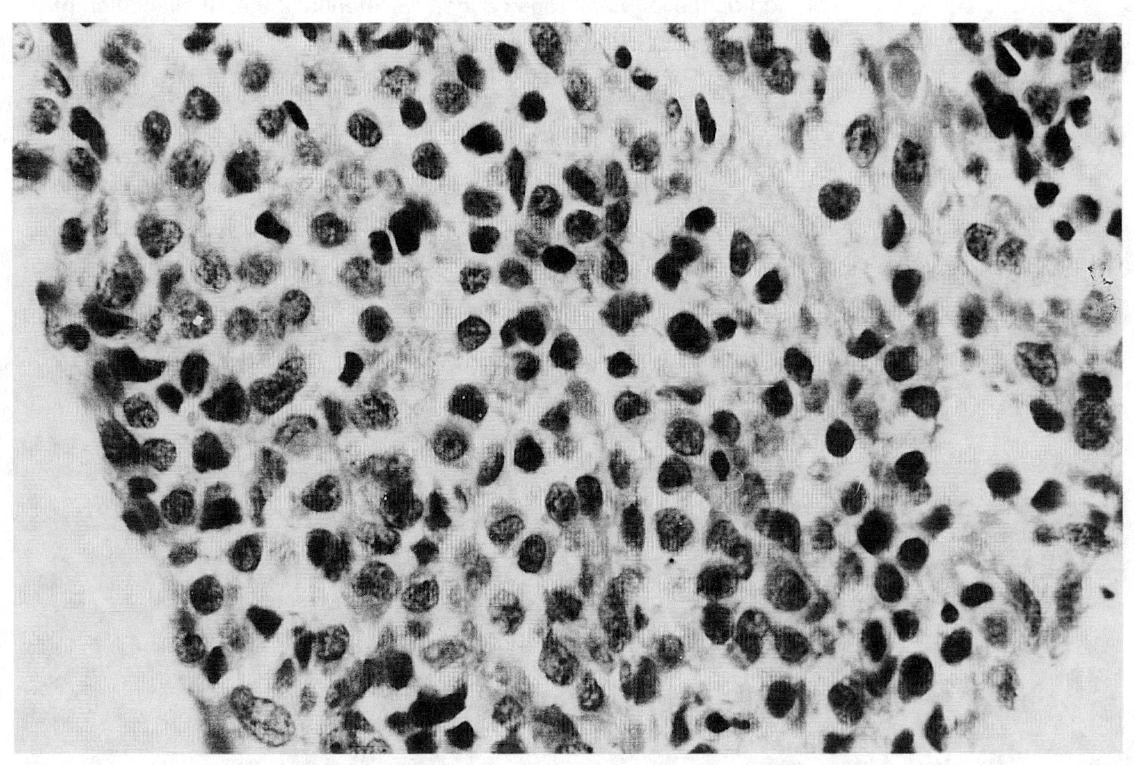

Figure 11-67. Synovial sarcoma. This tumor, removed from the knee, is
composed of 2 components—epithelial cells forming cleft spaces and
spindle cells resembling fibroblast type cells intimately surrounding the
epithelial cells. This is the biphasic type. The monophasic type has only
1 of the cell types. However, for a firm diagnosis, a biphasic pattern
should be visible, even if it is only in a single small area. Reticulin stain
outlines the epithelial areas when they are not easily discernible with H
& E stain. Mast cell infiltrates can also be readily seen with PAS stain
showing positive granules. PAS, alcian blue, and mucicarmine-positive
material—which are diastase and hyaluronidase resistant—are seen in
the cleft and pseudoglandular spaces. Differential diagnosis would include fibrosarcoma and malignant schwannoma when the tumor is
monophasic synovial sarcoma. Immunohistochemical stain using antiker-
atin and epithelial membrane antigen will identify the epithelial differentiation of this tumor. (H & E, X125)

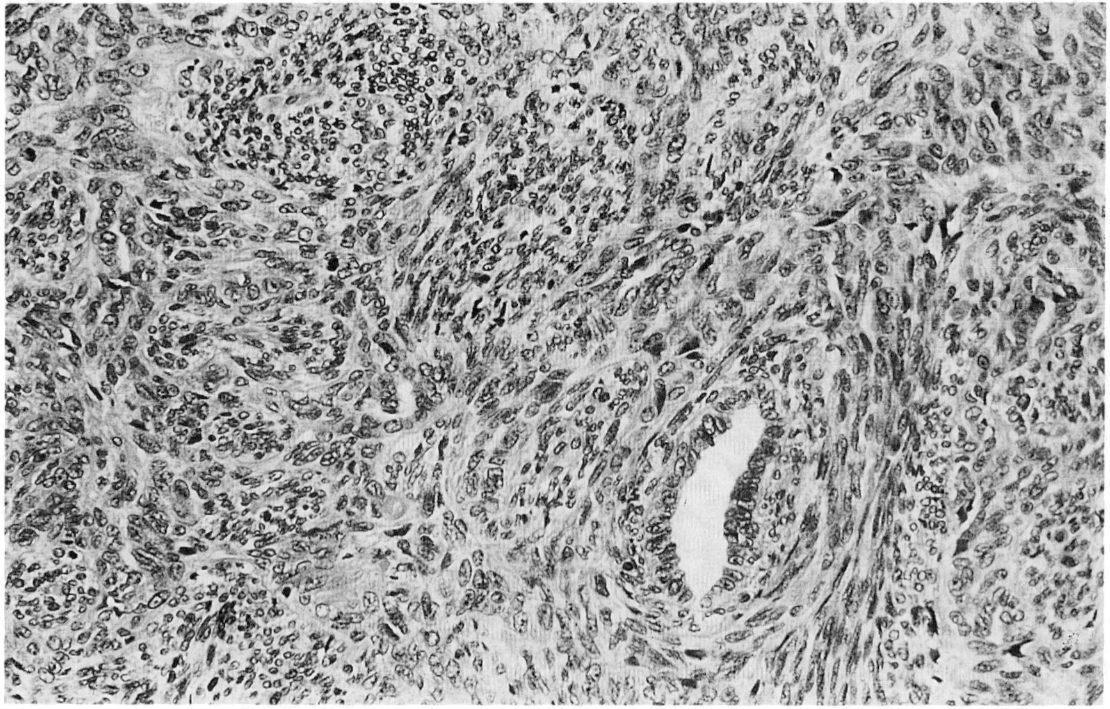

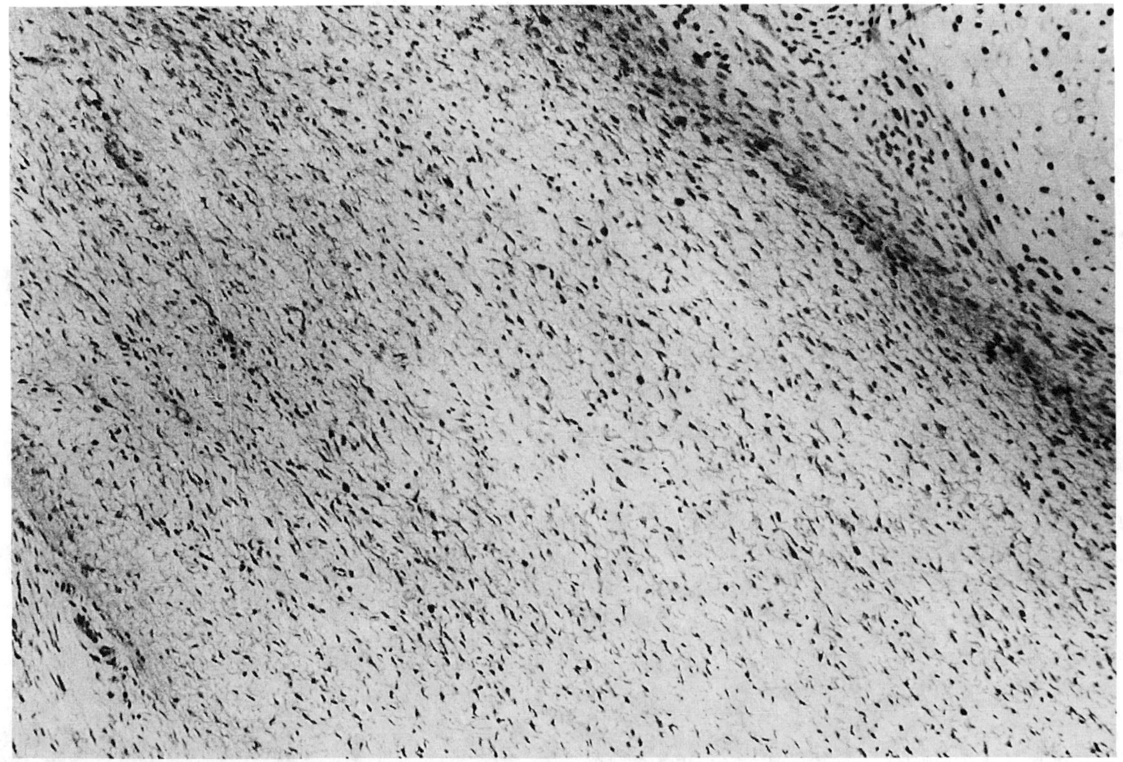

Figure 11-68. Malignant schwannoma. It is a variegated cellular tumor, in this case removed from the retroperitoneum, composed of spindle cells in fascicular pattern admixed with myxoid to hypocellular areas. The nuclei are elongated, wavy to undulating with indistinct cytoplasmic border. Nuclear regimentation (palisading), small whorled arrangement, and hyaline nodules with a wreath of cells may be seen. Mature sheets of cartilage or bone may be seen more often with this tumor than with other sarcomas. Skeletal muscle and mucin-secreting glands are rare. The tumor is frequently associated with Recklinghausen's disease. The combination of neural and skeletal muscle elements has been called Triton tumor (named after Triton Salamander).* It is often applied to malignant schwannoma with rhabdomyosarcoma. Differential diagnosis includes fibrosarcoma and monophasic synovial sarcoma. This may be resolved by electron microscopy. S 100 protein gives variable positive results with the tumor. (H & E, X75)

---

*Masson P, Martin JF. Rhabdomyomes des Nerf. Assoc Franc Etude Cancer 1938; 27:751.

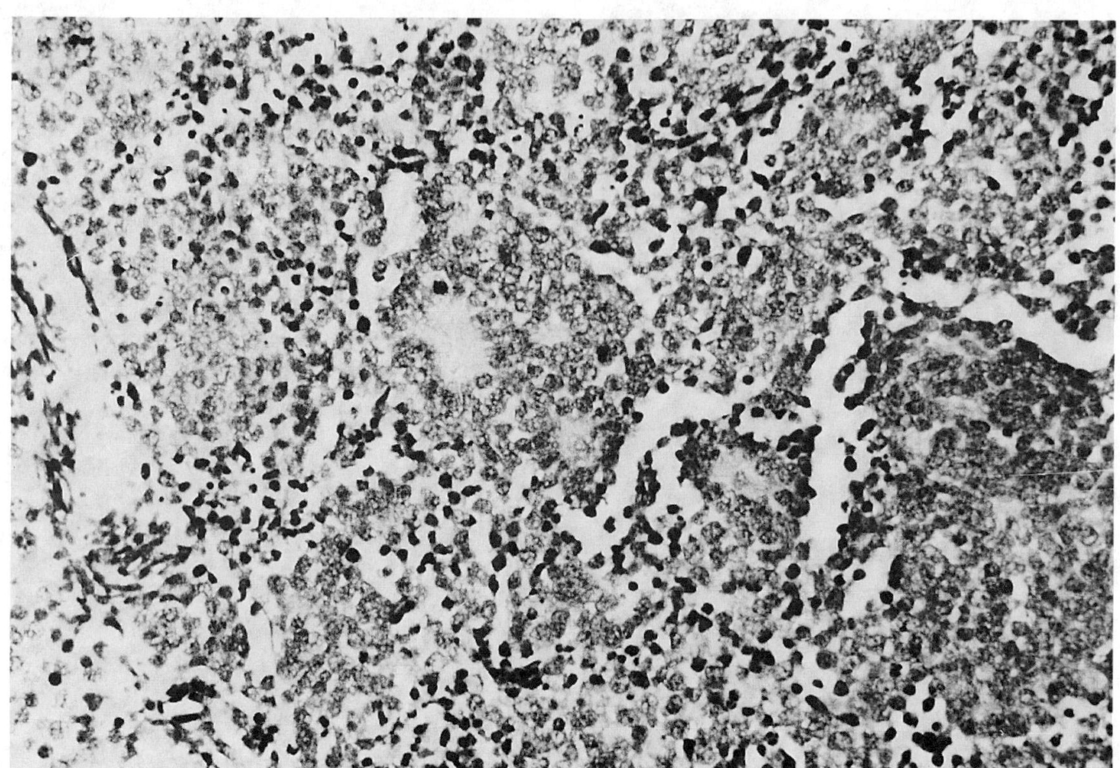

Figure 11-69. Neuroblastoma. The tumor is composed of lobules of small round cells with hyperchromatic nuclei and scant cytoplasm. The cells may display a perivascular arrangement or rosette pattern. Depending upon the degree of differentiation, the cells may have more cytoplasmic processes or present as fully mature ganglion cells. Ganglioneuroblastoma is the term applied to neuroblastoma with ganglion cell differentiation. Neuroblastomas showing no ganglion differentiation are considered grade III; those with partial ganglionic differentiation grade II; and those with mature ganglion cells grade I. Immunohistochemical stain using neurofilament protein antisera gives a strong reaction with this tumor. Some degree of variability may be noted due to fixation and, to some extent, to tumor cell differentiation. (H & E, X200).

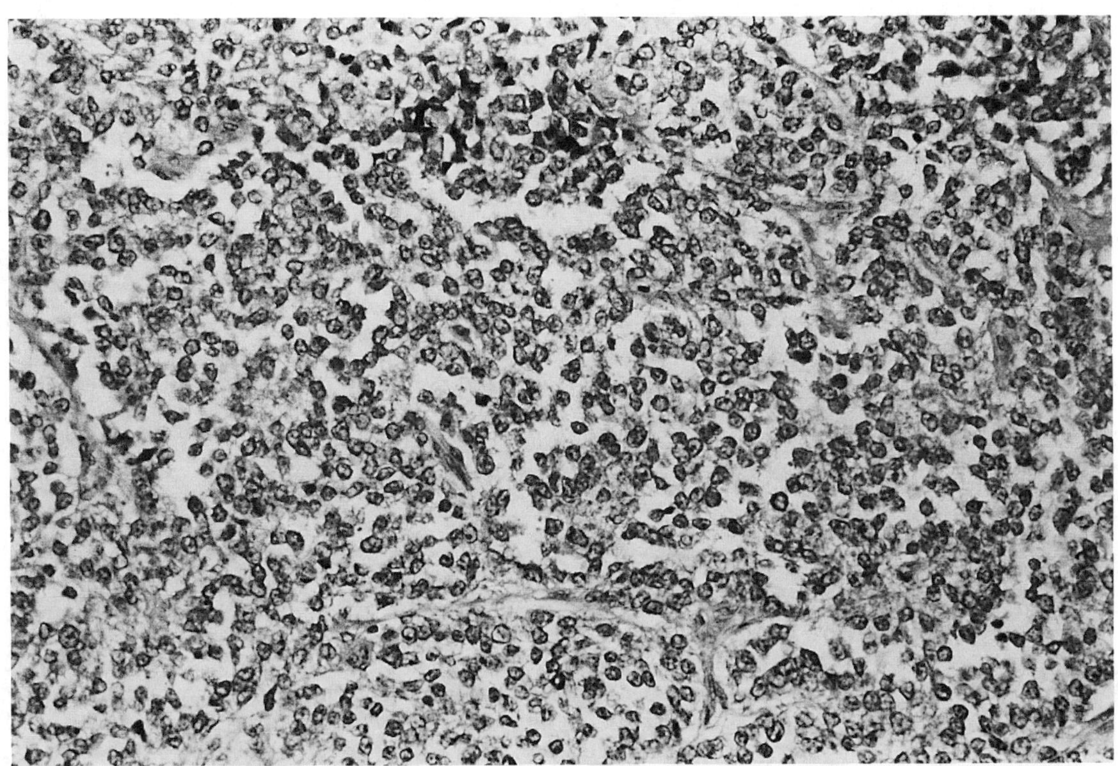

Figure 11-70. Ewing's sarcoma. This tumor, removed from the femur, is composed of lobules of conspicuously uniform small round cells having round-to-ovoid vesicular nuclei, distinct nuclear membrane, and fine chromatin pattern with a small nucleolus. Cytoplasm is scanty, often vacuolated, showing a moderate amount of glycogen demonstrated by PAS-positive material, which can be removed by prior diastase treatment. Giant cells are not seen, nor is pleomorphism a feature of this tumor. Mitoses are infrequent. Differential diagnosis includes rhabdomyosarcoma, neuroblastoma, and malignant lymphoma. (H & E, X200)

Figure 11-71. Myxoma (intramuscular). The striking feature of this tumor, removed in this case from the thigh, is the paucity of stellate cells, which are small and have hyperchromatic nuclei with several cytoplasmic processes. Vascular structures and fibrocollagenous areas are scanty. Macrophage may be positive for "oil red 0" stain showing small red droplets. The small lipid droplets and absence of hyperchromatic scalloped nuclei differentiate this tumor from lipoblast. Recurrence is rare, even in cases with a narrow margin of resection. (H & E, X200)

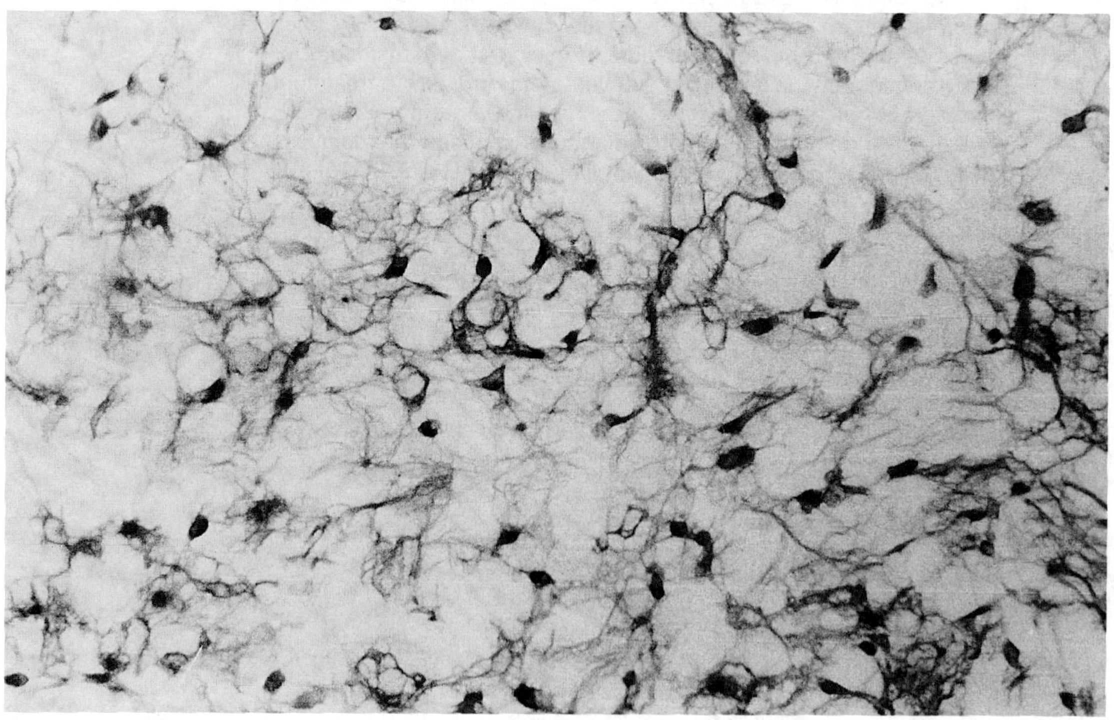

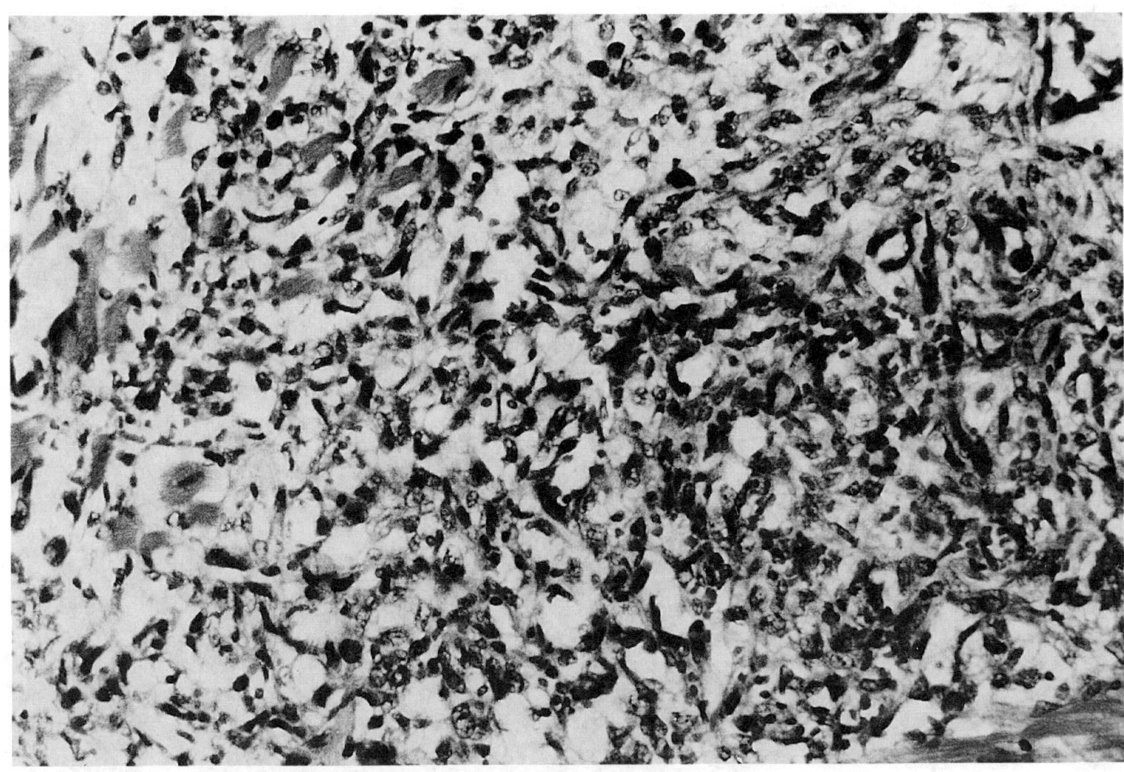

Figure 11-72. Angiosarcoma. The tumor may display distinct vascular channels lined by plump hyperchromatic cells, with some cellular tufting or poorly defined vascular channels resembling high-grade fibrosarcoma. Factor VIII-associated antigen has been demonstrated in this tumor in variable amounts. (H & E, X200).

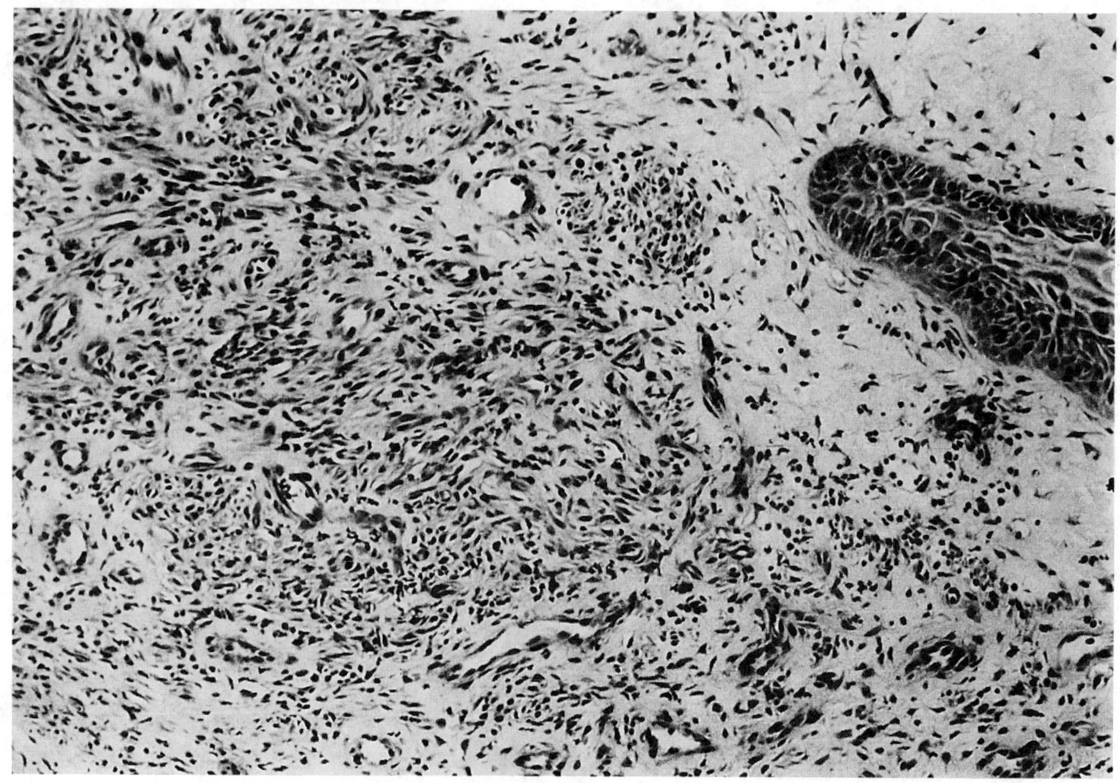

Figure 11-73. Kaposi's sarcoma. The histological features of this tumor, which originates in the skin, varies with the course of the disease and the host's immunocompetence. It ranges from a mere granulation of tissue to features simulating a well-differentiated fibrosarcoma bearing slit-like spaces containing red blood cells. Hemosiderin deposits and inflammatory reaction may be conspicuous. (H & E, X125)

Figure 11-74. Hemangiopericytoma. This solid tumor is composed of compact vascular channels surrounded by tumor cells bearing round-to-ovoid nuclei and a moderate amount of cytoplasm with distinct borders. When the tumor exhibits more cellularity and pleomorphism with >4 mitotic figures per 10 high-power fields, it is then classified as malignant hemangiopericytoma. (H & E, X200).

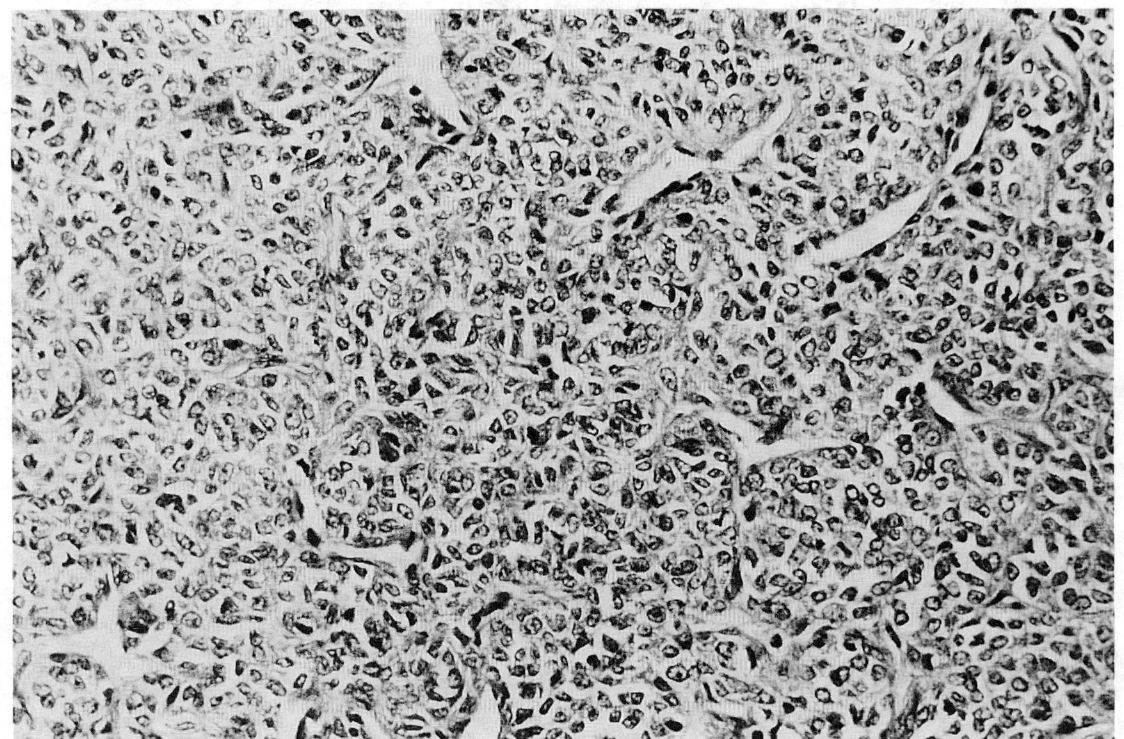

Figure 11-75. Osteogenic sarcoma. Generally, in all bone tumors, correlation of x-ray, gross, and histologic features is necessary in order to arrive at the correct diagnosis. This tumor, removed from the thigh, consists of pleomorphic spindle cells and occasional osteoid or woven bone structures formed by these cells directly. Mitosis is frequent. A malignant cartilage component may be noted. (H & E, X125)

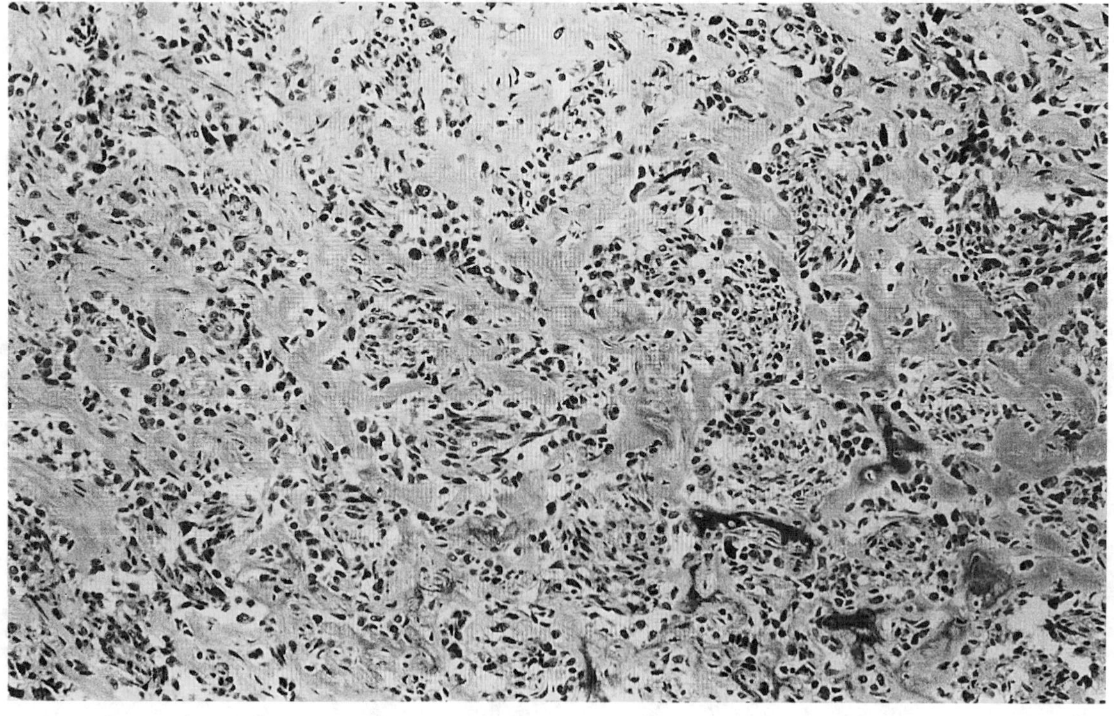

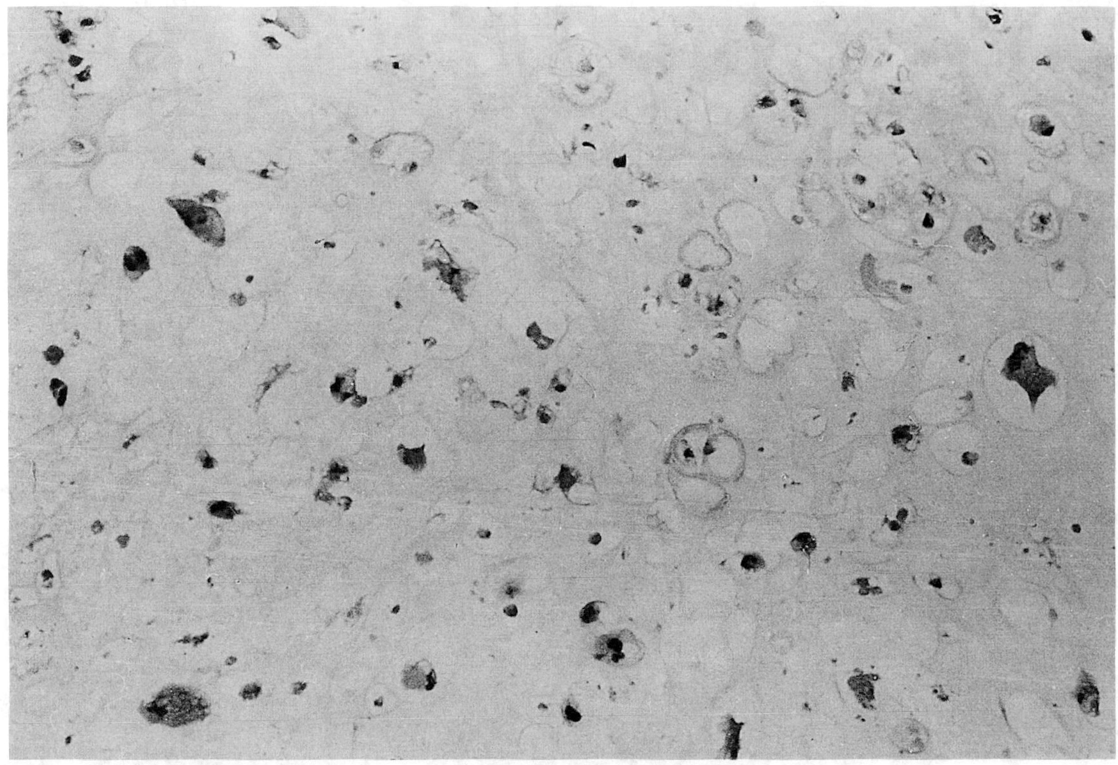

Figure 11-76. Chondrosarcoma. This tumor presentation ranges from a well-differentiated structure, with chondrocytes indistinguishable from those seen in benign chondromas, to an anaplastic pattern with chondrocytes showing hyperchromatic, multilobated and bizarre nuclei. (H & E, X125)

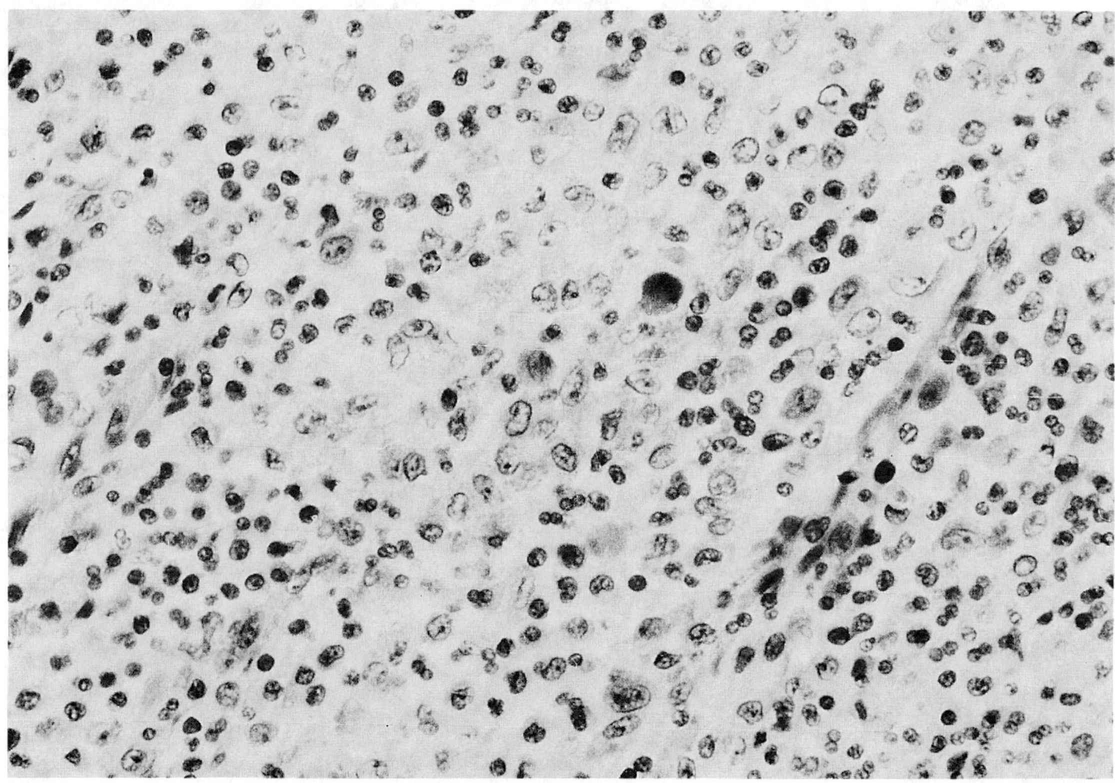

Figure 11-77. Histiocytosis X. The lesions, seen primarily in the skull, consist of eosinophils and histiocytes with some admixture of lymphocytes and plasma cells. The histiocytes may be mononuclear to multinuclear cells having characteristically benign-appearing nuclei with deep grooves and small nucleoli and abundant, pale cytoplasm. The cell population may vary from case to case and with duration of the disease. Electron microscopy of these histiocytes discloses that they are Langerhans cells showing Birbeck granules comprised of multilaminar rod-shaped structures with an expanded end (like a tennis racquet). The term *histiocytosis X* is used here to include the Hand-Schüller-Christian disease, the Letterer-Siwe disease, and eosinophilic granulomas. (H & E, X310)

Malignant Tumors of the Breast

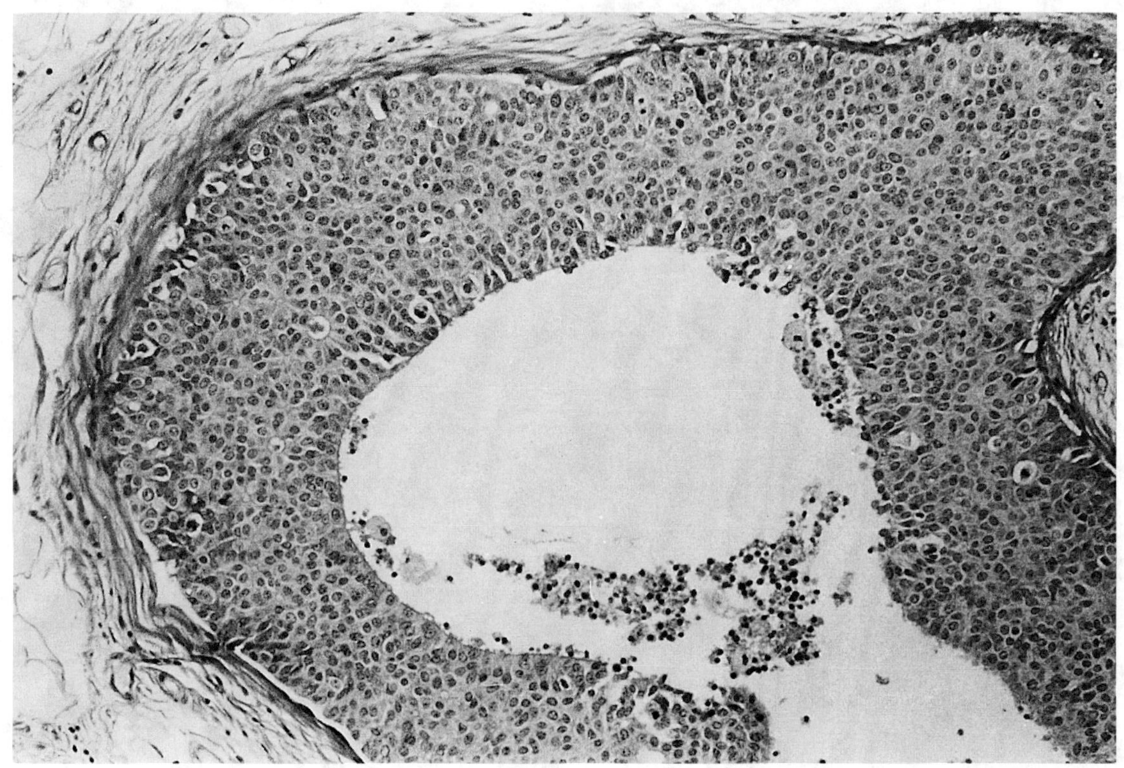

Figure 11-78A. Ductal carcinoma *in situ* of the breast (intraductal carcinoma). The tumor is distinctly confined within ductal structures. Tumor cells may be well-differentiated epithelial ductal cells homogenously similar to one another in size and shape, but may also be anaplastic in focal areas or sometimes throughout. The pattern may be cribriform, comedo (showing central necrosis), solid, or papillary. The lesion is frequently multicentric and may be confluent in some cases, particularly the comedo type. (H & E, X125)

Figure 11-78B. Invasive ductal carcinoma of the breast. The tumor cells are more pleomorphic, showing varied forms of nests, glandlike structures, and cords with conspicuous desmoplastic reaction. This is the most common breast carcinoma. Intraductal carcinoma may also be noted. If the intraductal carcinoma is the predominant feature, it should be stated in the diagnosis, inasmuch as there is an impression that this is less aggressive than the usual predominant invasive ductal carcinoma. (H & E, X75)

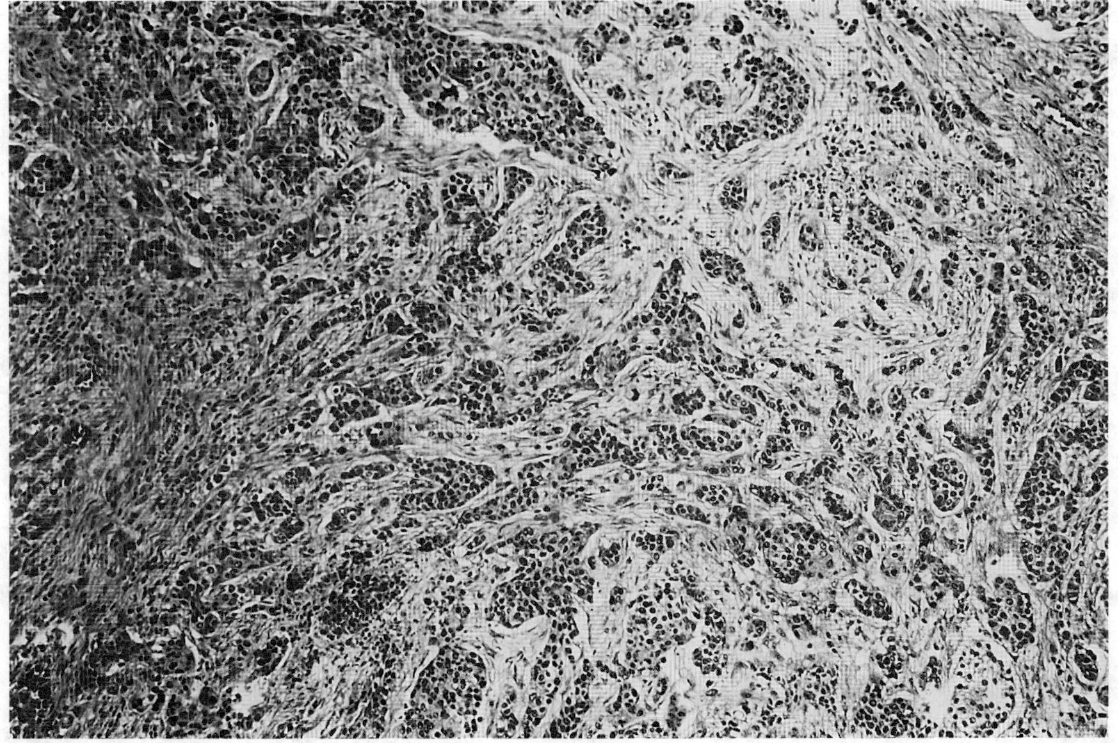

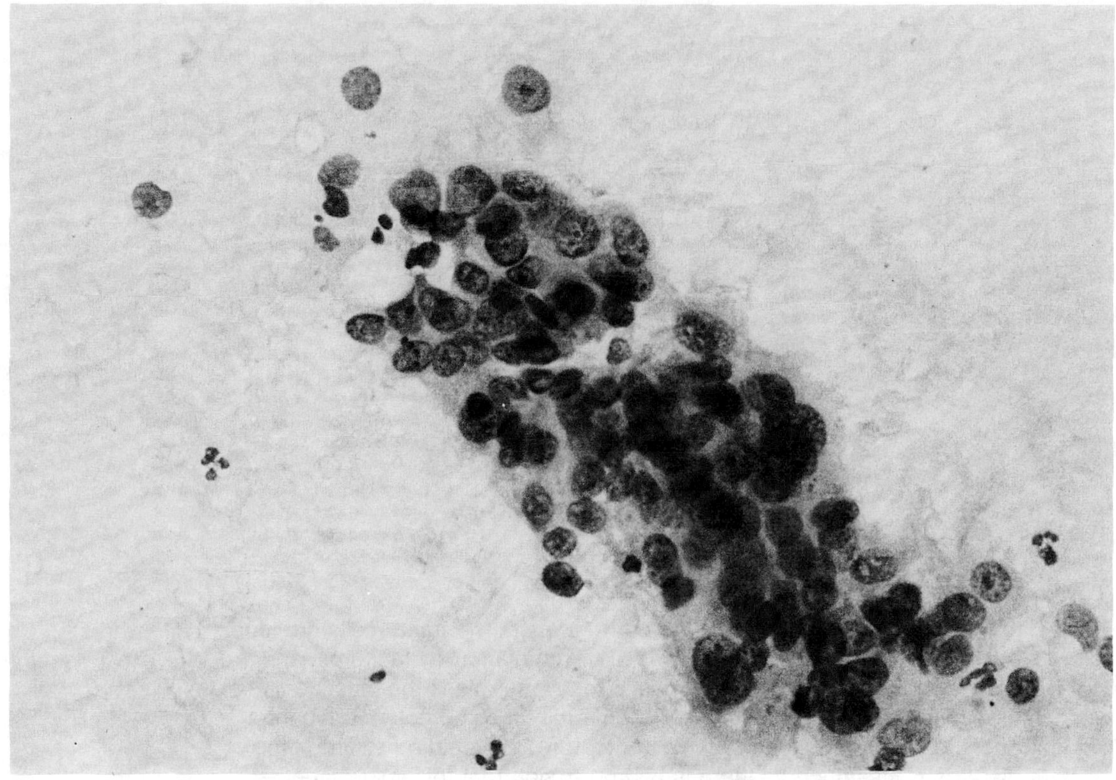

Figure 11-79. Ductal carcinoma of the breast (fine-needle aspirate cytology). The aspirate yields a cellular smear composed of poorly cohesive cells exhibiting a moderate degree of pleomorphism. The nuclei are irregular in size and shape, with coarse chromatin clumps. Nucleoli may be prominent. (Pap, X310)

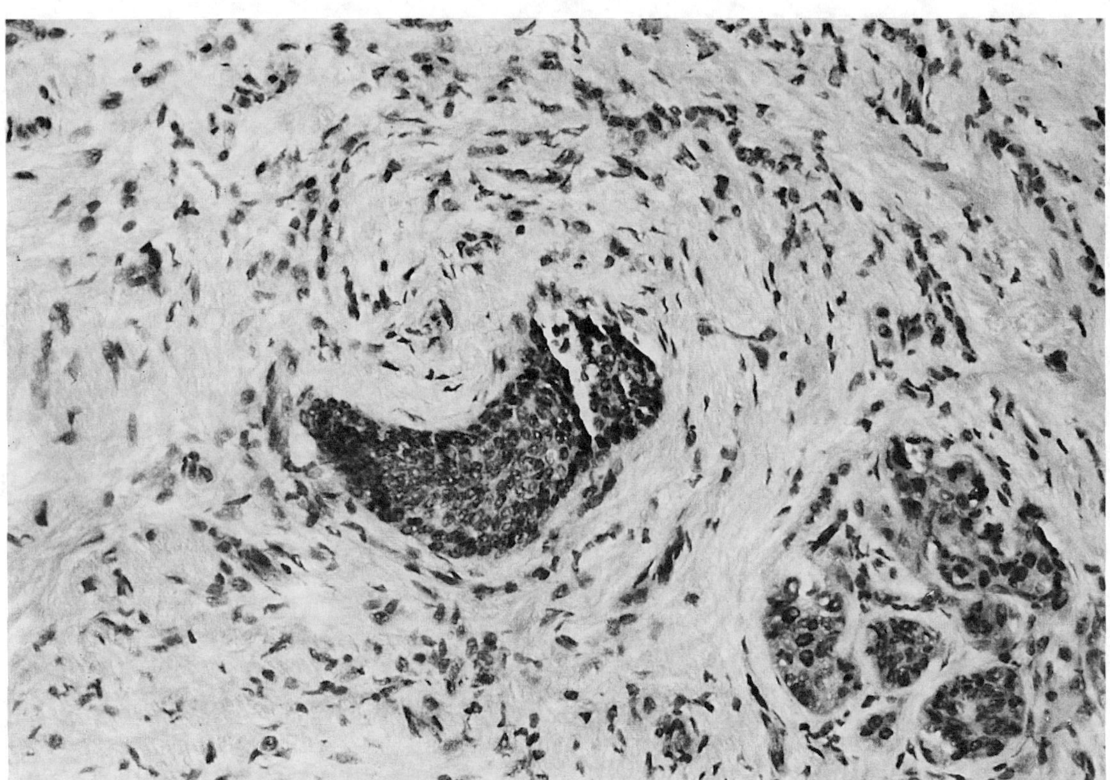

Figure 11-80A & B. Lobular carcinoma of the breast (invasive). The tumor consists of uniform, small/round-to-ovoid cells, loosely cohesive with hyperchromatic nuclei, and small nucleoli having scant cytoplasm. The cells typically have a linear arrangement and tend to infiltrate around normal ducts, forming a targetlike pattern (photo A, above). In some cases, lobular carcinoma *in situ* filling up and expanding the acini and terminal ducts with pagetoid cells in adjacent interlobular ducts may also be noted (photo B, opposite page). The periductal infiltrate-producing targetoid pattern has been overemphasized, since it can also be seen in benign inflammatory lesions and leukemic infiltrate. To rely on this pattern alone could be hazardous, particularly during intraoperative consultation with frozen section. Lymph node metastases from this carcinoma may mimic malignant lymphoma. (H & E, 80A X200; 80B X125)

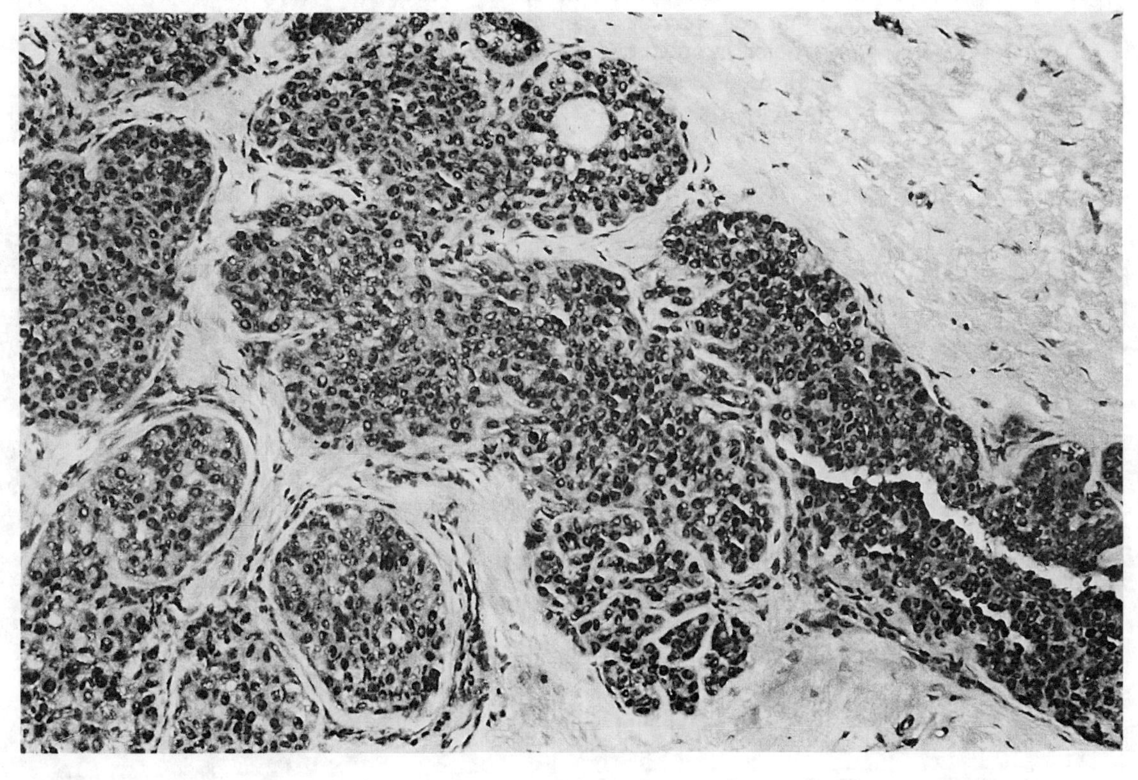

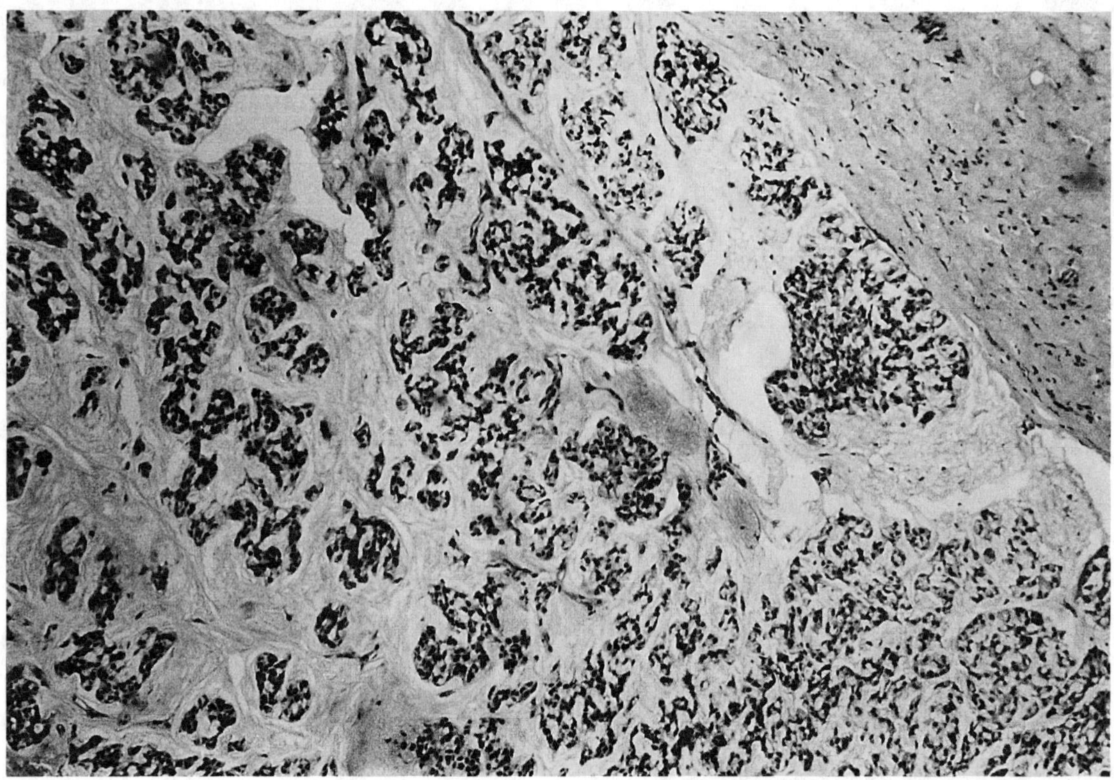

Figure 11-81. Mucinous carcinoma of the breast (colloid carcinoma). Nests of columnar cells having vesicular nuclei with pale and vacuolated cytoplasm are noted in pools of mucin; sometimes they form glandular structures. This is considered to have a better prognosis than invasive ductal carcinoma. (H & E, X75)

Figure 11-82. Medullary carcinoma of the breast. The tumor is composed of large anaplastic cells with vesicular nuclei and prominent nucleoli forming trabecular anastomosing cords of cells accompanied by extensive lymphoid infiltrate. The tumor is well circumscribed; the borders often compress adjacent tissue by expansion rather than by infiltration. (H & E, X75)

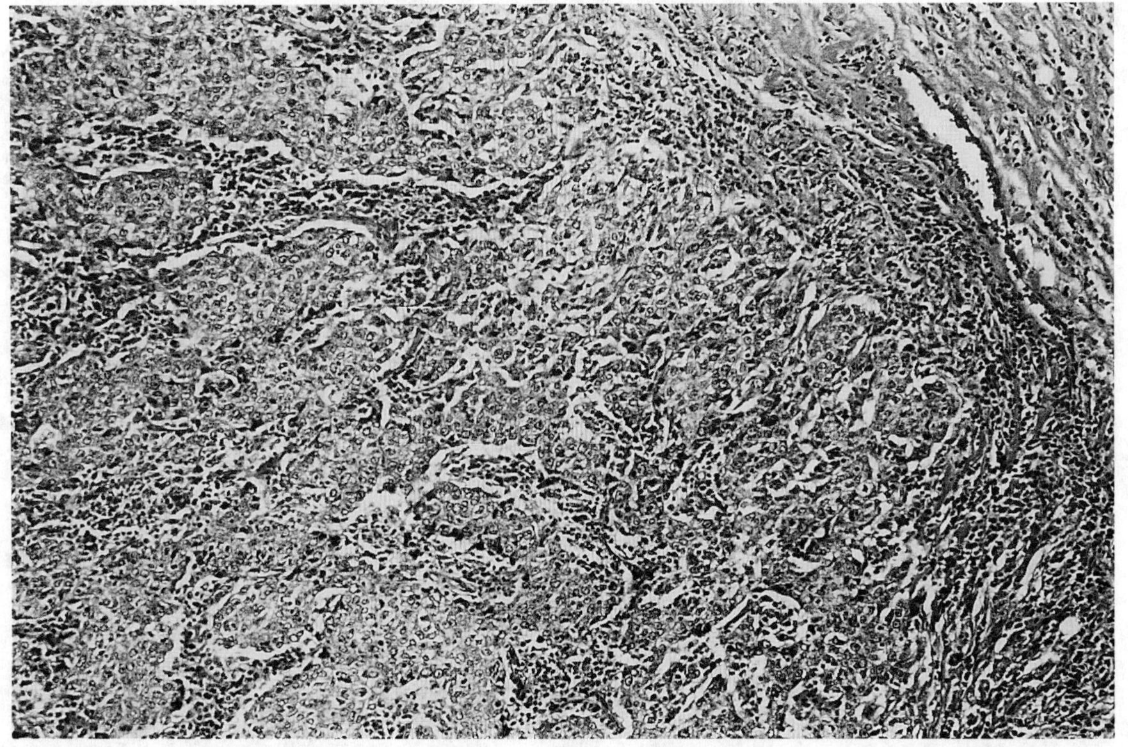

Figure 11-83. Medullary carcinoma of the breast (cytology fine-needle aspirate). The smear of the aspirate is cellular, with large pleomorphic cells having vesicular nuclei with prominent nucleoli and some coarse chromatin clumps. Nuclear cytoplasmic ratio is decreased. There is an abundant admixture of lymphocytes and plasma cells. (Pap, X310)

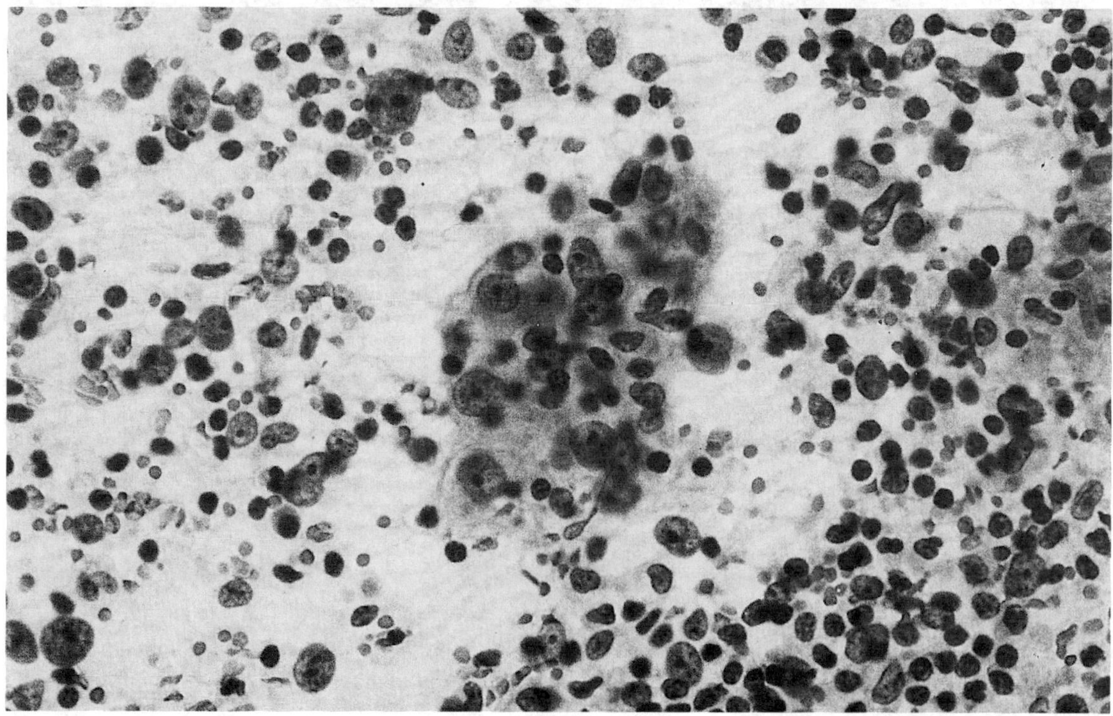

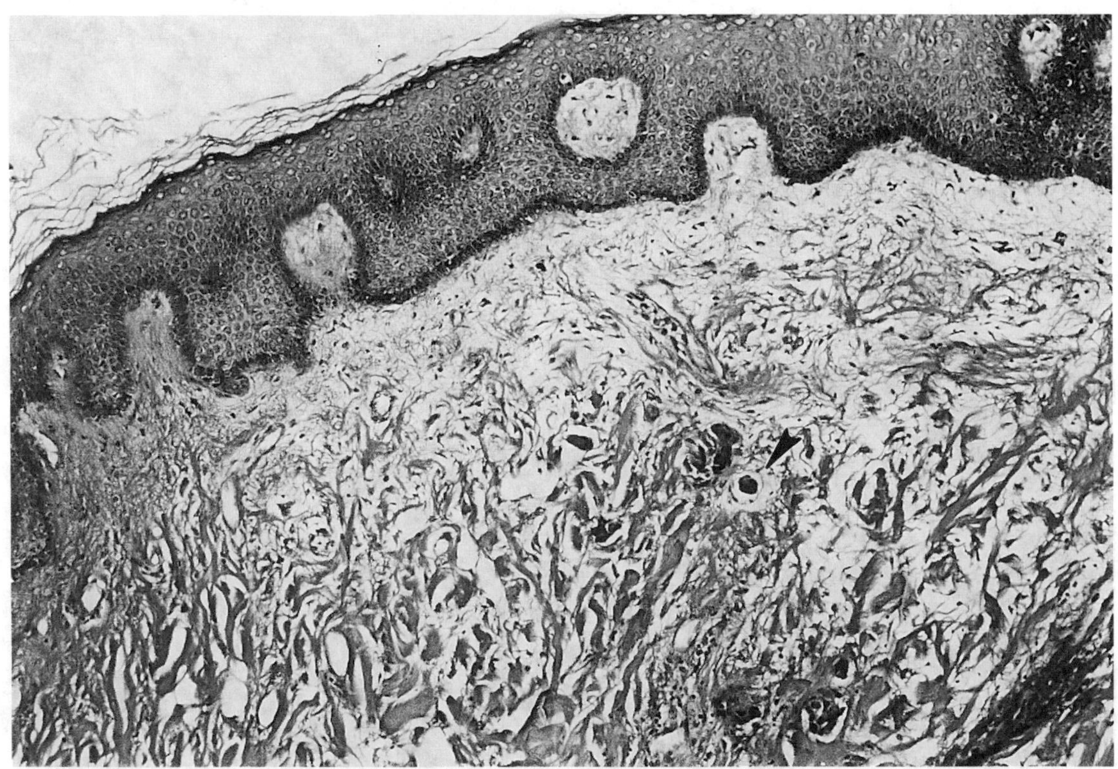

Figure 11-84. Inflammatory carcinoma of the breast. Superficial and deep dermal lymphatics are permeated by clusters of malignant cells composed of cohesive round-to-ovoid cells with hyperchromatic nuclei and scant cytoplasm. This is a clinical entity characterized by rapid enlargement of the breast due to edema and erythema. (H & E, X75)

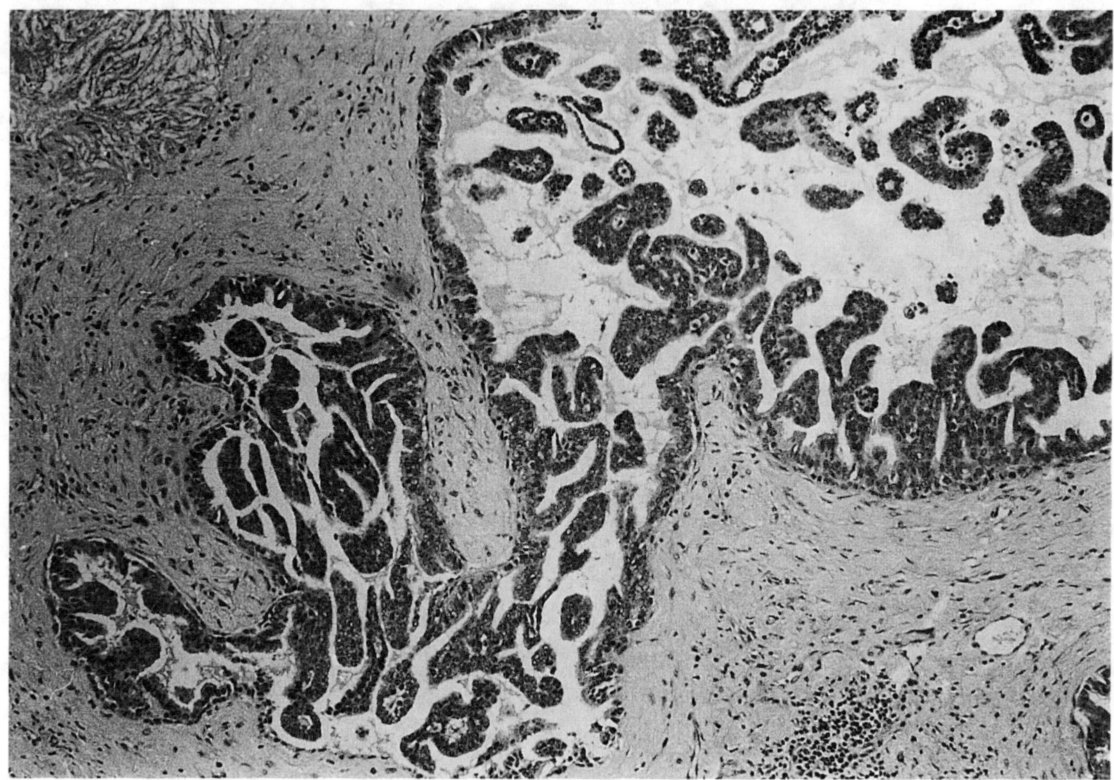

Figure 11-85. Mammary papillary carcinoma. The tumor is comprised of low columnar and cuboidal cells forming a papillary pattern even in the invasive and metastatic foci. The photo illustrates papillary carcinoma in a cystic structure. This rare tumor is usually seen in elderly women. Aspiration of the lesion may yield only hemorrhagic fluid. (H & E, X75)

Figure 11-86. Mammary tubular carcinoma. The tumor is composed of low columnar and cuboidal cells forming a distinct tubular structure with fibrous stroma. It has a good prognosis. (H & E, X75)

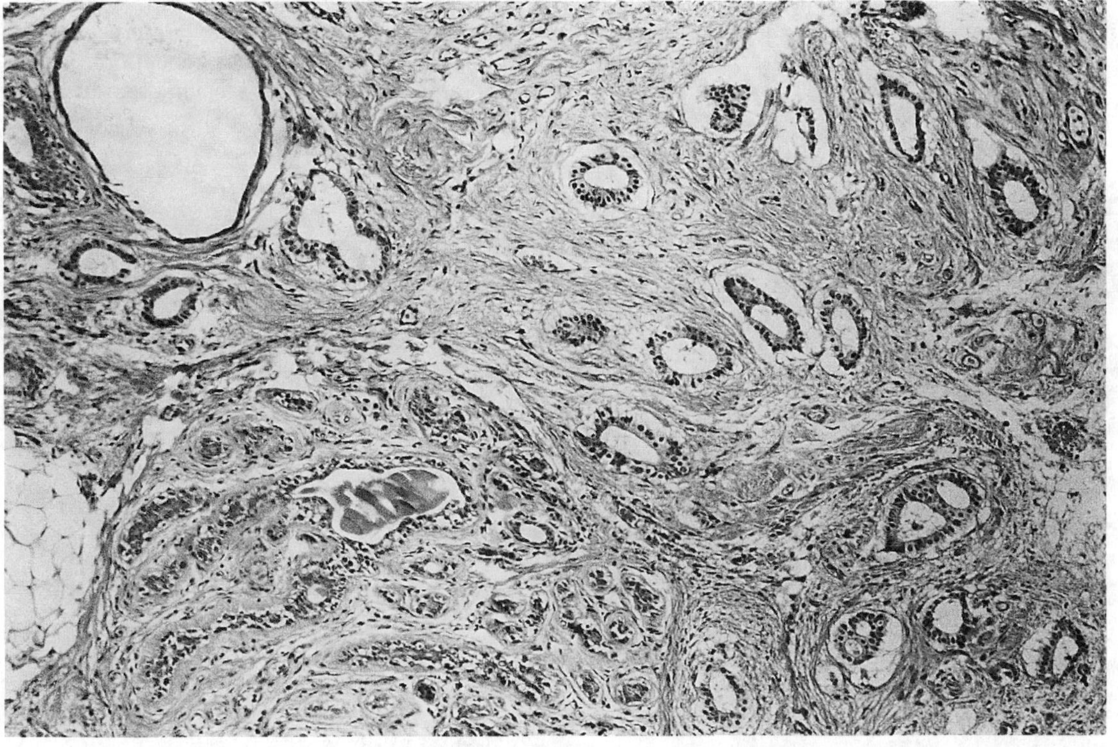

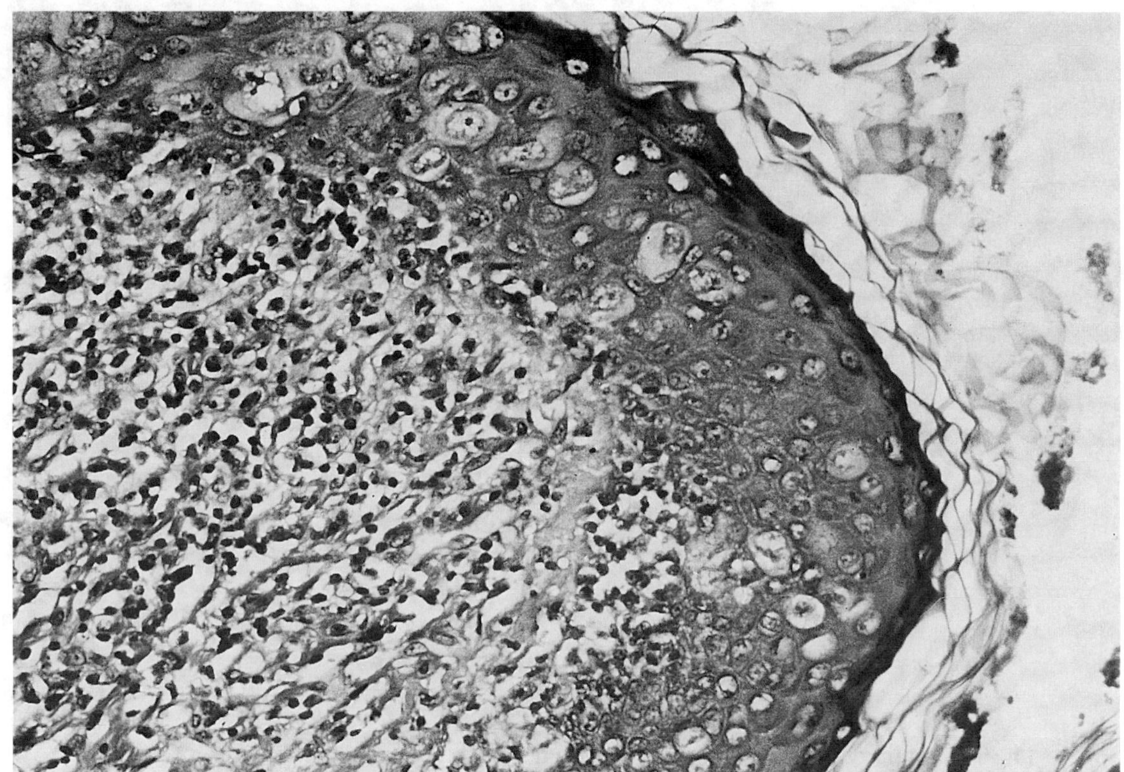

Figure 11-87. Mammary Paget's disease of the nipple. The lesion consists of large, pale staining cells surrounded by a halo noted within the epidermis; it is positive for mucin stain. When melanin granules are present, superficial malignant melanoma must be ruled out. The concept of Paget's disease occurring as *in situ* rather than as an extension of an underlying carcinoma is gaining some ground.* (H & E, X125)

*Lagios MD et al. Paget's disease of the nipple. Cancer 1984; 54:545–51.

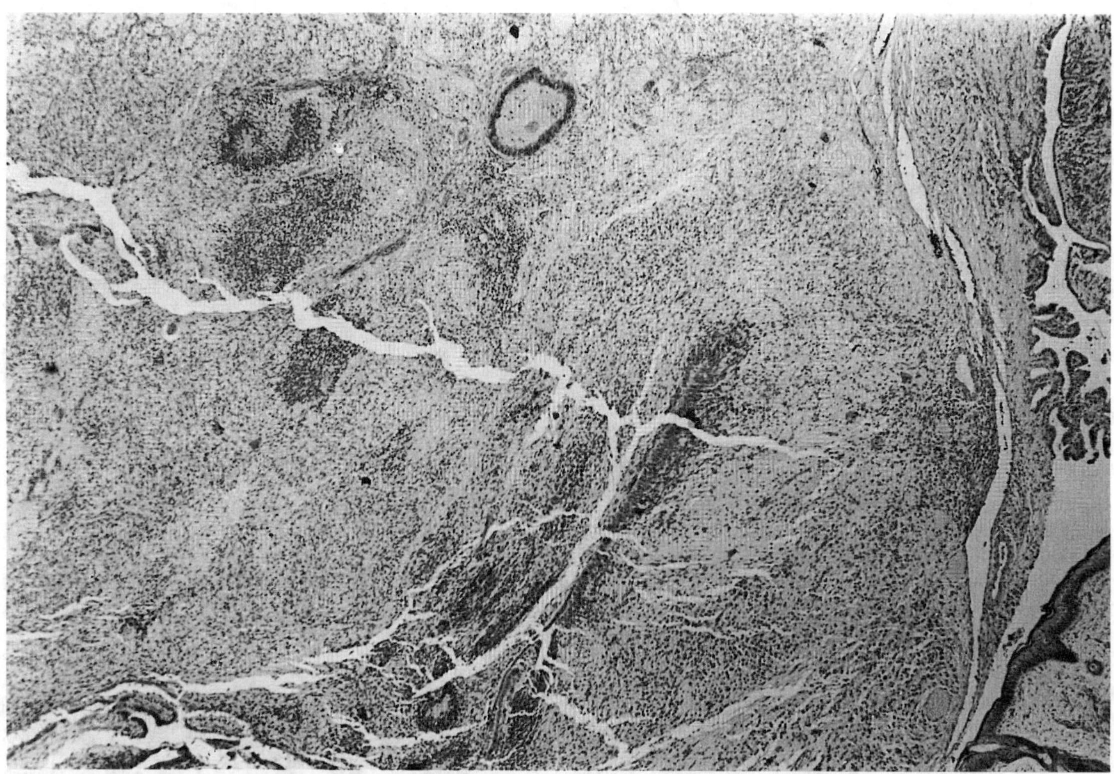

Figure 11-88. Malignant cystosarcoma phylloides of the breast. The tumor mimics a fibroadenoma except that the stroma is quite cellular and pleomorphic. The degree of stromal cellularity ranges from low-grade fibrosarcoma to a high-grade sarcoma. Size, mitosis, and infiltrating tumor border are some of the criteria to be considered in classifying this lesion as malignant. In patients with tumor of >4 cm in diameter, the recurrence rate is about 40%. Metastases occur mainly via the hematogenous route and are often found in the lungs. The metastatic foci are only of stromal elements. Lymph node metastases are rare. (H & E, X75)

Malignant Tumors of the Skin

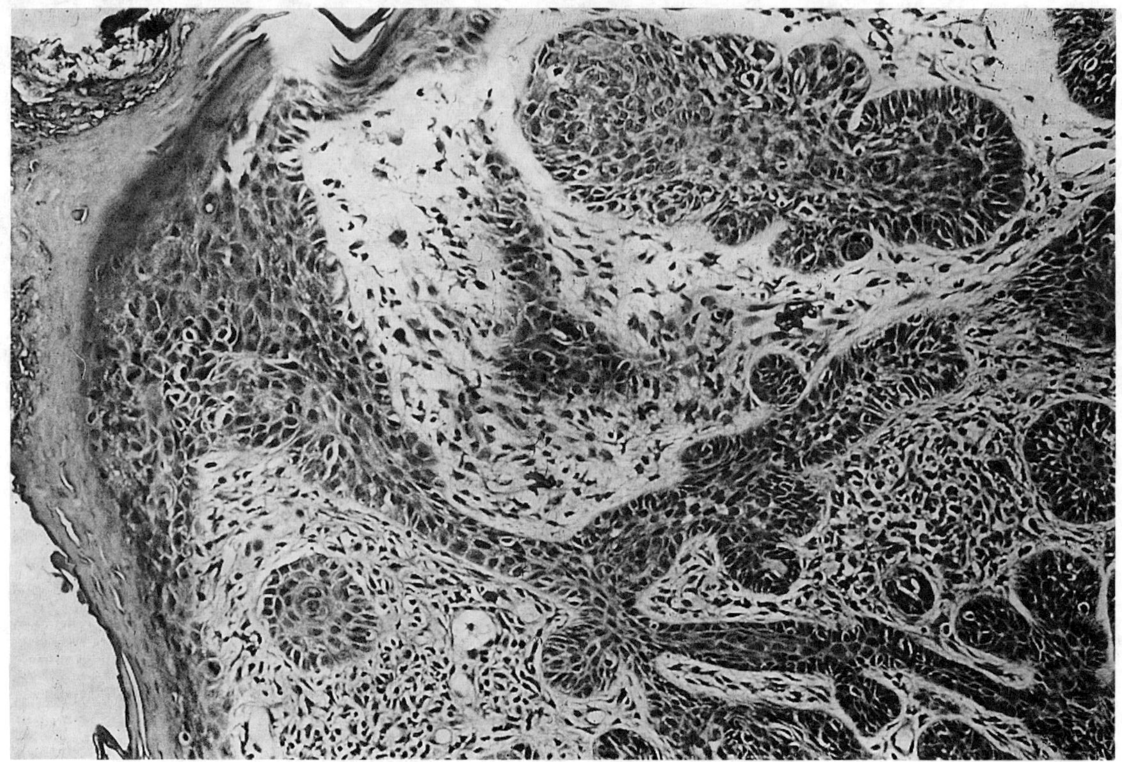

Figure 11-89. Basal cell carcinoma of the skin. The cells are ovoid or elongated, with uniform hyperchromatic nuclei and indistinct cytoplasmic border. The tumor grows in solid sheets or forms a lacelike pattern, sometimes accompanied by extensive fibrosis. The tumor is easily seen arising from the basal layer of epidermis. (H & E, X125)

Figure 11-90. Merkel cell carcinoma of the skin (neuroendocrine carcinoma, trabecular carcinoma). Tumor cells are quite uniform in size and shape, having round-to-ovoid nuclei with distinct nuclear membrane, finely dispersed chromatin with small nucleoli, and a narrow rim of pale cytoplasm. The tumor forms anastomosing cords of cells, a trabecular pattern in the dermis, and may extend into subcutis. The tumor is not attached to the epidermis. Electron microscopy discloses membrane-bound, dense-core granules 125–210 nm in diameter (like the neurosecretory granules seen in cells derived from the neural crest). It is an aggressive tumor. Differential diagnosis includes malignant lymphoma (immunoblastic) and metastatic small-cell carcinoma. (H & E, X125)

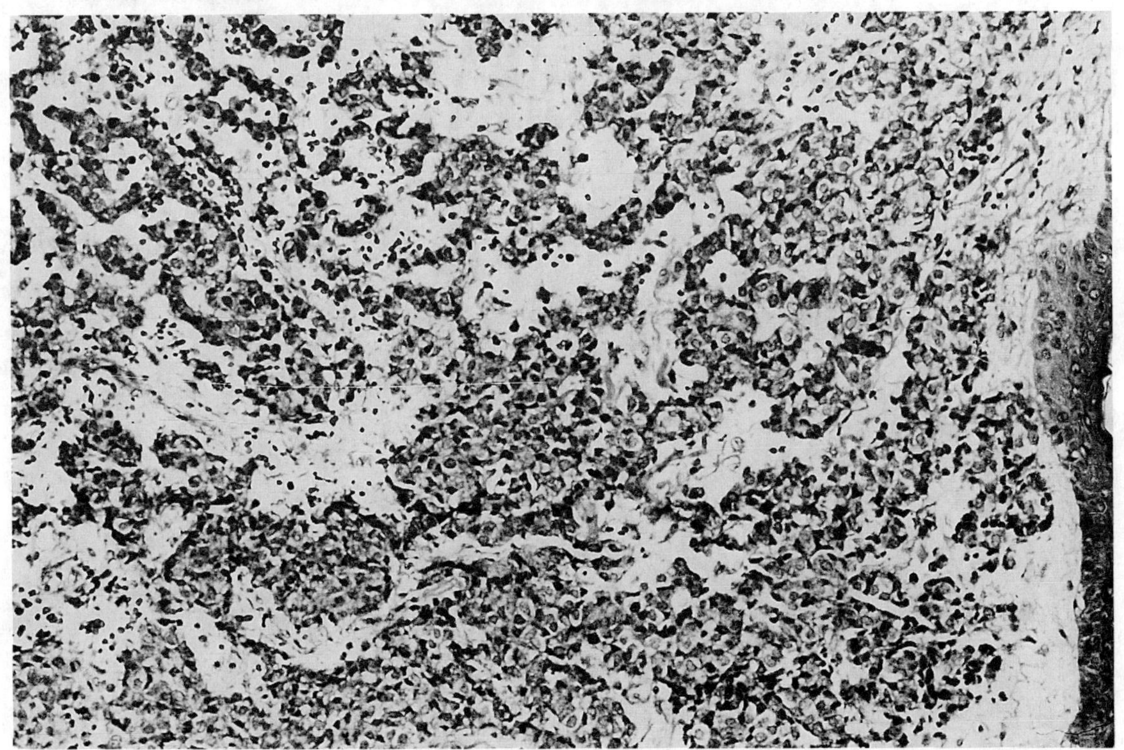

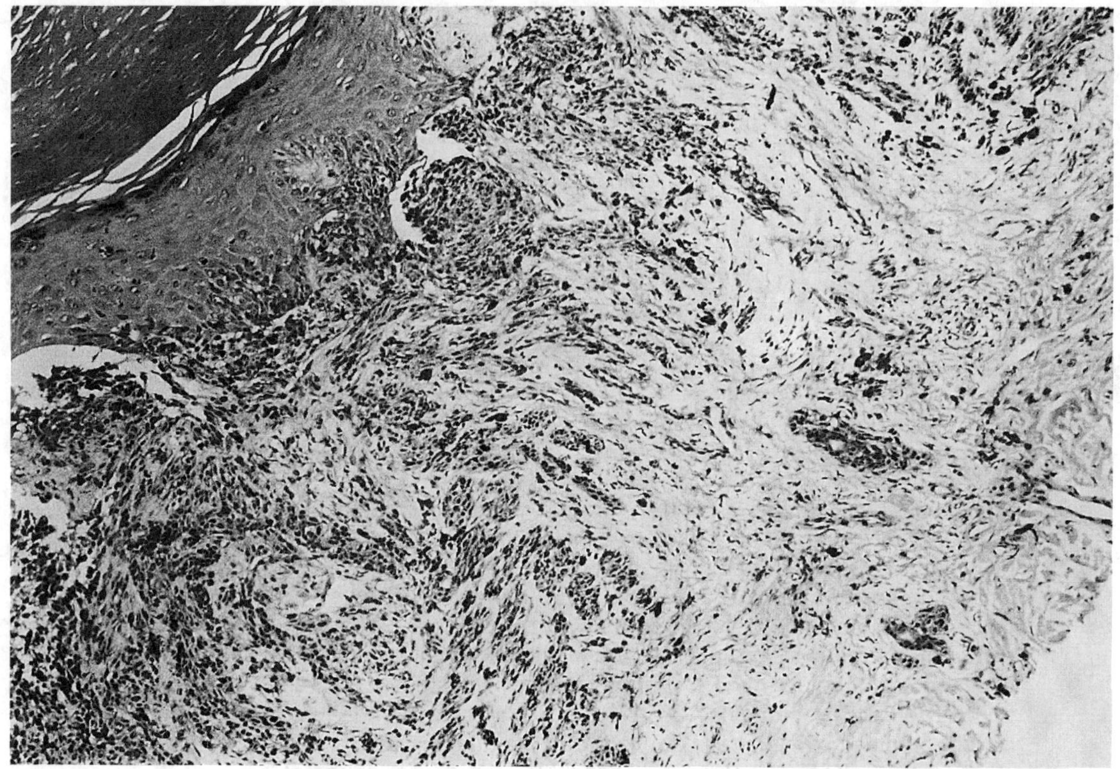

Figure 11-91. Malignant melanoma. This lesion at the dermoepidermal junction shows downward growth of melanocytes into deep dermis. The cells are polygonal but may be spindle form. Mitosis is frequent. Melanin pigment also varies in amount, but it can be absent. (H & E, X75)

Malignant Tumors of the Endocrine and Chemoreceptor System

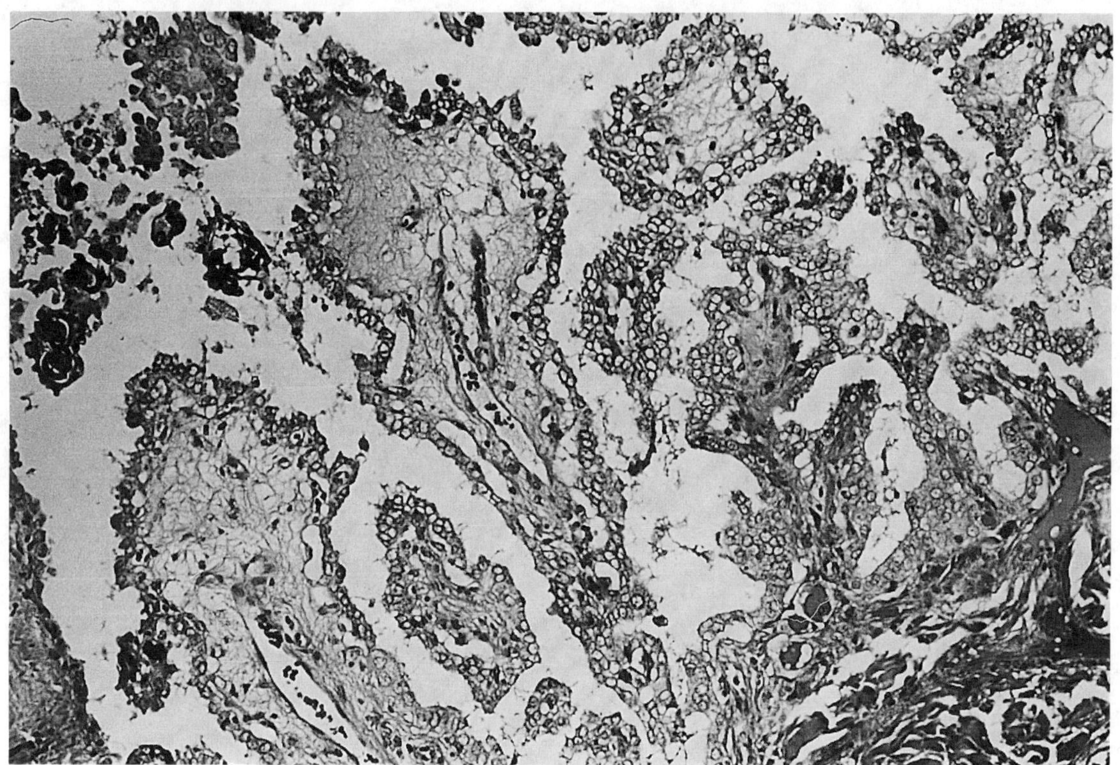

Figure 11-92A & B. Thyroid papillary adenocarcinoma. The nuclei have a characteristic ground glass ("Orphan Annie eye") nuclei and lack nucleoli. The tumor may form a papillary (photo A, above) and follicular pattern (photo B, opposite page). Psammoma bodies (laminated calcified body) are frequent. This is rarely seen in the absence of carcinoma. (H & E, X125)

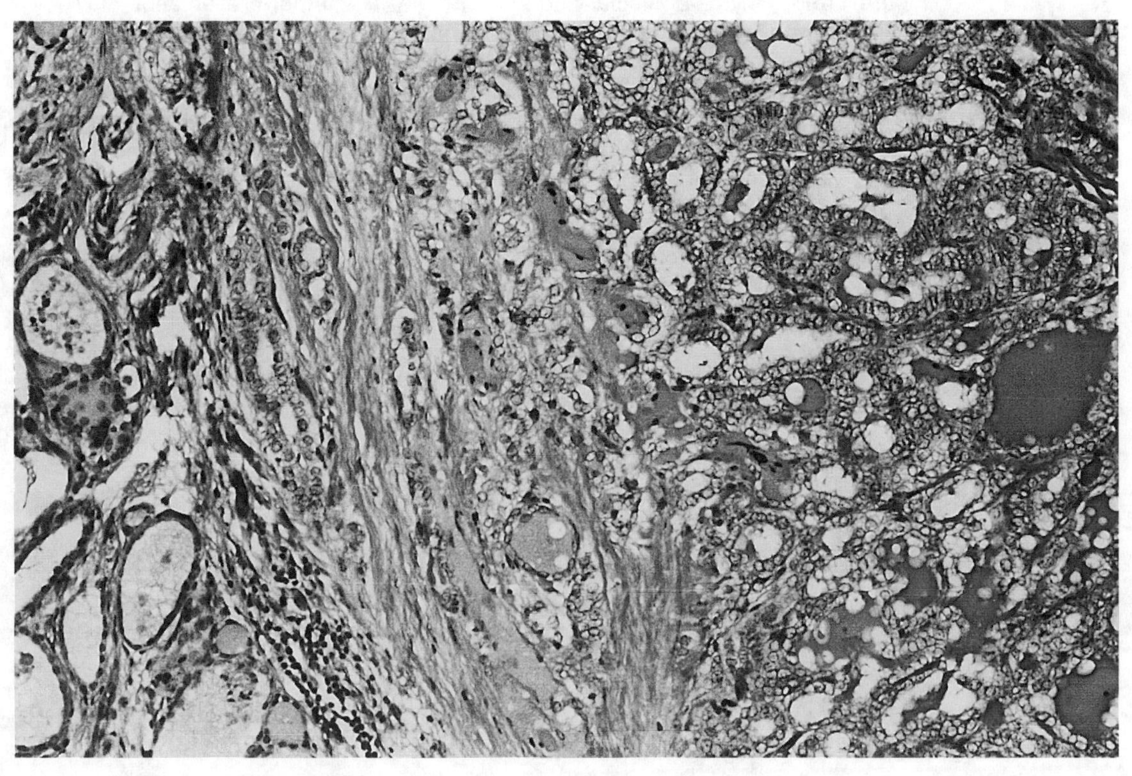

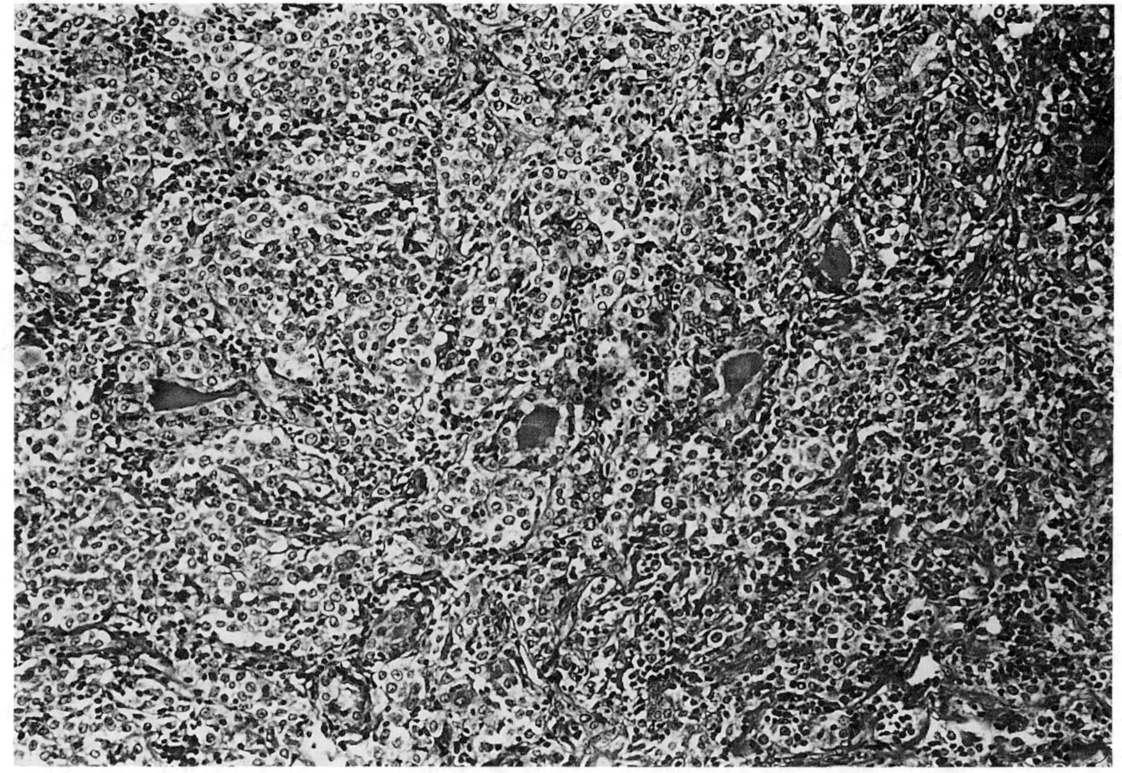

Figure 11-93. Thyroid follicular adenocarcinoma. The tumor presentation may range from that of a mass with normal-looking follicles to a poorly differentiated carcinoma with very few small follicles. Aspirate may show few follicles, with atypia of the epithelial cells. This is dangerous, however, because adenoma may have atypical cells. For this reason, in some cases biopsy is needed to supplement aspirate findings. This tumor may be encapsulated with capsular invasion or it may be an outright invasive lesion. (H & E, X125)

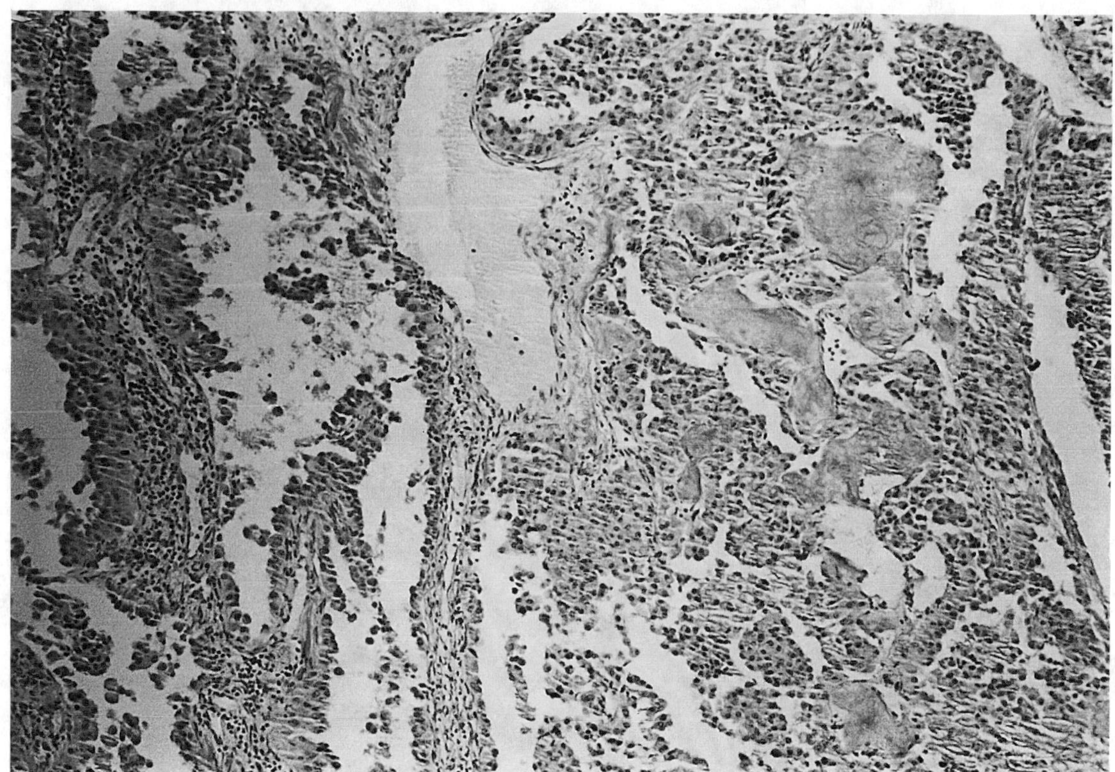

Figure 11-94A & B. Thyroid medullary carcinoma. Tumor cells are round to spindle shaped, with copious amphophilic cytoplasm, and grow in solid tumor nests. Papillary and aborted follicles may be noted (photo A, above). Amyloid deposition is variable. A rare variant of medullary carcinoma resembles the undifferentiated spindle and giant cell carcinomas (photo B, opposite page). (H & E, X75)

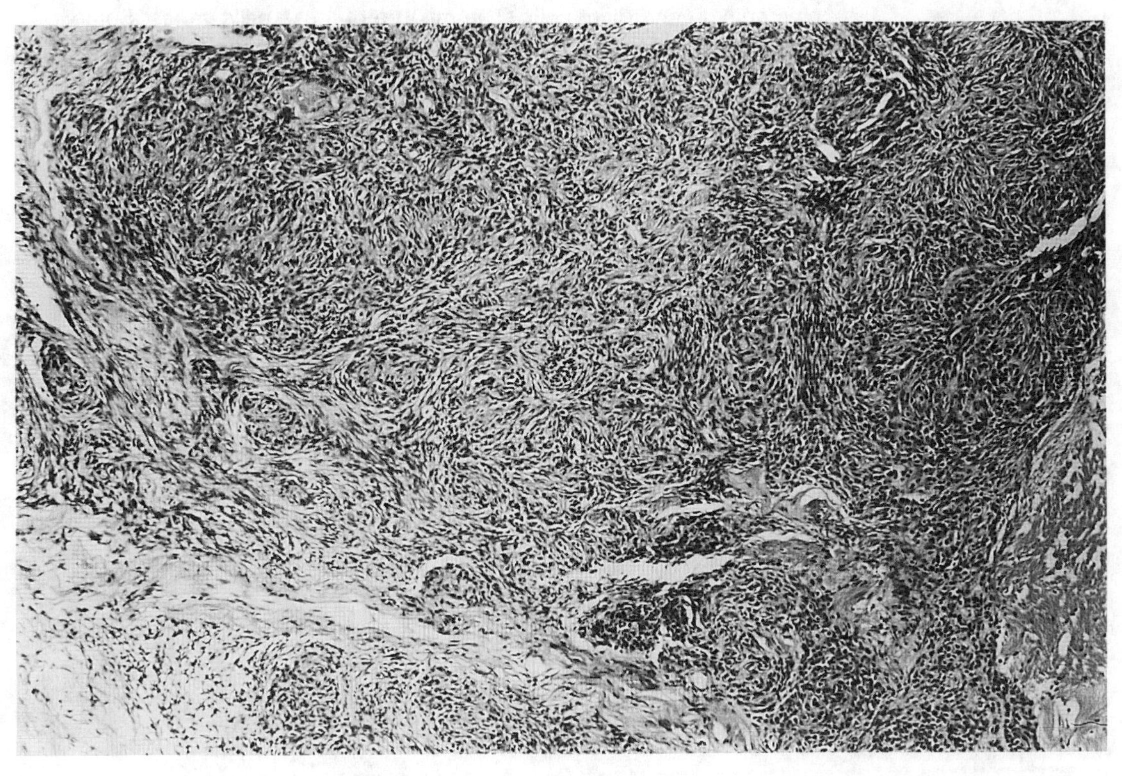

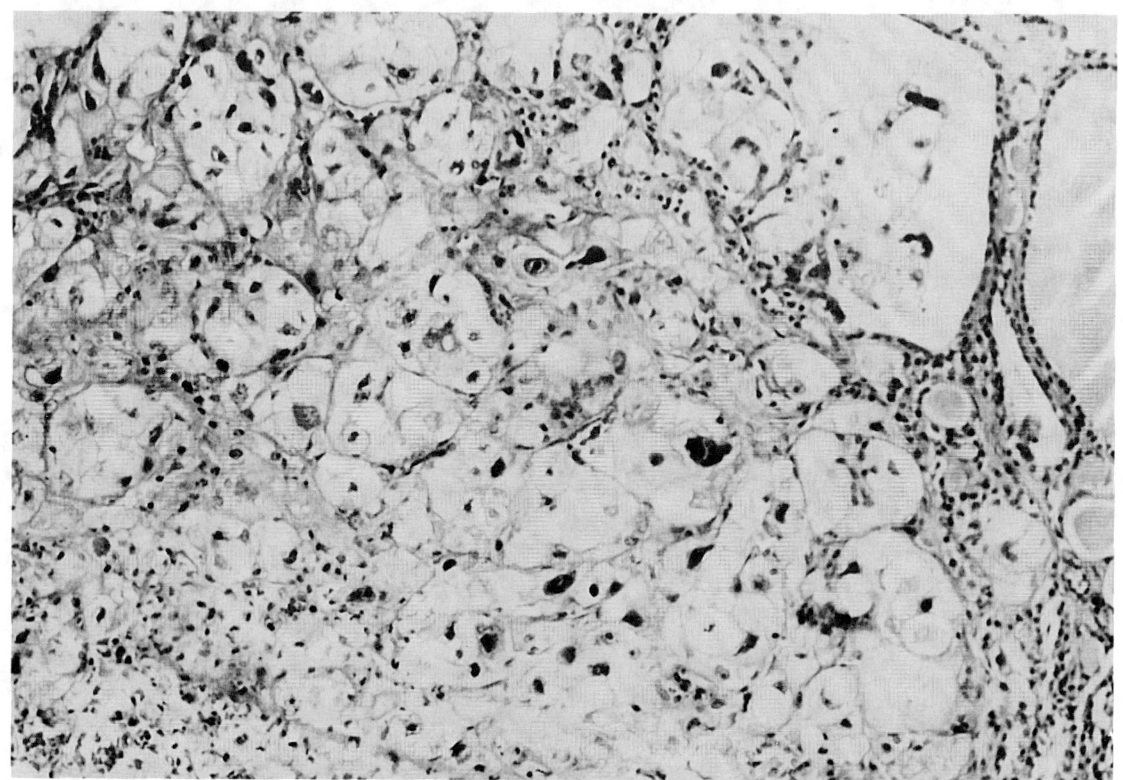

Figure 11-95. Thyroid undifferentiated carcinoma. Tumor cells consist of pleomorphic spindle and giant cells. The mixture of these cells varies. Some small-cell undifferentiated carcinoma lesions have been reclassified as truly malignant lymphoma. (H & E, X125)

Figure 11-96. Parathyroid carcinoma. Tumor cells are like chief cells with granular cytoplasm, exhibiting some palisading arrangement and having a trabecular pattern with broad fibrous bands. However, mitosis is the most valuable single criterion in the absence of vascular invasion or metastases. Adenoma often displays more pleomorphic chief cells than carcinoma cells. (H & E, X75)

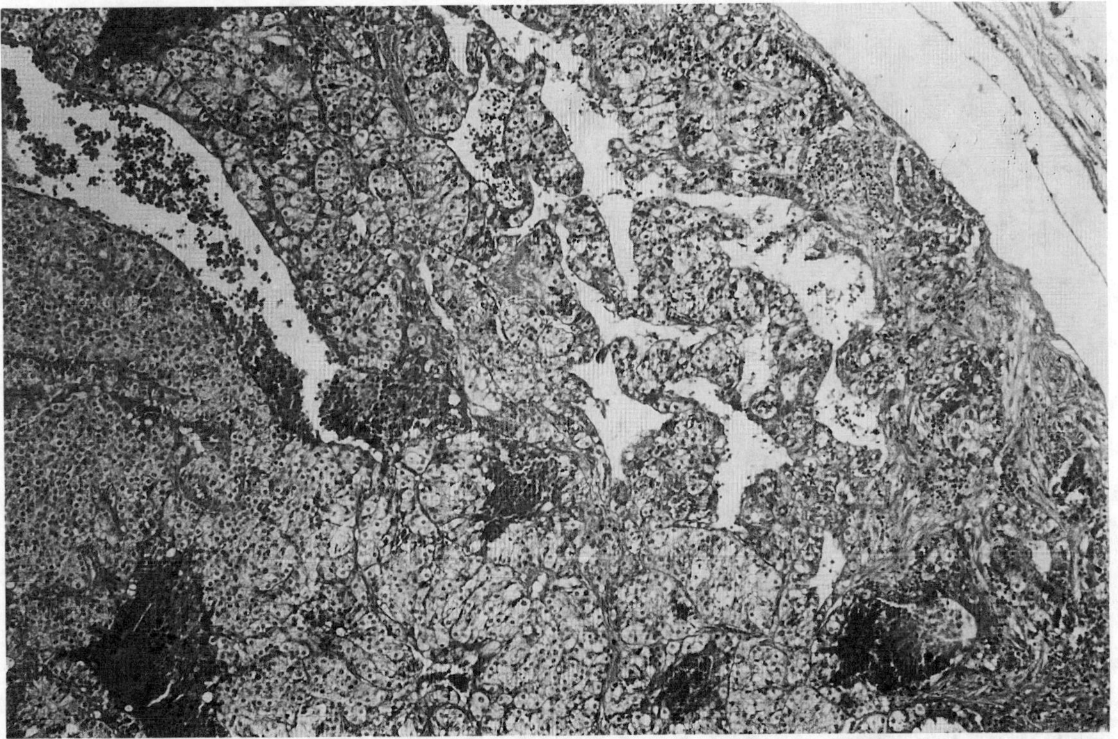

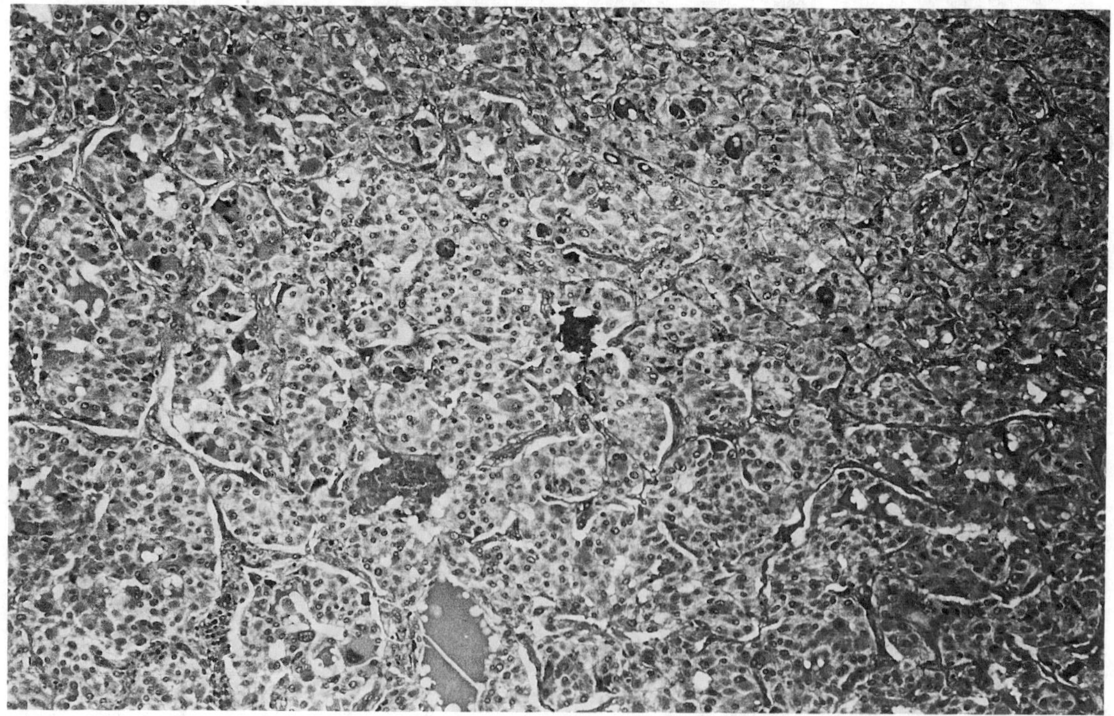

Figure 11-97. Pheochromocytoma of the adrenal gland. The tumor consists of pleomorphic cells similar to pheochromocytes occurring in clusters and nests divided by thin fibrovascular septae. Dichromate fixative imparts brownish stain to the cytoplasm. Argentaffin reaction is positive. The only absolute criterion for malignancy is the presence of metastases. (H & E, X75)

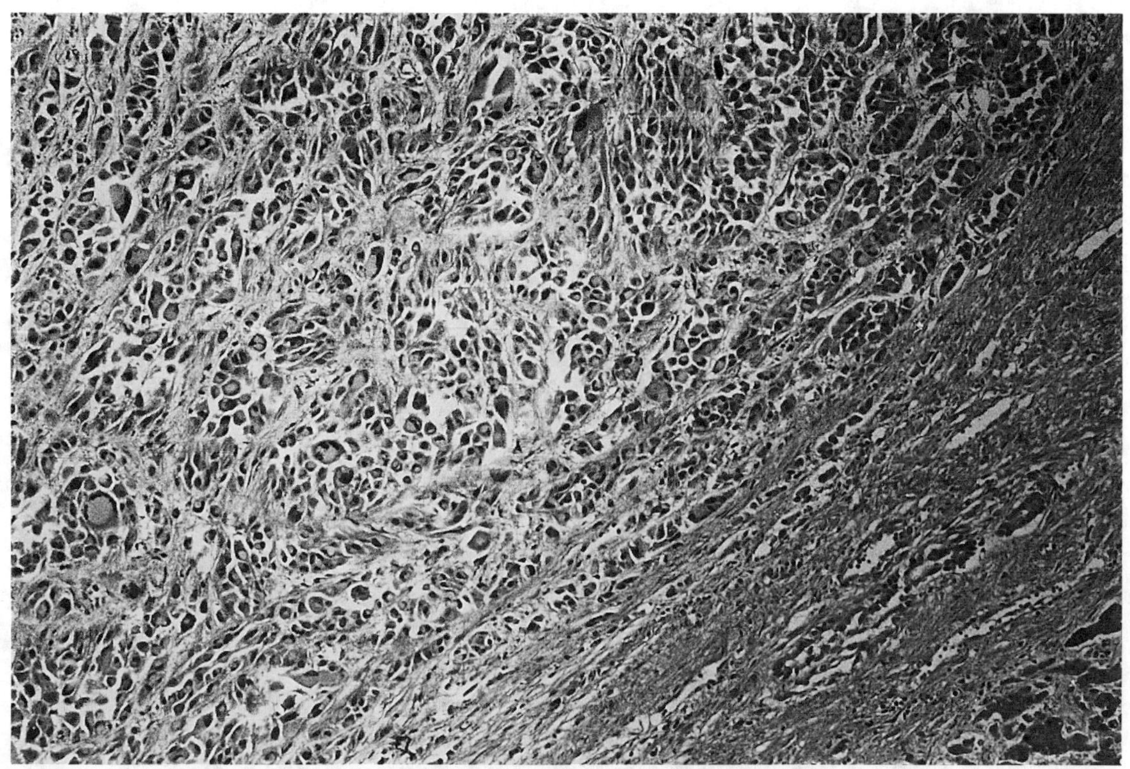

Figure 11-98. Paraganglioma of chemoreceptors. Tumor cells are arranged in nests around a network of vascular channels. The cells vary from oval to polygonal to plump spindle cells forming lobules or cell nest (zellballen). Histologic criteria for malignancy are lacking. Metastasis is the only absolute criterion at this time. Photo shows metastasis to liver. Neurofilament proteins are often expressed by paragangliomas and pheochromocytomas. (H & E, X75)

Lymphomas

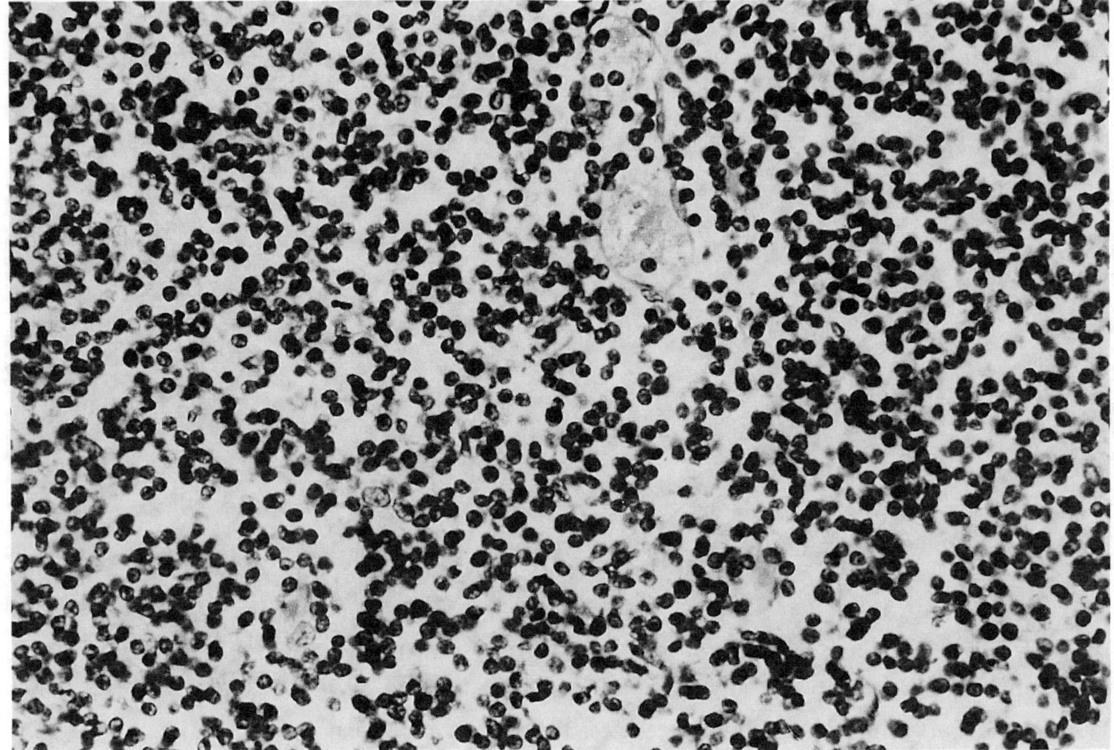

Figure 11-99. Malignant lymphoma, small lymphocytic (well differentiated). This tumor is characterized by diffuse pattern composed of lymphocytes averaging 6–7 μ with rounded dense hyperchromatic nuclei, rarely recognizable nucleoli, scant cytoplasm, and infrequent mitosis. This is equivalent to chronic lymphocytic leukemia. Those showing some plasmacytic differentiation may be associated with monoclonal gammopathy. Waldenstrom macroglobulinemia, heavy- and light-chain disease would fall in this category, (plasmacytic, lymphocytic, lymphoma, or well-differentiated lymphocytic lymphoma with dysproteinemia). This is a low-grade lymphoma. (H & E, X310)

Figure 11-100. Malignant lymphoma, follicular predominantly small cleaved cell (poorly differentiated lymphocytic lymphoma of Rappaport's). The cells average 7–12 μ. The nuclei are angulated, twisted and cleaved, with homogenous chromatin and inconspicuous nucleoli. The same type of cells are noted in the interfollicular zone. This is the most frequent form of follicular lymphoma (working formulation). In practice, all nodular lymphomas are B cells. (H & E, X310)

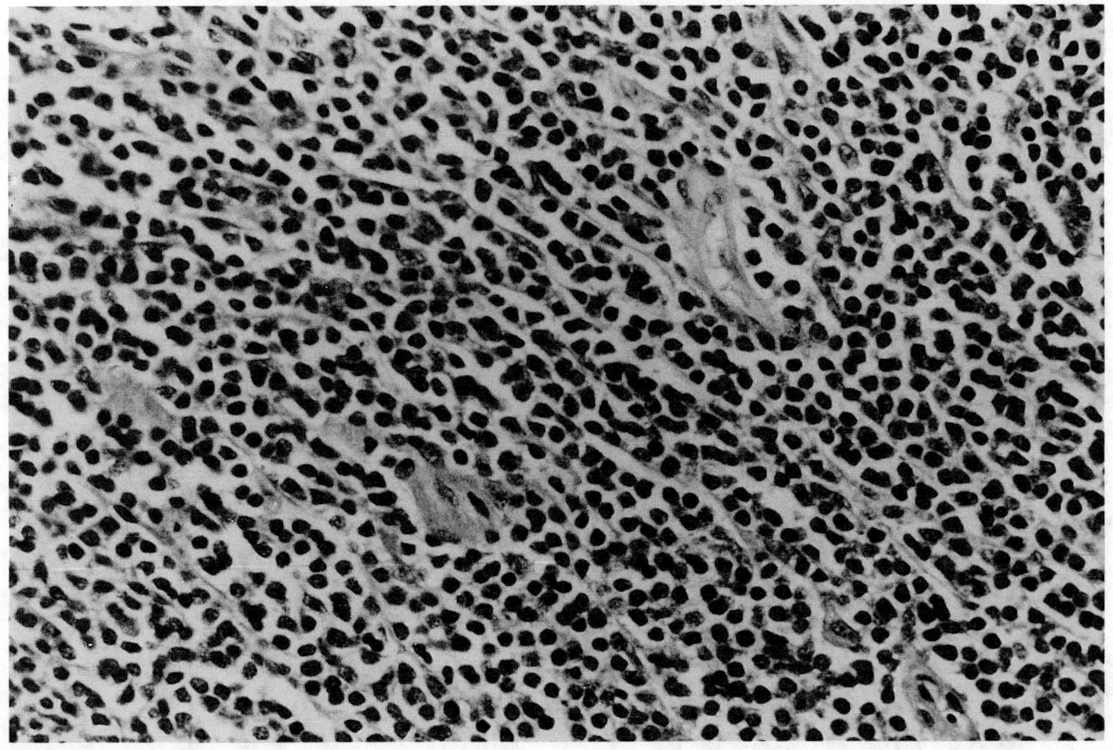

Figure 11-101. Malignant lymphoma, follicular mixed small-cleaved and large-cell. There is an admixture of small-cleaved lymphocytes and large cells, 2–3 times the diameter of small normal lymphocytes, having round, ovoid or irregular nuclei, with 2–3 nucleoli apposed to the nuclear membrane. It has been suggested that the large cells should be 20–50% of the cell population to classify for mixed cell type. Others accept this diagnosis after seeing at least 5 large noncleaved cells per high-power field. Those showing a follicular pattern are considered low grade, whereas those with diffuse pattern are classified as intermediate grade. (H & E, X310)

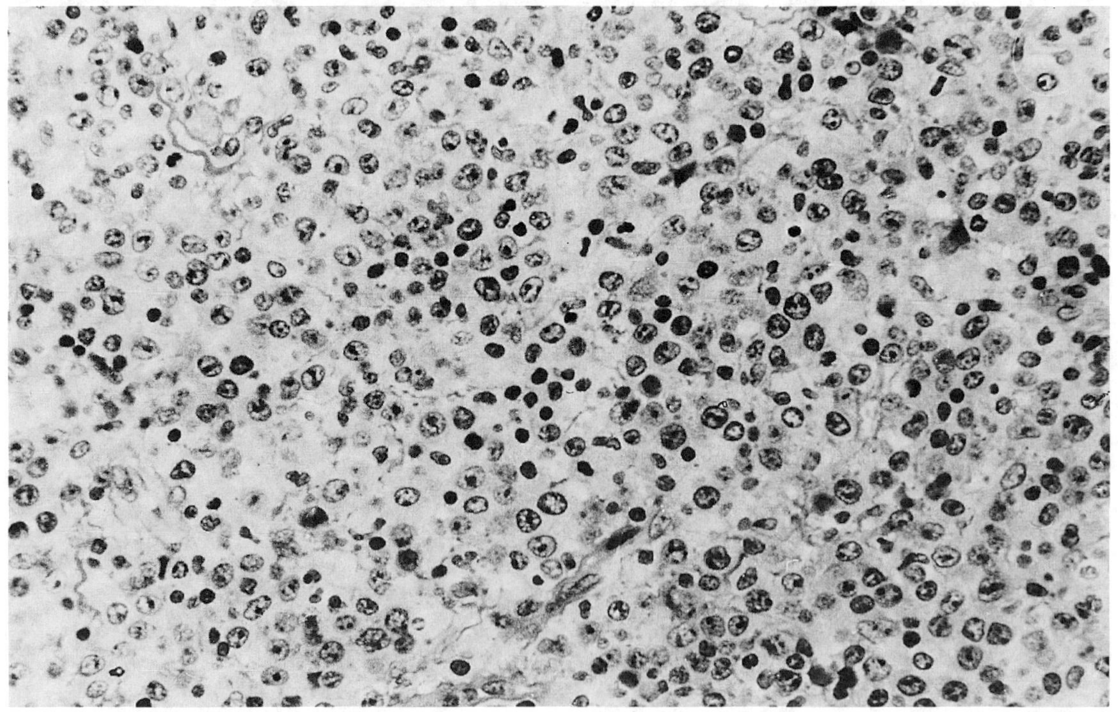

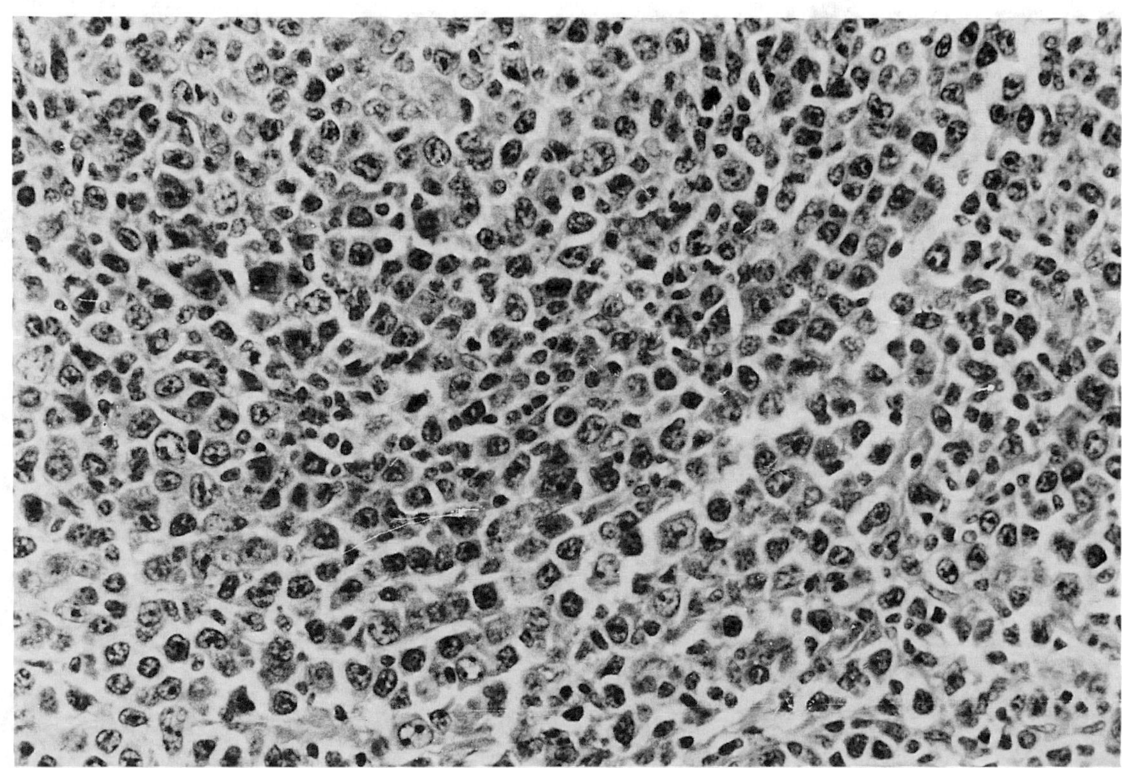

Figure 11-102. Malignant lymphoma, follicular predominantly large-cell type. The cells range from 20 to 40 μ and their nuclei may be rounded, ovoid or angulated, twisted and cleaved with inconspicuous nucleoli and scant cytoplasm. Both follicular noncleaved and diffuse pattern are considered intermediate grade. There is usually an admixture of small-cleaved lymphocytes. (H & E, X310)

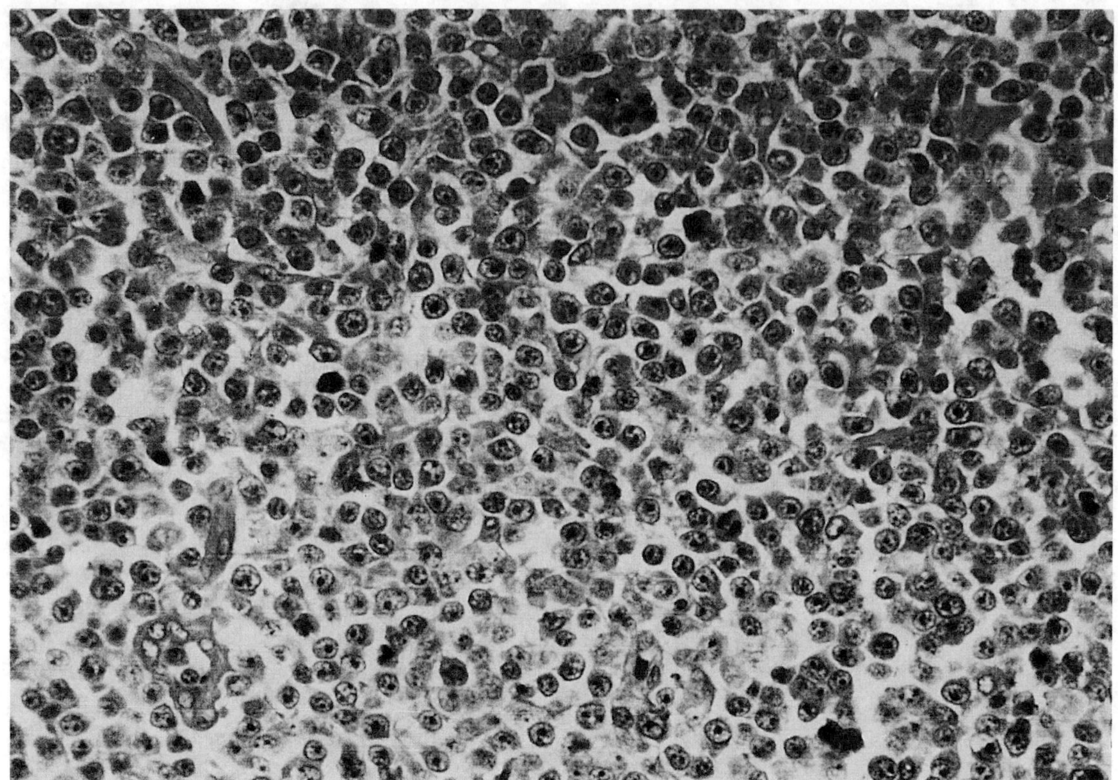

Figure 11-103A & B. Malignant lymphoma—diffuse large-cell immunoblastic type. The cells average more than 20 μ and have nucleoli varying from immunoblast to intermediate forms. Some cases may show homogenous population of large cells with plasma-cytoid features. Cytoplasm is strongly pyroninophilic. Mitosis is frequent. Small necrotic areas may be noted (photo A, above). In some cases, the degree of pleomorphism is quite marked, with multinucleation simulating Hodgkin's disease (mixed type) (photo B, opposite page). (H & E, X310)

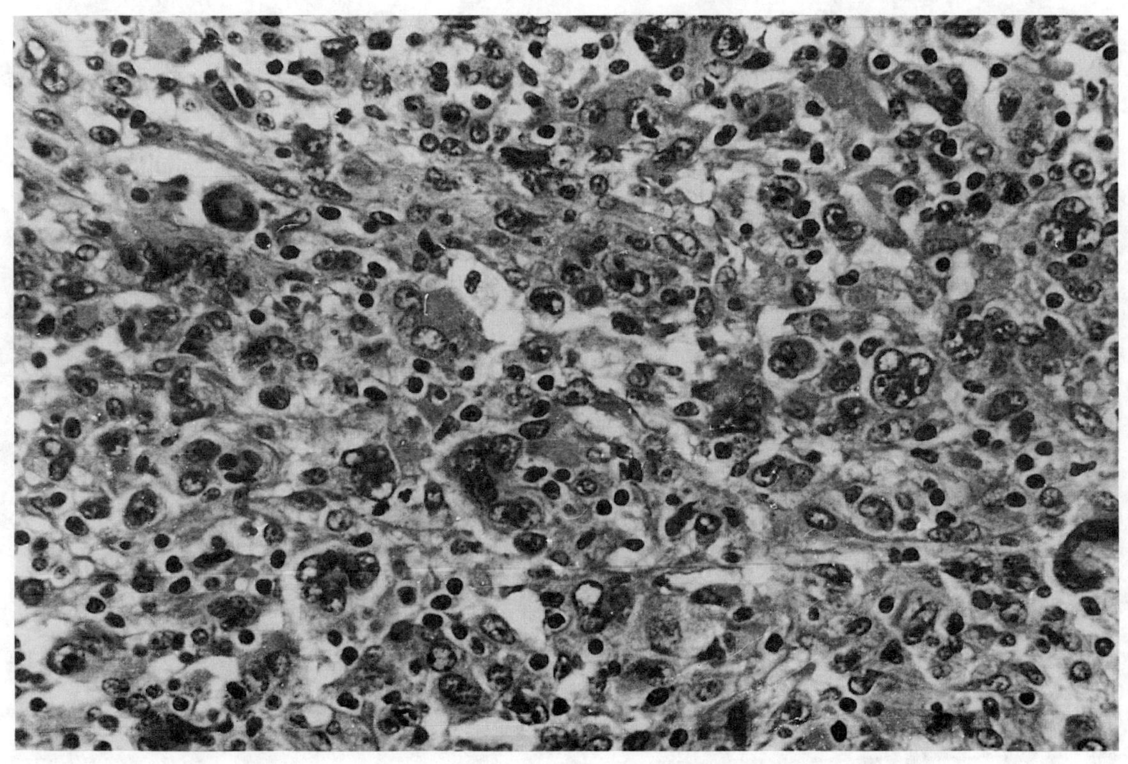

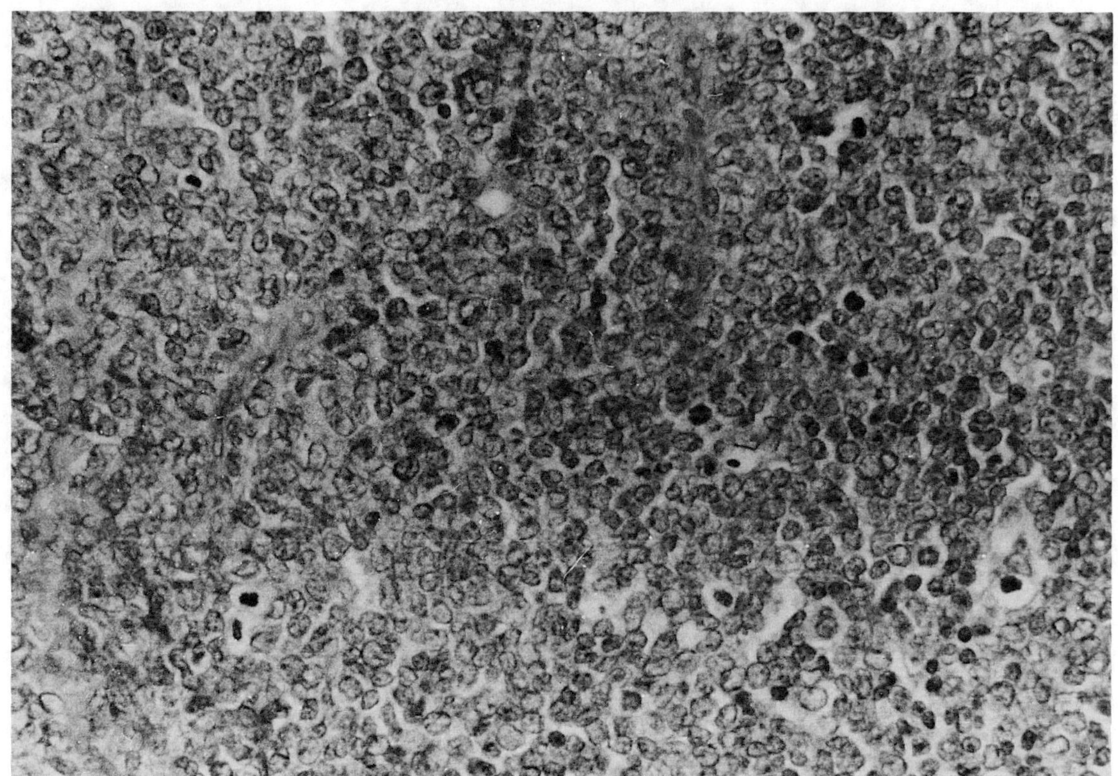

Figure 11-104. Malignant lymphoma, lymphoblastic type. Cells range between 10–15 μ with irregular nuclear contours often indented, giving a convoluted impression with fine chromatin and absent or small nucleoli; a small rim of cytoplasm is weakly pyroninophilic. Some cases may be composed of nonconvoluted cells positive for intranuclear TdT. When the bone marrow becomes involved, the lymphoma progresses to the leukemic phase, making this type indistinguishable from acute lymphoblastic leukemia. This type occurs commonly among adolescents and frequently involves the mediastinum and the CNS; it accounts for a third of all childhood lymphoma. Mitosis is frequent and "starry sky" pattern may occasionally be seen. (H & E, X310)

Figure 11-105. Malignant lymphoma, small noncleaved cell (Burkitt's). The cells
range between 15–20 μ. Nuclei are uniform, with a small rim of
cytoplasm that is deeply pyroninophilic. Nucleoli are distinct and multiple. Mitoses are numerous. A "starry sky" pattern is frequent. Both endemic and nonendemic forms of Burkitt's lymphoma often involve the
head and neck areas in younger patients, whereas in older children abdominal tumors are more frequent. In small noncleaved cell lymphoma
(non-Burkitt's), the cells are similar to Burkitt's lymphoma except that the
cell population is less uniform in nuclear sizes and shapes and multinucleation is also noted. This type occurs in an older age group, with a
mean average in the early 30s. (H & E, X310)

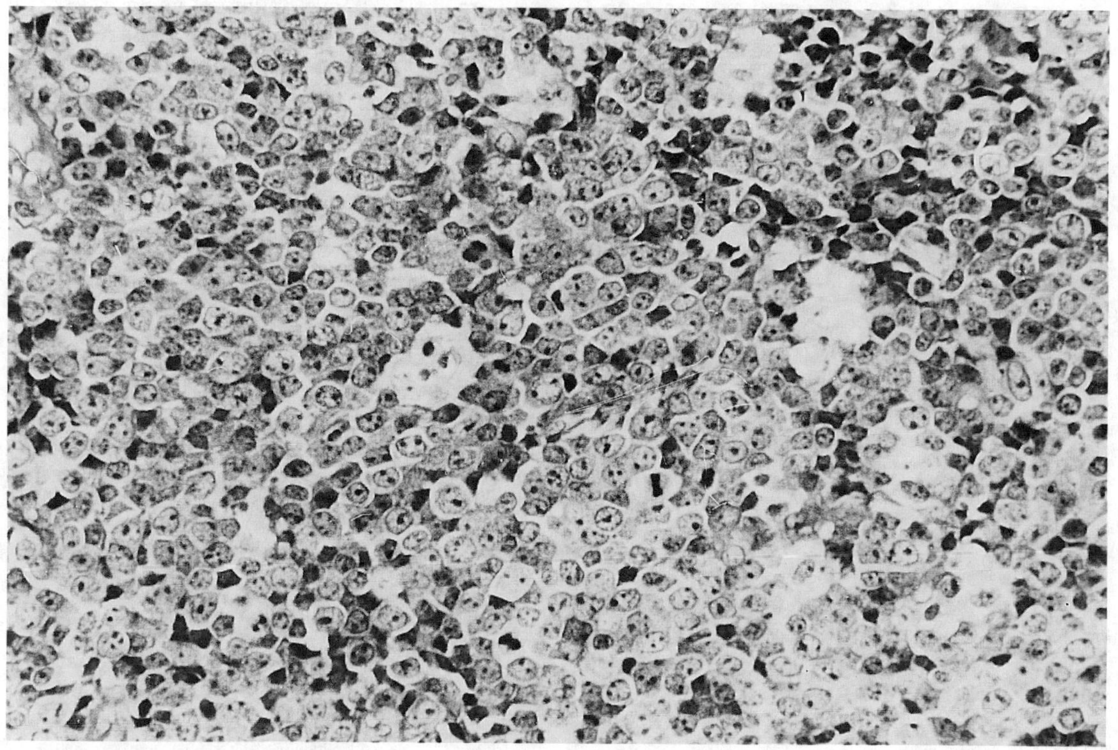

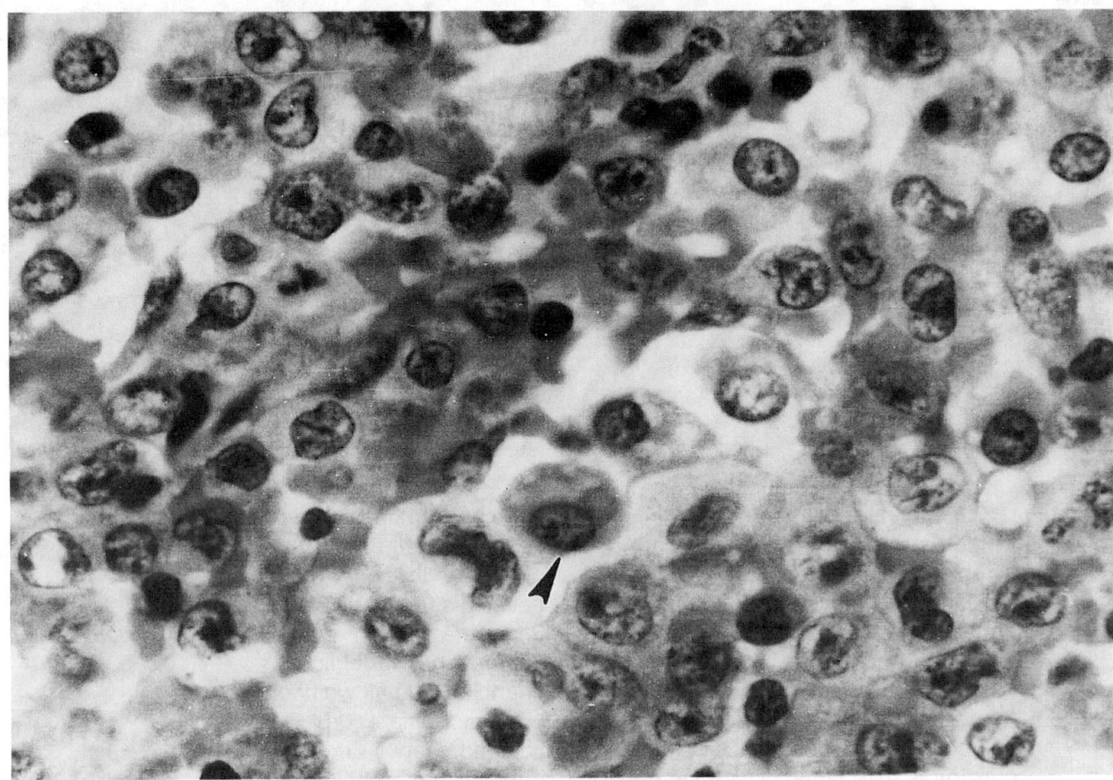

Figure 11-106. Malignant lymphoma, true histiocytic type. The cells are large, sometimes reaching 50 μ in diameter, and have abundant acidophilic cytoplasm with a large vesicular nucleus and prominent nucleoli. Erythrophagocytosis may be noted. Monoclonal antisera has been less helpful in true histiocytic lymphoma than with T or B cell markers. (H & E, X240)

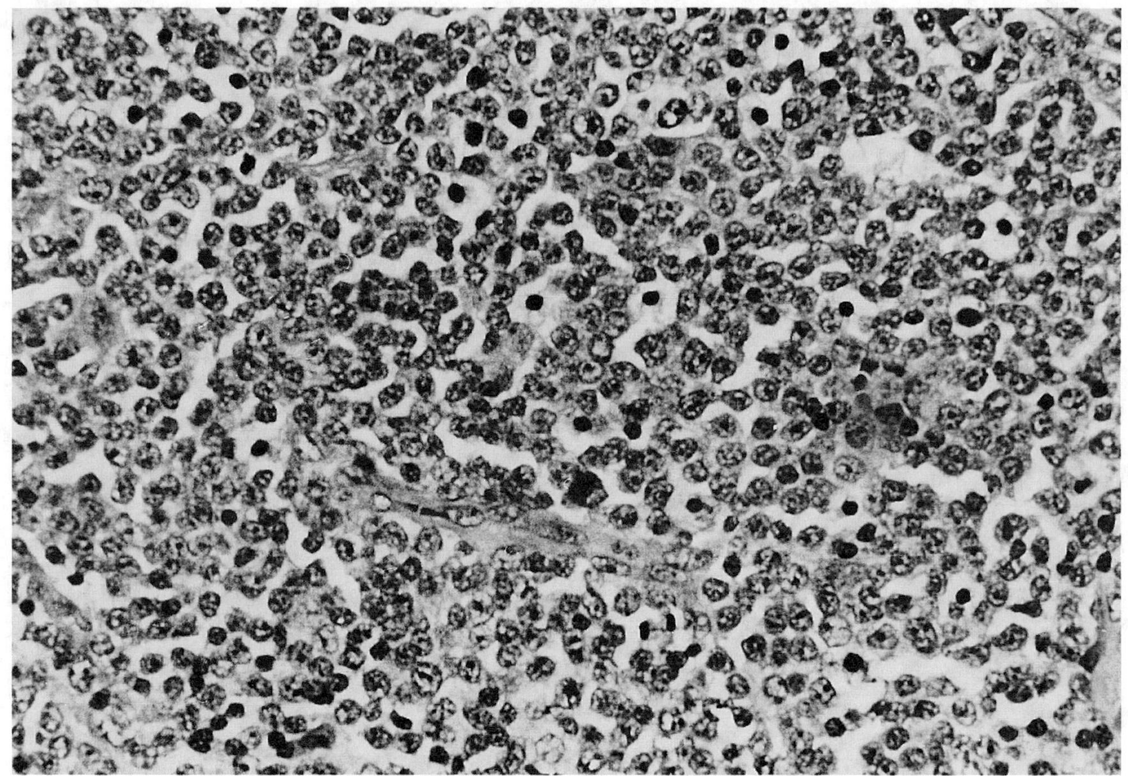

Figure 11-107A & B. Granulocytic sarcoma. The entire lymph node may be involved, and replacement by myeloblast may mimic non-Hodgkin's large-cell lymphoma (photo A, above). The presence of eosinophilic myelocyte is diagnostic for granulocytic sarcoma. Myeloperoxidase staining is helpful because it does not stain lymphocytes (photo B, opposite page). (H & E, 11-107A X310; PX, 11-107B X310)

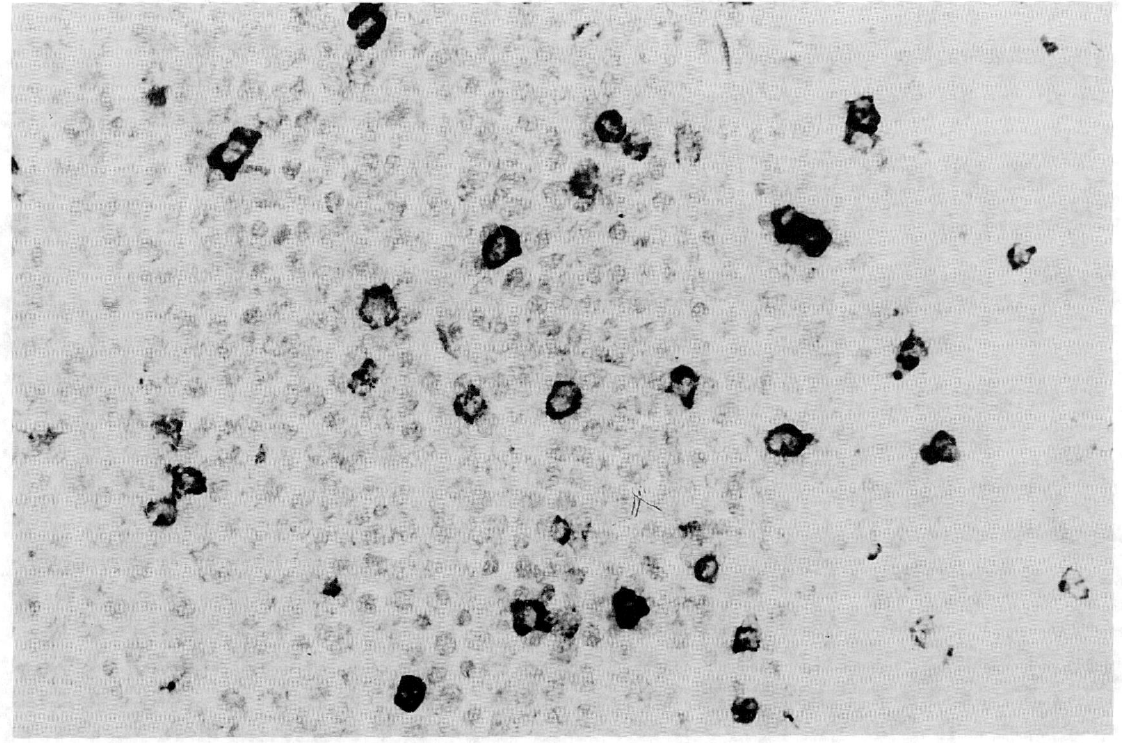

Figure 11-108. Hodgkin's disease, lymphocytic predominance type. It is characterized by predominance of mature lymphocytes admixed with some histiocytes, rare Reed-Sternberg cells, and convoluted large cells. Due to a predominance of small lymphocytes and effacement of normal lymph node architecture, this tumor must be differentiated from well-differentiated lymphocytic lymphoma and infectious mononucleosis. (H & E, X125)

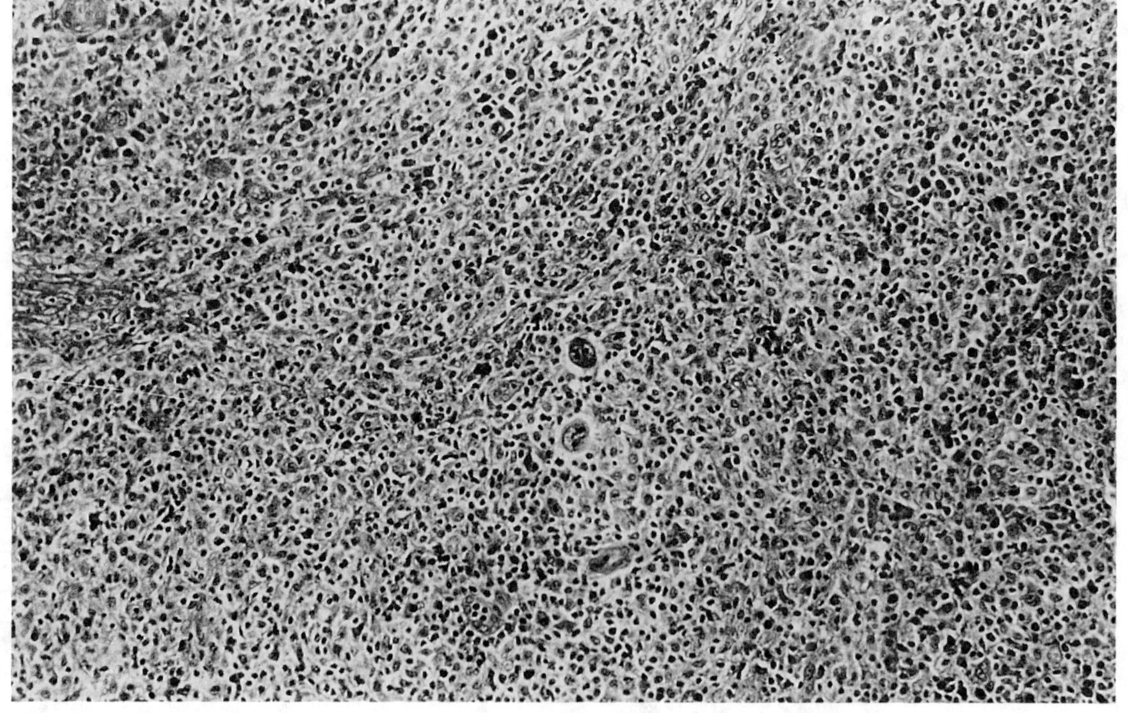

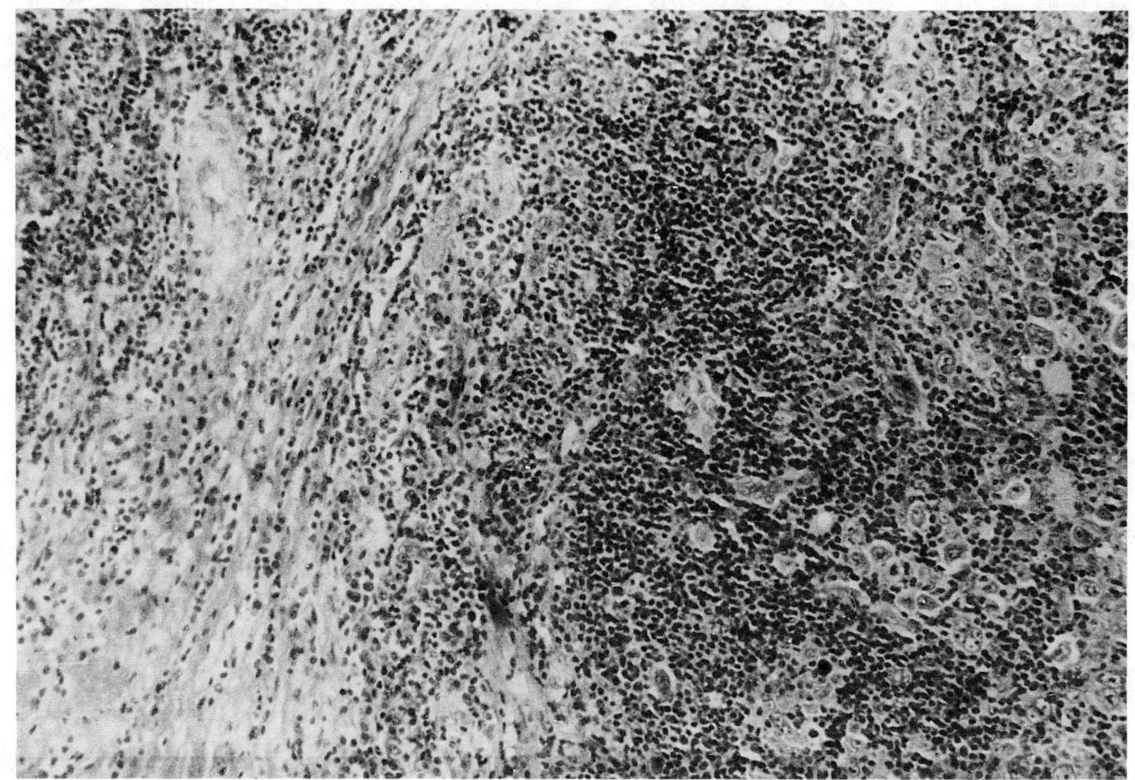

Figure 11-109A,B,C. Hodgkin's disease, nodular sclerosis type. This lesion is characterized by collagen bands forming incomplete nodules (photo A, above), lacunar cells (photo B, opposite page, top), and the presence of diagnostic Reed-Sternberg cells (photo C, opposite page, bottom). (H & E, 11-109A X125; 11-109B & C X310)

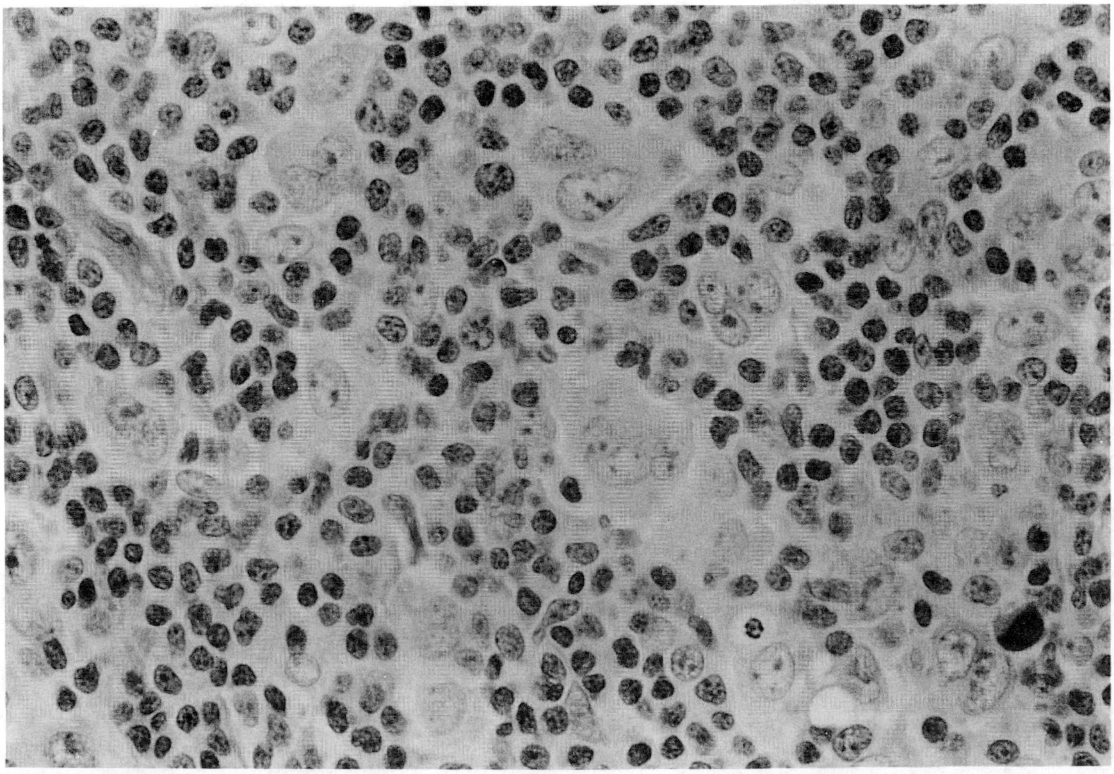

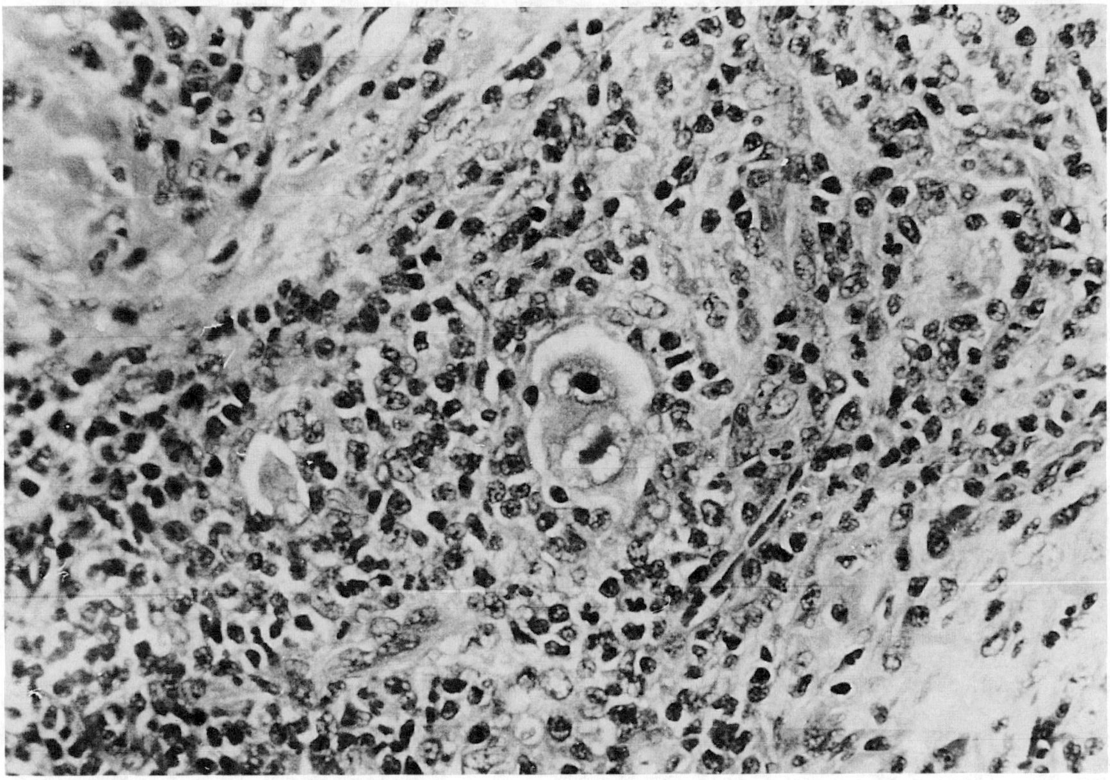

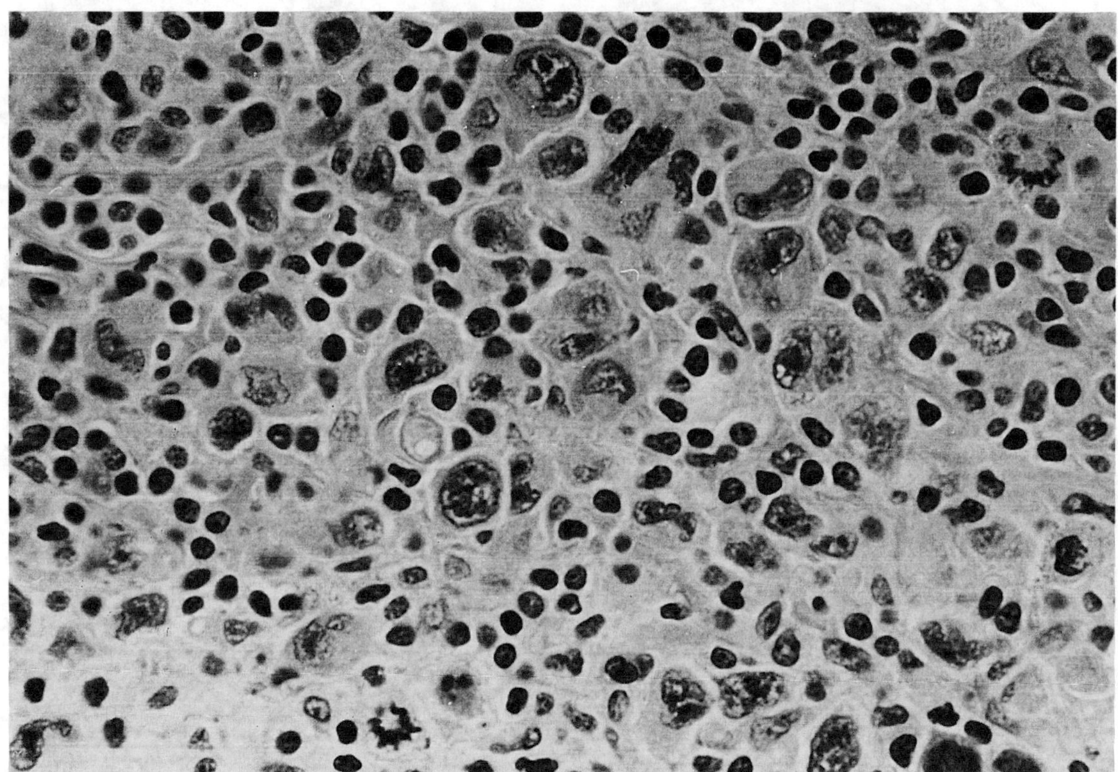

Figure 11-110. Hodgkin's disease, mixed cellularity (MC). Reed-Sternberg cells are numerous besides the usual milieu of Hodgkin's disease represented by lymphocytes, histocytes, plasma cells, eosinophils, and a few atypical angular lymphocytes. It has been suggested that a more strict quantitative criterion for MC would require at least 5–15 Reed-Sternberg cells and mononuclear Hodgkin's cells per high-power field and anything less than 5 per high-power field should be categorized as lymphocyte predominance (LP) Hodgkin's disease. More than 15 Reed-Sternberg cells and mononuclear Hodgkin's cells would be lymphocyte depleted (LD). Differential diagnosis for MC would include the diffuse non-Hodgkin's lymphoma with mixed T cells displaying predominant angular lymphocytes of various sizes admixed with large pleomorphic cells and epithelioid histiocytes. Plasma cells and eosinophils may also be seen. (H & E, X500)

Figure 11-111. Hodgkin's disease, lymphocyte depleted reticular type. It is composed of abundant Reed-Sternberg cells, sometimes bizarre (sarcomatous-like variants of RS cells), admixed with fibroblastic proliferation. (H & E, X200)

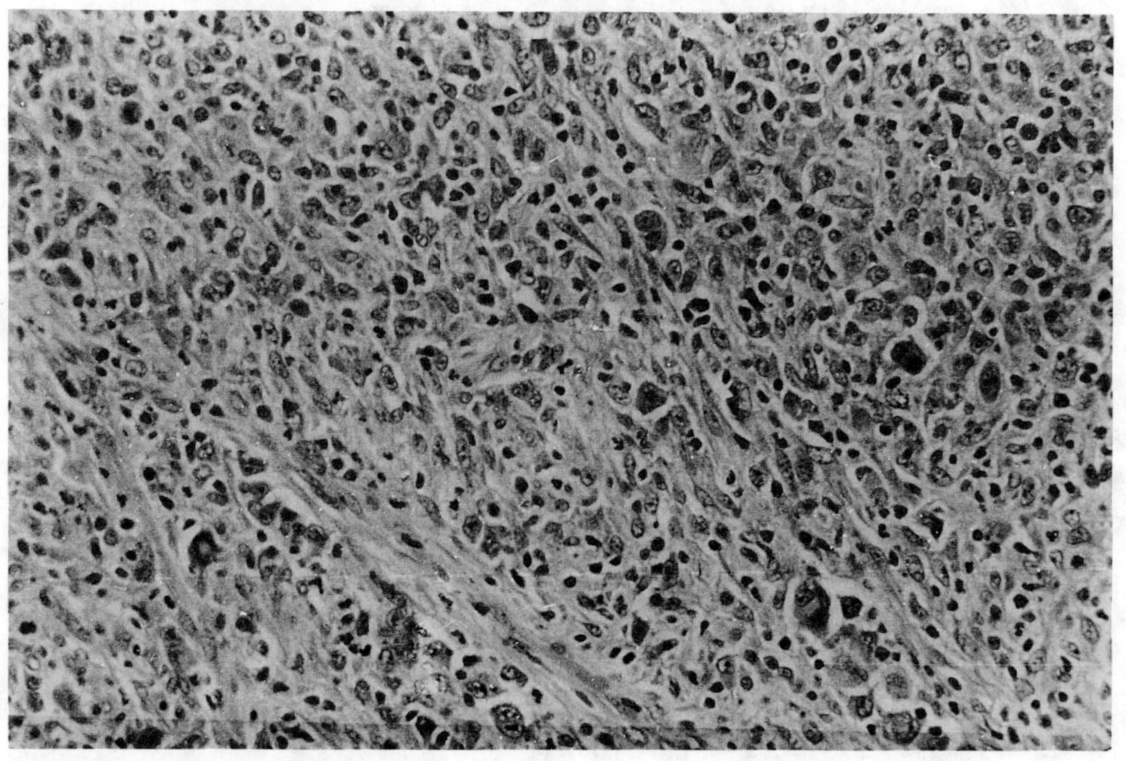

Figure 11-112. Hodgkin's disease, lymphocyte depleted diffuse fibrotic type. It shows extensive fibrosis with variable numbers of RS cells. For both entities, a pleomorphic large-cell lymphoma has to be ruled out. The nuclei of the mononuclear cells are more atypical and are irregular. There is also a display of large and small cells. Distinguishing Hodgkin's disease from T cell non-Hodgkin's lymphoma may require cell marker studies. In general, RS cells do not stain with LCA but often are positive with Leu MI (antigranulocytic marker). (H & E, X200)

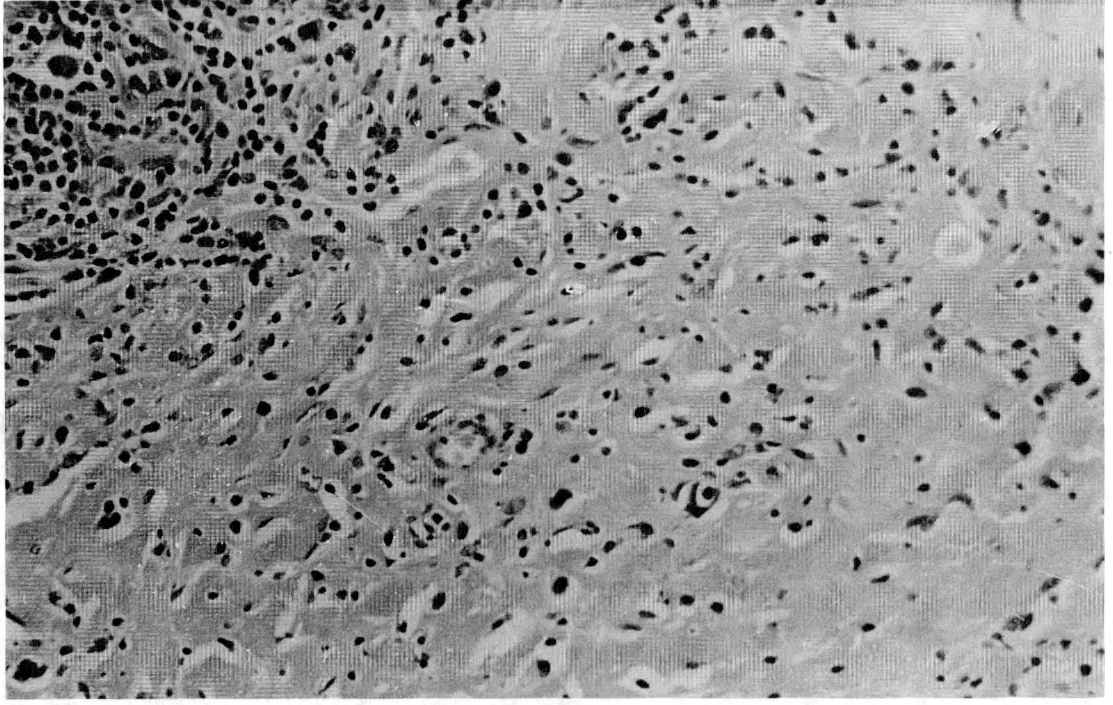

Hematopoietic Malignancies

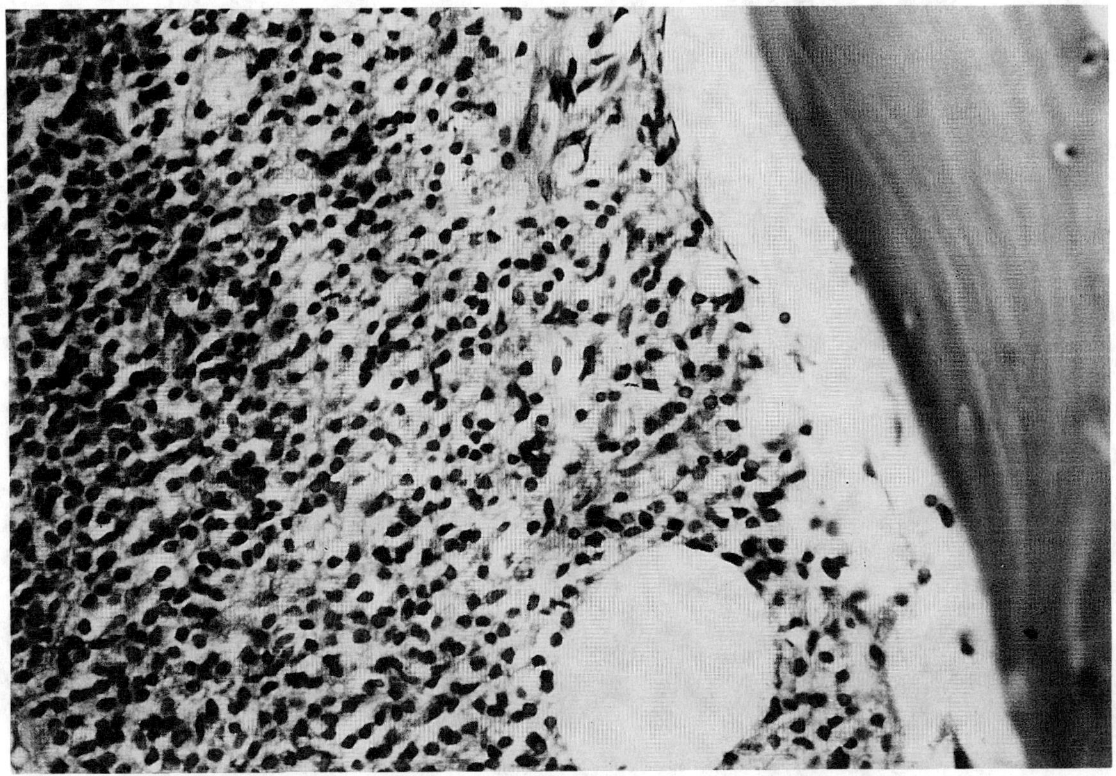

Figure 11-113. Hairy cell leukemia (bone marrow biopsy). The marrow is focally
    or diffusely hypercellular due to mononuclear cells. The cells are ovoid
    to slightly indented, with clear to pale cytoplasm. Nuclear chromatin is
    finely granular with inconspicuous nucleoli. Mitosis is rare. (H & E, X780)

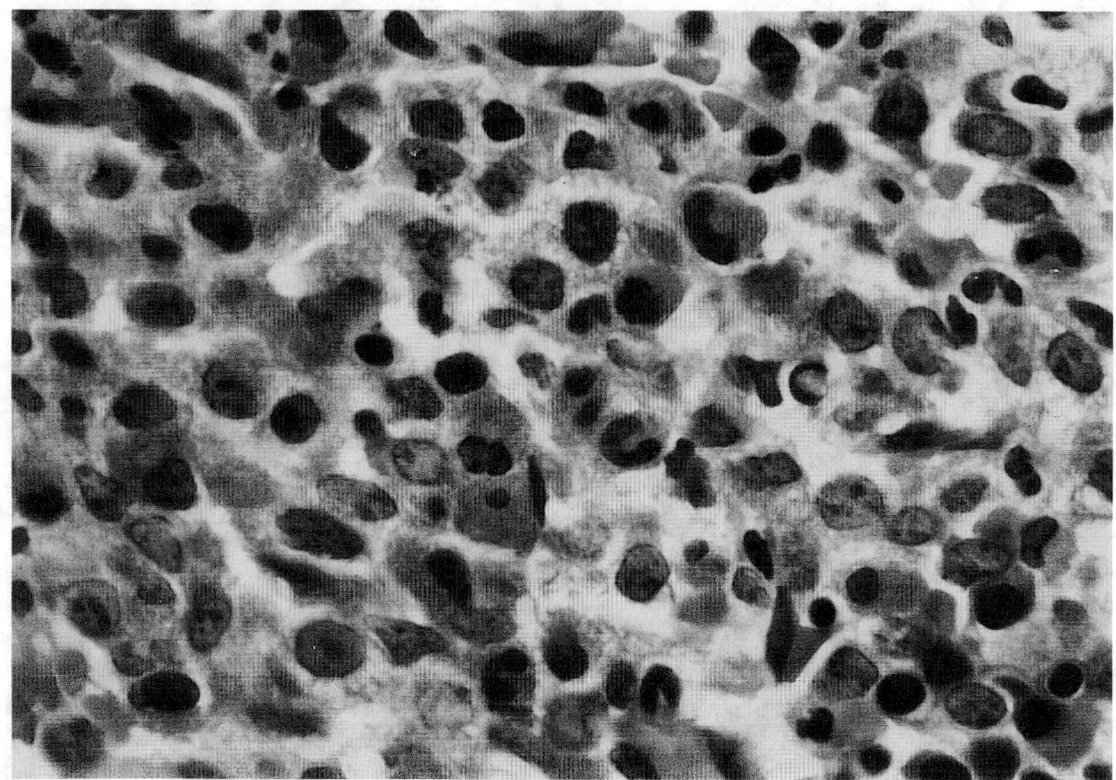

Figure 11-114. Chronic myelogenous leukemia (bone marrow biopsy). The marrow is hypercellular, packed with hematopoietic cells. Myelocytes tend to be paratrabecular, and the segmenters are scattered in the middle. Myeloblasts usually do not exceed 5% of the granulocytic population. Erythroid series is normal. Megakaryocytes may be increased in 20% of cases. A few macrophages simulating Gaucher cells may also be seen. (H & E, 78)

Figure 11-115. Acute myeloblastic leukemia (bone marrow biopsy). The marrow
   displays homogenous and dense cell population. The cells have round-
   to-ovoid nuclei with conspicuous nucleoli, while others have indented or
   folded nuclei and inconspicuous nucleoli. There is a moderate amount of
   granular cytoplasm. Nuclear chromatin is coarse. In contrast, the lymphoblast has an irregular to indented nucleus with finely dispersed chromatin. Nucleoli are absent or very small. Cytoplasm is hardly visible. For
   acute leukemia, there should be a minimum 30% of blast cells (French-
   American-British classification). (H & E, X780)

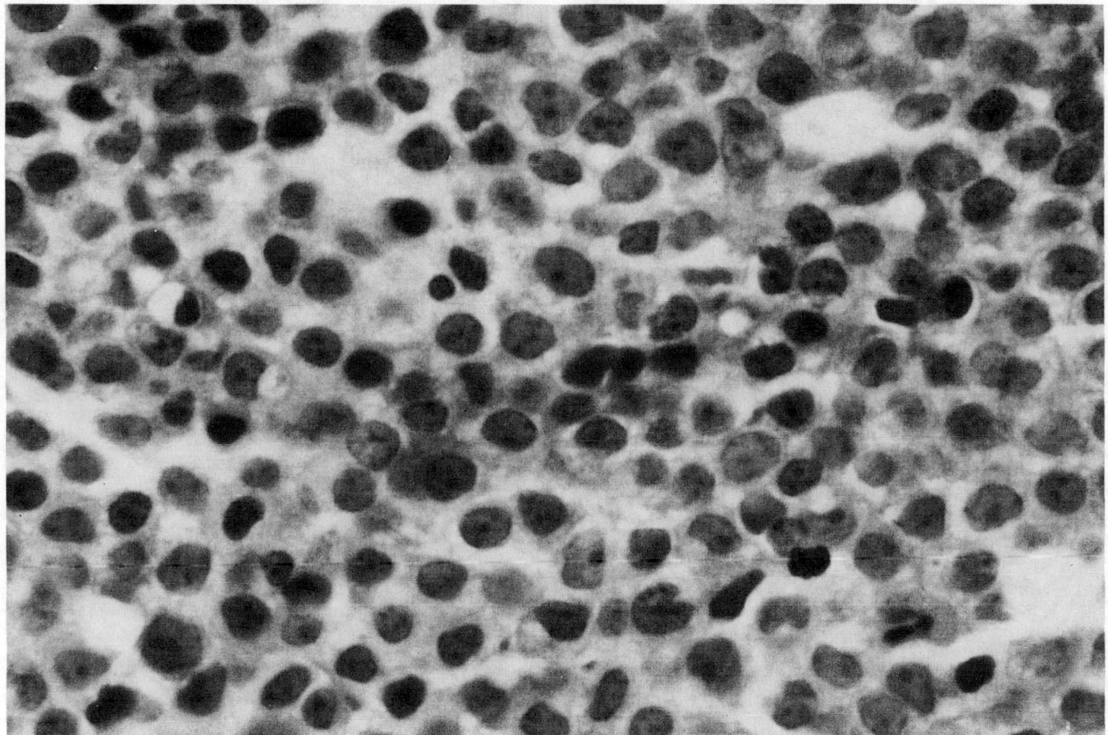

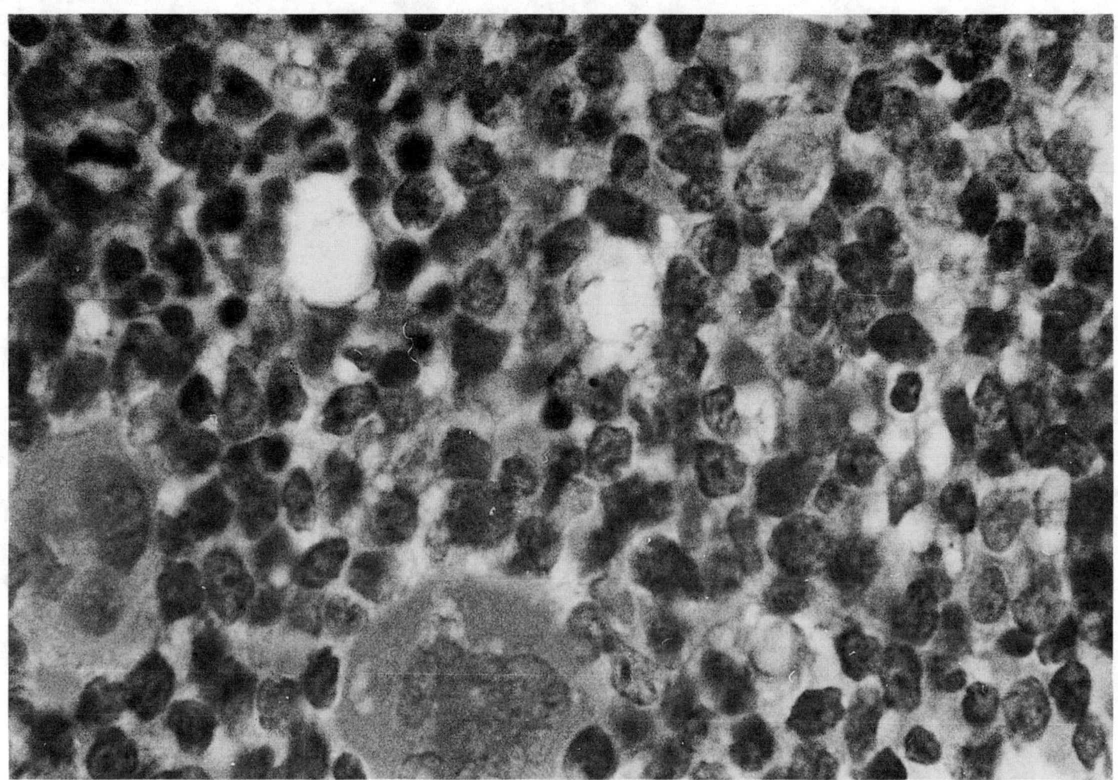

Figure 11-116. Acute lymphoblastic leukemia (bone marrow biopsy). The cells almost invariably replace all marrow elements; they range from uniformly round nucleus, distinct nuclear membrane with no visible nucleoli (L-1 type, French-American-British classification) to pleomorphic cells with indented to convoluted nuclei and inconspicuous nucleoli (L-2 type, FAB classification). The third group of lymphoblasts has a uniformly round nucleus with conspicuous nucleoli and visible amphophilic cytoplasm. (H & E, X780)

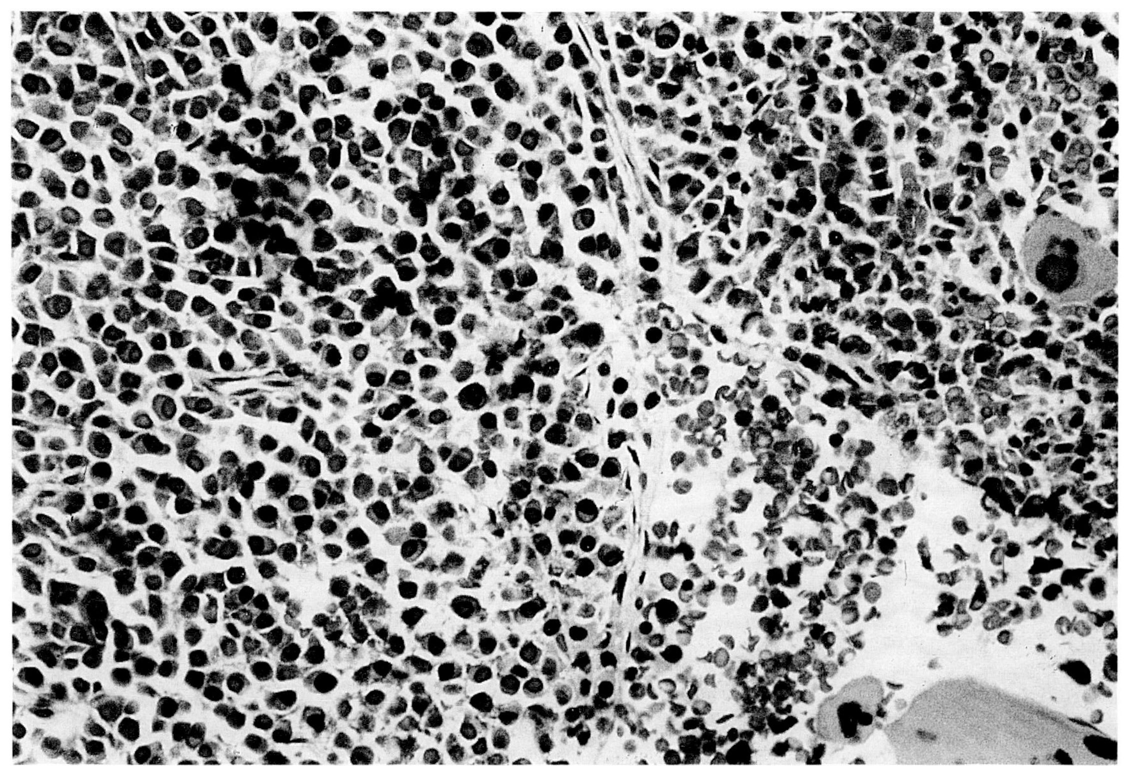

Figure 11-117. Multiple myeloma (bone marrow biopsy). The cells may be in clusters or (rarely) in sheets composed of readily recognizable plasma cells showing eccentric nucleus, with amphophilic cytoplasm and paranuclear clearing. The nuclear chromatin is coarse and peripherally dispersed to the nuclear membrane. Nucleoli are surrounded by coarse chromatin. The plasma cells are usually seen in various stages of maturation. Reactive plasmacytosis is most difficult to eliminate as a differential diagnosis. Russell bodies and Dutcher bodies are seen in both conditions, therefore are not helpful. Phenotypic staining with either lambda or kappa antisera would favor monoclonality of the cells supporting neoplasia. (H & E, X310)

Figure 11-118. Acute lymphocytic leukemia (bone marrow aspiration) (subtype L-1, French-American-British classification). The abnormal cells replace all marrow elements; they are relatively uniform in size, have a round nucleus and no visible nucleoli or just 1 nucleolous. This type is common in childhood ALL. (J-G, X100)

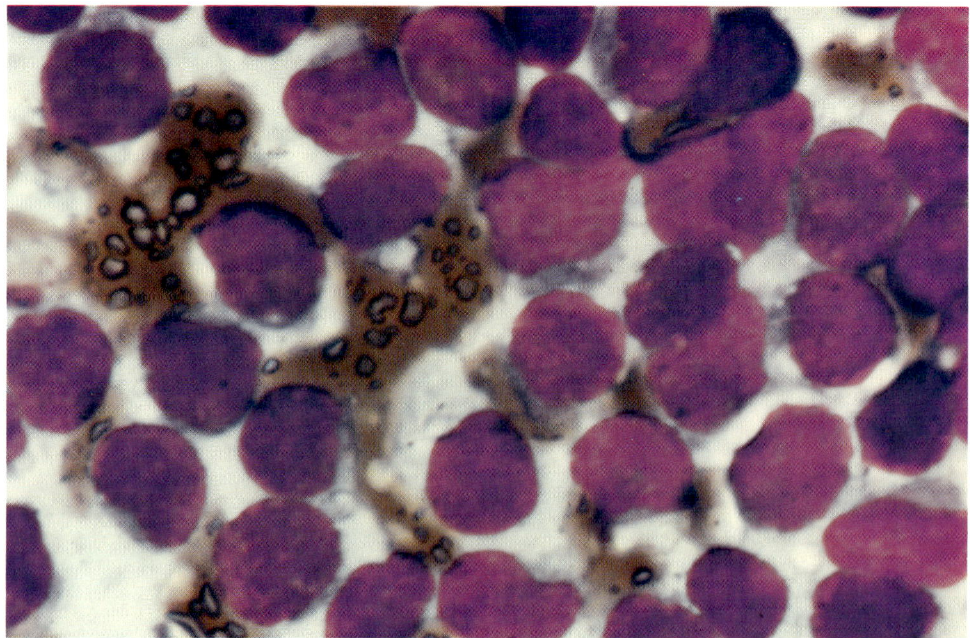

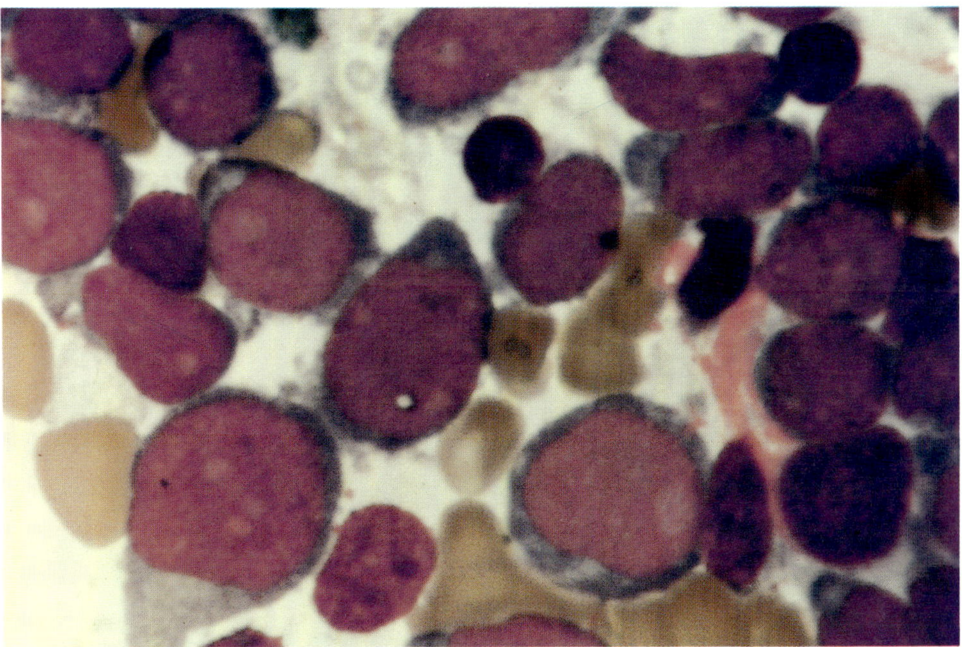

Figure 11-119. Acute lymphocytic leukemia (bone marrow aspiration) (subtype
L-2, French-American-British classification). The leukemic cells are pleomorphic, with a mixture of large and small cells; they all have at least 1
and a maximum 3 well-defined nucleoli. This type is common in adult
ALL. (J-G, X100)

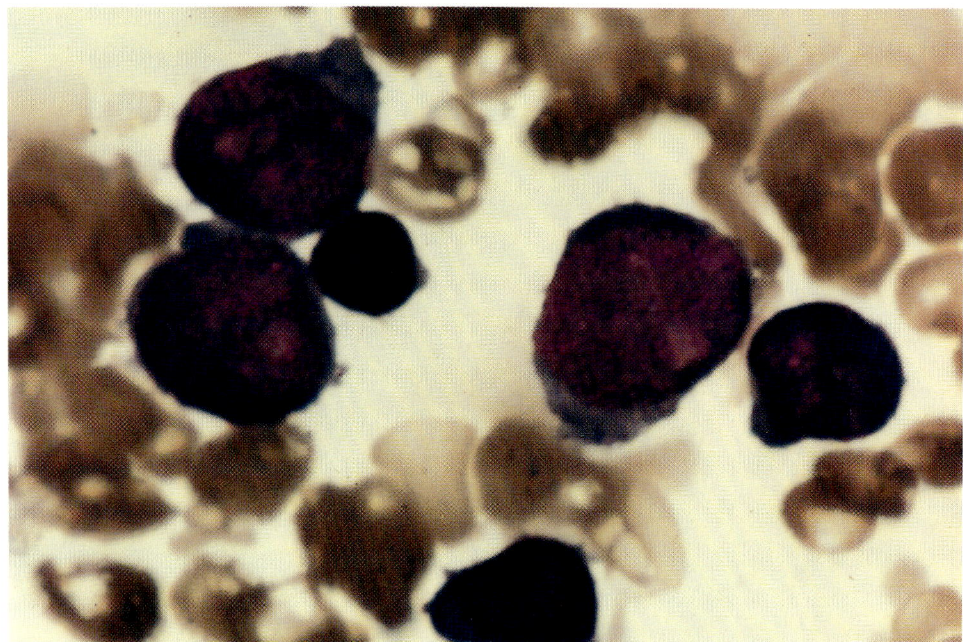

Figure 11-120. Acute lymphocytic leukemia (peripheral blood) (subtype L-2, French-American-British classification) with T cells ("T cell ALL"). Characteristically, the nucleus of the lymphoblasts is frequently indented or can be convoluted or cerebriform, with a folded chromatin mimicking the cerebral convolutions. (J-G, X100)

Figure 11-121. Acute lymphocytic leukemia (peripheral blood) (subtype L-3). The leukemic cells are generally uniform in size and have a nucleus with somewhat more clumped chromatin; nucleoli are frequently absent. Instead, numerous vacuoles are present in the cytoplasm as well as in the nucleus. (J-G, X100)

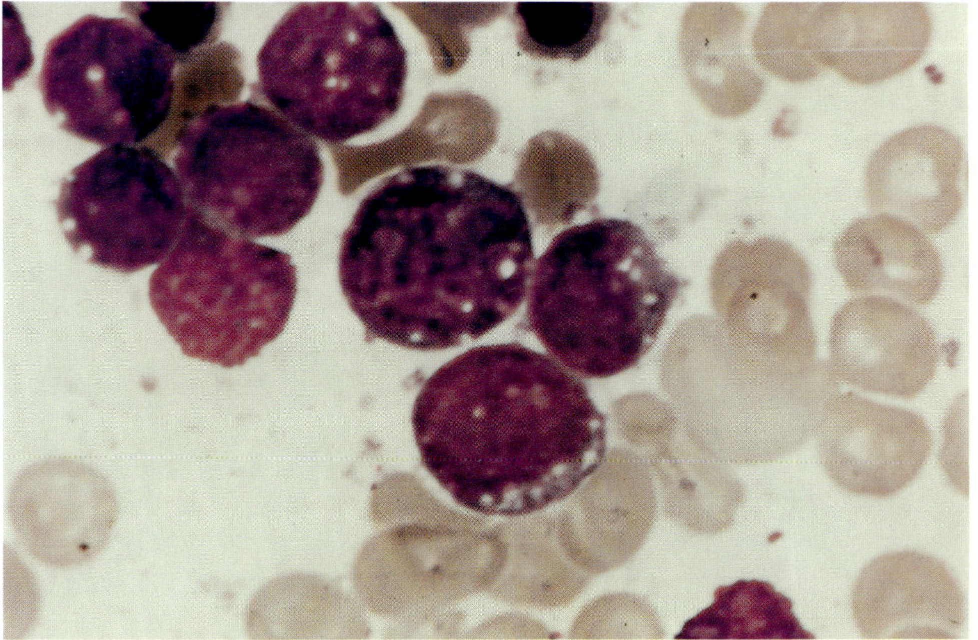

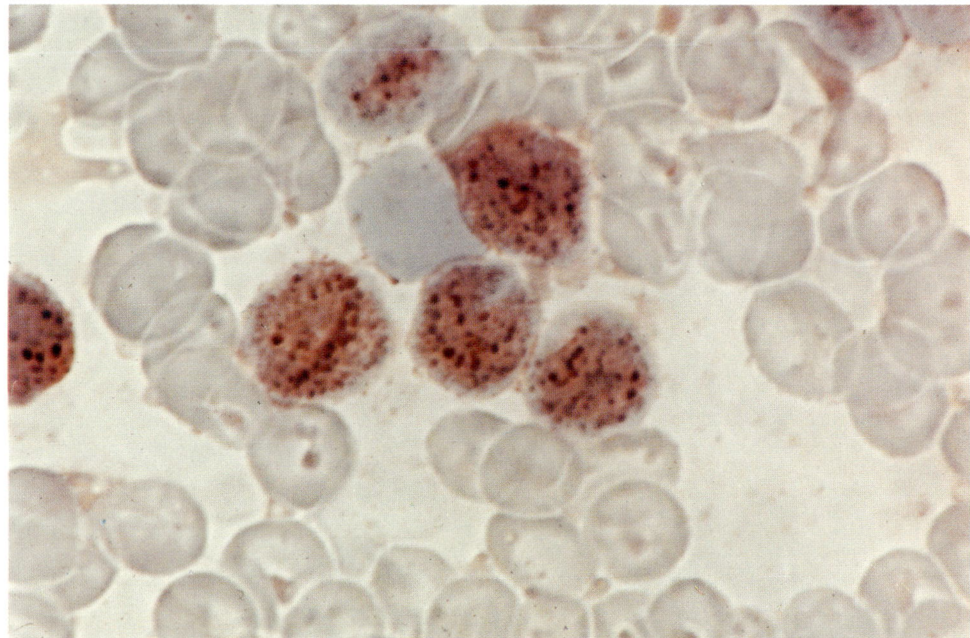

Figure 11-122. Acute lymphocytic leukemia (bone marrow aspiration) (subtype L-2). This enzyme is present in leukemic cells with T antigens as well as in the CALLA (common acute lymphocytic leukemia antigen)-positive leukemic cells encountered in the childhood and adult ALL (L-1 and L-2 subtypes). The nucleus of these cells stains generally diffusely. (TdT, X100)

Figure 11-123. Acute myelogenous leukemia, Auer rod (peripheral blood). A leukemic cell characteristic for many of the AML subtypes is presented; it is large ($<$40 μ in diameter) and has a large polygonal nucleus, many times eccentrically located. A clearly distinct rod (Auer rod) can be seen in its cytoplasm; this is present in $<$25% of cases of myelocytic and myelomonocytic leukemia.
(J-G, X100)

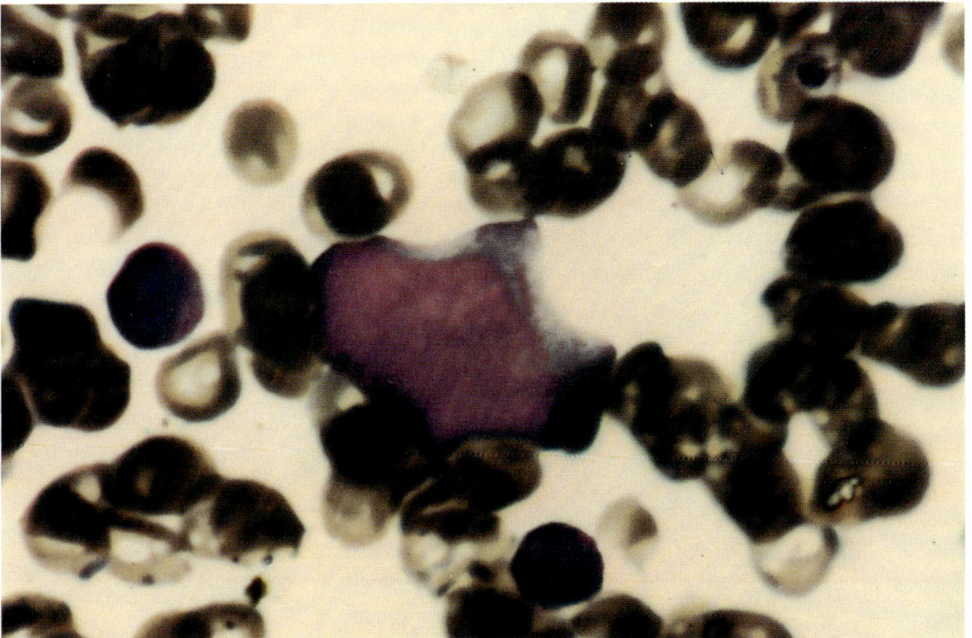

Figure 11-124. Acute myelogenous leukemia, Auer rod (peripheral blood). In this smear, 2 characteristic leukemic blast cells stained with SBB are contrasted with a normal myelocyte; the secondary granules stained by SBB are less well represented in the leukemic cells than in the normal myelocyte. An Auer rod present in the lateral blast is well stained by SBB; several nucleoli present in the blastic cells are readily visible; a giant platelet can be seen close to the white cell in the middle. (SBB, X100)

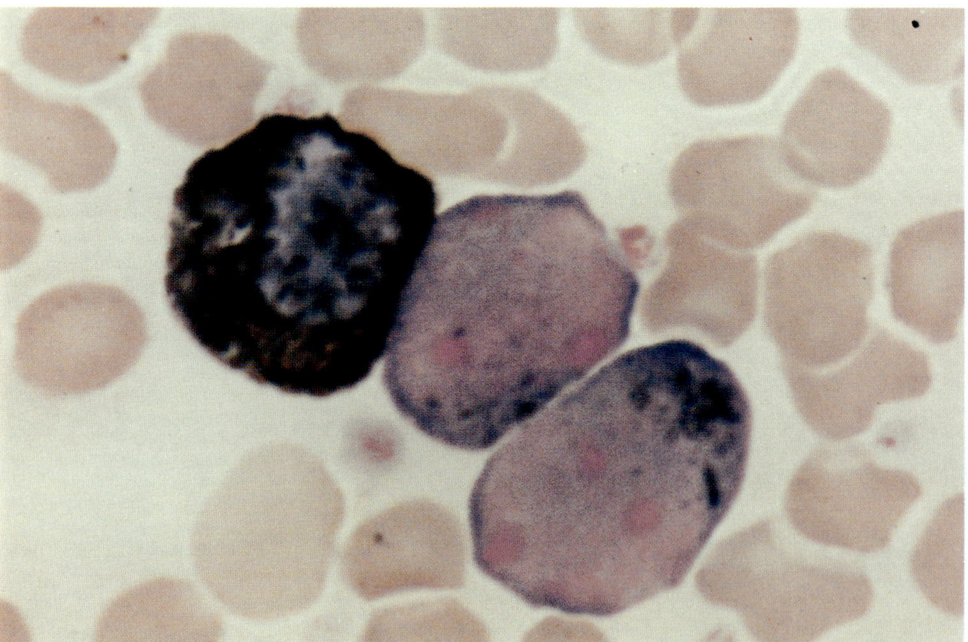

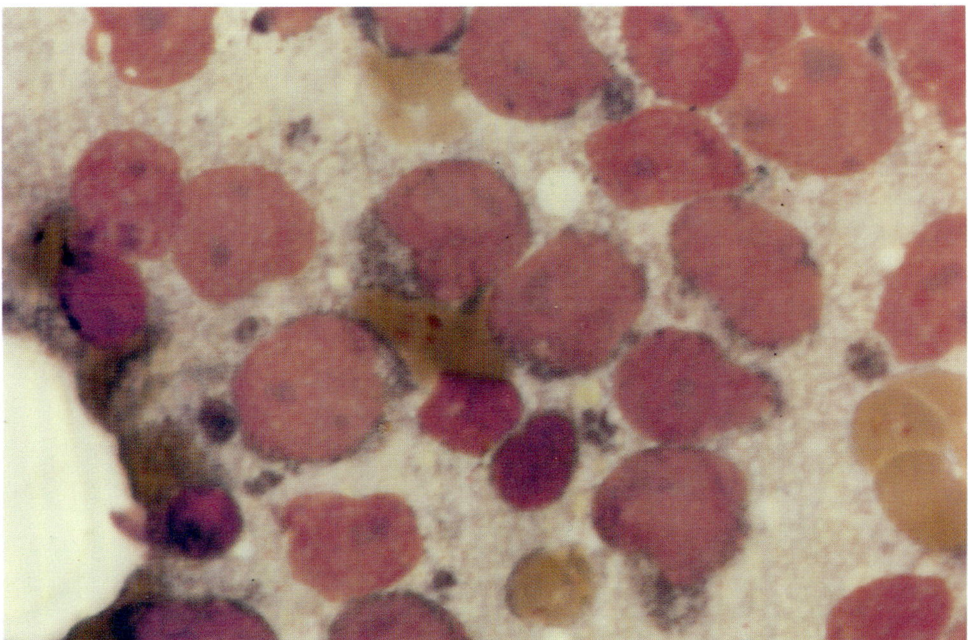

Figure 11-125. Acute myelogenous leukemia (AML) (bone marrow aspiration) (French-American-British classification). The marrow displays in this type a relatively homogenous and dense cell population, with large polygonal-shaped nuclei whose chromatin is uniformly dispersed. Several nucleoli are recognizable in each nucleus; they are uniquely stained with a bluish discoloration darker than the surrounding chromatin. Similarly to nucleoli in normal histiocytes, these leukemic cells are the most undifferentiated cells among AML cells and are difficult to differentiate from ALL cells without histochemical stains. (J-G, X100)

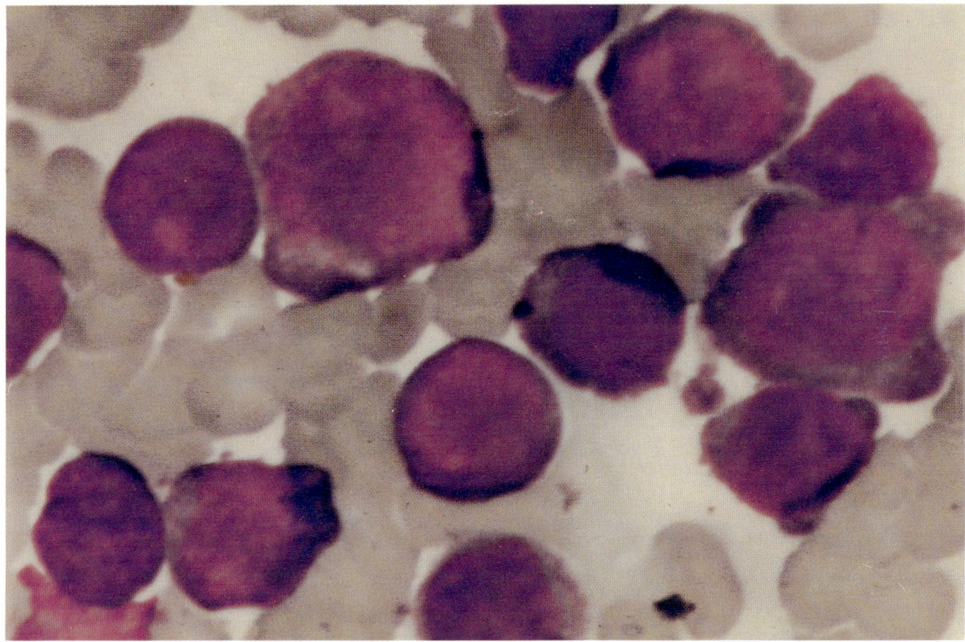

Figure 11-126. Acute myelogenous leukemia (peripheral blood) (subtype M-1, FAB classification). The leukemic cells are pleomorphic; regular-size blasts with a relatively round-shaped nuclei alternate with huge cells with polygonal-shaped nuclei, uniformly dispersed chromatin, and several large less well-stained nucleoli. (J-G, X100)

Figure 11-127. Acute myelogenous leukemia (bone marrow aspiration) (subtype M-1). As in figure 11-126, the cells are pleomorphic; large cells with polygonal nuclei alternate with normal-size cells with round nuclei. The nucleoli are less visible than on the peripheral blood smears. (J-G, X100)

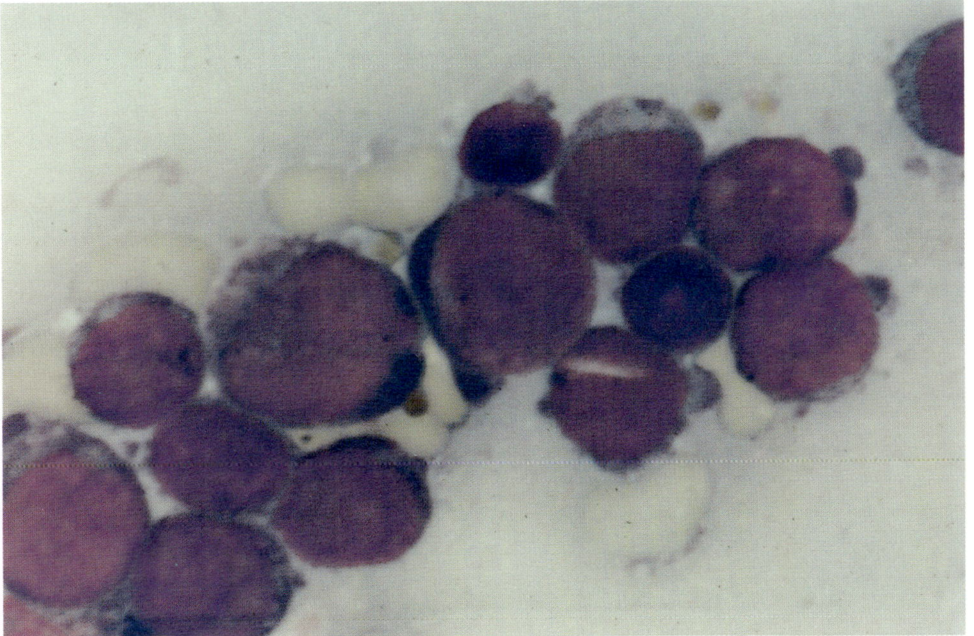

Figure 11-128. Acute myelogenous leukemia (bone marrow aspiration) (subtype M-3). The large leukemic cells usually have an eccentric nucleus with 1 or 2 nucleoli; their cytoplasm is greatly occupied by relatively large granules staining in orange with the J-G stain; these granules are releasing thromboplastin-like substances, which may trigger a disseminated intravascular coagulation process. (J-G, X100)

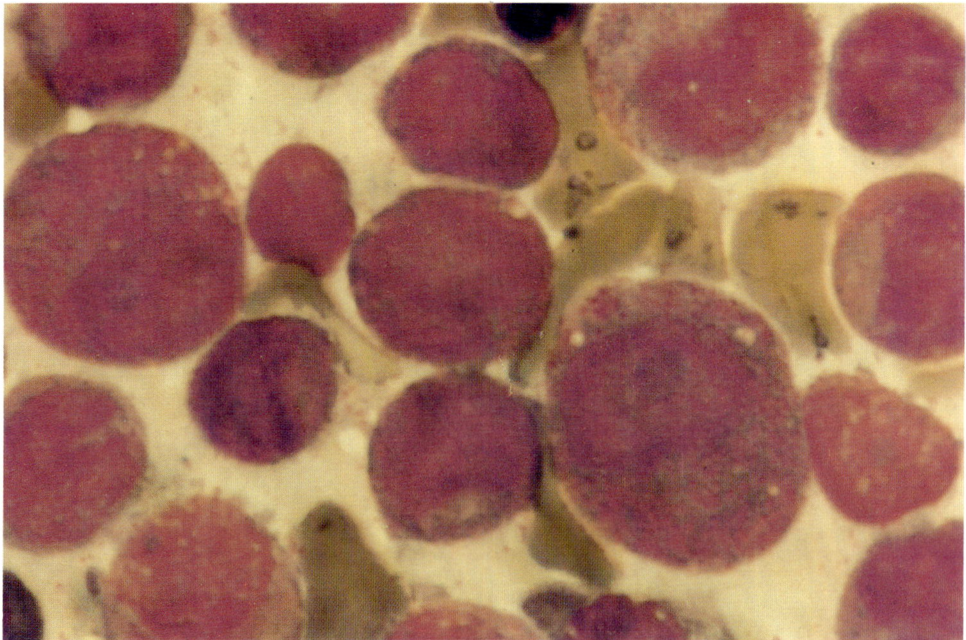

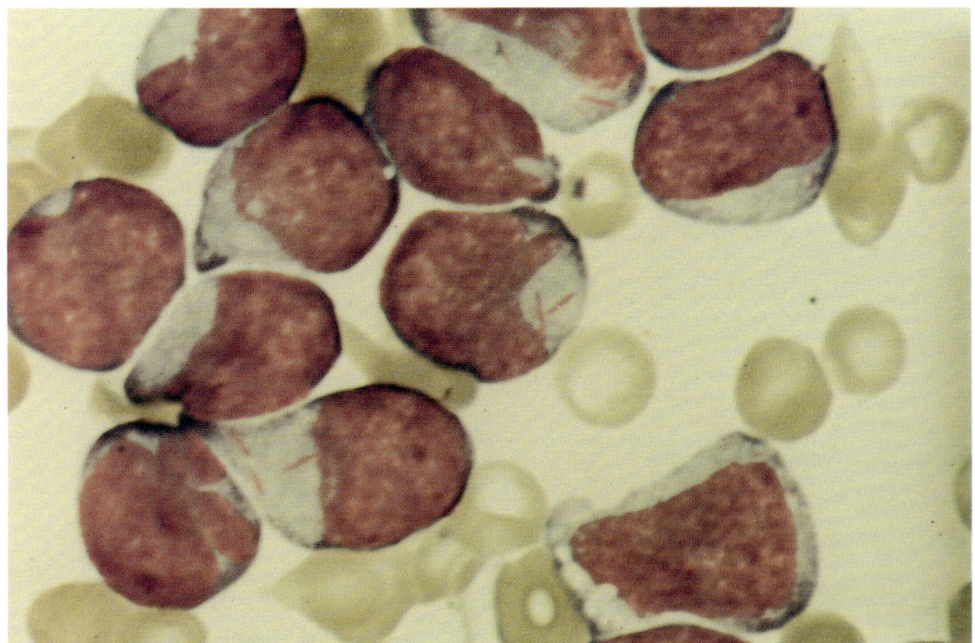

Figure 11-129. Myelomonogytic (peripheral blood) (AML subtype M-4). Large leukemic cells with horseshoe-like nuclei (monocyte lineage) alternate with leukemic cells with round or polygonal-shaped nuclei (granulocytic lineage). All nuclei have a relatively clumped chromatin seen also in patients with AML subtype M-2 not depicted in this chapter. Several cells contain Auer rods; they are present in the cells of the monocytic as well as granulocytic lineage. (J-G, X100)

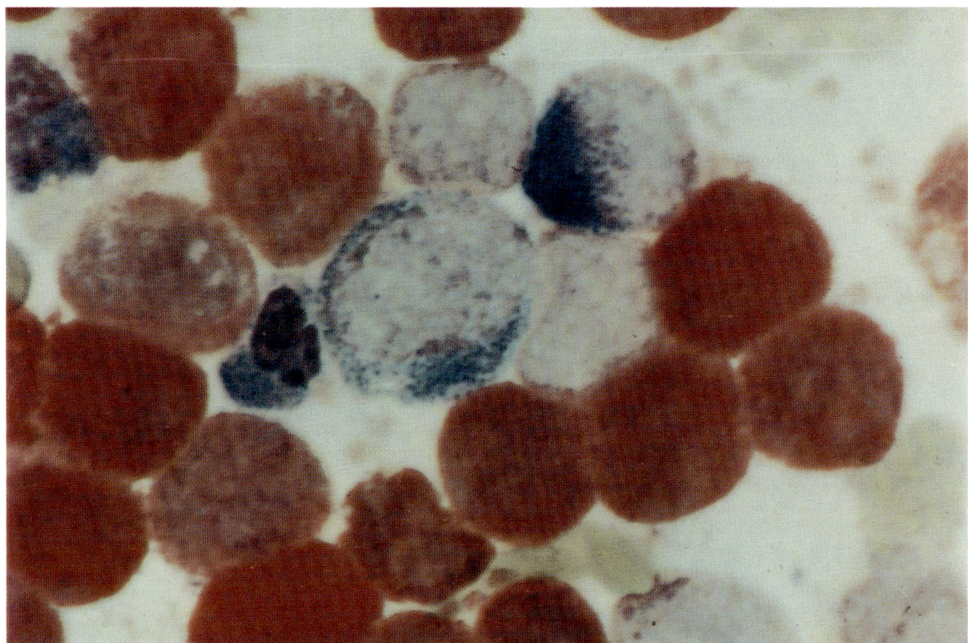

Figure 11-130. Myelomonocytic (bone marrow aspiration) (AML subtype M-4). The monocytic leukemic cells are stained with the combined esterase stain, which helps distinguish the 4 leukemic cells of the monocytic lineage from the middle of the cell aggregate from the surrounding myelocytic blasts and granulocytes whose cytoplasmic granules are vividly stained in red-brown. The monocytic series blast staining is inhibited by the sodium fluoride added to the acetate esterase in the combined esterase stain. (CE, X100)

Figure 11-131. Pure monocytic (peripheral blood) (AML subtype M-5). All leuke-
    mic cells are large and have irregularly shaped nuclei with clumped
    chromatin. The nuclei are cleaved or folded; these cells should be differ-
    entiated from acute lymphocytic leukemia T blasts, which occasionally
    can present similar folding but are usually smaller. (J-G, X100)

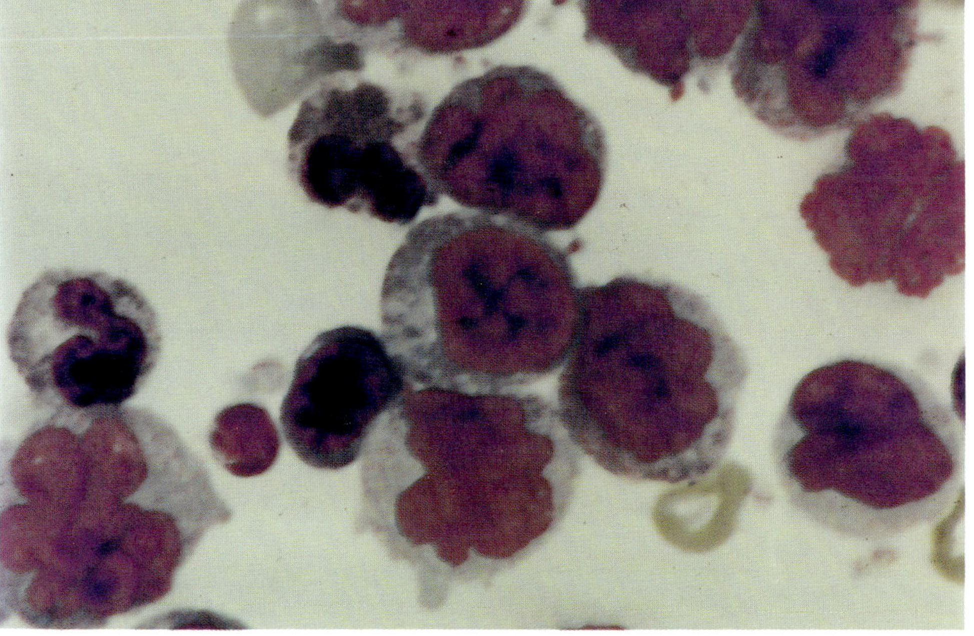

Figure 11-132. Erythroleukemia (Di Guglielmo's disease) (AML subtype M-6).
(bone marrow aspiration). Two giant erythroid precursors with double nuclei, intensely stained cytoplasm, and dispersely granular chromatin in
their nuclei similar to that of megaloblasts in the bone marrow of mega-
loblastic anemia cases. These cells accompany myeloblasts similar to
those present in AML subtype M-2. (J-G, X100)

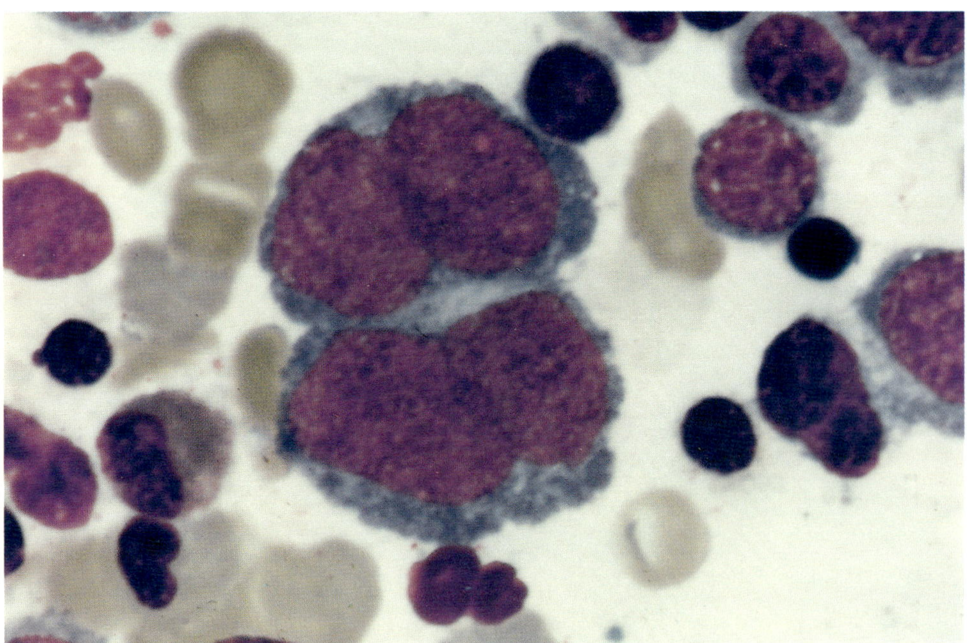

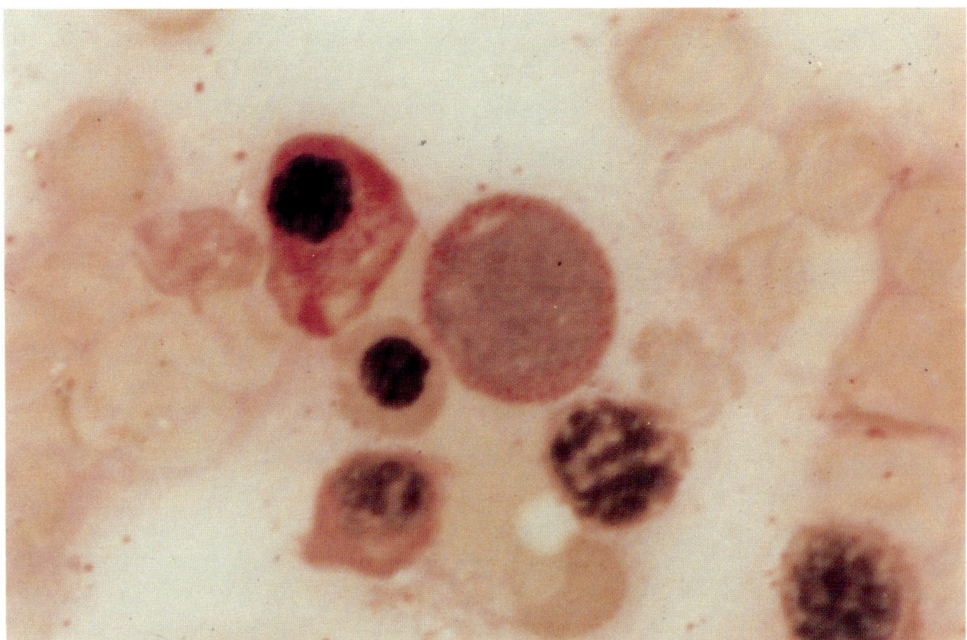

Figure 11-133. Erythroleukemia (AML subtype M-6) (bone marrow aspiration). On this slide, a red cell precursor at the level of basophilic normoblast at the top of the cell aggregate is seen with its cytoplasm intensely stained in red due to the reaction of the stain with glycogen. Although this stain is positive in most of the leukocyte lineages, it is negative among red cell precursors with the exception of those present in patients with erythroleukemia and paroxysmal nocturnal hemoglobinuria. (PAS, X100)

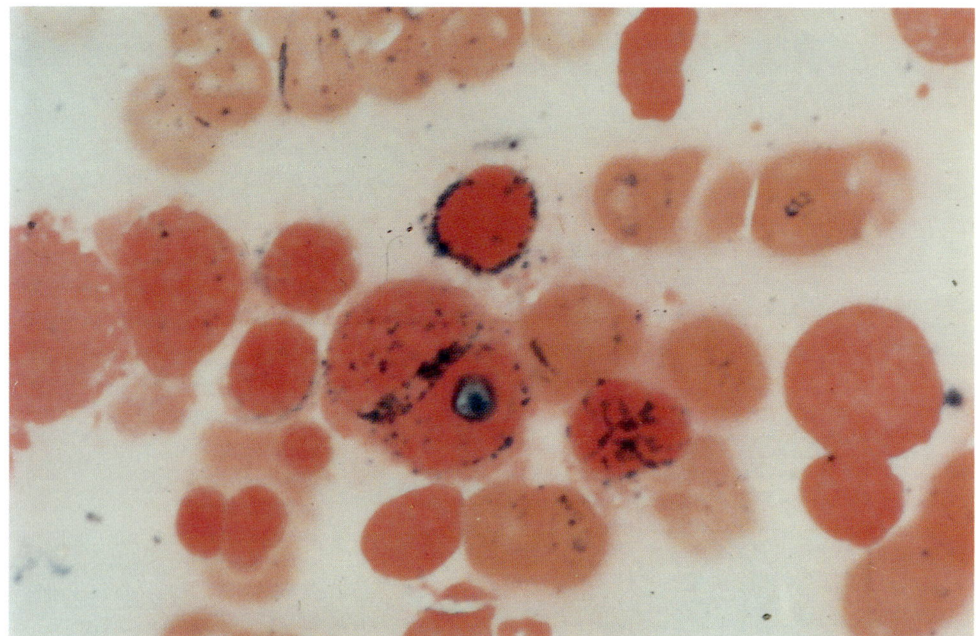

Figure 11-134. Erythroleukemia (AML subtype M-6) (bone marrow aspiration). On this slide, excessive iron deposits frequently forming rings are seen in all erythroid precursors. (FE, X100)

Figure 11-135. Chronic myelogenous leukemia (peripheral blood). This figure depicts 2 myelocytes with numerous basophilic granules. The presence of myelocytic basophiles in the peripheral blood along with more mature granulocytes is highly suggestive of chronic myelogenous leukemia. (J-G, X100)

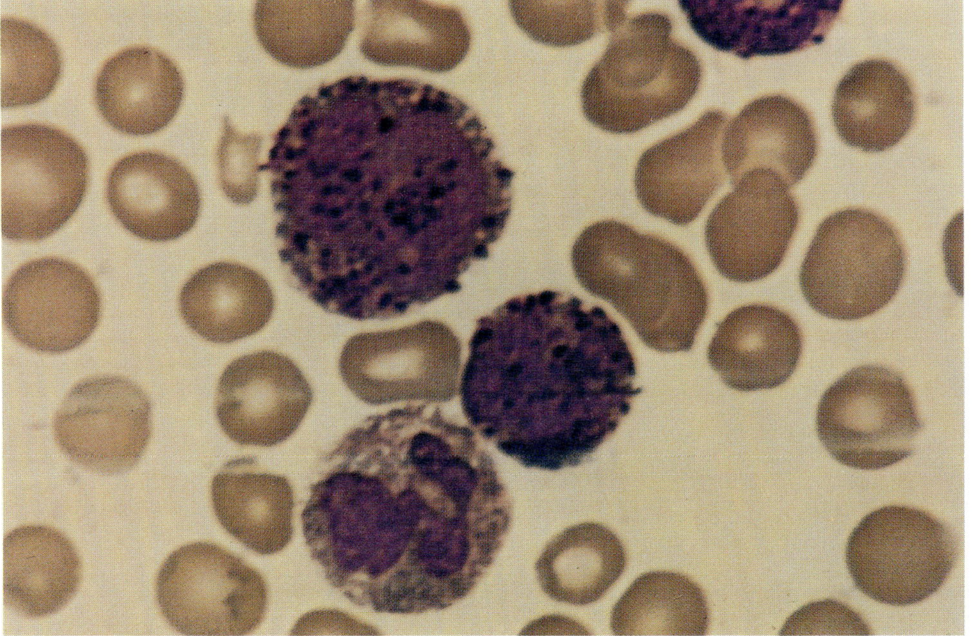

Bibliography

1. Coulson WF. Surgical pathology. Philadelphia: Lippincott, 1988.
2. Berard CW, Dorfman RF, Kaufman N. Malignant lymphoma. Int Acad Pathol monogr. Baltimore: Williams & Wilkins, 1987.
3. Enzinger FM, Weiss SW. Soft tissue tumors, St. Louis: Mosby, 1988.
4. Gompel C, Silverberg SG. Pathology in gynecology and obstetrics. Philadelphia: Lippincott, 1985.
5. Silverberg SG. Principles and practice of surgical pathology. New York: John Wiley, 1990.

12

THE PHYSICAL AND RADIOBIOLOGICAL BASES OF RADIATION THERAPY

Hassan Aziz, M.D., and Glaister Ayr, M.Sc.

R ADIOTHERAPY (XRT) IS THE treatment of malignant and some nonmalignant diseases with radiation; it is mainly concerned with the application of ionizing radiation. The biological effects of radiation are due to ionization of molecules and atoms of tissues when radiation interacts with them. To fully describe the clinical practice of radiotherapy, this chapter will first briefly review the physics of the atom, the types of radiation used, and the implications of radiobiology before describing the major forms of XRT and their clinical applications.

Physics

Atoms consist of a central nucleus, closely packed with protons and neutrons, and electrons orbiting the nucleus forming "shells" at specific distances from the nucleus (figure 12-1).[6,12] Protons have 1 unit of positive electric charge, $+1.6 \times 10^{-19}$ coulombs and electrons have 1 unit of negative charge. A proton and a neutron have about the same mass (1.672×10^{-24} g and 1.675×10^{-24} g, respectively). Electrons have very little mass (9.11×10^{-28} g). The number of protons in an atom is equal to the number of electrons and is known as the atom's atomic number. The sum of the number of neutrons and protons is the mass number of the atom.

Electrons orbit the nucleus in concentric shells designated K,L,M,N,O,P,Q in the order of their increasing distance from the nucleus.[6,12] K shell electrons, being nearest to the nucleus, are more firmly bound to the nucleus by electrical force than are electrons further from the nucleus. For this reason, they require

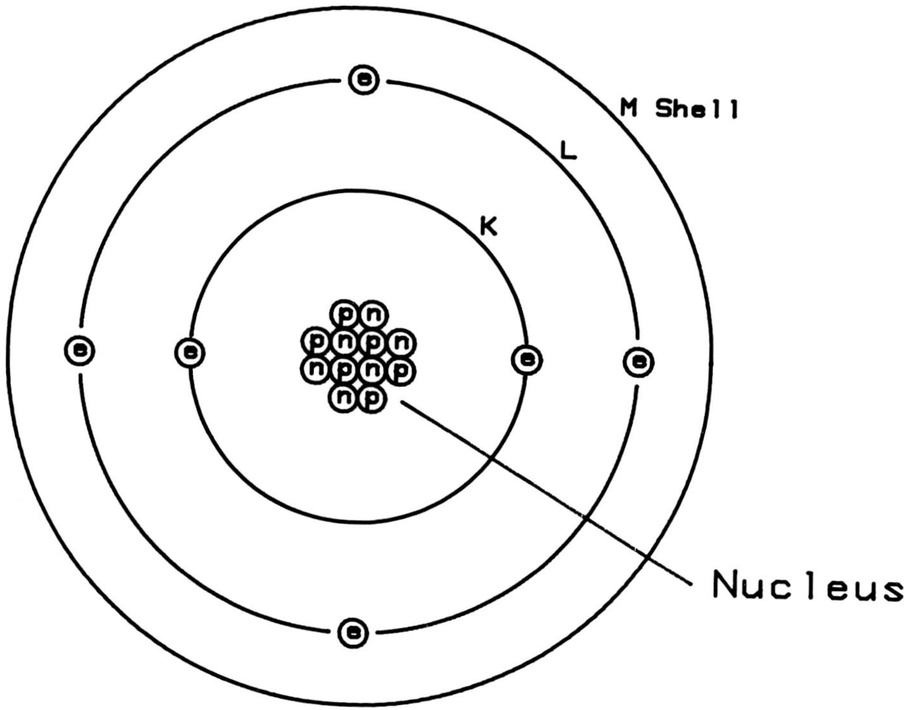

Figure 12-1. Diagram of an atom; mass number of 12, atomic number of 6; M shell is empty.

more energy to be removed from the atom than electrons in shells farther from the nucleus. Electrons in outer orbits require little energy to be removed from the atom and give the atom its chemical properties. Radiation ionizes matter by removing electrons from its atoms.

Outer-orbit electrons are more energetic than inner-orbit electrons. The outer electrons shed their extra energy as X rays and/or light when they move to inner orbits.

The *nucleus* of the atom can exist because the neutrons cause protons and neutrons to get close enough to one another to become bound by the extremely strong attractive short-range nuclear force. Nuclei with low mass numbers are stable if the numbers of neutrons and protons are equal.[12] Nuclei with high mass numbers require more neutrons than protons for stability. A given type of atom (element), with its fixed number of protons in each nucleus, may have a different number of neutrons in each nucleus. Nuclei with varying degrees of stability therefore occur, giving rise to isotopes. Isotopes of an element have the same chemical properties but a different mass number. Some isotopes of the same element are stable and some are unstable, i.e., radioactive. The characteristic of the particular isotope, a nuclide, is determined by the number of neutrons and the number of protons in the nucleus.

Ionization is the basis of XRT effect. When 1 or more orbital electrons are removed from an atom by radiation, a positive ion is produced. The expelled electron/electrons may attach themselves to other atoms producing negative ions. Alternatively, they may expel electrons from other atoms, producing several positive and negative ions and thus forming a chain reaction of ionization. Ionization of atoms in the DNA molecules seems to be the basis of clinical radiotherapeutic effect and is of primary interest to radiation oncologists.

Ionizing radiation can be divided into 2 classes: (1) X and gamma (γ) radiation and (2) particulate radiation. X and γ electromagnetic radiation consists of an electric and a magnetic field perpendicular to each other as the radiation travels from its source. X and γ radiation exists in discrete packets (quanta) of energy called *photons*. X rays differ from γ radiation only in source of origin; γ-rays result from radioactive decay (described below). X rays are produced either by decelerating electrons or from cascading orbital electrons. They ionize matter by removing electrons from atoms.

Production of X Rays

An energetic electron, traveling at almost the speed of light, is slowed down when it interacts with an atomic nucleus. It therefore loses kinetic energy, which is transformed into electromagnetic radiation of a certain energy. The energy lost by the electron is equal to the energy of the photon and depends on the distance of approach of the electron to the nucleus. X rays are produced when the electrons interact with the nuclei of target atoms and are slowed down, producing bremsstrahlung, a continuous spectrum of X rays that consists of millions of photons.[7] These bremsstrahlung photons have energies equal to or less than the maximum energy of the electrons. Alternatively, some energetic electrons may expel inner shell electrons from the atoms, producing

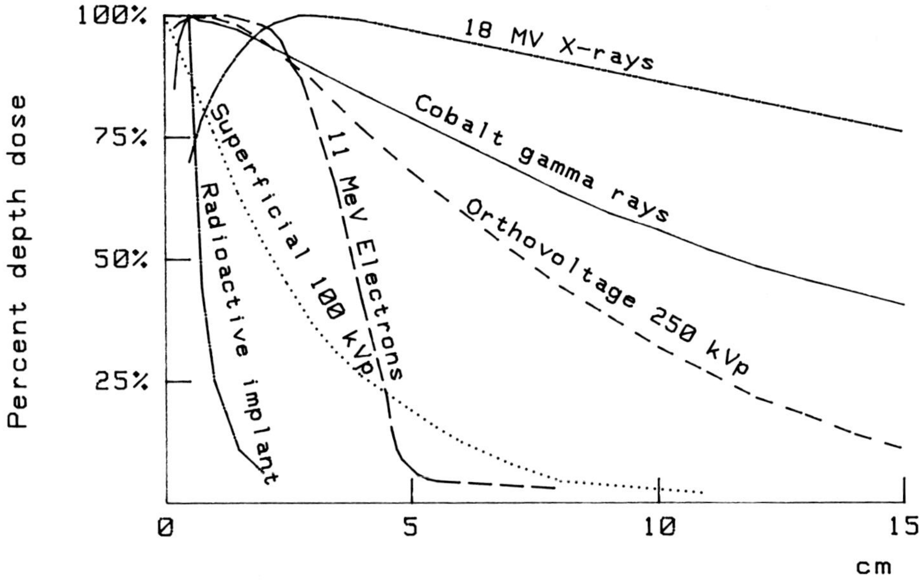

Figure 12-2. Dose in percentage versus depth below the skin or distance from the implant for radiation commonly used in radiotherapy.

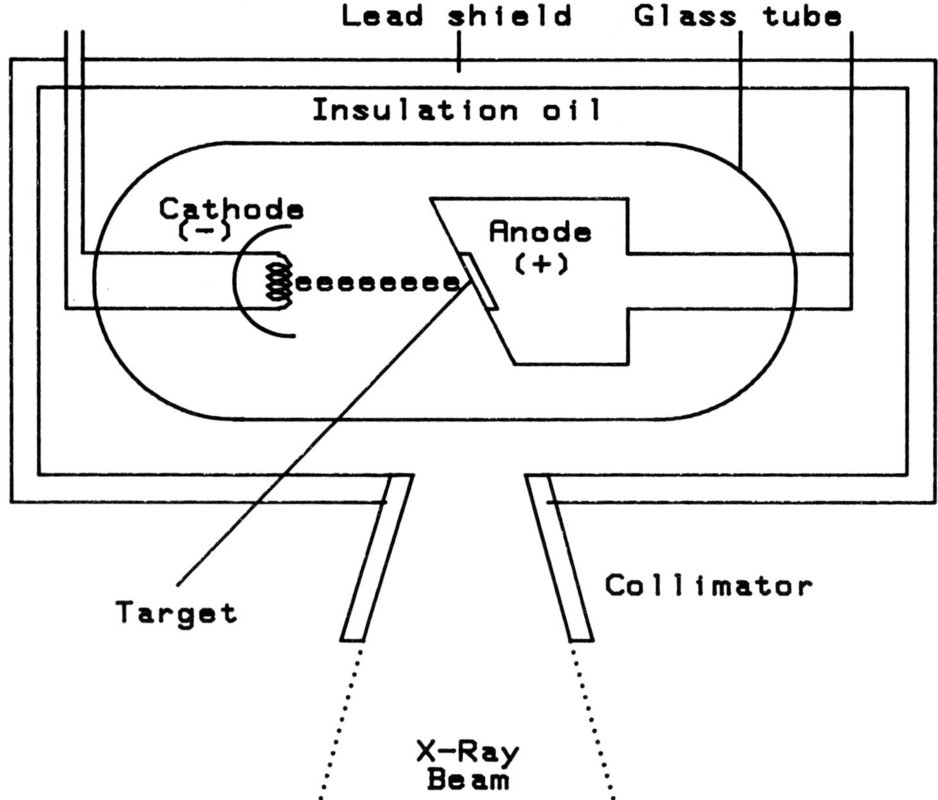

Figure 12-3. The x-ray tube head.

inner shell vacancies. Electrons from the outer shells shed their excess energy as they move to the empty space created in the inner shell. Their excess energy is released as characteristic X rays, whose photon energy is characteristic of the atom from which it was produced. The energetic electrons may also interact with orbital electrons, producing heat.

X-Ray Machines

The penetrating power of the types of radiation used in radiotherapy is shown in figure 12-2. Superficial and orthovoltage x-ray machines are contained in a lead-shielded glass tube (figure 12-3). Inside this tube, electrons are produced by an electrically negative filament heated by thermionic emission. The electrons are accelerated toward an electrically positive anode to hit a tungsten target, where X rays are emitted. The X rays are collimated, i.e., their dimensions and direction are defined, and filtered so that they are suitable for clinical use.

Higher energy photons and/or electrons are produced by the betatron and the linear accelerator.[8] The linear accelerator produces higher dose rates than the betatron and is in wide use today.

High-energy X rays and electrons used in XRT are usually produced by an electron *linear accelerator*.[10] Essentially, an electron gun supplies electrons (figure 12-4). A klystron or a magnetron supplies 3,000 MHz microwaves to accelerate the electrons. The microwaves are transported from the source through a smooth-surfaced metal tube known as a wave guide. They then travel through another wave guide consisting of corrugated metal tubing. In this wave guide, the corrugation of the tube and the microwaves interact to produce a strong electric field, which accelerates the electrons produced by the electron gun in small groups. A modulator rapidly switches the high-voltage supply of the electron gun and the microwave source in the proper sequence. The final energy the electrons attain is determined by the strength of the electric field and the length of the accelerating wave guide. A magnet is used to direct the electrons toward the patient.

The electrons then strike a water-cooled metal target of high atomic number (e.g., tungsten) where the electron's energy is converted into (1) X rays by bremsstrahlung and (2) heat. The X rays are filtered by a flattening filter and collimated, producing a clinically useful beam.

To produce the treatment electron beam, the target and flattening filter are removed. The electrons are scattered by thin metal foil to produce a broad, uniform electron beam that can be collimated for clinical use.

Linear accelerators are heavily shielded with lead, uranium, or heavy metal alloys to reduce their radiation leakage to safe levels. They produce very high radiation dose rates, varying from 100 to 1,000 cGy (1–10 grays) per min. Linear accelerators are equipped with sophisticated electrical and mechanical monitoring devices to ensure their safe operation. The machines have isocentric gantries that permit rotation of the radiation beam around the patient.

The advantages of treating with linear accelerators are that more of the high energy X rays penetrate deep into the tissue; the beam's penumbra is very small; high-energy X rays deliver low doses to the skin, thus having a significant skin sparing effect; and electron treatment is available for superficial and shallow tumors.

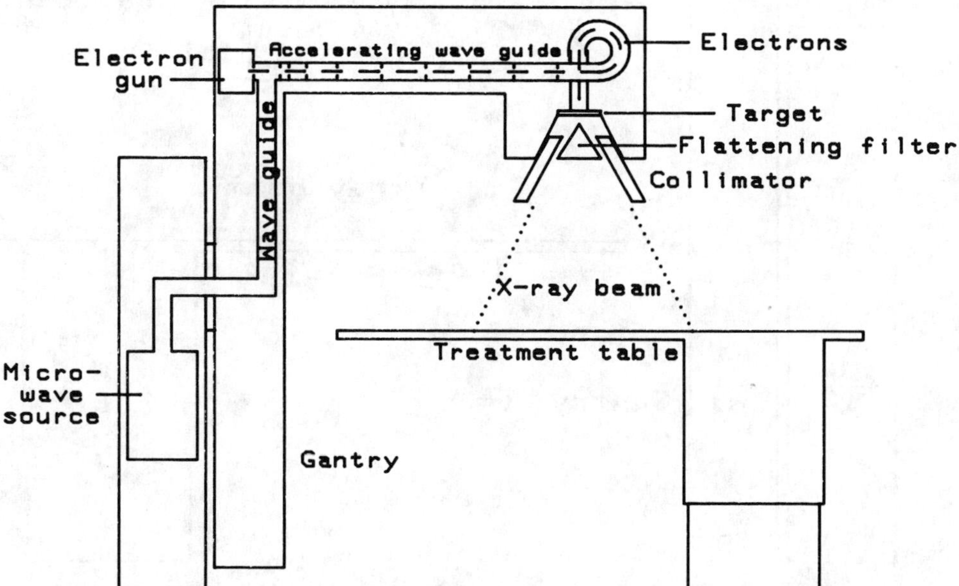

Figure 12-4. Schematic diagram of a linear accelerator.

Radioactivity

Radioactive decay may produce particulate radiation as well as photons in the form of γ radiation by mechanisms including alpha, beta and gamma (α, β, γ) decay. Alpha particles have a very short range and are not clinically useful. Those disintegrations of use in XRT are described below.

Beta decay can result in the emission of a β^+ or β^- particle. The clinically useful β^- particle is produced when an atomic neutron transforms into a proton, an electron, and a neutrino. The electron, or β particle, and the neutrino are emitted from the nucleus. The atomic number of the atom increases by 1, while mass number is unchanged; ^{90}strontium-yittrium and ^{32}phosphorus are examples.

Gamma decay. Some β emission leaves behind a nucleus with more energy than is required for its stability. The excess energy is emitted as a γ ray photon whose energy is characteristic of the atom. There is no change in atomic or mass number during γ ray decay (e.g., ^{60}cobalt, or ^{137}cesium).

Production of isotopes. Some radioisotopes are naturally occurring; these include ^{226}radium and ^{226}radon. ^{60}Cobalt, ^{32}phosphorus, and ^{198}gold are artificially produced by neutron bombardment of suitable stable target elements. ^{90}Strontium and ^{137}cesium are the result of uranium fission. The

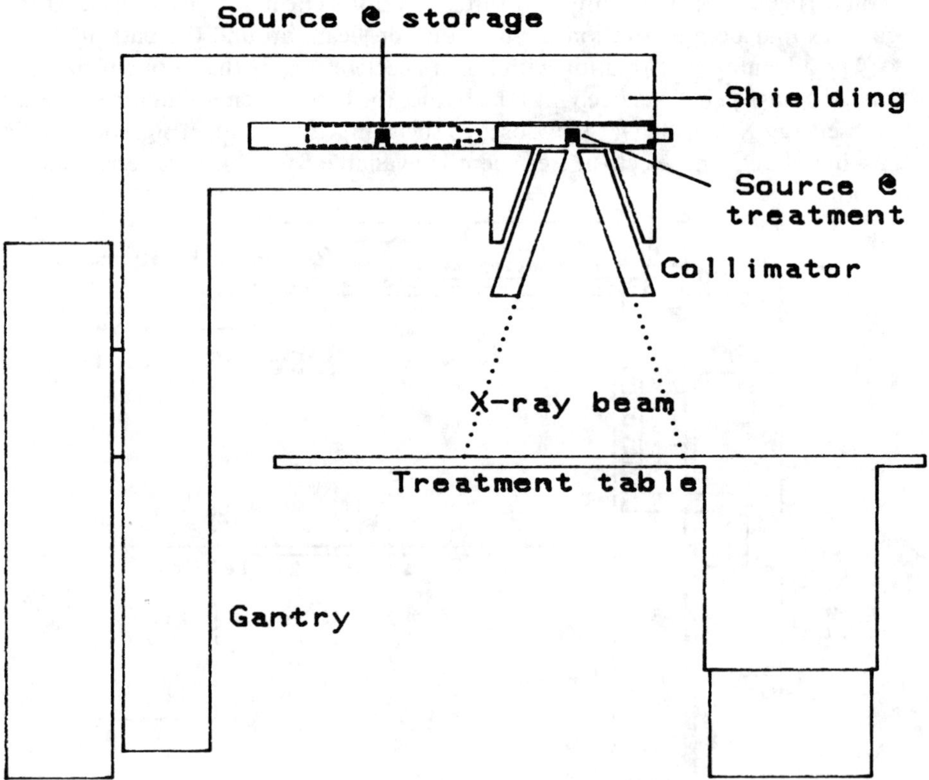

Figure 12-5. Schematic diagram of a cobalt isocentric teletherapy unit.

radioisotopes are usually sealed in a capsule so that only the emission, i.e., β or γ radiation, escapes. Unsealed radioactive material is sometimes used (e.g., radioactive chromium). The amount of radioactive material in a sample is measured in curies (Ci) or becquerels (Bq); 1 curie of radioactive material produces 37×10^{10} disintegration per sec; one bequerel of radioactive material produces 1 disintegration per sec.

The time taken for the number of curies to decay to one-half its initial value is characteristic of the neuclide and is referred to as its half-life (t½). Long t½ materials (e.g., ^{226}radium, 1,600 yr; ^{137}cesium, 30 yr; and ^{192}iridium, 74 days), are applied in brachytherapy to deliver a specific dose of radiation and are then removed. Short t½ materials (e.g., ^{125}iodine, 60 days; ^{198}gold, 270 days; and ^{131}iodine, 8 days) are implanted permanently to give the full dose at complete decay.

External γ rays. Five to 12 kilocuries of ^{60}cobalt or ^{137}cesium is placed in a sealed container so that only the radiation emanates from the container.[8] This container is placed inside a heavily shielded container equipped with a collimating system so that the radiation may be directed to the patient for treatment. The ^{60}cobalt machine is the most commonly used teletherapy machine (figure 12-5).

High-LET radiation. Radiation with high LET (linear energy transfer) interacts with matter to produce dense ionization. Such radiation, presently too costly for routine use, includes protons, neutrons, and ($-$) pi mesons. Cyclotrons are used to accelerate charged particles such as protons in spiral paths to high energies. These protons can be used for XRT or can be used to produce neutrons or negative pi mesons ($-$ mesons) for clinical purposes. The high-energy protons or deutrons are made to bombard a beryllium target to produce neutrons for XRT. Similarly, π mesons are obtained by bombarding targets of low atomic number of carbon with protons of extremely high energy produced in a large circular accelerator. High LET radiation has a high radiobiological effect.

Interaction of radiation with matter.[4] Biological effect is mainly produced when dense ionization occurs in tissue. The X and γ radiation "indirectly" ionize matter and do not produce dense ionization. X and γ radiation must first produce charged particles, which in turn will produce the dense ionization. Each ionization by X and γ radiation produces an electron that may ionize 10–100 other atoms in a short distance. The processes by which the photons produce the initial electron are: the *photoelectric effect;* the *compton interaction,* and the *pair production.*

Photons of low energy (0.01 to 0.15 Mev) usually interact with high-atomic-number material by the photoelectric effect. This is an energy absorption process because the photon interacts with an inner shell electron and disappears. Its energy dislodges the electron from its atom and gives the electron kinetic energy to ionize other atoms.

Photons of a wide range of energy (0.01–100 Mev) usually interact with matter of up to moderate atomic number by dislodging outer shell electrons. This electron will then produce dense ionization. The bombarding photon loses only some of its energy, but suffers a change in direction. After traversing some distance, the scattered photon may interact again by compton interaction, or if it has degraded enough, by photoelectric effect.

Pair production predominates at high energy only. The incident photon interacts with the atomic nucleus and is absorbed. Two types of electrons—a negatron, the usual electron with unit negative charge and a positron, an electron with unit positive charge—are produced. The negatron will produce dense ionization. The positron will interact with an electron in the material and annihilate to produce 2 photons of 0.51 Mev energy in opposite directions. These photons may further interact by compton and photoelectric effect; therefore, the threshold energy for pair production is 1.02 Mev.

Electrons and charged particles ionize matter densely, efficiently stripping electrons from atoms. Electrons that have too little energy to remove other electrons will become attached to atoms. A large number of positive and negative ions are produced, and these in turn may form very reactive chemical radicals.

Radiobiology

Mechanism of Cell Killing

The cellular damage may be the result of direct or indirect effect of radiation.

Direct effect. Nuclear DNA is considered to be the critical target in cell killing. Many complex reactions with DNA take place, the most important of which is the formation of free radicals due to ionization, with cross links among themselves with other free radicals. They interact with the DNA molecule to produce damage. High-LET radiation produces biological radiation damage by the direct effect.

Indirect effect. X and γ radiation is associated with the indirect effect of biological radiation damage. Damage of the cell is the result of ionization of water molecules, which constitute 80–85% of cellular material, producing very reactive $OH°$ and H ions that interact with DNA molecules and inactivate them.

Molecular linkage of free radicals with DNA, whether produced by direct ionization or through water, is unstable. The presence of oxygen during ionization tends to render the inactivation of DNA permanent.

Some cells are not critically damaged when irradiated, escaping death at the same time others are critically damaged. Radiation deposits energy to all sites randomly so that 2 adjacent sites may receive radiation dose at a fractionally different time from the same radiation exposure. The target theory postulates that there are 1 or more critical sites within each cell that must be damaged at the same time to inactivate the cell. The number of critical targets per cell is equal to the extent of DNA site damage required to inactivate the cell; otherwise, cell repair is possible. Deactivation occurs if one DNA-damaging event occurs in a cell containing 1 critical target. Such cells demonstrate an exponential survival curve, not commonly found in mammalian cells. Most mammalian cells exhibit an initial "shoulder" indicating repair of sublethal damage when irradiated with a low dose of X or γ radiation.[14] For this reason, multiple radiation hits are required to inactivate most mammalian cells, which must have multiple critical targets.

Two types of radiation cell death are possible in relation to their cell cycle: mitotic cell death and interphase death. Proliferating tissues (e.g., tumor cells, intestinal mucosa, and skin and bone marrow cells) demonstrate mitotic cell death. These cells fail to go beyond the mitotic phase when irradiated, thus suffer mitotic death. Mitotic cell death occurs in rapidly dividing cells and is responsible for acute reaction in XRT.

Large doses of radiation produce interphase death. Except when they are used against very radiosensitive cells (e.g., small lymphocytes and spermatogonia), radiotherapy doses are not high enough to produce interphase death. In interphase cell death, the cells do not progress through the cell cycle and do not reach the mitotic phase. Moderate radiation doses to proliferating tissue produce a delay in the G-2 phase, depending on 2 factors: (1) the dose received and (2) whether the cell was irradiated in the early or late phase of the cell cycle.

Irradiation early in the cell cycle causes a shorter G-2 phase delay than irradiation in later phases of the cell cycle. A moderate radiation dose to cells in random cell phases will synchronize all the cells to the same phase by this mechanism. The cells will then repeat the cell cycles in synchrony. Maximum biological effect in XRT is achievable by irradiating such synchronized cells in the G-2 and the M phases, when the cells are more radiosensitive.

Modifiers of Radiation Effect

The radiation effect can be enhanced by 4 types of different agents or can be inhibited by radioprotectors.[16]

The oxygen effect. Radiosensitivity of cells increases with their molecular oxygen concentration. This ability of oxygen to increase radiosensitivity is known as the oxygen effect. Oxygen enhances the response by fixation of damage produced by radiation-induced, chemically active radicals. Oxygen modifies the quantitative amount of radiation damage but does not alter it qualitatively. It reduces the dose required to achieve a certain radiobiological effect. Oxygen concentration and thus radiosensitivity of the cells increases as the partial pressure of oxygen in blood increases. Radiosensitivity increases rapidly from a partial pressure of 15 mm Hg and is maximum at 40 mm Hg. Radiosensitivity increases by a factor of 2 to 3. The increase in sensitivity is due to the presence of oxygen enhancement ratio (OER).

In an effort to overcome the hypoxic problem in tumors, hyperbaric oxygen has been used. During XRT, the patient lies in a hyperbaric chamber and the oxygen pressure is raised to 2–3 atmospheres. Benefit from this technique has been very limited.

Hypoxic sensitizers. Certain electron-affinic compounds, known as hypoxic sensitizers, act in the same way as oxygen. They act by fixation of the damage produced by the active radicals, preventing chemical restoration of these molecules to their undamaged state. The hypoxic sensitizers metronidazole and misonidazole were found to be capable of diffusing to hypoxic regions of tumors in animals, raising the sensitization effect about 2-fold. However, several clinical trials have shown either very little benefit or none at all from combined treatment with misonidazole and radiation.

True sensitizers: halogenated pyrimidines. These compounds are classified as true sensitizers because they become incorporated into the structure of DNA and render the DNA more radiosensitive. They include 5-iododeoxyuridine (IUdR), 5-bromodeoxyuridine (BUdR), 5-chlorodeoxyuridine, and 5-fluorodeoxyuridine (FUdR). The first 3 substitute the thymine in DNA and the last, FUdR, prevents the initiation of new DNA synthesis. These agents have been tried clinically, but because of rapid dehalogenation in the liver, are of limited value.

Apparent sensitizers. Several drugs have been found to enhance the effect of radiation. Prominent among these are actinomycin-D (ACT), methotrexate (MTX), and 5-fluorouracil (5-FU). ACT has been shown to depress DNA-dependent RNA synthesis. Repair of sublethal damage may also be inhibited. MTX prevents the synthesis of thymidine and therefore of DNA, producing enhanced cell killing. 5-FU inactivates the cells in the DNA synthetic phase and also possibly inhibits sublethal damage, producing radiosensitization. Recently, concomitant use of 5-FU infusion and XRT has increased in clinical practice, achieving encouraging results in the treatment of esophageal, anal, and bladder carcinoma. Similarly, concomitant use of cisplatin (DDP) and XRT is being seen with increasing frequency in the treatment of esophageal and advanced head and neck carcinoma.

Radioprotectors. The sulfhydryl compounds (e.g., cysteine, cysteamine, and 2-mercapto-ethyl-guamidine) operate primarily by hydrogen donation to prevent the stabilization of molecule damage by oxygen. Other compounds, including butanol, glycerol, and dimethyl sulfoxide, act by "scavenging" the active free radicals to prevent molecular damage. It is thought that the sulfhydryl group of these drugs is differentially taken up by well vascularized normal tissues, thus protecting the normal tissues while giving no protection to tumor cells. Hypoxic cells have reduced ability to absorb the sulfhydryl group of drugs. Toxicity has prevented their use beyond research.

Basis for Fractionation

The fractionation of the radiation dose facilitates the occurrence of 4 processes: *reoxygenation, cell cycle redistribution, repopulation,* and *damage repair.* During a course of fractionated XRT, the well-oxygenated tumor cells are sterilized first, diminishing their demand for oxygen. Oxygen is then able to diffuse farther into the tumor and reach cells that were previously hypoxic, a process defined as reoxygenation. Additionally, blood vessels that may have been compressed by the tumor mass may reopen due to the response of the aneated tumor cells, producing revascularization of the tumor. Revascularization can take place as quickly as 24 hr after irradiation, a phenomenon that is difficult to explain in terms of reoxygenation alone. However, reoxygenation remains of great importance in XRT.[9]

When rapidly dividing cells of either normal or tumor tissues receive the first fraction of radiation, cells in the sensitive phases of the cell cycle (M and G-2) are inactivated first, leaving a population of cells in resistant phases. These cells progress in cell cycle at different rates, resulting in rapid desynchronization toward the original cell phase distribution. This redistribution results in production of even more cells in sensitive phase at the time of the second fraction. The extent of radiosensitization due to redistribution has been completed before the second fraction is given. It should be emphasized here that redistribution occurs in rapidly dividing cells and forms the basis of fractionation and hyperfractionation.

Depopulation of tumor or normal cells by radiation stimulates regeneration of cells. Rapidly proliferating cells (e.g., intestinal mucosa, bone marrow, and skin) regenerate and repopulate faster than slowly proliferating cells (e.g., CNS, bone, and connective tissues). The presence of stem cells is necessary for regeneration to occur. The repopulation provides an effective means of achieving improved therapeutic ratio, as normal tissues repopulate faster than tumor tissue. Fractionated XRT makes use of this effect, and hyperfractionation applies it to an even greater extent.

The target theory suggests that damage to each target is required to kill cells with multiple hits. This may not happen in XRT. At low radiation doses, some critical targets are not completely damaged, leaving cells with sublethal damage;[2] therefore, the shoulder of the mammalian survival curve depicts a threshold dose before the exponential part of the curve begins (figure 12-6). By delivering fractionated doses, an enhancement of cell survival over that expected when the total dose is given in 1 fraction is observed. The increase in cell survival obtained by a fractionated course of radiation is due to repair of sublethal damage. This increased cell survival is of great importance to XRT in

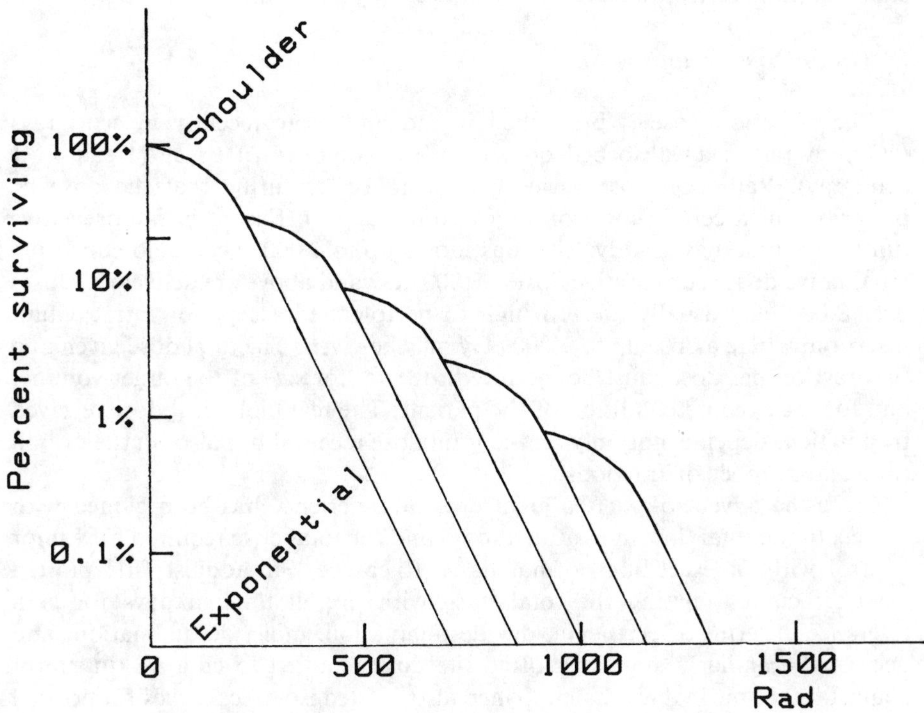

Figure 12-6. Typical mammalian survival curve: 0.1% survives a single dose of 600 rad; 0.1% survives 1,200 rad in 5 fractions.

terms of producing an acceptable therapeutic ratio because repair of the normal tissue is more efficient than repair of tumor tissue.

Certain cellular damage produced by radiation is only potentially lethal. Cells with such damage require an unfavorable condition for the damage actually to become lethal. If these cells progress in the cell cycle to the synthetic phase, their damage becomes "permanent." On the other hand, if potentially lethally damaged cells do not progress in cell cycle due to inhibition of metabolism, they may repair themselves, and in so doing may produce radioresistance. Because certain radioresistant tumors are known to contain viable but growth-inhibited cells, such tumors may be better treated with high LET radiation rather than X rays.

The number of neoplastic or normal cells killed increases with radiation dose, with very high doses killing all cells. The relationship between dose and the probability of cell killing is sigmoidal. Because of differences in the radiosensitivity of different types of tumors and normal tissues, several sigmoidal curves exist. The therapeutic ratio is favorable if the tumor can be destroyed without excessive normal tissue damage. Favorable therapeutic ratio is possible only if the sigmoid curve for tumor tissue lies to the left of that for normal tissue. A favorable therapeutic ratio is not achievable with a single large radiation dose because sterilization of tumor cells is less likely, and a tremendous amount of normal tissue damage will occur. Favorable therapeutic ratio is achievable with fractionated radiation doses. A fractionated XRT regimen allows reoxygenation, redistribution, repopulation, and repair of sublethal damage, producing a favorable therapeutic ratio.

Time/Dose Relationship

The radiation dose is prescribed in rad and more recently in centigrays (cGy). A rad is an absorbed dose of 1/100 joule/kg of tissue (1 rad = 1 centigray). Radiation dose varies with distance, requiring that the dose be prescribed at a certain location (e.g., 10 cm depth). Except in radiosensitive tumors, seminomas, and lymphomas, doses up to 4,000 cGy would constitute a palliative dose. For curative doses, 5,000 cGy and above are delivered. Doses over 8,000 cGy usually are too high to be tolerated except for intracavitary insertion, where a dose up to 9,000 cGy may be given. The total dose given and the fraction per dose must be modified for site, for size of the target volume, and for the age and condition of the patient. The real biological dose received by a patient depends not only on the total dose received but also on the overall time and number of fractions.

Since the advent of XRT, a great deal of experience has been gained with respect to the total time in treatment days and the total dose required for tumor control without exceeding normal tissue tolerance. Strandquist first plotted isoeffect curves relating the total dose with overall time in days for skin tolerance in terms of erythema, dry desquamation, moist desquamation, and necrosis.[15] Similarly, he also plotted the dose required to cure a skin tumor against total time in days. Later, Cohen also plotted isoeffect curves for normal skin tolerance as well as for various squamous cell carcinomas.[1] In plotting isoeffect curves, Strandquist and Cohen both used only 2 factors: the overall dose in rad plotted against the overall time in days. In their experimentation with pig skin, Fowler and Stern determined various fractionation schemes resulting in similar erythema.[5] Their experiments defined isoeffects from various fractionation schemes. Once the isoeffect information concerning total dose, total time in days, and fractionation was available, Ellis in 1969 formulated the following equation after some modifications:[3]

$$D = (NSD)\ T^{0.11} \times N^{0.24}$$

where D is the total tolerated dose, T is overall time in days, and N is the number of fractions of a treatment regimen. NSD (nominal single dose) in the equation is a number that indicates the biologically effective dose for the treatment regimen. The NSD value is a measure of the effectiveness of the given treatment regime. Known as the rad equivalent therapy, it can be used to compare the effectiveness of various treatment schemes. This equation does not, however, take into account 3 other important factors: tumor radiosensitivity, radiobiological effectiveness (RBE), and different ionizing radiations used. All of these factors must be considered when a treatment regimen is being planned so that a favorable therapeutic ratio is achieved.

Tissue radiosensitivity is high in neoplasms with rapidly dividing stem cells of hematapoeitic lymphoid tissue and spermatogenic epithelium; examples are lymphomas, leukemia, and seminomas. Patients suffering from these tumors do not require surgery, and the diseases are quite controllable with small or moderate doses of radiation. Radiosensitivity is moderate in basal cell and squamous cell carcinomas. These also are controlled with XRT alone, using slightly higher doses and longer fractionation. Next in the spectrum of radiosensitivity is adenocarcinoma. These tumors are removed surgically along with their regional lymph nodes, and XRT is used either pre- or postoperatively as an adjunct therapy in high-risk cases.

Other tumors, such as those arising from interstitial tissues (e.g., soft-tissue sarcomas) or from neurological tissues (gliomas), are radioresistant and must be removed surgically. In these cases, XRT is given in high doses and in many fractions as an adjunct therapy. Tumors arising from cartilage and bone (e.g., chondrosarcoma and ostosarcoma) are very radioresistant. Pre- or postoperative radiation may be used in conjunction with chemotherapy to control these tumors.

The volume of the treatment area has an impact on the patient's tolerance to treatment, which decreases as the treated volume increases. Large doses, therefore, cannot be delivered to large volumes. For example, in ovarian carcinoma or G.I. tract tumor where intraperitoneal spread has occurred, only small doses delivered in multiple fractions can be given. Smaller volumes, however, tolerate XRT better; if required, large doses in fewer fractions can be given.

The RBE (relative biological effectiveness) is different for different ionizing radiations. The RBE of 250 kv X rays is taken as the basic unit, and other radiation is compared relative to the effect of 250 kv. Megavoltage or supervoltage is about 85% as compared to 250 kv, whereas high-LET radiation from neutrons or protons may have a RBE of 1.5–2.0. For this reason, the dose must be adjusted according to the RBE of the type of radiation used.

New Approaches in Radiation Therapy

Failure to control the tumor locally is still a major cause of cancer deaths. This is especially true in cases of large local tumor with a large hypoxic cell component. A greater understanding of radiobiology now makes it possible to use XRT in ways that more effectively control local disease, resulting in greater cure rates. These techniques include the following:

Hyperfractionation. Hyperfractionation is the delivery of smaller than conventional doses (in the range of 110–120 cGy) 2 or 3 times a day. A higher total dose thus is given in the same time period as the conventional treatment. Hyperfractionated treatment with smaller doses may be considered as continuous irradiation, resulting in a decreased OER.[17] Reoxygenation is enhanced, but probably there is less dependence on oxygen for cell killing. The radiobiological effect is due mainly to an increased rate of redistribution, causing an increased radiosensitization of the tumor cells. With this method of treatment, more repair of the sublethal damage and repopulation may take place in normal tissues, allowing delivery of higher doses to the tumor. Because redistribution primarily affects rapidly dividing cells, hyperfractionation does not affect the slowly dividing cells, which are mainly responsible for late radiation complications. This type of treatment therefore allows a higher dose of radiation to be given for the same degree of late complications as with the conventional therapy.

Accelerated fractionation. This is a treatment regime in which 2 or 3 large-dose fractions are delivered to give the same total dose as in conventional therapy but over a shorter overall time. Here the repopulation and proliferation of rapidly dividing cells is curtailed by the high dose per fraction. Redistribution gives rise to a favorable therapeutic ratio. This type of treatment is especially suitable for the treatment of large, rapidly growing radioresistant tumors.

Hyperthermia. Heat with or without radiation has been used to treat advanced cancers for many years. The combined use of hyperthermia and radiation has been an area of recent interest. Hyperthermia may be localized or systemic, where the temperature is raised to 40–42 C. Local heating may be achieved by hyperthermic perfusion, radiofrequency, microwaves, and ultrasound techniques. Whole body temperature may be raised by hot air, hot water, hot wax, and/or by a thermally controlled space suit. A combination of heat and radiation may produce synergistic killing of tumor cells, as heat can sensitize cells in the S phase of the cell cycle that are normally radioresistant. Heat also inhibits the repair of the sublethal and potentially lethal damage. In addition, OER is low in the presence of heat. This mode of treatment may become popular and effective, but at present the techniques for applying hyperthermia are suboptimal and produce inhomogeneous temperatures.

Radiation particles with high LET neutrons. Neutrons are high-LET radiation, hence have a definite advantage over photons in XRT.[11] When neutrons are used, there is significantly less change in radiosensitivity in the various phases of the cell cycle than when photons are used. Recovery from sublethal damage is also less likely to occur, and the neutron's low OER makes hypoxic cells very vulnerable. With more than 20 yr of experience with neutron therapy to draw from, reports of higher local control rates of radioresistant tumors are common, but complication rates are higher. A better neutron therapeutic ratio may be obtained with a greater understanding of neutron dosimetry, RBE, and treatment techniques. To reduce complications, mixed beam therapy using photons and then neutrons is used as a means of increasing the tolerance of normal tissue. The sharp Bragg peak portion of the *proton beam* indicates a very dense ionization area.[13] It can differentially deliver high doses to tumors and relatively low doses to normal tissue. This is desirable in the treatment of the pituitary gland and certain eye tumors such as choroidal melanoma. The Bragg peak can be broadened with peak-shifting devices so that larger target volumes (e.g., prostatic carcinoma and soft-tissue sarcoma) can be treated with protons. Therapy using *negative mesons* offers improved physical dose distribution as well as increased biological effect. The negative mesons travel a greater range into tissue and exhibit a higher Bragg peak than protons. Negative mesons are used to treat tumors of the head and neck, lung, and abdomen. The use of particle radiation is extremely complex and costly. Small increases in local and regional control—but accompanied by increased complications—have been obtained with their use.

Practical Aspects of Radiation Therapy

External Beam Therapy

Tissue diagnosis and knowledge that XRT will be of benefit are prerequisites for a course of XRT treatment. Superficial tumors are palpated to determine their location and size and are treated with superficial X rays of 80–140 kvp energy or with electrons. Deep-seated tumors must be visualized by 1 or more of today's diagnostic imaging techniques (figure 12-7). The radiotherapist will then be able to use this information to determine the target volume, i.e., the tumor, its regional lymph nodes, and adequate margins, to be treated. The

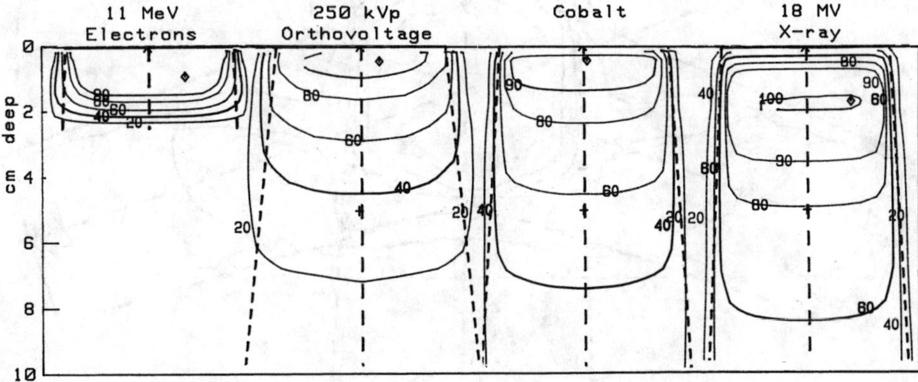

Figure 12-7. Radiation distribution of various radiotherapy treatment beams, showing 20%, 40%, 60%, 80%, 90%, and 100% isodose. Tumors receive non-uniform dose. Intervening tissues receive a much higher dose.

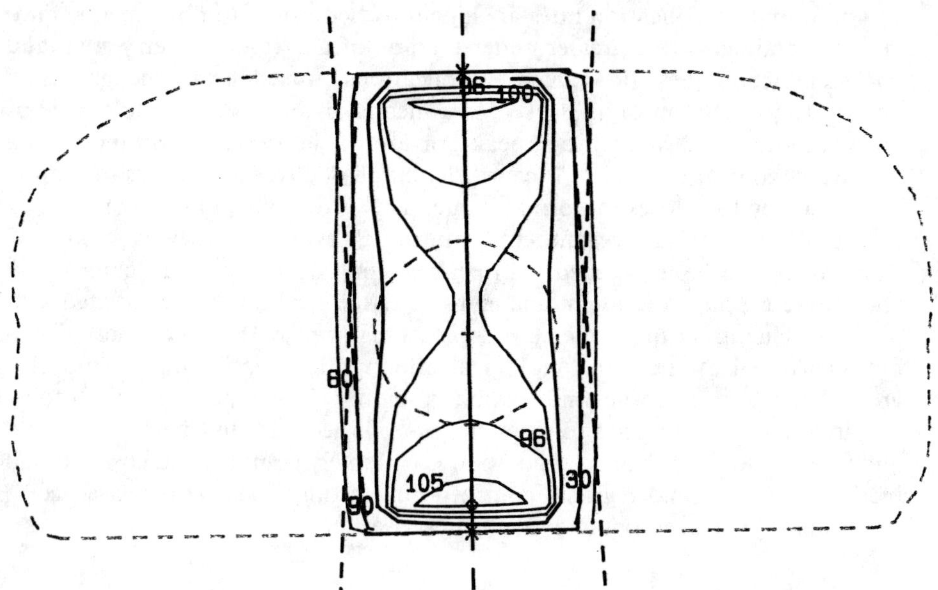

Figure 12-8. Radiation distribution using 2 parallel opposing beams gives a uniform target dose, but intervening tissues receive a high dose.

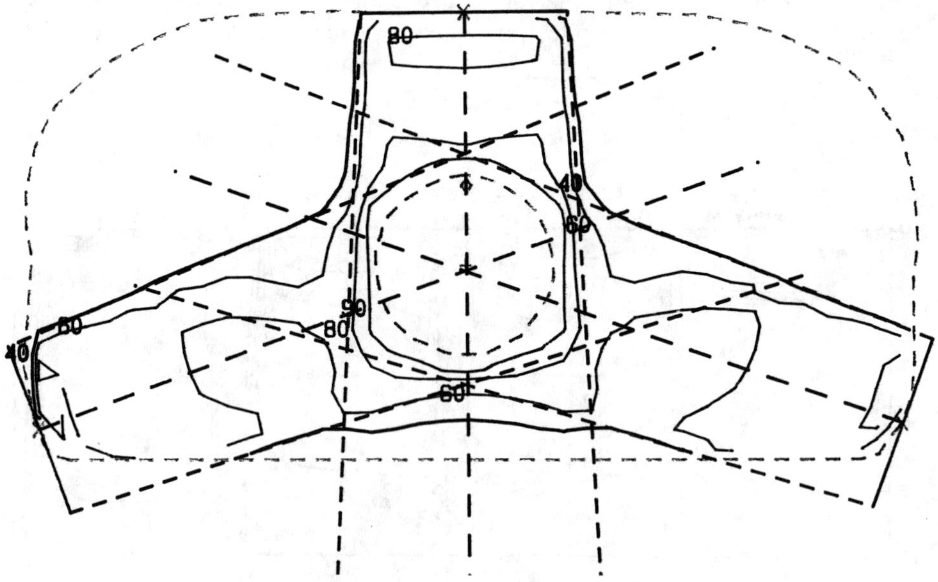

Figure 12-9. Radiation distribution using 3 beams produces a uniform target dose; intervening tissues receive a lower dose.

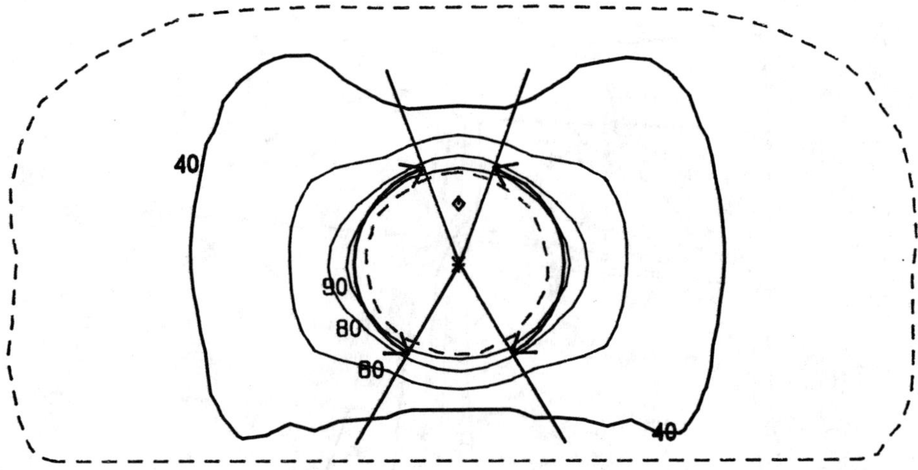

Figure 12-10. Radiation distribution using 2 arcing beams producing a uniform target dose; intervening tissues receive a much lower dose.

exact location and dimensions of the target volume and its position relative to the skin is determined by use of a simulator x-ray machine, a procedure requiring that the patient assume the treatment position for fluoroscopy and radiography. The simulator has special delineators visible on the patient's skin and on the radiograph that determine location and size of the target volume. Upon radiographic indication that the delineator demarks the target volume, its position is marked on the skin and is included on a cross-sectional drawing of the patient's body contour. Lateral and anterior/posterior simulation radiographs, in combination with the CT, MRI, and ultrasound images, enable the clinician to localize on the body contour or on CT the area to be treated, anatomical landmarks, and radiosensitive structures, and to choose the type of radiation.

In the treatment of deep-seated tumors, orthovoltage x-ray machines (200–250 kv) have been replaced by supervoltage machines, the cobalt machine and the linear accelerator. Supervoltage machines, which produce high-energy radiation, have definite advantages over orthovoltage machines. These advantages include sparing of the skin and bones, a sharp beam edge, and greater beam penetration.

An XRT treatment plan is then developed with the aid of a treatment planning computer. Along with other data, the simulation information and the CT or the body contour containing the location of target volume are entered into the computer. The machine then determines the most appropriate direction to apply the radiation in order to achieve a uniform radiation dose to the target volume without endangering radiosensitive tissues. Finally, the computer draws an isodose plan showing the expected radiation distribution within the patient. XRT is then based on the accepted computer treatment plan following simulation and port film radiographic verification.

Single ports are commonly used to treat the superficial lesions of skin or tumors that are nearer the surface. The dose delivered with a single port is not

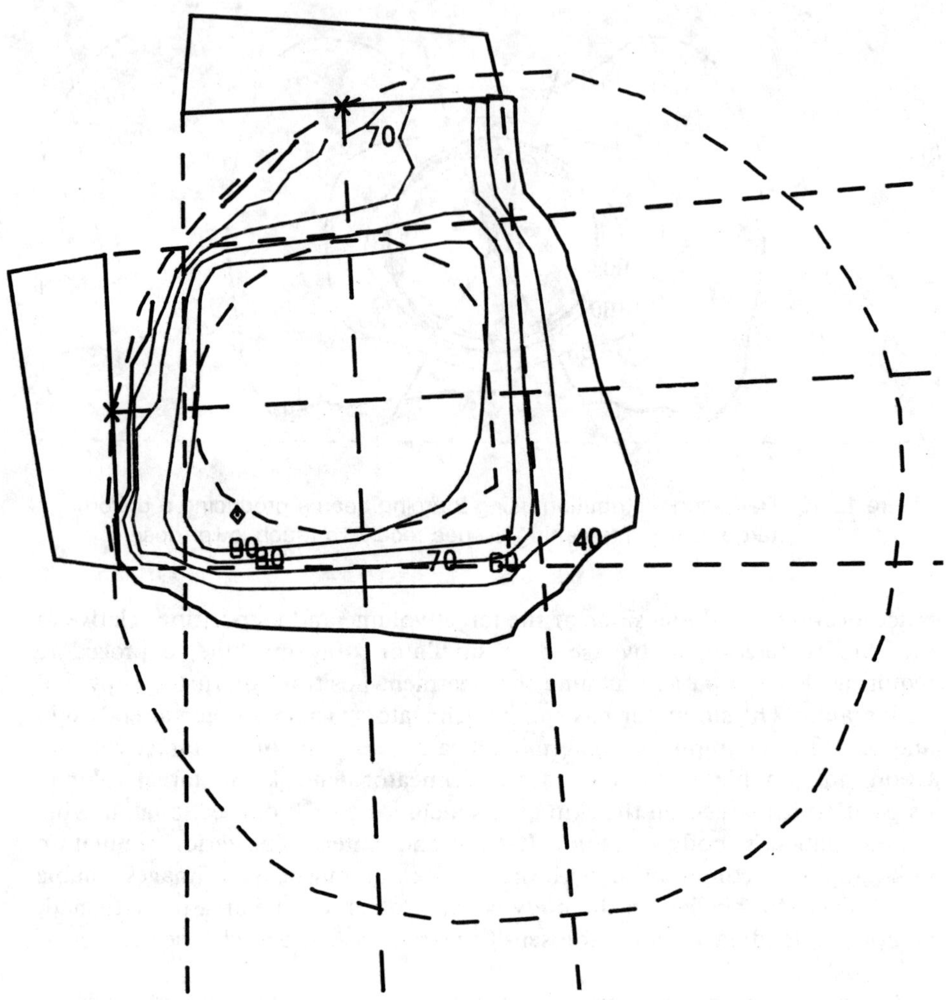

Figure 12-11. Radiation distribution using 2 beams at 90° and 2 lead wedges producing a uniform target dose; intervening tissues receive a lower dose.

uniform, and except for skin tumors its use is usually for palliation. The use of parallel opposed ports, in which the radiation encompasses the entire intervening tissue, is also common (figure 12-8). Both normal and tumor tissue receive a relatively high dose. Parallel opposed ports are usually used for palliation or in the initial part of a curative treatment.

The use of 2 oblique ports, 3 or more ports (figure 12-9), or arcing ports (figure 12-10) results in low doses to normal tissue but high uniform doses to the tumor. These techniques are usually used for curative treatments. Often due to bodily contours, the dose to the target volume cannot be made uniform without the use of triangular lead wedges. Wedges will homogenize the dose distribution (figure 12-11).

Brachytherapy

Radioactive materials deliver an intense radiation dose when placed near the site of a tumor but have a rapid dose "fall off" with distance. Advantage can be taken of this characteristic of radioactive materials by placing them at the tumor site so that they deliver a high dose of radiation to the tumor but only a small dose to distant tissues, thus sparing normal tissue. There are 3 brachytherapy techniques:

- *Intracavitary insertions.* In treatment of carcinoma of the cervix, endometrium, or vagina, applicator tubes are placed in the cavity and then loaded with ^{226}radium or ^{137}cesium.
- *Interstitial treatment.* Interstitial treatment of carcinoma of the mouth, pancreas, bladder, or prostate is commonly achieved by placing needles of ^{226}radium, ^{192}iridium, or ^{125}iodine seeds into the tumor bed. A very high tumor dose is delivered, but only a low dose to normal tissues.
- *Surface applicators (molds).* The mold consists of radioactive tubes of ^{137}cesium or ^{226}radium on wax, perpex, or plastic so that the radioactive material is at a suitable distance from the surface to achieve a uniform dose. Molds deliver a high dose to the treatment area and very little beyond. Superficial tumors of mouth and skin can be treated in this way.

References

1. Cohen L. Estimation of biological dosage factors in clinical radiotherapy. Br J Cancer 1951; 5:180–94.
2. Elkind MM, Sutton H. Radiation response of mammalian cell growth in culture. Repair of x-ray damage in surviving chinese hamster cells. Radiat Res 1960; 15:556–93.
3. Ellis F. Dose, time and fractionation: a clinical hypothesis. Clin Radiol 1969; 20:1–7.
4. Evans RD. X-ray and = ray interactions in radiation dosimetry. 2nd ed. Attix FH, Roesch WC, eds. New York: Academic Press, 1968; 94–144.
5. Fowler J, Stern BE. Dose rate effects: some theoretical and practical considerations. Br J Radiol 1960; 33:389–95.
6. Johns HE, Cunningham JR. The nucleus. In: The physics of radiology. 4th ed. Springfield Ill.: Thomas, 1983; 13–15.
7. Johns HE, Cunningham JR. Production and properties of x ray. In: The physics of radiology. 4th ed. Springfield Ill: Thomas 1983; 36–39.
8. Johns HE, Cunningham JR. High energy machines. In: The physics of radiology. 4th ed. Springfield Ill.: Thomas, 1983; 106–11.
9. Kallman RF. The phenomenon of reoxygenation and its implications for fractionated radiotherapy. Radiology 1972; 103:135–42.
10. Karzmark CJ, Pering NC. Electron linear accelerator for radiation therapy: history, principles and contemporary developments. Phys Med Biol 1973; 18:321–54.
11. Kelsey CA. Current status of D. T. targets for cancer therapy. Med Phys 1975; 2:185–90.

12. Lapp RE, Andrew HL. Atomic structure and structure of the atomic nucleus in nuclear physics. 3rd ed. Englewood Cliffs, N.J.: Prentice Hall, 1963; 21–61.
13. Lapp RE, Andrew HL. Particle accelerators in nuclear radiation physics. 3rd ed., Englewood Cliffs, N.J.: Prentice Hall, 1963; 213.
14. Puck TT, Markus P. Action of x-rays on mammalian cells. J Exp Med 1956; 103:653–66.
15. Strandquist M. Studien uber die kumulative wirkung der roentgenstrahlen bei fraktionierring. Acta Radiol (Supp) 1944; 55:287.
16. Coleman CN. Modification of radiotherapy by radiosensitizers and cancer chemotherapy agents. I. Radiosensitizers. Semin Oncol 1989; 16:169–75.
17. Peters LJ, Brock WA, Travis EL. Radiation biology at clinically relevant fractions. In: Important advances in oncology 1990. Philadelphia: Lippincott, 1990; 65–83.

13

PRINCIPLES OF CHEMOTHERAPY

*Michael Green, M.D., Ruth Oratz, M.D., and
Abraham Chachoua, M.D.*

ALTHOUGH SURGERY AND RADIATION remain the mainstays of cancer treatment for localized tumors, the role of cytotoxic chemotherapy has become more prominent in recent years. Increased understanding of tumor biology, mechanisms of action, and interactions of cytotoxic drugs, as well as improved staging techniques, has allowed the use of effective chemotherapy earlier in the course of disease, either alone or as an adjunct to surgery or radiation therapy (XRT).

The primary aim of therapy is to eradicate all viable tumor cells, therefore effecting a cure without prohibitive toxicity. Short-term aims such as symptomatic palliation and improvement in disease-free and overall survival may also be beneficial to the patient if toxicity is not extensive.

Cell Kinetics and Chemotherapy

The basis for the rational development of chemotherapy treatment regimens, whether they be single or combinations of drugs, lies in the relationship between the pharmacokinetics of drug action and the kinetics of tumor growth and the cell cycle. As outlined in a previous chapter, the dividing cell progresses through several phases. In the synthetic phase (S phase), triphosphate nucleotide DNA precursers are incorporated into DNA, and during the mitotic phase (M phase), the cell divides. The phase between the end of mitosis and the beginning of DNA synthesis is known as the first gap (G-1), and the phase

The authors wish to acknowledge the assistance of Margaret Nixdorf in manuscript preparation.

between the end of DNA synthesis and beginning of mitosis is termed the second gap (G-2). Dividing cells can also pass into a quiescent or resting phase known as the G-0 phase.

Cytotoxic drugs can be classified in 2 groups according to their phase-specificity.[1,2] Phase-specific agents kill cells only during specific proliferative phases of the cell cycle. They do not affect G-0 or G-1 cells. Examples include the antimetabolites, such as methotrexate and 5-fluorouracil, and the vinca alkaloids vincristine and vinblastine.

Nonphase-specific agents are equally toxic to both proliferating and non-proliferating cells. Examples are alkylating agents such as nitrogen mustard cyclophosphamide, and certain antibiotics such as mitomycin-C and doxorubicin. The precise mechanisms of drug action are discussed below.

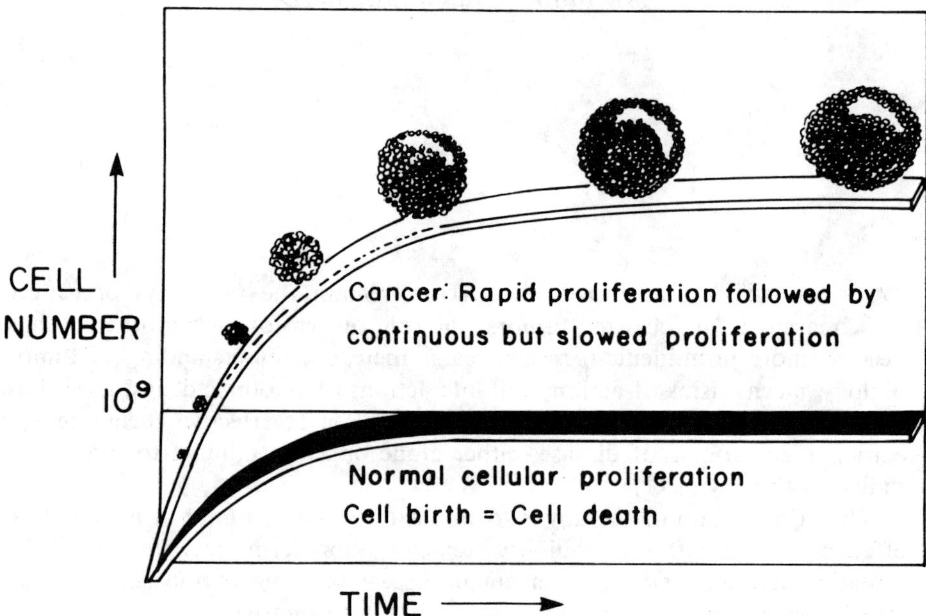

Figure 13-1. Gompertzian function.

The growth of a malignant neoplasm generally follows a Gompertzian function (figure 13-1).[3] As a tumor increases in size, the time it takes to double its volume also increases. This can be explained at the cellular level by an increase in cell cycle time (time from 1 mitosis to the next), increase in the number of dividing cells, and an increase in tumor cell loss due to factors such as a decrease in nutrients caused by the loss of vascular supply. Conversely, the smaller the tumor, the shorter its doubling time, due to more rapid cellular division. As a tumor shrinks with treatment, its doubling time decreases, and as a result a greater number of cells begin to divide. The larger percentage of dividing cells increases the sensitivity of the tumor to phase-specific chemotherapy. This reasoning provides a rationale for the sequential use of nonphase-specific agents to reduce tumor size, followed by phase-specific drugs to kill dividing cells. By virtue of their small size and relatively rapid growth, tumor metastases may be more sensitive to phase-specific chemotherapy than the primary tumor. The insensitivity of the primary tumor to a drug regimen might not necessarily predict responses to the same regimen in the case of metastases. Difficulties arise, however, when an attempt is made to rely solely on kinetic phenomema as the basis for drug sensitivity. Although data from preclinical systems suggest a direct relationship between growth rate and curability of tumors, clinical experience does not illustrate this. Burkitt's lymphoma, one of the most rapidly growing human cancers, is not the most highly curable. The growth rates of a relatively responsive solid tumor such as breast carcinoma overlap with much less responsive tumors such as melanoma. Adenoid cystic carcinoma, a slow-growing tumor, may display sustained responses to chemotherapy, but an extremely rapidly growing tumor, chronic myelogenous leukemia in blast crisis, is generally very refractory to drug treatment. These observations suggest that factors other than kinetics play a role in tumor responses to chemotherapy. These may include tumor cell heterogeniety and vascular supply.[4]

The Biochemical Basis for Drug Action

Chemotherapeutic drugs exert their effects by interfering with a variety of essential cellular processes, leading to inhibition of cell division. Targets for drug action include nucleic acids, DNA and RNA, cellular proteins such as tubulin, and such enzymes as dihydrofolate reductase. Because these targets are not unique to cancer cells, these drugs may also damage normal host tissues. Knowledge of the sites and mechanisms of drug action is therefore important in the understanding of the mechanisms of toxicity. In addition, the combination of cytotoxic agents with different sites of action may enhance tumor cell kill without a concomitent increase in toxicity. Mechanisms of cytotoxic drug toxicity will be explored more fully in a separate section.

Antimetabolites

Because of their structure, antimetabolites compete with normal cellular substrates in enzymatic reactions and disrupt essential metabolic pathways. Antifolates inhibit dihydrofolate reductase, the enzyme necessary for maintaining the intracellular pool of reduced folates. Inhibition of this enzyme leads to the intracellular accumulation of inactive oxidized folates, which in turn inhibit thymidylate and purine synthesis. As a result, DNA synthesis is arrested.[5]

The most widely used antifolate is methotrexate (MTX). Other antifolates undergoing clinical investigation include triazinate (Bakers antifol) and trimetrexate. MTX crosses the cell membrane by means of a carrier-mediated mechanism and then undergoes polyglutamation intracellularly.[6] The polyglutamated form is an active metabolite that itself inhibits enzymes other than dihydrofolate reductase (e.g., thymidylate synthetase). MTX is usually given I.V. by a variety of dose regimens that range from conventional ($25-100$ mg/m^2) to high ($1.5-7.5$ g/m^2) doses. The use of high-dose MTX attempts to maximize the dose/response relationship of cancer as well as overcome resistance as outlined below. Results of clinical trials in various malignancies have, however, been disappointing. MTX can also be administered orally and is well absorbed in low doses. Because the major mechanism of drug clearance is the kidney, compromised renal function leads to prolonged drug clearance and an increase in toxicity, particularly mucositis and myelosuppression. The effects of MTX can be reversed by the administration of a reduced folate such as leucovorin (LCV).[7] MTX is effective as a single agent in choriocarcinoma and, in combination with other chemotherapy, against breast cancer, head and neck cancer, and lymphoma.

Fluoropyrimidines

5-Fluorouracil (5-FU),[6] a pyrimidine analogue, is converted intracellularly to fluorouridine monophosphate (FUMP). FUMP may be converted to fluorouridine triphosphate (FUTP), which is incorporated in RNA and subsequently inhibits RNA function.[8] Another metabolic product of FUMP, 5-FdUMP, inhibits thymidylate synthetase, with the eventual depletion of deoxythymidine triphosphate (dTTP), one of the nucleosides necessary for the synthesis of DNA. In its native form, 5-FU is also incorporated into DNA, and may in this way contribute to its cytotoxic effects. 5-FU is usually administered I.V., but may be administered intraperitoneally.[9] Because it is metabolized by the liver, 5-FU may be infused into the hepatic artery or portal vein for the treatment of hepatic metastasis, with only small amounts of drug reaching the systemic circulation.[10] I.V. bolus administration is complicated mainly by myelosuppression occurring in 4–7 days, with full recovery usually within 2 wk. Stomatitis and diarrhea are also side effects. On the other hand, continuous I.V. infusion, although it has equivalent therapeutic results, has a different pattern of toxicity. Myelosuppression is usually mild, whereas such G.I. symptoms as stomatitis and diarrhea are the predominant toxicity. This illustrates that the method of administration of cytotoxic drugs may alter their pattern of toxicity. 5-FU is used extensively in the treatment of G.I. cancer and in combination therapy for breast cancer.

Cytosine arabinoside (ara-C), an arabinosine nucleoside, penetrates cells by carrier-mediated mechanisms. It is metabolized to the active form ara-CTP, which inhibits DNA polymerase and interferes with DNA replication.[11] Ara-C is also incorporated in DNA, leading to defects in ligation of fragments of newly synthesized DNA.[12] As an inhibitor of DNA synthesis, ara-C kills cells selectively during the S phase of the cell cycle. It is rapidly metabolized by cytidine deaminase, an enzyme found in plasma and in granulocytes. Because of rapid inactivation and its phase-dependent killing, ara-C is usually administered as a continuous infusion or in multiple bolus doses. Ara-C is useful in the treatment of acute myeloid leukemia, either alone or in combination with anthracyclines.

Alkylating Agents

Alkylating agents exert their cytotoxic action by forming covalent bonds with nucleic acid. The main sites of DNA attack are the N_7 position of guanine, the 1, 3, and 7 positions of adenine, and the N_3 position of cytosine. Consequences of base alkylation include misreading of the DNA code, cross-linking of DNA and single- and double-strand breaks. These actions may be responsible for the increased incidence of secondary leukemias in patients treated with alkylating agents.

Cyclophosphamide (CTX) is converted to 4-hydroxycyclophosphamide in the liver. 4-Hydroxycyclophosphamide is spontaneously converted to aldophosphamide, which is hydrolyzed within the target cells to the active compound phosphoramide mustard.[13] CTX can be administered orally and IV. Nausea and vomiting and alopecia are common. In addition, active metabolites (possibly acrolein) excreted in the urine can cause hemorrhagic cystitis due to bladder irritation, a side effect that is particularly common with high-dose regimens or prolonged oral administration.[14] Instillation of thiol compounds into the bladder or systemic administration of N-acetyl cysteine or sodium-2-mercaptoethane sulfonate (MESNA) prevents this toxicity.[15] CTX is useful in the treatment of lymphoma and small-cell lung cancer.

Cisplatin

Cisplatin (DDP) is a water-soluble square planar coordination complex containing a central platinum atom surrounded by 2 chloride atoms and 2 ammonia groups. The antitumor activity of the complex is much greater when the chloride and ammonia groups are in the *cis* position compared to the *trans* position. The chloride ions dissociate in water to create an active complex, which in turn interacts with DNA, RNA, or proteins.[16] This interaction causes changes in DNA conformation and inhibition of DNA synthesis. DDP is excreted in the form of free platinum via glomerular filtration.[17,18] Impaired renal function leads to a prolonged serum half-life, exacerbating its toxicity. DDP has activity against testicular and ovarian cancer and can effect a cure in these tumor types. In addition, DDP is active against small-cell lung and squamous cell cancer of the head and neck. Recently, interest has been focused on the ability of DDP to inhibit repair of radiation-induced sublethal DNA damage. This property, which makes it valuable as a potential radiation sensitizer, is being explored in concurrent DDP-irradiation regimens.[19]

Antibiotics

Anthracyclines. These compounds do not have a clearly defined single mechanism of cytotoxic action. Doxorubicin (ADR) and daunorubicin can act as intercalators between strands of the DNA double helix, resulting in inhibition of DNA, RNA, and protein synthesis.[20]

Anthracyclines can cause single-strand DNA breaks and also inhibit DNA repair. This may be due to the ability of anthracyclines to produce free radicals, to cause the generation of hydroxyl radicals, or to cause DNA intercalation.[21] The generation of radicals is thought to be responsible for the cardiotoxicity that complicates treatment with anthracyclines.[22] In addition, anthracyclines react directly with cell membranes and alter their function, a characteristic that may also contribute to their cytotoxic activity.[23] Renal clearance of anthracyclines is minor; dose modification is not necessary if renal function is impaired.

ADR and daunorubicin are metabolized chiefly in the liver, and dosages are modified in patients with liver impairment. Anthracyclines are effective against a wide range of tumors, including small-cell lung cancer, soft-tissue sarcomas, lymphomas, and leukemias.

Bleomycin (BLM) produces single- and double-strand breaks in DNA, an action mediated by the formation of superoxide and hydroxyl radicals.[24] BLM is active in the combination therapy of lymphomas, and testicular cancer and as single agent in the treatment of epidemic Kaposi's sarcoma. A BLM-inactivating enzyme is found in normal and malignant cells and is prominent in the liver.[25] This enzyme is not found in the lung or skin, perhaps explaining the main toxicities associated with BLM therapy.

Plant Alkaloids

The *vinca alkaloids* include vincristine (VCR) and vinblastine (VLB). They cross the cell membrane by an active transport process and bind to tubulin, a protein that is essential for spindle formation during mitosis.[26] As a result, affected cells are arrested in the metaphase of mitosis. Renal excretion is minimal in both drugs; clearance is mainly by hepatic metabolism.[27-29] VCR causes little myelosuppression; in contrast, the primary toxicity of VLB is found in the bone marrow. Leukopenia is usually dose-limiting. Vinca alkaloids are used extensively in the treatment of hematologic malignancies.

Epipodophyllotoxins: Etoposide (ETO, VP-16) and teniposide (VM-26) are epipodophyllotoxins. These compounds have no discernable effect on microtubular assembly and cause cellular arrest in G-2 rather than mitosis.[30] Their exact mechanism of action is unknown. ETO is administered either orally or I.V. Bioavailability by the oral route, however, is variable.[31] VM-26 is given only I.V. The clearance of VM-26 and ETO is both metabolic and renal. Both agents have important clinical activity in lymphomas, small-cell lung cancer, and testicular cancer.

Nitrosoureas

These compounds include carmustine (BCNU), lomustine (CCNU), and methyl CCNU (MeCCNU). Cytotoxic activity includes DNA alkylation, producing strand breaks and cross-links. In addition, metabolic products of nitrosoureas yield isocyanates, which inhibit DNA repair and alter maturation of RNA.[32] Because of their high lipid solubility, nitrosoureas can penetrate the blood/brain barrier and are useful in the treatment of neurological malignancies.

Enzymes

L-Asparaginase is an enzyme that catalyzes the conversion of L-asparagine to L-aspartic acid. The antitumor effects of L-asparaginase relate to the depletion of L-asparagine. Tumor cells that lack L-asparagine synthetase—and consequently must obtain L-asparagine from the circulating amino acid pool—are susceptable to the actions of L-asparaginase.[33] L-Asparaginase is effective in such lymphoid malignancies as childhood acute lymphatic leukemia.

Resistance

Drug resistance continues to be the major factor limiting the effectiveness of cancer chemotherapy. Resistance may be natural (occurring prior to exposure to chemotherapy) or acquired through exposure to cytotoxic drugs. A hypothesis advanced by Goldie and Coldman proposes that the occurrence of natural resistance relates to the genetic instability of tumor cells.[34] This accounts for the spontaneous generation of variant forms characterized by different phenotypic and genotypic properties. Genetic changes include mutations, deletions, transpositions, gene amplifications, chromosomal rearrangements, and translocations. These changes may be associated with altered, diminished, or increased gene products that can be involved with the generation of phenotypic drug resistance. Selection pressures caused by exposure to cytotoxic agents can lead to similar genetic changes, with subsequent selection of resistant cell lines. The use of combination chemotherapy may prevent or delay the emergence of resistant cell lines.

Biochemical mechanisms of resistance include:

- *Defective transport.* Decreased carrier-mediated transport is seen in vitro and in vivo with the development of MTX resistance. This can be overcome with high extracellular drug concentrations that promote uptake of drug by diffusion. Impaired uptake, also seen with ara-C resistance, is thought to relate to a decrease in membrane-binding sites. Increased drug excretion seen with in vitro resistance to anthracyclines is mediated by an active transport mechanism; the specific enzymes, however, have not been identified. Calcium antagonists such as verapamil can circumvent in vitro and in vivo resistance to anthracyclines. However, the high doses of verapamil required for this action are associated with significant side effects, making the clinical applications impractical.
- *Defective drug metabolism to active species.* Decreased activating enzymes, including uridine kinase, orotic acid phosphoribosyltransferase, and uridine phosphorylase have been described in in vitro cells resistant to 5-FU. Decreased deoxycytidine kinase activity is associated with ara-C resistance, and defective polyglutamation may play a role in MTX resistance.
- *Increased drug inactivation.* Increased intracellular drug inactivation due to the induction of intracellular enzymes is important in BLM resistance because of increased BLM hydrolase activity, in ara-C resistance because of increased cytidine deaminase, and possibly in DDP and ADR resistance because of increased intracellular metalothionine and glutathione, respectively.
- *Altered DNA repair.* In normal and malignant cells, intracellular enzymes are capable of repairing sublethal DNA damage. The ability to rapidly repair DNA damage caused by cytotoxic drugs may be important in the development of tumor resistance. This mechanism is seen in DDP and alkylator-resistant cell lines.
- *Altered target proteins* (extensively studied as a mechanism of MTX resistance). MTX-resistant cells in which dihydrofolate reductase has a decreased affinity for drug have been isolated in animal and human cells in vitro. The change is mediated by amino acid substitutions at the

enzymatic active site, and can lead to a 2.5- 270-fold decreased affinity for MTX. Other altered target proteins implicated in resistance to cytotoxic drugs include tubulin, in the case of VCR, and thymidylate synthetase, in the case of 5-FU.

Genetic alterations can cause quantitative as well as qualitative changes in proteins targeted by chemotherapy. This phenomenon was first documented as a mechanism of resistance to MTX due to increased cellular production of dihydrofolate reductase secondary to amplification of its coding gene. Gene amplification occurs independently of drug exposure, but confers a survival advantage only in the presence of a drug that interacts with the amplified gene product. Gene amplification may also play a role in resistance to 5-FU and ADR.

As a consequence of a single mutation, tumor cells may display significant orders of resistance to a number of antineoplastic agents. This finding, referred to as pleiotropic drug resistance, represents a common mechanism of resistance directed against a variety of antineoplastic drugs of large molecular size. One example is the anthracyclines, vinca alkaloids, and actinomycin-D (ACT). In this case, resistance is associated with decreased cellular accumulation of drug. This is due to increased active outward transport by mechanisms common to all 3 drugs and is the consequence of a single mutation leading to the amplification of the gene coding for the P32 glycoprotein.[35] Several of the above mechanisms may occur simultaneously.[35]

Toxicity

Toxicity is the injury of normal host tissues as an adverse side effect of antineoplastic therapy. Damage or killing of host cells is caused by the same mechanisms of drug action as against tumor cells. Chemotherapy-mediated toxicity may be caused either by the parent compound or by its metabolites. In general, such toxicity is self-limited, and host tissues return to normal within a few weeks after chemotherapy administration. Usually, little more than routine supportive care is necessary in the management of patients receiving anticancer chemotherapy. Some agents, however, can cause cumulative damage, which becomes irreversible despite cessation of the drug. Examples of this include the cardiomyopathy induced by anthracyclines and the pulmonary fibrosis caused by BLM. Table 13-1 lists some commonly used drugs and their specific toxicities.

Myelosuppression

The rapidly proliferating cells of the normal bone marrow are susceptible to the toxic effects of drugs that act by interfering with DNA synthesis and cell replication. Cytotoxic drugs impair the replication, maturation, and release of hematopoietic stem cells from the marrow, leading to decreases in the number of circulating white blood cells (WBC) and platelets. Usually, myelosuppression first appears 7–14 days after administration of the last dose of chemotherapy because the marrow has a reserve storage compartment that can supply mature cells to the periphery up to that time. The lowest peripheral WBC and platelet

Table 13-1. Several Commonly Used Drugs and Their Specific Toxicities

Class	Route of administration	Elimination	Toxicity
Vinca alkaloids	I.V.	Metabolic	Myelosuppression, neuropathy, mucositis
Anthracycline	I.V.	Metabolic	Myelosuppression, alopecia, cardiomyopathy
Antimetabolites	p.o. I.V. Intrathecal	Renal	Myelosuppression, stomatitis, neurotoxicity
Alkylating agents	p.o.	Metabolic	Myelosuppression, cystitis/renal failure, pulmonary fibrosis, leukemia
Bleomycin	Subcutaneous I.M. I.V. Intracavitary	Renal	Pulmonary, cutaneous hypersensitivity
Cisplatin	I.V.	Renal	Nephrotoxic, ototoxic, peripheral neuropathy, myelosuppression

counts are known as the *nadir* counts. The *absolute neutrophil count* (ANC) is a measure of the total number of mature granulocytes and segmented band forms. It is calculated by adding the products of the percent of each cell in the differential and the total WBC count. For example:

$$
\begin{aligned}
\text{WBC count} &= 1.5 \\
\text{Differential: polys} &= 70\% \\
\text{bands} &= 10\% \\
\text{lymphs} &= 20\% \\
\text{ANC} &= (.70)(1.5) + (.10)(1.5) \\
&= 1.05 + .15 \\
&= 1.2
\end{aligned}
$$

In the treatment of solid tumors, effective doses of chemotherapeutic drugs may result in nadir WBC counts of about $2.0 \times 10^3/\text{mm}^3$ and platelet counts of $50\text{--}100 \times 10^3/\text{mm}^3$. Although infection and hemorrhage are potential complications of chemotherapy, they are uncommon; however, nadir counts below these levels are more likely to be complicated by infection or hemorrhage, usually necessitating dose reductions in subsequent cycles of chemotherapy. On the other hand, more intense treatment of hematologic neoplasms such as leukemia and lymphoma is required to eradicate malignant clones of hematopoietic stem cells. Severe damage to normal marrow cells is an unavoidable consequence, resulting in aplasia and life-threatening levels of neutropenia and thrombocytopenia. Profound neutropenia may lead to infection, often with opportunistic organisms, and thrombocytopenia may result in hemorrhage. Intensive medical support, with transfusion of blood products and treatment of infections, should be available to these patients. Full recovery of normal peripheral counts may be expected within 14 days following the nadir as normal stem cells recover.

The time taken to reach peripheral blood nadirs and the time needed for subsequent recovery may vary for each chemotherapy drug. Some drugs, such as the nitrosoureas and mitomycin-C (MIT), cause prolonged myelosuppression and thrombocytopenia, necessitating a recovery period of up to 6 wk. In addition, prolonged chemotherapy can lead to a depletion of bone marrow reserves. This can be manifested as low nadir counts and slower marrow recovery.

Gastrointestinal Toxicity

Nausea and vomiting are common side effects seen during chemotherapy administration; although it is uncommon, they may continue for up to 24 hr. Two regions in the brain have been identified as important in the neurohumoral mechanisms of nausea and vomiting. The vomiting center, deep in the reticular formation of the brain, coordinates the somatic reflex of vomiting. A second area, known as the chemoreceptor trigger zone (CTZ) is located in the dorsolateral reticular formation. Both blood and cerebrospinal fluid (CSF) are in contact with the CTZ. The vomiting center may be stimulated directly by afferent input from the upper G.I. tract via the vagus and sympathetic nerves. XRT, invasion of the G.I. tract by tumor, and a few drugs may act in this manner. Most emetogenic chemotherapeutic agents probably act by direct stimulation of the CTZ, which in turn releases neurotransmitters that activate the vomiting center.[36] The vomiting center may also be stimulated by messages from the vestibular apparatus of the middle ear or from higher brain stem or cortical areas.[37] The latter mechanism offers a possible explanation for the occurrence of psychogenic and anticipatory vomiting, i.e., nausea and vomiting provoked by the thought of chemotherapy or expectation of treatment before the actual administration of drugs. In addition to being subjectively unpleasant for patients, vomiting may cause significant fluid and electrolyte imbalance and represent a dose-limiting toxicity. Table 13-2 is a partial listing of antineoplastic drugs arranged according to emetogenic potential. Several antiemetic drugs and combinations have been developed for the prevention and treatment of chemotherapy-induced emesis. They are outlined in table 13-3.

Table 13-2. Severity of Nausea and Vomiting Induced by Cancer Chemotherapeutic Drugs

Severe	Moderate	Mild
Cisplatin	Cyclophosphamide	Vinca alkaloids
Adriamycin	Cytarabine	5-fluorouracil
Dacarbazine	Methotrexate	Bleomycin
Nitrogen mustard	Nitrosoureas	

Table 13-3. Some Antiemetic Agents Useful in Chemotherapy-Induced Vomiting

Drug	Dosing	Side Effects	Comments
Prochlorperazine	10 mg p.o. q. 6 h 10 mg I.M. q. 4 h 25 mg rectal suppository b.i.d.	Sedation, Possible hypotension Extrapyramidal	*Pretreatment
Trimethobenzamide	250 mg p.o. q. 6 h 200 mg I.M. q. 6 h 200 mg rectal supp. q. 1 d	Extrapyramidal	
Haloperidol	2 mg p.o. q. 3 h × 8 doses 1–2 mg I.M. q. 4 h × 3 doses	Sedation/hypoactive Extrapyramidal	
Dexamethasone	10 mg I.M. × 2 doses 25 mg I.V. q. 6 h × 4 doses		*Pretreatment
Lorazepam	2–8 mg p.o. q. 4 h × 2 doses 2–4 mg I.V. × 1 dose	Sedative	*Pretreatment
Dephenhydramine	25–50 mg p.o. q. 3 h 25–50 mg I.M. q. 3 h	Sedative	*Pretreatment
Metoclopramide	20 mg p.o. q. 8 h 10 mg I.V. q. 2–4 h for 4 doses	Extrapyramidal	*Pretreatment

*Many of these drugs are useful in preventing nausea and vomiting or decreasing emetic response to chemotherapy if administered 15 min prior to treatment. Combinations may be more effective than single drugs. Treatment should be tailored to the individual patient unless participating in a research protocol studying efficacy of antiemetic regimens.

Anticancer drugs are also toxic to the rapidly multiplying cells of the G.I. epithelium. Mucositis and stomatitis range in severity from mild erythema to severe ulceration that may prevent eating and drinking. It occurs in about the same time frame as myelosuppression. Oral infections caused by candida albicans, herpes simplex, and varicella are not unusual and may confuse the clinical picture. Their diagnosis is important because they require specific treatment. Severe involvement of the G.I. tract may lead to diarrhea and/or G.I. bleeding. Paralytic ileus secondary to autonomic nervous dysfunction may complicate treatment with vinca alkaloids or DDP.

In general, the G.I. side effects of drugs are mild and self-limited, but at times, because of decreased food intake and increased G.I. losses of nutrients and fluids, patients may become malnourished or dehydrated. Hospitalization, I.V. hydration, supplemental feedings, or even parenteral nutrition may sometimes be necessary.

Nephrotoxicity

Renal damage may be caused by different mechanisms of a variety of antineoplastic drugs. MTX and its metabolites precipitate in the tubules and cause acute renal failure.[38] Vigorous hydration and alkalization of the urine may prevent this complication. DDP toxicity is due to coagulative necrosis of distal tubular epithelium and collecting ducts.[39] In addition, decreased renal perfusion and glomerular filtration are seen.[40] Vigorous hydration, along with mannitol and furosemide diuresis, has been used to limit the nephrotoxicity of DDP. More recently, it has been shown that simpler programs of saline hydration and diuresis have been as effective in maintaining glomerular filtration and preventing renal damage, especially if the dose of DDP is divided over several consecutive days. Intensive diuresis with drugs or osmotic agents may actually worsen fluid and electrolyte imbalances and increase toxicity. Cumulative renal toxicity may occur after several courses of DDP. Doses must be adjusted according to blood urea nitrogen, creatinine, and 24-hr urinary creatinine clearance. Because of potential additive renal damage, the concomitant use of nephrotoxic antineoplastics such as DDP with other nephrotoxic agents such as the aminoglycosides is contraindicated.

Hepatotoxicity

Hepatoxicity is most often reflected in elevated liver enzymes (SGOT, SGPT, alkaline phosphatase) and hyperbilirubinemia. Liver damage caused by MTX and L-asparaginase may be related to impairment of choline synthesis, leading to an inability to mobilize lipids and subsequent fatty infiltration.[41] As in renal failure, hepatic insufficiency may necessitate dose adjustments for drugs that are metabolized by the liver (e.g., ADR).

Pulmonary Toxicity

Subacute chronic pneumonitis and interstitial fibrosis is a dose-related pulmonary toxicity of BLM chemotherapy seen in up to 10% of patients who have received total doses of >450 mg.[42,43] This result may be related to the absence in lung of an enzyme that mediates the degradation of BLM in other tissues.[24] Progressive decline in diffusion capacity causes cough and dyspnea. Diffuse pulmonary fibrosis has also been seen following treatment with busulfan and MIT.[44,45] High levels of oxygen tension, which exacerbate pulmonary toxicity, may be mediated by the production of reactive oxygen radicals. The combination of XRT and chemotherapy with drugs such as BLM may also lead to increased pulmonary toxicity.

Cardiac Toxicity

Cardiac toxicity is seen predominantly with the anthracyclines ADR and daunorubicin. A rare early, acute syndrome, unrelated to dose, is manifested by dysrhythmias, conduction abnormalities, and pump failure within the first few hours after administration.[46] EKG findings include supraventricular tachyarhythmia, ventricular tachycardia, and heart block. Severe myocarditis and pericarditis with pericardial effusion have also been reported.[47] More common, however, is a cumulative dose-dependent, chronic cardiomyopathy that develops in patients who receive total doses of >550 mg/m^2.[48] Ejection fraction and pump function may be irreversibly diminished. Mortality may reach 45–50% of affected patients. Although <10% of patients who receive this total dose develop clinically apparent cardiac failure, the outcome is serious enough to militate against treating anyone beyond a total dose of 550 mg/m^2. In addition, a drop in ejection fraction of 10–15% from baseline, even at cumulative doses of <550 mg/m^2, is an indication to discontinue therapy.

One mechanism of this cardiac toxicity is related to the inability of myocardial cells—because they lack the enzyme catalase—to eliminate hydrogen peroxide and superoxide radicals produced after anthracycline exposure.[21] These chemicals are directly toxic to cells. Another possible mechanism of cell damage is related to the binding of anthracycline to components of the cell membrane—spectrin and the phospholipid cardiolipin.

Risk factors that may potentiate this cardiotoxicity include underlying cardiovascular disease, uncontrolled hypertension, mediastinal radiation, or coadministration of either CTX or MIT. Very high dose CTX as a single agent is cardiotoxic and may cause hemorrhagic myocardial necrosis.[49]

Neurotoxicity

The peripheral or central nervous system may be adversely affected by cancer chemotherapy. The vinca alkaloids cause a progressive and disabling peripheral neuropathy that is manifested in the early stages by decreased deep tendon reflexes progressing to paresthesias and weakness. Cranial nerve and laryngeal nerve palsies appear less commonly. Autonomic neuropathy, which may also be seen, is evidenced by dysfunctional G.I. motility/constipation, obstruction or paralytic ileus, and symptomatic postural hypotension.[50] Older patients, and patients with diabetes or medical problems that predispose to neuropathy, are at higher risk for developing such complications from the plant alkaloids. Treatment with DDP may also lead to distal sensory and autonomic neuropathy. A peripheral neuropathy that is milder but similar in nature may follow administration of ETO. 5-FU can cause acute neurological symptoms that include confusion and lethargy and also ataxia, particularly among elderly patients or those receiving intracarotid infusions.

CNS toxicity has been well described following intrathecal and high-dose systemic administration of drugs such as MTX and ara-C.[51] Acute symptoms of arachnoiditis, seizures, altered mental status, confusion, ataxia, and increased intracranial pressure may occur. Long-term side effects include cerebral atrophy, leukoencephalopathy with degenerative disease, and dementia. Concurrent whole brain irradiation and intrathecal chemotherapy, particularly with MTX, can lead to more severe neurological symptoms. Such side effects have been seen especially in children with acute lymphoblastic leukemia who have been treated with both of these modalities.

Other Toxicities

Among other side effects seen in patients receiving chemotherapy are allergic reactions, including hypersensitivity, urticaria, wheezing and hypotension, mild rashes, and fever. BLM and L-asparaginase are the 2 agents most frequently associated with these reactions. Some drugs have unique toxicities: Hemorrhagic cystitis is associated with CTX, ototoxicity with DDP, conjunctivitis with 5-FU, and unusual cutaneous reactions with BLM. Irritants, or drugs that cause burning or minor inflammation if extravasated during I.V. administration, include BCNU and dacarbazine (DTIC). The vesicants, or agents that can lead to local skin and subcutaneous tissue necrosis if extravasated, include the anthracyclines, vinca alkaloids, and nitrogen mustard. Extreme care must be taken to ensure proper administration.

A common side effect of chemotherapy is hair loss. It, too, is the result of drug action on rapidly proliferating cells, in this case the hair roots. Although it is not threatening to the patient's health, hair loss is often quite distressing and may be responsible for patient noncompliance with therapy.

In general, most drugs can cause a variety of toxicities, but changes in doses or schedules may prevent some of them. Clinicians who administer antineoplastic chemotherapy must be familiar with the range of possible toxicities and their appropriate medical management.

Pharmacodynamics

Dose/Response and Therapeutic Index

In general, tumor cell kill, or cytotoxicity (K), is a function of the concentration of drug (C) and the time of exposure to the drug (T):

$$K = C \times T$$

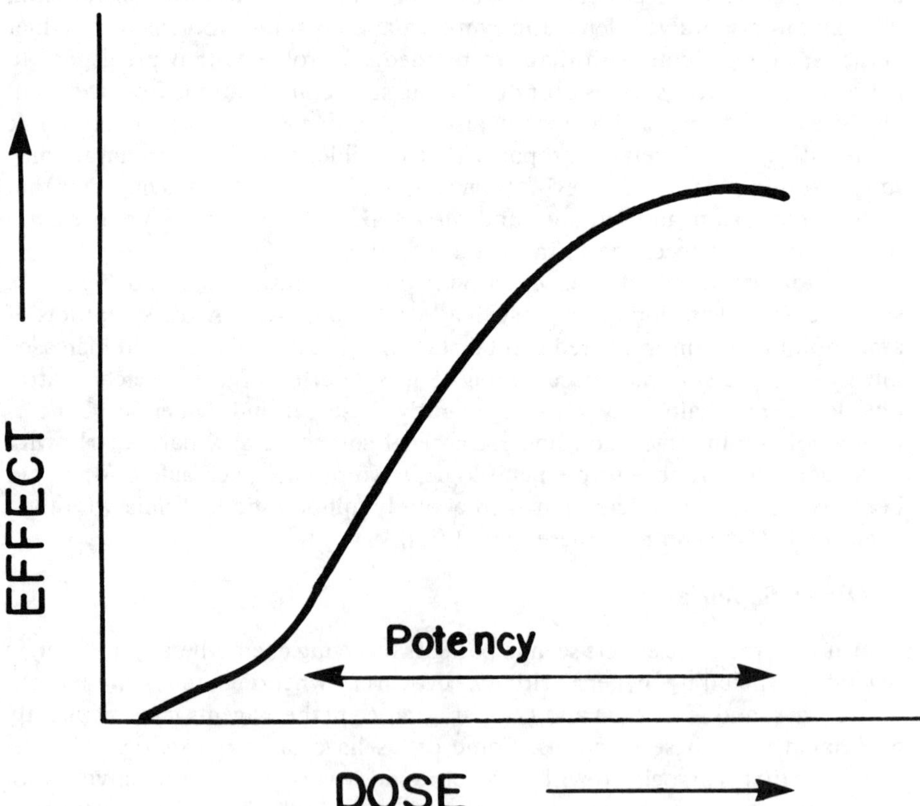

Figure 13-2. The dose/effect relationship.

For many drugs, this relation is applicable over a wide range of both concentrations and times. Increased cytotoxicity and therapeutic effect can be achieved by altering either the dose or the time of exposure to the drug. Because the mechanisms of action that account for an antineoplastic effect also damage normal cells, host toxicity may also be related to the concentration and time of drug exposure. Very high doses or prolonged drug exposure may lead to unacceptable toxicity and limit the clinical usefulness of certain chemotherapeutic regimens.

The dose/response curve of most anticancer drugs relates the effect of the drug—on both the host and the tumor—to the dose administered. This relation is determined by several factors, including characteristics of the drug itself, the target tissue, and the metabolic status of the host. The dose/response relationship applies over a wide range of drug doses; small changes in dose result in significant changes in effect. This is known as a *linear-log* dose/response effect. For example, doubling the dose increases the tumor cell kill by 10 times (1 log) (figure 13-2). Numerous examples of this principle are found in experimental animal studies,[52] and clinical studies in humans show the same relationship. In lymphomas, doubling the dose of the alkylating agent and the antimetabolite can lead to up to a 5-fold increase in tumor response rates.[53,54]

Two hypotheses have been advanced to explain the kinetics of cytotoxic drug cell kill. The principal hypothesis, proposed by Skipper et al, considers that a given dose of drug kills a constant fraction, not a constant number of tumor cells.[55] For example, a dose that reduces tumor cell mass from 10^9 to 10^7 cells will also reduce a mass of 10^6 cells to 10^4 cells. This hypothesis provides a rationale for the use of multiple cycles of cytotoxic chemotherapy. An

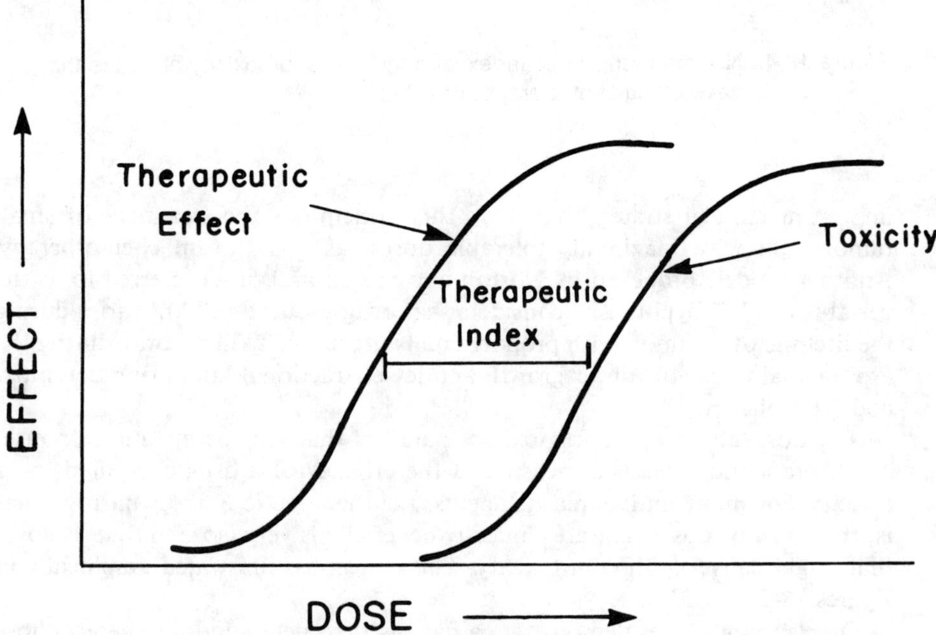

Figure 13-3. Wide therapeutic index with tolerable levels of toxicity at doses that have significant therapeutic effect.

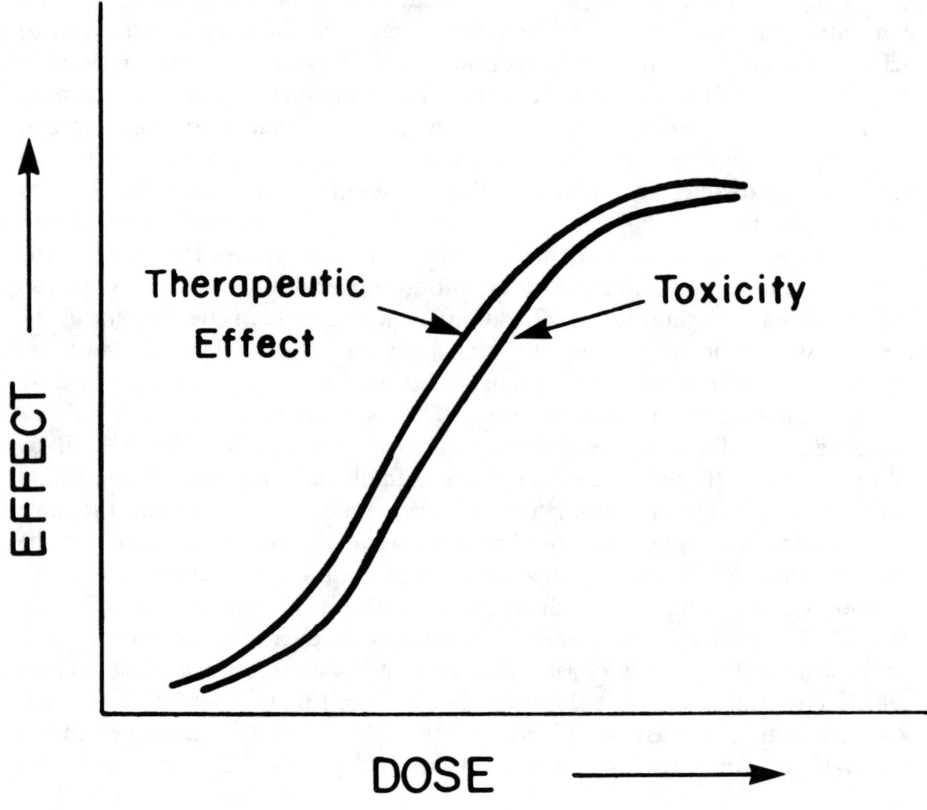

Figure 13-4. Narrow therapeutic index with high level of toxicity at doses that have significant therapeutic effect.

important clinical strategy based on this principle is the treatment of small tumor bulk with maximally tolerable doses, as in adjuvant chemotherapy. Another model, proposed by Norton and Simon and often referred to as the variable cell kill hypothesis, considers that drug-induced cell kill varies during the lifetime of a tumor, with proportionally greater cell kill midway during the exponential phase of tumor growth and lesser fractional kill during the initial and later phases.[56]

The dose/effect curve for toxicity parallels that for therapeutic response. The therapeutic index is a measure of the efficacy of a drug compared to its toxicity. For many antineoplastic agents, the therapeutic index is narrow; that is, the range of doses that are clinically beneficial is very close to that of doses that might cause significant toxicity. This concept is illustrated graphically in figures 13-3 and 13-4.

Overlapping curves demonstrate a narrow therapeutic index, whereas those that are widely separated demonstrate a more favorable index. In figure 13-3, maximum therapeutic effect is obtained by doses that produce little if any toxicity. On the other hand (figure 13-4), dose/response curves for therapeutic and toxic effects lie so close together that significant toxicity is also seen at every effective dose.

Doses for antitumor drugs are calculated on the basis of body surface area rather than weight. Body surface area (m^2), a function of both weight and height, correlates with cardiac output, an indirect measure of the rate of drug delivery to the kidneys and liver (principal organs of drug metabolism and elimination). The therapeutic effect, as well as the toxicity of equivalent doses based on body surface area, has demonstrated greater reproducibility between species as well as between individuals.

Table 13-4. Summary of Pharmacologic Principles

1. K = C × T

2. Dose/response curve for both therapeutic effect and toxicity follows first-order kinetics and a linear-log relationship

3. A constant fraction, not a constant number of cells, is killed with a given dose

4. Importance of maintaining dose/rate

5. Adjustment of schedules and/or dose if necessary to limit toxicities

6. Pharmacokinetics of absorption, distribution, metabolism, and elimination of drugs

Schedule Dependence

Generally, chemotherapy is administered in several cycles over periods of time lasting months to years. The periodic administration of drugs in this fashion constitutes the schedule of treatment. Manipulation of the schedule of drug administration provides one means of controlling toxicity without diminishing response. The dose rate is a reflection of both the amount of drug given at any one time and the interval between administration. The interval between doses allows recovery of host tissues from toxicity. The optimum dose rate should be maintained; lowering doses or prolonging treatment intervals may allow tumor regrowth and diminish therapeutic effect. This principle has been demonstrated in the analysis of clinical trials in breast cancer and Hodgkin's disease. Three drugs, CTX, MTX, and 5-FU (CMF), have been shown to be effective in the adjuvant treatment of breast cancer in premenopausal women. In patients who received <85% of the protocol dose over time, disease-free survival was significantly reduced.[57] Similarly, in the treatment of Hodgkin's disease, reductions in the dose rate of the MOPP combination (mechlorethamine + VCR + prednisone + procarbazine) led to decreases in tumor response and overall survival.[58]

Pharmacokinetics

Although the dose/effect curve for antineoplastic agents is largely determined by the kinetics of host cell and tumor cytotoxicity, other factors must be taken into account in the design of clinical chemotherapeutic regimens. The specific details of the regimen, not only the biochemical reactivity of the drug, but also the drug's bioavailability, distribution, metabolism, and excretion, have an impact on the regimen's therapeutic potential. The route of administration, whether oral, subcutaneous, intramuscular, intravenous, or intra-arterial, affects the rate of absorption into the circulation and subsequent plasma levels. Distribution into extravascular spaces, such as pleural effusions and ascites, may lead to prolonged effect and delayed toxicity as a result of delayed reentry of drugs into the circulation. For example, elevated serum levels and severe toxicity have been seen in patients with ascites or pleural effusions 2-3 wk after receiving conventional doses of MTX. The ability to cross the blood/brain barrier and achieve therapeutic levels in the CSF depends on the lipid solubility of a drug as well as the concentration gradient between serum and CSF. This determines the utility of systemically administered antineoplastic agents against primary and metastatic CNS malignancies. If therapeutic CSF levels cannot be attained, intrathecal or intraventricular administration may provide an alternative. Both MTX and ara-C have been shown to be effective against CNS disease and may be given either directly into the CSF or systemically in high doses.

The liver is essential to the activation or degradation of many commonly used chemotherapeutic agents. Abnormal liver function may require appropriate adjustments of certain drug doses. An example of this is ADR, which is partially eliminated by the liver. In patients with impaired liver function receiving ADR, plasma concentrations of the drug and its metabolites were 4–5 times higher than in patients with normal liver function, and they experienced more toxicity manifested by mucositis and myelosuppression.[59]

Similarly, abnormal renal function and inability to eliminate some drugs may lead to excessive and toxic levels of either the parent compound or metabolites. For example, DDP is excreted in the urine as the result of glomerular filtration. In patients with impaired renal function, the nephrotoxicity of DDP is further potentiated, and systemic toxicity, including myelosuppression, nausea and vomiting, and neurotoxicity, is worse.

Special methods of administration may be used to circumvent problems of systemic toxicity while achieving high levels of drug in localized sites. Intracavitary installation of drug directly into the peritoneal space to treat widespread intra-abdominal disease has been used in the treatment of ovarian cancer. Drugs with high molecular weight (e.g., DDP), are preferred because they do not readily diffuse into the systemic circulation. Concentrations of DDP in ascitic fluid reached 15 times those attained by I.V. administration, and systemic toxicity is acceptable.[60] Similarly, cytotoxic drug installation into the pleural and pericardial spaces has been used to control malignant effusions. Local tumor perfusion by arterial infusion is another means of maximizing drug delivery. Hepatic artery infusion with 5-FU and carotid artery infusion with DDP have been effective in the treatment of tumors localized to the liver or brain.[61,62]

Finally, the therapeutic index of antineoplastic drugs, like that of any pharmacologic agent, must be interpreted in the context of the patient's overall condition. A patient with poor performance status, such as an elderly, malnourished patient with multiple medical problems, will not tolerate antineoplastic therapy as easily as a relatively healthy younger patient. Even though expected response rates might be similar for both patients' tumors, the likelihood of toxicity and medical complication is clearly higher in the first case.

Combination Chemotherapy

The concept of combination chemotherapy evolved in response to both theoretical and practical considerations. In principle, improved therapeutic results can be obtained by combining several noncross-resistant drugs rather than a single agent. This concept had been successful in designing antibiotic combinations in the treatment of virulent infectious diseases. In oncology, combining drugs with different mechanisms of action might enhance antitumor activity as well as provide a means of overcoming tumor resistance. One strategy is to select agents that act at different points in vital biosynthetic and metabolic pathways of malignant cells; another is to select drugs that act against cells in different phases of the cell cycle.

In practice, the clinical utility of such combinations would be limited by toxicity. The selection of individual drugs that do not have overlapping toxicities is critical to the design of combination regimens. The 2-drug regimen of VLB + BLM used in the treatment of testicular carcinoma demonstrates the principles. These drugs show synergistic activity based on complementary mechanisms of action. VLB arrests cells in the mitotic phase of the cell cycle, then BLM kills them during mitosis. Furthermore, BLM is usually not myelosuppressive and does not add to the marrow toxicity of VLB. This combination regimen has produced complete response rates on the order of 40–50%, representing a significant advance in therapy.[63]

Although combination therapy has resulted in dramatic improvements in response rates of some tumors, later relapse is not uncommon. Attempts to prolong the duration of remissions and improve overall survival led initially to the concept of maintenance chemotherapy. Maintenace therapy is the continued administration of active anticancer drugs—at lower doses and longer intervals—for extended periods of time after initial induction of remission. The rationale for this practice is the notion that steady but low-level chemotherapy might eradicate any recurrence while tumor volume was still low, as predicted by the Gompertzian model of cell growth. Studies of maintenance treatment programs, however, have failed to show benefit except perhaps in the case of childhood acute lymphoblastic leukemia.

Late-intensification chemotherapy argues that active drugs are most effective when used at full intensity, a rationale based on the Norton and Simon hypothesis of variable cell kill outlined above. Unlike maintenance therapy, late-intensification protocols call for the repeated administration of full dose rates of agents used in induction treatment. The utility of this approach is under investigation in clinical trials in lymphoma and breast cancer.

To avoid the emergence of pleiotropic drug resistance, other efforts to increase patient survival include the use of alternating cycles of noncross-resistant combinations as proposed by Goldie and Coldman. This concept is currently being tested in Hodgkin's disease with the use of alternating cycles of MOPP with ABVD (ADR + BLM + VLB + DTIC). In one randomized clinical trial, complete remission rates and relapse-free survival were better at both 5- and 7-yr follow-ups in patients treated with MOPP/ABVD when compared to MOPP alone.[64] Similarly designed studies are underway for chemotherapy of solidtumors such as small-cell lung cancer and breast cancer.

In tumors that may be sensitive to hormonal manipulation, the combination of hormonal and systemic chemotherapy may have additive effect. The precise mechanisms of hormone action are poorly understood. Possible mechanisms include direct inhibition of tumor cell growth or recruitment of resting cells from the G-0 phase to the G-1, S or G-2 phases, thereby rendering them more susceptible to phase-specific cytotoxic agents. This relationship is currently being studied in postmenopausal women with breast cancer undergoing treatment with estrogens and drug combinations such as CTX + MTX + 5-FU (CMF).

Cytotoxic drug effect may also be enhanced by biochemical modulation of tumor cell metabolism. Dipyridamole inhibits the facilitated membrane transport of extracellular nucleotides, therefore preventing salvage from MTX-induced damage. Certain human cancers such as colorectal carcinoma show increased salvage enzyme activity. Combined treatment of these tumors with MTX and dipyridamole is currently under study in phase 1 and 2 trials.[65] Similarly, N-(phosphonacetyl)-L-aspartic acid (PALA), by inhibiting pyrimidine biosynthesis, can potentiate the cytotoxic effects of 5-FU.[65] However, although clinical trials so far have demonstrated increased antitumor activity using this approach, severe toxicities have been encountered. Other combinations being tested include 5-FU and LCV. In addition, recent in vitro studies demonstrate that alteration of intracellular glutathione (GSH) levels modulate the action of some chemotherapeutic drugs. For example, GSH depletion by addition of buthionine sulfoxamine sensitizes mouse tumor cells to phenylalanine mustard.[66] Clinical correlation is pending.

Adjuvant Chemotherapy

Adjuvant chemotherapy is the use of drugs in conjunction with potentially curative treatment for the primary tumor, usually surgery or XRT. The rationale for its use derives from the concept that microscopic metastatic disease is already present at the time of treatment for the primary tumor. In patients with primary breast cancer who have lymph node metastasis, the incidence of systemic recurrence is about 75% within 10 yr. Because antineoplastic agents are most effective against small tumor volume, the use of systemic chemotherapy immediately following primary tumor therapy leads to a greater chance of cure. In this context, chemotherapy probably has its maximum curative potential.

A good example of effective adjuvant chemotherapy is the postoperative use of regimens such as CMF in premenopausal women with breast cancer. Controlled clinical trials have shown an advantage in disease-free and overall survival for the treated women.[67] Similarly, the Gastrointestinal Tumor Study Group has demonstrated the benefit of postoperative XRT and 5-FU in the treatment of localized rectal cancer.

Multimodality Treatment

When chemotherapy is to be used as a single modality in the treatment of advanced disease, the principles outlined above pertain. The use of chemotherapy as part of a multimodality approach (along with surgery and/or XRT) requires other considerations. In combined modality treatment, the therapeutic index of each treatment should be optimized, rather than allowing decreases in the doses of either the radiation or the drugs. Regional irradiation and systemic chemotherapy have different mechanisms for cell kill and may have additive or synergistic effects. The simultaneous use of chemotherapy and XRT has been shown to enhance the radiation effect on experimental tumors.[68] For some drugs, this appears to be due to the reduction in the ability of cells to repair radiation damage. One mechanism of DDP activity is to inhibit repair of DNA damage, thus making this agent of use as a potential radiation sensitizer. In carcinomas of the head and neck, early studies of the concomitant use of XRT and DDP suggest possible improvement in responses. ACT inhibits repair of radiation-induced DNA damage and also adds to cytotoxicity. Combining preoperative XRT therapy and chemotherapy with MIT and 5-FU in the treatment of epidermoid cancer of the anal canal has been successful in achieving a high proportion of long-term survivors.[69] Other drugs act specifically to enhance radiation response by sensitizing hypoxic cells. Compounds such as metronidazole and misonidazole were shown both in vivo and in vitro to act as potent radiosensitizers. They mimic oxygen in their ability to release electrons and produce free radicals, which then damage DNA. Clinical trials to date have been inconclusive. The lack of benefit for misonidazole-treated groups may be related to the low cumulative doses of drug used.

An advantage to combined modality treatments lies in the complementary distribution their effects. Systemic chemotherapy is widely distributed in the body and may be effective against occult or micrometastases, whereas radiation is directed locally and may be applied to sanctuary sites such as the CNS. In Hodgkin's disease, for example, relapse-free survivals are higher in patients with stage I and IIa disease treated with both chemotherapy and XRT when compared to either modality alone. In acute lymphoblastic leukemia, both systemic chemotherapy and craniospinal irradiation produce long-term disease-free survival.[70]

Careful attention must be paid to potential additive toxicity of chemotherapy and radiation. Severe myelosuppression and mucositis are not uncommon in combined modality treatment. Furthermore, reactivation of radiation-induced tissue damage, or so-called recall toxicity, has been described for MTX, ACT, ADR, and BLM in a variety of tissues, including bone marrow, G.I. epithelium, and lung.

Clinical Development of Anticancer Drugs

After in vitro and early in vivo studies are completed, antineoplastic drugs must be evaluated for safety and efficacy in a sequence of clinical trials:[71]

- *Phase 1.* When a new drug is first tested in humans, it is done in the setting of a phase 1 trial. These trials are conducted in patients with advanced disseminated malignancies for whom standard treatment does not exist or is ineffective. Employing a schedule of dose escalation, the main scientific aim is to define the toxicity associated with drug treatment, in turn determining the maximum dose of the drug that can be administered without severe side effects. This is known as the maximum tolerated dose (MTD). For most clinically useful compounds, bone marrow toxicity is dose-limiting. When myelosuppression is the dose-limiting toxicity, treatment of 6–10 patients at or near the MTD is sufficient to establish a safe phase 2 dose. Toxicities other than myelosuppression may be more difficult to quantitate and may make determination of the MTD more difficult.
- *Phase 2.* Phase 2 studies have 2 distinct goals: the assessment of antitumor activity of the drug and the further definition of patterns of acute toxicity in patients who are less debilitated by their malignancies. Phase 2 studies also provide a mechanism for monitoring of chronic side effects.
- *Phase 3.* The endpoint of phase 3 studies is the comparison of efficacy of a single drug or a combination of drugs with that of standard treatment. These studies are usually conducted in a randomized fashion, with 1 group of patients randomly chosen to receive standard treatment (the control group) and the other receiving the study drug(s). Responses, response duration, and survival are assessed in phase 3 trials. The ultimate aim is to define the specific role of a given treatment in the therapy of a particular cancer.

Criteria for Tumor Response

Objective tumor responses are associated with improved patient survival. Standard criteria have been developed to evaluate results of clinical trials.[72] In the case of 2-dimensionally measurable disease such as pulmonary nodules on chest x-ray or cutaneous metastasis, the following definitions apply:

1. *Complete response* is defined as complete disappearance of all lesions for at least 1 mo.

2. *Partial response* is defined as a 50% decrease in the product of the greatest perpendicular diameters of 1 or more measurable lesions for at least 1 mo and not associated with new or increasing lesions elsewhere.

3. *Progressive disease* represents a 25% increase in the product of the greatest perpendicular diameters of measurable lesions or the development of new lesions.

4. *No change* or *stable disease* implies no measurable difference in tumor dimensions.

The criteria for response become more obscure when clearly defined and easily measurable lesions do not exist (e.g., bone metastasis). Patients are said to have "evaluable disease." Response criteria for evaluable disease include: (1) regression, defined as definite decrease in tumor size with no new lesions as judged by the investigators; and (2) progression, defined as definite increase relative to the smallest measurement or the occurrence of new lesions.

Most clinical trials require the presence of measurable disease to evaluate responses. In addition, the definition of *complete response* has become more strict, often requiring pathologic confirmation. This may in part explain changes seen in response rates observed with some treatment combinations used over a period of time.

Conclusion

Understanding the principles of chemotherapy requires an understanding of the interrelationships between tumor cell kinetics and cytotoxic drug pharmacology.

By predicting an increase in the number of dividing cells as a tumor shrinks in size, the Gompertzian model provides a rationale for the sequential use of nonphase-specific and phase-specific agents. The Skipper hypothesis of constant tumor cell kill suggests that maintenance treatment may be of benefit, whereas the Norton and Simon hypothesis of variable cell kill argues for continued intensive chemotherapy. In experimental systems, a steep dose/response relationship is seen for most anticancer drugs. In these systems, the maximum dose of drug compatible with host survival appears to be the optimum for achieving maximum tumor cell kill. Clinical approaches using this concept include intraperitoneal chemotherapy and selective tumor perfusion.

The limitations to chemotherapy are host toxicity and the emergence of tumor resistance. Host toxicity, which may be acute or chronic, arises because the mechanisms of cytotoxicity can affect both normal and malignant cells. The therapeutic index of a particular drug provides an estimate of its clinical efficacy compared to its systemic toxicity. Tumor drug resistance occurs by a variety of biochemical mechanisms, including defective transport, defective metabolism, and increased inactivation of cytotoxic drugs, as well as by increased DNA repair and altered target proteins. These mechanisms are induced by genetic changes, either occurring naturally or emerging due to selection pressures posed by cytotoxic drugs. Several strategies to overcome tumor resistance have evolved, including treatment with combinations of drugs acting at various sites of the tumor cell metabolism, biochemical modulation, and the combination of different treatment modalities. Future directions lie in the development of newer classes of cytotoxic drugs and combinations with other modalities such as biological response modifiers.

References

1. Bruce WR, Meeker BE, Valeriote FA. Comparison of the sensitivity of normal hematopoietic and transplanted lymphoma colony-forming cells to chemotherapeutic agents administered in vivo. J Natl Cancer Inst 1966; 37:233.
2. Hill BT, Baserga R. The cell cycle and its significance for cancer treatment. Cancer Treat Rev 1975; 2:159.
3. Tannock IF. Biology of tumor growth. Hosp Pract 1983; 81–93.
4. Goldie J, Coldman A. The genetic origin of drug resistance in neoplasms: implications for systemic therapy. Cancer Res 1984; 44:3643–4215.
5. Zaharko DS, Fung WP, Jang FM. Relative biochemical aspects of low and high doses of methotrexate in mice. Cancer Res 1977; 37:1602–07.
6. Schilsky RL, Bailey BD, Chabner BA. Methotrexate polyglutamute synthesis by cultured human breast cancer cells. Proc Natl Acad Sci USA 1980; 77:2919–22.
7. Pinedo HM, Zaharko DS, Bull JM, Chabner BA. The relative contribution of drug concentration and duration of exposure to mouse bone marrow toxicity during continuous methotrexate infusion. Cancer Res 1977; 37:445–450.
8. Mandel HG. Incorporation of 5-fluorouracil into RNA and its molecular consequences. Prog Mol Subcell Biol 1969; 1:82–135.
9. Speyer JL, Collins JM, Dedrick RL, et al. Phase I and pharmacologic studies of intraperitoneal 5-fluoruracil. Cancer Res 1980; 40:567–72.
10. Ensminger WD, Rosowsky A, Raso V. A clinical pharmacological evaluation of hepatic arterial infusion of 5-fluoro 2′-deoxyuridine and 5-fluorouracil. Cancer Res 1978; 38:3784–92.
11. Cohen SS. The lethality of ara nucleotides. Med Biol 1976; 54:299–326.
12. Fridland A. Inhibition of DNA chain initiation by 1-B-D-arabino furanosylcytosine (ara-C) in human lymphoblasts. J Supramol Struct 1978; 771:331.
13. Colvin M. A review of the pharmacology and clinical use of cyclophosphamide. In: Pinedo HM, ed. Clinical pharmacology of antineoplastic drugs. Amsterdam: Elsevier/North Holland, 1978; 245–61.
14. Cox PJ. Cyclophosphamide cystitis. Identification of acrolein as the causative agent. Biochem Pharmacol 1979; 28:2045–49.
15. Brock N, Pohl J, Stekar J. Detoxification of urotoxic oxazaphosphorines by sulfhydryl compounds. J Cancer Res Clin Oncol 1981; 100:311.
16. Scovell WM, O'Connor T. Interaction of aquated cis-[NH$_3$)$_2$PtII] with nucleic acid constituents: 1. Ribonucleosides. J Am Chem Soc 1977; 99:120–26.
17. Patton TF, Himmelstein KJ, Belt R, Bannister SJ, Sternson LA, Repta AJ. Plasma levels and urinary excretion of filterable platinum species following bolus injfection and I.V. infusion of cis-dichlorodiammine-platinum (II) in man. Cancer Treat Rep 1979; 63:1359–1361.
18. Jacobs C, Kalman SM, Tretton M, Weiner MW. Renal handling of cis-diamminedichloroplatinum (II). Cancer Treat Rep 1980; 64(12):1223–26.
19. Douple E, Richmond R. Radiosensitization of hypoxic tumor cells by cis- and trans-dichlorodiammine platinum II. Int J Rad Oncol Biol Phys 1979; 5:1369–72.
20. Pigram WJ, Fuller W, Amilton LDH. Stereochemistry of intercalation: interaction of daunomycin with DNA. Nature 1972; 235:17–19.
21. Lown JM, Sim S, Majumdar KC, Chung R. Strand scission of DNA by bound Adriamcyin and daunomycin in the presence of reducing agents. Biochem Biophys Res Commun 1977; 79:705–10.

22. Doroshow JH, Locker GY, Myers CE. Enzymatic defenses of the mouse heart against reactive oxygen: alterations produced by doxorubicin. J Clin Invest 1980; 65:128–35.

23. Murphree SA, Cunningham LS, Hwang KM, Sartorelli AC. Effects of Adriamycin on surface properties of sarcoma 180 ascites cells. Biochem Pharmacol 1976; 25:1227–31.

24. Takeshita M, Grollman AP, Ohtsubo E, Ohtsubo H. Interaction of bleomcyin with DNA. Proc Natl Acad Sci USA 1978; 75:5983–87.

25. Umezawa H, Hori S, Sawa T, Yoshioka T, Takeuchi T. A bleomycin-inactivating enzyme in mouse liver. J Antibiot 1974; 27:419–24.

26. Owellen RJ, Hartke CA, Dickerson RM, Hains FO. Inhibition tubulin-microtubule polymerization by drugs of the vinca alkaloid class. Cancer Res 1976; 36:1499–1502.

27. Castle MC, Margileth DA, Oliverio VT. Distribution and excretion of ^{3}H-vincristine in the rat and the dog. Cancer Res 1976; 36:3684–89.

28. Jackson DV, Castle MC, Bender RA. Biliary excretion of vincristine. Clin Pharmacol Ther 1978; 24:101–07.

29. Owellen RJ, Harke CA, Hains FO. Pharmacokinetics and metabolism of vinblastine in humans. Cancer Res 1977; 37:2567–2602.

30. Drewinko B, Barlogie B. Survival and cycle-progression delay of human lymphoma cells in vitro exposed to VP–16–213. Cancer Treat Rep 1976; 60:1295–1306.

31. D'Incalci M, Farina P, Sessa C, et al. Pharmacokinetics of VP16–123 given by different administration methods. Cancer Chemother Pharmacol 1982; 7:141.

32. Hann HE Jr. Comparison of biochemical and biological effects of four nitrosoureas with differing carbamoylating activities. Cancer Res 1978; 38:2363–66.

33. Ohnuma T, Holland JF, Sinks LF. Biochemical and pharmacological studies with L-asparaginase in man. Cancer Res 1970; 30:2297–2305.

34. Goldie JH, Coldman AJ. The genetic origin of drug resistance in neoplasms: Implications for systemic therapy. Cancer Res 1984; 44:3643–53.

35. Deuchars KL, Ling V. P-glycoprotein and multiple drug resistance in cancer chemotherapy. Semin Oncol 1989; 16:156–65.

36. Wang SC. Emetic and antiemetic drugs. In: Root WS, Hofmann FE, eds. Physiological pharmacology. vol 2. New York: Academic Press, 1965; 255–328.

37. Wang SC, Renzi AA, Chinn SI. Mechanism of emesis following X-irradiation. Am J Physiol 1958; 193:335–39.

38. Bleyer WA. The clinical pharmacology of methotrexate. Cancer 1978; 41:36–51.

39. Gonzalez-Vitale JC, Hayes DM, Cvitkovic E, Sternberg SS. The renal pathology in clinical trials of cis-platinum (II) diamminedichloride. Cancer 1977; 39:1362–71.

40. Madias NE, Harrington JT. Platinum nephrotoxicity. Am J Med 1979; 65:307–14.

41. Dahl MGC, Gregory MM, Scheuer PJ. Liver damage due to methotrexate in patients with psoriasis. Br Med J 1971; 1:625–30.

42. DeLena M, Guzzon A, Monfardini S. Clinical, radiologic, and histopathologic studies on pulmonary toxicity induced by treatment with bleomycin. Cancer Chemother Rep 1972; 56:343–56.

43. Luna MA, Bedrossian CW, Lichtiger B. Interstitial pneumonitis associated with bleomycin therapy. Am J Clin Pathol 1972; 58:501–10.

44. Littler WA, Ogilvie C. Lung function in patients receiving busulfan. Br Med J 1970; 4:530–32.

45. Andrews AT, Bowman HS, Patel SB. Mitomycin and interstitial pneumonitis. Ann Intern Med 1979; 90:127.

46. Cortes EP, Lutman G, Wanka J, et al. Adriamycin cardiotoxicity: a clinicopathologic correlation. Cancer Chemother Rep (pt 3) 1975; 6:215–25.

47. Bristow MR, Thompson PD, Martin RP, et al. Early anthracycline cardiotoxicity. Am J Med 1978; 65:823–32.

48. Von Hoff DD, Rozencweig M, Layard DW, et al. Daunomycin-induced cardiotoxicity in children and adults. A review of 110 cases. Am J Med 1977; 62:200–10.

49. Buckner CD, Rudolph RH, Fefer A, et al. High-dose cyclophosphamide therapy for malignant disease. Cancer 1972; 29:357–65.

50. Weiss HD, Walker MD, Wiernik PH. Neurotoxicity of commonly used antineoplastic agents. N Engl J Med 1974; 291:127–33.

51. Bleyer WA, Drake JC, Chabner BA. Neurotoxicity and elevated cerebrospinal-fluid methotrexate concentration in meningeal leukemia. N Engl J Med 1973; 289:770–73.

52. Schabel FM Jr, Simpson-Herren L. Some variables in experimental tumor systems which complicate interpretation of data from in vivo kinetic and pharmacologic studies with anticancer drugs. Antibiot Chemother 1978; 23:113–27.

53. Brindley CO et al. Further comparative trial of thio-phosphoramide and mechlorethamine in patients with melanoma and Hodgkin's disease. J Chron Dis 1964; 17:19.

54. Frei E III, Spurr Cl, Brindley CO, et al. Clinical studies of dichloromethotrexate (NSC 29630). Clin Pharmacol Ther 1965; 6:160–71.

55. Skipper ME, Schabel FM Jr, Wilcox WS. Experimental evaluation of potential anticancer agents. XII. On the criteria and kinetics associated with "curability" of experimental leukemia. Cancer Chemother Rep 1964; 35:3–11.

56. Norton L, Simon R. Tumor size, sensitivity to therapy and design of treatment schedules. Cancer Treat Rep 1977; 61:1307–17.

57. Bonadonna G, Valagussa P. Dose-response effect of CMF in breast cancer. Proc Am Soc Clin Oncol 1980; 21:413.

58. DeVita VT. The consequences of the chemotherapy of Hodgkin's disease. Cancer 1981; 47:1–13.

59. Benjamin RS. Pharmacokinetics of Adriamycin in patients with sarcomas. Cancer Chemother Rep 1974; 58:271–73.

60. Howell SB, Pfeifle L, Wung WE, et al. Intraperitoneal cisplatin with systemic thiosulphate protection. Ann Intern Med 1982; 97:845.

61. Feun LG, Wallace S, Steward DJ, et al. Phase I-II trial of intracarotid cisdiamminedichloroplatinum (CDDP) in patients with intracerebral tumors (abstr). Proc Amer Soc Clin Oncol 1982; 1:197.

62. Ensminger WD, Rosowsky A, Raso V. A clinical pharmacological evaluation of hepatic arterial infusion of 5 fluoro 2'-deoxyuridine and 5-fluorouracil. Cancer Res 1978; 38:3784–92.

63. Samuels ML, Johnson DE, Holoye PY. Continuous intravenous bleomycin therapy with vinblastine in stage III testicular neoplasia. Cancer Chemother Rep 1975; 59:563–70.

64. Bonadonna G, Viviani S, Bofante V, et al. Alternating chemotherapy with MOPP/ABVD in Hodgkin's disease: updated results. Proc Am Soc Clin Oncol 1984; 3:254.

65. Muggia FM. Personal communication.

66. Washington Phase I Meeting, 1985. Unpublished data.

67. Henderson IC, Canellos GP. Medical progress, cancer of the breast: the past decade. N Engl J Med 1980; 302:17–30, 78–90.

68. Looney WB, Hopkins HA. Modifications of radiotherapy by radiosensitizers and cancer chemotherapeutic agents. II. Cancer chemotherapeutic agents. Semin Oncol 1989; 16:176–79.

69. Nigro ND, Seydel HG, Considine B, et al. Combined preoperative radiation and chemotherapy for squamous cell carcinoma of the anal canal. Cancer 1983; 51:1826–29.

70. Willoughby MLN. Treatment of overt CNS leukemia. In: Mastrangelo R, Poplack DG, Riccardi R, eds. Central nervous system leukemia: prevention and treatment. Boston: Martinus-Nijhoff. 1983; 113–22.

71. Piantadosi S. Principles of clinical trial design. Semin Oncol 1988; 15:423–33.

72. Marsoni S, Wittes R. Clinical development of anticancer agents. A National Cancer Institute perspective. Cancer Treat Rep 1984; 68:77–84.

73. Livingston R, Carter S. Experimental design and clinical trials: clinical perspectives. Clinical Perspectives. In: Carter S, Glatstein E, Livingston R, eds. Clinical perspectives. New York: McGraw Hill, 1982.

14

SUPPORTIVE CARE OF THE
CANCER PATIENT

Thomas J. Forlenza, M.D., F.A.C.P.

DURING THE USUALLY LENGTHY course of the disease, the patient with cancer experiences many complications of treatment and of progressive disease. Treatment modalities are necessarily aggressive, bringing with them not only social and psychological problems that are too easily ignored in a highly scientific environment but also medical complications of multiple organ system failure.[22]

This chapter takes up the topic of supportive care of the cancer patient, giving special attention to problems associated with nutritional support, control of pain, and the use of blood and blood components. It is the role of the oncology team to support the cancer patient throughout all phases of a disease that more than 60% of the time ends in death.

Nutritional Support

Cachexia, which leads to much debility in the oncology patient, is not simply an effect of anorexia and decreased intake;[24] tumor factors not yet identified play a role.[1] Much controversy surrounds nutritional support in the treatment of cancer patients, but most authors agree that it is indicated only when there is good evidence that the treatment will be effective and potentially curative—e.g., the patient undergoing bone marrow transplantation who develops severe enteritis, or the young male with severe vomiting from the treatment of testicular carcinoma.[2,3] Parenteral nutrition has been shown to decrease the rates of postoperative wound infection, pneumonia, major

399

complications, and mortality.[5,6,12] If treatment is not curative, enteral or parenteral supplementation may render the treatment slightly more effective,[4] but the overall benefit to the patient is minimal and may be detrimental.[29]

One should keep in mind, however, that the patient's well-being and self-esteem may be boosted by concern for his eating habits and caloric intake. Withdrawal of enteral support may be interpreted by the patient as abandonment.

It is understood that controlling nausea and vomiting when present is the first step toward improving the patient's nutritional status. A significant number of agents belonging to 7 different pharmacologic classes of compounds are currently available (see Appendix). A new agent, ondansetron (GR38032F), is now available.[30] These agents can control and possibly prevent such symptoms in patients receiving chemotherapy agents known for their frequent emetic effect. However, these measures are often expensive, not available, or inconvenient to the patient, and in any case will not have a bearing on the overall outcome of the disease.[11] Indeed, a clinician would not decide to initiate nutritional support based on any of the above-mentioned variables; they would serve merely to place the patient's nutritional status in perspective. Short-term nutritional support probably does not have a significant effect on tissue repletion.[3]

Pain Control

Pain is the subjective experience of discomfort. Among the many reasons for pain in the cancer patient are direct tumor infiltration of various anatomical regions; pain associated with the side effects of chemotherapy; and noncancer-related causes of pain, such as osteoarthritis and nonspecific headache.[13] The patient's mood and perception of the pain and what it does or might mean will color his experience.[14] Pain represents a significant problem in 33% of patients undergoing active therapy and in 60–80% of patients with terminal illness.[15] Two-thirds of pain is the result of direct tumor involvement and one-fourth results from cancer therapy.[16]

Understanding the multiple reasons for cancer pain will, it is to be hoped, lead to a rational approach to pain control. Mechanical problems should be addressed first:

- Is the patient comfortable in bed? Many patients are confined to bed and are unable to move on their own. Decubital ulcers can be prevented by repositioning, providing a water bed, or asking the patient to roll from side to side during daily physical examinations or other care procedures.
- Does the patient have a fracture? Repair of a fracture and treatment of a painful bone lesion with radiation may greatly improve the overall well-being of the patient.
- Does the patient have normal bowel function? Pain medications frequently cause constipation, but very effective bowel cathartics are available (e.g., milk of magnesia, cascara, lactulose). The patient should use these to be as regular as he was before he became ill.

Psychological factors are very important. The clinician should be cheerful when visiting a patient, giving good news whenever possible, and being especially caring when a poor result must be reported. How are family members interacting with the patient? How are they responding to his illness? How does the patient perceive his family and the new relationship he has taken on with them?[23]

These lists and questions could go on and on. The basic message is that the clinician must know the patient's medical, social, family, and psychological status at all times and think about these each day. It may not be necessary to act on these data each day, but an attempt should be made to view the patient as a whole human being and not a "breast case" or a "gastric cancer." Why emphasize the diseased part of the person and forget about the rest of his being that is not diseased?

There are specific, stepwise approaches to analgesia once the above factors have been considered. If a remediable cause of pain or discomfort is not identified, it is not unreasonable to start with prostacyclin inhibitors such as aspirin or a nonsteroidal anti-inflammatory agent such as ibuprofen or acetaminophen with codeine. Communication with the patient will be the guide as to when to advance to the next line of treatment. Hydromorphine and meperidine, and then methadone, should be tried (see Appendix). Medications should be given regularly, not p.r.n. The patient should not be awakened at night for the administration of pain medications. Various routes of administration are available. The intramuscular route may provide quick relief of pain and should be used in extreme circumstances; however, liquid preparations may be better tolerated. If a patient cannot swallow, most medications are available for rectal administration or can be compounded. Long-acting preparations that are also available have better compliance.

Use of nonnarcotic agents, such as phenytoin for specific nerve syndromes, phenothazines for their sedative and antiemetic effect, haloperidol for its antipsychotic effect, and amitriptyline for its use in peripheral nerve syndromes, should be considered.[17]

One of the best combinations of agents used to control persistant pain in patients with malignant tumors consists of:

- A long-acting narcotic given around the clock (e.g., long-acting morphine sulfate 60 mg p.o. q. 8 hr or methadone 5 mg p.o. q. 6 hr)
- A nonsteroidal, nonnarcotic analgesic (e.g., ibuprofen 400 mg p.o. q. 4–5 hr)
- A hypnotic sedative such as lorazepam 1 mg p.o. q. 12 hr
- Finally, a short-acting narcotic analgesic (e.g., hydromorphone 4 mg p.o. q. 4 hr or meperidine 100 mg p.o. q. 4 hr) should also be prescribed p.r.n.

More complicated procedures (e.g., continuous epidural[27] and intrathecal morphine infusions and—extremely rarely—hypophysectomy or surgical and chemical cordotomy) should be considered only in very specific instances. Adequate relief is usually possible with narcotic analgesics given in adequate doses.[28]

Behavioral modification modalities such as hypnosis, cognitive behavior training, and biofeedback are interesting and deserve consideration, but are not available to or appropriate for the typical cancer patient with a pain control problem.

Keeping the overall well-being of the patient in mind will dictate which treatment modality to use.

Use of Blood and Blood Products

The same guidelines for the use of blood and blood components apply in the cancer patient as in any other patient. Red blood cells are given to increase the oxygen-carrying capacity of the blood, platelets to aid hemostasis, and fresh frozen plasma to replace coagulation factors.

Metastatic cancer and cancer therapies can cause bone marrow suppression. Treatment-induced cytopenias can be predicted fairly well with normal bone marrow reserve. Nadirs in the WBC and platelet count are predictable 7–10 days after the administration of chemotherapy. Quite often, treatment-induced cytopenias will require the transfusion of packed red blood cells and platelets. Leukocyte transfusions are rarely required. Specific stimulating factors (e.g., erythropoitin and GM-CSF) are now available to treat cytopenias.

Red Cell Transfusion

It may be difficult to assess oxygen requirements, but in the presence of sepsis, acute surgery, and fever, the demand will be greater, and maintaining a hematocrit of 25–30% will make the patient feel better. Rubenstein et al suggest that there is a higher incidence of retinal hemorrhage in the presence of both thrombocytopenia and anemia; they recommend keeping the hemoglobin >8 mg/100 ml.[18] In a chronic setting, there is an increase in erythrocyte diphosphoglycerate, and oxygen is more easily released at any given level of PaO2, therefore eliminating the acute need for transfusion in many instances.[1,3]

Platelet Transfusion

A decrease in the platelet count predictably will prolong the bleeding time, which measures in vivo platelet function. In the presence of normal platelet function, no aspirin intake, and normal renal functioning, there should be adequate hemostasis with a platelet count of $\geq 100,000$/ml. Major surgery requires a platelet count of $>100,000$/ml and should not be undertaken with values less than this in a nonemergency setting.

During the induction phase of acute leukemia or while waiting for engraftment after bone marrow transplantation, it is necessary to keep the platelet count at $\geq 20,000$/ml. Gaydos found a quantitative relationship between the platelet count and the occurrence of hemorrhage in the leukemia patient, especially when the count was $<20,000$/ml.[19] Platelet counts of 5,000–20,000/ml were, however, not associated with intracranial bleeding. Because of the decreased survival time of platelets in the presence of fever, hemorrhage, and antibiotic usage and the increased incidence of bleeding, it is good practice to monitor the platelet count on a daily basis and maintain a level of $>20,000$/ml.

The use of HLA (histocompatibility leukocyte antigen)-matched platelets is required only when there is evidence of refractoriness to platelet transfusion manifested by an insignificant rise in the platelet count after transfusion. Under normal circumstances, there should be a rise of 5,000–7,000/ml in the platelet count per unit of platelets transfused. For example, the transfusion of 10 U of platelets should raise the platelet count to 50,000–70,000/ml. This does not hold in the face of fever, sepsis, acute hemorrhage, hypersplenism, or diffuse intravascular coagulation (DIC).

Plateletpheresis provides a single donor source for platelets. This is not indicated unless there is refractoriness to platelet transfusion and an HLA-compatible donor is available. Usually, a family member is the most likely donor.

Regardless of the source of the platelets, a platelet count should be obtained at 1 hr and 24 hr post-transfusion to help ascertain the presence of alloimmunization. This "quick method" to determine refractoriness will hold only if there is no hypersplenism, acute hemorrhage, fever, sepsis, or DIC. In the absence of these clinical settings, the count does provide an estimate of post-transfusion platelet survival and should be used as a guideline for using HLA-matched platelet transfusions.

Granulocyte Transfusion

A quantitative relationship exists between the number of circulating granulocytes and the incidence of infection.[20] When the absolute granulocyte count is <500/ml, the patient is at increased risk for infection. Reverse isolation, consisting of strict handwashing and masks for visitors or staff members with upper respiratory infections, is recommended. The patient should not be placed in strict isolation because it is inconvenient for the staff to visit him and his care will suffer.

Granulocyte transfusions are associated with major toxicities of fever, pulmonary infiltrates, and an increased incidence of cytomegalovirus infection. It is difficult to obtain leukocytes for transfusion, and voluntary donors must take either steroids or hydroxyethyl starch to increase the yield.

It is strongly believed that there is no role for the routine use of granuylocyte transfusions, and their therapeutic efficacy has been questioned.

Bone Marrow Transplantation

It is now possible to cryopreserve autologous bone marrow for salvage after high-dose chemotherapy. This procedure requires a staff well acquainted with the method and with access to the equipment needed to preserve the bone marrow. The procedure is limited to specialized centers. To date, it led to lasting complete remissions after failures to aggressive conventional therapy in patients with Hodgkin's lymphoma, acute myelogenous leukemia without HLA match, and in a few cases of aggressive carcinoma of the breast and glioblastoma multiforme.[21]

Allogeneic bone marrow transplantation offers the only known method of cure for chronic myelogenous leukemia, aplastic anemia, and certain cogenital deficiencies. The equipment and staff required are more sophisticated than for autologous transplantation, and the use of this technique requires serious discussion between the patient and his or her physician. The procedure carries a 40–50% mortality 3 mo post-transplant and is associated with significant morbidity. It is, however, the only known cure for the above diseases. Autologous bone marrow transplantation is associated with less mortality but significant morbidity.

References

1. Theologides A. Pathogenesis of cachexia in cancer. Cancer 1972; 29:484–88.
2. Brennan MF. Total parenteral nutrition in the cancer patient. N Engl J Med 1981; 305 (7):375–82.
3. Nixon DW, Moffitt S, Lawson DH, et al. Total parenteral nutrition as an adjunct to chemotherapy of metastatic colorectal cancer. Cancer Treat Rep 1981; 65 (suppl 5):121–28.
4. Buzby GP, Mullen JL, Stein PT, Miller EE, Hobbs CL, Rosato EF. Host-tumor interaction and nutrient supply. Cancer 1980; 45:2940–48.
5. Muller JM, Brenner U, Dienst C, Pichlmaier H. Preoperative parenteral feeding in patients with gastrointestinal carcinoma. Lancet, 1982.
6. Mullen JL, Buzby GP, Mathews DC, et al. Reduction of operative morbidity and mortality in combined preoperative and postoperative nutritional support. Ann Surg 1980; 192:604.
7. Shetty PS, Watrasiewicz KE, Jung RT, James WPT. Rapid-turnover transport proteins: an index of subclinical protein-energy malnutrition. Lancet 1979; 2:230.
8. Grant JP, Custer PB, Thurlow J. Current techniques of nutritional assessment. Surg-Clin-North Am 1981; 61:437.
9. Ingenbleek Y, Van Den Schrieck HG, De Nayer P, DeVisscher M. Albumin, transferrin and thyroxine-binding prealbumin/retinol-binding protein (TBPA-RBP) complex in assessment of malnutrition. Clinica Chimica Acta 1975; 63:61–67.
10. Wilson RE, Christensen C, LeBlare LP. Oxygen consumption in critically ill surgical patients. Ann Surg 1972; 176:801.
11. Nixon DW, Heymsfield SB, Cohen AE, et al. Protein-calorie undernutrition in hospitalized cancer patients. Am J Med 1980; 68:683–90.
12. Harvey KB, Bothe A, Blackburn GL. Nutritional assessment and patient outcome during oncological therapy. Cancer 1979; 43:2065–69.
13. Payne R, Foley K. Advances in the management of cancer pain. Cancer Treat Rep 1984; 68:173–83.
14. Spiegel D, Bloom JR. Pain in metastatic breast cancer. Cancer 1983; 52:341–45.
15. Foley KM. Pain syndromes in patients with cancer. In: Bonica JJ, Ventafriddo V, eds. Advances in pain research and therapy. vol. 2. New York: Raven Press, 1979.
16. Kanner RM, Foley KM. Patterns of narcotic drug use in a cancer pain clinic. JN research development in drug alcohol use. Ann N.Y. Acad Sci 1981; 362:162–82.
17. Watson PC, Evans RJ, Reed K, Merskey H, Goldsmith L, Warsh J. Amitriptyline versus placebo in posttherpetic neuralgia. Neurology (NY) 1982; 32:671–3.
18. Rubenstein RA, Ranoff M, Albert DM. Thrombocytopenia, anemia, and retinal hemorrhage. Am J Opththalmol 1968; 65:435–49.
19. Gaydos LS, Freireich EJ, Mantel N. The quantitative relation between platelet count and hemorrhage in patients with acute leukemia. N Engl J Med 1962; 266:905–09.
20. Bodey GP, Buckley M, Sathe YS, et al. Quantitative relationships between circulatory leukocytes and infections in patients with acute leukemia. Ann Intern Med 1966; 64:328–40.
21. Appelbaum FR, Buckner CD. Overview of the clinical relevance of autologous bone marrow transplantation. Clin Hematol 1986; 15:1–18.
22. Levy M, Catalano B. Control of common physical symptoms other than pain in patients with terminal disease. Semin Oncol 1985; 12(4):411–30.
23. Taylor AG, Lorentzen LJ, Blank MB. Psychologic distress of chronic pain sufferers and their spouses. J Pain Sympt Manage Feb 1990; 5(1):6–10.

24. Bruera E, Brennis C, Michaud M, et al. Association between asthenia and nutritional status, lean body mass, anemia, psychological status and tumor mass in patients with advanced breast cancer. J Pain Sympt Manage Jun 1989; 4(2):59–63.
25. Bruera E, Brennis C, Michaud M, MacDonald RN. Influence of the pain and symptom control team (PSCT) on the patterns of treatment of pain and other symptoms in a cancer center. J Pain Sympt Manage Sept 1989; 4(3):112–16.
26. Dorrepaal KL, Aaronson NK, et al. Pain experience and pain management among hospitalized cancer patients: a clinical study. Cancer 1989; 63:593–98.
27. Wermiling DP, Foster TS, et al. Drug delivery for intractable cancer pain: use of new disposable parenteral infusion device for continuous outpatient epidural narcotic infusion. Cancer 1987; 60:875–78.
28. Swanson G, Smith J, et al. Patient-controlled analgesia for chronic cancer pain in the ambulatory setting: a report of 117 patients. J Clin Oncol 1989; 7:1903–08.
29. Baron PL, Lawerence W Jr, et al. Effects of parenteral nutrition on cell cycle kinetics of head and neck cancer. Arch Surg 1986; 121:1282–86.
30. Cubeddu LX, Hoffman IS, et al. Efficacy of ondansetron (GR38032F) and the role of serotonin in cisplatin-induced nausea and vomiting. N Engl J Med 1990; 322:810–16.

15

PSYCHOLOGICAL DISORDERS IN CANCER PATIENTS

Ramaswamy Viswanathan, M.D., D.Sc.

ATTENTION TO PSYCHOSOCIAL FACTORS in the care of cancer patients is an important aspect of care. Such attention is necessary because of the high degree of stress faced by the patient, the family, and health care personnel, and the high incidence of psychological disorders in these patients.[1,2] In a study involving inpatients and outpatients in 3 cancer centers (excluding patients with a high degree of physical disability or whose condition was terminal), 47% of the subjects were found to have a diagnosable psychiatric disorder.[3] This incidence is twice the rate typically reported for medical patients and 3 times the estimate for the general population. Of the total studied, 32% were found to have adjustment disorder with significant anxiety or depression, 6% had major depression, and 4% had an organic mental disorder.

For most psychiatric disorders, it is best that the physician seek psychiatric consultation. Nevertheless, the primary physician should be familiar with the nature of the disorder and its treatment so that he or she can play an active treatment role even when a psychiatrist or another mental health professional is the primary care giver for the psychological disorder. Using this focus, this chapter will cover the diagnostic issues and the principles of psychological and pharmacological treatment as they pertain to common disorders in cancer patients.

Psychodynamics of Stress in Cancer Patients

Stressors Affecting the Cancer Patient

In order to help the patient, the physician must understand the nature of stressors the patient faces and those faced by the family and the treatment staff,

406

Table 15-1. Losses and Threatened Losses Faced by Cancer Patients

- Life
- Sense of well-being, bodily integrity, bodily functions
- Intellect
- Self-esteem, autonomy, sense of usefulness and purpose
- Family and social roles and relationships
- Financial
- Control over life, health, and relationships

as well as be familiar with the resources available for coping with these stressors.[1,4] The diagnosis of cancer raises the specter of death in most people's minds. Even though great strides have been made in the treatment and cure of various cancers, the fear of death remains a major factor. In addition, depending on the nature of the disease, the stage, and the treatment, as well as the patient's life situation, the patient must face many losses or threats of loss (table 15-1). To this must be added the stress of pain and other physical distress and the fear of the unknown. Underlying it all is the distress produced by a sense of lack of control.[5,6]

Coping Mechanisms

Coping and defense mechanisms are protective mechanisms instituted by the mind to reestablish equanimity when faced with a stressor, just as the body mobilizes some defensive physiological processes to maintain homeostasis when faced with a stressor. Coping refers to conscious attempts by the individual to ward off dysphoria (anxiety and depression), whereas defense mechanisms refer to unconscious mental mechanisms. Because a mechanism often has both conscious and unconscious aspects, the 2 terms will be used somewhat interchangeably in this discussion.

Coping mechanisms can be divided into instrumental and palliative coping mechanisms (figure 15-1). In instrumental coping, the person takes action on the environment to correct the situation causing the dysphoria. In palliative coping, the individual engages in a mental mechanism that changes his perception of a situation but does not change the situation itself. Instrumental coping is somewhat analogous to curative surgery, whereas palliative coping could be compared with taking analgesics for cancer pain. Both kinds of coping are important for proper functioning, and often both are required.

A coping or defense mechanism may be adaptive or maladaptive. A maladaptive mechanism is characterized by one or more of the following:

1. It fails to contain the distress or may even increase the distress.

2. It interferes with proper treatment.

3. It interferes unduly with everyday functions (work, interpersonal relationships, sources of gratification).

4. It results in psychosis (severe impairment of reality testing).

Instrumental coping should be used whenever it is appropriate. A woman noticing a lump in her breast and immediately arranging an appointment with

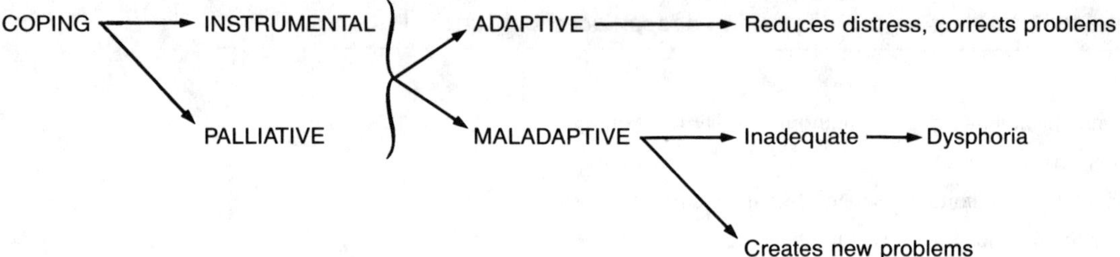

Figure 15-1. Coping mechanisms.

a physician is an example of adaptive instrumental coping. If she ignores it, thinking it will go away, she is engaging in maladaptive palliative coping. In many situations, not much can be done to partially or entirely correct the situation; in these cases, the patient has to mitigate suffering by palliative coping mechanisms. In some cases, severe dysphoria due to failure of palliative coping can interfere with whatever instrumental coping mechanisms are called for in the situation. For example, a 40-year-old woman with suspected pituitary tumor was so emotionally distraught that she fled from a scheduled radiological examination.

Following are some defense or coping mechanisms found in cancer patients: Denial or minimization, suppression, distraction, selective attention (e.g., optimism and faith), compartmentalization, rationalization, displacement, projection, delusions, seeking relevant information, learning specific procedures, setting concrete and limited goals, rehearsing alternative outcomes, anticipatory mourning, sharing of emotions, use of support systems, focus on living, altruism, and finding meaning and purpose in life.[4-7] Of these, only denial and displacement are discussed here because of space limitations. The reader is referred to references 4–7 for discussion of other mechanisms.

Denial is an unconscious defense mechanism by which the full available information is kept from conscious awareness and the patient behaves as if that information were not true. Denial may be cognitive or affective. An example of cognitive denial is a patient denying the fact that he has cancer or is seriously ill, even after being presented with information to the contrary. In affective denial, even though a person intellectually accepts a fact, at an emotional level he does not believe in it, i.e., he behaves as though that information is not really true, at least for him at that time. An example of affective denial is a physician smoking. Denial can be partial, and there are varying degrees of denial. For example, a patient may cooperate with surgery or radiotherapy or chemotherapy and still maintain that he does not have lung cancer but only pneumonia or flu. Another may acknowledge that he has leukemia and cooperate with treatment but at the same time employ partial affective denial so that he does not become overly distraught and is able to maintain equanimity in day-to-day function. Another might engage in too much denial and not come in for treatment or start making unrealistic plans for the future.

Displacement denotes transfer of feelings toward one object to another object. An example is a 45-year-old woman with recently diagnosed cancer of the cervix who displayed considerable anger toward the house staff, nursing staff, and her family. Exploration revealed that she was angry at having developed the cancer, but instead of acknowledging it, she had (unconsciously) directed this feeling toward others. It is also important to remember that coping is a process, and that it often takes time for people to adapt to new stressors.

A psychological symptom or collection of symptoms becomes a disorder when the individual experiences significant distress or when an important area of functioning becomes impaired.[8] The cardinal features of psychological disorders are anxiety, depression, conduct disturbance, disorganized thinking, and perceptual distortion. These can be due to psychological stress or an organic cause. Common psychiatric syndromes in cancer patients are described below; their treatment is discussed in a subsequent section.

Common Psychiatric Syndromes

Adjustment Disorders

The commonest psychiatric diagnosis in cancer patients is adjustment disorder, a maladaptive reaction to an identifiable psychosocial stressor that occurs within 3 mo of the onset of the stressor. The maladaptive nature of the reaction is indicated by impairment in social or occupational functioning or by symptoms that are in excess of a normal and expectable reaction to the stressor.[8] Depending on the predominant manifestation, adjustment disorders can be subdivided as follows: with depressed mood, with anxious mood, with mixed emotional features, with disturbance of conduct, with mixed disturbance of emotions and conduct, with work or academic inhibition, with withdrawal, and with physical complaints.

If the disorder meets the criteria for another mental disorder or is an exacerbation of a preexisting mental disorder, then that diagnostic label and not that of adjustment disorder should be used. Examples are patients who develop major depression, brief reactive psychosis, phobic disorder, or an exacerbation of preexisting schizophrenic disorder in reacting to a psychosocial stressor.

Major Depression

Major depression is characterized by the presence of at least 5 of the following symptoms not clearly due to a physical condition, occurring during the same 2-wk period.[8] At least 1 of the symptoms is either (1) a depressed mood, defined as a depressed or irritable mood most of the day, nearly every day; or (2) loss of interest or pleasure, i.e., markedly diminished interest or pleasure in almost all activities most of the day, nearly every day.

Other symptoms:
- Significant weight loss or weight gain, or a decrease or increase in appetite, nearly every day
- Insomnia or hypersomnia, nearly every day
- Psychomotor agitation or retardation, nearly every day
- Fatigue or loss of energy, nearly every day

- Feelings of worthlessness or excessive or inappropriate guilt, nearly every day
- Recurrent thoughts of death, suicidal ideation, or a suicide attempt or plan.

As can be seen, somatic symptoms such as fatigue and loss of appetite and weight can also be due to cancer itself; these symptoms can be used to support the diagnosis of depression when they are severe, out of proportion to the medical illness, and temporally related to the affective and cognitive symptoms. The most useful features are the affective and cognitive symptoms, namely the depressed mood, anhedonia (diminished interest or pleasure in almost all activities), feelings of worthlessness or guilt, and thoughts of death.[9] If the depression is due to an organic mental disorder or is superimposed on schizophrenia, then that diagnostic label is used.

Organic Mental Disorders

Organic mental disorders are those in which a transient or permanent dysfunction of the brain due to known or presumed organic (biochemical or physical) changes leads to a psychological or behavioral abnormality. Organic mental syndromes can be divided into delirium, dementia, amnesic syndrome, organic hallucinosis, organic delusional syndrome, organic mood syndrome, organic anxiety syndrome, organic personality syndrome, substance intoxication and withdrawal, and organic mental syndrome not otherwise specified.[8]

Delirium is characterized by:
- Reduced ability to maintain attention to external stimuli and to appropriately shift attention to new external stimuli (This is the main feature that distinguishes delirium from other organic mental syndromes.)
- Disorganized thinking
- At least 2 of the following:
  —Reduced level of consciousness—e.g., difficulty keeping awake during examination
  —Perceptual disturbance (misinterpretations, illusions, or hallucinations)
  —Disturbance of sleep/wake cycle, with insomnia or daytime drowsiness
  —Increased or decreased psychomotor activity
  —Disorientation to time, place, or person
  —Memory impairment
- Clinical features that develop over a short period (usually hours to days) and tend to fluctuate over the course of a day.

Dementia is characterized by:
- Impairment of short- and long-term memory
- At least 1 of the following:
  —Impairment in abstract thinking
  —Impaired judgment
  —Other disturbances of higher cortical function, such as aphasia, apraxia, agnosia, and constructional difficulty
  —Personality change
- The disturbances in short- and long-term memory and any of the 4 symptoms just given interfere with work or usual social activities or relationships with others.

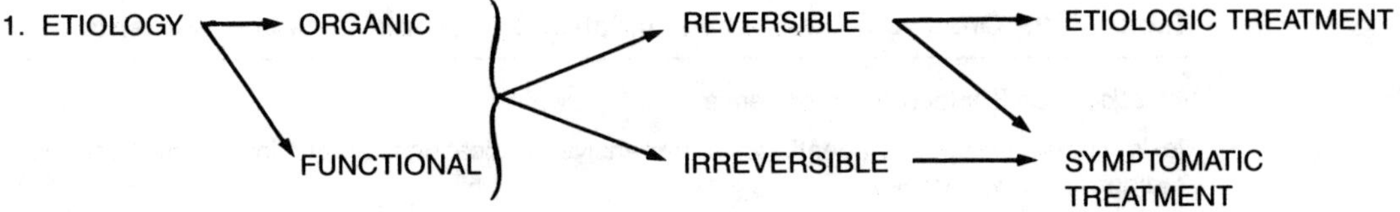

2. DANGER to self or others ⟶ Restraints (chemical, physical) and observation

Figure 15-2. Treatment issues.

In dementias uncomplicated by coexisting delirium, the patient is alert. Because of the loss of higher cortical control, both delirium and dementia can be associated with anxiety, agitation, socially unacceptable behavior, incontinence, hallucinations, and delusions.[10]

Amnesic syndrome is an organic impairment in both short- and long-term memory without other features of delirium and dementia.

Organic mood syndrome is a prominent and persistent depression or elevation in mood without delirium. Likewise, the other organic mental syndromes are characterized by the disturbances their names suggest that are not part of delirium or dementia.

Psychosis connotes gross impairment in reality testing, as suggested by delusions, hallucinations, grossly disorganized speech or behavior, or catatonia. It can accompany organic mental syndrome, major depression, or a manic episode, or it can be a manifestation of brief reactive psychosis or schizophrenia.[8]

Diagnostic Approach

An important task for the physician is to determine whether the disorder is caused by organic or psychological causes and whether the cause is reversible or irreversible (figure 15-2). Symptoms of depression, anxiety, and psychosis may be due to psychological (functional) or organic factors or a combination of both. The sudden onset of a psychiatric disorder in a previously mentally healthy individual, without any clear psychological precipitant, should especially alert one to look for an organic mental disorder. The physician should especially look for chronological relationship to changes in medical status, changes in medications or their dosage, any index of sepsis (e.g., fever), and any neurological findings. Knowledge of some commonly encountered organic causes of psychiatric disorders in cancer patients (table 15-2) should help the physician in doing an appropriate workup.[11-13]

In most organic mental syndromes when causes other than medications are suspected, tests to be considered include CT or MRI scans of the head, spinal tap (infection, meningeal carcinomatosis), CBC, BUN, serum calcium, other electrolytes, glucose, B_{12} and folate levels, arterial blood gas, liver function tests, blood ammonia, thyroid function tests, bacterial blood cultures (if septicemia is suspected), and EEG. The EEG can be of value if uncertainty exists about the

Table 15-2. Organic Causes of Psychiatric Symptoms in Cancer Patients

Infectious: CNS infections, septicemia

Toxic: chemotherapeutic agents, antihypertensive medications, anticholinergic medications, digoxin, corticosteroids

Metabolic: hypercalcemia, hypokalemia, other electrolyte disturbances, hypoxia, hypo- or hyperglycemia, uremia, hepatic encephalopathy, vitamin deficiency (B_{12}, folate, niacin, thiamine)

Endocrine (native or ectopic psychoactive hormonal substances): hypo- or hyperthyroidism, hypo- or hyperadrenocorticalism, endorphins

Structural: intracranial neoplasms (primary or secondary), cerebral abscess, hydrocephalus

Vascular: cerebral infarction

Miscellaneous: withdrawal from sedative-hypnotics, pyrexia, depression as a manifestation of malignancy (e.g., carcinoma of the pancreas) or viral illness, encephalopathy due to radiotherapy, degenerative dementias

clinical diagnosis of organic mental syndrome, because all deliriums—other than delirium tremens—show a generalized slowing of the EEG.[14] The EEG also may show some focal abnormalities not picked up by other measures. In addition, the EEG is useful in identifying seizure activity.

Treatment

Treatment can be etiologic, symptomatic, or both (figure 15-2). A brief outline of salient treatment principles targeted toward specific psychological symptoms or syndromes is given in this section, along with detailed information on some specific treatment approaches and medications.

1. Is the patient acutely agitated, assaultive, or suicidal, or is there a potential for it? If so, the situation constitutes an emergency requiring prompt and aggressive treatment. In anticholinergic delirium, physostigmine 2 mg I.M. or I.V. should be administered, repeating it every 30 min until clinical status improves or cholinergic toxicity is seen (etiologic treatment).[15] In case of delirium tremens, lorazepam 2–4 mg I.M. q. 1 hr (or another agent cross-tolerant with alcohol) should be used until the patient is sleepy but arousable, thereafter repeating it q. 4–6 hr (etiologic and symptomatic treatment).[10] Lorazepam may also be given by slow I.V. infusion, as needed. In all other cases, a neuroleptic should be administered parenterally for rapid neuroleptization (for dosages, see section below on pharmacological treatment); if necessary, an I.V. benzodiazepine can be added (symptomatic treatment). Restraints and 1:1 nursing observation should be used until the patient is medicated to the point of being sleepy but arousable; thereafter, frequent nursing observations should be continued, taking precautions to prevent the patient from hurting self or others.

2. The patient is not imminently dangerous, but is very anxious. If the patient is psychotic, a neuroleptic should be used I.M. or p.o., as the urgency of relief warrants. If the patient is not psychotic, a benzodiazepine should be

used. A neuroleptic can be used if addiction is of concern or if anxiety is very intense. Psychotherapy should be offered in addition.

3. The patient is suffering from a major depression. Antidepressant medication and psychotherapy are indicated. If the patient is also psychotic, a neuroleptic should be added, and electroconvulsive therapy can be considered. Suicidal and delusional patients should be hospitalized.

4. The patient exhibits mild to moderate anxiety or depression and adjustment disorders. Primarily, psychological intervention should be used. Antianxiety agents or antidepressants may be used as adjuncts in some cases when necessary; for example, a benzodiazepine may be used to deal with a time-limited stressor such as upcoming surgery or to contain the anxiety so that the patient is more amenable to psychotherapy.

5. The patient has organic mental syndrome. The anxiety, depression, or psychotic thinking should be treated as above, depending on the degree of anxiety and depression. In addition, the underlying causes should be investigated and corrected to the extent possible. Delirium connotes acute cerebral insufficiency, and one should promptly search for and correct the causes to prevent or minimize permanent cerebral damage, which can cause dementia. In both delirium and dementia, it is also important to provide the patient with cues to orient himself. A calendar, clock, and radio or television should be kept at the bedside, constancy of environment (avoiding changes of nurses, other health care personnel, or room) should be provided, the patient should be regularly informed about the environment, and adequate illumination at night should be provided. Also, appropriate protective measures should be taken to prevent the patient from walking off the ward, falling out of bed, etc. If possible, a companion or relative should stay with the patient around the clock.

6. The patient shows conduct disturbance. The underlying anxiety or cognitive disturbance needs to be recognized and dealt with as above. In addition, clear limits must be set on behavior and firmly imposed in a nonpunitive manner.

Psychological Treatment

The most important thing the physician can do in providing treatment for psychological disorders is to be available and show interest in the patient as a person. It has been found that genuineness, accurate empathy, and unconditional positive regard for the other person are important ingredients of any helping relationship.[16] In every case, the physician should explore the patient's feelings about the illness, the issues troubling him, and how he is coping. The physician must help the patient ventilate feelings, listen attentively in an empathic manner, offer emotional support, correct misconceptions, and help in the development and use of effective coping mechanisms. Specific stressors that bother a patient the most should be identified and addressed. This basic scheme of intervention will be of enormous help to most patients. Behavioral interventions such as relaxation training, desensitization, coping skills training, and hypnosis can be of help in dealing with anxiety, depression, pain, and anticipatory nausea and vomiting associated with chemotherapy.[5,17,18] An example is a 26-year-old woman with Hodgkin's lymphoma (stage IV) who was noncompliant with chemotherapy because of anticipatory nausea and anxiety. Even I.V. dextrose in water infusions, gallium scan and antiemetic medications such as prochlorperazine elicited nausea and anxiety (stimulus generalization). She was successfully treated using imaginal desensitization and hypnosis. The procedure involved her imagining various situations that were associated with anxiety and nausea, reducing the anxiety with relaxation and some cognitive coping mechanisms, and counteracting the nausea with imagery of her stomach being filled with ice-cold water or of eating a favorite food.

Family members are an important resource in helping the patient cope with the stressors: they should be guided in being optimally helpful to the patient. Emotional needs of the family also should be addressed. Support and educational groups can be helpful to the patient and the family. When referring a patient to a psychiatrist or other mental health professional for consultation or treatment, it is important for the primary physician to educate the patient about the consultation, emphasizing that he or she as the primary physician will continue to care for the patient and show interest in his or her physical and emotional well-being. (For more discussion on psychological care of cancer patients, see refs 4, 6, 11, 19, 20.)

Communicating the Diagnosis of Cancer

To promote proper emotional adjustment, it is important to keep both patient and family adequately informed regarding the diagnosis, nature of the illness, and its treatment.[4,20,21] Withholding the diagnosis from the patient loads unnecessary emotional burdens onto the family, the patient, and the health care team. Also, a well-informed patient is easier to manage than one kept in ignorance. Studies have shown that most patients want to be told the truth regarding their diagnosis of cancer.[4,20,21] But patients vary in the amount of information they want or are able to tolerate at a given time and in the degree of denial they use. The physician must be sensitive to these variances and careful of words used in communicating with patients on these matters. Many patients may automatically equate cancer with death, without realizing the tremendous advances made in the treatment of many cancers, or may have unrealistic fears that may lead to anxiety or an unnecessarily pessimistic mood. For this reason, the physician should explore the patient's views on his cancer, correct any misconceptions, and provide adequate emotional support.

Refusal of Diagnostic or Therapeutic Procedures

It can be puzzling and frustrating when a patient refuses important diagnostic or therapeutic procedures even after the procedure has been explained. In these situations, the physician should first explore with the patient the reasons for the refusal and listen attentively. In some cases, the refusal may be justifiable. An example is an 83-year-old woman with carcinoma of the esophagus who refused to have a feeding gastrostomy and radiotherapy because she knew that she would die soon anyway and felt that the procedures would simply prolong her agony.

In some instances, the patient's value system may be different from the physician's, and the physician must recognize this and accept it. If the refusal seems unreasonable or unadaptive, the physician should explore the patient's understanding of his illness, the nature of the procedure, and the consequences of having the procedure or not having it. If the patient possibly has organic mental syndrome or a psychotic disorder that impairs understanding and judgment in this area, a psychiatric consultation should be obtained to determine his or her competence to refuse; the physician should then proceed through the legally indicated means. In the author's experience, in most instances the patient is mentally competent to refuse, but denial, anxiety, misconceptions, anger, and a power struggle with the staff underlie the refusal.

If the patient is given an opportunity to ventilate his feelings, if caregivers are empathetic and attempt to clarify misconceptions, and if the patient is given a sense of being in control, many will change their minds and agree to the procedure. An example is a 64-year-old man admitted for evaluation of an intrathoracic mass found on chest roentgenogram. He refused mediastinoscopy, saying that he felt well and wanted to return to work. He resented an intern's aggressive attempts to change his mind. In interviews with the psychiatric consultant, the patient initially expressed anger at the staff, but then began expressing his anxiety about what might be wrong with his body and about surgical procedures. Then, without the consultant's ever making an overt attempt to change his mind, the patient agreed to the mediastonoscopy and subsequently cooperated in treatment for adenocarcinoma of the lung. In this case, the maladaptive denial, anxiety over loss of control, displaced anger, and power struggle that interfered with care were dealt with by giving the patient an opportunity to ventilate his feelings in a nonthreatenting atmosphere and respecting the patient's need for control.

The Terminally Ill Patient

Thanatology refers to the study of death and the matters leading up to it and following it. Death is not only a finite event, but there is also a process surrounding it—namely, its anticipation and the events following it. Kubler-Ross has popularized the stages of the anticipatory process as denial, anger, bargaining, depression, and acceptance.[22] Although this scheme is of value as in helping to identify the various features of the process, it must be recognized that many patients go back and forth among the various stages and may show signs of more than one stage at a time. Many physicians tend to avoid or disengage from terminally ill patients because of a sense of hopelessness, powerlessness, inadequacy, or failure. This reaction leads to a painful feeling of isolation in the patient. The physician must anticipate and avoid this disengagement, examining and coming to terms with these feelings and keeping in mind that he can still do a lot for the patient by mitigating his suffering and just by being with the patient. If the family tends to disengage from the patient, this also should be dealt with in a similar manner.

If a patient dies when the family is not present and if the death was expected, news of the death can be conveyed to the family by telephone. If the death is unexpected, it is generally preferable to inform the family of the death in person.[23] Usually, this entails telling the family over the telephone that the patient is critically ill and requesting that the family come to the hospital immediately. In either case, the physician should meet with the family in person to answer their questions and provide emotional support.

Dealing with Children

All of the above discussion is fully applicable when the patient is a child. In children, one should keep in mind the stage of development and cognitive maturity and take care to explain things at their level. Many children are much more psychologically perceptive than generally thought, and it is important to be honest with them just as with adults.[4,21] Special developmental needs of children such as play and education should be addressed. (For detailed discussions of psychological and pharmacological approaches, see refs 4, 19, 24, 25.)

Pharmacological Treatment

This section is limited to discussion of antidepressants, neuroleptics, and benzodiazepines that are used most frequently, and dosages given are those for adults. (The reader is referred to psychiatric textbooks—refs 10, 26, 27—for more detailed coverage.)

Antidepressants

These agents are indicated in the treatment of major depression. They are also effective in the treatment of panic disorder and as adjuvants to conventional analgesics in the treatment of chronic cancer pain.[27] The therapeutic effect of many antidepressants is thought to be due to their action of blocking the reuptake of norepinephrine and serotonin by the presynaptic neuron. Imipramine, desipramine, amitriptyline, nortriptyline, doxepin, and protriptyline are some of the tricyclic antidepressants (TCAs) that have been in use for several years. Fluoxetine, trazodone, bupropion, and maprotiline are not tricyclic. All antidepressants are equally efficacious when employed in the appropriate dosage, and the choice depends mainly on their possible side effects and the physician's familiarity with a particular medication. The side effects of the antidepressants are as follows:

- *Anticholinergic.* All of the TCAs have significant anticholinergic side effects; they can cause dry mouth, blurred vision, tachycardia, constipation, urinary hesitancy, and mental confusion. They are contraindicated in untreated narrow-angle glaucoma. Among the TCAs, desipramine is the least anticholinergic, and amitriptyline is the most anticholinergic. Fluoxetine, trazodone, and bupropion do not have significant anticholinergic effects.
- *Sedation.* Almost no sedation is seen with bupropion, fluoxetine, and protriptyline; a mild effect is seen with desipramine; moderate with

imipramine, nortriptyline, and maprotiline; and pronounced with amitriptyline, doxepin, and trazodone. Sedation may be an advantage or disadvantage; tense or agitated patients may find the sedation beneficial; others may experience undesirable daytime drowsiness.

- *Cardiovascular effects.* TCAs are associated with orthostatic hypotension, tachycardia, and quinidine-like effects on the heart. If a patient has a cardiac conduction defect, TCAs pose the danger of impairing the conduction further. Fluoxetine and bupropion do not seem to have significant cardiovascular side effects.
- *Lowering of seizure threshold.* This is seldom a problem except in overdose or in seizure disorder patients with inadequate anticonvulsant blood levels. Bupropion and maprotiline should be avoided in patients prone to seizures.
- *Other side effects.* Nausea, gastrointestinal upset, headaches, and agitation are frequent reasons for discontinuance of fluoxetine, which otherwise has a good side effects profile. These side effects also can occur with other antidepressants. There have been reports of priapism with trazodone.

Dosage

Fluoxetine has a simple dosing regimen of 20 mg p.o. o.d. Desipramine, imipramine, doxepin, and amitriptyline should be started with 25 mg p.o. h.s., increasing the daily dosage by 25 mg increments every 2 days until a dosage of 2 mg/kg per day is reached, or the patient develops significant side effects. Patients generally develop tolerance to the side effects within a few days, making it possible to gradually increase the dosage. In the beginning, the daily dosage may be divided (b.i.d. or t.i.d.) to reduce the severity of side effects, but later the entire dose can be given at bedtime.

Generally it takes 3 wk for the antidepressant effect of these drugs to become significantly manifest, although some improvement may be noted earlier. If the patient does not show significant improvement, the plasma level of the drug after the patient has been on the same dosage for 7 days should be measured; if it is less than the optimal level, the dosage should be increased accordingly. The same dosage can result in significantly different blood levels in different individuals, and inadequate blood level is a common reason for lack of response.

With desipramine, the proportion of patients responding grows with increases in blood levels until a level of 125 ng/ml is reached; beyond this level, further increases do not increase therapeutic efficacy but only increase the side effects.[28] The optimal plasma level for imipramine is 225 ng/ml. Nortriptyline has a therapeutic window of 50–150 ng/ml; if the plasma level exceeds 150 ng/ml, efficacy is actually reduced. Optimal plasma levels for other antidepressants have not been firmly established.

Patients who show improvement should be kept on the medication for 6 mo in order to minimize the chances of relapse. Dosages of TCAs should be reduced gradually because the abrupt discontinuance of these drugs can cause cholinergic rebound symptoms.

Neuroleptics

Neuroleptics are indicated in the treatment of intense anxiety, agitation, and psychosis, and for chemical restraint in an assaultive or suicidal patient (especially on an open medical ward). They decrease psychomotor activity, correct psychotic process (hallucinations and delusions), are sedative, and are also antiemetic. Prochlorperazine, a phenothiazine, is frequently used as an antiemetic agent in cancer patients. The antipsychotic action of neuroleptics is thought to be due to their blockade of dopaminergic receptors. They also block noradrenergic receptors. Some commonly used neuroleptics are chlorpromazine, thioridazine, trifluoperazine, fluphenazine, perphenazine, thiothixene, and haloperidol.

The side effects of neuroleptics include:
- Postural hypotension
- Sedation
- Anticholinergic effect (mainly with thioridazine and chlorpromazine)
- Lowering of the seizure threshold
- Extrapyramidal effects such as acute dystonia and dyskinesia (muscular spasms, including locked jaw, cervical torticollis, opisthotonos, oculogyric crisis), akathisia (restlessness), and Parkinsonian symptoms (akinesia, cogwheel rigidity, and tremors). These effects should be treated with antiparkinsonian agents such as benztropine, diphenhydramine, or trihexyphenidyl (e.g., benztropine 2 mg I.V. or I.M. or p.o. stat, and thereafter 2 mg p.o. h.s.), while continuing the neuroleptic medication as required. Acute laryngospasm is a rare complication that requires prompt recognition and treatment with I.V. benztropine and discontinuance of the neuroleptic.
- Neuroleptic malignant syndrome (muscle rigidity, hyperthermia, clouded consciousness), agranulocytosis, and aplastic anemia are also rare but serious complications.
- Tardive dyskinesia (involuntary rhythmic movements of the tongue, facial, and other muscles), which may appear after months or years of therapy, is thought to be due to compensatory dopaminergic rebound.
- Increased prolactin levels (this may be of importance in patients with prolactin-sensitive tumors), cholestatic jaundice on a hypersensitivity basis, photosensitivity sunburns (chlorpromazine), retrograde ejaculation, ECG changes, and cardiac arrhythmias (thioridazine).

Even though they differ in antipsychotic potency per milligram (e.g., 1 mg of haloperidol is equivalent to about 50 mg of chlorpromazine), all neuroleptics are equally efficacious in the treatment of psychosis when used in appropriate dosage, and the choice of an agent is based primarily on the side effect profile. Of the neuroleptics mentioned above, chlorpromazine and thioridazine are the least potent per milligram, most sedative, and most anticholinergic. The 2 drugs are more likely to cause hypotension but are less likely to cause extrapyramidal side effects. For a given medication, there is a wide dose/response range: dosage is determined primarily by clinical response or side effects.

When a patient is dangerous, potentially dangerous, or extremely agitated, it is important to rapidly tranquilize the patient, both on humanitarian grounds (to spare the patient prolongation of the intense anxiety experience) and as a precaution to avert mishaps such as assaults on other patients and staff, self-injury, or pulling out I.V. lines. Haloperidol is preferred in this setting because of the greater risk of orthostatic hypotension with chlorpromazine, considering the fact that high doses of the neuroleptic probably will need to be given rapidly and parenterally.[10,29] Initially, 3 mg haloperidol should be given I.M.; injections should be hourly, increasing the subsequent doses if necessary up to 10 mg until the patient is sleepy but arousable. Thereafter, the last effective dose should be repeated q. 4 hr. Alternatively, one can give haloperidol by I.V. infusion (mixed with dextrose or saline solution) at the rate of 10 mg/hr, starting and stopping the infusion as required to keep the patient in a calm state. After 24 hr, a switch to oral administration can be made.

Less highly agitated patients can be managed by oral haloperidol or another neuroleptic, starting with haloperidol 2 mg b.i.d. or t.i.d. and gradually increasing the daily dosage by 2 mg every 2 days until the patient is calm. Or chlorpromazine can be used, 50 mg b.i.d. or t.i.d., increasing the daily dosage by 50 mg every 3 days as desired. Many patients require a much lower daily dosage of a neuroleptic for maintenance of behavioral control than the amount they required for its induction. For this reason, the daily dosage should be gradually reduced, matching it to the needs of the patient. Once the patient has been stabilized, the entire daily dose can be given at bedtime, taking advantage of the sedative effect at night.

Benzodiazepines

Benzodiazepines are useful as adjuncts to psychological treatment in the management of anxiety, as adjuncts to neuroleptics in the rapid control of agitation, as hypnotics, for producing amnesia and tranquility during invasive procedures or chemotherapy, and in the treatment of alcohol withdrawal. Their antianxiety effect seems to be due to enhancement of gamma aminobutyric acid (GABA) activity in the CNS. Benzodiazepines in clinical use include alprazolam, chlordiazepoxide, clorazepate, diazepam, lorazepam, and oxazepam. The choice of an agent is guided by its half-life, metabolic pathway, and drug interaction effects. For I.M. administration, lorazepam is preferred over diazepam or chlordiazepoxide because of its better absorption.

For the rapid control of the acutely agitated patient, lorazepam can be administered I.V. or I.M. in conjunction with haloperidol, starting with 0.5 mg of lorazepam and increasing the hourly dosage as required.[29] The effective haloperidol-lorazepam combination dose is then repeated q. 4 hr; lorazepam is discontinued after 12–18 hr, and haloperidol alone is continued thereafter. Caution must be used in giving I.V. benzodiazepines because of the potential for respiratory depression; emergency resuscitative equipment and personnel should be readily available. I.V. lorazepam has also been used along with chemotherapy infusions to produce amnesia, thereby inhibiting the development of conditioned nausea.

For the management of nonpsychotic anxiety, benzodiazepines can be useful in conjunction with psychotherapy, especially when time-limited stressors are part of the picture. Alprazolam has antidepressant and antipanic effects in addition to its antianxiety effect; it is especially useful in the management of the patient with both anxiety and depression or the patient with panic attacks. Typical dosage range is 0.25 mg p.o. t.i.d. to 4 mg/day, in divided doses. Benzodiazepines can also be used sporadically on a p.r.n. basis to deal with expected anxiety situations (e.g., alprazolam 0.5–1 mg p.o., or lorazepam 1–2 mg p.o. or I.M., 1 hr before an anxiety-inducing procedure or situation).

The major side effects of benzodiazepines are sedation and (at higher doses) ataxia and respiratory depression. They should be used with caution in the presence of liver disease, as they are metabolized primarily in the liver. Because abrupt withdrawal of benzodiazepines after prolonged high doses can induce rebound anxiety, seizures, and delirium similar to delirium tremens, dosage should be gradually reduced before discontinuance. Because they carry the risk of drug dependence, the smallest dose possible for the shortest possible period should be used. Benzodiazepines should not be used as a substitute for psychotherapy or personal attention.

Conclusion

As can be seen, the approach to the psychological problems in cancer patients requires a blend of biological and psychosocial knowledge, scientific approach, and human concern. Although complex psychiatric problems require psychiatric consultation, the primary physician's familiarity with the issues discussed above will help to implement the consultant's recommendations and increase the physician's involvement in the total care of the patient.

References

1. Noyes R Jr, Kathol RG, Debelius-Enemark P, et al. Distress associated with cancer as measured by the illness distress scale. Psychosomatics 1990; 31:321–30.
2. Massie MJ, Holland JC. Overview of normal reactions and prevalence of psychiatric disorders. In: Holland JC, Rowland JH, eds. Handbook of psycho-oncology: psychological care of the patient with cancer. New York: Oxford University Press, 1989; 273–282.
3. Derogatis LR, Morrow GR, Fetting J, et al. The prevalence of psychiatric disorders among cancer patients. JAMA 1983; 249:751–57.
4. National Cancer Institute. Coping with cancer. Bethesda, Md.: the institute, 1980 (NIH pub no. 80–2080).
5. Viswanathan R, Kachur EK. Development of agoraphobia after surviving cancer. Gen Hosp Psychiatry 1986; 8:127–32.
6. Weisman AD. Coping with illness. In: Hackett TP, Cassem NH, eds. Massachusetts General Hospital handbook of general hospital psychiatry. 2nd ed. Littleton, Mass.: PSG Publishing, 1987: 297–308.
7. Inderbitzin L, Luke CM, James ME. Psychoanalytic psychology. In: Stoudemire A, ed. Human behavior: an introduction for medical students. Philadelphia: Lippincott, 1990; 51–84.
8. American Psychiatric Assoc. Diagnostic and statistical manual of mental disorders. 3rd ed (revised). Washington, D.C.: the association, 1987.
9. Cavanaugh S. Diagnosing depression in the hospitalized patient with chronic medical illness. J Clin Psychiatry 1984; 45(3,sec.2):13–16.

10. Glickman LS. Psychiatric consultation in the general hospital. New York: Marcel & Decker, 1980.
11. Goldberg RJ. Management of depression in the patient with advanced cancer. JAMA 1981; 246:373–76.
12. Patchell RA, Posner JB. Cancer and the nervous system. In: Holland JC, Rowland JH, eds. Handbook of psycho-oncology: psychological care of the patient with cancer. New York: Oxford University Press, 1989, pp 327–341.
13. Goldberg ID, Bloomer WD, Dawson DM. Nervous system toxic effects of cancer therapy. JAMA 1982; 247:1437–41.
14. Engel GL, Romano J. Delirium, a syndrome of cerebral insufficiency. J Chron Dis 1959; 9:260–77.
15. Granacher RP, Baldessarini R. Physostigmine: its use in acute anticholinergic syndrome with antidepressant and antiparkinson drugs. Arch Gen Psychiatry 1975; 32:375–80.
16. Rogers CR, Sanford RC. Client-centered psychotherapy. In: Kaplan HI, Sadock BJ, eds. Comprehensive textbook of psychiatry. 4th ed. Baltimore: Williams & Wilkins, 1985; 1374–1388.
17. Spiegel D. Hypnosis with medical/surgical patients. Gen Hosp Psychiatry 1983; 5:265–77.
18. Viswanathan R. Management of phobias. Compr Ther 1983; 9(6):53–58.
19. Holland JC, Rowland JH, eds. Handbook of psycho-oncology: psychological care of the patient with cancer. New York: Oxford University Press, 1989.
20. Cassem NH. The dying patient. In: Hackett TP, Cassem NH, eds. Massachusetts General Hospital handbook of general hospital psychiatry. 2nd ed. Littleton, Mass.: PSG Publishing, 1987; 332–352.
21. Goldberg RJ. Disclosure of information to adult cancer patients: issues and update. J Clin Oncol 1984; 2:948–55.
22. Kubler-Ross E. On death and dying. New York: Macmillan, 1980.
23. Viswanathan R, Clark JJ, Viswanathan K. Physicians' and the public's attitudes on communication about death. Arch Intern Med 1986; 146:2029–33.
24. Pfeffer CR. Children's reactions to illness, hospitalization, and surgery. In: Kaplan HI, Sadock BJ, eds. Comprehensive textbook of psychiatry. 4th ed. Baltimore: Williams &Wilkins, 1985; 1836–1842.
25. Rapoport JL, Kruesi MJP. Organic therapies. In: Kaplan HI, Sadock BJ, eds. Comprehensive textbook of psychiatry. 4th ed. Baltimore: Williams & Wilkins, 1985; 1793–1798.
26. Kaplan HI, Sadock BJ, eds. Comprehensive textbook of psychiatry. 4th ed. Baltimore: Williams & Wilkins, 1985.
27. American Psychiatric Association Task Force on Treatments of Psychiatric Disorders. Treatments of psychiatric disorders. Washington, D.C.: the association, 1989.
28. Nelson JC, Jatlow P, Quinlan DM, Bowers MB. Desipramine plasma concentration and antidepressant response. Arch Gen Psychiatry 1982; 39:1419–22.
29. Adams F. Neuropsychiatric evaluation and treatment of delirium in the critically ill cancer patient. Cancer Bull 1984; 36:156–60.

16

ONCOLOGIC EMERGENCIES

Albert S. Braverman, M.D., F.A.C.P., and
C. Julian Rosenthal, M.D., F.A.C.P.

EMERGENCIES MAY ARISE IN patients with cancer in 3 distinct clinical settings, each requiring a somewhat different approach.[1] First, a patient not known to have cancer may present with severe life-threatening complications. In this case, the examining physician must combine the initial diagnosis and staging with appropriate emergency treatment. Second, an emergency may arise during the course of treatment of a known cancer patient; whenever possible, in this situation it is important to avoid any compromise in the therapeutic regimen already selected. Third, an emergency may arise with a terminal patient, in which case the decision to intervene with the full force of modern technology must be based only on the need to palliate the patient's symptoms rather than attempt to prolong his/her life.

The decision concerning the best therapeutic approach in oncologic emergencies must be individualized to each patient. This decision must take into account:

- Tumor histologic type and stage
- Previous therapy
- Existence of any other therapeutic regimen likely to produce a good remission
- Plan of treatment for the patient after the emergency has passed.

It is extremely important to establish the tumor histologic diagnosis before the emergency treatment is instituted because on many occasions, the latter can induce cellular changes that will make an accurate histologic diagnosis very difficult.

The list of emergencies in patients with cancer is relatively long, but a list of some of the more frequent ones would include: superior vena cava syndrome,

"

neoplastic cardiac tamponade, spinal cord compression, seizures and cerebral herniation due to brain lesions, airway obstruction, obstructive uropathy, hypercalcemia and other electrolytic abnormalities,* acute renal failure due to kidney infiltration, and thrombotic and hemorrhagic manifestations of malignancies.

Among all emergency situations caused by malignant neoplasms, only 3 require therapeutic procedures not used when similar situations arise during the course of other diseases. These are superior vena cava syndrome, cardiac tamponade, and spinal cord compression.

This chapter will first review these syndromes, then will present a few data on specific aspects of other emergencies occurring in patients with malignant tumors.

Superior Vena Cava Syndrome

Superior vena cava syndrome (SVCS) occurs in 3–8% of patients with bronchogenic carcinoma and malignant lymphoma.

Anatomical and Etiological Factors

The superior vena cava descends in the right paratracheal location to enter the superior mediastinum. Just above the pericardium, the left innominate vein joins the right to form the superior vena cava, which empties into the right atrium.

The location of lymph node groups within the mediastinum plays an important role in the pathophysiology of SVC obstruction. Three main groups are located there: anterior, intermediate (tracheal-bronchial) and posterior. The anterior nodes are located in the upper half of the thorax and are distributed on the anterior surface of the great vessels of the thorax, including the aortic arch and vessels arising from it and the superior vena cava. On the right side, nodes are situated between the vena cava and the trachea. These nodes lie medial to the right phrenic nerve and communicate with the right paratracheal nodes. The superior vena cava, with a thin wall and low intravascular pressure, is a collapsible vessel surrounded by solid structures such as the trachea, vertebral bodies, sternum, and lymph nodes, which are relatively rigid.

Conditions leading to SVC obstruction include a variety of benign and malignant disorders. The most common benign causes, encountered in about 20% of all cases, include aortic aneurysm, vein thrombosis due to central vein catheterization (pacemaker, indwelling catheters), substernal thyroid, sarcoidosis, and pericarditis.

The most common malignant causes of SVCS, encountered in 80% of all cases, include bronchogenic carcinoma in 77% of cases (the small-cell histology is the most frequent, whereas adenocarcinoma rarely causes SVC), lym-

---

*See chapter 9 for hypercalcemia and other electrolytic abnormalities.

phoma in 17%, and other cancers (testicular, sarcomas, adenocarcinoma of the breast) in 6%.

Pathophysiology and Clinical Manifestations

Three mechanisms can account for the occurrence of SVC syndrome: (1) occlusion due to extrinsic pressure, (2) invasion of the vein wall by neoplasm, and (3) intraluminal thrombosis.

The clinical picture is due to venous hypertension (usually >150 mm saline) in areas normally drained by the SVC or its tributaries. Delayed circulation time, development of venous collaterals and, in more advanced cases, development of cerebral edema, are all consequences of SVC obstruction. Symptoms are typically increased when the patient bends forward or lies down.

The most common symptoms, listed in order of frequency, include dyspnea, facial swelling, swelling of the trunk and upper extremities, chest pain, cough, dysphagia, and hoarseness.

The most common physical findings seen in SVCS include, in order of frequency, distension of thoracic veins, distension of neck veins, edema of face, plethora of face, cyanosis, edema of upper extremities, paralysis of true vocal cord, and Horner's syndrome (myosis, ptosis, enophthalmos).

Diagnosis and Treatment

Of some concern to physicians with patients who have developed SVCS is the often-stated opinion that diagnostic procedures carry with them significant hazard in terms of excessive bleeding. However, recent data show that such concern is generally unjustified.

The major invasive and semiinvasive procedures performed in patients with SVCS are listed in sequence of a logical stepwise approach: contrast venogram or nuclear venogram, lymph node biopsy if superficial enlarged nodes are palpable, bronchoscopy with biopsy, mediastinoscopy with biopsy, and thoracotomy with biopsy.

Radiation therapy (XRT) is the major modality of treatment in all cases of SVCS.[2] It should be initiated on the day of diagnosis, but only after an appropriate biopsy to establish a correct histologic diagnosis is performed.[3] It is recommended that 3–4 high-dose fractions of 400 cGy tumor dose per daily session be administered first, followed by 180–200 cGy per session per day up to the completion of a total tumoricidal dose of 4,000–6,000 cGy for patients with solid tumors and 2,000–4,000 cGy for patients with lymphoma. The radiation portals encompass the mediastinal, hilar, and any adjacent pulmonary parenchymal lesions as well as the supraclavicular nodes when enlarged.

Chemotherapy, usually with a single alkylating agent given I.V. (nitrogen mustard or cyclophosphamide), is recommended for administration concurrently with XRT only in cases of lymphoma or leukemia known to generally respond promptly to these drugs. In cases of other solid tumors, it is usually recommended that the most appropriate combination chemotherapy regimen for the respective tumor be started 3–4 wk after the termination of radiation in order to avoid side effects generated by the "recall" phenomenon.

The overall results of this treatment indicate that symptomatic relief can be achieved in 80% of all cases somewhat faster in patients receiving initially high fractions of radiation.[2] Recurrence of severe SVCS has been seen in 10–20% of patients with bronchogenic carcinoma but was not encountered in patients with lymphoma.[2] The most common side effects of this treatment are dysphagia and (in patients also receiving chemotherapy) transient leukopenia and thrombocytopenia.

Neoplastic Cardiac Tamponade

Neoplasia is the most common cause of cardiac tamponade, being the etiologic agent in nearly 60% of all cases.[4]

Pathophysiology

Cardiac tamponade describes a state of compression of the heart that leads to a rise of the intrapericardial pressure that interferes with the function of the heart as a pump; this causes overt impairment of the systemic circulation. The severity of cardiac tamponade depends on (1) the rate of pericardial fluid accumulation, (2) the distensibility of the pericardium, (3) the fluid volume, and (4) the tempo of compression of the heart. The specific aspects of cardiac tamponade in patients with neoplastic diseases refer to the specific causes and the therapy of cardiac tamponade in these patients.

Etiology

Malignant tumors of the pericardium may be primary or secondary. Primary neoplasms of the pericardium, which include mesotheliomas and sarcomas, represent about 5–10% of all cases of neoplastic cardiac tamponade. Their clinical course is generally that of a rapid accumulation of massive amounts of bloody pericardial fluid.

Cardiac metastases (secondary neoplasms) in patients with cancer were reported in several autopsy series with a greatly variable incidence of 1–21%. Seven percent of metastases were found only in the myocardium, 5–7% in the parietal pericardium, and 2% in both myocardium and pericardium. The most common malignant tumors causing pericardial involvement are carcinoma of the lung, adenocarcinoma of the breast, leukemias, Hodgkin's disease, non-Hodgkin's lymphomas, melanomas, and soft-tissue sarcomas. The pericardial involvement can be manifested as an extension of the surrounding tumor to the pericardium or as diffuse or nodular infiltration of the pericardium not connected to the surrounding tissues.

Finally, radiation pericarditis leading to cardiac tamponade can be seen in patients with cancer receiving XRT to the mediastinum. Its incidence varies between 3 and 30%, depending on the amount of radiation given and the portals used. Generally, it occurs when >4,000 cGy have been administered.

Radiation pericarditis can be manifested as (1) an acute form, either inflammatory or effusive, appearing during the XRT or within weeks to up to

12 mo after the end of XRT (mean 14 wk); or (2) a chronic form, either effusive or constructive, that appears from a few months up to 20 yr after treatment.

Distinguishing radiation pericarditis from progressive neoplastic pericarditis is very difficult, because both present as exudates that can be bloody and may not present neoplastic cells in the pericardial fluid.

Treatment

In cardiac tamponade, the possibility of sudden death is always present. The only immediately effective treatment of tamponade is removal of the fluid through pericardiocentesis after supportive therapy to expand the venous blood volume has been started.[4] The pericardial puncture should be done under electrocardiographic and blood pressure monitoring and, if the effusion is loculated, under CT scan guidance.

If the fluid reaccumulates, 3 approaches are available:

- Pericardiectomy (pericardial stripping), followed by radiation therapy to the mediastinum ($\sim$ 3,000 cGy). This the most commonly used approach.
- Draining the pericardial fluid a second time and instilling chemotherapeutic agents in the pericardial space. Quinacrine, nitrogen mustard, thio-tepa, 5-fluorouracil, and methotrexate were used in various studies, with effective control in 30% of cases but also with an occasional death following the instillation.
- Instillation of radioactive material in the pericardial space after partial drainage. ^{32}Phosphorus, ^{90}ytrium, and ^{198}gold have been used, with best results reported for phosphorus.

Despite treatment, the prognosis of patients with neoplastic pericardial tamponade is very poor: They survive only a few weeks after diagnosis. Survival is significantly better (mean: 12.5 mo) in patients in whom the malignant pericardial effusion is diagnosed and treated before tamponade develops.

Spinal Cord Compression

Spinal cord compression due to invasion by malignant tumors is an emergency clinical situation whose prompt evaluation and treatment is essential in preventing permanent neurological sequelae. Once complete paraplegia develops, the likelihood of meaningful recovery is small.

Pathophysiology

Spinal cord compression in cancer patients may result from epidural metastases (by far the most common cause); intramedullary metastases; vertebral subluxation, usually atlantoaxial due to pathologic fractures of the odontoid process and subsequent anterior dislocation of the atlas (C-1) on the axis (C-2); or spinal subdural hematoma, an occasional complication of lumbar puncture in thrombocytopenic patients.

Metastatic tumor to the spinal epidural space can develop via several pathophysiologic mechanisms, including the following:

- Metastases to the vertebral bodies, with invasion of the anterior epidural space (by far the most common mechanism). Cancers that frequently follow this mechanism are carcinoma of the breast, prostate, and lung.
- Invasion of the spinal canal through the intervertebral foramina by direct extension of neoplasms located in the paravertebral space (seen in patients with lymphomas).
- Hematogenous metastases to the epidural space or to the spinal cord itself, which are very rare (seen in patients with soft-tissue sarcomas).

Intramedullary metastases occur in <4% of all cases with spinal cord dysfunction due to metastatic disease. Tumor cells may reach the interior of the cord by hematogenous spread; growth along the roots from paravertebral tumor masses; or, in patients with leptomeningeal metastases, invasion from the Virchow-Robin spaces.

The spinal cord may be compressed at any level, although the thoracic region is the most common site. The level of compression varies somewhat with the primary tumor; i.e., colon cancer metastasizes more frequently to involve the lumbar spine, whereas metastases from carcinoma of the breast and lung are more frequently encountered in the thoracic region.

Etiology and Clinical Manifestations

Primary tumors causing epidural spinal cord compression with increasing frequency are slightly variable in several published reports of clinical trials.[5] The most common tumors spreading in the epidural space in the Memorial Sloan-Kettering Cancer Center series are breast, lung, and prostate.[5] This is a reflection of both the prevalence of these tumor types in the patient population and the tendency for these tumors to metastasize to the spine. Lymphomas, which 20 yr ago accounted for 17% of all cancers causing cord compression (second only to breast cancer), now account only for 5% of all cancers. This trend possibly is the result of vigorous early treatment that frequently includes radiation of the paravertebral spaces. Other tumors causing spinal cord compression, listed in descending order of frequency, include multiple myeloma, sarcomas, kidney tumors, G.I. tract malignancies, and thyroid carcinoma.

Regardless of the primary tumor, clinical presentation of spinal cord compression is fairly consistent; it is separable into *prodromal* and *compressive* phases. The prodromal phase is characterized by back pain with or without radicular pain, the latter consisting of pain radiated to various parts of the trunk or extremities along the territory of distribution of various nerves. The compressive phase can follow the prodromal pain after a few days (high-grade lymphomas, seminomas) or up to several months later (low-grade sarcoma, breast carcinoma, etc.).

As has been shown in a dog experimental model, the neurological deficit that develops progresses from initial motor loss to paresthesias and then to sensory loss; appreciation of pain and ability to detect a pinprick are the last functions lost. The return of function after release of the mechanical pressure occurs in reversed order.

Some patients describe unilateral weakness or foot drop in addition to difficulty maintaining balance. This can be followed abruptly by paraparesis, with inability to walk, and loss of sphincter control. Compression of the cervical cord above C-5 can lead to pain (frequently unilateral, high in the neck), aggravated by lateral rotation of the head and radiating to the shoulder or occiput; respiratory failure; loss of sphincter control; and quadriplegia preceded by sensory loss.

Compression of the conus medullaris and cauda equina are characterized by saddle anesthesia (sensory impairment in the lumbosacral dermatomas), with loss of urethral, vaginal, and rectal sensations and impaired control of micturition. Hesitancy and urgency in micturition may represent early signs of cord compression.

Diagnosis and Treatment

Diagnostic procedures should be performed at an early stage. A 1981 study showed that when a myelogram was performed when only back pain was present, incomplete occlusion of the spinal canal was found in 17% of cases.[6] If a myelogram was performed at the time radicular pain was present, 35% of patients showed almost complete occlusion. This number increased to 80% when compressive neurologic symptoms were present. Four diagnostic tests are currently available: roentgenogram of the spine, myelogram, CT scan of the spine with mitrizamide contrast, and MRI scan of the spine.[7]

In the absence of any neurologic abnormalities, a negative x-ray study of the spine is sufficient to eliminate the presence of epidural masses. The cancer patient with back pain should continue to be closely observed, however.

In the presence of any neurologic abnormality (radiculopathy or myelopathy), a myelogram should always be performed. It has been found positive in 10% of cases with normal x-ray of the spine. CT scan of the spine can better define a lesion that causes only radicular pain due to minimal bony destruction not evident on plain x-ray nor on a myelogram. An MRI study is frequently the only test that can reveal an intramedullary lesion and can also accurately define neoplastic lesions in the epidural space and bony structures; it appears to be superior to other modalities.[9]

The appropriate treatment for any spinal cord compression due to neoplastic lesions depends on the histology of the primary tumor, the level of the block, the rapidity of onset, and the degree and duration of the block.

XRT accompanied by dexamethasone therapy (4–8 mg p.o. q. 6 hr) and furosemide (given to mitigate the edema caused by the tumor and by radiation) should be instituted at once in patients with minimal or slowly progressive symptoms, with incomplete block, with epidural metastases to the cauda equina, or with complete block of < 6 hr in cases of tumors extremely sensitive to radiation (e.g., multiple myeloma, certain lymphomas, seminomas).

In these cases, laminectomy is restricted to patients who failed to respond to XRT. Laminectomy is the treatment of choice in all patients with rapidly progressing neurologic deficit or acute deficit consistent with spinal cord compression. In these cases, it must be performed < 24 hr from the development of paraplegia. Beyond this time limit, the spinal cord lesions are irreversible even if the compression is relieved. For this reason, in one study laminectomy resulted in partial remission of neurologic deficit in only about 10% of cases with complete blocks due to tumors resistant to radiation. This result was not statistically different from that obtained with radiation alone.[5] Nonetheless, laminectomy is the only chance these patients have for remission of some of their neurologic deficit and for pain relief.

Although most epidural masses are anterior, posterior laminectomy can usually provide acute decompression and tissue diagnosis. The procedure does not preclude radiation within a few days of surgery. Modern orthopedic spine surgery techniques make it possible to resect multiple vertebral bodies by an anterior approach. The role of this procedure in neoplastic vertebral disease has not yet been defined, but it may be indicated in patients with recurrent, slowly growing, and localized disease.[8]

Although laminectomy achieves prompt relief of any cord compression, it rarely results in complete removal of the tumor. For this reason, XRT should be administered postoperatively to prevent tumor regrowth and relieve pain.

Suitable doses of XRT for spinal cord compression are in the range of 3,000–4,000 cGy delivered over 2–4 wk. The outcome of the above outlined treatment of spinal cord compression differs with the type of primary tumor. Satisfactory remission of the neurologic deficit occurs in 50% of patients with lymphoma and multiple myeloma, but in only 30% of patients with breast and prostatic carcinoma and 10–14% of those with other solid tumors. These numbers can be significantly improved if the treatment is instituted before the neurologic deficit becomes apparent.

Other Oncologic Emergencies

In discussing other emergency conditions that can develop in cancer patients due to their neoplasm, a few comments will be made concerning aspects of these situations that are specific to patients with cancer.

Airway Obstruction

Upper airway obstruction, an obstruction of the trachea or larynx, is an exceedingly grave and emergent complication of bronchogenic neoplasms and primary mediastinal tumors. It is not invariably associated with stridor; dyspnea or diffuse wheezing may be the only symptom. Diagnosis may be verified by examining the tracheal air column pattern on routine chest film and by tomography, chest CT, and closed loop pressure studies.

Surgery and the induction of general anesthesias is exceedingly hazardous in such patients and can be fatal, particularly when the obstruction is below the level where intubation or tracheostomy are practicable. XRT is the treatment of choice. Bronchoscopic heat or laser fulguration may be used in refractory or previously irradiated patients. Tracheostomy is, of course, indicated in high obstruction.

Bronchial obstruction and atelectasis. This frequently can cause postobstructive pneumonia, which usually responds well to standard antibiotic therapy. Laser therapy, using the Nd:YAG laser that can be used through a bronchoscope, is the most rapid and efficient way to reduce the occlusive bronchial lesion.[10] Thereafter, treatment should be continued with chemotherapy or irradiation.

In obstruction due to nonoat cell carcinomas or to metastases from other tumors, radiation should be initiated immediately, preceding chemotherapy. The longer the obstruction persists, the more likely it is that the atelectatic lobe will sustain irreversible damage and not reexpand. Conversely, atelectasis documented for < 1 mo may be reversible by prompt radiation.

Vaso-Occlusive Emergencies other than SVC Obstruction

Large veins, rather than arteries, are commonly obstructed in patients with oncologic disease. Lymphatics are also frequently occluded. For the most part, these obstructive phenomena are due to direct impingment of tumors on vessels, but in the hypercoagulable states associated with certain mucin-producing adenocarcinomas (especially pancreatic carcinoma—Trousseau's syndrome) and in polycythemia vera, phlebothromboses at distant sites occur. Thrombosis can also occur with increased frequency in postsurgical patients, in patients treated with hormones or chemotherapeutic agents, and in association with bacterial sepsis.[11]

When a vein is encased by tumor, it is difficult to exclude thrombosis as part of the pathogenesis of the ultimate obstruction, since angiographic procedures usually do not reliably distinguish extrinsic compression, intraluminal tumor masses, or fibrin thrombi from one another. The reduced flow rate and endothelial changes induced by local tumor may promote thrombosis, which may precipitate acute venous obstruction. In such a situation, there may be a role for anticoagulation or even for fibrinolytic therapy while attempts are made to control the obstructing tumor mass. There are few data on such approaches, however, and control of the tumor mass remains the major goal of treatment.

Acute edema of an extremity may result from the occlusion of a major vein, possibly causing greater morbidity and disability than SVCS. In breast cancer, homolateral arm edema may be due to combined surgery and XRT, but is often the result of tumor recurrence deep in the axilla and supraclavicular space that may not be apparent on physical examination. Pelvic lymphoma or local recurrence of rectal or uterine cervical carcinomas may cause severe unilateral leg edema.

Venography is appropriate if the patient presents within a week of the acute development of edema; a trial of heparin or fibrinolytic therapy may be appropriate if the result is compatible with thrombosis and no contraindications are present. CT scanning may help to demonstrate the presence of tumor masses when they are not apparent on physical examination. Systemic chemotherapy—or hormonal therapy in breast cancer patients—should be initiated immediately in patients with potentially responsive tumors. Otherwise, the area should be irradiated regardless of whether a venous thrombosis is demonstrated or whether it responds to anticoagulation.

Hemorrhagic Emergencies

When technically feasible and if the patient can tolerate the procedure, surgery is the treatment of choice for intractable intraluminal bleeding. Otherwise, XRT in large fractions has an excellent styptic effect, usually controlling the problem within days.

Hemoptysis. Copious hemoptysis (persistent expectoration of >20 ml of bright red blood per day) is a grave emergency. Primary bronchogenic malignancies are the most common cause, but adenomas may also bleed heavily. Lobectomy may be considered in patients inoperable by other criteria. Rigid bronchoscopy provides the best opportunity for surgical control. Heat or laser fulguration have been effective, and angiographic embolization has drawn recent interest. XRT remains a definitive treatment if there is time to apply it.

Hematuria. The radiation of residual primary prostatic carcinoma in stage D (with distant metastases) patients is a good way of preventing this complication. Formalin instillation is occasionally effective in hematuria arising from the bladder. Embolization has been effective in controlling bleeding from inoperable renal cell tumors.

Vaginal bleeding. This bleeding may be massive and life-threatening in recurrent uterine or vaginal tumors or in metastatic vaginal implants. Packing usually will control the problem until effective radiation can be delivered.

Disseminated intravascular coagulation (DIC). Although chronic, low-grade DIC is common in a variety of disseminated malignancies, progressive DIC with severe thrombocytopenia and coagulopathy occurs infrequently as the primary result of malignancy. The complications are hemorrhagic rather than vaso-occlusive. This problem is particularly common in promyelocytic (hypergranular, microgranular, M-3) leukemia. It is observed sporadically in metastatic prostatic carcinoma and in metastatic mucin-producing carcinomas, such as gastric or bronchogenic adenocarcinoma.

Elevated fibrin split products, falling fibrinogen levels, elevated thrombin time, progressive coagulopathy, and falling platelet counts are diagnostic. Actual defibrination is not common, and fibrinogen levels may reflect the hyperfibrinogenemia commonly observed in oncologic patients.

This is one of the few types of DIC in which heparin therapy is effective. Full-dose heparin with vigorous clotting factor and platelet replacement should be employed. The presence of schistocytes on the blood smear is diagnostic but not specific. Their absence by no means rules out DIC.

References

1. Yarboro JW, Bornstein RS, eds. Preface. In: Oncologic emergencies. New York, London, Toronto: Grune and Stratton, 1981; 7–9.
2. Perez CA, et al. Management of superior vena cava syndrome. Semin Oncol 1978; 5:123–34.
3. Ahmann FR. A reassessment of the clinical implications of the superior vena cava syndrome. J Clin Oncol 1984; 2:961–69.

4. Theologides A. Neoplastic cardiac tamponade. Semin Oncol 1978; 5:181–92.
5. Cairncross JG, Posner JB. Neurological complications of systemic cancer. In: Oncologic emergencies. Yarboro WJ, Bornstein RS, eds. New York: Grune and Stratton, 1981; 73–96.
6. Rodichok LD, Harper GR, et al. Early diagnosis of spinal epidural metastases. Am J Med 1981; 70:1181–88.
7. Hagenau C, Grosh W, et al. Comparison of spinal MRI and myelography. J Clin Oncol 1987; 5:1663–69.
8. Sundaresan N, Galicich JH. Treatment of spinal metastases by vertebral body resection. Cancer Invest 1984; 2:383–97.
9. Willson JKV, Masaryk TJ. Neurologic emergencies in the cancer patient. Semin Oncol 1989; 16:490–501.
10. Spain RC, Whittlesey D. Respiratory emergencies in patients with cancer. Semin Oncol 1989; 16:471–89.
11. Ratnoff OD. Hemostatic emergencies in malignancy. Semin Oncol 1989; 16:561–71.

17

ACUTE MYELOID LEUKEMIA

Janet Cuttner, M.D., and Kevin M. Troy, M.D.

A CUTE MYELOID LEUKEMIA (AML) is a rare malignancy, with an incidence of 1 case out of 100,000 population; it is the most common type of acute leukemia seen in adults. Patients commonly seek medical attention because of bleeding manifestations or because of recurrent infections. A blood count will usually show anemia, thrombocytopenia, and a variable white blood cell count with a differential showing a predominance of lymphocytes, or mononuclear cells. The patient then is usually referred to a hematologist or medical oncologist for further evaluation. The diagnosis is confirmed by a bone marrow aspiration and biopsy (see chapter 11, figures 11-115, 11-123, 11-124).

Cytologic Classification and Clinical Presentation

AML is classified according to the French-American-British (FAB) classification (table 17-1). According to this classification, AML is subdivided into 8 subtypes, M-O–M-7, based primarily on cytochemical stains as shown in table 17-2. Acute megakaryocytic leukemia (M-7) must be diagnosed by the use of immunological testing.[1] Chapter 10 shows photomicrography of some of these subtypes.

Patients with acute promyelocytic leukemia (M-3) usually present with bleeding; they have the highest incidence of disseminated intravascular coagulation (DIC) as evidenced by low fibringen and increased fibrin degradation products. This diagnosis is usually very easy to make, usually not requiring the use of cytochemical stains. The bone marrow is replaced by predominantly promyelocytes with many auer rods (see chapter 11, figure 11-128). These

Table 17-1. Acute Myeloid Leukemia, FAB* Classification

M-0	Acute undifferentiated leukemia (AUL)
M-1	Acute myeloid leukemia (AML) without maturation
M-2	AML with maturation
M-3	Acute promyelocytic leukemia (APL)
M-4	Acute myelomonocytic leukemia (AMML)
M-5a	Acute monocytic leukemia (AMOL) without maturation
M-5b	AMOL with partial maturation
M-6	Acute erythrocytic leukemia (AEL)
M-7	Acute megakaryocytic leukemia

*French-American-British classification

Table 17-2. Cytochemical Stains*

	PX	SBB	PAS	ABE	NSE	NSE-F	Fe
M-0	0	0	0 to ±	0 to ±	±	±	0
M-1	± to +	± to +	0	± to +	±	±	0
M-2	+ +	+ +	0	± to +	± to +	± to +	0
M-3	+ + + +	+ + + +	0	+	+	± to +	0
M-4	+ +	+ +	0 to ±	+ + to + + +	+ + +	+	0
M-5a	0 to ±	0	±	+ + to + + +	+ + + +	+	0
M-5b	0 to ±	0 to ±	±	+ + to + + +	+ + + +	+	0
M-6	+ to + +	+ to + +	+ (NRBC)	±	±	±	+ to + + sideroblasts
M-7[†]	0	0	± to +	0	+ to + +	0 to ±	0

*PX = myeloperoxidase
 SBB = Sudan black B
 PAS = periodic acid Schiff
 ABE = acetyl butyrate esterase
 NSE = nonspecific esterase
 NSE-F = nonspecific esterase with fluoride inhibition
 Fe = Prussian blue
[†]Must use monoclonal antibodies to make definitive diagnosis

patients must be followed by daily coagulation tests for the first 7–10 days after chemotherapy is begun. It is at this time that the patients are at the greatest risk of developing DIC. The prophylactic use of low-dose or regular-dose heparin remains controversial. They do require support with platelets, fresh frozen plasma, and cryoprecipitate. These patients have a characteristic chromosomal derangement, t(15;17). Table 17-3 shows chromosomal abnormalities, arranged by FAB subtypes, that have been found in AML.

Patients with myelomonocytic and monocytic leukemia (M-4, M-5) may first consult a dentist because of swollen and tender gums; they may present with hyperleukocytosis (see chapter 11, figures 11-129, 11-130, 11-131). These patients have the highest incidence of CNS leukemia.[2] In addition to having gingival hypertrophy, these patients may have hepatosplenomegaly. The diagnosis is made by means of cytochemical stains and, if available, monoclonal antibodies. A group of patients with M-4 acute leukemia and eosinophilia has been reported with q16 abnormality on cytogenetic analysis. These patients appear to have a better prognosis with a longer remission duration and survival.

Table 17-3. Chromosome Abnormalities in AML

M-1	t(9;22) (q34; q11)
	inv (3) (q21; q26)
M-2	t(6;9) (p23; q34)
	t (8;21) (q22; q22)
M-3	t (15;17) (q22;q21)
M-4	t (16;16) (p13; q22)
	inv (16) (p13; q22)
M-4	t (9;11) (p22; q23)
M-5	
M-1, M-2	del (5) (q13–q31)
M-4, M-5	del (7) (q31–q36)
	+8

Patients with acute erythroid leukemia (M-6) may present with a refractory anemia or a myelodysplastic syndrome before progressing to erythroleukemia (see chapter 11, figures 11-132, 11-133). Many patients have been treated with vitamin B_{12}, folic acid, and iron for anemia without response before a correct diagnosis is made.

Acute megakaryocytic leukemia (M-7) is the most recent addition to the FAB classification. These patients commonly have fibrosis present on bone marrow biopsy. It should be noted that this diagnosis requires the use of monoclonal antibodies, which is a departure from the other categories that rely on cytochemical stains.

Prognosis and Therapy

Many studies of prognostic factors in AML have been published purporting to show that one or another factor is important. Among the most important factor in all studies is the age of the patient at diagnosis.[3] The younger the patient, the better the outcome—both in remission induction and in remission duration and survival. Patients over 60 have a poorer prognosis than younger patients, and patients over 70 have an even worse prognosis. Patients who present with hyperleukocytosis (WBC $>100,000$ /μl) have a lower remission induction rate and a shorter remission duration.[4] Patients having multiple chromosomal abnormalities at diagnosis have a poorer prognosis. Patients who develop AML after receiving therapy for another cancer, so-called secondary leukemias, have a very poor prognosis in almost all reported studies. Patients who have a history of a myelodysplastic syndrome before the development of acute leukemia fair poorly.

Supportive Treatment

Before discussing chemotherapy, it is appropriate to discuss supportive therapy, because the latter is vital to a good outcome. All patients aged ≤ 45 yr who have siblings should receive only irradiated blood products until a decision is made on bone marrow transplantation. Patients and siblings should be HLA typed. Patients with a WBC of $> 100,000 /\mu$l should undergo leukapheresis, if it is available, as a means of preventing the complications of leukostasis. Unless there is a history of allergy, all patients should be placed on allopurinol at diagnosis. Dosage can usually be stopped 7–10 days after the start of chemotherapy. All patients should have an indwelling I.V. catheter such as a Broviac or Hickman inserted before chemotherapy is begun. The nursing and medical staff should be familiar with the care of these catheters. Platelet transfusions should be given if there are signs of bleeding. They should also be given prophylactically for platelet counts of $\leq 20,000/\mu$l. Platelet concentrates are usually available from a blood center; administration of 6 U/day is recommended. Single-donor platelets are preferred if they are available. Granulocyte transfusions are usually available only at centers specializing in the treatment of acute leukemia. The indications for granulocyte transfusions are proven sepsis in a granulocytopenic patient or suspected sepsis in a granulocytic patient undergoing chemotherapy who is unresponsive to broad-spectrum antibiotics.

Therapy of Infection in a Compromised Host

Infections remain the commonest cause of death in patients with acute leukemia.[5] With the use of more intensive chemotherapy regimens, patients are severely granulocytopenic for prolonged periods of time, thus making them vulnerable to infectious complications. Bacterial infections, especially those caused by gram-negative organisms, account for most cases of proven sepsis. Gram-positive infections, especially with staphylococcal organisms, are a cause of many I.V. catheter infections, and fungal infections are increasing in incidence. At our institution (Mount Sinai Medical Center, New York), we treat all leukemia patients undergoing chemotherapy with clotrimazole troches to prevent oral candida infections. Even more serious are such invasive fungal diseases as aspergillus and mucor; they are treated with amphotericin B. Herpetic infections of the mouth can now be treated with oral acyclovir, but if the infection is extensive, I.V. acyclovir should be used. All granulocytopenic patients with AML undergoing chemotherapy who develop a fever must be treated promptly. A history and physical examination should be performed to look for an infection; blood cultures, throat cultures, urine cultures, and a chest x-ray also should be performed. If no obvious infection is found, patients should be empirically treated with broad-spectrum bactericidal antibiotics. The regimens will vary, but they usually include a cephalosporin and an aminoglycoside or a cephalosporin, aminoglycoside, and a third-generation penicillin derivative.

Antineoplastic Therapy

Induction chemotherapy with cytosine arabinoside (ara-C) and an anthracy-cline (either daunorubicin or Adriamycin) produces 50–70% remission rates.[6] The most experience has been with a 7-day infusion of ara-C and 3 days of daunorubicin (7 + 3) (see Appendix). Certain centers will add a third drug such as 6-thioguanine. Comparative randomized studies have not shown a that the addition of a third drug is beneficial.

The median remission duration in most studies is between 15–18 mo. Many groups are showing a 5-yr 15–30% relapse-free survival. The goal of newer treatments is to increase this percentage. It appears that "standard" mainten-tance consisting of monthly courses of ara-C with other drugs (e.g., cyclophos-phamide, 6-thioguanine, or an anthracycline) does not achieve this. Research groups such as the Cancer and Leukemia Group B are now involved in randomized studies comparing multiple consolidation courses of chemother-apy with either infusional ara-C at 200 mg/m^2 or with high-dose ara-C (HiDAC) to see if this will produce a longer relapse-free survival. Other groups are using HiDAC chemotherapy for remission induction and consolidation (see Appendix).[7] These types of treatment should be used only in centers where good supportive therapy is available. CNS prophylaxis with intrathecal ara-C should be considered for patients who present with elevated WBCs of 100,000/ μl or with M-4, M-5 type AML, as these patients are at greater risk of developing CNS leukemia.

In the past few years, bone marrow transplantation has become an important consideration in AML therapy. Very few randomized studies are available comparing chemotherapy and bone marrow transplantation, but certain generalizations can be made. The procedure is done when the patient is in remission, with the best results being obtained when the patient is in the first remission.[8] The immediate (first 60 days) mortality is very age-dependent. The best results are in patients under 20.[9]

The mortality of the procedure increases with each decade of life; very few transplant centers will treat patients over 50. The initial mortality is usually due to acute graft-versus-host disease (GVHD) or to infections, especially viral infections. The Seattle transplant group believes that chronic GVHD may have an antileukemic effect. Patients with AML transplanted in first remission who survive the first 100 days have a longer relapse-free survival than do patients treated with chemotherapy. The overall survival of age-matched patients receiving chemotherapy may not be different because of the early mortality seen in transplantation. Randomized studies are needed in age-matched patients to determine the best treatment. All patients younger than 40 should be HLA typed, and if they are not a participant in a study, bone marrow transplantation would be a therapeutic option if an HLA-identical sibling were available.

A newer therapy for AML in patients who do not have an HLA-identical sibling is the use of autologous marrow transplantation.[10] Bone marrow harvested from the patient in remission is purged with monoclonal antibodies or drugs in an attempt to remove residual leukemic cells. The "purged" marrow is then reinfused after the patient is given myeloablative therapy. Autologous bone marrow transplantation should be considered for relapsed patients who have been reinduced into remission and who do not have a suitable allogeneic donor. It should also be considered for high-risk, first-remission patients.

References

1. Bennett JM, Catovsky D, Daniel MT, et al. Criteria for the diagnosis of acute leukemia of megakaryocyte lineage (M7). A report of the French-American-British Cooperative Group. Ann Intern Med 1985; 103:460–62.
2. Meyer RJ, Ferreira PPC, Cuttner J, Greenberg M, Goldberg J, Holland JF. Central nervous system involvement at presentation in acute granulocytic leukemia: a prospective cytocentrifuge study. Am J Med 1980; 68:691–94.
3. Delmer A, Marie JP, Thevenin D, Cadious M, Viguie F, Zittoun R. Multivariate analysis of prognostic factors in acture myeloid leukemia: value of clonogenic leukemic cell properties. J Clin Oncol 1989; 7:738–46.
4. Cuttner J, Conjalka MS, Reilly M, Goldberg J, Meyer RJ, Holland JF. Association of monocytic leukemia in patients who present with extreme leukocytoses. Am J Med 1980; 60:555–58.
5. Bodey GP, Buckley M, Sathe YS, Freireich EJ. Quantitative relationships between circulating leukocytes and infection in patients with acute leukemia. Ann Intern Med 1966; 64:328–40.
6. Preisler HD, Anderson K, Rai K, Cuttner J, Yates J, DuPre E, Holland JF. The frequency of long-term remission in patients with acute myelogenous leukaemia treated with conventional maintenance chemotherapy: a study of 760 patients with a minimal follow-up time of 6 years. Br J Haematol 1989; 71:189–94.
7. Wolff SN, Marion J, Stein RS, et al. High-dose cytosine arabinoside and daunorubicin as consolidation therapy for acute nonlymphocytic leukemia in first remission: a pilot study. Blood 1985; 65:1407–16.
8. Appelbaum FR, Dahlberg S, Thomas ED, et al. Bone marrow transplantation or chemotherapy after remission induction for adults with acute nonlymphoblastic leukemia. Ann Intern Med 1984; 101:581–88.
9. Petersen FB, Buckner D. Allogeneic and autologous bone marrow transplantation for acute leukemia and malignant lymphoma: current status. Hematol Oncol 1987; 5:233–43.
10. Yeager AM, Kaizer H, Santos GW, et al. Autologous bone marrow transplantation in patients with acute nonlymphocytic leukemia, using ex vivo marrow treatment with 4-hydroperoxycyclophosphamide. N Engl J Med 1986; 315(3):141–7.

18

CHRONIC MYELOCYTIC LEUKEMIA

Janet Cuttner, M.D., and Kevin M. Troy, M.D.

Pathophysiology

CHRONIC MYELOCYTIC LEUKEMIA (CML) was the first hematologic neoplasm to be associated with a consistent cytogenetic abnormality—the Philadelphia (Ph′) chromosome. The Ph′ chromosome usually results from a balanced translocation of the long arms of chromosomes 9 and 22 t(9;22) (q34.1; q11.21). Very recently, molecular biology techniques have shown that the breakpoint of the translocation does vary among patients but occurs within a small region on chromosome 22, resulting in the translocation of the proto-oncongene c-abl (usually on chromosome 9) to chromosome 22; and c-sis, which is usually on 22, goes to chromosome 9.[1] Groffen et al identified this small region, known as the breakpoint cluster region (bcr), on chromosome 22.[2] This region contains the chromosomal breakpoints in all patients with CML who are Ph′ positive. They have shown that the bcr is part of a gene, the bcr gene. As a consequence of the Ph′ translocation, part of the gene is translocated to chromosome 9 and the rest remains on the Ph′ chromosome. As a consequence of the translocation, a novel DNA sequence is created on chromosome 22 composed of c-abl plus a portion of the bcr region. Transcription of this sequence leads to the production of a tyrosine kinase that may possibly play a role in the pathogenesis of CML.

Through glucose -6- phosphate dehydrogenase (G6PD) isoenzyme studies and cytogenetic analysis, Fialkow et al have shown that CML is a clonal disorder of the pluripotent hematopoietic stem cell.[3]

Natural History and Clinical Presentation

Although enormous progress has been made in understanding CML, largely through molecular biology and cytogenetics, the natural history of the disease itself has changed only slightly. Patients usually present because of symptoms due to anemia or because of symptoms referable to an enlarged spleen. Weakness, fatigue, increasing abdominal girth, early satiety, or left upper quadrant pain are common presenting symptoms. Patients are usually found to be mildly anemic (Hgb 10–12 gm/dl) and have an elevated WBC, with a differential resembling bone marrow (see chapter 11, figure 11-135) i.e., myelocytes, meta-myelocytes, stabs, segs, occasional basophils, and a rare promyelocyte and myeloblast. Physical examination usually shows only pallor of the mucous membranes and splenomegaly. The WBC is always elevated. The platelet count is usually normal or mildly elevated. The diagnosis is confirmed by a bone marrow aspiration, biopsy (see chapter 11, figure 11-114), cytogenetic studies, and/or molecular studies. The Ph′ chromosome is found in 85–90% of patients. Appropriate additional studies would include serum B_{12}, which is characteristically sharply elevated; leukocyte alkaline phosphatase (LAPA), which is low to absent; and serum uric acid, which may be elevated.

Most patients with CML present in what is known as the chronic phase of the disease. After an average time of 3 yr, half of these patients will progress to either an accelerated or blastic phase of CML that is typically highly resistant to therapy. Thus, the median survival in CML is 38–44 mo, with most patients deceased at 5 yr.

Prognosis and Therapy

Several groups have looked at prognostic factors in CML. Age is an important factor, with older patients having a worse prognosis. Patients with a cytogenetic abnormality in addition to the Ph′ have a very poor prognosis. Patients with increasing basophilia or a spleen size of >6 cm have shortened survival,[4,5] as also do patients who lack the Ph′ chromosome.

Conventional therapy for patients in the chronic phase of CML is busulfan or hydroxyurea (HYD). Currently, HYD would be the chemotherapeutic agent of choice. Both agents are given orally; hydroxyurea has few side effects other than bone marrow depression. Initially, allopurinol is given to prevent hyperuricemia from cellular breakdown. Because side effects are few, almost all patients can continue to lead normally active lives until they enter an accelerated phase. In our experience, patients who present with greatly elevated WBC and/or platelet counts, respond better to cyclical treatment with cytosine arabinoside and 6-thioguanine. A few groups have used aggressive multiagent chemotherapy in an effort to decrease the Ph′ chromosome and prolong the chronic phase of the disease.[6] Unfortunately, to date they have been able to induce only a 6-mo prolongation at best, and this has been with a marked increase in toxicity. Because most patients with CML have splenomegaly—and marked splenomegaly has been found to be a indicator of shortened survival—splenectomy has been advocated by some groups. Several randomized studies have shown no increase in survival with splenectomy.

Bone marrow transplantation is being tried in many centers. Patients are usually pretreated with chemotherapy and total body irradiation. Virtually all patients who engraft will lose their Ph′ chromosome. As with acute leukemia, age is the most important prognostic factor. Younger patients have the longest survival and the lowest mortality. Initial results appear promising, but it is still too early to say if a significant improvement in survival will be obtained. Patients with an identical twin, however, have been shown to have a very significantly improved survival and should be transplanted within the first year of diagnosis.[7]

The newest treatment for CML is the use of the biological modifier alpha interferon. This treatment was first reported by the group at the University of Texas M.D. Anderson Cancer Center and has been confirmed by other groups. The initial Anderson report on 14 patients with CML showed that 13/14 had a hematologic response. Of greater importance, however, was that in 6 of the patients with hematologic remission, a complete suppression of the Ph′ chromosome was observed in at least 1 examination period. This is the first form of treatment other than bone marrow transplantation in which there has been a decrease—and in some cases, complete loss—of the Ph′ chromosome. Long-term results from these studies are awaited.

Alpha interferon is given subcutaneously on a daily basis. The main toxicity is fever and a flulike syndrome that usually subsides in several weeks' time. Whether this will translate to prevention of blast crisis is unknown at present, but this is an area of active research.

The *blastic phase* of CML is characterized by fever, anemia, leukocytosis, marked splenomegaly, and increased numbers of blasts and promyelocytes. About 30% of these patients will have a lymphoblastic transformation with TdT positivity. This group of patients will respond for a time to the same treatment given for acute lymphoblastic leukemia. They have a median survival of 6–8 mo. The 70% of patients with myeloblastic transformation respond very poorly to chemotherapy and have a median survival of 3 mo.

References

1. De Klein A, Geurts van Kessel A, Grosveld G, et al. A cellular oncogene is translocated to the Philadelphia chromosome in chronic myelocytic leukemis. Nature 1982; 300:765-7.
2. Groffen J, Stephenson JR, Heisterkamp N, de Klein A, Bartram CR, Grosveld G. Philadelphia chromosomal breakpoints are clustered within a limited region, bcr, on chromosome 22. Cell 1984; 36:93-9.
3. Fialkow PJ, Jacobson RJ. Papayannopoulou T: chronic myelocytic leukemia: Clonal origin in a stem cell common to the granulocyte, erythrocyte, platelet and monocyte/macrophage. Am J Med 1977; 63:125-30.
4. Kantarjian HM, Smith TL, McCredie KB, et al. Chronic myelogenous leukemia: A multivariate analysis of the associations of patient characteristics and therapy with survival. Blood 1985; 66:1326-35.

5. Sokal JE, Cox EB, Baccorani M, et al. Prognostic discrimination in "good-risk" chronic granulocytic leukemia. Blood 1984; 63:789–99.
6. Clarkson B. Chronic myelogenous leukemia: is aggressive treatment indicated? J Clin Oncol 1985; 3:135–38.
7. Fefer A, Cheever MA, Thomas ED, et al. Disappearance of Ph'-positive cells in four patients with chronic granulocytic leukemia after chemotherapy, irradiation and marrow transplantation from an identical twin. N Engl J Med 1979; 300:333–37.
8. Talpaz M, Kantarjian HM, McCredie K, Trujillo JM, Keating MJ, Gutterman JU. Hematologic remission and cytogenetic improvement induced by recombinant human interferon alpha in chronic myelogenous leukemia. N Engl J Med 1986; 314:1065–69.

19

ACUTE LYMPHOBLASTIC
LEUKEMIA

Kevin M. Troy, M.D., and Janet Cuttner, M.D.

Incidence and Pathophysiology

ACUTE LYMPHOBLASTIC LEUKEMIA (ALL) is a malignant disorder arising in lymphoid progenitor cells. It is characterized by the accumulation of poorly differentiated lymphoblasts within the bone marrow, with consequent marrow replacement and suppression of normal hematopoiesis. ALL can occur at any age. Its overall incidence is about the same as AML, but its peak incidence is in children aged 2–10. Great progress has been made in the treatment of childhood ALL, with about 50% of children now expected to be long-term survivors. Although improved induction chemotherapy and supportive care have now enabled most adults with ALL to enter remission, the percentage of long-term survivors remains disappointingly small. Predisposing factors are less readily identified in ALL than in AML. Studies in twins suggest some genetic predisposition to ALL in childhood, with the identical twin of a child with ALL having a 20% chance of developing the disease within the next year. An increased incidence of ALL has been noted in survivors of atomic bomb explosions. In general, however, ALL is not associated with prior identifiable injury to stem cells and is rarely preceded by a "preleukemic" phase. The exception to this is Burkitt's-type ALL, which has been associated with Epstein-Barr virus infection.

443

Clinical Presentation and Diagnosis

The presenting symptoms of ALL are usually referable to suppression of normal hematopoiesis and less commonly due to tissue infiltration. Thus, symptoms of fatigue, weakness, and dyspnea secondary to anemia; mucosal bleeding and bruisability due to thrombocytopenia; and infections related to granulocytopenia are common. Bone pain and arthralgias may occur, but are more common in children.

Lymphadenopathy and hepatosplenomegaly are not uncommon physical findings, but usually are not marked. CNS involvement is not common at presentation, but if it occurs it is manifested by signs of increased intracranial pressure (headache, blurred vision, and vomiting) and cranial nerve palsies. T cell ALL is associated with male predominance, high initial WBC, and high incidence of mediastinal mass.

Table 19-1. Acute Lymphoid leukemia, FAB* Classification

L-1	Cells are small, uniform in appearance, scanty cytoplasm, nucleoli are inconspicuous (childhood type)
L-2	Cells are large and heterogenous in appearance, nuclei may be irregular in shape and indented, nucleoli are often prominent, cytoplasm may be abundant (adult type)
L-3	Cells are large and homogenous, cytoplasm is deeply basophilic, cytosplasmic vacuolation is prominent (Burkitt-like)

*French-American-British classification

Laboratory examination usually reveals anemia and thrombocytopenia. The WBC is usually elevated, often strikingly so, but is normal or low in one third of the patients. The diagnosis of ALL is confirmed by examination of the peripheral blood and bone marrow for blast cell morphology, cytochemistry, and immunophenotyping. Morphologically, ALL is subdivided according the the French-American-British (FAB) classification shown in table 19-1.[4] L-1 represents the predominant type of ALL found in childhood (see chapter 11, figure 11-118). L-2 (chapter 11, figure 11-119) displays more heterogenous features and is the type of ALL most commonly seen in adults. L-3 (chapter 11, figure 11-121) has a distinctive morphology, represents Burkitt's-type ALL, and is rare. It has characteristic immunologic and cytogenetic features described below.

Cytochemical studies may be useful in confirming a diagnosis of ALL suspected on morphologic grounds. In most cases, the leukemic cells will show some PAS (periodic acid Schiff) positivity, which is often present in a blocklike pattern. Myeloperoxidase activity and Sudan black B positivity are absent. T cell ALL (see chapter 11, figure 11-120) may demonstrate dotlike positivity in ANBE (alpha-naphthyl butyrate esterase) as well as acid phosphatase positivity.

More critical to the diagnosis of ALL than cytochemistry is the use of immunophenotyping techniques. Terminal deoxynucleotidyl transferase (TdT) is an enzyme that can be demonstrated by either cytochemical or immunofluorescent techniques. TdT activity is normally present in the thymus and in lymphoid progenitor cells in the bone marrow. Significantly increased activity is associated with ALL. Specifically, TdT activity is present in T cell and "common" ALL. It is not found in B cell (surface immunoglobulin positive) ALL. The presence of TdT activity is not specific for ALL, being found in about 30% of cases of blast crisis CML, in lymphoblastic lymphoma, and in a certain subset of patients with AML (so-called "biphenotypic" cases).

Immune surface markers are of critical importance in ALL, both diagnostically and prognostically. In the past, the use of E rosette formation and surface immunoglobulin has shown that 20–30% of patients with ALL have T cell disease. Surface immunoglobulin is found in most patients with Burkitt's but very rarely in other forms of ALL. Newer techniques, including the use of monoclonal antibodies, have shown that some E rosette-negative patients possess other T cell markers and that other "null cell" ALL patients have cells containing cytoplasmic immunoglobulin and thus represent pre-B cell ALL. Immune markers have shown that most ALL cases are of B cell lineage. A 1985 study reported the results of monoclonal antibody studies on 90 adult patients with ALL.[2] The patients fell into 4 groups. Most of the patients (58/90) had evidence of B cell lineage by CALLA or B1, B2, B3, B4 positivity. None had surface immunoglobulin (true B cell ALL); 12/90 had evidence of T cell ALL (T+, BA-1–); 8/90 had true null cell ALL (ALL monoclonal antibodies negative); and 6 were classified as having myeloid antigen ALL. The remaining 6 patients could not be classified.

Cytogenetic analysis can be prognostically useful in ALL and diagnostically important in Burkitt's. The most common cytogenetic abnormality in ALL is the presence of the Philadelphia (Ph′) chromosome t(9;22), which is found in about 20% of patients. Its presence is associated with a significantly worse prognosis. Most patients with Burkitt's have a specific cytogenetic abnormality: t(8;14).[1]

The role of molecular genetics in the evaluation of acute leukemia remains to be established. However, 2 important findings have been made with respect to ALL: (1) the finding of immunoglobulin gene rearrangements in the majority of patients with CALLA + ALL, confirming the B-cell lineage of this leukemia; and (2) the possible role of the c-myc oncogene in Burkitt's lymphoma. The c-myc oncogene is normally found on the distal end of chromosome 8. In the 8;14 translocation characteristic of Burkitt's, the c-myc oncogene is normally found on the distal end of chromosome 8. In the 8;14 translocation characteristic of Burkitt's, the c-myc oncogene is brought into proximity of the gene coding for the heavy chain of immunoglobulin. Under the influence of the immunoglobulin heavy chain promotor, there is increased transcription of c-myc, with consequent increase in the DNA-binding protein that is the product of c-myc. This in turn may play a role in malignant transformation.[1]

Prognosis and Therapy

Prognostic factors have been clearly delineated for childhood ALL. Adverse prognostic factors include age (<2 or >10 yr); presence of initial high WBC, T cell, B cell, or true null cell disease; L-2 or L-3 morphology; or the presence of cytogenetic abnormalities. More controversy surrounds the prognosis for adults, but advanced age, presence of non-"common" ALL and initial high WBC are poor prognostic factors for remission achievement and remission duration in most studies, with age being the most important. The presence of the Ph' chromosome at diagnosis signals a very poor prognosis.

The role of supportive therapy in acute leukemia has been reviewed in the chapter on AML. Initial effective therapy for ALL in adults was based on the childhood ALL experience with the use of vincristine (VCR) and prednisone in induction therapy (see Appendix). Only about 40% of patients enter remission with this regimen. The addition of L-asparaginase increases the frequency of complete response (CR) to about 50%. With the use of an anthracycline in addition to VCR and prednisone, the CR rate can be increased to 75–85%.[3] Unfortunately, although the addition of an anthracycline has led to greatly increased CR rates in adults, its use in induction therapy has not led to an increase in long-term survivors. Using maintenance therapy (see Appendix) with methotrexate (MTX) and 6-mercaptopurine with periodic reinforcement with VCR and prednisone, the median duration of remission is about 15 mo, irrespective of anthracycline use in induction. Only 15–20% of patients achieve long-term CR. A variety of strategies have been revised in an attempt to improve long-term survivorship, the best results having been obtained with regimens using intensive multidrug consolidation. The success of these regimens has varied considerably from study to study. The L-10 protocol demonstrated a 39% continuous CR at 5 yr.[5] Unfortunately, not all similar regimens have produced such dramatic results.[7] The optimal intensity and duration of postremission induction therapy in adult ALL remain uncertain at present. The Cancer and Leukemia Group B is currently studying the use of 3 intensification courses given over a period of about 6 mo.

The incidence of CNS involvement is much higher in adult ALL than in AML. Although only about 10% of patients have overt CNS disease at presentation, ≤50% of patients will develop this complication during the course of the disease if prophylactic treatment is not given. Prophylactic therapy, usually given shortly after CR is achieved, usually consists of cranial radiotherapy (2,400 cGy in 12 fractions) accompanied by 5 to 6 doses of intrathecal MTX (12 mg/m^2, with a maximum of 15 mg/dose). An alternative approach is the use of high-dose systemic MTX in combination with intrathecal MTX. The use of high-dose systemic MTX following cranial irradiation has been associated with an increased incidence of leukoencephalopathy and should be avoided if possible. It is clear that prophylactic CNS treatment can decrease the risk of CNS relapse in ALL; therefore, it is recommended that every patient with ALL receive such treatment.

Allogeneic bone marrow transplantation has been used as an alternative strategy to prolong survival in ALL patients who achieve remission and have a suitable (usually sibling) donor. In addition to problems with graft-versus-host disease that preclude its use in older patients, there is a higher risk of leukemic relapse following bone marrow transplantation in ALL than in AML. For this reason, transplantation should be reserved for patients in second remission or for those in first remission with particularly adverse prognostic features (e.g., Ph' chromosome positivity) or high initial white count.

References

1. Bartram CM. Activation of proto-oncogenes in human leukemias. Blut 1985; 51:63–71.
2. Sobol RE, Royston I, Lebien TW, et al. Adult acute lymphoblastic leukemia phenotypes defined by monoclonal antibodies. Blood 1985; 65:730–35.
3. Gottlieb AJ, Weinberg V, Ellison RR, et al. Efficacy of daunorubicin in the therapy of adult acute lymphocytic leukemia: a prospective randomized trial by Cancer and Leukemia Group B. Blood 1984; 64:267–74.
4. Bennett JM, Catovsky D, Daniel MT, et al. Proposals for the classification of acute leukemias. Br J Haematol 1976; 33:451–58.
5. Schauer P, Arlin ZA, Mertelsmann R, et al. Treatment of acute lymphoblastic leukemia in adults: results of the L-10 and L-10M protocols. J Clin Oncol 1983; 1 (8):462–70.
6. Champlin R, Gale RP. Acute lymphoblastic leukemia: recent advances in biology and therapy. Blood 1989; 73:2051–66.
7. Hoelzer D, Thiel E, Loffler H, et al. Intensified therapy in acute lymphoblastic and acute undifferentiated leukemia in adults. Blood 1984; 64:38–47.

20

ADULT T CELL
LEUKEMIA/LYMPHOMA

Muthuswamy Krishnamurthy, M.D., F.A.C.P., and
Harvey Dosik, M.D., F.A.C.P.

ADULT T CELL LEUKEMIA/LYMPHOMA (ATLL) was first described in 1977 as a rapidly progressive fatal lymphoproliferative disorder affecting adults in Southwestern Japan. It has unique clinical, morphological, immunophenotypic, and epidemiological features and is associated with infection by a type C human retrovirus (HTLV-1).[2,3] The disease is endemic in circumscribed geographic regions of Japan and the Caribbean basin.[1,4] It has also been found in Southern United States[5,7] and is reported in sporadic clusters worldwide.[6-11]

Clinical and Laboratory Features

ATLL generally occurs in young to middle-aged adults of either sex. Japanese patients tend to be older (median 56 yr) than patients from the United States and the Caribbean area (median age: 34 and 40 yr). In the United States, almost all patients are black. There is an increased familial disposition for ATLL in affected families. Characteristic clinical features include generalized lymphadenopathy with sparing of the mediastinum, hepatosplenomegaly, frequent skin infiltration, hypercalcemia with or without destructive bone lesions, interstitial pulmonary infiltrates, and the presence of leukemic cells with distinct morphological features. The leukemic cells are mature T cells of the helper inducer type showing prominent pleomorphism with polylobulated and irregular nuclei (see chapter 11, figure 11-120). Opportunistic infections and infiltration of organs—especially of the pulmonary and central nervous system—and renal failure are common. The disease usually runs an aggressive course.[1,4-7,11-20]

Clinical diversity of this aggressive disorder has been recognized. Acute, chronic, smoldering, crisis, and lymphoma types of ATLL have been described according to clinical behavior. Crisis is the transformation of the chronic and smoldering type into the acute type.[13] Although no seasonal incidence was found in a large study of ATLL from Japan,[21] one study from the United States noted progression to the aggressive phase or onset of illness occurring during the coldest months of the year.[11]

Cutaneous manifestations, which are diverse and not pathognomonic, may take the form of erythematous or purpuric papules, discrete or confluent nodules, and plaques with or without ulceration. There may be vesicular and pruritic eruptions,[5,6,12-15,20] and generalized maculopapular, erythematous, or parapsoriatic lesions are also described.

Hypercalcemia is frequently associated with ATLL, and the patient may present with signs and symptoms related to this disorder. The mechanism of hypercalcemia is poorly understood and seems diverse. Serum phosphate levels are usually within the normal range. Serum parathormone levels are usually normal or appropriately low. Serum calcitriol levels are either low or normal.[11,12] Most patients demonstrate evidence of osteoclast activation and increased bone turnover. Bone scans show increased uptake of radionucleotide throughout the skeleton, most prominently in the skull and joints. These so-called "super scans" are unusual in other lymphomas. Serum alkaline phosphatase levels are increased in most patients. Skeletal surveys may show destructive bone lesions. The neoplastic cells may produce a bone resorption stimulating factor.[22] Calcium seems to play an important role in the growth of ATLL cells. The growth of ATLL cells and the expressions of interleukin-2 receptors (Tac antigens) on ATLL cells in vitro are enhanced by calcium and inhibited by calcium antagonists.[23] Thus, the hypercalcemia triggered by the disease may in turn accelerate the disease process.

The presence of typical neoplastic cells in the peripheral blood, cutaneous infiltrates, and hypercalcemia may be present at diagnosis or develop some time during the course of the illness. Opportunistic infections, notably pneumocystis carinii, fungi, and viruses, frequently occur. This is the result of T cell dysfunction secondary to the disease itself and chemotherapy treatment.[5,6,10,12,15,19,24]

ATLL should be distinguished from the following conditions: mycosis fungoides, Sézary syndrome, related cutaneous T cell lymphomas, and T chronic lymphocytic leukemia.[6] In addition, ATLL should be considered in non-Hodgkins lymphomas with unusual features such as hypercalcemia and skin infiltration.

Pathology

ATLL is characterized by a broad range of morphological features.[25,26] Although characteristic ATLL cells are present in most patients, in some cases the nuclear irregularities are less extreme, and differentiation from Sézary syndrome on a morphological basis alone may be difficult.[7,12] The neoplastic cells are T cells and express OK-4, Leu 3 phenotype with absence of OKT-8, and

Leu 2 cell surface markers. Anti-Tac (antigen—T cell growth factor receptor) is prominent.[27,28]

The histopathological spectrum is broad, encompassing several diffuse histological subtypes in the Rappaport classification, the working formulation, and the classification of the lymphoma study group.[25] No correlation can be made between the clinical course and the histological subtypes.[26] Pathologically, ATLL cannot be distinguished from virus negative lymphomas on morphological grounds.[12]

Cutaneous involvement occurs in most ATLL patients.[1,4-7,9-15] Focal epidermal infiltration or Pautrier's microabscesses are common, but acanthosis and hyperkeratosis are usually absent, thus mimicking cutaneous T cell lymphomas. Other sites of involvement include bone marrow, lungs, and meninges.[5,10,12] Bone marrow may not be involved, even in patients with peripheral blood involvement. but if such involvement is present, it usually is of a lesser degree than one would expect, given the high level of circulating neoplastic cells. Biopsy of lytic bone lesions usually fails to demonstrate involvement by tumor, showing only microscopic resorption and increased osteoclastic activity.[10,12,25,26] These findings support the concept of lymphokinin production by neoplastic cells, which is believed to be responsible for osteoclastic activation.

The single most characteristic pathological finding in ATLL is the presence of the typical neoplastic cells. When these are not prominent, the disease can be mistaken for other types of non-Hodgkin's lymphomas. A high index of suspicion, along with clinical correlation in endemic areas, will aid correct diagnosis.

Cytogenetic studies in ATLL reveal several abnormalities.[29-32] The most frequently involved chromosomes are 3, 6, 10, 13, 14 and X. They are observed most frequently in unstimulated cultures of peripheral blood or bone marrow. Cytogenetic abnormalities may be detected in peripheral blood even when there are no morphologically detectable abnormal cells in the peripheral blood. They include trisomy 3, 7, partial deletion of the long arm of chromosome 10 and 4q, 14q, 14q +, 7p, and loss of the X chromosome in female patients. In a recent study, the loss of the short arm of chromosome 10 (10p −) was found to be predominent.[29]

More severe manifestations of ATLL seem to correlate with the most extensive karyotypic abnormalities. The presence of a 6q deletion tends to be associated with a more indolent course,[30] and a strong correlation seems to exist between the presence of 7q abnormality and the expression of Tac antigen.[31]

The interleukin-2 receptor (IL-2R or Tac antigen), encoded by a gene located on 10p (band p14–p15), is known to be overexpressed in this type of leukemic cell. Recent observations using the Southern blot technique revealed rearrangement of the IL-2R gene that correlated with 10p abnormalities.[29a]

Etiology and Epidemiology

The studies of ATLL by Gallo and co-workers provided the most convincing evidence of the viral etiology of human cancer.[2] ATLL is caused by human leukemia/lymphoma virus (HTLV-1), a unique, exogenously acquired human type C retrovirus with distinct nucleotide sequence of the provirus genome.[33] HTLV-1 (originally isolated from a cutaneous T cell lymphoma) adult T cell leukemia virus ATLV (isolated later from an ATLL patient in Japan),[34] and the Caribbean HTLV all have been proven to be the same.[35]

The viral association is also borne out by clinical and extensive seroepidemiological work. Antibodies to the viral core protein have been demonstrated in more than 90% of patients with ATLL from various areas.[37-38] The association of the virus is also demonstrated by detecting the provirus genome in ATLL cells.[39] Antibodies were not detected in most non-ATLL T cell malignant disorders and nonlymphoid neoplasms.

Population surveys for the presence of the HTLV-1 antibody revealed a low incidence in nonendemic areas and a high incidence in endemic areas. The prevalence increases with age in endemic areas. The prevalence of HTLV-1 antibodies in close family members of patients with ATLL is 3–4 times more than in normal populations in the area.[40-43] Close, prolonged, and intimate contact seems to be essential for production of disease. The development of frank ATLL in antibody-positive healthy carriers is of low incidence, but the incidence is higher in the older age group.[42-43]

The prevalence of HTLV antibodies seems to be high in individuals who received multiple blood transfusions in endemic areas where the incidence of antibody-positive individuals is greater among blood donors.[41,44,45] HTLV-1 infection has been shown to be transmitted by blood transfusion, by seroconversion, and by demonstration of proviral DNA of HTLV-1 in recipients. HTLV-1 antibodies are not present to a greater extent in individuals receiving multiple transfusions in nonendemic areas.[46-47] Of interest is the presence of antibodies to HTLV-1 in association with HTLV-3 antibodies in a significant number of I.V. drug abusers and patients with AIDS.[48]

The virus appears to be transmitted through sexual intercourse, transfusion of contaminated blood products, sharing of needles during I.V. drug abuse, and perinatally during the birth process.

Recently, a small number of patients (5) with typical ATLL, but with no evidence of integration of HTLV-1 into the leukemic cells or presence of HTLV-1 antibody in their sera, have been reported from a nonendemic area, suggesting that factors other than HTLV-1 infection may be involved in ATLL leukemogenesis.[49]

Biology of HTLV-1

HTLV-1 can transform primary human T cells in vitro. Because transformed T cells show similarity to HTLV-1–positive primary ATLL cells, this system affords an opportunity to learn about the detailed molecular mechanism of transformation, also relevant to the situation in nature.

HTLV-1 is a human T lymphotropic virus that directly infects the lymphocytes and, by using reverse transcriptase, makes a DNA copy that subsequently integrates into a host cell DNA to form a "provirus." This HTLV integration into the target cells is a prerequisite for the development of ATLL.[50] The provirus then interacts with host cellular genes and also directs the synthesis of proteins encoded by the viral gene.

ATLL is associated with abnormal expression of IL-2R. ATLL cells spontaneously and continuously express IL-2R. They contain 5–10 times more IL-2R than lymphoblasts maximally stimulated with phytohemagglutinin. Unlike normal T lymphocytes, ATLL cells on long-term culture with IL-2R do not demonstrate a rapid decline of the receptors. Some ATLL cells also have aberrant IL-2 receptors.[51-54] Unlike normal activated T cells, IL-2R of ATLL cells are not down-regulated by the addition of anti-Tac. IL-2R in ATLL cells remain spontaneously and persistently phosphorylated, whereas the IL-2R of mitogen-activated T cells are phosphorylated only in the presence of IL-2R.[55] This nonregulatory phosphorylated state may relate to the leukemogenesis of ATLL by HTLV-1.

The mechanism of IL-2R expression by HTLV-1 has been studied, and it has been found that HTLV-1 genomes do not contain cell-derived "onc" genes. The virus contains the gag, pol, env, and long-terminal repeat (LTR) common to all retroviruses. It has an additional unique genomic region, known as PX, which encodes a 42-kd protein and acts as a transcriptional transactivator (tat). The tat protein acts on promotor and regulatory sequences of HTLV-2, stimulating transcription of mRNA. The tat proteins may turn on the host genes for IL-2 and IL-2R.[55] Rearrangement of the IL-2R gene seems to correlate with the abnormalities of the short arm of chromosome 10.[29]

Another possible mechanism in the leukemogenesis of ATLL has been suggested: Many ATLL cells constitutively produce a non-IL-2R lymphokinin known as ATLL-derived factor (ADF), which induces expression of high affinity IL-2R and its gene by enhancing the transcription of IL-2R mRNA.[55]

Prognosis and Treatment

ATLL is invariably fatal; however, a few prognostic factors seem to emerge. Poor prognostic factors include higher leukocyte count, hypercalcemia, and elevated serum lactic dehydrogenase level.[14] Patients with the above features have a median survival of about 3 mo; those without any of the poor prognostic factors have a median survival of about 8 mo. Various modalities of treatment do not seem to alter the clinical course. Death is attributable to recurrent disease, with multiple organ infiltration and failure, hypercalcemia, and opportunistic infections.

So far, no effective treatment for ATLL has been found, even though various combination chemotherapeutic regimens have been tried.[5] Most patients respond well to initial treatment with chemotherapy, but these responses unfortunately are short-lived. The higher rate of clinical response in American patients as compared to Japanese and Caribbean patients is attributed to more intensive combination chemotherapy.[1,4,5]

On the speculation that anti-Tac monoclonal antibody would interfere with the interaction between IL-2 and its receptor on malignant cells, destroying IL-2 and its receptor while sparing other mononuclear cells, anti-Tac has been used in a small number of patients.[51,54] Preliminary results, although they were short-lived, were encouraging.

Arming the anti-Tac with more powerful agents such as pseudomonas endotoxins or conjugating anti-Tac to [212]bismulth, an alpha-emitting isotope, adds to the efficacy of anti-Tac on ATLL cells in vitro. These approaches are currently being evaluated.[54]

Large granular lymphocytes with natural killer activity have been shown to protect T cells from infection by HTLV-1, indicated by lack of transformation and expression in vitro. Studies are under way to evaluate the adoptive transfer of IL-2R–activated lymphocytes in patients with ATLL.[57] Preliminary results of treatment with the adenosine deaminase inhibitor 2-deoxycoformycin in patients refractory to conventional chemotherapy is encouraging.[58]

References

1. Uchiama T, Yodoi J, Sagawa K, Takatsuki I, Uchino H. Adult t-cell leukemia: clinical and hematological features of 16 cases. Blood 1977; 50:481.
2. Poiesz BJ, Ruscetti FW, Gazdar AF, Bunn PA, Minna JD, Gallo RC. Detection and isolation of type C retrovirus particles from fresh and cultured lymphocytes of a patient with cutaneous T cell lymphoma. Proc Nat Acad Sci USA 1980; 77:7415.
3. Posner LE, Robert-Guroff M, Kalyanaraman VS, et al. Natural antibodies to the human T-cell lymphoma virus in patients with T-cell lymphomas. J Exp Med 1981; 154:333.
4. Catovsky D, Rose M, Goolden AWG, White JM, et al. Adult T-cell lymphoma—leukemia in blacks from the West Indies. Lancet 1982; 1:639.
5. Bunn Jr PA, Schechter GP, Jaffe E, et al. Clinical course of retro-virus-associated adult T-cell lymphoma in the United States. N Engl J Med 1983; 309:257.
6. Blattner WA, Takatsuki K, Gallo RC. Human T-cell leukemia-lymphoma virus and adult T-cell leukemia. JAMA 1983; 250:1074.
7. Blayney DW, Blattner WA, Robert-Guroff M, et al. The human T-cell leukemia—lymphoma virus in the Southeastern United States. JAMA 1983; 250:1048.
8. Manzari V, Gradilone A, Barillari G, et al. HTLV-1 is endemic in Southern Italy: detection of the first infectious cluster in a white population. Int J Cancer 1985; 36:557.
9. Su IH, Chan HL, Kuo TT, et al. Adult T-cell leukemia/lymphoma in Taiwan. A clinicopathologic observation. Cancer 1985; 56:2217.
10. Urba WJ, Longo D. Clinical spectrum of human retroviral-induced diseases. Cancer Res (suppl) 1985; 45:4637S.
11. Dosik H, Denic S, Patel N, Krishnamurthy M, Levine PH, PH, Clark JW. Adult T-cell leukemia/lymphoma in Brooklyn. JAMA 1988; 259:2255–57.

    Khan F, Warman J, Krishnamurthy M, Dosik H. Prevalence and etiology of hypercalcemia in leukemia/lymphoma associated with human T-cell virus (abstr). Endocrine Soc annu meet 1986.
12. Broder S, Bunn Jr PA, Jaffe ES, et al. T-cell lymphoproliferative syndrome associated with human T-cell leukemia/lymphoma virus. Ann Intern Med 1984; 100:543.
13. Takatsuki KT, Yamaguchi K, Kawano F, et al. Clinical diversity in adult T-cell leukemia-lymphoma. Cancer Res (suppl) 1985; 45:4644S.
14. Tamura K, Nagamine N, Araki Y, et al. Clinical analysis of 33 patients with adult T-cell leukemia (ATL)—diagnostic criteria and significance of high and low risk ATL. Int J Cancer 1986; 37:355.
15. Kikuchi M, Mitsui T, Takeshita M, Okamura H, Naitoh H, EiMoto T. Virus associated adult T-cell leukemia (ATL) in Japan: clinical histological and immunological studies. Hematol Oncol 1986; 4:67.

16. Ichimaru M, Kinoshita K, Kamihira S, et al. Familial disposition of adult T-cell leukemia and lymphoma. Gann monogr on cancer research 1982; 28:185.
17. Miyamoto Y, Yamaguchi K, Nishimura H, et al. Familial adult T-cell leukemia. Cancer 1985; 55:181.
18. Ichimaru M, Kinoshita K, Kamichira S, et al. Familial disposition of adult T-cell leukemia and lymphoma. Hematol Oncol 1986; 4:21.
19. Yoshioka R, Yamaguchi K, Yoshinaya T, Takatsuki K. Pulmonary complications in patients with adult T-cell leukemia. Cancer 1985; 55:2491.
20. Chan HL, Su IJ, Juo TT, et al. Cutaneous manifestations of adult T-cell leukemia/lymphoma. Report of three different forms. J Am Acad Dermatol 1985; 13:213.
21. T and B-Cell Malignancy Study Group. Statistical analysis of clinocopathological, virological and epidemiological data on lymphoid malignancies with special reference to adult T-cell leukemia/lymphoma: a report of the second nationwide study of Japan. Jpn J Clin Oncol 1985; 15:(3):517.
22. Fujinara T, Eto S, Sato K, et al. Evidence of bone resorption factor in adult T-cell leukemia. Jpn J Clin Oncol 1985; 15:385.
23. Shirakawa F, Yamashita U, Oda S, Chiba S, Eto S, Suzuki H. Calcium dependency in the growth of adult T-cell leukemia cells in vitro. J Cancer Res 1987; 46:658–61.
24. Shirakawa F, Tanaka Y, Oda S, Chiba S, Suzuki H, Eto S and Yamashita U. Immunosuppressive factors from adult T-cell leukemia cells. Cancer Res 1986; 46:4458.
25. Jaffe ES, Blattner WA, Balyney DW, et al. The pathological spectrum of adult T-cell leukemia/lymphoma in the United States. Am J Surg Pathol 1984; 8:263.
26. Jaffe ES, Clark J, Steis R, Blattner W, Macher A, Lango DL, Reichert C. Lymph node pathology of HTLV and HTLV-associated neoplasms. Cancer Rese (suppl) 1985; 45:4662S.
27. Waldmann T, Broder S, Gree W, et al. A comparison of the function and phenotype of Sézary T-cells with human T-cell leukemia/lymphoma virus (HTLV)-associated adult T-cell leukemia. Clin Res 1983; 31:5474.
28. Yamada Y. Phenotypic and functional analysis of leukemic cells from 16 patients with adult T-cell leukemia/lymphoma. Blood 1983; 61:192.
29. Verma RS, Macera MJ, Krishnamurthy M, Abramson J, Kapelner S, Dosik H. Chromosome abnormalities in adult T-cell leukemia/lymphoma (ATLL). J Cancer Res Clin Oncol 1987; 113:192.

    Macera MJ, Szabo P, Verma RS, Weksler ME, Dosik H (1986). An aberrant interleukin-2 receptor (IL-2R) in adult T-cell leukemia (ATL) (presented at 28th annu meet of Ame Soci Hematol, San Francisco). Blood 1987; 68(5 suppl 1):260s.
30. Whang-Peng J, Bunn PA, Knutsen T, et al. Cytogenetic studies in human T-cell lymphoma virus (HTLV)-positive leukemia/lymphoma in the United States. JNCI 1985; 74:357.
31. Britto-Babaplle V, Matutes E, Parreira L, Catovsky D. Abnormalities of chromosome 7q and TAC expression in T-cell leukemias. Blood 1986; 67:516.
32. Rowley JD, Haren JM, Wong-Staal FW, Franchini G, Gallo RC, Blattner W. Chromosome pattern in cells from patients positive for human T-cell leukemia/lymphoma virus. In: Human T-cell leukemia/lymphoma viruses. Cold Spring Harbor Laboratory 1984; 85.
33. Seiki M, Hattori S, Yoshida M. Human adult T-cell leukemia virus: molecular cloning of the provirus DNA and the unique terminal structure. Proc Natl Acad Sci USA 1982; 79:6899.
34. Yoshida M, Miyoshi I, Hinuma Y. Isolation and characterization of retrovirus from cell lines of human adult T-cell leukemia and its implication in the disease. Proc Natl Acad Sci USA 1982; 79:2031.
35. Watanabe T, Seiki M, Yoshida M. HTLV type I (US isolate) and ATLV (Japanese isolate) are the same species of human retrovirus. Virology 1984; 133:238.
36. Hinuma Y, Komoda H, Chosa T, et al. Antibodies to adult T-cell leukemia virus associated antigen (ARLA) in sera from patients with ATL and controls in Japan: a nation-wide sero-epidemiologic study. Int J Cancer 1982; 29:631.
37. Robert-Guroff M, Nakao Y, Notake K, Ito Y, Sliski A, Gallo RC. Natural antibodies to human retrovirus HTLV in a cluster of Japanese patients with adult T-cell leukemia. Science 1982; 215:975.
38. Blattner WA, Kalyanaraman VS, Robert-Guroff M, et al. The human type C retrovirus, HTLV in blacks

from the Caribbean region, and the relationship to adult T-cell leukemia/lymphoma. Int J Cancer 1982; 30:257.

39. Wang-Staal R, Hahn B, Manzari V, et al. A survey of human leukemias for sequences of a human retrovirus. Nature 1983; 302:626.

40. Robert-Guroff M, Kalyanarman VS, Blattner WA, et al. Evidence for human T-cell lymphoma-leukemia virus infection of family members of human T-cell lymphoma-leukemia virus infection of family members of human T-cell lymphoma-leukemia virus positive T-cell leukemia-lymphoma patients. J Exp Med 1983; 157:248.

41. Gallo RC, Kalyanaraman VS, Sarngadharan MG, et al. Association of the human type C retrovirus with a subset of adult T-Cell cancers. Cancer Res 1983; 43:3892.

42. Gallo RC. The human T-cell leukemia/lymphotropic retroviruses (HTLV) family: past, present and future. Cancer Res (suppl) 1985; 45:4524S.

43. Tajima K, Kuroishi T. Estimation of rate of incidence of ATL among ATLV (HTLV-I) carriers in Kyushu, Japan. Jpn J Clin Oncol 1985; 15:429.

44. Okochi K, Sato H. Adult T-cell leukemia virus, blood donors and transfusion. Experience in Japan. Infection, immunity and blood transfusion. New York: Alan R Liss, 1985; 245.

45. Hino S, Kawamichi T, Funakoshi M, Kanamura T, Miyamoto T. Transfusion-mediated spread of the human T-cell leukemia virus in chronic hemodialysis patients in a heavily endemic area, Nagasaki. Gann 1984; 75:1070.

46. Okochi K, Sato H, Hinuma Y. A retrospective study of transmission of adult T-cell leukemia virus by blood transfusion: seroconversion in recipients. Vox Sang 1984; 46:245.

47. Sato H, Okochi K. Transmission of human T-cell leukemia virus (HTLV-1) by blood transfusion: demonstration of proviral DNA in recipients' blood lymphocytes. Int J Cancer 1986; 37:395–400.

48. Robert-Guroff M, Weiss SH, Giron J, et al. Prevalence of antibodies to HTLV-1, -11 and -111 in intravenous abusers from an AIDS endemic region. JAMA 1986; 255:3133.

49. Shimoyama M, Kagami Y, Shimontohno K, et al. Adult T-cell leukemia/lymphoma not associated with human T-cell leukemia virus type I. Proc Natl Acad Sci USA 1986; 83:4524.

50. Yoshida M, Seiki M. Human T-cell leukemia virus: causative roles in development of adult T-cell leukemia and virus integration into leukemic cell DNA. Hematol Oncol 1986; 4:13.

51. Waldmann TA, Longo DL, Leonard WJ, et al. Interleukin 2-receptor (Tac-antigen) expression in HTLV-1 associated adult T-cell leukemia. Cancer Res (suppl) 1985; 45:4559S.

52. Uchiyama T, Hori T, Tsdo M, et al. Interleukin-2 receptor (Tac-antigen) expressed on adult T-cell leukemia cells. J Clin Invest 1985; 76:446.

53. Hatanaka M. Molecular approach to adult T-cell leukemia. Hematol Oncol 1986; 4:3.

54. Waldmann TA, Tsudo TA. Interleukin 2-receptors: biology and therapeutic potentials. Hosp Practice 1987; 22:1, 77.

55. Haseltine WA, Sodroski J, Patarca R, Briggs D, Perkons D, Wong-Staal F. Structure of 3' terminal region of type II human T lymphotropic virus: evidence for new coding region. Science 1984; 225:419.

56. Yodio J, Uchiyama T. IL-2 receptor dysfunction and adult T-cell leukemia. Immunol Rev 1986; 92:135.

57. Ruscetti FW, Mikovits JA, Kalyanaraman VS, et al. Analysis of effect or mechanisms against HTLV-1, and HTLV-III/LAV lymphoid cells. Immunol 1986; 136:10, 3619.

58. Yamaguchi K, Yul LS, Oda T, et al. Clinical consequences of 2 deoxycoformycin treatment in patients with refractory adult T-cell leukemia. Leuk Res 1986; 10:8, 989.

21

CHRONIC LYMPHOCYTIC
LEUKEMIA

Robert L. Stahl, M.D., and Robert Silber, M.D.

CHRONIC LYMPHOCYTIC LEUKEMIA (CLL) is a malignant clonal proliferation and accumulation of small, well-differentiated lymphocytes in blood, bone marrow, lymph nodes, and (sometimes) other tissues. In more than 95% of the cases, the lymphocytes are B cells.

Epidemiology and Pathophysiology

As the most common leukemia of adults in Western society, CLL accounts for 25–40% of all leukemias. In Japan and elsewhere in the Orient, where CLL is rare, it comprises only 2.5% of all leukemias.[1] CLL is primarily a disease of the elderly, with 90% of patients older than 50 and the majority over 60 at time of diagnosis. CLL is rarely observed in children or young adults; males are affected twice as often as females. Although some families have been found to have an increased incidence of CLL, no clear genetic pattern has been established,[2,3] and a viral etiology has not been proven. There appears to be no relationship to prior radiation exposure.[4] The advent of readily available complete blood profiles and the greater proportion of an elderly population in our society may likely lead to an apparently increasing incidence of this disorder.

In B cell CLL, the leukemic lymphocytes are monoclonal—i.e., they have arisen from a single clone of B lymphocytes and express surface immunoglobulin of 1 light chain class (either kappa or lambda). The surface immunoglobulin is usually IgM, although IgD or light chains alone can be seen. In 5% of cases, the immunoglobulin present on the cell surface is found in the serum and

456

can be detected as a monoclonal protein or M spike on serum protein electrophoresis. Rarely, crystalloid intracytoplasmic inclusions of IgM have been seen in these lymphocytes.[5,6]

Within the spectrum of B cell ontogeny, CLL B cells appear to represent a relatively immature stage of development. Although the cells are no longer CALLA (+) (CD10) or TdT (+), as would be seen in pre-B cell acute lymphoblastic leukemia, they have other markers of immaturity. These properties include the presence of mouse erythrocyte receptors (MRBC-R) and only a low-density surface immunoglobulin. Indeed, the ability to form rosettes with mouse red blood cells is relatively specific for B cell CLL. HLA-DR (Ia) antigens are also seen. Paradoxically, CLL B cells have the pan-T antigen CD5 (T101, Leu-1), a 67 kilodalton surface protein. CLL lymphocytes are therefore weakly surface immunoglobulin (+), CD5 (+), MRBC-R (+), C3d (+), and CD 19, 20, 24 (+). A counterpart with many features of the CLL B cell has been detected at the periphery of lymph nodes, tonsil,[66] and fetal spleen.[67]

Recently, chromosomal analysis of CLL lymphocytes has been achieved. Because CLL lymphocytes generally are nondividing cells, banding analysis previously had been difficult. With the use of such mitogens as lipopolysaccharide, pokeweed mitogen, and Epstein-Barr virus, sufficient numbers of metaphases have been obtained in about 80% of analyses; roughly 50% of these were found to be abnormal. The percentage of abnormal metaphases correlates with disease stage in that only 20% of early disease patients have anomalies, compared to 80% among advanced patients. The most common finding is trisomy 12, which is seen alone or in association with other abnormalities in 50–60% of patients with abnormal metaphases.[7,8,68] Also frequently seen are structural changes of chromosome 14, such as t 11, 14, or 14 q$^-$. The gene for the α chain of the human T cell receptor has been mapped to a region on chromosome 14 that is abnormal in some cases of T cell CLL.[9] The karyotype appears to be of prognostic value in that patients with trisomy 12 alone do as well as those with normal karyotypes, whereas those with multiple abnormalities such as trisomy 12 in association with other anomalies have poorer survival.[10] It is of speculative interest that most of the abnormal karyotypes in CLL involve chromosomes that contain either immunoglobulin-encoding genes such as 14 (heavy chain) or oncogenes such as 12 (c-ras-Harvey) and 11 (c-ras-Kirsten).

Comparison of normal and CLL lymphocytes has revealed multiple abnormalities of CLL membrane composition and function. These abnormalities include the following:

- Absent or decreased blood group antigens[11]
- Lower sialic acid content[12,13]
- Differences in lipid composition[14]
- Reduced number of catecholamine hormone receptors[15]
- Anomalous cap formation in response to lectins[16]
- Fewer receptor sites for phytohemagglutinin[12] or Concanavalin A[17]
- Diminished immunoglobulin density[18]
- Abnormal surface protein glycosylation[19]
- Absence of membrane 5′-nucleotidase in 70% of patients[20]
- Absence of a 185,000-dalton macromolecular insoluble cold globulin found in normal B cells[21]

- Differences in the behavior of membrane-associated filamentous structures (intramembranous particles) in response to lectins[22]
- Decreased actin[23] and alpha-tocopherol contents[24]
- Occurrence of membrane podosomes[25]
- A rudimentary L system for amino acid transport[26,27]
- Decreased velocity of dehydroascorbic acid uptake[28] in association with increased cellular contents of ascorbic acid[29] and dehydroascorbic acid.[30]

Clinical Features

More than 25% of patients are asymptomatic when diagnosed following routine physical examination or blood count. When present, the most frequent symptoms initially are fatigue, malaise, and decreased exercise tolerance. Because CLL usually occurs in an elderly population that is likely to have concomitant medical problems, exacerbation of existing conditions such as coronary artery or cerebrovascular disease may be the initial presentation. Enlarged lymph nodes or abdominal discomfort and early satiety due to splenomegaly may be noted by the patient. Lymphadenopathy is more often cervical, supraclavicular, or axillary, whereas inguinal lymph node enlargement is less common. Splenomegaly is found in 50% of patients at presentation. The most common site of visceral involvement is the liver, although lymphocyte infiltration can occur in any organ. Unusual places include skin, gums, pleura, lung parenchyma, and G.I. or respiratory tract mucosa. Jaundice most often suggests hemolysis, although periportal lymph node enlargement with biliary tract obstruction may also be seen. Purpura due to thrombocytopenia signals an advanced disease stage. Fever is almost always secondary to infection. Clinical hyperviscosity is rarely encountered unless the leukocyte count exceeds 0.8×10^6 per μl.[31]

Laboratory Findings

Diagnosis of CLL requires the demonstration of sustained lymphocytosis and bone marrow lymphocyte infiltration in the absence of other causes. The absolute lymphocyte count is generally $>15,000/\mu$l, although the demonstration of a monoclonal B cell lymphocytosis of $5,000/\mu$l is probably sufficient. These cells are mature in appearance and are usually indistinguishable from normal lymphocytes, although they are slightly smaller,[32] with a mean corpuscular volume (MCV) of 170.[28] Late in the disease, larger cells occasionally with nucleoli are seen. CLL lymphocytes tend to smudge in the preparation of the blood smear. Although in B-CLL the predominant cell is a B cell, the absolute number of T cells is also increased. These T cells show an inverted ratio of helper to suppressor cells, a phenomenon that has been thought to play a role in the development of a pure red cell aplasia described in a few patients.[33]

Although most CLL patients are of the B cell type, about 1% of cases have lymphocytes that form rosettes with sheep red blood cells. In these patients, classified as having T cell CLL, clonality cannot be demonstrated by currently available techniques. Both helper (T4 +) and suppressor (T8 +) forms of T-CLL are seen. A subset of T cell CLL has become known as the large granular lymphocyte syndrome, which appears to be a proliferation of the natural-killer-cell and antibody-dependent, cell-mediated cytotoxicity populations.[34-36] These patients often have severe neutropenia and occasionally have pure red cell aplasia. Bone marrow infiltration is modest, and splenomegaly may be mild to massive. A high concurrence with rheumatoid arthritis is seen.[35] Whereas in some patients rapid progression with an unfavorable outcome is seen, most cases have an indolent course. It has recently been questioned whether this truly represents a malignant proliferation,[35] although clonality has been demonstrated in many cases.[36]

Examination of the blood smear in CLL shows that the red blood cell morphology is usually normal. Anemia is found in 10–20% of patients and most often is normochromic/normocytic. Bone marrow replacement, hypersplenism, or suppressor mechanisms may be contributory factors. The Coombs' test shows IgG coating of red blood cells in about 20% of all patients; however, an immune hemolytic anemia with microspherocytes is seen in only 8%.[37] Thrombocytopenia is found in 10–20% of cases and is related to bone marrow replacement, hypersplenism, or antiplatelet antibodies.

Because morphology is an indicator of clinical status, bone marrow aspiration and biopsy should be obtained at presentation. Interstitial or nodular lymphocytic infiltration is seen in early disease, whereas diffuse infiltration is found at advanced stages.[38,39]

In addition to cell surface marker immunologic studies, several tests should be obtained as part of the initial laboratory evaluation of patients with CLL. The serum protein electrophoresis shows a monoclonal paraprotein in 5% of cases. A positive direct Coombs' test may herald an immune hemolytic anemia. Quantitative serum immunoglobulins are important as a means of documenting the depression of IgG, IgA, and IgM that correlates with disease stage. Skin tests with purified protein derivative (P.P.D.) and control recall antigens may show anergy. The frequency of this T cell defect increases with advanced stages. Patients with a positive P.P.D. should receive prophylactic antituberculous treatment with isoniazid at the initiation of chemotherapy for CLL.

Differential Diagnosis and Variant Forms of CLL

Reactive lymphocytosis is transient, occurring with a number of viral illnesses, including infectious mononucleosis and cytomegalovirus. It is also seen with *Bordetella pertussis* and *Toxoplasma gondii* infections. These reactive lymphocytes are mostly T cells, and the B cells are not monoclonal. In CLL, the lymphocytosis is sustained.

Although CLL is the most common leukemia of adults, some less common disorders can be confused with it. *Prolymphocytic leukemia* is characterized by massive splenomegaly and minimal or absent lymphadenopathy. An aggressive clinical course with a median survival of <3 yr is usual.[40] The malignant cell is large with distinct nucleoli, and the white blood cell count (WBC) generally exceeds 100,000/μl. Both B and T cell forms are seen. The B cell type is more common and has strongly positive surface immunoglobulin. The cells do not form mouse rosettes. A serum M spike is seen in 30% of cases. Recently, characteristic and possibly specific chromosomal anomaly t 6, 12, has been described.[41]

Hairy cell leukemia is characterized by pancytopenia, modest splenomegaly, difficulty in obtaining bone marrow aspirates (dry tap) (see chapter 11, figure 11-113), and a variable clinical course. Leukemic cells are larger than CLL cells (MCV 400) and have fine cytoplasmic projections. These cells have a strongly positive acid phosphatase stain that is tartrate-resistant (TRAP positivity). Hairy cell leukemia appears to be sensitive to therapy with alpha-interferon.[42] Two new agents, 2'-deoxycoformycin[43,69] and 2-chlorodeoxyadenosine[70] appear to be highly effective as well.

"Lymphosarcoma cell" leukemia is a term that should be abandoned; it generally connotes the blood involvement by small cleaved cell lymphomas. This variant may present with marked adenopathy and (occasionally) massive splenomegaly. The leukemic cells are large and stain intensively for surface immunoglobulin, in contrast to the weak reaction found in CLL. The nuclei are cleaved and have well-delineated nucleoli. Biopsy of a lymph node will confirm follicular or diffuse small cleaved cell (poorly differentiated lymphocytic) lymphoma.

Well differentiated lymphocytic lymphoma with blood involvement is often indistinguishable morphologically from CLL. Two other techniques may serve to distinguish these entities: CLL lymphocytes form rosettes with mouse erythrocytes, whereas lymphoma cells do not; CLL lymphocytes do not form caps when exposed to multivalent ligands, whereas lymphoma cells cap normally.

Sézary syndrome, the leukemic form of mycosis fungoides, has a helper T cell phenotype and must be differentiated from T4+ cases of CLL. It is accompanied by a generalized scaling erythema of the whole body. The lymphocytes have a cerebriform nucleus and infiltrate the skin diffusely,

Table 21-1. Rai Clinical Staging in CLL

Stage	Definition
0	Lymphocytosis only; peripheral count usually 15,000 per cu mm, marrow population >40%; median survival >150 mo
I	Lymphocytosis with palpable lymphadenopathy; median survival 101 mo
II	Lymphocytosis with hepatomegaly or splenomegaly or both; nodes may or may not be enlarged; median survival 71 mo
III	Lymphocytosis with anemia (hemoglobin <11 g/dl); nodes, spleen, or liver may or may not be enlarged; median survival 19 mo
IV	Lymphocytosis with thrombocytopenia (platelets <100,000 per μl); anemia or organomegaly may or may not be present; median survival 19 mo

Table 21-2. International Workshop on CLL

Stage	Definition
A	No anemia or thrombocytopenia and <3 areas of lymphoid enlargement Median survival >7 yr
B	No anemia or thrombocytopenia, with 3 or more involved areas Median survival <5 yr
C	Anemia (Hgb <10 g/dl) and/or thrombocytopenia (<100,000/μl) regardless of the number of areas of lymphoid enlargement Median survival <2 yr

including the epidermis, where "Pautrier's abscesses" are formed at an early stage and only later invade the bone marrow and other organs. Leukapheresis, as well as the treatment of the lymphocytes or of the whole body skin with psoralen under ultraviolet light (PUVA), was found temporarily effective in inducing partial remission or stabilization of disease in patients with Sézary leukemia.

Staging and Prognosis

A clinical staging system based on examination and complete blood count was advanced by Rai and Sawitsky in 1975 (table 21-1).[44] Stages 0 and I constitute a favorable prognostic group, whereas patients with stages III and IV have a relatively short survival; prognosis in stage II is intermediate. Overall median survival in CLL is 71 mo. The International Workshop on CLL has recently proposed a revised system that considers total lymphoid mass (table 21-2).[45] Patients in groups A and B have ≤2 or 3 sites involved, respectively, with these sites including cervical, axillary, or inguinal lymph nodes or liver or spleen. Group C patients, who have anemia or thrombocytopenia, represent the ultimate compromise of marrow function by the accumulation of lymphocytes. Generally, disease progression follows a step-wise pattern from earlier to later stages.

The difficulty with these staging systems is that patients in intermediate prognostic groups, i.e., Rai stage II, are hetergeneous and may have variable clinical courses. For example, patients with lymphocytosis and isolated splenomegaly in the absence of lymphadenopathy may have a favorable prognosis.[46] In contrast, some patients will have a rapidly progressive course; therefore, other prognostic factors should be considered.

The pattern of bone marrow involvement is of prognostic value. Diffuse replacement of the bone marrow carries a poorer prognosis than a nodular or interstitial pattern.[47,48] The median survival for stage C patients with a diffuse pattern was 20 mo, as opposed to 30 mo for the nondiffuse pattern in one series[48] and 21 mo versus 51 mo, respectively, in another.[47] Similarly, stage B patients with a diffuse pattern had about 30 mo median survival; for the nondiffuse group, it was 80 mo.[48] For this reason, it has been recommended that a bone marrow trephine biopsy be included in the routine staging procedure for all new cases of CLL.

Karyotype may be of prognostic significance. The association of trisomy 12 with other chromosomal anomalies carries a worse prognosis than trisomy 12 alone or a normal karyotype. These other abnormalities include 14q⁻, trisomy 3, and t11, 14, with the last being associated with a particularly poor prognosis. Patients with trisomy 12 alone do not appear to do worse than patients with a normal karyotype.

A less clear relationship between the surface immunoglobulin phenotype and prognosis has been reported. Cells whose surface immunoglobulin is IgM may carry a worse prognosis than those with IgD.[49]

Treatment

Although survival in CLL is often prolonged, overall 5-yr survival is only about 50%, and 20% of patients (group C) have a very limited life expectancy (2 yr). This wide spectrum of life expectancy emphasizes the importance of separating those patients with indolent disease in whom treatment is likely to be of no benefit from those with aggressive disease for whom early therapy may be indicated. It is generally agreed that patients with Rai stage 0 disease do not require treatment; this is usually extended to stage I patients as well. Treatment for these early-stage patients has not been investigated in any large studies because such treatment may actually be deleterious: Complications of chemotherapy can be immediate, such as infections, or long-term, most notably acute nonlymphocytic leukemia.

A major cause of morbidity and mortality in CLL is infection. Patients should be instructed to seek medical attention promptly in the presence of fever. Infections usually respond adequately to antibiotics early in the disease; however, at later stages the response is less satisfactory and more often associated with systemic complications. Prolonged administration is often required. The use of high-dose I.V. gammaglobulin (400 mg/kg/mo) in patients with recurrent bacterial infections has been shown to decrease the risk of subsequent infections.[71]

In patients with autoimmune hemolytic anemia or thrombocytopenia, therapy may be initiated with corticosteroids as a single agent. Prednisone 1 mg/kg/day generally will control autoimmune phenomena and can be tapered to the minimum dosage necessary.

When prednisone is used as a single agent to control nonimmune manifestations of CLL, a response rate of 11% can be achieved.[50] Blood lymphocytosis may be seen on initiation of therapy. Although a striking decrease in lymphadenopathy or hepatosplenomegaly can occur, the complete response (CR) rate is limited. For this reason, the use of corticosteroids alone should be restricted to those with autoimmune cytopenias only.

Treatment for CLL, which has centered on the use of noncycle-specific agents to reduce the leukemic mass, includes alkylating agents, radiation therapy (XRT), and corticosteroids. This treatment approach is based on thymidine labeling studies indicating that most cells were noncycling, with an overall incorporation rate of 0.65–1.4%.[51]

Chlorambucil (CLB), a derivative of nitrogen mustard, has been the main alkylating agent used for CLL. It induces CR rates of 10–20% and partial responses (PRs) of 50–80%.[52] CLB may be given 0.08–0.2 mg/kg/day or intermittently at 0.4–0.8 mg/kg every 4 wk. Pulse CLB is at least as effective as continuous administration, and is less myelotoxic (see Appendix).[50] The addition of prednisone has been reported to increase the response rate; however, a change in the survival rate has not yet been demonstrated.[52] Cyclophosphamide (CTX) is probably as effective as CLB.[53] However, a comparison of different alkylating agents in a controlled, randomized trial has been done, and the results are pending. Recently, the combination of CTX, vincristine (VCR), and prednisone (CVP) has been shown to be effective in previously untreated and also refractory CLL patients.[54] Comparison of the regimen CLB + prednisone with CTX + VCR + prednisone has shown no survival difference between the 2 arms.[72] Prolonged therapy over 12–18 mo may actually prolong survival.[72,73] The use of CHOP (CTX + doxorubicin + VCR + prednisone) for advanced stages has been suggested but is unproven.[74]

XRT is often used for localized bulky disease, especially for nerve impingement, vital organ compromise, or painful bone lesions. Total body[55] and mediastinal irradiation[56] are palliative procedures that have been described as too toxic in some reports.[57] Extracorporeal irradiation of blood has not been associated with sustained control.[58]

In the evaluation of a patient's response to therapy, certain criteria should be reviewed. A CR requires the demonstration of normal blood counts, resolution of lymphadenopathy or organomegaly, a decrease in bone marrow lymphocytes to <30%, and a normalization of depressed serum immunoglobulins. A PR is considered a 50% improvement in the above parameters. When the response to therapy is complete, treatment is generally continued for 1 yr, whereupon the patient is observed for recurrence. For PRs, treatment should be continued only if necessary to maintain a desired response without untoward toxicity.

Although alkylating agents have been useful in controlling CLL, they do not cure it. Three drugs are currently being evaluated on an investigational basis. Fludarabine (fluoro-ara-AMP) has been administered as an I.V. bolus 20 mg/m^2/day × 5.[75] Clinical improvements were noted in >50% of patients. Deoxycoformycin, a potent inhibitor of adenosine deaminase, has been given I.V. bolus 4 mg/m^2 every 14 days, producing an overall response rate of 25%.[76] 2-Chlorodeoxyadenosine, an adenosine deaminase-resistant analogue of adenosine, produces a response rate of about 50% in patients with advanced CLL, with only minor marrow suppression.[77] Novel approaches are being considered for future clinical investigation. The B cell has been shown to have greater susceptibility to H_2O_2 toxicity that T lymphocytes.[59] Recent areas of research involving biological response modifiers include the use of alpha-interferon;[60] monoclonal antibodies such as T 101, which reacts with normal T lymphocytes and malignant B cells;[61,62] and anti-idiotype monoclonal antibodies.[63]

Transformations and Second Malignancies

Disease progression to an acute leukemia blast crisis, as occurs in chronic myelogenous leukemia, is rarely reported in CLL. More commonly, as the disease progresses, a prolymphocytic transformation is seen in about 10% of patients. This is manifested by a sequential decrease in the number of mouse rosetting cells in parallel with an increase in larger forms with nucleoli and intense surface immunoglobulin density. The 6,12 translocation has been reported to be seen as an acquired abnormality in prolymphocytic transformation as well.[41] The development of fever, weight loss, rapid lymph node enlargement, abdominal symptoms, splenomegaly, CNS symptoms, and clinical deterioration is suggestive of Richter's syndrome,[64] which is a transformation to an aggressive large-cell lymphoproliferative disorder resembling diffuse histiocytic lymphoma. Lymph node biopsy is essential to document this. Response to chemotherapy is generally disappointing, and survival is poor.

In addition to lymphoproliferative transformations, the occurrence of an increased incidence of second malignancies has been documented as well.[37,65] Of 4,869 patients with CLL followed by the National Cancer Institute, a 10% increased risk was observed.[65] The tumors most frequently reported were melanomas, soft-tissue sarcomas, and lung carcinomas. An altered immune surveillance mechanism was thought to play a role. Rai and Sawitsky, who followed patients with CLL from 1960–79, found a 9% incidence of second malignancies, as compared to 2% in an age-matched control population of patients with other malignancies.[37] Prominent tumors included skin, colorectal, and lung cancers. Careful monitoring of patients for a new malignancy is therefore in order.

References

1. Weiss NS. Geographical variation in the incidence of the leukemias and lymphomas. In: Henderson BE, ed. Second symposium on epidemiology of cancer registries in the Pacific Basin. Natl Cancer Inst monogr 53. NIH pub no. 79–1864, 1978; 139.
2. Schweitzer M, Melief CJM, Ploem JE. Chronic lymphocytic leukemia in 5 siblings. Scand J Haemat 1973; 11:97.
3. Gunz FW. The epidemiology and genetics of the chronic leukemias. Clin Haematol 1977; 6:3.
4. Bizzozero OJ Jr, Johnson KG, Ciocc A, et al. Radiation-related leukemia in Hiroshima and Nagasaki 1946–1964. II. Observations on type-specific leukemia, survivorship, and clinical behavior. Ann Intern Med 1967; 66:522.
5. Cohnen G, Douglas SD, Konig E, et al. Crystalloid intracytoplasmic inclusions in lymphocytes of a patients with CLL. Mt Sinai J Med (NY) 1973; 40:249.
6. Hurez D, Flandrin G, Preud'homme JL, et al. Unreleased intracellular monoclonal macroglobulin in CLL. Clin Exp Immunol 1972; 10:223–34.
7. Juliusson G, Robert KH, Ost A, et al. Prognostic information from cytogenetic analysis in chronic B-lymphocytic leukemia and leukemic immunocytoma. Blood 1985; 65:134–41.
8. Han T, Ozer H, Sadamori N, et al. Prognostic importance of cytogenetic abnormalities in patients with CLL. N Engl J Med 1984; 310:288–92.

9. Croce CM, Isobe M, Palumbo A, et al. Gene for alpha-chain of human T-cell receptor location on chromosome 14 region involved in T-cell neoplasms. Science 1985; 227:1044.

10. Han T, Emrich LJ, Ozer H, Sandberg AA. Prognostic implication of trisomy 12 and non-trisomy 12 karyotypes in B-cell CLL. Blood 1985; 66:470–73.

11. Brody JI, Beizer LH. Alteration of blood group antigens in leukemic lymphocytes. J Clin Invest 1965; 44:1582–89.

12. Kornfeld S. Decreased phytohemagglutinin receptor sites in chronic lymphocytic leukemia. Biochim Biophys Acta 1969; 192:542–45.

13. Speckart SF, Boldt DH, MacDermott RP. Chronic lymphatic leukemia (CLL): cell surface changes detected by lectin binding and their relation to altered glycosyltransferase activity. Blood 1978; 52:681–95.

14. Peel WE, Thomson AER. The fatty acyl chain composition of human normal and leukaemic lymphocytes and its modulation by specialized hydrogenation. Leuk Res 1983; 7:193–204.

15. Sheppard JR, Gormus R, Moldow CF. Catecholamine hormone receptors are reduced on chronic lymphocytic leukaemic lymphocytes. Nature 1977; 269:693–95.

16. Cohen HJ. Human lymphocyte surface immunoglobulin capping. Normal characteristics and anomalous behavior of chronic lymphocytic leukemic lymphocytes. J Clin Invest 1975; 55:84–93.

17. Novogrodsky A, Biniaminov M, Ramot B, et al. Binding of concanavalin A to rat, normal human, and chronic lymphatic leukemia lymphcytes. Blood 1972; 40:311–16.

18. Shevach EM, Herberman R, Frank MM, et al. Receptor for complement and immunoglobulin on human leukemic cells and lymphoblastoid cell lines. J Clin Invest 1972; 51:1933–38.

19. Andersson LC, Gahmberg CG, Slimes MA, et al. Cell surface glycoprotein analysis: a diagnostic tool in human leukemias. Int J Cancer 1979; 23:306–11.

20. Lopes J, Zucker-Franklin D, Silber R. Heterogeneity of 5′ nucleotidase activity in lymphocytes in chronic lymphocytic leukemia. J Clin Invest 1973; 52:1297–1300.

21. Simmonds MA, Sobczak G, Hauptman SP. Chronic lymphocytic leukemia cells lack the 185,000-dalton macromolecular insoluble cold globulin present on normal B-lymphocytes. J Clin Invest 1981; 69:624–31.

22. Zucker-Franklin D, Liebes LF, Silber R. Differences in the behavior of the membrane and membrane-associated filamentous structures in normal and CLL lymphocytes. J Immunol 1979; 122:97–107.

23. Stark R, Liebes LF, Nevrla D, Conklyn M, Silber R. Decreased actin content of lymphocytes from patients with CLL. Blood 1982; 59:536–41.

24. Kayden HJ, Hatam L, Traber MG, Conklyn M, Liebes LF, Silber R. Reduced tocopherol content of B cells from patients with CLL. Blood 1984; 63:213–15.

25. Caligaris-Cappio F, Bergui L, Tesio L, Corbascio G, Tousco F, Marchisio PC. Cytoskeleton organization is aberrantly rearranged in the cells of B chronic lymphocytic leukemia and hairy cell leukemia. Blood 1986; 67:233–39.

26. Segel GB, Lichtman MA. Decreased L-system for amino acid transport in chronic lymphocytic leukemia. J Biol Chem 1982; 257:9255–57.

27. Segel GB, Simon W, Lichtman MA. Multicomponent analysis of amino acid transport in human lymphocytes. Diminished L-system transport in chronic leukemic B lymphocytes. J Clin Invest 1984; 74:17–24.

28. Stahl RL, Farber CM, Liebes LF, et al. Relationship of dehydroascorbic acid transport to cell lineage in lymphocytes from normal subjects and patients with CLL. Cancer Res 1985; 45:6507–12.

29. Liebes LF, Krigel R, Kuo S, et al. Increased ascorbic acid content in chronic lymphocytic leukemia B lymphocytes. Proc Nat Acad Sci USA 1981; 78:6481–84.

30. Farber CM, Kanengiser S, Stahl RL, et al. A specific high-performance liquid chromatography assay for dehydroascrobic acid shows an increased content in CLL lymphocytes. Anal Biochem 1983; 134:355–60.

31. Lichtman MA, Rowe IM. Hyperleukocytic leukemias: rheological, clinical and therapeutic considerations. Blood 1982; 60:279–83.

32. Liebes LF, Pelle E, Zucker-Franklin D, et al. Comparison of lipid composition and 1,6-Diphenyl-1,3,5-hexatriene fluorescence polarization measurements of hairy cells with monocytes and lymphocytes from normal subjects and patients with CLL. Cancer Res 1981; 41:4050–56.

33. Mangan KF, Chikkappa G, Farley PC. T gamma cells suppress growth of erythroid colony-forming units in vitro in the pure red cell aplasia of B-cell CLL. J Clin Invest 1982; 70:1148–56.

34. Brouet JC, Flandrin G, Sasportes M, et al. CLL of T-cell origin: Immunologic and clinical evaluation in 11 patients. Lancet 1975; 2:890–93.

35. Newland AC, Catovsky D, Linch D, et al. Chronic T cell lymphocytosis: a review of 21 cases. Br J Haematol 1984; 58:433–46.

36. Chan WC, Link S, Mawle A, Check I, Brynes RK, Winton EF. Heterogeneity of large granular lymphocyte proliferations—delineation of two major subtypes. Blood 1986; 68:1142–53.

37. Rai KR, Sawitsky A. Studies in clinical staging, lymphcoyte function, and markers as an approach to the treatment of CLL. In: Silber R, Gordon AS, Lobue J, Muggia FM, eds, Contemporary hematology/oncology. Vol. 2. New York: Plenum, 1981; 227–62.

38. Carbone A, Santoro A, Pilotti S, et al. Bone marrow patterns and clinical staging in CLL. Lancet 1978; 1:606.

39. Charron D, Dighiero G, Raphael M, et al. Bone marrow patterns and clinical staging in CLL. Lancet 1977; 2:819.

40. Galton DAG, Goldman JM, Wiltshaw E, et al. Prolymphocytic leukemia. Br J Haematol 1974; 27:7–23.

41. Sadamori N, Han T, Minowada J, et al. Possible specific chromosome change in prolymphocytic leukemia. Blood 1983; 62:729–36.

42. Golomb HM, Fefer A, Golde DW, et al. Report of a multi-institutional study of 193 patients with hairy cell leukemia treated with interferon alpha 2b. Semin Oncol 1988; 15 (suppl 5):2–6.

43. Spiers ASD, Parekh SJ, Ramnes CR, Cassileth PA, Oken MM. Hairy cell leukemia: pentostatin (dCF, 2'-deoxycoformycin) is effective both as initial treatment and after failure of splenectomy and alpha interferon. Blood 1985; 66:208a.

44. Rai KR, Sawitsky A, Cronkite EP, et al. Clinical staging of CLL. Blood 1975; 46:219–34.

45. Binet J-L, Catovsky D, Chandra P, et al. CLL: proposals for a revised prognostic staging system. Br J Haematol 1981; 48:365–67.

46. Baccarani M, Cavo M, Gobbi M, et al. Staging of CLL. Blood 1982; 59:1191–96.

47. Bartl R, Frisch B, Burkhardt R, et al. Assessment of marrow trephine in relation to staging in CLL. Br J Haematol 1982; 51:1–15.

48. Rosman C, Montserrat E, Rodriquez-Fernandez JM, et al. Bone marrow histological pattern—the best single prognostic parameter in CLL: a multivariate survival analysis of 329 cases. Blood 1984; 64:642–48.

49. Ligler FS, Kettman JR, Smith G, et al. Immunoglobulin phenotype on B cells correlates with clinical stage of CLL. Blood 1983; 62:256–63.

50. Sawitsky A, Rai KR, Glidewell O, et al. Comparison of daily vs. intermittent chlorambucil and prednisone therapy in the treatment of patients with CLL. Blood 1977; 50:1049–59.

51. Theml H, Trepel F, Schick P, et al. Kinetics of lymphocytes in CLL. Studies using continuous ^{3}H-thymidine infusion in two patients. Blood 1973; 42:623–36.

52. Han T, Ezdinli EZ, Shimaoka KS, et al. Chlorambucil vs. combined chlorambucil-corticosteroid therapy in CLL. Cancer 1973; 31:502–08.

53. Huguley CM. Treatment of CLL. Cancer Treat Rev 1977; 4:261–73.

54. Oken MM, Kaplan ME. Combination chemotherapy with cyclophosphamide, vincristine, and prednisone in the treatment of refractory CLL. Cancer Treat Rep 1979; 63:441–47.

55. Johnson RE. Total body irradiation of CLL. Cancer 1976; 37:2691–96.

56. Sawitsky A, Rai KR, Aral I, et al. Mediastinal irradiation for CLL. Am J Med 1976; 61:892–96.

57. Rubin P, Bennett JM, Begg C, et al. The comparison of total body irradiation vs. chlorambucil and prednisone for remission induction. In: Active CLL: an ECOG study. Part I: Total body irradiation response and toxicity. Int J Radiat Oncol Biol Phys 1981; 7:1623–32.

58. Chanana AD, Cronkite EP, Rai KR. The role of extracorporeal irradiation of blood in the treatment of leukemia. Int J Radiat Oncol Biol Phys 1976; 1:539–48.
59. Farber CM, Liebes LF, Kanganis DN, et al. Human B lymphocytes show greater susceptibility to H_2O_2 toxicity than T lymphocytes. J Immunol 1984; 132:2543–46.
60. Foon KA, Bottino GC, Abrams PG, et al. Phase II trial of recombinant leukocyte A interferon in patients with advanced CLL. Am J Med 1985; 78:216–20.
61. Dillman RO, Shawler DL, Sobol RE, et al. Murine monoclonal antibody therapy in two patients with CLL. Blood 1982; 59:1036–45.
62. Foon KA, Schroff RW, Bunn RA, et al. Effects of monoclonal antibody therapy in patients with CLL. Blood 1984; 64:1085–93.
63. Miller RA, Maloney DG, Warnke R, et al. Treatment of B-cell lymphoma with monoclonal anti-idiotype antibody. N Engl J Med 1982; 306:517–22.
64. Foucar K, Rydell RE. Richter's syndrome in CLL. Cancer 1980; 46:118–34.
65. Greene MH, Hoover RN, Fraumein JF Jr. Subsequent cancer in patients with chronic lymphocytic leukemia: a possible immunologic mechanism. J Natl Cancer Inst 1978; 61:337.
66. Freedman AS, Nadler LM. B cell development in CLL. Semin Hematol 1987; 24:230–39.
67. Fredman AS, Boyd AW, Bieber FR, et al. Normal cellular counterparts of B cell CLL. Blood 1987; 70:418–27.
68. Han T, Henderson ES, Emrich LJ, et al. Prognostic significance of karyotypic abnormalities in B-cell CLL: an update. Semin Hematol 1987; 24:257–63.
69. Kraut EH, Bouroncle BA, Grever MR. Low-dose deoxycoformycin in the treatment of hairy cell leukemia. Blood 1986; 73:38–46.
70. Piro LD, Carrera CJ, Carson DA, Beutler E. Lasting remissions in hairy cell leukemia induced by a single infusion of 2-chlorodeoxy adenosine. N Engl J Med 1990; 322:1117–21.
71. Cooperative Group for the Study of Immunoglobulin in CLL. Intravenous immunoglobulin for the prevention of infection in CLL. A randomized, controlled clinical trial. N Engl J Med 1988; 319:902.
72. Bennett JM, Raphael B, Moore D, et al. Comparison of chlorambucil and prednisone vs total body irradiation and chlorambucil: prednisone vs cytoxan, vincristine, prednisone for the therapy of active CLL. A longterm followup of two ECOG studies. In: Gale RP, Rai KR, eds. Chronic lymphocytic leukemia: recent progress and future direction. New York: Liss, 1987; 317.
73. Keller JW, Knospe WH, Raney M, et al. Treatment of CLL using chlorambucil and prednisone with or without cycle active consolidation chemotherapy. A Southeastern Cancer Study Group trial. Cancer 1986; 58:1185–92.
74. French Cooperative Group on CLL. Prognostic and therapeutic advances in CLL management: the experience of the French cooperative group. Semin Hematol 1987; 24:275–90.
75. Keating MJ, Kantarjian H, Talpaz W, et al. Fludarabine: A new agent with major activity against CLL. Blood 1989; 74:19–25.
76. Grever MR, Leiby JM, Kraut EH, et al. Low dose deoxycoformycin in lymphoid malignancy. J Clin Oncol 1985; 3:1196.
77. Piro LD, Carrera CJ, Beutler E, et al. 2-chlorodeoxy adenosine: an effective new agent for the management of CLL. Blood 1988; 72:1069–73.

22

MULTIPLE MYELOMA

C. Julian Rosenthal, M.D., F.A.C.P.

MULTIPLE MYELOMA IS THE most common disease of a group of *monoclonal gammopathies,* disorders characterized by the proliferation of a clone of cells derived from a putative primordial plasma cell or lymphocyte producing a monoclonal immunoglobulin. Each monoclonal protein spike consists of only one class of heavy chains and light chains, whereas the polyclonal immunoglobulins consist of one or more heavy chain classes and both light chain types (kappa and lambda).

Monoclonal gammopathies can be classified as follows:

A. Malignant monoclonal gammopathies

1. Multiple myeloma (IgG, IgA, IgD, free light chains and an exceptional IgM type). Can present as (1) overt multiple myeloma, (2) smoldering multiple myeloma, or (3) nonsecretory myeloma

2. Plasma cell leukemia, which could be of the essential type or could represent the end stage of a multiple myeloma case

3. Plasmacytoma, which can present as (1) solitary plasmacytoma of the bone, (2) multiple plasmacytomas of the bones without bone marrow involvement, or (3) extramedullary plasmacytoma of the soft tissues, solitary or multiple

4. Amyloidosis of the AL (light chain type), which could be primary or accompanying multiple myeloma. (Other types of amyloidosis—secondary, familial and localized—are not accompanied by monoclonal proteins in their serum.)

5. Waldenstrom macroglobulinemia, a lymphoproliferative disorder accompanied by circulating IgM monoclonal protein (IgM monoclonal proteins and sometimes IgG paraprotein may also be found occasionally in the blood of patients with various types of malignant lymphomas).

Table 22-1. Relative Incidence of Various Monoclonal Gammopathies

Type of monoclonal gammopathy	% of total cases
Plasma cell myeloma	
Multiple myeloma—symptomatic	50
Multiple myeloma—asymptomatic and indolent	3
Localized plasmacytoma (1–2 lesions)	2
Waldenstrom's macroglobulinemia	10
Heavy chain diseases	1
Idiopathic monoclonal peak	30
Primary amyloidosis (without myeloma)	5

Table 22-2. Functional Features of Immunoglobulin Classes

	IgG	IgA	IgM	IgD	IgE
Electrophoretic mobility	to	to B	to		to
Sedimentation coefficient	6.7S	7–15S	19S	7S	8S
Molecular weight (x10^3)	150	170–500	900	180	200
Serum concentration, mg/ml	12.4	2.5	1.2	0.03	0.0003
Metabolism					
Half-time (days) in					
circulating plasma	21	5.8	5.1	2.8	2.2
% Catabolized/day	6	25	18	37	
% Intravascular	45	42	76	75	
Synthetic rate, mg/kg/day	30	25	6	0.4	0.02
External secretions	+	+ + +	+		
Placental transport	+ + +	0	0	0	0
Skin sensitization (P-K test)	+	0	0	0	+ + +
Agglutination efficiency	1		100		
C' fixation	+	Alt.pathway	+	–	Alt.pathway

B. Monoclonal gammopathies of undetermined significance
1. Biclonal gammopathies
2. Benign gammopathies
3. Transient monoclonal gammopathies that could be associated with neoplasms not derived from plasma cells nor from B lymphocytes that normally produce immunoglobulins (e.g., carcinoma of the bowel, breast, and biliary tract) or be the consequence of drug hypersensitivity reaction (e.g., sulfonamides).

The approximate relative incidence of these various monoclonal gammopathies is shown in table 22-1; the main characteristics of the immunoglobulin classes that constitute the monoclonal gammopathies are given in table 22-2.

Pathophysiology

The immunoglobulin secreted by plasma cells in patients with neoplastic gammopathies, especially in those with multiple myeloma and macroglobulinemia, generally have the structure of one of the normal Igs. However, they are secreted by one clone of plasma cells or, respectively, lymphocytes (in macroglobulinemia); for this reason, they are homogeneous and localized sharply in their electrophoretic migration. Normal Igs, on the other hand, are heterogenous, consequently are electrophoretically distributed from the β to the slow γ regions. Occasionally, as in patients with heavy chain disease, the monoclonal paraproteins produced are Ig molecules that are missing the light chains and have significant deletions. Similarly, in light chain myeloma cases, the molecule is represented exclusively by 1 of the 2 light chains not attached to its heavy chain.

Of note is the fact that in most cases of multiple myeloma, an excess production of the light chain attached to the monoclonal heavy chain is noted.[2] The supplemental monoclonal light chain circulates freely in the blood and is excreted in the urine, where it exceeds the ability of the proximal tubule to catabolize it; thus, it can be picked up in the urine by the Bence Jones protein test or by immunoelectrophoresis. It is also known that in normal individuals, immunoglobulin light chains are synthesized in slight excess of their counterpart heavy chain; for this reason, trace amounts (5–40 mg/24 hr) of polyclonal heterogenous light chains are detected in the urine of healthy individuals. In case of renal tubular dysfunction, the amount of polyclonal light chain picked up by the Bence Jones protein test will be significantly increased (e.g., in Fanconi's syndrome of children and adults and in combined light chain nephropathy). In these cases, the polyclonal nature of the excreted light chains can be easily established by urine immunoelectrophoresis.

The incidence of various monoclonal immunoglublins in patients with plasma cell or plasma cell precursor neoplasms is shown in table 22-3.

Incidence and Etiology

Patients with multiple myeloma represent about 1% of all patients with malignant tumors and slightly more than 10% of patients with hematologic malignancies.[1] The death rate from multiple myeloma is 2–3 per 100,000 population. The disease occurs in all geographic sites and in all races, but the incidence in blacks is double that in whites. Multiple myeloma is more common among males (61% vs. 39% in females). Occasional clusters of patients have been described in small communities. Multiple myeloma usually has its onset between the ages of 40 and 70 yr, with a peak incidence in the seventh decade of life; it is exceptionally rare before the age of 40.

The etiology of the disease is unknown. The possibility of a viral, chemical, or physical (radiation) cause of multiple myeloma in humans is slight. Repeated antigenic stimulation of the reticuloendothelial system could contribute to the development of myeloma.[1] A genetic factor was incriminated in multiple myeloma in a report on 23 familial clusters of 2 or more first-degree relatives who had myeloma.[3] Chromosomal abnormalities are found in more than half of the cases, most of them in chromosome 14, where a 14q marker occasionally can be identified.[4] In half of the cases, karyotype analysis shows hyperdiploidy.

Table 22-3. Frequency of M Protein Classes Produced by Plasma Cell Neoplasms

	%
A. M proteins containing both H and L chains	
1. IgG	52
Majority are tetramers (HL)	
Half-molecule,	
HL disease has been reported	
2. IgA	18
3. IgM	11
Majority are 19 S polymers	
7 S IgM has been also reported	
4. IgD	1
5. IgE	0.01
B. M proteins containing only L chains (k or λ)	15
C. M proteins containing only H chains (μ, γ and α)	1
D. 2 or more M proteins	1
E. No M protein in serum or urine	1
	100

Diagnosis

The clinicopathologic definition of multiple myeloma includes 3 criteria: (1) the presence in the bone marrow of $>5\%$ plasma cells, (2) the presence in the blood or urine of a monoclonal immunoglobulin or part of it, and (3) the presence in the bones of lytic or osteoparotic lesions due to plasma cell infiltration. In just one condition, the rare nonsecretory multiple myeloma, one of these criteria—the monoclonal immunoglobulin—is missing.

The presence of 2 or just 1 of these clinicopathologic criteria can also be seen in a variety of other pathologic conditions that are included in the differential diagnosis of multiple myeloma. For instance, patients with benign monoclonal gammopathies (monoclonal gammopathy of unknown significance, or MGUS) have an increase in the number of plasma cells in their bone marrow ($\leq 10\%$) and a circulating monoclonal immunoglobulin (<2 g/dl) but do not have bone lesions. Macroglobulinemia patients have circulating monoclonal IgM, but they do not present bone lesions; their bone marrow is infiltrated by monoclonal B lymphocytes, not by plasma cells.

In primary amyloidosis (not accompanying multiple myeloma), a monoclonal paraprotein is present in the urine and sometimes in the blood, but there are no bone lesions, and the percentage of plasma cells in the bone marrow is $<15\%$. There are many conditions (acute or chronic infections, nonhematologic neoplasms, hypersensitivity reaction) in which patients may have in their serum a transient monoclonal immunoglobulin that disappears with the resolution of the primary disorder.

Clinical Presentation

Multiple myeloma patients may present with symptoms related to the main pathologic process of bone marrow infiltration by monoclonal plasma cells with secondary osteolysis. These include bone pain, primarily in the back and ribs, that is exacerbated by movements (present in 70% of cases at time of diagnosis); generalized weakness and fatigue, also present in almost all patients due primarily to their progressive anemia; and weight loss and anorexia encountered primarily in patients with advanced disease.

Most of the symptoms are related to the multiple complications that can occur during the course of this disease; they include the following:

- Pathologic fractures causing sudden onset of localized persistent pain
- Increased incidence of infections due to B lymphocyte suppression by monocyte (macrophage) suppressor cells[5]
- A decrease in the level of normal immunoglobulins and a decrease in the absolute number of circulating polymorphonucleated neutrophiles due to bone marrow infiltration by plasma cells
- Hypercalcemia due to the release by leukocytes of the osteoclast activating factor (OAF)[6]
- Renal failure, which could be caused by (1) the obstruction of the distal convoluted tubules and collecting tubules by large laminated casts composed of precipitated Bence Jones protein, albumin, immunoglobulins, and Tamm-Horsfall mucoprotein, which normally coats the tubules (these precipitates may occur due to the encounter of positively charged Bence Jones proteins at a pH of <5.5 with the negatively charged Tamm-Horsfall mucoprotein); (2) the amyloid deposition in the kidneys; (3) the development of interstitial nephritis due to recurrent infections; or (4) the development of nephrocalcinosis caused by hypercalcemia.

Other complications include:

- Neurologic abnormalities represented by spinal cord compression (encountered in 5% of cases),[1] root compression, peripheral polyneuropathy, and multifocal leukoencephalopathy
- Amyloid deposition of the light chain type (AL) in the kidney and other tissues and organs, frequently accompanied by the carpal tunnel syndrome due to compression of the median nerve and by orthostatic hypotension due to autonomic nervous system involvement
- Bleeding dyscrasia due to thrombocytopenia or fibrin monomer aggregation or the presence of a circulating anticoagulant to factor VIII or factor X deficiency.
- Development of blood hyperviscosity due to the presence of some of the monoclonal paraproteins i.e., IgM and (rarely) IgA and IgG (this disorder can cause blurred vision, dizziness, oronasal bleeding, and other neurologic symptoms)
- Finally, second malignancies can develop in up to 15% of cases; the most commonly reported are carcinoma of the colon, breast, biliary ducts, and myelomonocytic leukemia (the last usually after melphalan treatment).

Laboratory Findings

Laboratory data are crucial in establishing the diagnosis of multiple myeloma. Bone marrow findings are among the most characteristic: The marrow is generally hypercellular due to its infiltration by plasma cells, which usually have normal morphology, but in 20% of cases can appear immature—without perinuclear hallo, with a pale cytoplasm, and a nucleus devoid of the usual clumps of chromatin. Plasma cells generally comprise $\geq 10\%$ of all nucleated cells in myeloma, whereas they represent $< 5\%$ of nucleated cells in a normal bone marrow. The range of variation of plasma cell number and distribution in multiple myeloma is great; plasma cells can be $< 5\%$ or almost 100% of the marrow cells, they may present diffusely, or they may appear in small clumps or in large sheets. Because marrow involvement is often focal at the time of diagnosis, specimens may vary significantly. Occasionally, unusual plasma cells can be seen. Some contain Russell bodies in their cytoplasm—acidophilic hyaline structures consisting of stored proteins. Others contain intranuclear inclusion bodies or present as flaming plasma cells characterized by intense, diffuse eosinophilic discoloration of the cytoplasm—seen more frequently but not exclusively in patients with IgA myeloma.

Identification of a monoclonal immunoglobulin in plasma cells of multiple myeloma patients can be achieved with immunoperoxidase staining, using an antibody directed to the specific monoclonal immunoglobulin thought to be stored in the respective plasma cell. In patients with advanced disease, all cells will stain with the same antibody, indicative of monoclonality; however, in cases of benign marrow plasmacytosis (encountered in some cases of carcinoma, connective tissue diseases, liver diseases, hypersensitivity states, and viral and bacterial infections), different plasma cells will stain with different antibodies to each of the major immunoglobulin classes and to both light chain types, which indicates polyclonality.

Electron microscopy of the plasma cell demonstrates a prominent, well-developed endoplasmic reticulum, the primary site of immunoglobulin synthesis and storage, and a prominent Golgi apparatus, the site of immunoglobulin chains assembly, which is also the cause of the perinuclear hallo seen on light microscopy after Wright staining.

With respect to the plasma cell morphology and growth in patients with multiple myeloma, a number of features have been analyzed to permit the differentiation between patients with overt active multiple myeloma and those with smoldering myeloma, or monoclonal gammopathy of undetermined significance. The nucleoli size is generally greater in overt myeloma patients; they also have more frequent plasma cell asynchrony (which means more undifferentiated plasma cells without perinuclear hallo and clumped chromatin). The most effective test in distinguishing overt myeloma cases from the other more benign forms is the determination of plasma cell labeling index by high-speed autoradiography, which determines the percentage of plasma cells that actively synthesize DNA.

Bone marrow of more advanced (stage III) myeloma patients also shows a decrease in the normal precursors of all 3 lineages of hematopoiesis.

Patients with multiple myeloma usually have a normochromic, normocytic anemia due to inadequate production. The anemia may appear more severe than the real decrease in red cell mass because of the increase in the plasma volume caused by the osmotic effect of the monoclonal protein. In many cases of myeloma, the red cells on the peripheral smear formed "rouleaux" (stacks of cells). Also, a blue-gray staining of the background of the peripheral blood is often present; it is attributed to the increased protein content of the serum.

Leukopenia and thrombocytopenia are encountered in the more advanced stages of the disease. A few immature granulocytes often can be found in the peripheral blood. In 15% of patients, plasma cells may also be present. When >20% plasma cells are seen in the peripheral blood, the disease is called plasma cell leukemia.

Immunologic studies are first directed at detecting a tall, sharp peak on the densitometer tracing serum protein electrophoresis corresponding to a dense, localized band on the cellulose acetate strip; this is seen in 75% of myeloma cases. However, in 15% of myeloma patients having light chain disease, hypogammaglobulinemia is instead present on serum protein electrophoresis. Meanwhile, a large monoclonal peak seen in the urine is caused by the presence of a monoclonal light chain that can be detected as a Bence Jones protein. These proteins are generally determined in a 24-hr urine sample. They were first described as pathognomonic for all cases of multiple myeloma, but as previously mentioned, they actually are present in all cases when there is an excess of light chains, (monoclonal or polyclonal), due to their hyperproduction or lack of degradation at the level of the proximal tubules. They precipitate better in the presence of sulfosalycylic acid and by gradual heating at 40°–60°C; they dissolve at 100°C and reprecipitate on being cooled to 40°C.

In order to identify the monoclonal immunoglublin detected by electrophoresis, immunoelectrophoresis is performed to determine the heavy chain class and its light chain type. In this procedure, the serum specimen is placed on microscope slides covered with 1% agarose having a trough in the middle and a well above and below it in the center. Two different sera can be placed in each of the 2 wells; their protein components are separated electrophoretically, usually over a 4-hr run. Six to 8 such slides are run for each pair of sera. After the electrophoretic run, each trough is filled with a monospecific antiserum, which is allowed to diffuse overnight and react with the specific immunoglobulin antigen it recognizes from the serum sample placed in the well and previously separated according to its electrical charge. They form precipitin lines in the form of thin arcs. When a monoclonal paraprotein or a heavy chain is present, the precipitin line becomes very thick or presents a tail or a fragmentation of the arc.

In the case of monoclonal immunoglobulin, the arc of the precipitin line caused by the respective antibody to the specific gammaglobulin will overlap with only 1 of the 2 monospecific antibodies to the kappa or lambda light chains. In the case of a polyclonal gammaglobulin elevation, both precipitin lines for the kappa and lambda light chains will overlap with that for the respective heavy chain. Other immunologic tests are useful to further define the monoclonal gammopathies. The *quantitation of immunoglobulins* performed by radial immunodiffusion (Mancini's technique) is useful to monitor the progression of the disease and the response of the myeloma patient to therapy.

This test also indicates a marked decrease in the level of immunoglobulins other than the monoclonal paraprotein in cases of advanced myeloma. The presence of *cryoglobulins* among monoclonal gammopathies can be detected by cooling the serum to 0°C and keeping it at that temperature overnight. If a precipitate forms, it can be confirmed as being a cryoglobulin by heating the serum to 37°C and holding it at that temperature for 30 min; the cryoglobulin precipitates will completely dissolve.

Finally, in cases of IgM paraproteinemia encountered in cases of macroglo-binlinemias, or of large amounts of IgA or IgG monoclonal gammaglobulins (>4 g/dl), hyperviscosity of the serum can be determined using a *viscosimeter,* which compares the viscosity of the serum to that of distilled water. Symptoms usually develop when serum viscosity is >5. This reading generally is an indication for emergency plasmapheresis. The *Sia test* for euglobulin is another relatively crude but very simple test for detecting IgM gammaglobulin. Rarely, the test can also be positive in cases of monoclonal IgG or IgA. It is performed by adding a drop of serum to a tube of distilled water or tap water. A positive result consists of the formation of a precipitate or flocculent while the drop of serum falls to the bottom of the tube.

Among other serum tests, the erythrocyte sedimentation rate is increased to >50 mm in 1 hr in 75% of myeloma cases, but occasionally it can be normal. Serum alkaline phosphatase is generally normal, despite the extensive bone involvement; only in cases with fractures with calus formation does serum alkaline phosphatase become elevated. Occasionally, patients present with hypercalcemia or hyperuricemia. In about one-third of cases, hyperlipidemia is reported, usually accompanied by the development of skin xanthomas (yellowish or tannish areas of varied shape and size) on practically any part of the body. Most other cases of multiple myeloma are generally associated with a decrease in cholesterol level.

Another test helpful in diagnosing multiple myeloma is the *skeletal survey,* which will reveal the degree of bone involvement. Such involvement can present as one or several lytic (punched out) lesions in various bones (most frequently in the skull, ribs, pelvis, and spine) or as a diffuse osteoparotic process due to the bone marrow expansion caused by plasma cell infiltration.

Course, Staging, and Prognosis

Multiple myeloma is a fatally progressive disease. In untreated patients, median survival ranges from 3.5 to 8.5 mo. Chemotherapy has now extended it to 2½ yr; almost 20% of patients survive >5 yr. The major causes of death are infections and renal failure. Durie and Salamon devised a clinical staging system based on the correlation of a combination of factors with the myeloma cell mass, which they measured indirectly from the ratio of the total body monoclonal immunoglobulin synthesis rate and the immunoglobulin production per plasma cell in vitro:[7]

- Stage I (early disease) is clinically defined in this classification by all of the following characteristics: hemoglobin >10.0 g/dl, normal serum calcium (<10.2 mg/dl), IgG monoclonal <5 g/dl or IgA <3 g/dl, Bence

Jones porteinuria <4 g/day; no more than 1 lytic lesion detected by skeletal survey. Patients in this stage were calculated as having a cell mass of about $0.6 \times 10^{12}/m^2$.

- Stage II (intermediate disease) is defined by all of the following characteristics: Hgb >8.5 g/dl but <10.0 g/dl serum calcium >10.5 mg but <12 mg/dl serum IgG monoclonal component <7 g but >5 g/dl or serum IgA monoclonal components <5 gm but >3 g/dl or Bence Jones proteinuria <12 g but >4 g/day and more than 1 lytic lesion on skeletal survey without generalized involvement. This stage corresponds to a cell mass of $0.6–1.2 \times 10^{12}/m^2$.

- Stage III (advanced disease) is defined by the following characteristics: Hgb <8.5 g/dl not due to overt bleeding; serum calcium >12 mg/dl; serum IgG monoclonal component >7 g/dl or serum IgA monoclonal component >5 g/dl or Bence Jones proteinuria >12 g/day and diffuse lytic lesions on the skeletal survey. Patients in this stage have a plasma cell mass of $\geq 1.2 \times 10^{12}/m^2$.

Patients are subclassified by their serum creatinine value as A (≤ 2 mg/dl) or B (>2 mg/dl). Prognoses indicated by this classification revealed a median survival of 62.1 mo for stage Ia, 40.1 mo for stage IIIa, and only 14.7 mo for stage IIIb. In the last group, prognosis is even worse (median survival 4 mo) if the serum albumin level is <3 g/dl.[8] Renal insufficiency, which is common in patients with high tumor cell burden, remains the principal poor prognostic determinant of survival. Response to treatment is also an important predictor of survival.

Multiple myeloma is frequently a slowly proliferating tumor that seems to pause after 1–2 yr of rapid subclinical growth. In general, patients with high tumor cell mass have a lower labeling index than those with a lower cell mass. A high labeling index in patients with a large tumor cell mass carries a poor prognosis.

In 1980, a few cases were reported of patients who presented all characteristics of multiple myeloma in stage I without progressing for >5 yr.[9] The number of plasma cells in the bone marrow and the monoclonal protein in their serum and urine remained stable. This type of myeloma, in which plasma labeling is 0%, was named smoldering myeloma. After a clinical response to drugs, the plasma cell labeling index is still very low; for this reason, these cells are resistant to chemotherapy agents that are generally effective only on cells in cycle.

An aggressive preterminal phase may occur in many multiple myeloma patients. It is characterized by the appearance and rapid growth of soft-tissue masses, fever without demonstrable infection, and pancytopenia due to bone marrow infiltration. In this phase, patients are resistant to chemotherapy and survive a median of 3 mo.

Treatment

In view of the systemic distribution of malignant plasma cells in the bone marrow of patients with multiple myeloma throughout all body, the starting treatment of choice is chemotherapy. However, due to the existence of occasional cases of smoldering multiple myeloma, all patients who are in stage I at diagnosis should not be started on chemotherapy for at least 3 mo. Therapy is then started only if the quantitation of the monoclonal protein and the plasma cell labeling index show at least a slow growth.

The chemotherapy of choice consists of alkylating agents and prednisone. The efficacy of phenylalamine mustard in myeloma was first reported in 1958 by Blokhin, while Korst recognized the efficacy of cyclophosphamide (CTX).[10,11] When prednisone was added to either of these 2 drugs, improved responses were seen; prednisone alone produces short-term responses in ≤44% of good-risk patients with myeloma.[11] For many years, the only recommended therapy for multiple myeloma was melphalan (MEL) and prednisone in daily schedules after a loading dose of MEL or in intermittent schedules of various doses found to be slightly less leukemogenic.

During the past 15 yr, many combination chemotherapy regimens were tested in phase 2 studies as well as in many phase 3 controlled studies. The results of those studies are somewhat controversial. They were extensively reviewed in a 1986 report.[12] With the exception of that of the Southwestern Oncology Group (SWOG) of 1983, most large studies did not show any clear statistical survival advantage for the combinations versus the MEL-prednisone regimen. However, in these studies there has been a consistent reproducible small advantage in response rates for patient receiving the combination chemotherapy.

The SWOG study showed that a combination of vincristine (VCR), MEL, CTX, and prednisone (VMCP) alternating after 3 wk with VCR, doxorubicin (ADR), CTX (or carmustine [BCNU]) and prednisone (VACP or VABP) led to 54% responses and a median survival of 43 mo versus a 32% response rate with a 23-mo median survival for MEL-prednisone (MP) administered every 3 wk. The beneficial effect of combination chemotherapy was displayed primarily in 70% of patients in stage III disease (high tumor load), but no difference in the response rate was seen in patients with stage I and II disease. For these reasons, it appears appropriate to start stage I patients (after a 3-mo observation period) and stage II patients on MEL 8 mg/m^2/day p.o. ×4, CTX 100 mg/m^2/day p.o. ×4, and prednisone 60 mg/m^2/day p.o. ×4 q. 3 wk, or MEL 10 mg/day p.o. ×7 and prednisone 40 mg/day p.o. ×7 q. 3 wk, and to give stage III patients—or those who relapse after MEL + prednisone—a broader combination chemotherapy. The regimen with the highest response rates (76–87%), tested primarily in phase 2 studies or only against MEL + prednisone, is the one included in the Memorial Sloan-Kettering Cancer Center protocol: MEL 0.25 mg/kg days 1–4 (or 8 mg/m^2/day ×4), prednisone 1 mg/kg/day, days 1–7 (or 60 mg/m^2/day, days 1–4), VCR 0.03 mg/kg or 1.2 mg/m^2 on day 1, BCNU 0.5 mg/kg or 20 mg/m^2 on day 1, and CTX 10 mg/kg or 400 mg/m^2 I.V. on day 1 to be repeated every 3 wk.

An objective response in all these studies is defined according to the criteria of the Chronic Leukemia-Myeloma Task force as a ≥50% reduction in serum M protein concentration and/or ≥50% reduction in urinary M protein excretion; or >50% reduction in the cross-sectional area of a plasmacytoma; or recalcification of bone lesions without the appearance of new lesions.[12]

Noteworthy is the fact that the quality of supportive care, which may also influence the outcome of therapy, has gradually improved during the past decade.

Once response is attained and maintained for 3 mo at a level at which no further reduction of the tumor mass can be indirectly detected, it is now being recommended—in view of the leukemogenic potential of chemotherapy—that treatment be discontinued. The patients should be carefully monitored and re-treated at the first sign of relapse. Initial therapy can again induce a response in 40–60% of cases. When these patients relapse again, or in patients with disease initially refractory to alkylating agents and prednisone (about one third of the total), a regimen of VCR + ADR, administered by continuous infusion for 4 days, combined with high-dose oral dexamethasone (DEX), also for 4 days and repeated every 3 wk, has been shown to lead to a 25% response in previously refractory patients and a 65% response in patients who relapsed after an initial response to other agents.[13] The estimated median survival for responders in this study was an impressive 22 mo. Similar results for refractory cases but not for those relapsing after prior responses were obtained with intermittent high-dose DEX alone. Beyond this salvage regimen, a number of other drugs and modalities are currently under investigation.[14] These approaches include enhancing MEL with 2-nitromidazole misonidazole (an oxidant) or with verapamil, a calcium blocker found to enhance the cellular uptake of MEL. High-dose I.V. MEL (140 mg/m^2), followed by bone marrow transplantation (syngeneic or allogeneic), is still in investigational status and to date has given only limited results. Autologous bone marrow, used after purging with specific monoclonal antibodies, could also be feasible in the future.* Alpha interferon was recently tested and found to be occasionally effective in patients with myeloma resistant to treatment.[15] In a relatively small study (with only 38 evaluable patients), objective responses were seen in 10% of patients primarily refractory to chemotherapy and in 26% of those who had previous responses. So far, phase 2–3 studies suggest that interferon added to MEL + prednisone or to the Sloan-Kettering regimen can improve the overall efficacy of these regimens, especially in inducing complete remissions (CRs) in patients with refractory disease.[16] Interferon can also prolong the duration of remission when administered alone as maintenance therapy at a dose of 10 MU/m^2 subcutaneously 3 times/wk until relapse.[19]

Finally, hemibody or total body irradiation was tested in a few cases of relapsing multiple myeloma, with brief responses in 3/7 evaluable patients. Radiation therapy (XRT) is also used in a tumoricidal dose of 4,000–4,500 cGy to treat solitary bony plasmacytomas or localized extramedulary plasmacytoma. In multiple myeloma, only rarely—in cases of epidural masses or bone lesions causing pathologic fractures—is a curative tumoricidal dose administered. In all other cases, XRT is generally used to mitigate and control pain; this palliative intent can be achieved with 2,000–3,000 cGy. Thus, XRT is limited to the control of "focal lesions."

---

*A new technique of administration of autologous peripheral blood stem cell autografts to patients with refractory multiple myeloma after they have received high-dose chemotherapy has induced high remission rates in several studies.[17,18]

Among the many complications patients with multiple myeloma can develop, hypercalcemia and spinal cord compression deserve special attention due to the urgent need for corrective intervention and other specific aspects.

Hypercalcemia is treated sequentially with (1) saline hydration up to 6 L over 24 hr, preferably maintaining a central venous pressure of up to 12 cm H_2O, and (2) furosemide, usually 40 mg I.V. q. 6–8 hr, with close monitoring of electrolytes at least q. 12 hr. Steroids (prednisone 50 mg p.o. q. 12 hr or hydrocortisone 100 mg I.V. q. 6 hr) are used next due to their effect in inhibiting the osteoclostic activator factor and their ability to inhibit calcium absorption from the G.I. tract. Calcitonin 100–200 mg s.c. q. 12 hr is added to previous therapy when calcium still remains high. Diphosphonates I.V. represent the next step, with the enteric product being used as maintenance therapy. Gallium nitrate by continuous I.V. infusion (200 mg/m$^2 \times$5 days) can be effective in refractory cases. Finally, when nothing else works, mithramycin (25 μg/kg I.V. in 1 L of 5% dextrose ½ normal saline over 8–10 hr q. d. $\times$2–5 days) is cytocidal for osteoclasts and generally controls hypercalcemia rapidly. It has, however, the disadvantage of suppressing bone marrow activity, thus limiting the amount of chemotherapy that can be given.

In spinal cord compression in multiple myeloma, timing is very important. If the patient has only back pain and has little or no neurologic deficit, a myelogram or MRI study should first be done to confirm the presence of an epidural mass due to a plasma cell proliferation in an already established case. In this event, XRT and dexamethasone 4 mg q. 6 hr I.V. can first reduce perilesional edema and then, it is to be hoped, reduce and eliminate the plasma cell mass.

In patients with neurologic evidence of spinal cord compression (paraplegia, sphincter incontinence, sensory deficit level), in view of the fact that measures taken to reverse a neurologic deficit must be carried out within 24 hr, decompressive laminectomy must first be performed and I.V. dexamethasone administered. Thereafter, XRT is given in an attempt to eradiacate the epidural mass.

Variant Forms of Myeloma

Other forms of myeloma include disorders that present only 1 or 2 of the 3 major manifestations of multiple myeloma: (1) monoclonal immunoglobulin in the serum; (2) monoclonal proliferation of plasma cells; (3) infiltration of bones by plasma cells, causing lytic lesions or diffuse osteoporosis on x-ray. These variant forms include the following:

Plasma cell leukemia. This is a disorder in which plasma cells are released in the peripheral blood. It is defined as a state in which plasma cells represent 20% of the circulating nucleated cells or reach an absolute count of 2,000/mm^3. Plasma cell leukemia patients are of 2 types: The first group are younger and have a more aggressive form of the disease; they present the leukemic phase at time of diagnosis. Patients in the second group developed the leukemic phase after being treated for a few months for multiple myeloma. The clinical manifestations of this disease are identical with those of other acute leukemias.

Treatment of plasma cell leukemia is generally unsatisfactory. A combination of CTX + VCR + ADR + prednisone leads to temporary, partial, or complete remissions lasting a mean of 7 mo.

Nonsecretory myeloma. In about 1% of myeloma cases, no monoclonal immunoglobulin or immunoglobulin fragment can be found in either the serum or the urine. These cases are classified as nonsecretory myelomas. For a definitive diagnosis, the monoclonal protein should be identified in the plasma cells by means of immunoperoxidase staining. However, sometimes the plasma cells do not produce any protein. Generally, patients with nonsecretory myeloma have a more aggressive course, but have the same clinical manifestations as in other myelomas.

Solitary plasmacytoma of the bone. Diagnosis is made by biopsy of a painful lytic lesion of the bone. These solitary lesions frequently will progress toward full-blown myeloma (in 60–70% of cases) in an average of 5 yr; some cases progress to myeloma after 10–20 yr. Treatment of solitary bone plasmacytoma consists of curative supervoltage XRT (4,000–5,000 cGy).

Extramedullary plasmacytomas. These lesions arise outside the bones and the bone marrow and can be solitary or multiple. The most common site of involvement is the upper respiratory tract. Only 40–50% will evolve toward a multiple myeloma within 14–320 mo. The treatment of choice is again curative XRT.

Waldenstrom's macroglobulinemia (primary macroglobulinemia). This disease, described by Waldenstrom in 1944,[1] resembles multiple myeloma only with respect to the presence in the circulating blood of a monoclonal IgM immunoglobulin. Otherwise, the disease resembles more chronic lymphocytic leukemia. Patients have lymphadenopathy and hepatosplenomegaly and present with insidious symptoms consistent with the hyperviscosity syndrome (chronic nasal bleeding and oozing along the G.I. mucosa; flame-shaped retinal hemorrhages causing blurred vision; headache; nystagmus; impaired hearing; ataxia). Additional neurologic abnormalities, primarily peripheral neuropathy, are present in 25% of cases. Unlike myeloma, no lytic lesions of the bones are seen; occasionally, diffuse osteoporosis is present.

In the peripheral blood, characteristic rouleaux formation by red cells is noted, and the bone marrow is infiltrated by mature lymphocytes with basophilic cytoplasm. As in chronic lymphocytic leukemia (CLL), naked nuclei are also present. Occasional patients present hemolytic anemia.

The treatment of macoglobulinemia is similar to that of CLL, with the drugs of choice chlorambucil and prednisone. Plasmapheresis is helpful in patients with hyperviscosity syndrome. Median survival is 3 yr.

Heavy chain disease. This disorder was initially described by Franklin in a patient who presented with a lymphoma-like illness and with a circulating gamma heavy chain found to have a deletion of the Fd fragment and of the hinge region.[20] To date, the literature includes reports of 55 cases of gamma heavy chain, > 120 cases of alpha heavy chain, 15 cases of mu heavy chain, and 1 of delta heavy chain. Their clinical manifestations cover a broad spectrum from a lymphoma-like illness to classic myeloma, chronic lymphocytic leukemia manifestations, and an asymptomatic disorder. In alpha heavy chain disease patients, the intestinal mucosa is invaded by malignant lymphocytes, resulting in diarrhea, weight loss, and malabsorption. The course of these patients varies from a rapidly progressive fatal disease to a chronic, relatively benign illness. Treatment for the more aggressive cases is similar to that used for high-grade lymphomas.

References

1. Kyle RA. Plasma cell dyscrasia. In: Fundamentals of clinical hematology. 2nd ed. Spivak JL, ed. Philadelphia: Harper and Row, 1984; 289–338.
2. Solomon A. Clinical implications of monoclonal light chains. Semin Oncol 1986; 13:341–49.
3. Maldonado JE, Kyle RA. Familial myeloma: report of eight families and a study of serum proteins in their relatives. Am J Med 1974; 57:875.
4. Liang W, Hopper JE, Rowley JD. Karyotype abnormalities and clinical aspects of patients with multiple myeloma and related paraprotein disorders. Cancer 1979; 44:630.
5. Mundy GR, Zolla-Pozner S. Immunosuppression and infection in multiple myeloma. Semin Oncol 1986; 13:282–90.
6. Horton JE, Raisz LG, Simmons HA, et al. Bone resorbing activity in supernatant fluid from culture human peripheral blood leucocytes. Science 1972; 177:793–95.
7. Durie BGM, Salmon SE. A clinical staging system for multiple myeloma: correlation of measured myeloma cell mass with presenting clinical features, response to treatment and survival. Cancer 1975; 36:842.
8. Durie BGM. Staging and kinetics of multiple myeloma. Semin Oncol 1986; 13:300–09.
9. Kyle RA, Grepp PR. Smoldering multiple myeloma. N Engl J Med 1980; 302:1347.
10. Blokhin N, Larionov LF, Perevodochikovd NI, et al. Clinical experience with sarcolysin in neoplastic disease. Ann NY Acad Sci 1958; 68:1128–32.
11. Korst DR, Clifford GO, Fowler WM, et al. Multiple myeloma II. Analysis of cyclophosphamide therapy in 165 patients. 1964; JAMA 189:758–62.
12. Sporn JR, McIntyre RO. Chemotherapy of previously untreated multiple myeloma patients: an analysis of recent treatment results. Semin Oncol 1986; 13:318–25.
13. Barlogie B, Smith L, Alexaman R. Effective treatment of advanced multiple myeloma refractory to alkylating agents. N Engl J Med 1984; 310-1353–56.
14. Kyle RA, Grepp PR, Gertz MA. Treatment of refractory multiple myeloma and considerations for future therapy. Semin Oncol 1986; 13:326–33.
15. Constansi IJ, Cooper MR, Scarffe JH, et al. Phase II study of recombinant alpha 2 interferon in resistant multiple myeloma. J Clin Oncol 1985; 3:654–59.
16. Cooper MR. Interferons in the management of multiple myeloma. Semin Oncol 1988; 15 (suppl. 5): 21–25.
17. Ventura GD, Barlogie B, Hester JP, et al. High dose cyclophosphamide, BCNU and VP-16 with autologous blood stem cell support for refractory multiple myeloma. Bone Marrow Transpl 1990; 5:265–8.
18. Bell AJ, North J, Stevenson FK, Hamblin TJ. Peripheral blood stem cell autografts in myeloma. Bone Marrow Transpl 1990; 5:33–4 (suppl).
19. Mandelli F, Avvisati G, Amadori S, et al. Maintenance treatment with recombinant interferon alpha-2b in patients with multiple myeloma responding to conventional induction chemotherapy. N Engl J Med 1990; 322:1430–4.
20. Franklin EC, Lowenstein J, Bigelow B, et al. Heavy chain disease, a new disorder of serum globulin: report of first case. Am J Med 1964; 37:332.

23

MALIGNANT LYMPHOMAS: HODGKIN'S DISEASE AND NON-HODGKIN'S LYMPHOMAS

David J. Straus, M.D., and
C. Julian Rosenthal, M.D., F.A.C.P.

DURING THE PAST 2 DECADES, major progress has been made in the study and treatment of malignant lymphomas, which traditionally have been classified as Hodgkin's disease (HD) and non-Hodgkin's lymphomas (NHL). The latter classification, which includes a little more than two thirds of all cases, was first described as a disease apart from HD by Dreschfield in 1892, but it was only in the 1920s that its existence was widely accepted based on Ewing's histologic description distinguishing lymphosarcomas from reticulum cell sarcomas.[1] The past 20 yr have seen significant progress in understanding the pathogenesis of lymphomas. This new insight has led to continuous revision of the histologic classification of lymphomas as well as to significant progress in their therapy. Currently, 85% of HD patients and 30% of diffuse large-cell lymphoma (DLCL) patients can be cured, the latter disease once having had a mean survival period of only 7 mo.

Even though it represents only 5% of all oncologic diseases, lymphoma has special socioeconomic impact because it frequently is encountered in early life.[2] Lymphoma is the third most common malignancy of childhood and the second most common in the second and third decades of life. It is estimated that 0.7% of newborns (1 out of 130) will develop NHL at some time during their lives,[2] with fatal consequences in 75% of cases. About 12,000 NHL patients die each year in the United States, whereas deaths from HD have dropped to about 1,000 per year.

Etiology and Pathogenesis

During the past 20 yr, evidence has accumulated suggesting a viral etiology of malignant lymphomas and lymphoid leukemias, at least in mammalians. Conclusive data indicate that in mice, rats, chickens, and cats, RNA viruses with C-type morphology cause lymphoma.

An additional factor ("hit") usually is required to trigger the virus-induced lymphomas. Examples of this type of intermediate factor include x-ray radiation, the graft-versus-host reaction, other conditions associated with cellular immune depression (e.g., autoimmune disorder in the NZB × NZW hybrid mice, bursectomy in chickens, and thymectomy in AKR mice), and the existence of a certain genetic compatibility between the host cell and virus; i.e., the presence of a genetic locus linked to the major histocompatibility site is a key to the susceptibility of mice to leukemia viruses.

The recent discovery of oncogenes has reinforced the belief in a viral etiology of lymphomas. The genomes of retroviruses that cause rapid transformation in vertebrate cells include genes that determine their oncogenic property (viral oncogenes, or VOGs). Genes homologous to VOGs that have been found in the genome of host vertebrate species are termed cellular oncogenes (COGs). These genes were shown to be highly conserved throughout vertebrate evolution, to be responsible for the control of proliferation and differentiation of normal cells (the reason they also are called proto-oncogenes), and to be capable of inducing transformation under appropriate conditions.[2] Preliminary findings indicate that malignant transformation requires the activation of at least 2 types of oncogenes: one that induces continuous active proliferation (usually the myc oncogene) and the other that acts to complete malignant transformation (frequently one of the ras oncogenes).

To date, these concepts appeared well demonstrated only in 2 subtypes of human lymphomas: (1) the Burkitt's lymphoma described in African children and young adults in Western Europe and the United States, consistently associated with Epstein Barr virus (EBV) infection and found to have predominantly an extranodal distribution with predilection for the facial bones; and (2) the low-grade follicular lymphomas presenting generally as a slowly progressive disease with transient response to therapy.

In both conditions, recurring chromosomal translocations with implications in tumorigenesis through oncogene deregulations were found.[3] In 90% of Burkitt's lymphomas, a translocation of the distal portion of chromosome 8 occurs, usually to the long arm of chromosome 14 [t(18;14) (q24; q32)] or sometimes to chromsome 22 [t(8;22) (q24; q11)] or to chromosome 2 [t(2;8) (p11; q24)]. This corresponds, in fact, with the translocation of the cellular homologue of the retroviral oncogene myc located on chromosome 8 band q24 into the encoding site for the heavy immunoglobin (IGH) chain on chromosome 14 band q32 or (less frequently) into those for lambda light chain on chromosome 22 or kappa light chain on chromosome 2. In 80–85% of follicular lymphomas, a t(14;18) (q32; q21) translocation was described representing a rearrangement of BCL2 oncogene from chromosome 18 q21 to the secondary site of IGH on chromosome 14q32. Thus, an oncogene rearrangement in these 2 types of lymphomas appears to trigger a chain of events leading to malignant transformation. Other frequently encountered translocations to one of the immunoglobulin gene sites are t(3;22) (q27; q11) and t(11;14) (q13; q32); the latter is encountered primarily in patients with diffuse small lymphocytic cell lymphoma and involving the locus of a new putative oncogene BCL-1.

Recently, a reciprocal translocation of the short arm of chromosome 2 (band p23) to the long arm of chromosome 5 (band q35) defined as t(2;5) (q23; q35) has been consistently associated with the Ki-1-anaplastic large-cell lymphoma (Ki-1-ALCL) clinically characterized by the invovlement of the skin and lymph nodes of young patients by bizarre large cells difficult to distinguish from anaplastic carcinoma. They are recognized by an antibody to the Ki-1 antigen (CD-30) originally raised against a Hodgkin's disease-derived cell line. The presence of the t(2;5) translocation helps distinguish ALCL from Hodgkin's disease and other lymphomas that also have cells with Ki-1 antigen.

Besides these recurrent translocations, data accumulated from pooling the information from 1,405 clinically abnormal cases of NHL[4] have also shown the existence of a number of numerical and structural nonrandom chromosomal aberrations. The most common are seen on chromosomes 6 (6q), 1 (1q or 1p) and 17 (trisomy 17). These aberrations were found to vary considerably in series from different countries; they were not found specific to any histologic subtype with the exception of the chromosome 14q32 aberration present in 70% of B cell lymphomas.[81] However, these aberrations were frequently associated with the transformation of some follicular lymphomas to a higher histologic grade. Thus, the trisomy 7, trisomy 3, deletion 13q32, or trisomy 18 in the presence of t(14;18) were found to accompany transformations from low to intermediate high grade lymphoma.

A number of karyotype parameters were found to adversely influence survival; examples are the presence of t(8;14) (q 24; q 32) abnormality and of abnormalities of chromosomes 1,7 and 17, as well as the presence of partially or completely unidentifiable chromosomes.[82] Conversely, the t (14;18) translocation was associated with a favorable prognosis.[84]

It was also found that immunologic abnormalities may predispose to the development of NHL in view of the fact that the incidence of NHL is 20–200 times higher in patients with a number of pathologic conditions accompanied by immune disregulation (table 23-1).

Table 23-1. Pathologic Conditions Associated with Immune Disregulation and Increased Incidence of NHL

- Acquired immunosuppression accompanying kidney transplantation
- AIDS
- Congenital immunodeficiency syndromes
    - Ataxia telangiectasia
    - Wiskott-Aldrich syndrome
    - Chédiak-Higashi syndrome
- Sjögren's syndrome
- Hydantoin-induced pseudolymphoma

Clinical Features

The clinical features of patients with lymphomas will be presented primarily in terms of their impact on prognosis. In NHL, the most accurate data concerning the prognostic value of various clinical and laboratory features were generated by studies that used the Rappaport's histologic classification as references (see below). For this reason, this classification is also primarily referred to in this chapter. (It can be converted to the most recently used NCI Working Formulation classification using table 23-2.)

Table 23-2. NCI Working Formulation Classification and Rappaport Classification Equivalents

NCI working formulation classification	Rappaport equivalent
Low-grade	
Small lymphocytic	Well-differentiated lymphocytic
Plasmacytoid	Plasmacytic
Follicular, predominantly small-cleaved	Nodular poorly differentiated (NPDL)
Follicular mixed, small-cleaved and large-cell	Nodular lymphocytic-histiocytic (NML)
Intermediate grade	
Follicular, predominantly large	Nodular histiocytic (NH)
Diffuse, small-cleaved cell	Diffuse poorly differentiated (DPDL)
Diffuse mixed, small and large	Diffuse lymphocytic-histiocytic (DM)
Diffuse large-cell	Diffuse histiocytic (DH)
High-Grade	
Diffuse immunoblastic	Diffuse histiocytic (DH)
Lymphoblastic (convoluted and nonconvoluted)	Lymphoblastic undifferentiated non-Burkitt's (DU)
Small, noncleaved cell (Burkitt's)	Burkitt's (BT)
Miscellaneous	
Histiocytic	—
Unclassifiable	—
Other	—

Age and sex. The median age at the time of diagnosis is 50 for NHL and 35 for HD. Age is not a prognostic factor in patients with DLCL. In other types of NHL, patients over 65 have a poorer prognosis than younger patients with just 2 exceptions: Patients with diffuse, small cleaved cell lymphoma and those with diffuse mixed lymphoma have a poorer prognosis if their disease is diagnosed when they are under 35. Adolescents with NHL often present with or develop a clinical picture that is identical to that of acute lymphocytic leukemia (lymphoblastic lymphoma).

Constitutional symptoms. The initial systemic manifestations that define stage B disease, such as night sweats, fever, and weight loss ($>10\%$ over a period of ≤ 6 mo), are encountered less frequently in patients with NHL than in those with HD, in whom they are present in 35% of cases at time of diagnosis. Their incidence is almost equal in patients with follicular NHL (16% of cases) and diffuse NHL (20% of cases). Pruritus is exceptionally rare in NHL, but is frequent in HD. The presence of constitutional symptoms in patients with NHL has much less significance for a poor prognosis than it does in patients with HD.

Lymphadenopathy. About 50% of patients with NHL will present with asymptomatic lymphadenopathy. The cervical, supraclavicular, axillary, and inguinal regions are most likely to be involved, similarly to the initial presentation of patients with HD. The epitrochlear nodes are involved in 11% of patients with follicular NHL; they rarely are enlarged in patients with diffuse NHL or HD. The lymphoid tissue of the Waldeyer's ring is involved in 11% of cases of diffuse NHL, 2% of cases of follicular NHL, and is extremely rare in cases of HD. Because of an association of Waldeyer's ring with G.I. tract involvement, the throat always should be examined thoroughly in patients suspected of NHL. Involvement of the mediastinal lymph nodes occurs in 18% of patients with follicular lymphomas and in 24% of those with diffuse NHL, in contrast with a 50–60% incidence in patients with HD. However, the superior vena cava syndrome, manifested by thoracic and neck vein distention, dyspnea, edema, and plethora of the face and upper torso, is seen more frequently in patients with NHL with mediastinal involvement (especially those with DLCL with elements of sclerosis) than in those with HD with mediastinal involvement.

Extranodal involvement. The bone marrow is the most common site of extranodal disease in patients with small cleaved cell NHL. Criteria used to diagnose bone marrow involvement include the presence of diffuse infiltrates or nodules with atypical lymphocytes and the "streaming" of lymphocytes along bone trabeculae. At least 2 bone core biopsies should be performed to assess bone marrow involvement. Overall, ≤70% of patients with follicular histology and 60% of those with diffuse histology have bone marrow involvement. However, among the latter, in only 15% of patients with DLCL has bone marrow been infiltrated. Also, the bone marrow is rarely infiltrated in patients with HD (10–12%).

The G.I. tract is the second most common extranodal site of involvement in patients with NHL. The most common histologic type is represented by DLCL; the stomach and small intestine are the most common sites of G.I. tract involvement. The most common symptoms of patients with gastric lymphoma are vague epigastric pain (in 90% of cases) similar to that of peptic ulcer disease; weight loss (50%); vomiting (25%); hematemesis (15%); and melena (10%). Occasionally, a palpable abdominal mass is present. On radiographic examination, the gastric lymphoma may appear as an ulcerative or polypoid lesion or as a giant rugal hypertrophy.

Primary lymphoma of the small intestine usually is confined to an intestinal segment of variable length. The small bowel also may be an associated site of involvement in patients with disseminated disease. In this situation, multiple sites in the small bowel may be involved, but frequently this involvement is unaccompanied by clinical symptoms unless bleeding or obstruction occurs. Patients with primary lymphoma of the small bowel usually present with pain, anorexia, vomiting, weight loss, and fever; an abdominal mass frequently is felt. Radiographic studies show thickening of the involved segment or a polypoid mass occupying the lumen; constrictive lesions are rarely seen. Malabsorption as a manifestation of small bowel lymphoma is seen in only 2% of NHL cases in Western countries. In these cases, the lesions are indistinguishable from celiac disease. A unique form of primary intestinal lymphoma with malabsorption is encountered in populations living around the Mediterranean Sea, especially in the Middle East. These patients are generally under 40 yr old. A lymphoid infiltrate of diffuse, histiocytic appearance infiltrates the small bowel and occasionally produces alpha-type heavy chain immunoglobulins.

The incidence of localized, primary G.I. tract lymphoma (stage I_E) is low (<5%); most patients have at least regional lymph node involvement (stage II_E) or dissemination (stage IV).

Parenchymal lung involvement is an unusual initial manifestation of NHL that is encountered in <0.5% of these patients and is seen in ≤2% of HD patients. Pericardial and myocardial involvement as an initial manifestation of NHL is extremely rare (<0.2%); it is more likely to occur in patients with advanced disease and prior mediastinal involvement.

CNS involvement is rarely seen as an initial manifestation in NHL (1–2% of cases), but it is commonly seen during the natural history of the disease. Especially prone to CNS involvement are patients with DLCL that already has invaded the bone marrow; 90% of these patients have CNS involvement characterized by diffuse leptomeningeal involvement or, rarely, by discrete tumor masses. Occasionally, NHL can present with orbital retrobulbar masses. CNS involvement is extremely rare in HD.

Cutaneous symptoms can be initially manifested in about 5% of all NHL cases, occurring more frequently in patients with DLCL and in those with T cell lymphomas. These manifestations generally present as nodular infiltrates of variable size. The T cell cutaneous lymphomas represent a rare type of NHL that has been studied extensively during the past decade due to its significance in clarifying some basic principles of the role of cellular immunity in human pathology. For purposes of this chapter, it is enough to mention that they are represented by a spectrum of malignant lymphomas, including the Sézary syndrome and mycosis fungoides (MF). They are characterized by the presence in the involved skin, lymph nodes, and various other organs of convoluted cells, frequently with serpentine ultrastructural appearance, and in some cases—especially in MF—of epidermal nests of large T cells known as Pautrier's microabscesses.

Intractable pruritus, erythematous lesions of the skin that can evolve toward the formation of intradermal plaques and fungating skin lesions, lymphadenopathy, and symptoms related to the involvement of various viscera are the major manifestations of cutaneous T cell lymphomas for which a special TNBV (tumor in skin, node, blood, visceral involvement) classification was developed.[6] They generally have a poor prognosis and respond only briefly to therapy.

Initially, NHL rarely involves the bones (1–2%), testis (<1%), kidney, larynx, salivary glands, or peritoneum. HD can initially involve bones in 1.5% of cases.

Staging

In a recent comprehensive analysis of the prognostic factors in NHL, it was found that the stage of the patient's disease has an impact on survival equal to that of its histopathology, while it is the most significant diagnostic factor in HD.

The current staging classification was established by the Ann Arbor Workshop in 1981.[7] The system includes both clinical staging (CS), which is all staging procedures short of staging laparotomy, and pathologic staging (PS), which refers to the findings at staging laparotomy during which liver biopsies, splenectomy, and excisional biopsies of retroperitoneal nodes are performed. An attempt is made by the surgeon to biopsy nodes that are suspicious on lymphangiogram. Some centers also perform open bone marrow biopsies from the iliac crest.

The Ann Arbor classification divides Hodgkin's lymphoma into 4 stages:
- *Stage I*—disease in a single lymph node or lymph node group
- *Stage II*—disease in 2 noncontiguous lymph node groups and/or spleen, either above or below the diaphragm
- *Stage III*—disease in 2 or more lymph node groups and/or spleen on both sides of the diaphragm
- *Stage IV*—disease in extranodal sites, usually lung, liver, bone or bone marrow, and (more rarely) other sites.

Extranodal involvement by extension from lymph node disease to such sites as the lung, bone, pleura, or skin may occur in stages I–III but is not considered to increase the stage to IV. Such disease is designated by a subscript E (I_E, II_E, III_E).

For each stage, the absence of systemic symptoms is designated by a subscript A, whereas the presence of unexplained fevers to 38°C or higher, night sweats, and/or weight loss of >10% over 6 mo are designated by a subscript B. In general, the prognosis worsens with higher stage, and, within each stage, the presence of B symptoms carries a worse prognosis than absence of such symptoms (A).

Staging procedures include chest x-ray, bipedal lower extremity lymphangiogram; liver/spleen scan; complete blood counts, including platelet and differential; bone marrow aspiration and biopsy; serum liver biochemistries, including alkaline phosphatase and 5′ nucleotidase; and erythrocyte sedimentation rate. The last test has been shown to carry prognostic significance.[8] A CT scan of the abdomen will show enlarged retroperitoneal, porta hepatis, and pelvic lymph nodes (see chapter 10, figures 10-13, 10-14–10-18). Some nodes involved by disease may not be enlarged but may show abnormalities on the filling pattern of lymphangiogram contrast material. Mesenteric node involvement at presentation in HD is much less common than in NHL. The accuracy of lymphangiography in determining the presence or absence of HD in retroperitoneal and pelvic nodes approaches 90% in experienced hands.

If there are abnormalities in the liver/spleen scan or gross abnormalities in serum liver biochemical studies, if a lymphangiogram indicates retroperitoneal or pelvic nodal disease, or if systemic B symptoms are present (see below), a liver biopsy should be performed. Slight elevations of serum alkaline phosphatase may be seen without liver involvement. Laparoscopy with direct visualization of the surface of the liver and biopsy of suspicious areas increases the yield of this procedure over blind percutaneous needle biopsy.[9] Gallium scanning may be a useful procedure for following mediastinal disease, but it is associated with a significant number of false negatives and false positives. CT scanning of the chest may show disease, particularly retrosternal disease, missed by plain chest x-ray. Although traditional radiotherapy (XRT) planning seems rarely to be affected by these findings, CT scanning may allow for refinements in XRT planning in the future.

The need for surgical staging is controversial,[10,11] but it is generally agreed that it is only performed if it makes a difference in treatment, usually between XRT alone or chemotherapy, either alone or in combination with XRT ("combined modality treatment"). As a consequence, it is also generally agreed that surgical staging is not necessary when treatment of even early-stage patients involves combination chemotherapy. It is controversial as to whether or not surgical staging is necessary when treatment for supradiaphragmatic stage I_A or II_A disease is XRT, including the mantle port (cervical, supraclavicular, mediastinal, and axillary regions), and para-aortic nodes, including the spleen or splenic pedicle if the spleen has been removed: "subtotal nodal irradiation." A large study using this type of treatment with either surgical or clinical staging showed no difference in overall survival, relapse-free survival, or pelvic recurrence rate between patients clinically and those surgically staged.[12]

The major finding at staging laparotomy has been that 20–30% of patients who are CSI_A or $CSII_A$ will have occult disease in the spleen and so will increase their stage to III_A.[10,13] It has been controversial as to whether disease in spleen or high para-aortic nodes carries a better prognosis following treatment with XRT only than does disease in the lower para-aortic nodes or pelvis.[14] Several research groups have found that minimal disease in the spleen (≤ 4 tumor nodules) carries a more favorable prognosis than more extensive disease in the spleen (≥ 5 tumor nodules) following treatment with XRT only.[15]

The problems associated with staging laparotomy must also be considered in the decision of whether or not it is to be performed. The overall mortality is 1.5% and has been as high as 3%. The morbidity is in the range of 6%, including wound infection, subphrenic abscess, intestinal obstruction from adhesions, and pulmonary embolus.[11] Late sepsis with pneumococcus or *Haemophilus influenzae* has also been reported. Pneumococcal vaccine may reduce the risk of pneumococcal sepsis. The discomfort caused by the surgery as well as its expense should also be considered.

In summary, staging laparotomy is indicated only when a potential treatment choice exists between XRT alone and combination chemotherapy with or without XRT.

The Ann Arbor staging classification devised for HD also has prognostic validity when applied, with some modifications, to NHL.[16] As with HD, patients with fevers, night sweats, and weight loss (B symptoms) have a shorter survival than asymptomatic patients (A). Stage I_E refers to a solitary extranodal presentation of NHL, including G.I. tract (most commonly stomach), skin, bone, thyroid gland, and breast. Such solitary extranodal presentations are extremely rare in HD. For gastric lymphomas, Mushoff has separated stage II_E

into 2 subgroups.[17] Stage II_{E1} refers to involvement of the gastric and regional perigastric lymph nodes. Stage II_{E2} refers to gastric involvement with distant abdominal node involvement, usually nodes in the celiac axis. Stage II_{E1} has a prognosis similar to stage I_E, whereas stage II_{E2} has a prognosis similar to stage III.

Among staging workup procedures, bone marrow biopsy is generally more sensitive than bone marrow aspiration because focal involvement may be detected on biopsy but missed on aspiration. In well-differentiated lymphocytic lymphoma/chronic lymphocytic leukemia and in lymphoblastic lymphoma, bone marrow aspiration may be more sensitive than biopsy. Bilateral posterior iliac crest bone marrow aspirations and biopsies may increase the yield by about 10% over unilateral aspirations and biopsies. Flow cytometry may detect a clonal excess of kappa or lambda light chains on the surface of lymphocytes in peripheral bloods or bone marrows that are not morphologically involved with lymphoma.[18] If the light chain is of the same type as those on the surface of tumor cells from other tissue, there may be lymphoma cells in the marrow or peripheral blood that cannot be detected morphologically. However, the clinical implications of these findings are still not completely clear.

Differences between HD and NHL in the sites typically involved at presentation have a number of implications in staging. CT scanning of the abdomen should be performed routinely in NHL patients to look for mesenteric as well as retroperitoneal node involvement. Lymphangiography is employed as a secondary procedure to look for involved nodes in the retroperitoneum when the CT scan is normal. As with HD, an abnormal filling pattern in the nodes with lymphangiogram contrast may suggest nodal involvement by lymphoma even if the nodes are of normal size. As noted above, because of the association of Waldeyer's ring involvement with G.I. tract involvement, patients with Waldeyer's ring involvement should have an upper G.I. series performed with a small bowel follow-through. Laparoscopically-directed liver biopsy is recommended, as in HD.

Staging laparotomy is not recommended routinely in NHL because 85–95% of patients will have disease beyond stage I or I_E with clinical staging. Staging laparotomy is only considered in relatively young stage I or I_E patients where a positive finding would lead to systemic treatment with chemotherapy rather than localized XRT.

Histopathology

The histopathology of lymphomas has been studied and extensively described since the first decades of this century; it has particular prognostic significance in NHL, but it has also prognostic value in HD.

Hodgkin's Disease

In HD, the Rye modification of the Lukes and Butler classification currently is in use throughout the world.[19] *Lymphocyte predominance* is characterized by an abundance of small lymphocytes with occasional, often atypical, Reed-

Sternberg cells of "lymphocytic-histiocytic" variety (see chapter 11, figure 11-108). The classic presentation is in a high cervical node in a young asymptomatic male. It carries the most favorable prognosis of the 4 histologic subtypes. *Nodular sclerosis* is the most common subtype in North America (see chapter 11, figure 11-109A,B,C). There is often abundant fibrosis in the node dividing tumor nodules containing inflammatory cells and the "lacunar cell" variant of Reed-Sternberg cells. The classic presentation would be in a young female with mediastinal involvement with or without symptoms. Although this finding has classically been believed to carry a relatively favorable prognosis, whether or not it does seems to depend on the stage of the disease, the bulkiness of the tumor masses, and the presence or absence of systemic symptoms. *Mixed cellularity* is characterized by a pleomorphic cellular infiltrate of plasma cells, eosinophils, lymphocytes, histiocytes, and Reed-Sternberg cells (see chapter 11, figure 11-110). Subdiaphragmatic and extranodal presentations and the presence of B symptoms may be somewhat more frequent than with the nodular sclerosis subtype. Mixed cellularity is the second most common histologic subtype in North America and is more common in the poorer parts of the world. It is also somewhat more common among older patients. Mixed cellularity has been associated with a worse prognosis than nodular sclerosis, but this may be due to the association of this subtype with the unfavorable clinical prognostic features mentioned above. The *lymphocyte depletion* subtype has a paucity of cellular elements and an increased reticular network (see chapter 11, figures 11-111 and 11-112). It is associated with advanced age, systemic symptoms, retroperitoneal node, and extranodal involvement. This subtype has the worst prognosis of the 4 histologic subtypes.

The origin of the cells thought to represent the hallmark of HD—the binucleated Reed-Sternberg cells and their large mononuclear counterparts, the Hodgkin's cells—is not yet fully known. Their apartenance to dendritic histiocytes[20] similar to those associated with normal lymphoid follicles or their representation of stimulated transformed T lymphocytes carrying IgM receptors is still subject of debate.[21]

Non-Hodgkin's Lymphomas

The NHL are a heterogeneous group of diseases. Cell marker studies over the past 10–15 yr have demonstrated that most adult lymphomas are of B lymphocyte origin while a minority are of T lymphocyte origin. They vary in their prognosis according to histologic and clinical features.

The Rappaport classification (table 23-3), which was introduced in 1966, divides NHL into 2 major categories.[22] In the nodular lymphomas, the follicular architecture of the lymph node is preserved. In the diffuse lymphomas, the follicular architecture is obliterated by infiltration with malignant cells. Within each category are several cell types: well-differentiated lymphocytic, poorly differentiated lymphocytic, histiocytic, and mixed lymphocytic and histiocytic. The "histiocytic" cells are large with large nuclei, vesicular chromatin, and distinct nucleoli (see chapter 11, figures 11-102 and 11-103A & B). They resemble tissue macrophages, but marker studies have shown that most cases are actually of B lymphocyte origin; some are of T lymphocyte

Table 23-3. Rappaport's Classification of NHL and its Clinical Significance*

Histologic type	Abbreviations	Incidence[†] (%)	Mean survival (mo)	5-yr survival (%)
Lymphocytic lymphoma				
Nodular well-differentiated	NWDL	1	—	—
Diffuse well-differentiated	DWDL	8	54	41
Nodular poorly differentiated	NPDL	18	75	58
Diffuse poorly differentiated	DPDL	14	36	40
Mixed (lymphocytic-histiocytic)				
Nodular	NM	15	84	58
Diffuse	DM	7	24	26
Histiocytic lymphoma				
Nodular	NH	4	86	50
Diffuse	DH	19	14	27
Undifferentiated Burkitt's type	BT	8	18	25
Undifferentiated non-Burkitt's	DU	5	12	20
Plasmacytic	—	1	—	—

*All values represent a mean of 4 series of cases published in the medical literature summing up a total of 2,225 patients.

[†]Incidence is expressed as a percentage of the total number of cases entered in these studies.

origin and a small minority are of monocyte-macrophage origin (see chapter 11, figure 11-106). The well-differentiated lymphocytic cases are virtually always diffuse; clinically and by cell marker analysis, they probably are part of the spectrum of the same disease as chronic lymphocytic leukemia (see chapter 11, figure 11-99). The poorly differentiated lymphocytic types are comprised of tumors with small lymphocytes with cleaved nuclei (see chapter 11, figure 11-100). The mixed types have a mixture of small lymphocytes with cleaved nuclei and large cells (see chapter 11, figure 11-101). The lymphoblastic subtype occurs most commonly in young adults, often with large mediastinal masses and either initial or eventual leukemic involvement and meningeal metastasis (see chapter 11, figure 11-104). Cell marker studies have shown that this type is very closely related to acute lymphoblastic leukemia and is of T cell or non-B, non-T cell origin. In most cases, the cells contain high levels of terminal deoxynucleotide transferase. The undifferentiated lymphomas are composed of small primitive cells with noncleaved nuclei. Often macrophages are interspaced between the malignant cells, which have phagocytized necrotic debris, giving the so-called "starry sky" appearance (see chapter 11, figure 11-105). The latter morphology is typical for Burkitt's lymphoma. The undifferentiated lymphomas also have been seen with increasing frequency in association with AIDS. The undifferentiated lymphomas are among the most rapidly growing malignancies in humans.

Separating patients into nodular and diffuse categories has been roughly equivalent to separating them according to prognosis. Survival in patients with nodular lymphomas has been longer than that in patients with diffuse histologies with minimal treatment.[23,24] Survival of patients with nodular histologies with minimal treatment has differed in various centers. Jones of Stanford reported median survivals of 8–9 yr for nodular poorly differentiated lymphocytic and nodular mixed varieties (NPDL, NML).[22] The National Cancer Institute (NCI)[24] and Memorial Sloan-Kettering Cancer Center[16] found the median survival to be 3–4 yr. The differences are difficult to explain, but may be due to differences in follow-up and in patient referral in the various centers. As described below, the different experiences of the different centers have influenced their current treatment philosophies.

Table 23-4. Immunologic Classification of NHL (Lukes-Collins)

Histologic type	Incidence (%)
B Cell lymphomas	
Small lymphocyte (B)	9.2
Plasmacytoid lymphocyte	6.8
Follicular center cell (FCC)	
Small-cleaved	28.0
Large-cleaved	4.9
Small noncleaved	6.8
Large noncleaved	5.7
Immunoblastic sarcoma (B)	3.5
Hairy cell leukemia	3.3
T Cell Lymphomas	
Small lymphocyte (T)	2.4
Convoluted lymphocyte	9.7
Cerebriform lymphocyte (Sézary syndrome, mycosis fungoides)	2.1
Immunoblastic sarcoma (T)	3.5
Lymphoepitheloid cell	1.0
Histiocytic lymphomas	0.2
Unclassifiable lymphomas	12.9

Several newer histopathologic classifications have been suggested in recent years, including the Lukes-Collins classification[25] (table 23-4) and the Kiel classification.[26] These both emphasize cell morphology correlated with surface marker studies over follicular or diffuse pattern. Recently, the Non-Hodgkin's Lymphoma Pathologic Classification Project compared the Rappaport, Lukes-Collins, Kiel, Dorfman, British National Lymphoma Investigation, and WHO classifications. All were found to have prognostic utility,[27] a finding that we have confirmed.[28] The new Working Formulation proposed by this group divides NHL into 3 prognostic groups: low-grade, intermediate grade, and high-grade lymphomas (table 23-2). These subdivisions also have prognostic utility.

The Lukes-Collins, Kiel, and Working Formulation classifications have added a few new categories not well recognized previously. One of these is the lymphoplasmacytic lymphomas, which were generally referred to in the Rappaport classification as diffuse well-differentiated lymphocytic lymphomas with plasmacytic features. Lymphomatous lymph nodes from patients with the clinicopathologic diagnosis of Waldenstrom's macroglobulinemia generally have this histologic appearance. Although monoclonal serum proteins are seen most frequently among patients with this type of lymphoma, they are not found in most patients. The incidence of bone marrow and splenic involvement is high. Also, a high proportion of patients presenting in the orbit, G.I. tract, and lung have this variety of lymphoma. It is included among the low-grade lymphomas.

Another contribution of the newer classifications is the recognition of various subtypes of large-cell lymphoma (diffuse histiocytic lymphoma in the Rappaport classification). One subtype, immunoblastic large-cell lymphoma, was included among the high-grade lymphomas in the Working Formulation, whereas the others were placed among those of intermediate grade. We have confirmed a worse prognosis for this subgroup for minimal treatment, although its prognostic importance for patients treated with current aggressive chemotherapy regimens is controversial.[28]

Two new histologic categories not included in the Working Formulation classification were recently described and reviewed:[85] (1) the intermediate lymphocytic/mantle zone lymphoma originated from B lymphocytes that express the CD5 antigen found in the mantle zone or corona of lymphoid follicles; and (2) the monocytoid B cell lymphoma, with generally large cells with pale cytoplasm and reniform nucleus, expressing B cell antigens as well as the CD 11c (Leu M5) antigen of monocytes similar to those of hairy cell leukemia. These cells usually originate from the parafollicular regions and sinuses. Both types are low-grade lymphoma, with the monocytoid B cell lymphoma added characteristic of being generally localized (stage I and II) and occasionally associated with Sjogren's syndrome.

Treatment

Therapy for lymphoma patients is much influenced in HD by the extent of their disease defined by their stage; in NHL, therapy is primarily related to the histopathologic presentation of the disease.

Hodgkin's Disease

Stages I_A and II_A. The work of Gilbert, Peters, and later Kaplan[11] demonstrated that recurrences rarely are seen within the treated areas with XRT doses of $\geq 3,500$ cGy. The use of the linear accelerator made it possible to deliver these doses to large fields. The mantle port (cervical, supraclavicular, mediastinal, and axillary regions), the "inverted Y" port (para-aortic nodes, spleen—depending on whether or not it was removed—and iliac, inguinal, and femoral nodes), and combinations of the 2 were developed in 1960s. Total nodal irradiation refers to combinations of the 2, which at times have also included low-dose irradiation of liver and lung. Subtotal nodal irradiation includes the mantle port with irradiation of para-aortic nodes and spleen if it was not removed, sparing the pelvis.

Local irradiation is probably adequate for high cervical stage I_A disease with a single tumor mass and lymphocyte predominant or nodular sclerosis histology in a young patient. It is also generally agreed that bulky mediastinal disease with a mediastinal mass over one-third of the chest diameter should be treated with combination chemotherapy or combined modality treatment with chemotherapy and XRT.[30]

The prognostic importance of extension of disease from hilar nodes into the lung parenchyma is controversial. Some centers that employ XRT only, generally with low-dose radiation also administered to the entire affected lung, report good results.[31] Others have had better success with combined modality treatment.[32]

Treatment options available for most patients with stage I_A and stage II_A HD include:

1. Subtotal nodal irradiation, which can include the spleen to doses of at least 3,500 cGy in 3½ wk, has resulted in a complete remission (CR) rate of >90% with a 20–40% relapse rate, probably depending upon XRT technique and/or patient selection. The salvage of these patients into second durable CRs may be >50%. The risks of leukemia and sterility are less than with combination chemotherapy. Long-term potential side effects of XRT include radiation lung fibrosis, pericarditis, premature coronary artery disease, and second solid tumor malignancies, particularly sarcomas.

2. Combination chemotherapy alone and combined with XRT has resulted in a CR percentage of >90% with <10% relapse rate.[33] This is achievable with 6 cycles of chemotherapy with the MOPP (nitrogen mustard, vincristine, [VCR], procarbazine [PCZ], prednisone) or similar regimens (see Appendix). One randomized trial has suggested that XRT may not be necessary with 6 cycles of CVPP (cyclophosphamide [CTX], vinblastine [VLB], PCZ, and prednisone).[34] When XRT is also used, fewer cycles of chemotherapy may give similar results.[35,36]

Azospermia occurs in about 80% of men with 6 cycles of MOPP, and another 10% are rendered oligospermic.[37] Sperm banking with cryopreservation is encouraged for male patients who may wish to have children in the future. Female patients under 30 are less likely to become permanently infertile than those over 30. Trials are in progress to attempt gonadal suppression in females with estrogens and progestins and in males with androgens in an attempt to preserve gonadal function.

The actuarial risk of acute leukemia or myelodysplastic syndrome has been estimated to be about 10% at 10 yr.[20]

Stage III_A. As mentioned in the section on staging, it has been proposed that patients with high retroperitoneal nodal or splenic disease (III_{A1}, III_{AS}) fare better with total nodal irradiation than those with disease in lower para-aortic or pelvic nodes (III_{A2}). This was true with respect to relapse-free survival.[14] With longer follow-up, other groups have noted an improved survival and relapse-free survival with combined modality treatment for III_A patients as compared to total nodal irradiation.[39] The only possible exception is in patients with minimal splenic involvement only (<5 nodules).[15,39]

Good results have been reported with 6 cycles of MOPP or modifications of MOPP alone without XRT, although numbers of patients are too small for definitive conclusions.

Stages II_B, III_B, and IV. The major advance for patients with advanced Hodgkin's disease came from the use of MOPP by DeVita and colleagues.[40] Of 198 patients, 80% achieved a CR, and 68% of these were free of disease 10 yr later; 90% of these patients had stage III_B or IV_B disease.[41]

Many modifications have been made in the MOPP regimen. One of these, carmustine (BCNU) + CTX + VLB + PCZ + prednisone (BCVPP) achieved a CR rate similar to that of MOPP—76% versus 73% in a randomized trial—and the duration of CR and the survival of patients achieving a CR was longer for patients on BCVPP than those on MOPP. Also, the neurologic and G.I. toxicity was reduced with BCVPP.[42]

The treatment of stage II_B disease is still not settled. The Stanford group has reported a 79% survival for PS I_B and II_B patients treated with total nodal irradiation, which often included irradiation of liver and lung. There was no improvement in survival with combined modality treatment.[43] Others have suggested that patients with pathologic stage II_B without bulky mediastinal masses (one-third the thoracic diameter) fare well with subtotal nodal irradiation, although the numbers of patients are small.[44]

Combined modality treatment of stage CS II_B using alternating potentially noncross-resistant drug combinations and low-dose XRT as described below has also been successful.[45] Excellent results obtained in clinically staged patients would seem to obviate the need for staging laparotomy for CS II_B patients if combined modality treatment is used.

The use of alternating potentially noncross-resistant drug combinations and low-dose XRT in advanced HD stages is currently under investigation. Bonadonna and his colleagues demonstrated that a drug combination differing with MOPP in the pharmacology and mechanism of action of the components could result in a CR rate similar to that of MOPP.[46] Also, it was demonstrated by Santoro et al that at least some patients relapsing after MOPP could achieve a second remission, although the duration of these remissions were not as long as with primary treatment.[47] This combination was doxorubicin (ADR), bleomycin (BLM), VLB, and dacarbazine (DTIC) (ABVD). These investigators suggested that this combination might be potentially noncross-resistant with MOPP in that tumor resistant to MOPP might be sensitive to ABVD (see Appendix). A protocol was designed in 1975 in which MOPP and ABVD were alternated monthly for 8 cycles. An interruption was made between cycles 4 and 5 for low-dose XRT to the involved lymph node regions—2,000 cGy in 2 wk—with an additional boost of 1,000 cGy to areas of bulky disease. The fifth cycle was resumed after a rest of 2–3 wk.[45]

In 1979, a new trial was started in which MOPP/ABVD/RT (8 drug regimens) was randomized against 3 alternating potentially noncross-resistant combinations (10 drug regimens) (see Appendix). The third combination was lomustine (CCNU), melphalan (MEL) and vindesine (VDS) (DVA), following phase 2 trials with VDS alone and in this combination for relapsed patients. DTIC was dropped from ABVD because it was most troublesome for patients. All patients received 6 cycles of chemotherapy with either 2 or 3 combinations (see Appendix). The results for the initial 8-drug/XRT protocol and the subsequent 8 versus 10-drug/XRT protocol are the same.[48]

Fifty-nine of 68 patients with CS III_B treated since 1975 on both protocols have achieved a CR (87%), 7 (10%) a partial remission (PR), and 2 patients have progressed (3%). There have been 16 deaths, and 11 patients have relapsed from a CR; thus, slightly less than 80% of the patients remain in CR at 10 yr.

Since 1975, of 50 patients with stage IV disease who have received these treatments, 38 (75%) achieved a CR, 11 (22%) a PR, and 12 patients (2%) progressed. About 70% of the patients remain in a CR at 10 yr. Thirteen patients have died, and 19 patients failed to achieve a durable CR as defined above. There have been 3 acute leukemias and 1 non-Hodgkin's lymphoma in 209 previously untreated patients at risk for up to 11 yr in the original 8-drug/XRT and the more recent 8- versus 10-drug/XRT protocols.

The most recent attempt to further optimize the initial chemotherapy regimen for patients with advanced Hodgkin's disease came from studies by Klimo and Conners at the University of British Columbia, Vancouver.[49] From the beginning, they administer the 2 most effective regimens for HD (see Appendix) found in previous studies—MOPP and ABVD at 1-wk intervals, with a few adjustments that made this combination tolerable and less toxic. PCZ was administered for only 7 days, whereas prednisone was administered for 14 days with each cycle of therapy. DTIC was eliminated from the original ABVD regimen because of its significant G.I. toxicity and based also on previous studies indicating that its absence did not decrease the efficacy of the regimen. A total of 6 cycles of this regimen, designated as MOPP/ABV hybrid, were administered to 79 patients between 1980 and 1984. XRT (3,500 cGy in 20 fractions) was also administered to a single area of residual lymph node-related abnormalities if still present after 6 cycles of chemotherapy. Of 76 available patients, 74 (97.5%) achieved CR; in 10 (13%), with assistance of involved field XRT, only 2 patients (2.5%) were primary treatment failures and only 7 (9.5%) relapsed, all within the first 24 mo. This treatment was generally well tolerated, with <10% of patients requiring hospitalization and >75% of them taking >90% of the calculated doses of drugs.

Salvage treatment. As mentioned above, about 50% of patients relapsing after XRT can successfully achieve durable CR with combination chemotherapy. Localized nodal relapses outside the irradiated portals may be treated with XRT alone. Although second CR rates with ABVD following primary chemotherapy vary between 4% and 59% due to patient selection, only ≤20% of these patients remain in ongoing unmaintained CR in even the best series. Results are similar with other "salvage" drug combinations. We have had our best success with MOPP/ABVD (8-drug) or CAD/MOPP/ABV (10-drug) in patients relapsing after other combination chemotherapy, with 40–50% of patients achieving a CR. With the unavailability of VDS, we have successfully substituted VLB 4 mg/m^2 for VDS 3 mg/m^2 in CAD (see Appendix). Factors predicting a favorable response include limited nodal sites of relapse, treatment in first (as opposed to subsequent) relapse, high performance status, absence of B symptoms, and, most important, a disease-free interval of at the least 11–12 mo.[50] Because of dissatisfaction with a high relapse rate following salvage chemotherapy after primary chemotherapy, some have advocated autologous bone marrow transplantation. The results are mixed and preliminary.[51] A high-dose regimen with CTX 6 g/m^2/day × 3 followed by autologous bone marrow transplantation (ABMT) has induced CRs in 47% of 62 treated patients; of these, 83% are disease-free after a mean interval of 19 mo.[52] Overall, a CR rate of 53%, with 36% rate of survival free of disease represents the relatively limited experience with ABMT of 3 other centers.[51]

Non-Hodgkin's Lymphoma

Non-Hodgkin's lymphomas vary in their prognosis according to histologic and clinical features.

Stage I and I$_E$. These patients may be approached in several ways; data are insufficient to recommend one approach over another. With regional treatment, XRT with or without surgery, about 30–50% of patients can be expected to recur, generally outside the XRT portals.[53] The local control rate with XRT doses of 4,400 cGy is 80–90%,[54] and we have seen few in-field relapses above a dose of 3,500 cGy. Our results have been similar for nodular and diffuse histologies and for nodal and extranodal presentations. For 17 pathologically staged I or I$_E$ patients, a University of Chicago group reported a 72% disease-free survival and a 70% overall survival at 10 yr with extended-field XRT.[55] As in our own experience, most pathologic stage II or II$_E$ patients relapsed following XRT only.

Our regional approach has included partial gastric resection in addition to abdominal XRT for patients with limited gastric I$_E$ or II$_E$ disease. This approach has decreased the incidence of catastrophic bleeding and perforation.[17] Total gastrectomy should not be performed because of the nutritional morbidity of the procedure. Limited resection can also be useful in the management of localized colonic or rectal lymphoma. Lymphomas involving the small bowel often are more extensive, making resection of large portions of the small bowel impractical because of short- and long-term morbidity.

Some support for the adjuvant therapy for stage I NHL can be found in 3 European studies that randomized patients to adjuvant chemotherapy following XRT.[56] All of these show an advantage for chemotherapy, but this is mostly among stage II patients, who probably should all be treated systemically with chemotherapy. It will take more patients and longer follow-up to determine whether or not adjuvant chemotherapy will be successful in curing an increased number of stage I patients as compared to those receiving regional treatment only.

Finally, promising early results have also been reported for the use of combination chemotherapy alone for stage I large-cell lymphoma, using CTX, ADR, VCR, and prednisone (CHOP) (see Appendix).[57] The number of patients is too small and the follow-up too short to warrant any definitive conclusions about this approach.

Stage II, III, and IV diffuse non-Hodgkin's lymphoma. Major advances in the treatment of large-cell lymphoma were the reports of DeVita et al and Berd et al of the achievement of long-term survival in patients teated with combination chemotherapy.[58,59] DeVita et al used CTX + VCR + PCZ + prednisone (C-MOPP) (see Appendix) and achieved long-term unmaintained remissions and survival in about 40% of patients. A group at Yale and later a group at the University of Chicago[60] employed a combination of CTX, VCR, intermediate-dose methotrexate (MTX) with leucovorin, and cytosine arabinoside (ara-C) (COMLA) (see Appendix). In these studies, 40–50% of patients achieved CRs; overall, about 35% were long-term survivors. The Southwest Oncology Group pioneered the use of CHOP with or without BLM. These studies resulted in CR rates of about 50%. In common with the other programs mentioned above, the long-term survival rate has been around 30%. Most relapses from CR in all of these studies tended to occur within the first 3 yr, but late relapses out to 6–7 yr have been seen.[60,61] It is not clear that BLM added to the CHOP regimen increased its efficacy.

The results at Sloan-Kettering were similar to those mentioned above for similar regimens.[62] We have recognized that certain prognostic features predict a poor outcome. Patients with bulky mediastinal presentations of large-cell lymphoma generally have done poorly with the type of regimen mentioned above. Bulky abdominal disease and multiple extranodal sites of involvement also have been associated with a poor prognosis, although not as strongly as mediastinal presentation. The most important prognostic factor in large-cell lymphoma with respect to both CR percentage and survival has been initial elevations of serum lactic acid dehydrogenase (LDH). There has been an inverse relationship of survival with the amount of elevation.[62]

Recently, several groups have reported an improvement in survival for patients with large-cell lymphoma of from 30–40% to 60–80%.[63-67] One of the simplest of these regimens is m-BACOD as reported by Skarin et al from the Dana Farber Cancer Center.[63] High-dose MTX was added to CHOP and BLM. The initial dose of MTX was 3 g/m^2 followed by leucovorin rescue,[63] but similar results with less toxicity apparently have been achieved with an intermediate dose of MTX 200 mg/m^2 followed by leucovorin[68] (see Appendix). A regimen consisting of prednisone + MTX + ADR + CTX + etoposide (ETO) + ara-C + BLM + VCR (ProMACE-CytaBOM)[64,67] (see Appendix) was found in a recent cooperative group study to induce CRs in 59% of diffuse large-cell lymphoma patients.

Recently, excellent early results have been reported with an intensive weekly schedule of CTX + ADR + VCR + BLM + prednisone and intermediate dose MTX for 12 wk by Klimo and Connors[66] (MACOP-B—see Appendix). In this study, 84% of patients achieved a CR, and 75% patients are surviving at a median follow-up of 2 yr. However, the morbidity of this regimen and a drug-induced mortality rate of 2–8% make this regimen better suited for administration in conjunction with autologous bone marrow transplantation.

It is possible that the improved results recently reported for large-cell lymphoma with more intensive chemotherapy regimens may be partly due to selection of patients with unfavorable prognostic features for therapy with supralethal total body irradiation and high-dose CTX followed by autologous bone marrow rescue in cases without initial bone marrow involvement.[69] This procedure also has had some success as a salvage regimen in relapsed patients.[51] Whether or not autologous bone marrow transplantation is superior to current intensive "conventional" chemotherapy for large-cell lymphoma patients with an unfavorable prognosis is currently under investigation.

The treatment of patients with small cleaved cell lymphoma and diffuse mixed lymphoma is still not satisfactory. With conventional combination chemotherapy, the percentage of remissions has been high, but they have been of shorter duration than those of patients with large-cell lymphoma.[70] Whether or not an increase in durable CRs will be obtained with more intensive chemotherapy regimens is not known.

Lymphoblastic lymphoma is closely related to acute lymphoblastic leukemia by clinical behavior and by cell marker analysis, as mentioned above. At Sloan-Kettering, about 40–50% of these patients have achieved long-term survival with the same intensive approach that has been used with the same results in adult acute lymphoblastic leukemia (ALL).[71] This approach involves a standard ALL-type induction with VCR and prednisone, with added pulses of CTX and ADR; an intensive, highly myelosuppressive consolidation; and 2½ yr of a rotating schedule of drugs given on an outpatient basis (see Appendix, LSA_2-L_2 regimen). Prophylactic intrathecal MTX is used throughout induction, consolidation, and maintenance. The meningeal relapse rate has been low, and it seems that continuous prophylactic intrathecal chemotherapy combined with intensive systemic chemotherapy has eliminated the need for phrophylactic CNS irradiation, with its associated morbidity. Results achieved with this approach are among the best reported. Cures also have been achieved with this approach in patients with undifferentiated lymphomas.

Patients with high and intermediate grade lymphoma who relapse early from CR or those who initially have less than a CR obtain only short-lived benefit from second-line chemotherapy.[86] Relapsed patients who enter a second remission or those whose lymphomas retain drug sensitivity may benefit from autologous bone marrow transplantation (ABMT).[87,88] Patients with intermediate or high-grade lymphoma with poor prognostic features may be considered candidates for ABMT as initial therapy.[87] ABMT results are optimal when the procedure is done during a first or second CR.[87]

The dose intensity of ABMT and of conventional chemotherapy may possibly be augmented by employing newly prepared recombinant growth factors—the granulocyte macrophage colony stimulating factor (GM-CSF) and the granulocyte colony stimulating factor (G-CSF). They are under intense scrutiny. Ongoing clinical studies will be needed to determine if the use of these growth factors can reduce the duration and severity of treatment-induced leukopenia without stimulating the lymphoma.[88]

Patients with measurable tumor resistant to second-line chemotherapy following relapse are unlikely to benefit from ABMT. In these patients, third-line salvage chemotherapy regimens have led to some favorable results. Some of these regimens, such as DHAP (dexamethasone, ara-C, and cisplatin [DDP]) and ESAP (ETO, methylprednisolone [steroid], ara-C and DDP), are based on the synergism between DDP and ara-C and have led to PRs and CRs in as many as 69% of cases.[89]

Diffuse small-cell lymphoma is probably part of a spectrum of the same disease as chronic lymphocytic leukemia (CLL), as mentioned above. With minimal treatment, these patients had a median survival of 76 mo in the Sloan-Kettering experience, a survival similar to that in patients with CLL.[16] There is no evidence that combination chemotherapy prolongs survival in these patients. Good palliative results have been reported with low-dose total body irradiation and with alkylating agents, often combined with prednisone. A randomized trial is in progress at Sloan-Kettering comparing CTX and prednisone alone and in combination with low-dose total body irradiation. Following is a convenient schedule for administering chlorambucil (CLB) and prednisone: CLB 30 mg/m^2 p.o. over 1–2 days with prednisone 30 mg/m^2/day × 4. This can be repeated every 2–3 wk until remission is achieved or until myelosuppression occurs. We have often continued treatment after remission has been achieved to give a total treatment period of about 1 yr even after a CR has been achieved. Despite the use of a large dose of CLB at once, nausea and vomiting do not occur or are minimal and can be controlled with antiemetics. Obviously, a risk exists for the development of acute leukemia with the long-term use of alkylating agents in this disease, so treatment is generally started only if the clinical situation warrants it.

Nodular or follicular lymphomas—stages II, III, and IV. Treatment of these lymphomas is controversial and not entirely satisfactory. As with the diffuse small cleaved cell and the diffuse mixed lymphomas, remissions are achievable with combination chemotherapy in about 60% of patients with follicular small cleaved cell and follicular mixed lymphomas. The NCI has reported that the CRs in the follicular large cell and follicular mixed lymphomas may be more durable than those for the follicular small cleaved cell lymphoma.[72,73] The variability of the manner in which pathologists classify patients as to whether they have follicular mixed or follicular small cleaved cell lymphoma has made it difficult to confirm these reports.

As previously noted, another major difficulty in the interpretation of treatment results for the nodular lymphomas has been the difference in natural history reported at various centers. Stanford investigators have reported median survival of 8–10 yr for the follicular small cleaved cell and follicular mixed lymphomas with some spontaneous remissions.[34,35] Groups at Sloan Kettering and the NCI have reported median survival of only 3–4 yr from the conservative treatment era. Using total nodal irradiation or low-dose total body irradiation, either alone or in combination with single alkylating agents or CTX, VCR, and prednisone (CVP), the Stanford investigators were unable to demonstrate an improvement in survival.[74] The one exception was a selected group of stage III patients who had an excellent survival following total nodal irradiation.[75] This has led the Stanford group to adopt a "watch and wait" approach for asymptomatic patients with follicular lymphomas, because they feel their survival would be long without treatment and that treatment would not prolong it.[74,76] Selected asymptomatic patients treated only when complications occurred had the same survival as symptomatic patients treated with the above modalities. It could be argued that this study shows advantage for treatment, because the survival of symptomatic patients was probably prolonged to that of asymptomatic patients by treatment.

Others have found that achievement of a CR has prolonged survival for patients with follicular lymphomas.[77] Our results with the combination of thio-tepa + VCR + CLB + prednisone followed sequentially by CTX + ADR + MEL + prednisone (NHL-4 protocol) has improved survival early on as compared to our previous results with minimal treatment. Although how many of these CRs will prove durable is not yet certain, some patients are certainly in remission, remaining off treatment for a number of years. Historic comparisons are difficult, of course, because treatment results might improve with time because of an overall improvement in medical care and a change in patient population with time rather than because of specific effects of treatment. Randomized trials of an intensive chemotherapy approach versus a conservative "watching and waiting" approach are currently in progress.

Biologic response modifiers (BRMs) have been also extensively studied in low-grade lymphomas and found to have good activity.[90] As a single agent, recombinant alpha interferon (r INF α) yielded objective PRs in about 25–42% of cases that lasted a median of 6–12 mo.[90,91] The response did not appear to be affected by patient stage, histology, by the presence of constitutional symptoms, bulky disease, or by prior therapy.[90] It also appears that low-dose (2 MU/m^2 3 times/wk) intermittent schedules achieved results similar to high-dose, more intensive regimens.

The best responses with r INFα therapy were seen in patients with low-grade cutaneous T cell lymphomas, including Sézary syndrome and mycosis fungoides. In these patients, PR and CR rates of 40–45%[91] were reported using higher doses of INFα (10–36 MU/m^2 3 times/wk). They also lasted a median of 6–12 mo.

Combinations of r INF-α with chemotherapy are under investigation. Myelosuppression appears to be the dose-limiting toxicity of these combinations, but this could be overcome with the addition of colony growth factors. Preliminary results of these combinations appear promising.[91] Other BRMs such as monoclonal antibodies, directed against tumor cell surface immunoglobulins (anti-idiotypic antibodies) or against B cell and T cell antigens, and used as single agents[92] or as radiolabeled immunoconjugates[93,94] have led only to partial transient responses in patients with low-grade lymphoma. Finally, recombinant interleukin-2 alone or in combination with INF and/or chemotherapy is currently being studied in the same group of patients.[91]

Until these problems are resolved, the current recommendation for stage II, III, and IV follicular lymphomas might be the following: For elderly patients who are asymptomatic, a "watch and wait" and ultimately conservative approach with single alkylating agents such as CLB or CTX or mild combination chemotherapy such as with CTX + VCR + prednisone (CVP) seems reasonable. Symptomatic elderly patients might be treated conservatively at time of diagnosis. Symptomatic younger patients definitely should be treated at time of diagnosis. Consideration could be given to one of the more aggressive combinations employed for large-cell lymphoma, inasmuch as it is possible that improving the likelihood for CR and the quality of the CR might improve chances for disease-free survival. Such treatment might also be considered either initially or after a period of observation for young asymptomatic patients, since the natural history of their disease is uncertain.

Combined modality treatment for non-Hodgkin's lymphomas. Addition of adjunctive XRT for localized, particularly bulky initial disease has been advocated, because these may be areas at particular risk as sites of relapse following combination chemotherapy. Whether or not such XRT will improve results needs to be addressed in large-scale randomized trials.

Treatment of meningeal disease. The role of prophylactic intrathecal MTX to prevent meningeal recurrence is unclear. Long-term survival is achievable with intrathecal or intraventricular treatment with or without whole brain irradiation in perhaps 25% of patients presenting with meningeal disease.[78] Patients who develop meningeal disease nearly always die of their disease, although autopsies have shown control of meningeal disease following treatment in 50% of such patients.[78]

Our recommendation is for biweekly intrathecal MTX, 6 mg/m^2, administered until the cerebrospinal fluid cytology becomes negative. Thereafter, it is administered at gradually increasing intervals. A decision to eventually stop treatment must be made only on an individual basis after prolonged treatment. Patients with cranial nerve palsies should immediately be started on high-dose dexamethasone to reduce edema and be given whole-brain XRT in addition to intrathecal treatment. It is important to start as soon as possible to try to reverse the neurological deficits. For patients in whom active systemic treatment is planned and for whom reasonably long-term survival is possible, placement of an Ommaya reservoir for direct intraventricular treatment is recommended. The pharmacokinetics of CSF MTX is improved over intrathecal administration, and there is some suggestion that clinical results may also be improved.[78]

Conclusion

XRT has resulted in cures in patients with localized HD and NHL. Combination chemotherapy also has achieved long-term unmaintained remissions in many patients. The role of adjuvant XRT needs to be clarified. Particular success has been seen in advanced HD and in diffuse large cell and lymphoblastic NHL. Further studies are needed to improve results in these patients and in patients with the other types of NHL.

References

1. Streuli RA, Ultman JE. Non-Hodgkin's lymphomas: historical perspective and future prospects. Semin Oncol 1980; 7:223–33.
2. Silverberg E. Leukemias and lymphomas: statistical and epidemiological information. New York: American Cancer Society, 1977.
3. Chaganti RSK, Doucette LA, Offit K, et al. Specific translocations in non-Hodgkin's lymphoma. Cancer Cells 1989; 7:33–36.
4. Treat JM, Kaneko Y, Mitelman F. Report of the committee on structural chromosome changes in neoplasia. Cytogenet Cell Genet 1989; 51:533–562.
5. Lukes RJ, Collins RD. The Lukes-Collins classification and its significance. Cancer Treat Rep 1977; 61:1–9.
6. Broder S, Bunn PA Jr. Cutaneous T-cell lymphomas. Semin Oncol 1980; 7:310–31.
7. Chabner BA, Fisher RI, et al. Staging of non-Hodgkin's lymphoma. Semin Oncol 1980; 7:285–91.
8. Carbone PP, Kaplan HS, Mushoff K, Smithers DW, Tubiana M. Report of the committee on Hodgkin's disease classification. Cancer Res 1971; 31:1860–61.
9. DeVita VT, Bagley CM, Goodell B, O'Kieffe DA, Trujillo NP. Peritoneoscopy in the staging of Hodgkin's disease. Cancer Res 1971; 31:1746–50.
10. Kinsella TJ, Glatstein E. Staging laparotomy and splenectomy for Hodgkin's disease: Current status. Cancer Invest 1983; 1:87–91.
11. Lacher MJ. Routine staging laparotomy for patients with Hodgkin's disease is no longer necessary. Cancer Invest 1983; 1:93–99.
12. Tubiana M, Hayat M, Henry-Amar M, Breur K, Van Der Werf-Messing B, Burgers M. Five-year results of the EORTC randomized study of splenectomy and spleen irradiation in clinical stages I and II of Hodgkin's disease. Europ J Cancer 1981; 17:355–63.

13. Glatstein E, Guernsey JM, Rosenberg SA, Kaplan HS. The value of laparotomy and splenectomy in the staging of Hodgkin's disease. Cancer 1969; 24:709–18.

14. Stein RS, Golomb HM, Wiernik PH, et al. Anatomic substages of stage IIIA Hodgkin's disease: Follow-up of a collaborative study: Cancer Treat Rep 1982; 66:733–41.

15. Hoppe RT, Cox RS, Rosenberg SA, Kaplan HS. Prognostic factors in pathologic stage III Hodgkin's disease. Cancer Treat Rep 1982; 66:743–49.

16. Straus DJ, Filippa DA, Lieberman PH, Koziner B, Thaler HT, Clarkson BD. The non-Hodgkin's lymphomas I. A retrospective clinical and pathologic analysis of 499 cases diagnosed between 1958 and 1969. Cancer 1983; 51:101–09.

17. Weingrad DN, DeCosse JJ, Sherlock P, Straus D, Lieberman PH, Filippa DA. Primary gastrointestinal lymphoma: A 30-year review. Cancer 1982; 49:1258–65.

18. Weinberg DS, Pinkus GS, Ault KA. Cytofluorometric detection of B cell clonal excess: A new approach to the diagnosis of B cell lymphoma. Blood 1984; 63:1080–87.

19. Lukes RJ, Craver LF, Hall TL. Report of the nomenclature committee. Cancer Res 1966; 26:1311.

20. Curran RC, Jones EL. Dendritic cells and B lymphocytes in Hodgkin's Disease. Lancet II 1977; 349.

21. Hunter CP, Pinkus G, Woodward L, et al. Increased I lymphocytes and Ig MEA receptor lymphocytes in Hodgkin's disease spleens. Cell Immunol 1977; 31:193–98.

22. Rappaport H. Tumors of the hematopoietic system. In: Atlas of tumor pathology sect 34, fasicle 8. Washington DC: U.S. Armed Forces Inst Pathol, 1966.

23. Jones SE, Fuks Z, Bull M, et al. Non-Hodgkin's lymphomas IV. Clinicopathologic correlation in 405 cases. Cancer 1973; 31:806–23.

24. Anderson T, DeVita VT, Simon RM, et al. Malignant lymphoma II: prognostic factors and response to treatment of 473 patients at the National Cancer Institute. Cancer 1982; 50:2708–21.

25. Lukes RJ, Collins RD. New approaches to the classification of the lymphomata. Br J Cancer 1975; (suppl II) 31:1–28.

26. Lennert K, Mohri N, Stein H, Kaiserling E, Muller-Hermelink HK. Malignant lymphomas other than Hodgkin's disease, histology, cytology, ultrastructure immunology. Berlin Heidelberg New York: Springer-Verlag, 1978.

27. The Non-Hodgkin's Lymphoma Pathologic Project Writing Committee. National Cancer Institute-sponsored study of classifications of non-Hodgkin's lymphoma. Summary and description of a working formulation for clinical usage. Cancer 1982; 49:2112–35.

28. Lieberman DH, Filippa DA, Straus DJ, Thaler HT, Cirrincione C, Clarkson BD. An evaluation of malignant lymphomas using three classifications and the working formulation based on 482 cases with a median follow-up of 11.9 years. Am J Med 1986; 81:365–80.

29. Kaplan HS. Hodgkin's disease. 2nd ed. Cambridge, Mass London: Harvard University Press, 1980.

30. Mauch P, Gorshein D, Cunningham J, Helman S. Influence of mediastinal adenopathy on site and frequency of relapse in patients with Hodgkin's disease. Cancer Treat Rep 1982; 66:819–25.

31. Lee CK, Bloomfield CD, Levitt SH. Results of lung irradiation for Hodgkin's disease patients with large mediastinal masses and for hilar disease. Cancer Treat Rep 1982; 66:819–25.

32. Wiernik PH, Slawson RG. Hodgkin's disease with direct extension into pulmonary parenchyma from a mediastinal mass: a presentation requiring special therapeutic considerations. Cancer Treat Rep 1982; 66:711–16.

33. Koziner B, Myers J, Cirrincione C, et al. Treatment of stages I and II Hodgkin's disease with three different therapeutic modalities. Am J Med 1986; 80:1067–76.

34. Pavlovsky S, Dupont J, Jimenez E, et al. Combination chemotherapy with cyclophosphamide, vinblastine, prednisone and procarbazine (CVPP) alone vs CVPP plus radiation therapy in clinical stage I-IIA Hodgkin's disease. Proc Am Proc Clin Oncol (abstr) 1983; 2:233.

35. Ferme C, Teillet F, D'Agay MF, Gisselbrecht C, Marty M, Boiron M. Combined modality in Hodgkin's disease. Comparison of six versus three courses of MOPP with clinical and surgical restaging. Cancer 1984; 54:2324–29.

36. Andrieu JM, Montagnon B, Asselain B, et al. Chemotherapy-radiotherapy association in Hodgkin's disease, clinical stage IA, IIA: results of a prospective clinical trial with 152 patients. Cancer 1980; 46:2126–30.

37. Redman J, Bajorunas D, Goldstein M, et al. Semen cryopreservation and artificial insemination in Hodgkin's disease. Proc Am Soc Clin Oncol 1983; 2:219.

38. Petersen-Bjergaard J, Larsen SO. Incidence of acute nonlymphocytic leukemia preleukemia and acute myeloproliferative syndrome up to 10 years after treatment of Hodgkin's disease. N Engl J Med 1982; 7:965–71.

39. Mauch P, Goffman T, Rosenthal DS, Canellos GP, Come GE, Hellman S. Stage III Hodgkin's disease: Improved survival with combined modality therapy as compared with radiation therapy alone. J Clin Oncol 1985; 3:1166–73.

40. DeVita VT, Serpick AA, Carbone PP. Combination chemotherapy in the treatment of advanced Hodgkin's disease. Ann Intern Med 1970; 73:881–95.

41. DeVita VT, Simon RM, Hubbard SM, et al. Curability of Hodgkin's disease with chemotherapy. Long-term follow-up of MOPP-treated patients at the National Cancer Institute. Ann Intern Med 1980; 92:587–95.

42. Bakemeier RF, Anderson JR, Costello W, et al. BCVPP chemotherapy for advanced Hodgkin's disease: evidence for greater duration of complete remission, greater survival, and less toxicity than with a MOPP regimen: Ann Intern Med 1984; 101:447–56.

43. Rosenberg SA, Kaplan HS. The evolution and summary results of the Stanford randomized clinical trials of the management of Hodgkin's disease: 1962–1984. Int J Radiat Oncol Biol Phys 1985; 11:5–22.

44. Leslie NT, Mauch PM, Hellman S. Stage IA-IIB supradiaphragmatic Hodgkin's disease: Long-term survival and recurrence frequency. Cancer 1985; 55:2072–78.

45. Young CW, Straus DJ, Myers J, et al. Multidisciplinary treatment of advanced Hodgkin's disease by an alternating chemotherapeutic regimen of MOPP/ABVD and low-dose radiation therapy restricted to originally bulky disease. Cancer Treat Rep 1982; 66:907–14.

46. Bonadonna G, Zucali R, Monfardini S, DeLena M, Uslenghi C. Combination chemotherapy of Hodgkin's disease with Adriamycin, bleomycin, vinblastine and imidazole carboximide versus MOPP. Cancer 1975; 36:252–59.

47. Santoro A, Bonfante V, Bonadonna G. Salvage chemotherapy with ABVD in MOPP-resistant Hodgkin's disease. Ann Intern Med 1982; 96:139.

48. Straus DJ, Myers J, Lee BJ, et al. Treatment of advanced Hodgkin's disease with chemotherapy and irradiation: controlled trial of two versus three alternating potentially non-cross resistant drug combinations. Am J Med 1984; 76:270–78.

49. Klimo P, Connors JM. An update on the Vancouver experience in the management of advanced Hodgkin's disease treated with the MOPP/ABV hybrid program. Semin Hematol 1988; 25:34–40.

50. Straus DJ, Myers J, Koziner B, Lee BJ, Clarkson BD. Combination chemotherapy for the treatment of Hodgkin's disease in relapse. Results with lomustine (CCNU), melphalan (Alkeran), and vindesine (DVA) alone (CAD) and in alternation with MOPP and doxorubicin (Adriamycin), bleomycin and vinblastine (ABV). Cancer Chemother Pharmacol 1983; 11:80–85.

51. Canellos GP, Nadler L, Takvorian T. Autologous bone marrow transplantation in the treatment of malignant lymphoma and Hodgkin's disease. Semin Hematol 1988; 25:58–65.

52. Cabanillas F, Velasquez WS, McLauglin P, et al. Results of recent salvage chemotherapy regimens for lymphomas and Hodgkin's disease. Semin Hematol 1988; 25:47–50.

53. Lipton A, Lee BJ. Prognosis of stage I lymphosarcoma and reticulum cell sarcoma. N Engl J Med 1971; 284:230–33.

54. Fuks Z, Kaplan HS. Recurrence rates following radiation therapy of nodular and diffuse malignant lymphomas. Radiology 1973; 108:675–84.

55. Vokes EE, Ultmann JE, Golomb HM, et al. Long-term survival of patients with localized diffuse histiocytic lymphoma. J Clin Oncol 1985; 3:1309–17.

56. Landberg TG, Hakansson LG, Moller TR, et al. CVP-remission-maintenance in stage I or II non-Hodgkin's lymphomas. Preliminary results of a randomized study. Cancer 1979; 44:831–38.

57. Miller TP, Jones SE. Initial chemotherapy for clinically localized lymphomas of unfavorable histology. Blood 1983; 62:413.

58. DeVita VT, Canellos GP, Chabner B, Schein P, Hubbard SP, Young RC. Advanced diffuse histocytic lymphoma, a potentially curable disease. Results with combination chemotherapy. Lancet 1975; 1:248–50.

59. Berd D, Corneg J, DeConti RC, Levitt M, Bertino JR. Long-term remission in diffuse histiocytic lymphoma treated with combination sequential chemotherapy. Cancer 1975; 35:1050–54.

60. Gaynor ER, Ultmann JE, Golomb HM, Sweet DL. Treatment of diffuse histiocytic lymphoma (DHL) with COMLA (cyclophosphamide, oncovin, methotrexate, leucovorin, cytosine arabinoside): a 10-year experience in a single institution. J Clin Oncol 1985; 3:1596–1604.

61. Jones SE, Grozea PN, Miller TP, et al. Chemotherapy with cyclophosphamide, doxorubicin, vincristine and prednisone alone or with levamisole plus BCG for malignant lymphoma. A Southwest Oncology Group study. J Clin Oncol 1985; 3:1318–24.

62. Koziner B, Little C, Passe S, et al. Treatment of advanced diffuse histiocytic lymphoma: an analysis of prognostic variables. Cancer 1982; 49:1571–86.

63. Skarin AT, Canellos GP, Rosenthal DS, et al. Improved prognosis of diffuse histiocytic and undifferentiated lymphoma by use of high-dose methotrexate alternating with standard agents (m-BACOD). J Clin Oncol 1983; 1:91–98.

64. Fisher RI, DeVita VT, Hubbard SM, et al. diffuse aggressive lymphomas: increased survival after alternating flexible sequences of ProMACE and MOPP combination. Ann Intern Med 1983; 98:304–09.

65. Laurence J, Coleman M, Allen SL, Silver RT, Pasmantier M. Combination chemotherapy of advanced diffuse histiocytic lymphoma with the six drug COP-BLAM regimen. Ann Intern Med 1982; 97:190–195.

66. Klimo D, Connors JM. MACOP-B chemotherapy for treatment of diffuse large cell lymphoma. Ann Intern Med 1985; 102:596–602.

67. Miller TP, Dana BW, Weick JK, et al. Southwest Oncology Group clinical trials for intermediate and high grade non-Hodgkin's lymphomas. Semin Hematol 1988; 25:17–22.

68. Skarin A, Conellos G, Rosenthal D, et al. Moderate dose methotrexate (m) combined with bleomycin (B) Adriamycin (A), cyclophosphamide (C), oncovin (O) and dexamethasone (D), m-BACOD in advanced diffuse histiocytic lymphoma. Pro Am Soc Clin Oncol (abstr) 1983; 2:220.

69. Gulati S, Fredorciu B, Gopal A, et al. Autologous stem cell transplant for poor prognosis diffuse histiocytic lymphoma. In: Dicke KA, Spitzer G, Zander A, eds. Autologous bone marrow transplantation. Proc First Int Symp. Houston: University of Texas M.D. Anderson Hospital and Tumor Institute, at Houston 1985; 75–81.

70. Al-Katib A, Koziner B, Kurland E, et al. Treatment of diffuse differentiated lymphocytic lymphoma: an analysis of prognostic variables. Cancer 1984; 53:2404–12.

71. Slater DE, Mertelsmann R, Koziner B, et al. Lymphoblastic lymphoma in adults. J Clin Oncol 1986; 4:57–67.

72. Longo DL, Young RC, Hubbard SM, et al. Prolonged initial remission in patients with nodular mixed lymphoma. Ann Intern Med 1984; 100:651–56.

73. Osborne CK, Norton L, Young RC, et al. Nodular histiocytic lymphoma: an aggressive nodular lymphoma with potential for prolonged disease-free survival. Blood 1980; 56:98–103.

74. Hoppe RT, Kushlan P, Kaplan HS, Rosenberg SA, Brown BW. The treatment of advanced stage favorable histology non-Hodgkin's lymphoma: a preliminary report of a randomized trial comparing single agent chemotherapy and whole body irradiation. Blood 1981; 58:592–98.

75. Paryani SB, Hoppe RT, Cox RS, Colby TV, Kaplan HS. The role of radiation therapy in the management of stage III follicular lymphomas. J Clin Oncol 1984; 2:841–48.

76. Portlock CS, Rosenberg SA. No initial therapy for stage III and IV non-Hodgkin's lymphomas of favorable histologic types. Ann Intern Med 1979; 90:10–13.

77. Diggs CH, Wiernik PH, Ostrow SS. Nodular lymphoma. Prolongation of survival by complete remission. Cancer Clin Trials 1981; 4:107–14.

78. Straus DJ, Recht L, Rodgers LO, Posner JB. Central nervous system (CNS) involvement in non-Hodgkin's lymphoma (NHL): analysis of clinical features and treatment in 96 patients. Proc Am Soc Clin Oncol 1984; 3:247.

79. Croce CM, Nowell PC. Molecular basis of human B cell neoplasia. Blood 1983; 65:1–7.

80. Manolow G, Monolova Y. Marker band or chromosome 14 from Burkitt's lymphomas. Nature 1972; 234:33–34.
81. Bloomfield CD, Arthur DC, Erizzera G, et al. Nonrandom chromosome abnormalities in lymphomas. Cancer Res 1983; 43:2975–84.
82. Le Beau MM. Chromosomal abnormalities in non-Hodgkin's lymphomas. Semin Oncol 1990; 17:20–29.
83. Stein H, Mason DY, Gerdes J, et al. The expression of the Hodgkin's disease associated antigen Ki-1 in reactive and lymphoid tissue. Evidence that Reed-Sternberg cells and histocytic malignancies are derived from activated lymphoid cells. Blood 1985; 66:848–52.
84. Kaneko Y, Rowley J, Variakoijis D, et al. Prognostic implications of karyotype and morphology in patients with non-Hodgkin's lymphoma. Int J Cancer 1983; 32:683–92.
85. Burke JS. The histopathologic classification of non-Hodgkin's lymphomas: ambiguities of the working formulation and two newly reported categories. Semin Oncol 1990; 17:3–10.
86. Armitage JO, Cheson BD. Interpretation of clinical trials in diffuse large cell lymphoma. J Clin Oncol 1988; 6:1335–47.
87. Takvorian T, Canellos GP, Ritz J, et al. Prolonged disease-free survival after autologous bone marrow transplantation in patients with non-Hodgkin's lymphoma with poor prognosis. N Engl J Med 1987; 316:1499–1505.
88. Yi PI, Coleman M, Saltz L, et al. Chemotherapy for large cell lymphoma: a status update. Semin Oncol 1990; 17:60–73.
89. Cabanillas F, Hagemeister FB, McLaughin P, et al. Results of recent salvage chemotherapy regimens for lymphoma and Hodgkin's disease. Semin Hematol 1988; 25:47–50.
90. Portlock CS. Management of the low-grade non-Hodgkin's lymphomas. Semin Oncol 1990; 17:51–59.
91. Gilewski TA, Richards JM. Biologic response modifiers in non-Hodgkin's lymphoma. Semin Oncol 1990; 17:74–87.
92. Hale G, Clark MR, Marcus R, et al. Remission induction in non-Hodgkin's lymphoma with reshaped human monoclonal antibody. CAMPATH-IH. Lancet 1988; 2:1394–99.
93. Press O, Badger C, Eary J, et al. Radioimmunotherapy of refractory human malignant B-cell lymphoma. Blood 1987; 70–248a (abstr suppl I).
94. Rosen ST, Zimmer AM, Goldman-Leikin R, et al. Radioimmunodetection and radioimmunotherapy of cutaneous T cell lymphomas using a ^{131}I-labeled monoclonal antibody. J Clin Oncol 1987; 3:562–573.

24

TUMORS OF THE CENTRAL NERVOUS SYSTEM

George A. Vas, M.D.

THE SIGNIFICANCE OF CNS neoplasm is far greater than its epidemiology or statistics might imply. Even a small and relatively benign tumor can have devastating effects on cognition and may alter behavior and impair motor or autonomic functions, thus limiting one's independence. Early detection and treatment might reverse the condition, which would surely fail to improve if appropriate measures were delayed.

In the 1860s, the renowned Broca was the first to differentiate between the focal and so-called diffuse symptoms of brain tumors. Not until 1886 did the first patient survive an actual removal of a brain tumor, under Horsley's hands. It was Cushing (1869–1939) who laid down the principles of modern neurosurgery during a career that spanned 4 decades. His students included Dandy, who introduced both ventriculography and pneumoencephalography, and Bailey, who revised earlier classifications of brain tumors on a clinicopathological basis.

Etiology

No single etiology of brain tumor has been defined; there is no doubt that it is multifactorial, with genetic factors playing a role. Tumors appear in association with disorders of clear hereditary patterns, such as tuberous sclerosis, von Hippel-Lindau's hemangioblastoma, or Recklinghausen's neurofibromatosis. Susceptibility of certain animals to experimentally produced tumors also implies genetic factors. The role of carcinogens and viral infections, although established in experimental models, has never been proven in man. The occurrence of certain types of tumors in specific age groups suggests some hormonal influence, and the predilection of some neoplasms to appear in specific locations suggests the presence of some local factors as well. Malfunction of immunological mechanisms concerned with tumor surveillance is postulated to be as important a factor in etiology of brain tumors as in systemic malignancies.[1]

Incidence and Histologic Classification

Brain tumor statistics are more variable than most because of differences in selection methods of material by the individual authors. According to the American Cancer Society, in 1979 about 11,600 new primary brain tumors were reported in the United States and about 9,500 persons died from brain neoplasms. This incidence represented somewhat more than 2% of all malignancies and implied that primary brain tumors were slightly more common than Hodgkin's disease. A 1985 report, based on a 1973–74 national survey of short-term hospital admissions, estimated the incidence of primary intracranial neoplasms to be 17,000 and that of metastatic brain tumors 17,400.[2] All primary brain tumors occur slightly more often in men than women. Meningiomas represent an exception, with a 2:1 female/male ratio. Some statistics reveal higher female incidence of schwannomas and pituitary adenomas. The incidence of brain tumors rises with age, reaching its peak in 55- to 64-year-olds. On the other hand, they represent the second most common malignancy in children, only leukemia having a higher incidence. Specific histologic tumor types have their individual age incidence, growth characteristics, and even location. Almost 70% of childhood tumors are infratentorial; in contrast, >60% of adult brain neoplasms are supratentorial. Two-thirds of childhood posterior fossa tumors are either cerebellar astrocytomas or medulloblastomas.

Present-day classifications are derived from several previous proposals.[3-6] Improved histological staining, better visual amplification techniques, experimental tumor inductions, and cell cultures have shed further light on the possible cell origins and oncogenesis. Although controversies still persist, most classifications agree that (1) most tumors are of neuroectodermal origin; (2) well-differentiated neurons have limited growth or multiplication potential, and consequently tumors derived from supportive elements (i.e., glia) are much more common; and (3) a significant percentage of tumors originate from primitive neuronal cell precursors (medulloblastoma) and vestigal tissues (craniopharyngioma).

Gliomas are widely credited to account for 40–50% of all intracranial tumors (both primary and metastatic)[3] and for up to 62% of primary brain tumors for all age groups.[4] The enormous variability of brain tumor statistics is reflected in table 24-1.[2-4]

Metastatic brain tumor statistics have been even more variable and unreliable.[8] Their increased incidence of late is due to improved diagnostic techniques, better reporting, and, predictably, more effective systemic treatment. Once reaching the brain, the malignant cells are protected from systemic chemotherapy by the blood/brain barrier. In seeming contradiction, most

Table 24-1. Incidence of Brain Tumor by Site

Site of tumor	Incidence (%)
Neuronal elements (i.e., medulloblastomas)	3–4
Neuroglial elements	40–67
Meningeal elements	12–20
Perineural elements	<2
Lymphoreticular elements	<1
Vascular elements	2
Choroid plexus	<1
Pineal gland	<2
Pituitary	2–17.8

Sources: refs 2–4

tumor cells reach the brain by hematogenous spread, implying that the lung is a common source. Less often, they reach the brain by Batson's venous plexus or by direct invasion from the skull or dura. At time of diagnosis, nearly half of the patients appear to have a single mass on CT scan. They tend to present at the junction of the grey and white matter.

The most common metastases are from the lung, breast, melanocytes, and genitourinary (testis, renal) tract, in decreasing order of frequency. Carcinomas of lung and melanoma tend to metastasize to the brain, whereas those of the ovary, uterus, and prostate rarely do. Some tumors, such as melanomas, tend to have multiple metastases, whereas others, such as metastatic renal cell carcinoma, tend to be single. Most metastatic tumors are solid, and choriocarcinomas, testicular tumors, and melanomas are often hemorrhagic.[9]

Clinical Presentation and Pathogenesis

Clinical manifestations of tumors are determined mostly by their location and growth pattern. To better understand the evolution of these symptoms and signs, they can be divided somewhat artificially into 2 groups: those due to diffuse effects and those due to focal manifestations.

Generalized symptoms and signs are explained by progressively increasing intracranial pressure. This pressure can occur simply because of the growing size of the mass, for which displacement of cerebrospinal fluid (CSF) can no longer compensate. It is often stated that elevated intracranial pressure might not appear prior to an increase of 8–10% of the original brain volume. Other mechanisms include extensive cerebral edema, obstruction of the CSF pathways or blockages of CSF reabsorption, and obstruction of the venous drainage of the brain. It is the increased intracranial pressure that is postulated to bring on headaches, light-headedness, nausea and vomiting, nuchal rigidity, and changes in behavior and orientation.

Diffuse manifestations of most lesions, however, are often accounted for by their location at the so-called silent areas, which include the frontal lobes and the nondominant temporal lobe. These areas can harbor large lesions without obvious focal symptoms or signs. Behavioral or cognitive impairment often associated with these lesions is usually gradual and is frequently denied by the patient or his family or attributed to aging and stress. Uncommon as these presenting symptoms may be, on initial examination they are elicited in a large number of patients. Because headaches are initial symptoms in only about 20–53% of cases, a good share of patients do not present with this symptom. Eventually, nearly 70% will develop headaches that are mostly intermittent (typical on awakening) and that disappear rapidly (about 40% of headaches appear only in the morning). Focal headaches often localize the intracranial mass or at least identify the involved hemisphere.

Papilledema is less common in adults than in children, but occurs only in about one fourth of all patients. Focal manifestations, which include aphasia, hemiparesis, sensory loss, and ataxia, make up a long list of great variety. They are dependent on the exact location of the tumors, the quality, (often insidious) of their onset, and the rate of their progression. Hemiparesis, a rather obvious deficit, is the presenting symptom in 40% of patients, whereas it is a presenting sign in two thirds of the same group. Sudden onset of symptoms is reported by 5–15% of patients, a phenomenon for which no clear explanation has been found. Seizures occur in about 15% of tumor cases initially, and 33% of patients will develop seizures during the course of their illness.

Common Types of CNS Neoplasms

Description of most individual tumor types is beyond the scope of this chapter. The ones included here are selected for their very high relative incidence, for the extensive experience in their treatment, or for the diversity their natural history represents.

Glioblastoma multiforme comprises about 33–50% of all gliomas, with an incidence that is twice as common among men than women. In practical terms, this means that if an adult male develops a primary brain tumor, it is more likely to be a glioblastoma, the most malignant of gliomas, than any other type of tumor. The origin of the glioblastoma is uncertain and thus controversial. Some theorize that it arises as a "primary" neoplasm. Although the glioblast as a cell type does not exist, anaplastic cells could differentiate to multiple forms of cellular elements. Others hold that they more likely originate from well-formed glial cells (mostly astrocytes) or less malignant gliomas by aggressive dedifferentiation.[4] They are multicolored, necrotic, infiltrating, and often hemorrhagic masses, generally with blood vessels that are large, tortuous, and abnormal. They usually originate in the white matter but may extend into the cortex; they are least common in the occipital lobes. Pathological diagnosis is made by their histological appearance, which is characterized by the presence of excessive pleomorphic mitosis, necrotic and hemorrhagic elements, pseudopalisading, and endothelial proliferation (see chapter 11, figure 11-2).

Despite contradictory reports, <5% of glioblastomas are multicentric. In spite of their aggressive nature, they rarely metastasize. Metastasis is most often found at the operative site, in the CSF, in various sinuses, and, much less often, in the lung.

Meningioma is the second most common intracranial tumor (13–18%); together, gliomas and meningiomas comprise about 80% of all adult primary intracranial tumors. Although their exact origin is still debated, all classifiers agree that they arise from arachnoid elements. Their incidence increases with age, reaching its peak in the seventh decade.[10] Their prominence in women was mentioned earlier; they have a slightly higher incidence in women with breast carcinoma. Although the parasagittal site is the most common (25%), these tumors also occur over the convexity (18%), over the sphenoid ridge (18%), in the olfactory groove (10%), and in the suprasellar region, posterior fossa, peritorcular area, temporal fossa, falx, etc., in decreasing frequency. Their rich vascular supply is derived mostly from the meningeal circulation (external carotid supply). Usually they are well encapsulated, do not invade the brain but compress it, and irritate the cortex. The wide variation in histological appearance has been classified in a number of ways. Although most types are slow-growing, some grow extremely fast and are potentially malignant. The clinical behavior of a meningioma and its histological appearance have some correlation, but less than one would expect. The clinical course is more affected by the location and the growth rate of the tumor. The overall recurrence rate of these benign noninvasive tumors is about 11%.[3] Distant metastases are most unusual.

Medulloblastoma is a tumor that arises from persisting cells similar to, or even part of, the external granular layer of the cerebellum, which usually disappears within the first 20 mo of life.[11,12] Medulloblastomas may appear at any age, but >80% present under the age of 15, representing 1 of the 2 (with cystic astrocytoma) most common childhood brain tumors. Most arise at the neighborhood of the posterior medullary velum and develop into a mostly midline cerebellar mass that easily obstructs the CSF pathway. Despite its well circumscribed appearance, the tumor may invade and destroy the surrounding structures. It often sheds cells into the ventricular system, with subsequent metastases throughout the subarachnoid space. Even intracranial metastases are not uncommon.[13]

Diagnosis

The diagnosis of brain tumors is based on a thorough and accurate clinical history and a complete neurological examination. Such clinical evaluation will establish the absence or presence of signs and will localize the region of suspected dysfunction. Only then can the appropriate diagnostic tests be chosen with special attention to the suspected areas of involvement.

The CT scan has replaced most of the older invasive techniques. It is quick and reliable: If the lesion is ≥ 1 cm in diameter, the CT scan is reportedly 95% accurate when performed before and after the I.V. administration of a contrast agent (see chapter 10, figures 10-57 to 10-60). The emphasis on both pre- and postconstrast studies is made not only to differentiate hemorrhagic and calcified areas, but because some tumors, especially those that are metastatic, have the density of normal brain tissue before injection of the contrast material, whereas others enhance after contrast just enough to reach the density of normal brain tissue.[9] Parasagittal and pituitary tumors are better seen and localized with direct coronal or reformatted sagittal images.

MRI is the most recently developed of the widely available techniques. Important advantages of this modality are the lack of exposure to ionizing radiation and the exquisite anatomical detail displayed in axial, coronal, or sagittal views. For suspected brain stem and spinal cord tumors, MRI is undoubtedly the best choice (see chapter 10, figure 10-63). For other tumors, such as meningioma, contrast-enhanced CT scanning is more reliable.

Cerebral angiography is still useful. It gives information about the special relationship between a tumor and the adjacent structures (i.e., the exact location of the internal carotid arteries prior to pituitary surgery); it identifies the specific source of blood supply of a very vascular tumor (e.g., meningioma); it may differentiate between 2 suspected tumor types (e.g., schwannoma vs. meningioma); it identifies abnormal vascular patterns usually associated with a tumor type (e.g., glioblastoma).

Plain radiography is rarely helpful. It can identify bony changes caused by an adjacent tumor (e.g., meningioma) or calvarian metastases. With appropriate settings, CT scan is often a more sensitive tool.

Electroencephalography might suggest the presence of focal brain lesions during a seizure workup or give information of cortical dysfunction distant from the known brain lesion. However, it is not useful in specific tumor diagnosis.

Lumbar puncture is not only not useful, but should not be performed if CT scan or MRI can identify a large mass. A neoplasm involving the meninges, on the other hand, is diagnosed by cytological studies of the CSF.

The ultimate diagnostic tool is histological examination of the lesion in question. This cannot be accomplished without biopsy of the lesion. CT-guided stereotactic technique reduces morbidity in deep or poorly accessible lesions,[15] but the open surgical method can accomplish both diagnosis and treatment at the same time. A 1969 report found 12% of clinical and radiological diagnosis of brain stem gliomas to be incorrect by histological confirmation.[16] Although radiological techniques have improved, to accept diagnosis and therapy without surgical confirmation is generally inadvisable.

Treatment

Several treatment modalities are available. The choice of these is determined by (1) the general condition of the patient; (2) the absence or presence, the nature, and the rate of progression of specific neurologic deficits; (3) the degree of certainty of the exact diagnosis (i.e., availability of tissue diagnosis); (4) the prospects for useful recovery; and (5) the location of the mass lesions.[16]

Patients who present with signs of herniation should be treated immediately to reduce intracranial pressure. This is to include lower Pa CO_2 to 25–30 mm Hg by hyperventilation, administration of I.V. osmotic diuretics (e.g., an initial 1½–2 g/kg mannitol) if not contraindicated, and 100 mg I.V. dexamethasone. Most such patients stabilize enough to receive a more definitive treatment.

For primary brain tumors, the principal therapy is surgical excision or reduction. Shapiro defined 5 goals for this surgery: (1) to make a diagnosis (histological, rather than presumptive), (2) to perform cytoreductive therapy (both kill and remove), (3) to treat symptoms (eliminate local compression and reduce intracranial pressure), (4) to provide time to permit other therapy (if available or advisable) and (5) to alter tumor kinetics (increase susceptibility to radiation and chemotherapy).[17] Recent advances in neuroimaging, surgical techniques, instrumentation, and neuroanesthesia have reduced the potential harm of surgical excision and biopsy. Typically, the operative mortality of low-grade astrocytoma fell from 16% in 1945 to 2% by 1975.[18] Solid tumors elsewhere in the body are seldom "cured" without complete excision. Similarly, when the growth pattern and the location allow complete removal of a brain tumor—a cystic astrocytoma, for example—surgery may be curative. Patients whose brain tumors (especially malignant gliomas) underwent a subtotal resection seem to have a longer survival than those whose tumors were only biopsied. Even without an available unbiased study, the consensus is to remove as much of an intracranial mass as possible, and in selected patients, to reoperate on recurrent tumors.[20]

In the case of metastatic brain tumors, even when the metastasis is single, no controlled study has yet indicated that surgical extirpation is superior to radiation therapy (XRT) alone. Still, if the patient's general condition is good, an easily accessible, single metastasis should be removed. Suggested criteria for such therapy include (1) unknown primary site, (2) uncontrollable neurological symptoms (e.g., focal seizures or increased intracranial pressure), (3) recurrence of neurological symptoms after maximum radiation therapy, (4) high radioresistance, and (5) life expectancy of at least 1 yr.[9]

XRT has been used for brain tumor treatment since the 1920s. Improvement was noted early, particularly with medulloblastoma. Technical advances have provided better tissue penetration (<200 kv radiation was replaced by orthovoltage of 200–400 kv and supervoltage or megavoltage of >1 million volts), multiple portals reduced skin irritation, and smaller doses lessened the likelihood of cerebral edema. Guidelines appeared for selecting the best beam energy, field, or target volume, daily dose fraction, treatment frequency and total dose. In a large series of low-grade but infiltrative astrocytomas, where complete resection is not possible, 11% of patients without and 35% of patients with postoperative XRT survived 10 yr. Of those who had grade I tumors, 25% without and 58% with XRT were alive after 5 yr. None of the patients with a grade II astrocytoma who received no XRT and only 25% of radiated patients survived 5 yr.[21] Combined treatment of surgical resection and XRT of oligodendrogliomas resulted in a 5-yr survival of $>90\%$.[22]

Following subtotal excision of meningiomas, postoperative XRT will reduce the likelihood of recurrence, delay growth, or even cause regression of recurrent meningiomas.[23] Postoperative XRT is essential in treatment of medulloblastomas, which are not only locally infiltrative, but tend to disseminate within the CNS.[13] Irradiation to the entire neuraxis is recommended, to be followed by localized treatment to the posterior fossa and to identifiable metastatic lesions. Significant evidence has been acquired showing the benefit of XRT in treating medulloblastomas, ependymomas, oligodendrogliomas, brainstem gliomas, pituitary adenomas, glioblastomas and metastatic tumors. Radiation is recommended for postoperative treatment in these and even less radiosensitive tumors when they are only partially removed.

As with glioblastoma therapy, the proper target is still—or again—controversial. Most radiation oncologists advocate whole-brain radiation of about 4,500 cGy followed by local "boost," with a final tumor volume of 5,000–6,000 cGy. However, improved imaging techniques allow more precisely localized, well-circumscribed portals to target the entire mass with assurance. This obviates the need to radiate large volumes of normal brain, reduces XRT toxicity, and consequently improves the quality, if not the length, of survival.

XRT has been and remains the mainstay in treating metastatic brain tumors. In rare patients, such therapy results in sterilization of the intracerebral tumor and prevention of recurrence. Several studies have suggested that temporary remission of symptoms or response to therapy do occur in patients undergoing XRT.

The basic principles of chemotherapy are (1) the proper exposure of the malignant cells to the agent and (2) the high sensitivity of the tumor cells to the chemicals. Treatment is limited by systemic toxicity and the possible emergence of resistant forms of tumor. The neoplastic process best suited for such therapy is a widespread one, where surgical removal or local radiation are not feasible.

The restricted applicability of chemotherapy to CNS tumors is due to some unique situations: (1) the protective blood/brain barrier, which admits only small, nonionized, lipid-soluble, nonprotein-bound drugs; (2) ischemic regions of tumors (significant even in such vascular tumors as glioblastoma) with insufficient exposure to blood-borne chemicals; (3) large extracellular space through which drugs can reach the targeted cells only by diffusion; and (4) a massive population of cells with little "sensitivity" to many of the agents and a slow rate of proliferation.

Shapiro calls chemotherapy for brain tumors "still investigational."[17] None of the agents known so far have found useful clinical application in treating tumors with relatively low proliferative capacity. Even in such highly malignant tumors as grades III and IV astrocytomas, glioblastomas, or medulloblastomas, chemotherapy has been reported to be useful only as an adjuvant method to surgery and radiation or as the single mode of therapy for recurrent tumors for which the alternative modalities have already been exhausted. A vast number of agents have been tried, with successful results reported in individual cases or small series. Combinations of drugs with different mechanisms of action have been designed to attack heterogeneous cell populations and to reduce cumulative side effects. Oral lomustine, procarbazine, and vincristine have been recommended by Shapiro as a substitute for carmustine (BCNU) in treating malignant gliomas. Even when used alone, no drugs proved more efficacious than the nitrosoureas, most specifically BCNU, as an "adjuvant" in treatment of malignant gliomas (see Appendix).

The recommendation for multimodality therapy for malignant gliomas, a regimen that includes a combination of surgery, XRT, and chemotherapy, is based on a series of randomized studies.[24] These studies concluded that whole-brain radiation of 6,000 cGy improves the median postoperative survival from 14 wk to at least 36 wk. The addition of BCNU increases to 19% the proportion of patients who survive 18 mo, nearly 5 times the 4% survival rate for those who receive postoperative XRT or BCNU alone. The BCNU therapy should be initiated simultaneously with XRT, at a dose of 80 mg/m^2/day × 3 every 8 wk.[14]

Despite recent reports of some success, the role of immunotherapy in clinical treatment of CNS tumors is yet to be established. Attempts have been made both in stimulating the immune system to react specifically with the tumor and in passively transferring tumor-specific humoral and cellular elements.

New approaches to brain tumor treatment continue to appear; their potential efficacy will be realized only when their combined benefit outweighs their unwanted side effects. New methodologies include hyperthermia, radiation sensitizers, stereotactic interstitial irradiation (brachytherapy), fast neutron radiation, local inhibition of the blood/brain barrier, intra-arterial chemotherapy, and combined active and passive immunotherapy.[25,26]

Several clinical factors influencing survival of patients with malignant brain tumors have been identified. These include age (younger patients live longer), presence/absence of personality changes (death rate lower when absent), duration of symptoms (patients with symptoms of >6 mo live twice as long as those with symptoms of <4 mo), presence of seizures (longer survival, possibly because of immediate attention), postoperative condition, and presence of coma at time of diagnosis. These factors should be considered before treatment plans for the patient are final.

Technical advances have brought tremendous strides to the understanding, diagnosis, and therapy of CNS tumors. However, the greatest benefits are limited to those patients with relatively benign tumors; treatment of the most malignant neoplasms is still mostly palliative. In our approach to the individual patient, early and accurate diagnosis is the most important guiding principle.

References

1. Ausman JI, French LA, Baker AB. Intracranial neoplasms. In: Baker AB, Joynt RJ, eds. Clinical neurology, vol. 2. Philadelphia: Harper and Row, 1986.
2. Walker AE, Robins M, Weinfeld FD. Epidemiology of brain tumors: the national survey of intracranial neoplasms. Neurology 1985; 35:226.
3. Rubinstein LJ. Tumors of the central nervous system. Atlas of tumor pathology (2nd series, fascicle 6). Washington, D.C.: Armed Forces Institute of Pathology, 1972.
4. Russel DS, Rubinstein LJ. Pathology of tumors of the nervous system. 5th ed. Baltimore: Williams and Wilkins, 1989.
5. Zulch KJ. Brain tumors: their biology and pathology. New York: Springer, 1965.
6. Bailey P, Cushing H. Tumors of the glioma group. Philadelphia: Lippincott, 1926.
7. Kernohan JW, Mabon RF, Svien HJ, Adson AW. A simplified classification of the gliomas. Proc Staff Meet Mayo Clin 1949; 24:71.
8. Patchell RA, Posner JB. Neurologic complications of systemic cancer. In: Neurologic clinics: neuro-oncology. Philadelphia: Saunders, 1985; 3(4):729–50.
9. Posner JB. Neurologic complications of systemic cancer. Disease-A-Month XXV, (2), 1978.
10. Walsche FMR. Critical reviews: intracranial tumors. Quart J Med 1930–1931; 24:587.
11. Crue BL Jr. Medulloblastoma. Springfield, Ill.: Charles C. Thomas, 1958.

12. Raaf J, Kernohan JW. Relations of abnormal collections of cells in posterior medullary velum of cerebellum to origin of medulloblastoma. Arch Neurol Psychiatry 1944; 52:162.

13. Packer RJ, Finlay JL. Medulloblastoma: presentation, diagnosis and management. Oncology 1988; 2(9):35–44.

14. Whyte TR, Colby MY Jr, Layton DD Jr. Radiation therapy of brainstem tumors. Radiology 1969; 93:413.

15. Hirschfeld A. Stereotactic techniques in the management of cerebral neoplasms. Oncology 1989; 3(2): 25–32.

16. Salcman M. Resection and reoperation in neuro-oncology. Rationale and approach. Neurologic Clin 1985; 3(4):831–42.

17. Shapiro WR. Treatment of neuroectodermal brain tumors. Ann Neurol 1982; 12:231–37.

18. Laws Jr ER, Taylor WF, Clifton MB, et al. Neurosurgical management of low grade astrocytoma of the cerebral hemisphere. J Neurosurg 1984; 61:655–73.

19. Salcman M, Kaplan RS, Ducker TB, et al. Effect of age and reoperation on survival in the combined modality treatment of malignant astrocytoma. Neurosurgery 1982; 10:454–68.

20. Salcman M. Surgical resection of malignant brain tumors: who benefits? Oncology 1988; 2(8):47–59.

21. Leibel SA, Sheline GE, Wara WM, et al. The role of radiation therapy in the treatment of astrocytomas. Cancer 1975; 35:1551–57.

22. Chin HW, Hazel JJ, Kim THC, et al. Oligodendrogliomas: 1. A clinical study of cerebral oligodenrogliomas. Cancer 1980; 45:1458–66.

23. Wara WM, Sheline GE, Newman H, et al. Radiation therapy of meningiomas. Am J Roentgenol 1975; 123:453–58.

24. Shapiro WR. Therapy of adult malignant brain tumors. What have the clinical trials taught us? Semin Oncol 1986; 13(1):38–45.

25. Nelson DF, Urtasun RC, Saunders WM, et al. Recent and current investigations of radiation therapy of malignant gliomas. Semin Oncol 1986; 13(1):45–55.

26. Bullard DE, Gillespie GY, Mahaley MS, et al. Immunobiology of human gliomas. Semin Oncol 1986; 13(1):94–109.

25

MALIGNANT NEOPLASMS OF THE
HEAD AND NECK

Jose R. Marti, M.D., Ashok Shaha, M.D., and
C. Julian Rosenthal, M.D., F.A.C.P.

FORTUNATELY, CANCER OF THE head and neck is a rare disease, representing only 2% of all annual cancer deaths.* Still, about 34,000 new cases of head and neck cancer are reported annually.[1] Of these, early-stage disease can be cured with surgery and/or radiotherapy (XRT). However, despite advances in techniques of surgery and XRT, 5-yr survival in head and neck cancer patients improved only from 45% in 1960 to 54% in 1982.[2] This poor showing was due primarily to a relative lack of progress in treating locally advanced lesions (stages III and IV). It is seen more often in tertiary care centers but it carries serious implications for the patient and frequently complex dilemmas for the physician.

Epidemiology

In contrast to other tumors, certain well-known facts regarding the etiology of head and neck cancer have been accumulated from epidemiologic studies.[3] Prolonged exposure to alcohol and tobacco have been most frequently implicated in the development of head and neck cancer by clinical as well as experimental evidence. However, poor dental hygiene and other less well-known etiologic factors also must be taken into consideration; for example, chronic exposure to the sun has been frequently associated with epidermoid tumors on the skin of the head and neck area, particularly cancer of the lip.

---

*Tumors of the eye and orbit, as well as tumors of the ear, auditory canal, and mastoid are not only rare but require highly specialized treatment; they will not be reviewed in this chapter.

518

Exposure to sawdust, nickel, and leather-tanning products also has been linked to tumors of the paranasal sinuses.[4,5] The carcinogenic effect of low-dose radiation on the thyroid has received wide attention as well.[6] Unfortunately, most patients fall under the category of substance abuse, and a significant number of them will not change or give up smoking or drinking alcohol; thus, the incidence of second primary tumors in the upper aerodigestive tract, including lung cancer, is substantial, reaching about 15–20% at 5 yr after diagnosis of the original tumor.[3,7]

Pathogenesis

Various factors pertinent to the pathogenesis of head and neck malignancies may have an impact in their treatment. These therapeutic implications will be included in the description of the pathogenetic factors.

Gross and Microscopic Tumor Characteristics

Excluding tumors of the thyroid, the vast majority of all head and neck tumors are squamous cell carcinomas.[7] Some tumors of the paranasal sinuses, which occasionally can be adenocarcinomas, and tumors of the salivary glands (where only 8% of them are of epidermoid origin), form the few exceptions to this rule (see chapter 11, figures 11-8 and 11-9). With the exception of rhabdomyosarcoma in children, mesenchymal tumors in the head and neck region are rare.

Epidermoid cancer of the head and neck can be categorized as follows:

Carcinoma in situ probably represents the originating tumor in the mucosa at its earliest stages before it becomes infiltrating. Wide primary excision with adequate margins is the preferred method of treatment. This tumor occasionally can be associated with areas of leukoplakia, but this is a clinical term and is recognized as a white patch of mucosa. It remains unclear what fraction of these areas of leukoplakia will go on to become malignant or how soon. If wide local excision of these areas is not practical, close observation, provided that the lesion shows no features of infiltration on the biopsy, might be indicated.

Verrucal carcinoma, a clinical diagnosis, is characterized by an exophytic tumor of a wartlike appearance that is very well differentiated microscopically and is sometimes difficult to diagnose from a histological point of view (see chapter 11, figure 11-13). Depending on the location of this tumor, surgical resection has been the preferred form of treatment.

Exophytic carcinomas are lesions that are pendunculated and outgrowing, with sharp distinct edges and minimal deep infiltration. They are usually well differentiated and radiosensitive. Depending on the size and location of the tumor, surgical resection is usually the preferred mode of treatment.

Ulcerating or infiltrating carcinomas are perhaps the most common form of presentation of these tumors. Usually, they originate on the mucosal surface, which then ulcerates and infiltrates along the tissues and fascial planes. Treatment depends importantly on the stage of the disease and on the location of the tumor, but often combined treatment using more than one treatment modality is preferred.

Lymphoepitheliomas are poorly differentiated squamous cell carcinomas with lymphoid stroma. They occur typically in the nasopharynx, but they may present in the tonsillar area and (occasionally) in the base of the tongue. These are high-grade malignancies that present all too often with early lymph node metastases. The tumors are rather sensitive to radiotherapy, and the preferred treatment approach usually is a combination of XRT and chemotherapy. Surgery is used only for the initial biopsy or, less frequently, for local radiation failures or for recurrent disease.

Anatomic Site of the Primary Tumor

The anatomical regions that are commonly classified as representing the head and neck area are the oral cavity, oropharynx, nasopharynx, hypopharynx, and the larynx (figure 25-1). In addition to these areas, the following regions are traditionally managed by head and neck surgeons as well: the nasal cavity and paranasal sinuses; the salivary glands and the thyroid gland; the external auditory canal, middle ear, and mastoid; the skin of the face, including the lip; the orbital or periorbital region; and the mandible, including soft-tissue tumors.

The biological behavior of cancer of the head and neck is closely associated with the anatomical region where the tumor is located. This is true not only with reference to the growth of the lesion and the local extension, but—more significantly—to symptomatology and the pattern of regional spread.[9,10] For example, due to the lack of pain fibers in the affected areas, tumors of the pyriform sinus or of the base of the tongue often reach significant size before producing any symptomatology. In contrast, an ulcerated lesion of the lateral aspect of the anterior part of the tongue or a small tumor on the vocal cords will show early signs and symptoms and elicit early attention. Similarly, a tumor of the lower lip, which is readily seen, will receive relatively early treatment. This is not the case, however, in tumors of the paranasal sinuses or the nasopharynx, which may go unrecognized for a long time, producing only chronic nonspecific symptoms, before the gravity of the situation becomes evident.

Tumor Size

The extent of the primary tumor is one of the most difficult variables to assess, even among tumors having a similar histology. In concept, tumors of the head and neck tend to spread by direct extension through the mucosa and along normal fascial planes to the surrounding soft tissues and bone. The nerve pathways can be favorite routes of spread. Most tumors of this area also tend to metastasize to the regional lymphatics in a fairly predictable pattern.[9,10] In contrast, distant metastases occur only in about 30% of all patients, usually late in the disease and almost always in the presence of recurrent or residual cancer.[11] Direct tumor extension to the osseous structures requires surgical resection of the structure, either totally, segmentally, or locally. XRT is usually contraindicated in these circumstances because bone is extremely radioresistant

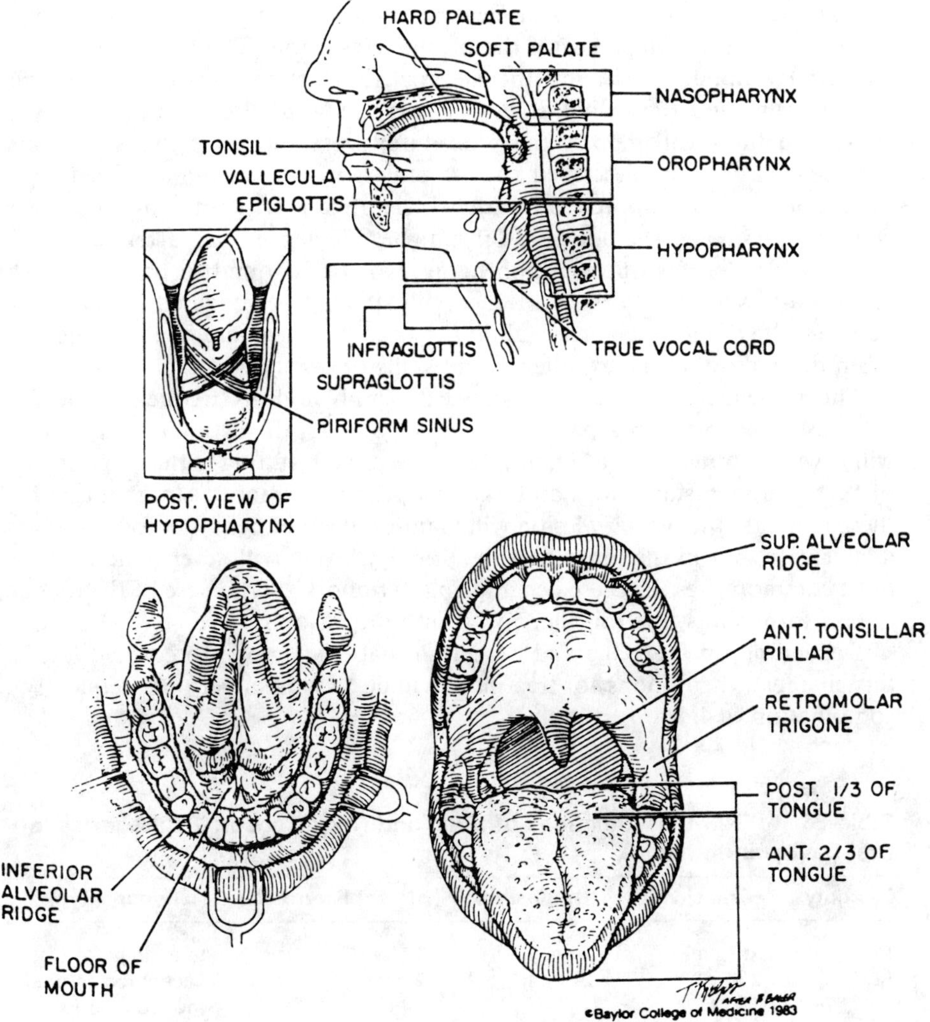

Figure 25-1. Schematic representation of anatomic regions of the head and neck in which primary cancers may arise. (Source: Calabresi P, Schein P, Rosenberg SA, eds. Medical oncology: basic principles and chemotherapy management of cancer)

and such treatment also carries a significant rate of complications, one of which is osteoradionecrosis, which is very painful and difficult to treat.

Involvement of Regional Lymph Nodes

Regional lymph nodes constitute the most frequent path for the of spread of head and neck cancer, and the spread follows a fairly predictable pattern.[9,10] Control of clinically obvious metastases is best approached surgically, and the classical concept of a radical neck dissection is still the preferred way of controlling this stage of disease. A classical radical neck dissection is most often done at the time of the surgical resection for the primary tumor, and it can be done in continuity with the primary resection. The term *radical neck dissection* implies sacrificing the sternocleidomastoid muscle, the internal jugular vein, and the spinal accessory nerve as well. Preservation of any of those structures will modify the procedure; preservation of the 3 structures together has been described by several authors as a modified neck dissection.[12,13] This approach has drawn significant criticism from those who claim that it creates the potential for a higher incidence of recurrent disease in the neck. If the metastatic lymph node involved is found to be fixed to the carotid artery or to the base of the skull, it may be rendered unresectable; however, the criteria of unresectability in head and neck are highly subjective, often depending on the experience and skills of the surgeon.

The presence of an enlarged cervical lymph node is frequently the first manifestation to alarm a patient. In some patients, the actual primary tumor will never be found, even after an extensive search, resulting in the classification of "cervical metastases with an unknown primary tumor."[14] In about half of these patients, the primary lesion will manifest itself either synchronously or at a later date, but in the other half the primary lesion will never be found. The most common sites for these occult primary tumors are the base of the tongue, the piriform sinus, the tonsillar fossa, and the nasopharynx.[8]

Depending on the stage and on certain patient factors (to covered later in this chapter), the options for treatment will be XRT or surgery or, frequently, a combination of both.

Table 25-1. TNM Classifications of Head and Neck Cancer: T Categories for Oral Cavity and Pharynx

Category	Oral cavity	Oropharynx	Nasopharynx	Hypopharynx
T1	<2 cm	2 cm	1 site	Site of origin
T2	2–4 cm	2–4 cm	2 sites	Adjacent region or site involved; no fixation of hemilarynx
T3	>4 cm	>4 cm	Extension to nasal cavity oropharynxnx	Extension to adjacent region or site with fixation of hemilarynx
T4	Massive with invasion	Massive with invasion	Skull and/or cranial nerves involved	Massive

Distant Metastases

Distant metastases represent an uncommon form of spread in head and neck cancer, occurring in only 18–25% of cases. Usually, they present late during the course of an uncontrolled primary tumor or in the presence of recurrent disease. The most common site of distant metastases is the lung parenchyma.[11] The only 2 exceptions to this are thyroid tumors and tumors of mesenchymal origin, which present distant metastases with a significantly higher incidence.

Staging and Clinical Evaluation

The currently used staging classification for head and neck tumors is the TNM system. T stands for tumor size and extension, which is classified following various criteria for neoplasms of the oral cavity and pharynx (table 25-1), for those of the larynx (table 25-2), and for those of the maxillary sinuses (table 25-3). N refers to lymph node involvement (table 25-4), and M is used to indicate the presence or absence of distant metastases (table 25-5). The stages are organized by counting together all 3 factors of the TNM classification (table 25-6).[15]

Most carcinoma of the head and neck should be assessed by physical examination. Before any therapeutic decision is made, patients suspected of having carcinoma of the head and neck should have a complete blood count and a complete serum chemistry (including renal and liver function tests) along with preliminary function tests—electrocardiogram, chest radiographs, and a lateral neck radiograph. Imaging studies might include a CT scan and, if

Table 25-2. TNM Classifications of Head and Neck Cancer: T Categories for Larynx

Category	Supraglottis	Glottis	Subglottis
T1	Confined to site of origin; normal mobility	Confined to glottis; normal mobility	Confined to subglottis
T2	Involves adjacent site—no fixations	Supra or subglottis extension; normal or impaired mobility	Extension to normal cords; normal or impaired mobility
T3	Limited to larynx with fixations and/or extention to post cricoid, medial wall of piriform sinus, pre-epiglottic space	Confined to larynx; cord fixed	Confined to larynx; cord fixed
T4	Massive—beyond larynx	Massive—beyond larynx and/or thyroid cartilage destruction	Massive—cartilage destruction and/or extension beyond larynx

Table 25-3. TNM Classifications of Head and Neck Cancer: T Categories for Maxillary Sinuses

Category	Description
T1	Confined to mucosa of infrastructure
T2	Confined to mucosa of suprastructure or infrastructure with medial or inferior wall destruction
T3	Invasion of skin of cheek, orbit, anterior ethmoid sinus or pterygoid muscles
T4	Massive invasion of cubiform plate, posterior ethmoids or sphenoid sinus, pterygoid plates or skull base

Table 25-4. TNM Classifications of Head and Neck Cancer: N Categories

Category	Clinical description of node(s)
N0	Nonpositive
N1	Single, homolateral 3 cm (dia)
N2	Single, homolateral 3–6 cm (dia) or multiple homolateral 6 cm
N2a	Single, homolateral 3–6 cm
N2b	Multiple, homolateral 6 cm
N3	Massive homolateral, bilateral or contralateral
N3a	Homolateral 6 cm
N3b	Bilateral
N3c	Contralateral only

Table 25-5. TNM Classifications of Head and Neck Cancer: M Categories

Category	Clinical description of metastases
M0	No (known) distant
M1	Distant present

Table 25-6. TNM Classifications of Head and Neck Cancer: Stage Groupings

Stage	TNM groups
I	T1, N0, M0
II	T2, N0, M0
III	T3, N0, M0, T1, T2, T3, N1, M0
IV	T4, N0, N1, M0, any T2, N3, N3, M0, any T, any N, M1

possible, an MRI scan of the head and neck and mediastinum. Depending on the clinical problem, special imaging required may include thyroid scanning, salivary gland scanning, tomography of the larynx, or laryngography.

Special imaging studies should precede endoscopy, because the latter may produce swelling of the affected part, perhaps leading to misinterpretations. The diagnosis of invasive carcinoma is almost always made histopathologically by biopsy at the time of endoscopy. Endoscopic evaluation of patients with head and neck cancer has other objectives: to determine the extent of the lesion and to exclude a second primary lesion (there is an incidence of $\leq 15\%$ of second primary cancers in the respiratory or upper alimentary tract in patients with head and neck malignancies).[8]

Direct hypopharyngoscopy and laryngoscopy are required for obtaining the biopsy and determining the extent of the primary lesion. Bronchoscopy with bronchial washing and esophagoscopy are useful to rule out a second primary neoplasm. In patients with a large mass that impinges upon the airway (especially at the level of the glottis), a tracheostomy might be necessary before the endoscopic examination in order to prevent the obstruction of the airway following the endoscopy due to edema.

Clinical Presentation and Treatment Approaches

Symptoms and physical findings of patients with head and neck cancer vary with the location of the tumor. Their detailed description is beyond the scope of this chapter, but common to all sites is the presence of pain that becomes severe and sometimes unbearable with the progression of the disease, requiring analgesia with narcotics and occasionally even neurosurgical intervention (rhysotomy). Depending on the location of their tumor, many patients will experience dysphagia at some stage of their disease. Consequently, they will also have a significant weight loss and other constitutional symptoms related to their poor nutritional status: lightheadedness, constipation, dryness of skin and mucosa, etc. These clinical factors also can have implications in the choice of treatment. In addition to the patient's general clinical condition, it is important to consider his/her habits and recent past history. If a patient is not willing to stop smoking during XRT, surgery might be the treatment of choice. In contrast, a patient who had a recent myocardial infarction and is a poor surgical risk might be a better candidate for XRT instead. Similarly, a patient who has 2 different synchronous tumors might derive an improved benefit from XRT plus chemotherapy.

Surgery and XRT have been used in the treatment of head and neck cancer for more then 5 decades, and chemotherapy has been tested with varying success for the past 2 decades.[11-13] Although the first 2 modalities can induce cures in most patients diagnosed in stage I or II, it is generally believed that for more advanced stages a combination of all 3 modalities—or at least of XRT with chemotherapy in a planned sequential or (more recently) concomitant fashion—gives better results than either modality alone, even though definitive controlled studies have not yet been carried out.[16,17] Considerable controversy prevails regarding the preferred sequence; although preoperative XRT received significant attention during the past decade, no evidence has been found that it provides better results than postoperative XRT.[12] Furthermore, due to the local nature of head and neck cancer, it is easy to understand why surgery and XRT occupy such competitive roles and why chemotherapy was once was used only in radiation failures in patients who were also inoperable. However, chemotherapy has now begun to figure in the quest for improved results as a primary modality of treatment. Recent reports on the use of chemotherapy in an adjuvant fashion prior to the use of surgery or XRT (neoadjuvant chemotherapy) are encouraging, and are covered later in this chapter.[18]

Details of surgical therapy of head and neck carcinoma will be covered briefly in this chapter. Some of its specific principles will be described during the presentation of the specific aspects of the cancer originating in the different regions of the head and neck. In general terms, the plan for surgical treatment should address the patient's entire problem, including the probability of the existence of nonpalpable metastasis. If this is likely and the operation cannot technically include the bed of the metastasis, XRT must be used following surgery to encompass these areas. The operative plan should include consideration of other disease states, age, and general health; rehabilitation of the patient in speech and deglutition should be compatible with a reasonable quality of life.[19]

Radiation Therapy

Radiation of head and neck malignancies has been practiced ever since the discovery of X rays in 1895, but it became a major part of the treatment of these tumors only after the use of megavoltage radiation equipment became practical.

Small lesions of the head and neck region (T1 and T2) can be treated effectively with XRT with excellent results and preservation of the organ being irradiated. In these early lesions, XRT is an effective alternative to surgery. The patient's general condition and preference must be considered in selecting the appropriate alternative. Of note is the fact that XRT failures sometimes can be effectively managed surgically.

Advanced lesions of the head and neck offer a significant therapeutic challenge because control rates and survival are moderately poor with either surgery or XRT alone. Currently, these advanced lesions are treated with a combination of XRT and surgery; in some investigational studies performed to date, chemotherapy seems to add further benefit to the XRT-surgery combination. The only multi-institution randomized investigation that compared the relative merits of preoperative versus postoperative XRT showed no significant differences in local control, complications, or survival between the 2 approaches in a study involving >300 patients.[21] Local regional success rates overall were 62%. Most patients died within 3 yr, and about 15% developed distant metastases without locally recurrent tumor.

When surgery is to be performed, many radiation therapists have favored the use of XRT before the procedure.[20] The rationale for this sequence is related to the fact that hypoxic tumor cells contained in the center of the tumor are less sensitive to irradiation and are much more effectively managed surgically, whereas the tumor cells at the periphery of the neoplasm and in its possible invisible peripheral extensions are more sensitive to XRT before surgery, when their vascular supply is intact. Preoperative XRT should encompass the primary tumor and all the draining lymph nodes at risk. The radiation fields typically include both sides of the neck as well as the supraclavicular nodes. Total doses have varied from 2,000 cGy in 1 wk, followed by immediate surgery, to 5,000 cGy in 5 wk, with surgery delayed for 3–6 wk.[20,21]

Postoperative XRT generally has been favored by the surgical community. The rationale of the sequence of surgery followed by XRT is that the tumor can be more adequately staged surgically, and the adverse effects of XRT or wound healing can be avoided.

The XRT dose is determined by the pathologic findings at the time of surgery; a dose of 5,000 cGy is adequate when all tumor has been grossly and microscopically removed and all margins are free of disease. An additional 1,000 cGy is recommended if microscopic residual disease is present or if the capsule of any of the lymph nodes has been transgressed. If gross residual disease remains following resection, the area of gross disease should be boosted to a total dose of 7,000 cGy in 7–8 wk, but in both instances, the prognosis for recurrence remains high.[17]

If less than maximum preoperative radiation is administered, postoperative radiation would also be indicated where there is transection of tumor or tumor spillage during the surgical procedure, involvement of multiple cervical lymph nodes with tumor or tumor extending through the capsules of lymph nodes, or where there is clinically detectable residual tumor in the neck.[17]

Finally, in accessible tumors such as those in the floor of mouth, anterior and posterior one-third of the tongue, and in the tonsillar regions, radioactive sources can be placed directly into the tumor by use of interstitial techniques. Techniques employing ^{226}radium or ^{192}iridium (as seeds or needles) require that the the radioactive source be removed after the calculated dose has been administered (usually in 3–7 days); those using radioactive seeds of ^{125}iodine or ^{198}gold, which have a short radiation emission life, represent permanent implants whose dose of radiation is calculated according to the effective life of the radioaction material. Small well-differentiated tumors may be treated with the use of an interstitial implant only, whereas larger tumors or those less well-differentiated are treated with a combination of external radiation and a supplemental boost to the tumor site using interstitial techniques.

Whatever technique is used, the volume of the irradiated site should include the site of the primary tumor as well as areas of potential lymph node involvement. When ipsilateral lymph nodes are palpable, the contralateral nodes also should be irradiated. The retropharyngeal nodes always should be irradiated when tumor arises in the piriform sinus or lateral hypopharyngeal nodes. All patients with N3 involvement as well as those with T3 and T4 piriform sinus tumors should have their upper mediastinal nodes irradiated.

Certain anatomic structures in the head and neck areas cannot tolerate high radiation doses. In all circumstances, the dose to the spinal cord should be limited to no more than 3,000 cGy, spread over 5 wk. Salivary glands, especially the parotid gland, should be excluded from the radiation field whenever possible because of the high incidence of dryness of the mouth after irradiation of head and neck carcinomas.

Another frequent side effect of XRT of these tumors is represented by frequent development of dental cavities due to chemical changes in the composition of the saliva; therefore, meticulous dental care is indicated for patients who are dentulous. Patients with teeth beyond repair require removal of all remaining teeth before irradiation and primary closure and surgical preparation of the alveolar ridges to support dentures. Those with salvageable teeth should have them repaired; like patients with normal teeth, they should then be instructed in dental prophylaxis with the use of a custom-made fluoride carrier (mouth guard) that permits the 5-min daily application of a commercially available fluoride solution that is then thoroughly rinsed. This program should continue indefinitely.

During the past decade, new XRT techniques have been explored in numerous studies, most of them conducted by the Radiation Therapy Oncology Group (RTOG). These studies, recently summarized by Marceol et al, included, among others, investigations of (1) the use of preradiation chemotherapy (methotrexate [MTX], cisplatin [DDP], 5-fluorouracil [5-FU] or DDP and 5-FU or cyclophosphamide-bleomycin [CTX-BLM] and vincristine [VCR]); (2) the administration of hypoxic cell tumor sensitizers (carbogen, nitroimidazole compounds, some of them still in the initial phase 1 developmental phase); (3) optimizing the radiation schedule (hyperfractionation); and (4) the use of hyperthermia to increase tumor radiosensitivity. Some of the results of these studies were initially disappointing but have become progressively favorable, with some techniques likely to enter routine clinical practice.[17,22]

Chemotherapy

Chemotherapy in head and neck cancer traditionally has been reserved for treatment of patients with recurrent or metastatic tumors. The response to chemotherapy is influenced by many prognostic factors, prominent among which are the patient's performance status and the presence of distant metastases. Patients with bulky disease, bone involvement with or without hypercalcemia, extensive skin involvement by lymphangitic spread, or persistent disease after XRT respond poorly to chemotherapy, and overall survival is short.[22]

Many single agents and combination regimens have been identified as active in patients with recurrent or metastatic head and neck cancer. Activity generally has been defined by the ability of the respective drug(s) to induce at least partial remission (PR) defined by the reduction of the measurable tumor volume by at least 50%. It is unfortunate that in head and neck cancer, achieving a PR does not improve the patient's overall poor survival. Survival is prolonged only in the few patients who achieve complete remission (CR).[22,23]

Among single chemotherapeutic agents, the most active drugs have been reported to be DDP, MTX, 5-FU, and BLM.[23,24] The overall response rate to each of these agents has ranged from 15 to 30% when used as first-line therapy; most of the responses were partial, with a median duration of 3–5 mo. When used as second-line chemotherapy, these agents induced PRs in <10% of cases (median duration about 3 mo).[22,25,26,27]

Due to these poor results, since the 1970s many of these drugs have been tested in various combination regimens in the treatment of recurrent and metastatic squamous cell carcinoma of the neck (see Appendix). These regimens included 1 or more of the 4 drugs previously mentioned as well as other drugs such as CTX, VCR, cytosine arabinoside (ara-C), and leucovorin. However, only a few combination chemotherapy regimens were tested in prospective randomized trials.[23,24]

In these trials, all regimens except 2 did not show differences in response rates and survival when compared with single-agent therapy. The first positive trial, from the Eastern Cooperative Oncology Group (ECOG), showed that a combination of MTX + BLM + DDP (see Appendix) induced a better response rate (48%, with 16% CR) than MTX alone—35% with only 8% CR. In the second positive trial, done by Al-Sarraf et al of Wayne State University, it was found that DDP 100 mg/m^2 and a 96-hr continuous infusion (C.I.) of 5-FU (1,000 mg/m^2/day) every 3 wk (PF regimen—see Appendix) induced an overall response rate of 72%, with 22% CRs.[22,24] This result compared favorably with the response rate of only 20% (with 10% CRs) in patients receiving the same combination chemotherapy but with the 5-FU given as an I.V. bolus.[24] For the first time, these results had an impact on survival: Most of the patients who achieved CR survived >3 yr. These studies were confirmed by others but not by all investigators who attempted to reproduce them. The 5-FU-DDP combination was found ineffective as second-line chemotherapy. Because the overall results of chemotherapy in metastatic and recurrent head and neck cancer are still poor, intensive efforts have been made to find effective new drugs as well as to test combination chemotherapy, especially as given by C.I. (DDP with 5-FU infusion) with concomitant XRT.[16,17]

Reports that the first combination chemotherapy regimens generated some positive results led to studies testing various multiagent regimens adjunctive to surgery and XRT and more frequently carried out before surgery (experimental data showed benefits of preoperative chemotherapy on a rat model[25,26]).

Despite relatively high response rates in nonrandomized studies, 7 randomized trials failed to show prolongation of survival in patients receiving preoperative chemotherapy.[22,26] They demonstrate, however, that (1) induction chemotherapy does not increase surgical or XRT complications, (2) initial response to chemotherapy predicts further response to XRT, (3) pathologic CR correlated with clinical CR in only 30 to 70% of cases, and (4) radical surgery could be omitted in patients who achieved pathologic CR. To date, best results have been reported from the Dana Farber Institute from 2 phase 2 studies in which a combination of DDP, BLM, and high-dose MTX with leucovorin (see Appendix) was compared with DDP and 5-FU administered by C.I.[16,17,22,27] The 2 combinations were found to be equally effective, including 26% CRs and 52% PRs before locoregional treatment (surgery or XRT was administered). The overall projected failure-free survival at 5 yr was 44% among the 80% of patients who were found to be disease-free after surgery and/or XRT. Locoregional recurrences were seen in 88% of cases that relapsed, whereas distant metastases occurred in only 30% of cases. It was found that most patients who achieved a clinical CR after chemotherapy could be successfully managed with XRT alone.[22-24]

In an attempt to improve these results, XRT is currently being used simultaneously with chemotherapy by C.I. (DDP and 5-FU alone or in combination), resulting in response rates of 52–94%. These overall results suggest that cure may be achievable in more than a third of recurrent head and neck cancer cases.[16,17,24]

Variations in Clinical Presentation and Therapy According to Site

Tumors of the Oral Cavity

The oral cavity is a well-defined anatomical region containing the buccal mucosa and the cheeks, the alveolar ridges (gingivae), the floor of the mouth, the mucosa of the hard palate, and the oral (anterior two-thirds) portion of the tongue.

Prolonged exposure to alcohol and tobacco, as well as ill-fitting dentures and poor oral hygiene, seems to play a predominant role in tumors of the oral cavity. Presenting symptoms can range from pain and loose teeth to the discovery of an ulcerated area. Sometimes the patient will discover the presence of a cervical lymph node. Quite often, the first medical person to discover this type of tumor is the dentist. In general, lesions in this area tend to be rather well differentiated and are quite amenable to treatment if discovered early. Except in far advanced cases, surgery is the preferred approach, but XRT gives equally good results in cases with small lesions (< 4 cm in diameter) without node involvement.[19] In early cases, the prognosis is generally good and the functional and cosmetic sequelae minimal. An exception to this is the tumor that has infiltrated the mandibular structures, a finding that makes surgery mandatory. In this circumstance, the wide excision of a tumor, which obviously will include mucosal and osseous structures en bloc with a radical neck dissection, will constitute a composite resection. The primary objective in these cases is to achieve adequate local control of the tumor; contrary to what one might expect, the functional and cosmetic sequelae are minimal provided that the anterior mandibular arch is not involved. The anterior mandibular arch, or mandibular symphysis, provides not only contour to the profile of the face but also gives support to the lower lip. Its absence will result in loss of the labial commissure competence, causing drooling and inability to control secretions; it will also alter the cosmetic aspect of the entire lower third of the face.

Tumors of the Pharynx

The pharynx can be divided in 3 different regions: nasopharynx, oropharynx, and hypopharynx.

Nasopharynx. Tumors in this region establish a very distinct group of patients. The etiologic factors in this area are less well understood, and in contrast to the previous group, the histology of these tumors is also less clear. Most of these tumors represent a combination of poorly differentiated squamous cell structures, often with no keratinization, and lymphoid elements. These tumors, known as *lymphoepitheliomas,* often cannot be traced to a specific etiologic factor. Although these patients might have some exposure to alcohol and tobacco, overall they tend to be younger than patients with other head and neck tumors.[2,3] This tumor appears to be more prevalent in Asia, particularly in some regions of China; the presence of the Epstein-Barr virus in the serum of these patients has led to speculation that this could be the etiologic agent of these tumors. Interesting features are found in their clinical presentation because they are among the few tumors that might present early with lymph node metastases to the posterior cervical triangle. Occasionally, a patient with such a tumor could also present with paralysis of the third cranial nerve due to its proximity to the base of the skull. This is a rather difficult area to explore surgically; fortunately, these tumors are quite sensitive to XRT, and, depending on their initial stage, the prognosis is generally good. Occasionally, well-differentiated squamous cell carcinoma can be encountered in this area, for which the therapeutic approach is also primarily XRT. The incidence of distant metastases in these patients is higher than in other head and neck malignancies.

Oropharynx. This area is best understood if one divides it into (1) the palatine arch, which is formed by the retromolar triangle, the anterior tonsillar pillar, the soft palate, and the uvula; and (2) the oropharynx proper, which includes the base of the tongue, the tonsillar fossa, and the pharyngeal walls to the level of the hyoid bone.

Tumors in this area are rather asymptomatic and may achieve significant size before they are discovered; however, this region has significant nerve supply and usually presents with pain. Ipsilateral lymphatic adenopathy, which may present early, usually represents a poorer prognosis.[12-14]

Although single modality treatment is preferred for early tumors, sequential multidisciplinary treatment is the best approach for late or advanced disease. Consideration must be given to the fact that this area is not easily accessible, and that removal of the tonsillar region necessitates the resection of the ascending portion of the mandible. The advantage of resecting the tumor in 1 stage but at the same time using a rather radical approach must be weighed against the advantage of XRT where no surgery is performed; however, this treatment requires 6–7 wk, and the side effects are considerable. The patient's reliability in completing the treatments and avoiding smoking and alcohol consumption during the course plays an important role.

Advanced tumors require not only a radical operation if the tumor is resectable but some form of neck dissection as well; this has to be coordinated with sequential XRT either before or after surgery.[19-21]

Hypopharynx. This area consists of the following structures: the valecula; the piriform sinuses; the postcricoid region, including the esophageal introitus; and the posterior pharyngeal wall from the level of the hyoid and upper cervical esophagus.

It is very important to keep in mind that these structures are located in the midline and that lymphatic drainage can go to either or both sides of the neck. The sparseness of nerve fibers in this region is another important consideration. Patients with these tumors usually present late in the disease, complaining of difficulty in swallowing or breathing, cervical lymphadenopathy, and changes in the quality of their speech, depending as to how advanced the tumor is or whether it is located in the piriform sinus, extending posteriorly toward the laryngeal region.[9,10] The major therapeutic objective other than tumor eradication is preservation of deglutition. Even though combined sequential therapy produces better results for these patients, the emphasis is heavily on surgery. Recent advances in surgical techniques, such as island flaps, free mucosal grafts, and even gastric transposition, have made this approach easier for the surgeon and more acceptable for the patient. All of these procedures can be accomplished in a single stage, and the need for any type of cervical stomas can be readily avoided. The overall prognosis for these patients is generally poor because presentation is usually late.

Tumors of the Larynx

This structure is divided into 3 areas: the glottic portion, formed by the vocal cord structures; the subglottic portion, inferior to the vocal cords; and the supraglottic portion, which includes the epiglottis, the aryepiglottic folds, and the false vocal cords.

Tumors in the larynx usually present early, with hoarseness the most frequent manifestation. Most tumors are suitable for XRT with good results.[20] Only late tumors or XRT failures are subject to laryngectomy. Conservative surgery with preservation of part of the larynx and some form of voice is being performed with increasing frequency, but not every patient is a candidate. Furthermore, the results, compared with those in patients receiving only postoperative XRT, have not yet been adequately evaluated. For early tumors, curative results with XRT alone can be expected to be near 90%. The voice quality is from acceptable to good in these patients. It is important to point out that the staging for laryngeal tumors, described earlier in this chapter, is somewhat special.

Tumors of the Nose and Paranasal Sinuses

These structures are grouped together for physiologic and etiologic reasons. These tumors are frequently related to the consumption of alcohol and tobacco; exposure to sawdust, nickel, and leather-tanning chemicals also has been associated with cancer in this area. Even though the overwhelming majority of these tumors are epidermoid, adenocarcinoma occasionally is encountered. This is not an uncommon site for tumors of the minor salivary glands, sarcomas, or lymphomas as well. The most common site of presentation is in the maxillary sinus, followed by the ethmoid sinus. The sphenoid sinus is only rarely the primary site of these tumors; however, it frequently might be involved as part of the local spread of an ethmoid or maxillary sinus tumor. The frontal sinus is virtually never the primary site of these tumors. Patients often present with nonspecific symptoms suggesting a chronic postnasal discharge or allergies for a prolonged period. Because of this, most patients will present late, and only an acute change will induce them to seek medical advice. Facial asymmetry, nasal bleeding, double vision, or dental complaints are among the most common symptoms before treatment. It is important to keep in mind that the staging system applied to this area is completely different from the usual TNM classification (table 25-1). Even though there are several classifications for tumors in this area, the most popular accepts the concept of the infrastructure and the suprastructure. It is important to understand the concept of Ohngren's line, an imaginary line that joins the medial canthus of the orbit with the angle of the mandible. The area caudad to this line is known as the infrastructure, and everything cephalic to this line—and therefore closely related to the floor of the orbit—is known as the suprastructure.[7] Tumors confined to the infrastructure, without bone destruction, are classified as T1. Similar tumors located in the suprastructure are classified as T2. If the lesion extends to the soft tissues or anterior ethmoid sinus cells or is approaching the pterygoid plate posteriorly, this is probably stage III disease. Anything beyond this must be considered as stage IV. A CT scan with sagittal and coronal cuts is probably the most efficient way to stage these patients today.

Among early tumors, the results of therapy are rewarding. This neoplasm spreads preferentially through tumor extension; lymph node metastases are rare and late. For these reasons, lymph node dissection is rarely performed, but sacrifice of the orbital structures, including the eye, is frequently necessary, particularly for tumors located in the suprastructure. A multidisciplinary approach, using radiation and surgery, yields the best results. Chemotherapy has been gaining in popularity, particularly for large tumors or recurrent disease.[17]

Tumors of the Salivary Glands

The salivary glands are generally divided into major and minor glands. The major glands are the parotid, submandibular, and sublingual glands. The minor salivary glands are an ubiquitous group of salivary secretion glands located throughout the buccal mucosa, hard and soft palate, lining of the sinus cavities, tongue mucosa, and pharyngeal tissue as far distally as the trachea. Tumors in this region can be benign or malignant; the incidence of malignant tumors is inversely proportional to the size of the glands. For instance, although two-thirds of all tumors in this area are found in the parotid gland, only 30% are malignant.

The most common neoplasms in this area are the pleomorphic adenomas, also called benign mixed tumors. Similarly, in the submandibular region, when a true neoplastic lesion of the submandibular gland arises, in 50% of the instances it is benign. In contrast, a tumor of a minor salivary gland is generally malignant (the incidence of benign disease in these glands is only 10%).

It is also important to keep in mind that benign salivary gland tumors should receive as much attention as their malignant counterparts for a number of reasons: The only way to establish an accurate diagnosis is through a surgical biopsy, and due to the relationship of these glands to important functional nerves in the head and neck area, this is always a major surgical procedure. Incisional biopsies under local anasthesia, either in the office or even in an ambulatory care setting, are contraindicated. Because these benign lesions tend to recur locally, they must be completely excised; this almost always means resection of the entire gland where the tumor is located. Inadequate resection of benign salivary gland tumors almost invariably will result in a local recurrence; in addition, surgery for these recurrences is more dangerous and carries a much higher complication rate, with frequent injury to the regional nerves.

The benign tumors of the salivary glands are classified as (1) benign mixed tumors (pleomorphic adenoma), (2) Warthin's tumor (papillary cystadenoma lymphomatosum), and (3) benign lymphoepithelial lesions.

Malignant lesions are separated into 2 groups—low- and high-grade malignancies. Tumors of low-grade malignancy are acinic cell carcinoma and low-grade mucoepidermoid carcinoma. Tumors of high-grade malignancy are high-grade mucoepidermoid carcinoma, malignant mixed tumors, adenoid cystic carcinoma, adenocarcinoma, squamous cell carcinoma, and poorly differentiated carcinoma (and/or anaplastic carcinoma).

As previously noted, most salivary gland neoplasms are benign. They appear more often in the parotid than in the other glands. They present most often in patients aged 20 to 40. With the exception of the Warthin's tumors, which occur more often in males, females are affected more frequently than males. These tumors may occur bilaterally, either synchronously or metachronously. Disregarding the size of these benign tumors, the incidence of facial nerve paralysis is negligible. Treatment requires resection of the entire lobe of the gland where the tumor is located. If it is the parotid gland, this implies a superficial parotidectomy in most cases. The operation turns out to be not only a diagnostic but also a therapeutic procedure; anything less than an anatomical resection has a significant incidence of local recurrence.

Malignant tumors are significantly less common than benign neoplasms, but as previously noted, the only way of arriving at this diagnosis is by surgical biopsy. Of the malignant tumors, the most common are the mucoepidermoid tumors, but these typically are of low-grade malignancy. These slow-growing lesions may affect any age group. They may be solid or cystic, but they are not encapsulated, even though they may appear well circumscribed. Wide excision with adequate margins is usually a curative procedure. However, this represents a superficial parotidectomy in most cases.

Acinic cell carcinomas are also slow-growing tumors of low-grade malignancy that occur most commonly in females. In contrast to the malignant mixed tumors, these have a well-recognized incidence for local recurrence and even distant metastasis. The recurrences may occur 25–30 yr after the initial resection; some authors consider them to be new primary tumors.

Tumors of high-grade malignancy are less common, but they may have ominous consequences if not recognized. High-grade mucoepidermoid carcinoma may widely infiltrate the salivary gland. Clinically, it may present with rapid growth and (frequently) early facial nerve paralysis. The incidence of lymph node invasion and even distant metastases is significant. If adequately treated, late recurrences are very late. A combination of surgery and XRT has been used with encouraging results.

Adenoid cystic carcinoma is common in the minor salivary glands but rather uncommon in the major ones. The rate of growth as well as the incidence of regional spread is similar to that of other tumors. However, perineural involvement is characteristic and very frequent. The mode of direct extension into the surrounding tissues represents a frustrating experience for surgeons because of the presence of skip areas and the frequency of involved margins. Because of this, the surgeon is frequently in a quandary regarding the amount of tissue to resect; recurrences many years after primary treatment are not infrequent.

Malignant mixed tumors are infrequent, accounting for only 5% of all salivary gland cancers. Some authors believe that at least some malignant mixed tumors arise from previous benign mixed tumors. These tumors progress to an obvious malignancy, demonstrating a very aggressive growth rate. The malignant component of the mixed tumors is usually epithelial in origin, possibly demonstrating features of an adenocarcinoma, squamous cell carcinoma, or even an undifferentiated tumor. Occasionally, all types may coexist in the same tumor. True squamous cell carcinomas most often end up being metastases to parotid lymph nodes from skin tumors of the head and neck or poorly differentiated high-grade mucoepidermoid carcinomas. Like true adenocarcinomas, these lesions are rare and appear late in life. They are usually very aggressive and often unresectable at time of presentation.

The most effective form of treatment for these tumors has been surgical; however, efforts to save the facial nerve by means of combination surgery and postoperative XRT have had encouraging results and are becoming increasingly popular.

Mesenchymal Tumors

These lesions, which are rare in the head and neck region, are more common among children. Ten percent of all pediatric neoplasms occur in the head and neck. As in the rest of the body, it is better to differentiate them as soft-tissue sarcomas and bone sarcomas. This does not take into consideration the lymphomas and tumors of the CNS, which should be reviewed under a separate category. Pediatric rhabdomyosarcoma, retinoblastoma, and Ewing's sarcoma are typical lesions of the head and neck in children. Combinations of XRT and chemotherapy have made significant advances in the prognosis of these patients, leaving surgery only for diagnosis. Among adults, bone sarcomas are slightly more frequent than soft-tissue tumors, but they are both rare. Even though presentation is usually late, most of these tumors are still treated primarily by surgery. Most common are the osteosarcomas of the mandible or the maxilla. When they present in association with Paget's disease of the bone, patients tend to be >60 yr old; however, when these tumors present as an independent lesion, the patients are most commonly in the second or third decade. Surgery is the main mode of therapy; XRT and chemotherapy play a secondary role either for palliation or in unresectable cases.

Tumors of the Skin of the Head and Neck

These tumors are considered the most common form of human cancer. However, because they are usually discovered early, they represent the most curable form. Less than 2% of all cancer-related deaths are due to skin cancer. Treatment of this disease is usually conservative, with surgical techniques the most common approach and cosmesis the underlying feature. The most common tumors in this area are epidermoid in origin and are closely associated with fair skin and prolonged exposure to ionizing radiation. Farmers, fishermen, and seamen are at high risk, but the underlying feature remains chronic exposure to the sun. The lower lip is almost always affected, whereas the upper lip is rarely affected. Squamous cell carcinomas and basal cell tumors are the most common. Melanoma is an infrequent disease and will not be covered in this chapter. These tumors respond well to surgery, but they also are highly sensitive to XRT, which should be seriously considered when surgery is likely to be deforming. It should be mentioned that with the exception of melanoma and certain syndromes such as the basal cell nevus syndrome, this disease carries an excellent prognosis.

References

1. Cancer Statistics 1988, New York: American Cancer Society, 1988.
2. Government Accounting Office Report: The war on cancer, a critical assessment. New York Times, Apr 16, 1987.
3. Blitzer PH. Epidemiology of head and neck cancer. Semin Oncol, 1988; 15:2–9.
4. Acheson ED, Cowdell RH, Rang E. Adenocarcinoma of the nasal cavity and sinuses in England and Wales. Br J Int Med 1972; 29:21–30.
5. Hadfield EH. A study of adenocarcinoma of the paranasal sinuses in woodworkers in the furniture industry. Ann R Coll Sing Engl 1970; 46:301–19.
6. Anletty JM, Guansing AR, Engbring NH. Radiation-related thyroid carcinoma. Arch Surg 1978; 1072–76.
7. Zarbo RJ, Grissman JD. The surgical pathology of head and neck cancer. Semin Oncol 1988; 15:10–20.
8. Shabra A, Hoover E, Marti JR, Krespi Y. Routine triple endoscopy; is it cost effective in head and neck cancer? Am J Surg 1988; 155:750–53.
9. Lindberg R. Distribution of cervical lymph node metastases from squamous cell carcinoma of the upper respiratory and digestive tracts. Cancer 1972; 29:1446–50.
10. Shah J. Patterns of cervical lymph node metastases from squamous cell carcinomas of the upper aerodigestive tract. Am J Surg 1990; 160:405–09.
11. Spaulding MB, Lore JM, Sundquist A. Longterm follow-up of chemotherapy in advanced head and neck cancer. Arch Otolaryngol Head Neck Surg 1989; 115:68–73.
12. Byers RM. Modified neck dissection: a study of 967 cases from 1970 to 1980. Am J Surg 1985; 150:414–21.
13. Khafil RA, Gelbfish GA, Attie JR, Tepper P, Fingale R. 35 year experience with 457 radical neck dissections in cancer of the mouth, pharynx and larynx. Am J Surg 1989; 158:303–07.
14. Spiro RH, DeRose G, Strong EW. Cervical node metastases of occult origin. Am J Surg 1989; 196:441–4.
15. American Joint Committee for Cancer Staging and End Results Reporting. 1980 manual for staging of cancer. Chicago: the Committee, 1980.
16. Cummings BJ, Keane TJ, Harwood AR, Thomas GM. Combined modality therapy with 5-Fluorouracil, Mitomycin-c and radiation therapy for squamous cell cancers. In: Rosenthal CJ, Rotman M, eds. Clinical applications of continuous infusion chemotherapy and concomitant radiation therapy. New York: Plenum Press, 1986.
17. Rotman M, Choi K, Isaacson S. Rosenthal CJ, Braverman A, Marti JR. Treatment of recurrent carcinoma of the paranasal sinuses using concomitant infusion Cis-Platinum and radiation therapy. In: Rosenthal CJ, Rotman M, eds. Clinical applications of continuous infusion chemotherapy and concomitant radiation therapy. New York: Plenum Press, 1986.
18. Minseyed A, Mahil-Tabatabai, Hill GJ, Raina S. Rush BF, Ohanian M. Multi-modality pre-operative treatment for advanced stage IV (M_o) cancer of the head and neck. Am J Surg 1990; 160:370–72.
19. Snow BJ. Surgical management of head and neck cancer. Semin Oncol 1988; 15:20–28.
20. Brody LW, Davis LW. Treatment of head and neck cancer by radiation therapy. Semin Oncol 1988; 15:29–38.
21. Snow JB, Gelber RD, Kramer S, et al. Randomized preoperative and postoperative therapy for patients with carcinoma of the head and neck: preliminary report. Laryngoscope 1980; 90:930–45.
22. Al-Sarraf M. Head and neck cancer: chemotherapy concepts. Semin Oncol 1988; 15:70–85.
23. Vogl SE, Schoenfeld DA, Kaplan BH, et al. A randomized prospective comparison of methotrexate with methotrexate, bleomycin and cisplatin in head and neck cancer. Cancer 1985; 56:432–42.
24. Kish JA, Ensley JF, Jacobs J, Al-Sarraf M. A randomized trial of cisplatin (CACP) and 5-Fluorouracil (5-FU) infusion and CACP and 5-FU bolus for recurrent and advanced squamous cell carcinoma of the head and neck. Cancer 1983; 56:2740–44.

25. Brock N. Neue experimentelle Ergebnisse mit. N-host-Phosphamidestern. Strahlen Therapie 1959; 41:347-54.
26. Choksi AJ, Dimery IW, Hong WK. Adjuvant chemotherapy of head and neck cancer: the past, the present and the future. Semin Oncol 1988; 15:45-59.
27. Clark JR, Fallon BG, Frei E III. Induction chemotherapy as initial treatment for advanced head and neck cancer: a model for the multidisciplinary treatment of solid tumors. In: DeVita VT, Hellman S, Rosenberg SA, eds. Important advances in oncology. Philadelphia: JB Lippincott, 1987; 175-95.

26

CARCINOMA OF THE LUNG

C. Julian Rosenthal, M.D., F.A.C.P.

Incidence and Etiology

FOR A LONG TIME, carcinoma of the lung has been the most common malignancy in males (55 new cases each year per 100,000 population) and in recent years the progressively higher incidence among females is nearly that of breast cancer.[1] Overall, it has become the second most common malignancy in the United States, with 161,000 new cases in 1990 (101,000 males and 60,000 females). Lung cancer accounted for 15% of all cancers (19% in males and 11% in females) and 28% of cancer mortality in 1990 (34% in males and 21% in females). The incidence may be increasing among blacks and decreasing among Mexican-Americans. The epidemiology of carcinoma of the lung has clearly indicated that tobacco smoking is by far the most common etiologic factor responsible for the steady increase in this disease during the past century. The impact of tobacco on the bronchial carcinogenetic process was proven in a multitude of studies recently summarized.[2] The effect of tobacco is supported by the fact that the incidence of lung cancer is 50 times higher in smokers of 2 packs of cigarettes daily for >20 yr; the risk gradually decreases when smoking is discontinued, with a return to the level of that for nonsmokers within 16 yr.

There is a dose/response relationship to the number of cigarettes smoked over a certain period of time. Experimentally, it was possible to induce carcinoma of the lung in >80% of hamsters and dogs kept in an environment with dense tobacco smoke. It was proven that 2 substances in tobacco are especially carcinogenic: nitrosamines, present in a liquid phase, and antracene in a solid phase. Other chemicals such as uranium, chromate, nickel, and asbestos were found to increase the incidence of bronchogenic carcinoma by

≤ 10 times that of a control population among miners living in an environment consistently polluted with these substances.

Chronic bronchitis and tuberculosis were also thought to induce a higher incidence of bronchogenic carcinoma, but by only 2–4 times the incidence seen in a control population.

Vitamin A deficiency as a predisposing cause of bronchogenic carcinoma was suggested by a number of experimental and clinical studies. Such deficiency decreases the number of goblet cells located on the basal membrane of the epithelium of all mucosae due to a decrease in the biosynthesis of L-fucose. This can occur only in the presence of retinol, a major constituent of vitamin A.[3] As a consequence of the loss of goblet cells, the ciliated cells exfoliate and expose the basal cells to the endobronchial environment, which in time leads to metaplesia and possibly to carcinogenesis. A deficiency of vitamin A also has been found to increase the binding of benzopyrine to tracheal DNA in hamsters.

Administration of high-dose vitamin A has been shown to inhibit the development of squamous cell tumors of the respiratory tract in hamsters. In a large epidemiologic study in Finland, the incidence of carcinoma of the lung was found to be 8 times higher in humans with dietary deficiency of vitamin A. For these reasons, retinoids (the major component of vitamin A) were tested in the prophylaxis of lung cancer until the trial had to be discontinued because of the development of peripheral neuropathy by a few individuals.

A deficiency of the enzyme aryl-hydrocarbon hydroxylase—a mixed-function oxidase—has been found with much higher frequency in smokers developing carcinoma of the lung than in those not developing it; this may explain why only 10–15% of smokers develop bronchogenic carcinoma.[4]

Oncogene amplification and point mutation have been found in lung cancer cell lines maintained in culture. The amplification of the myc oncogenes (C,N and L) and a deletion of the short arm of chromosome 3 in the 3p14–23 region have been found consistently in small-cell carcinoma DNA extracts.[5] In the same carcinoma cell line cultures, several peptides have been consistently found released in the supernatant (bombesin, vasopressin, neurotensin, ACTH, phys-alamin, calcitonin, transferrin-like peptide, epidermal growth factor, etc.). Among them, a bombesin-like peptide, the gastrin-releasing peptide (GRP) for small-cell lung carcinoma (SCLC) and the epidermal growth factor (EGF) for nonsmall-cell lung carcinomas (NSCLC), have the role of autocrine growth factors that can play an important role in growth deregulation leading to malignant transformation.[5]

Histology

The histologic classification of lung cancer as proposed by the Working Party for Therapy of Lung Cancer includes 5 major types:[6] (1) epidermoid (squamous cell carcinoma), (2) small-cell carcinoma, (3) adenocarcinoma with a bronchioalveolar subtype, (4) large-cell carcinoma, and (5) mixed types.

The histologic features of well-differentiated tumors can be described as follows: Epidermoid or squamous cell carcinoma consists of epithelial bronchial cells that grow in stratified or pseudoductal patterns and may form small whorls of nests containing keratin (see chapter 11, figure 11-14); this is also present in the cell cytoplasm and can be detected by a special stain (see chapter 11, figure 11-15). Squamous cells are connected by intercellular bridges that give the cells a prickle appearance. They may coalesce to form epithelial pearls, which are small foci composed of degenerated and malignant cells and keratotic debris.

Adenocarcinoma, when arising from bronchial mucous glands, tends to form lobules of neoplastic glands which may be mucin producing or may be arranged in a complicated cribriform pattern (see chapter 11, figures 11-21 and 11-22). When arising from bronchioles or alveoles, the tumors generally form subpleural nodules and are frequently multicentric.

Small-cell or oat cell carcinoma is composed of cells with nuclei that are small and round or oval or spindle and have a scant, indistinct cytoplasm; the cells are almost twice the size of lymphocytes and are arranged in clusters, ribbons, trabeculae or small nests; they are supported by a thin vascular fibrous matrix (see chapter 11, figures 11-16, 11-17, and 11-18).

Large-cell carcinoma has anaplastic features, being composed of large, polygonal, spindle, or oval cells with abundant cytoplasm and large, irregular pleomorphic nuclei with prominent nucleoli (see chapter 11, figures 11-19 and 11-20).

The growth rates of malignant tumors of the lung vary according to their histologic types and whether they are primary or secondary lesions.[7] The median doubling time of primary squamous cell carcinoma is 80 days; that of its metastatic lesions is 56 days. The median doubling time of primary adenocarcinoma is 207 days, whereas the lung metastases from adenocarcinoma double their size over a median of 89 days. The median doubling time of primary large-cell carcinoma is 32 days, whereas that of primary SCLC is only 33 days.

Clinical Manifestations

The clinical manifestations of bronchogenic carcinoma include a wide variety of symptoms that could be classified as symptoms due to the local lesion, those due to intrathoracic (regional) spreading of the primary lesion, and systemic manifestations.[8] Local symptoms due to central and endobronchial tumor growth include cough, dyspnea, chest pain, hemoptysis, wheezing or stridor, and postobstructive pneumonia with fever and productive cough. Other symptoms may result from the peripheral tumor growth: pain due to invasion of the pleura or chest wall and dyspnea from restriction of lung volume.

Symptoms caused by the intrathoracic dissemination of the primary lesions can be classified in relation to specific involvement of various anatomic sites (table 26-1).

Systemic manifestations of lung cancer are seen in <5% of cases. They can include any of the following disorders:
- Coagulation disorders presenting as thrombotic manifestations (e.g., migratory thrombophlebitis or nonbacterial thrombotic endocarditis) or

as hemorrhagic manifestations (e.g., disseminated intravascular coagulation, microangiopathic hemolytic anemia, or thrombotic thrombocytopenic purpura)
- Cutaneous and connective tissue disorders (e.g., acanthosis nigricans, dermatomyositis, tylosis [hyperkeratosis palmaris et plantaris], or scleroderma)
- Neurologic and muscular disorders (e.g., cortical or cerebellar degeneration, peripheral neuropathies, encephalopathy, myositis, or the reversed myasthenia-like syndrome or Eaton-Lambert's syndrome [encountered only in SCLC])
- Miscellaneous disorders (e.g., anorexia, weight loss, fever without any other origin, weakness, fatigue).

Finally, other objective and subjective manifestations of lung cancer are attributed to the release by the neoplastic cells of peptides with a structure identical to that of physiologic hormones (phenomenon possible through cell dedifferentiation). These manifestations, generally defined as endocrine paraneoplastic syndromes, are summarized in table 26-2.

Table 26-1. Symptoms Due to Intrathoracic Dissemination of Carcinoma of the Lung

Cause	Symptom
Nerve entrapment	
Brachial plexus due to chest wall involvement	Pancoast's syndrome: pain in shoulder and arm
Recurrent laryngeal nerve	Hoarseness
Phrenic nerve	Hemidiaphragm elevation with dyspnea
Vascular obstruction	Superior vena cava syndrome
Pericardial or cardiac extension	Tamponade
	Arrhythmia
	Cardiac failure
Mediastinal extension	Esophageal compression with dyspnea
	Lymphatic obstruction with pleural effusion
	Horner's syndrome: myosis, ptosis, and enophtalmos

Table 26-2. Endocrine Paraneoplastic Syndromes in Carcinoma of the Lung

Clinical syndrome	Substance or hormone produced	Most common cell type in which encountered	Percent of cases with syndrome
Osteoarthropathy	HGH (human growth hormone)	Adenocarcinoma, epidermoid	9
Hypercalcemia	PTH (parthyroid hormone)	Large-cell, epidermoid	7
Cushing's syndrome or hypokalemia	ACTH (adenocorticotropic hormone)	Small-cell	3
Inappropriate ADH	ADH (antidiuretic hormone)	Small-cell epidermoid, adenocarcinoma	1
Carcinoid syndrome	Serotonin	Small-cell	0.6
Gynecomastia	HCG (human chorionic gonadotropin)	Large-cell	0.5

The radiographic presentation of lung cancer may vary in early stages with the various histologic types previously described; they have a relatively consistent distribution in the lung parenchyma at the time of their early detection. The epidermoid and small-cell histologic types have a centripetal distribution (close to the hilum), whereas adenocarcinoma and large-cell anaplastic carcinoma have a centrifugal distribution (close to the pleura). With time, all lesions expand, and differences among histologic types vanish. The radiographic features of the various histologic types of lung cancer are summarized in table 26-3.

Table 26-3. Radiographic Features of Major Histologic Types of Lung Carcinoma

Histology	Approx. frequency (%)	Parenchymal abnormality	Intrathoracic or extrapulmonary involvement	Comments
Epidermoid	35–60	Central large or small ill-defined mass	Pleural effusion	Grows by direct invasion Cavitation Obstructive pneumonia and collapse Late metastases
Small-cell anaplastic	35	Hilar mass	Mediastinal widening	Grows by submucosal lymphatic extension Early metastases Obstructive pneumonia and collapse
Adenocarcinoma	15–20	Peripheral small or large ill-defined mass	Uncommon	Early hematogenous metastases Rare cavitation Scar carcinoma
Large-cell anaplastic	5–15	Peripheral large ill-defined mass	Occasional mediastinal mass	Very rapid growth Early lymphatic and hematogenous metastases Infrequent cavitation
Bronchial adenoma	5–10	Central, sharply marginated mass	Uncommon	Low-grade malignancy Infrequent metastases Bronchial obstruction Hemoptysis

Diagnosis and Staging

Diagnosis of lung cancer can be reached through stepwise performance of the following procedures: a correct and complete history and physical examination, followed by a chest radiogram and the cytologic examination of at least 3 sputum specimens (obtained with the help of a vaporizer).[9] In rare instances, cytology can be conclusive enough to firmly establish the diagnosis of malignancy, but the histologic type usually cannot be defined by this means.

Fiberoptic bronchoscopy is the procedure of choice for obtaining a suitable bioptic specimen that will permit definition of the tumor histology and assessment of the extent of the bronchial lesion. A CT scan of the chest should then be carried out to define the overall extent of the primary lesion, the possible presence of other small metastatic lesions missed by plain x-ray, and the possible involvement of the mediastinum (see chapter 10, figures 10-37–10-40). If mediastinal involvement is not seen, a gallium scan focused on the thorax is recommended because it can reveal areas of increased uptake in the mediastinum missed by the CT scan, which cannot discriminate lesions of <0.5 cm in diameter. Mediastinoscopy is currently recommended only in patients with abnormal upper mediastinal nodes on CT scan or gallium scan. Their biopsy showing infiltration by malignant cells would make thoracotomy unnecessary; no patients have survived 5 yr after resections attempted when high paratracheal nodes were involved.

The metastatic workup of patients with lung cancer should include a bone scan, abdominal CT scan, and a CT head scan, the last only for patients with SCLC or adenocarcinoma, which can present early lesions not accompanied by neurologic deficit (see chapter 10, figures 10-24A-D). Neurologic deficit can be sometimes prevented if small brain lesions are immediately irradiated.

The staging classification of patients with lung cancer is based on the TNM system, which defines 3 major parameters: tumor size (T), node involvement (N), and the presence or absence of metastases (M) (table 26-4). Based on these TNM parameters, a staging classification was developed and recently modified to reflect new progress and approaches in the treatment of carcinoma of the lung.[10]

Table 26-4. TNM Staging of Carcinoma of the Lung

Category	Description
TX	Tumor proven only by positive sputum cytology
T1	A bronchial tumor with greater diameter ≤3 cm or with bronchial invasion not proximal to a lobar bronchus
T2	A bronchial tumor with greater diameter >3 cm or bronchial invasion further than 2 cm from carina
T3	tumor invading mediastinum, pleura, diaphragm, or pericardium without invading other anatomic formations of the mediastinum; or a tumor located <2 cm from carina; or tumor associated with atelectasis of entire lung
T4	A tumor of any size involving heart, great vessels, trachea, esophagus, vertebral bodies or carina or accompanied by a malignant pleural effusion
N0	No lymph node involvement
N1	Involvement of ipsilateral hilar nodes or the ipsilateral peribronchial nodes
N2	Involvement of ipsilateral mediastinal nodes or subcarinal nodes
N3	Involvement of contralateral mediastinal or hilar nodes
M0	No distant metastases
M	Distant metastases, including scalene and cervical and ipsilateral lymph nodes

Stage Groupings

Stage	
Occult carcinoma	TX, N0, M0
I	T1 or T2, N0, M0
II	T or T2, N1, M0
IIIa	T3, N0 or N1, M0
IIIb	Any T, N3, M0, or T4, any N, M0
IV	Any T, any N, M1

Treatment

Three therapeutic modalities have been administered with various degrees of success to patients with lung cancer: surgical resection, radiation therapy (XRT), and combination chemotherapy. Immunotherapy, a fourth modality, was found ineffective in a number of recent studies. Introduction of bacille Calmette-Guerin (BCG) into the pleural space 4 days after surgical resection of the tumor initially was found to be effective in prolonging survival in patients with stage I disease, but this was not confirmed by other studies nor found to reduce the overall mortality rate among responders.

With the exception of cases of SCLC in which the current staging classification has little impact on patient management, the patient's tumor stage is the single most important prognostic factor.

The early hematogenous and lymphatic spread in SCLC can lead to the presence of occult metastatic lesions at the time of diagnosis; this explains the failure of radical surgery to cure patients with clinical and pathologic stage I disease. However, the extent of metastatic disease, which reflects the total tumor mass, is still the most important prognostic factor in patients with SCLC. Other prognostic factors with somewhat lesser impact on survival include: age, the concomitant presence of chronic obstructive lung disease, history of lung tuberculosis, and the rapidity of tumor response to initial therapy.

Currently, the recommended general approach to the treatment of lung cancer related to its histology and staging classification is as follows:

1. For SCLC, combination chemotherapy is the major primary treatment, complemented successfully by XRT when bulky disease is present.

2. For NSCLC cases in stage I, surgical resection has been found to be sufficient; no trial of adjuvant chemotherapy, XRT, or immunotherapy to date has shown any survival advantage.

3. NSCLC cases in stage II respond best to a combined modality regimen represented by initial extensive radical resection followed by adjuvant XRT.

4. For NSCLC cases in stages III and IV, various combination chemotherapy regimens are the therapeutic modality that could induce a temporary partial remission (PR) of short duration reflected in a brief prolongation of survival for responding patients. In the early 1980s, it was found that patients with stage III NSCLC with involvement only of the low mediastinal nodes can also be successfully resected.[9,11]

Due to the short duration of the response and of the fact that no combination chemotherapy has been found clearly superior, it has been recommended that eligible patients with stage III and IV NSCLC be enrolled in one of the numerous ongoing clinical trials.

The surgical treatment of operable lung cancer consists of lobectomy or pneumonectomy; the latter is indicated if hilar nodes are involved (stage II). Before surgery, pulmonary function tests should be carried out to verify that the patient can function with only 1 lung.

The results of several surgical studies of patients thought to be operable after staging workup are summarized in table 26-5 by histologic type and by 2 special patient groups, those with Pancoast's syndrome and those with lower medias-

Table 26-5.   Results of Surgical Therapy of Carcinoma of the Lung

Type of tumor	Unresectable (%)	Survival at 5 yr (%)
Squamous cell	7.5	35
Large-cell undifferentiated	25	30
Adenocarcinoma	21	40
Oat cell carcinoma	50	0
Pancoast's syndrome in patients with squamous cell or adenocarcinoma (resection en bloc of upper lobe and chest wall after XRT)	40	25
Stage III nonsmall-cell carcinoma with low mediastinal node involvement	30	15–25

tinal node involvement. Unresectability at time of surgery is because of infiltration of major vessels or other mediastinal formations or because of dissemination to the upper mediastinal nodes. In patients with stage IIIa NSCLC with low mediastinal lymph node infiltration by malignant cells, the mean percentage of survivors at 5 yr varied between 15 and 25%, depending on the groups of lymph nodes involved (periaortic, low paratracheal).[10]

Surgical and anesthesiologic procedures are occasionally indicated in stage III unresectable carcinoma of the lung for palliation of symptoms. For intractable pain, a nerve block with formaldehyde or rhisotomy could permanently eliminate pain. Other recent procedures used in the therapy of intractable pain include (1) the administration by continuous I.V. infusion of morphine sulfate via indwelling devices inserted in a central vein to which portable controlled pump delivery systems for morphine sulfate are attached and (2) the continuous delivery of morphine sulfate in the epidural space through an indwelling device connected with the epidural space by a special catheter.

For the lysis of unresectable bronchial masses that cause the collapse of a lobe or a segment of the lung or could be the indirect cause of persistent postobstructive pneumonia, laser therapy is currently recommended.

XRT of lung cancer is used primarily for control of loco-regional disease but can also be used as adjuvant therapy to surgery or for palliation of symptoms caused by distant metastases.[12]

The use of XRT can be subdivided as:

- Irradiation with curative intent as an adjunct to surgery after resection in cases in which ipsilateral lymph nodes were infiltrated by tumor (it improved results in one series from 2% to 28% survival at 5 yr when an average dose of 5,500 cGy was delivered postsurgically to the hilum and mediastinum[8])
- Irradiation with palliative intent administered for 1 of 2 major purposes: (1) to control the growth of unresectable tumors limited to one lung or (2) to palliate symptoms.

When administered to control the growth of tumors limited to one hemithorax, XRT leads to a fair number of complete responses (CRs), but these unfortunately are of short duration and have little effect on survival.

Data compiled from 5 studies published during the past 10 years are

Table 26-6. Results of Radiation Therapy Delivered to Possibly Eradicated Primary Carcinoma of the Lung Lesions

Histologic type	Complete response (%)	Survival at 1 yr	
		With radiation (%)	Without radiation (%)
Squamous cell	36	23	13
Adenocarcinoma	32	18	10
Large-cell	25	20	11
Small-cell	82	7	2

summarized in table 26-6. The 4 major histologic types are shown, along with the percentage of CRs after 5,500-6,000 cGy XRT to the involved area and mean survival at 1 yr as compared with that of matched patients who did not receive XRT. Despite the poor results of XRT in SCLC patients as shown in this table, a recent study indicated that XRT of the primary lesion in patients with SCLC limited to the chest (intrathoracic disease), administered sequentially to an effective combination chemotherapy, led to a definite survival advantage and better control of intrathoracic disease in comparison with a group of patients who received only combination chemotherapy.[13]

XRT is also administered for palliation of symptoms in patients with advanced metastatic disease. In these cases, the dose is usually less than optimal in order to avoid potential radiation complications. It was found successful in controlling hemoptysis in 84% of cases, pain in Pancoast's syndrome and at the site of distant bone metastases in 73%, superior vena cava syndrome in 88%, chest pain in 67%, dypsnea in 60%, and atelectasis in 23%.[12] XRT also was found successful in temporarily controlling the growth of lung cancer metastases to the brain as well as in largely preventing the development of metastases to the brain in patients with SCLC limited to the chest. In a group usually receiving 3,500 cGy to the whole brain, the incidence of brain metastases during the course of their disease was decreased from 70% to 5–10%.

Chemotherapy has clear indications in all cases of SCLC as well as in cases with stage III and IV NSCLC. However, with respect to the latter group, chemotherapy can lead only to PR and a brief prolongation of survival. For this reason, this approach in patients with stage III and IV NSCLC could be offered as an alternative to strictly supportive care aiming primarily at pain control and psychological comfort. However, the enrollment of patients in well-conceived and conducted studies should be highly encouraged because they are the most rational way to achieve progress in the treatment of advanced neoplastic diseases.

During the past 2 decades, progress made in the use of chemotherapy agents has been especially gratifying in the treatment of SCLC (see Appendix). The presence of distant metastases and regional nodal spread in $\leq 80\%$ of SCLC cases at the time of initial clinical presentation is consistent with the more aggressive biologic behavior of this type of lung cancer in relation to other histologic types. This pattern is confirmed by a higher mitotic index and a shorter doubling time and explains the better response of SCLC to chemotherapeutic agents and XRT. Because most SCLC patients were already in advanced stages III and IV at time of diagnosis, a 2-stage system for advanced disease was developed for SCLC that has more meaningful prognostic significance than the conventional staging system used for other histologic types. Limited disease, comprising about a third of cases, is defined as disease confined to one hemithorax, the mediastinum, and supraclavicular fossae that can be encompassed in a single tolerable radiotherapy portal. In extensive disease, tumor is found beyond the confines of the limited stage.

Among single agents identified in phase 2 trials as effective in inducing PRs ($>50\%$ reduction in tumor size) and CRs in SCLC patients are cyclophosphamide (CTX), doxorubicin (ADR), vincristine (VCR), methotrexate (MTX), etoposide (ETO, VP-16), teniposide (VM-26); vindesine (VDS), nitrogen mustard (HN_2), hexamethylminelamine (HMM), procarbazine (PCZ), and cisplatin (DDP) and its analogue carboplatin (CARB). These agents were found to induce a reasonable percentage of objective responses varying between 20 and 60% in untreated patients but only marginal responses (10–15%) in previously treated patients.[14] Combination chemotherapy regimens in SCLC were found clearly superior by historical comparison to single agents, producing CRs in 25–50% of cases and total objective responses in limited disease of 70–90% of all cases. Among the most successful combination chemotherapy regimens and one of the most commonly used: CTX 1,000 mg/m^2, ADR 50 mg/m^2, and VCR 2 mg every 3 wk (CAV). It induces PRs and CRs in 75–90% of patients with limited-disease SCLC but in only 15–20% of patients with SCLC with distant metastases. The duration of remission averages 15 mo for limited disease and 7 mo for extensive disease. Due to the potential significant cardiac and neurologic toxicity of the CAV regimen, variant regimens—CAE, in which ETO has replaced VCR (see Appendix), and CEV, in which ETO has replaced ADR—have led to results similar to those of CAV but lower neurologic and cardiac toxicity, respectively. When compared with other regimens in phase 2 trials, CAE showed a slight superiority to CAV in prolonging response duration (by 9 wk) in patients with extensive disease. A combination of DDP (60–80 mg/m^2) and ETO (180–375 mg/m^2 in 3 divided daily doses) was found to be the best salvage therapy in patients relapsing after CAV therapy, showing a 40–50% response rate.[14]

The use of alternating combination chemotherapy (CAV) followed 3 wk later by ETO-DDP (see Appendix) as an outgrowth of the Goldie-Coldman model of tumor growth reflecting its phenotypic and genotypic heterogeneity led to the best results reported to date: 95% objective remissions in patients with limited disease and 90% in extensive disease, with a median duration of 18 and 12 mo, respectively. However, this small study, which was performed in a single institution, now must be confirmed by randomized studies.[15]

In SCLC patients with bulky disease, the addition of XRT to chemotherapy was found to be beneficial only in those with limited disease, prolonging the duration of their remission and their survival.[12] Various studies of the duration of combination chemotherapy in SCLC patients suggest that it can be limited to 5–12 mo and that maintenance therapy after attaining remission is generally not useful in prolonging survival.

The experimental approach of resecting the primary lung lesion in patients with limited-disease SCLC who achieved CR after chemotherapy to date has not led to prolongation of survival as compared with similar patients who received chemotherapy and XRT without resection.[14]

Combination chemotherapy is less successful in patients with stage III or IV NSCLC. Various combinations have led to PRs but to very few CRs.[16] The most popular among these combinations are: CAMP (CTX + ADR + MTX + PCZ), CAP (CTX + ADR + DDP), BPVM (bleomycin, DDP + VLB + MTX), and MVP (mitomycin-C, VLB + DDP). Detailed schedules and dosages of several currently tested regimens are listed in the Appendix. Recently, carboplatin,[17] a derivative of DDP with significantly less nephrotoxicity but more bone marrow suppression effect, and ifosfamide,[18] a derivative of CTX requiring protection of urothelial mucosa with MESNA during its infusion, were administered in clinical trials alone and in combination with other drugs. They were found to induce encouraging preliminary results, but the results were not significantly superior to those with previous regimens.[19]

The usual measurable response rate varies between 30–45%, and mean duration of response varies between 5 and 9 mo. All these regimens have side effects, including nausea and vomiting, bone marrow suppression, and potential renal and ototoxicity. For this reason, only patients with fair or good performance status (out of bed >50% of the time) should be treated. Their treatment is indicated because it leads to palliation of symptoms, to a modest overall prolongation of survival,[20] and to some unequivocal objective responses. A few patients have a significant prolongation of survival: 10–15% survive >3 years and 3–5% >5 years. There are no methods to predict the long-term survivors. It is recommended that prolonged chemotherapy—up to 8–10 monthly cycles—be given only to patients who achieve objective responses after 2 mo of therapy. At that time, nonresponders should no longer receive chemotherapy.

New approaches are currently being investigated in the therapy of carcinoma of the lung. They include specific monoclonal antibodies, monoclonal antibodies coupled with cytotoxic agents, concomitant radiation with continuous infusion of chemotherapy agents found to have synergistic effects on the tumor cells, new radiosensitizers, fast neutron irradiation, and hyperthermia.

References

1. Boring CC, Squires TS, Tong T. Cancer statistics 1991. CA 1991; 41:19–36.
2. Weiss W, Alton S, Rosenzweig M, et al. Lung cancer type in relation to cigarette dosage. Cancer 1977; 39:2586–72.
3. Gazdar A, Carney D, and Minna J. The biology of non small cell carcinoma of the lung. Semin Oncol 1983; 10:3–16.
4. Carney DN, DeLeij L. Lung cancer biology. Semin Oncol 1988; 15:199–215.
5. Birrer MJ, Minna JD. Molecular genetics of lung cancer. Semin Oncol 1988; 15:226–35.
6. Mathews M, Mackay B, Lukerman J. The pathology of non small cell carcinoma of the lung. Semin Oncol 1983; 10:34–55.

7. Straus M. Growth characteristics of lung cancer. In: Straus MJ, ed. Lung cancer. New York: Grune and Stratton, 1977; 19–33.
8. Cohen MH. Signs and symptoms of bronchogenic carcinoma. In: Straus MJ, ed. Lung cancer. New York: Grune and Stratton, 1977; 85–95.
9. MacMahon H, Courtiney JV, Little A. Diagnostic methods in lung cancer. Semin Oncol 1983; 10:20–33.
10. Mountain CF. Prognostic implications of the international staging system for lung cancer. Semin Oncol 1988; 15:236–45.
11. Martini N, McCormack P. Therapy of stage III (non metastatic disease) carcinoma of the lung. Semin Oncol 1983; 10:95–110.
12. Cox J, Byhardt R, Komaki R. The role of radiotherapy in squamous cell large cell and adenocarcinoma of the lung. Semin Oncol 1983; 10:81–94.
13. Perry MC, et al. Chemotherapy with or without radiation therapy in limited small cell carcinoma of the lung. N Engl J Med 1987; 316:912–17.
14. Seifter EJ, Ihde DC. Therapy of small cell lung cancer: a perspective on two decades of clinical research. Semin Oncol 1988; 15:278–299.
15. Natale R, Shank B, Hilaris B, et al. Combination cyclophosphamide, Adriamycin and vincristine rapidly alternating with combination cis-platin and VP-16 in treatment of small cell lung cancer. Am J Med 1985; 79:303–308.
16. Hoffman P, Bitran J, Golomb H. Chemotherapy of metastatic non small cell carcinoma of the lung. Semin Oncol 1985; 10:111–22.
17. Gatzemeier U, Heehmayr M, Neuhauss R, et al. Phase II studies with carboplatin in non small cell lung cancer. Semin Oncol 1990; 17 (suppl 2):25–31.
18. van Zandwigk N, teu Bokkel Huniuk W, Wanders J, et al. Dose finding studies with carboplatin, ifosfamide, etoposide and mesna in non small cell lung cancer. Semin Oncol 1990; 17 (suppl 2):16–19.
19. Klastersky J, Sculier JP, Daboun G, et al. A randomized trial of two platinum combinations in patients with advanced non small cell lung cancer: a preliminary report. Semin Oncol 1990; 17 (suppl 2):20–24.
20. Evans WK. Combination chemotherapy confers modest survival advantage in patients with advanced non small cell lung cancer. Report of a Canadian multicenter trial. Semin Oncol 1988; 15 (suppl 7):42–45.

27

MEDIASTINAL TUMORS

Richard S. Stark, M.D.

PRIMARY MEDIASTINAL TUMORS, ALTHOUGH uncommon, can arise from any of the varied structures found within the mediastinum. They are of particular interest in that mediastinal neoplasms are associated with a wide range of paraneoplastic syndromes and unusual presentations. Because these tumors are rare, little is known about true incidence, epidemiology, or etiology.[1]

Anatomic Structures

The mediastinum is defined by the thoracic outlet superiorly, the diaphram inferiorly, the sternum anteriorly, and the vertebral bodies and ribs posteriorly. Because of the propensity for certain tumors to occur predominantly in certain regions of the mediastinum, attempts have been made to subdivide the mediastinum into anatomical compartments. Several classifications have been proposed, but in general, a superior compartment can be defined by the area from the thoracic outlet to a line drawn from the fourth vertebral body to the sternal angle of Louis. Major structures normally found in this region are the transverse aorta and other great vessels. The boundaries of the anterior compartment are the sternum anteriorly and the anterior pericardium. This region contains the ascending aorta, vena cava, thymus gland, and lymph nodes. The posterior mediastinum, which extends from the vertebral bodies and posterior rib cage to the posterior portion of the pericardium, contains the esophagus, descending aorta, and sympathetic and vagus nerves. The middle mediastinum contains the heart, pericardium, trachea, major bronchi, and

Table 27-1. Usual Locations of Mediastinal Masses*

Superior	Anterior	Middle	Posterior
Thymoma	Thymoma	Bronchogenic cysts	Neurogenic tumors
Thyroid masses	Thyroid	Pericardial cysts	Bronchogenic cysts
Posterior mediastinal	Teratoma	Lipoma	Enteric cysts
tumors	Germ cell	Epicardial fat pad	
	Neoplasms	Metastatic disease	Esophageal mass and
	Lipoma		diverticuli
	Aortic aneurysms		Hiatal hernia
			Meningocele
			Paravertabral
			abscess

*Lung cancers and lymphomas can occur anywhere in mediastinum.

Table 27-2. Systemic Syndromes Associated with Primary Mediastinal Tumors

Syndrome	Tumor
Myasthenia gravis	Thymoma
Pure red cell aplasia	Thymoma
Hypogammaglobulinemia	Thymoma
Other autoimmune diseases	Thymoma
Cushing's disease	Thymoma, carcinoid
Multiple endocrine adenomatosis	Thymoma, carcinoid
Gynecomastia	Germ cell tumors
Hypertension	Pheochromocytomia, ganglioneuroma
Diarrhea	Ganglioneuromas
Hypercalcemia	Parathyroid adenoma, lymphoma
Thyrotoxicosis	Intrathoracic goiter
Osteoarthropathy	Neurofibroma, neurilemoma
	Mesothelioma
Opsoclonus	Neuroblastoma
Hypoglycemia	Teratoma, mesothelioma, neurosarcoma

lymph nodes. The various types of abnormal structures that can present as mediastinal masses, subdivided by the compartment in which they most commonly occur, are listed in table 27-1.

Clinical Presentation and Diagnosis

About half of patients presenting with mediastinal masses are asymptomatic, and the majority (90%) of asymptomatic patients have benign lesions. Symptoms, when present, can be nonspecific, secondary to compression of mediastinal structures, secondary to abnormal endocrine function, or secondary to poorly characterized systemic syndromes (table 27-2).

With the advent of CT scanning, many of the diagnostic procedures used in the past are no longer needed.[2] The CT scan (see chapter 10, figures 10-36A&B)

can define precisely the anatomy of the mediastinum as well as make a definitive diagnosis of vascular lesions and excessive fat deposition. In evaluating posterior mediastinal lesions, plain films of the spine and ribs are useful to detect rib erosions and widened vertebral foramina. If the latter are present, myelography is mandatory to rule out an intraspinal component, although CT and MRI scanning of the adjacent spine will likely replace this. A barium swallow is of value in assessing the posterior mediastinum to demonstrate primary esophageal neoplasms, hiatal hernia, or esophageal diverticulum. Urinary catecholomines and VMA are useful markers in the preoperative assessment of posterior mediastinal lesions.

Preoperative assessment of anterior mediastinal lesions should include a thyroid scan (particularly if there is a superior mediastinal component), examination of the peripheral blood and bone marrow biopsy for evidence of lymphoma, and the markers alpha-fetoprotein and beta-human chorionic gonadotropin. In a male under 40, the elevation of one of these markers in association with a compatible needle biopsy should be sufficient to establish the presense of a mediastinal germ cell neoplasm. Bronchoscopy should be performed in males and females aged 40+ with a smoking history. Because of the relatively high incidence of thymoma in this age group, careful preoperative evaluation for myasthenia gravis should be made.

The role of skinny-needle biopsy in the diagnosis of mediastinal masses is controversal.[3] Although there is increasing experience and success with this technique, significant ambiguity and error remain. Many neoplastic lesions have similar cytological features that make it difficult to distinguish among thymoma, lymphoma, germ cell neoplasms, carcinoid tumors, and certain undifferentiated carcinomas, even when large pieces of tissue are available for histological examination. In the younger age group, in which lymphomas and germ cell tumors are relatively more common, mediastinoscopy is an important diagnostic procedure because aggressive surgical resection is of questionable value with these tumors. In older patients, the likelihood of finding a tumor requiring aggressive surgical resection for optimal cure is greater. Thoracotomy with frozen section is thus advisable as the first diagnostic procedure, because the patient likely will require definitive surgery.

Thymoma

Neoplasms thought to arise from the thymus gland include thymoma, lymphomas, germ cell tumors, endocrine tumors ("carcinoids"), carcinomas, and thymolipomas. The most common of these, the thymoma, is the most common primary tumor arising in the anterior-superior mediastinum in adults. Thymoma results from neoplastic transformation of the thymic epithelium. Although lymphocytic infiltration is frequently found, these are not thought to be malignant. Several classifications for thymomas that have been devised are based on histopathologic features. In one, based upon the predominant cell type, the tumor is classified as either epithelial, lymphoid, or mixed.[4,5] Most thymomas (42%) are epithelial. Some pathologists recognize a spindle cell variant of epithelial thymoma.[6] In general, the prognosis is most favorable in lymphocytic and spindle cell variants.[6] Little correlation has been found between histologic type and malignant potential or associated paraneoplastic syndromes.

The malignant potential of thymoma correlates with its invasive characteristics rather than histologic appearance. The most practical staging system is based upon the extent of invasion.[5] For stage I (40% overall), the tumor is confined by an intact capsule. In stage II (19%), pericapsular growth extends into mediastinal fat. Stage III (41%) is marked by invasive growth into surrounding organs or intrathoracic metastasis. Metastases from thymoma are almost exclusively intrathoracic, with pleural involvement being the most common. Distant metastases are rare, but have been reported in liver, bone, colon, kidney, brain, and spleen.

Clinical Features

In 30–40% of cases, thymoma is discovered in asymptomatic patients receiving a chest x-ray for unrelated reasons. When present, symptoms are usually vague and include cough, chest tightness, dyspnea, or chest pain. Myasthenia gravis and other systemic syndromes also lead to presenting symptoms (see below). Most patients are between 40 and 60 yr old. Males and females are equally affected.

Thymoma is associated with a wide range of other syndromes and diseases (table 27-2) that can be broadly classified as autoimmune, endocrine, neoplastic (nonthymic), and infectious. In most cases (70%), associated diseases are immunologically related. The most common of these is myasthenia gravis, accounting for 40–50% of patients with associated syndromes. Red cell aplasia, other cytopenias, and hypogammaglobulinemia are the next most commonly associated syndromes, accounting for about 5% each.

Myasthenia gravis is a disorder characterized by weakness and fatigability or—more specifically—by development of voluntary muscle weakness after repeated muscle stimulation. It is widely held to be an autoimmune disorder, with autoantibodies directed against acetylcholine receptors.[7] Symptoms are relieved by drugs that inhibit acetylcholinesterase. About 80% of patients with myasthenia gravis have associated abnormalities of the thymus gland, most have thymic lymphoid hyperplasia, and 15–50% have thymoma. Thymectomy will lead to remission of myasthenia gravis in 20–36% of patients, and most of the others will show some improvement.[7] Patients with thymic hyperplasia are more likely to have a remission after thymectomy (50%) than those with thymoma (25%). Treatment of myasthenia gravis entails complete excision of the thymus gland, including as complete an excision as possible of any invasive thymoma. Most patients have some response to corticosteroids or azathioprine. Recognition of myasthenia gravis in patients with mediastinal tumors undergoing thoractomy is of great importance, because these patients are at risk for serious exacerbations during anesthesia and the postoperative period.

Therapy and Prognosis

The mainstay for treatment of thymoma is complete surgical excision whenever possible. The optimal surgical approach is through a midline sternal-splitting incision. Encapsulated thymomas are easily resected. If adjacent structures have been invaded, an aggressive surgical approach is advocated that may call for resection of involved structures, including lung, pleura, pericardium, diaphragm, and major veins (including superior vena cava with grafting). Resections should be considered for local recurrences as well as metastasis to pleura and pericadium.

Radiation therapy (XRT) is important in the treatment of thymoma because these tumors are generally radiosensitive. Postoperative XRT should be given to all patients with invasive thymoma. About 3,500–4,500 cGy should be delivered to the mediastinum over 3–6 wk. Using postoperative radiation, a local control rate approaching 100% is expected for totally resected cases with invasive thymoma.[8]

Chemotherapy has had limited trials in the treatment of thymoma, generally having been reserved for use in failures of surgery and XRT. A number of active agents have been reported, including corticosteroids, doxorubicin (ADR), cisplatin (DDP), and alkylating agents. Combinations with demonstrated partial responses (PRs) include cyclophosphamide (CTX) + vincristine (VCR) + prednisone + procarbazine; and bleomycin (BLM) + ADR + DDP + prednisone.[9] Using lomustine (CCNU) + CTX + VCR + prednisone, one group reported complete responses (CRs) in 4/9 patients, with a median response duration of 37 mo.[10] In a recent large series of 32 patients with invasive thymoma, a total response rate of 91% with 47% CRs was obtained using DDP + ADR + VCR + CTX.[11]

The prognosis for patients with thymoma is relatively favorable, with a 10-yr survival of about 60%.[12,13] The 10-yr survival for encapsulated, noninvasive tumors is 65–85%. For invasive tumors, 10-yr survival falls to 30%. The worst prognosis is for patients with myasthenia gravis and invasive tumors, where the 10-yr survival is <10%.

Neurogenic Tumors

Neurogenic tumors arise from intercostal nerves or sympathetic ganglia. As primary mediastinal tumors, they occur almost exclusively in the posterior mediastinum, accounting for 20% of all mediastinal tumors and cysts in adults.[1] They are more common in children, accounting for nearly 40% of all mediastinal masses.[14] Most neurogenic tumors are benign. In adults, these tumors most commonly present as an incidental finding on chest x-ray. The most common symptoms are chest pain secondary to compression of intercostal nerves or erosion of adjacent bone. Pleural effusions can be found with both benign or malignant tumors. If the effusion is bloody, the tumor is more likely to be malignant. These tumors can present as Pancoast's tumors, with associated brachial plexus dysfunction, Horner's syndrome, or spinal cord compression. About 10% of posterior mediastinal neurogenic tumors present with extension through an intervertebral foramen into the epidural space (dumbbell tumor).[15] A myelogram should be part of the evaluation of posterior mediastinal masses prior to surgery, particularly if neurologic symptoms suggest spinal cord compression or evidence of eroded vertebral pedicles or enlarged intervertebral foramina appears on spine x-rays. Less commonly, these tumors can produce symptoms caused by endocrine products. Ganglioneuromas and neuroblastoma may be associated with diarrhea, abdominal distention, flushing, excessive sweating, or hypertension thought to result from excessive catecholamine production and (in some cases) from production of vasoactive intestinal peptide.[16] Neurosarcomas rarely have produced hypoglycemia associated with elevated insulin levels.

The most common neurogenic tumor in adults is the neurilemoma, or schwannoma, which arises from Schwann cells of the neural sheath. This tumor presents most commonly in the third to fifth decade of life. Because it is well encapsulated, simple excision is the only treatment required. Neurofibromas arise from both nerve elements and sheath cells. They are the tumors most commonly associated with generalized neurofibromatosis (von Recklinghausen's disease). Although benign, they are generally poorly encapsulated and difficult to excise. When tumors arising from intercostal nerves undergo malignant change they are referred to as neurosarcomas. The incidence of neurosarcoma is increased in generalized neurofibromatosis. Neurosarcomas are associated with rapid growth and poor survival. These tumors are generally treated with an aggressive approach that combines surgery, XRT, and chemotherapy, using the principles for treating soft-tissue sarcomas.

Tumors that arise from sympathetic ganglia and nerves include ganglioneuromas, ganglioneuroblastoma, and neuroblastoma. These tumors occur more commonly in the younger age group. Ganglioneuromas are benign, encapsulated tumors that arise from sympathetic ganglion cells and appear as aggregates of mature ganglion cells and nerve fibers. Ganglioneuroblastoma is a malignant tumor composed of immature elements of the sympathetic nervous system. Although it is infrequent in adults, widespread metastasis frequently occurs. Neuroblastomas occur most commonly in children <4 yr old. Ten percent of neuroblastomas occur in the mediastinum. These highly malignant tumors, which metastasize early to bone, brain, liver, and regional lymph nodes, are associated with increased catecholamine production. An unusual neurological syndrome associated with neuroblastoma is known as opsoclonus or acute cerebellar ataxia, characterized by nonrhythmic horizontal or vertical oscillations of the eyes. This can be a presenting syndrome in patients with occult and localized tumors, thus is associated with a relatively good prognosis. An unusual feature of neuroblastomas is their tendency to undergo spontaneous regression and differentiation. Visceral metastases have been found composed of mature ganglion cells. Survival has been described in children with metastatic disease in the absence of any treatment. Neuroblastomas are radiosensitive. Those arising in the mediastinum have a better prognosis than other sites, with an expected long-term survival of 85%.

Mediastinal Germ Cell Neoplasms

Between 5 and 10% of mediastinal tumors are classified as germ cell neoplasms. Because in almost all cases these are of extragonadal origin, there is little indication for testicular biopsy unless the testes are abnormal on physical examination or high-resolution ultrasonography or there is evidence of retroperitoneal adenopathy on CT scan or lymphangiogram. Mediastinal germ cell neoplasms can be classified into 3 broad groups: benign teratomas, pure seminomas, and nonseminomatous pure and mixed germ cell tumors.

Teratomas are found largely in the anterior-superior mediastinum and are frequently calcified. They occur most frequently in young adults, affecting males and females equally. Teratomas are benign in 80% of cases. Pathologically, they usually contain representations of all 3 germ layers. When they are cystic and contain hair and teeth they are referred to as dermoid cysts. Most of these tumors are asymptomatic, although symptoms may occur if they grow large. Appropriate therapy entails simple excision.

About half of mediastinal germ cell tumors are seminomas. These occur primarily in men between 20 and 40. Symptoms occur as a result of compression of normal mediastinal structures. Most of these tumors are unresectable because of great vessel invasion. Like their gonadal primary counterpart, mediastinal seminomas are highly radiosensitive. All patients should receive XRT to a dose of 4,500 cGy over 5–6 wk.[17] Prophylactic radiation to the para-aortic and supraclavicular regions is frequently given, although the value of this is controversial. With this approach, the 5-yr survival rate is 58–82%.[17,18]

Metastases from seminoma are common and may involve bone, liver, spleen, thyroid, skin, and the CNS. Factors predictive of distant metastasis include older age, hilar or neck nodal involvement, and superior vena caval obstruction.[19] Although experience with chemotherapy is limited, these tumors are sensitive to alkylating agents and combinations of agents used for nonseminomatous germ cell neoplasms. The combination of vinblastine (VLB) + BLM + DDP produced a CR rate of 58% in one series.[18] For this reason, some authors recommend chemotherapy in the absense of extramediastinal spread, particularly if poor prognostic factors are present.

Nonseminomatous and mixed germ cell neoplasms of the mediastinum include all histological types encountered with testicular carcinomas. They may contain seminomatous, embryonal, trophoblastic, teratomatous, and endodermal sinus elements. Most patients are males between 15 and 35. Symptoms result from compression by the growing mass. Patients with tumors producing beta human chorionic gonadotropin may present with gynecomastia. As with testicular carcinoma, most patients have elevations of the beta-human chorionic gonadotropin (60%) or alpha-fetoprotein (70%). These markers are crucial for following response to therapy and documenting a CR.

The nonseminomatous and mixed germ cell neoplasms are highly sensitive to chemotherapy. Combinations used in the treatment of testicular carcinoma, including DDP + vinblastine (VLB) + BLM (PVB, see Appendix); and VLB + actinomycin-D + BLM + DDP + CTX (VAB-6, see Appendix), have been most successful.[20,21] CR rates of 65% have been reported.[20] The overall prognosis is worse than for testicular carcinoma, very likely because of initial bulkier disease at presentation. XRT and surgery are of limited value. The mainstay of treatment is intensive chemotherapy as soon as the diagnosis is confirmed. Some authors advocate resection of tumor after chemotherapy if there is minimal residual disease.[21,22]

References

1. Silverman NA, Sabiston DC Jr. Primary tumors and cysts of the mediastinum. Curr Probl Cancer 1977; 2:5.
2. Livesay JJ, Mink JH, Fee HJ. The use of computed tomography to evaluate suspected mediastinal tumours. Ann Thorac Surg 1979; 27:305–11.
3. Adler OB, Rosenberger A, Haran P. Fine-needle aspiration biopsy of mediastinal masses: evaluation of 135 experiences. AJR 1983; 140:893–96.
4. Rosai J, Levine GD. Tumors of the thymus. Atlas of tumor pathology, fascicle 13. Washington D.C.: Armed Forces Institute of Pathology, 1976.
5. Bergh NP, Gatzinsky P, Larsson S, Lundin P, Ridell B. Tumors of the thymus and thymic region: I. Clinicopathological studies of the thymomas. Ann Thorac Surg 1978; 25:91–98.
6. Verley JM, Hollmann KH. Thymoma. A comparative study of clinical stages, histologic features, and survival in 200 cases. Cancer 1985; 55:1074–86.
7. Drachman DB. Myasthenia gravis. N Engl J Med 1978; 298:136–42, 186–93.
8. Curran WJ, Kornstein MJ, Brooks JJ, Turrisi AT III. Invasive thymoma: the role of mediastinal irradiation following complete or incomplete surgical resection. J Clin Oncol 1988; 6:1722–27.
9. Hu E, Levine J. Chemotherapy of malignant thymoma. Case report and review of the literature. Cancer 1986; 57:1101–04.
10. Daugaard G, Hansen HH, Rørth M. Combination chemotherapy for malignant thymoma. Ann Intern Med 1983; 99:189–90.
11. Fornasiero A, Daniele O, Ghiotto C, et al. Chemotherapy of invasive thymoma. J Clin Oncol 1990; 8:1419–23.
12. Bernatz PE, Khonsari S, Harrison EG, Taylor WF. Thymoma: factors influencing prognosis. Surg Clin North Am 1973; 53:885–92.
13. Verley JM, Hollmann YH. Thymoma: a comparative study of clinical stages, histologic features, and survival in 200 cases. Cancer 1985; 55:1074–85.
14. Gale AW, Jelihovsky T, Grant AF, Leckie BD, Nicks R. Neurogenic tumors of the mediastinum. Ann Thorac Surg 1974; 17:434–43.
15. Akwari OE, Payne WS, Onofrio BM, Dines DE, Muhm JR. Dumbbell neurogenic tumors of the mediastinum. Mayo Clin Proc 1978; 53:353–58.
16. Cooney DR, Voorhass ML, Fisher JE, et al. Vasoactive intestinal peptide producing neuroblastoma. J Pediatr Surg 1982; 17:821–825.
17. Bush SE, Martinez A, Bagshaw MA. Primary mediastinal seminoma. Cancer 1981; 48:1877–82.
18. Clamon GH. Management of primary mediastinal seminoma. Chest 1983; 83:263–67.
19. Hurt RD, Bruckman JE, Farrow GM, Bernatz PE, Hahn RG, Earle JD. Primary mediastinal seminoma. Cancer 1981; 49:1658–63.
20. Hainsworth JD, Einhorn LH, Williams SD, Stewart M, Greco FA. Advanced extragonadal germ cell tumors: successful treatment with combination chemotherapy. Ann Intern Med 1982; 97:7–11.
21. Vugrin D, Martini N, Whitmore WF, Golbey RB. VAB-3 combination chemotherapy in primary mediastinal germ cell tumors. Cancer Treat Rep 1982; 66:1405–07.
22. Economou JS, Trump PL, Holmes EL, Eggleston JE. Management of primary germ cell tumors of the mediastinum. J Thorac Cardiovasc Surg 1982; 83:643–49.

28

ESOPHAGEAL CARCINOMA

Richard S. Stark, M.D.

Incidence and Epidemiology

CARCINOMA OF THE ESOPHAGUS accounts for 1.5% of all cancers and 7% of gastrointestinal cancers; it is the cause of between 7,000 and 8,000 deaths per year in the United States. It affects men 3–4 times more often than women and blacks 3 times more often than whites. The 5-yr survival rate is <5%.[1]

Alcohol and tobacco consumption are thought to be important risk factors in Western countries. Esophageal carcinoma is more common in lower socioeconomic groups and there is some evidence that this might be related to poor nutrition, including a predominantly corn- and wheat-based diet and deficiencies in riboflavin, nicotinic acid, zinc, and magnesium. Conditions associated with an increased incidence of esophageal carcinoma include lye stricture, where there is a 5% chance for developing this cancer; achalasia, which is associated a 7% risk after 25 yr, tylosis (hyperkeratosis of palms and soles); and papillomata of the esophagus, which is associated with a 75% risk. Other conditions with a possible association include esophageal diverticula and webs. There is a clear etiological relationship between Barrett's esophagus and adenocarcinoma.

Pathology and Patterns of Spread

The most common histological type is squamous cell carcinoma, which accounts for >90% of cases. These can be subclassified as well-, moderately, or poorly differentiated, although this does not provide useful prognostic information. Spindle cell carcinoma, verrucous carcinoma, and carcinosarcoma are thought to be variants of squamous carcinoma (see chapter 11, figure 11-27).

Adenocarcinomas occur most frequently in the distal esophagus, arising from the columnar epithelium in that region. Adenocarcinoma may rarely occur at other sites, likely arising from glandular elements located throughout the esophagus. Less common pathological types include adenoid cystic carcinoma or cylindroma, small-cell carcinomas with apudoma characteristics, and leiomyosarcomas.

Carcinoma of the esophagus is generally characterized by extensive local growth and nodal metastasis rather than early metastatic spread to distant sites. Although metastases to distant organs eventually occur in $\leq 90\%$ of patients (based on autopsy series), it is unusual for these to be of major clinical significance. Distant metastases most commonly involve lymph nodes, lung, or liver, but may involve just about any other site, including bone, brain, peritonium, adrenals, kidney, and stomach.

The proximity of the thoracic esophagus to such vital structures as the trachea, left main stem bronchus, and aortic arch partly accounts for the poor prognosis of patients with esophageal cancer. The rapid loco-regional spread is explained by the lack of serosal membrane.

The complex lymphatic network draining the esophagus results in unpredictable lymph node metastasis and skip areas with tumor involvement. In the esophagus, 2 systems of lymphatics, those draining the mucosa and submucosa and those draining the muscularis, form a complex network draining longitudnally for variable distances before draining into regional lymph nodes. Thus, metastases can arise in any nodal group from the cervical to celiac region from just about any primary site. For example, celiac nodal metastases are found in 10% of cases in which the primary tumor arises in the upper third of the esophagus, and in 44% of cases when the primary tumor is in the middle third. Nodal sites frequently involved by esophageal cancer include internal jugular, cervical, supraclavicular, paratracheal, hilar, subcarinal, para-aortic, gastric, and celiac nodes. The presence of microscopic metastatic disease within the esophageal wall several centimeters from the site of gross tumor ("skip areas") can be accounted for by this unusual lymphatic drainage.

Clinical Presentation and Diagnosis

Most patients with esophageal carcinoma present with dysphagia and weight loss. The swallowing difficulty initially is encountered with coarse foods but eventually progresses to liquids as well. The average duration of symptoms is 3–4 mo. Patients with more advanced lesions may present with aspiration pneumonia, hematemesis, melena, cough secondary to tracheobronchial fistula, superior vena caval obstruction, Horner's syndrome, or recurrent laryngeal nerve paralysis. Hypercalcemia may occasionally be present in the absence of bone metastasis.

A barium swallow is routinely performed for the initial evaluation of dysphagia. With most large lesions (>3.5 cm), the radiographic appearance is usually diagnostic of malignancy. With smaller lesions, the diagnostic accuracy decreases to 60%.[2] After the barium studies, upper endoscopy is generally performed to obtain a tissue diagnosis. About 70% of direct biopsies are positive. Difficulties may arise because of heaped-up normal mucosa obscuring more deeply situated tumor that cannot be reached by the biopsy forceps. Brushings for cytology are generally more accurate, with a true-positive rate of 90%. The combination of multiple biopsies plus brushings should be diagnostic in essentially all patients.[3]

Staging and Prognosis

It is essential to assess the extent of the disease, whenever possible using noninvasive methods, prior to initiating therapy. The physical examination should be focused on searching carefully for evidence of supraclavicular and cervical adenopathy, Horner's syndrome, phrenic or recurrent laryngeal nerve paralysis, hepatomegaly, or bony tenderness. A chext x-ray is obtained to exclude lung metastasis, pleural effusions, and infiltrates caused by repeated aspirations or by tracheobronchial fistula. If these procedures provide no evidence for distant spread, then the local (mediastinal) or intra-abdominal extension should be assessed, using CT scans of both chest and abdomen (see chapter 10, figure 10-35). The chest CT scan is recommended for all patients being considered for surgery, even though there can be a significant false-negative rate for detecting mediastinal nodal metastasis or invasion of the trachea, bronchus, and aorta.[4] The abdominal CT scan can provide evidence for liver, adrenal, celiac nodal, or peritoneal involvement. Prior to resection, other studies that should be considered are a bone scan, bronchoscopy to exclude tracheal involvement or second lung primaries, pulmonary function tests, and a laparatomy for celiac nodal biopsy.

Staging for esophageal carcinoma most commonly uses a TNM classification (see table 28-1). Stage I includes noncircumferential lesions <5 cm in length, without evidence of extraesophageal spread. Stage II lesions are >5 cm or circumferential, without extraesophageal spread, and stage III lesions are those with tumor extension to involve mediastinal structures, nodal metastasis, or distant metastasis. Generally, stage I and II tumors are considered for surgical resection. If the patient is inoperable by virtue of being a poor surgical candidate, consideration is given for curative therapy using radiation (XRT). The long-term prognosis for patients with esophageal carcinoma remains poor. The 5-yr survival is 2% for men and 6% for women. Five-year survival after surgical resection is 2–20% and following XRT with curative intent, 1–20%.

Treatment

Therapy for esophageal cancer, including surgery, XRT, and chemotherapy, can have a palliative or curative goal. The major aim of palliation is to permit

Table 28-1. TNM Staging of Carcinoma of Thoracic Esophagus

Clinical staging in use prior to 1988	
I	T1, N0, M0
II	T2, N0, M0
III	T3 or N1 or M1

T1	Length <5 cm, nonobstructive, noncircumferential
T2	Length >5 cm, obstructive or circumferential
T3	Outside esophagus and invading mediastinal structures
N1	Nodal involvement
M1	Distant metastasis (including nodes outside mediastinum)

American Joint Committee on Cancer Staging, 1988	
I	T1, N0, M0
IIa	T2 or T3 N0 M0
IIb	T1 or T2 N1 M0
III	T3, N1, M0
	T4, any N, M0
IV	any T, any N, M1

T1	Tumor invades lamina propria or submucosa
T2	Tumor invades muscularis propria
T3	Tumor invades adventitia
T4	Tumor invades adjacent structures
N1	Regional nodal metastasis
M1	Distant metastasis

as near normal swallowing as possible and, although less of a problem, to alleviate pain. Combined modality therapy is being increasingly applied to the treatment of loco-regional disease.

Surgery

Optimal surgery for lesions of the thoracic esophagus requires a subtotal or near total esophagectomy that includes a cuff of stomach and extends up into the neck. Reconstruction is best accomplished by anastomosing the stomach to the cervical esophagus through a retrosternal tunnel. This procedure gives excellent palliation of dysphagia. Operative mortality is 4–30%. In patients with prior gastrectomy, a colonic interposition is required. The major cause of morbidity and mortality are anastomatic leaks and cardiopulmonary complications such as respiratory insufficiency, congestive heart failure, and pulmonary embolization. Five-year survival rates after surgery alone are 3–18%.[5]

Radiation

Radiation with curative intent is appropriate for patients with stage I or II disease who are not surgery candidates. It is used with palliative intent in patients with more advanced disease. Palliation of dysphagia can be achieved in ≤80% of patients, although most will have recurrence of symptoms.

Palliation generally requires the delivery of 4,000–5,000 cGy over 4–6 wk. Therapy with curative intent generally involves the delivery of 5,000–6,500 cGy over 4–7 wk. Complications of XRT, which include fistula formation and hemorrhage in 10–20%, generally occur when tumors have invaded the major airways or the aorta. Stricture formation can occur, but when present is more likely to result from residual or recurrent tumor. When therapy with curative attempt is given, 2-yr survival is 8–28% and 5-yr survival 1–20%.[6]

Chemotherapy

Chemotherapy generally has been considered to be of palliative value, although more recently has been used in combination with XRT and surgery with curative intent.[7] Single agents with significant response rates include bleomycin (BLM), 15%; mitomycin-C (MIT), 26%; cisplatin (DDP), 22%; 5-fluorouracil (5-FU), 17%; doxorubicin (ADR), 18%; vindesine (VDS), 15%; and methyl-GAG, 20%. The responses with single agents are mostly partial and of short duration (2–5 mo). Combinations of agents may have a higher response rate with a slightly more prolonged duration. Active combinations include DDP + BLM, DDP + methotrexate (MTX) + BLM, and DDP + 5-FU infusion (see Appendix). Although the numbers of patients studied have been small, complete response (CR) rates in the range of 10–20% and partial responses (PRs) in the range of 20–60% have been reported. Median response durations are 6–8 mo. As yet, no studies have compared single agents to combinations or compared different combinations of agents.

Combined Modality Therapy

Numerous studies have been performed combining XRT and surgery in the treatment of esophageal carcinoma.[8] Uncontrolled trials using preoperative XRT have demonstrated complete clearance of tumor in the surgically resected specimen in about 15% of cases and have suggested increased resectability rates with modestly improved survival. However, 2 randomized studies have failed to demonstrate either an increased resectability rate or an improvement in survival.

Postoperative XRT has been less extensively evaluated. Several small series described long-term survivors in groups with residual disease following surgery. One study demonstrated improved survival with postoperative XRT in patients without evidence of mediastinal nodal involvement; no benefit was seen for those with mediastinal node involvement, however. Overall, 35% receiving XRT and 20% receiving surgery alone were alive at 5 yr.

Several trials have been reported using preoperative chemotherapy. In one such trial, DDP + VDS + BLM was given. This resulted in a response rate of 60%, a resection rate of 82%, an acceptable operative mortality of 5.6%, and 3-yr disease-free survival of 24%. Other trials have used preoperative chemotherapy and XRT. MIT + 5-FU infusion or DDP + 5-FU infusion have been given concomitantly with XRT to a dose of 3,000 cGy. These initial studies suggested a high resectability rate, complete clearance of tumor in ≤33% of cases, and a survival of >2 yr in about 20%. There was, however, a treatment-related mortality of 30%. A larger study using DDP + 5-FU infusion and concomitant XRT was reported in 1987.[9] The resectability rate was 49% and surgical mortality was 11%. Complete eradication of tumor by the preoperative treatment alone was achieved in 17%. The rates for 2- and 3-yr survival were 28% and 16%, respectively. Because these results are no better than those achieved with XRT and surgery alone, these approaches must be considered investigational at this time.

Finally, for patients who are not surgical candidates or for those who refuse surgery, XRT and chemotherapy have been used in combination. Both single agents and various combinations have been tested. In the only randomized trial, no advantage was seen in using BLM with XRT over XRT alone. Uncontrolled studies using combination chemotherapy and XRT achieve results equal to those of surgery for stages I and II disease.[10]

Palliation

Because dysphagia is such a distressing symptom and because of the need for nutritional support in patients with esophageal cancer, many palliative procedures have been devised.[11] These include dilatation, endoprosthesis placement, laser therapy, surgical bypass, and XRT. Advocates of each of these procedures claim successful palliation in >80% of patients. As a practical approach, the initial procedure should be that chosen for the primary treatment. Thus, where primary resection is planned, surgical palliation is most reasonable. Esophagogastrostomy is the procedure of choice in most cases. Relief of dysphagia is achieved in >90% of patients, with an associated 7% operative mortality and a 33% complication rate. For the majority of patients who are not candidates for surgical resection, XRT should be used as the primary theraputic and palliative modality. Palliation is achieved in 70–80% of patients, and life-threatening complications are uncommon. The other modalities should be used where these primary modalities fail. Dilatation is a highly successful procedure with a low complication rate and should be considered for use just prior to XRT in patients with severe dysphagia. Endoprosthesis placement should be reserved for radiation and dilatation failures, but is probably the procedure of choice when an esophageal-pulmonary fistula is present.

References

1. Schottenfeld D. Epidemiology of cancer of the esophagus. Semin Oncol 1984; 11:92–100.
2. Moss AA, Koehler RE, Margulis AR. Initial accuracy of esophagrams in detection of small esophageal carcinoma. Am J Roetgenol 1976; 127:909.
3. Graham DY, Schwartz JT, Cain GD, Gorkeg F. Prospective evaluation of biopsy number number in the diagnosis of esophageal and gastric carcinoma. Gastroenterology 1982; 82:228.
4. Halvorsen RA, Thompson WM. Computed tomographic staging of gastrointestinal tract malignancies. I. Esophagus and stomach. Invest Radiol 1987; 22:2–16.
5. Skinner DB. Surgical treatment for esophageal carcinoma. Semin Oncol 1984; 11:136–43.

6. Hancock SL, Glatstein E. Radiation therapy of esophageal cancer. Semin Oncol 1984; 11:144–58.
7. Kelsen D. Chemotherapy of esophageal cancer. Semin Oncol 1984; 11:159–68.
8. Kelsen D, Bains M, Hilaris B, Martini N. Combined-modality therapy of esophageal cancer. Semin Oncol 1984; 11:169–77.
9. Poplin E, Fleming T, Leichman L, et al. Combined therapies for squamous cell carcinoma of the esophagus. A Southwest Oncology Group study. J Clin Oncol 1987; 5:622–28.
10. Coia L, Engstrom P, Paul A. Nonsurgical management of esophageal cancer: report of a study of combined radiotherapy and chemotherapy. J Clin Oncol 1987; 5:1783–90.
11. Cox J, Bennett JR. Light at the end of the tunnel? Palliation for oesophagal carcinoma. Gut 1987; 28:781–85.

29

GASTRIC CANCER

Richard S. Stark, M.D.

Incidence and Epidemiology

DESPITE A REMARKABLE DECREASE in incidence over the past 40 years in the United States, gastric carcinoma remains a major health problem. About 25,000 new cases are diagnosed yearly; with an expected mortality of 90%, it is the seventh leading cause of cancer death. In several countries, including Chile, Japan, Iceland, China, Poland, and Finland, the incidence is significantly higher than in this country, where the number of cases has fallen from 30/100,000 in 1930 to 8/100,000 in 1980. Within individual countries, the incidence is highest in lower socioeconomic groups. In the United States, the incidence is twice as high in blacks an in whites, and about twice as high in males as in females. The striking geographic diversity and decreasing incidence in certain countries suggest that environmental factors play a major causative role.

Pathogenesis and Histopathology

A considerable body of data suggests the likelihood that food components are chiefly responsible for gastric carcinoma. Most work has focused on nitrosamides, or N-nitroso compounds, which are produced in the stomach from food-derived amides and nitrite. The evidence in support of this has been reviewed extensively.[1] Briefly, the hypothesis is that nitrate from the diet is converted to nitrite by oral flora (or stomach flora in achloryhdric states). The nitrite then reacts with various amine compounds in the stomach to form short-lived but highly reactive and presumably carcinogenic substances. The specific amine precursors have not been identified, but may include methylguanidine and methylurea found in high concentrations in certain fish and fried food. Formation of N-nitroso compounds is catalyzed by acidic pH and certain bacteria, and is inhibited by vitamin C (ascorbic acid) and vitamin E. The decreased incidence of gastric cancer in the United States might be explained by the widespread use of refrigeration, which has lowered the use of nitrates as food preservatives and the increased the availability of fresh fruits and vegetables containing vitamins C and E.

Several conditions have been identified as being associated with an increased risk of gastric cancer. These include pernicious anemia, chronic atrophic gastritis, intestinal metaplasia, and postgastrectomy states. These conditions have in common varying degrees of achlorhydria, with the potential for intragastric proliferation of nitrate-reducing bacteria. In patients with pernicious anemia, the age-adjusted incidence of gastric carcinoma is 10- to 20-fold higher than in the control population. Following a Billroth II gastrojejunostomy, about 15% of patients will develop "stump cancer" in the gastric remnant after a mean interval of 24 yr. There is some evidence that adenomatous polyps in the stomach are precursors of carcinoma. Finally, the increased incidence of gastric carcinoma reported in relatives of patients with gastric cancer and in certain "cancer families" suggest that genetic factors may be operative.

The most common malignant neoplasm of the stomach is adenocarcinoma, which accounts for 95% of all malignant lesions.[2] (See chapter 11, figures 11-28 and 11-29.) Other histological types include lymphomas, leiomyosarcomas, squamous cell carcinoma, and carcinoid tumors (see chapter 11, figure 11-29). Among the adenocarcinomas, pathological factors of prognostic value include gross appearance, site, degree of differentiation, degree of local invasion, and histological type. Two major types of gastric adenocarcinomas are recognized: intestinal and diffuse or anaplastic. The intestinal type has a glandular or papillary pattern and tends to be well defined. Diffuse carcinomas lack a glandular pattern, being composed instead of separated single cells or small clusters of cells. They are less well defined and have increased fibrous tissue proliferation. The diffuse type is associated with a younger age group, early evidence of intraperitoneal spread, and a poorer prognosis.

The gross appearance of gastric carcinomas falls into 1 of 4 classifications. The most common is the ulcerative type, accounting for 75% of all gastric carcinomas. An additional 10% are polypoid and tend to be well differentiated or of the intestinal type. The third type is the scirrhous pattern resulting from diffuse infiltration of the gastric wall with anaplastic, diffuse cells. This pattern is associated with a fibrotic reaction, giving the gastric wall a stiffened appearance generally referred to as linitis plastica. The scirrhous pattern accounts for 10% of gastric carcinomas and is associated with the worst prognosis (5-yr survival of 2%). The fourth type is the superficial variety characterized by sheetlike collections of cells.

The degree of differentiation is also of some prognostic value. Using Broders's classification, 4 grades are identified ranging from well-differentiated grade 1 to anaplastic grade 4. The median survival of grade 1 and 2 lesions is 7 mo, and that of a grade 3 and 4 lesions is 4 mo.

Gastric carcinoma can spread to other organs by a variety of routes. Direct extension with invasion can occur to any adjacent structures including omentum, liver, diaphragm, pancreas, transverse colon, and liver. Intramural spread can lead to the involvement of the esophageal or duodenal wall. Lymphatic metastasis can occur to any of 3 collecting systems: the left gastric chain, the splenic chain, and the hepatic chain. There can be spillage of cells through the gastric serosa, resulting in intraperitoneal seeding. Finally, hematogenous spread can result in metastasis to several organs. The most common metastatic site is the liver (see chapter 10, figures 10-5 and 10-6), followed by peritoneum, lungs and pleura, pancreas, adrenal glands, and bone.

Clinical and Laboratory Presentation

The presenting symptoms of gastric carcinoma are typically vague and nonspecific. Weight loss, ill-defined abdominal pain, and nausea and vomiting are symptoms most commonly present, although it is not unusual for patients to present with physical findings of advanced disease. When physical signs of cancer are present, patients are incurable. Lymphadenopathy in the supraclavicular fossa (Virchow's nodes), periumbilical area, and left axilla (Irish's node) should be carefully searched for, as their presence allows for a simple tissue diagnosis. Other physical findings, including hepatomegaly, palpable abdominal mass, an enlarged ovary (Krukenberg's tumor), Blumer's shelf on rectal exam, and ascites, may be present and imply extensive disease. Massive upper G.I. bleeding is uncommon, although mild blood loss detectable as occult blood in the stool is common.

A number of paraneoplastic syndromes, although rare, have been associated with gastric cancer. It is the most common visceral malignancy associated with acanthosis nigricans and dermatomyositis. Microangiopathic hemolytic anemia with or without disseminated intravascular coagulation, migratory superficial thrombophlebitis, deep venous thrombosis with pulmonary emboli, and marantic endocarditis have been described.

Generally, diagnosis of gastric carcinoma is easily achieved using the upper G.I. series and fiberoptic endoscopy with biopsy.[3] The upper G.I. series (see chapter 10, figure 10-34) leads to a correct diagnosis in 80% of cases, with an additional 15% misdiagnosed as benign ulcers. Diagnostic accuracy is increased when a double contrast study is performed, although this is not routinely done in the United States. The success rate for upper endoscopy in diagnosing gastric cancer is variable, depending on a number of factors. Exophytic tumor masses are successfully diagnosed >90% of the time. However, the success rate for infiltrative or ulcerative tumors falls to 50%. The chances for successful diagnosis of malignancy are decreased for tumors of <3 cm, tumors located in the cardia or lesser curvature, and recurrent tumors. It is recommended that at least 4–6 biopsies be obtained during endoscopy.

Although not of value in the diagnosis, CT scanning, ultrasonography, and radionuclide scanning of the liver are of value in assessing preperatively the extent of disease in the abdomen.[4] The CT scan is of particular value because it can detect the presence of local extension, intraperitoneal spread, liver metastasis or ascites (see chapter 10, figure 10-33). Tumor markers are not of value in the diagnosis of gastric cancer, although the carcinoembryonic antigen (CEA) is elevated in $\leq 50\%$ of patients with advanced gastric cancer and the alpha-fetoprotein is elevated in 10–20% of patients.

Application of mass screening techniques can be successful when applied to high-risk populations. Such an approach has been evaluated in Japan.[5,6] The incidence of early gastric cancer, i.e., cancer confined to the mucosa, increased from 4% in 1955–56 to 35% in 1966 because of the widespread use of screening procedures. The survival rate of patients with early gastric cancer exceeds 90%.

Staging and Prognosis

The staging of gastric carcinoma is best accomplished using the TNM system devised by the American Joint Committee on Cancer Staging and End Results Reporting (table 29-1).[7,8] The 5-yr survival for tumors confined to the mucosa without lymphatic or distant metastasis was 85% (T1,N0,M0). For tumors penetrating through the serosa but lacking lymph node metastasis (T1 or 2, N0, M0), the 5-yr survival was about 50%. With involvement of regional lymph nodes (T1-3, N1 or 2, M0), survival decreased to 17%. With more distant nodal metastasis, 5-yr survival was 5%.

From a practical viewpoint, an older informal staging system is still of value. Three recognized stages dictate the most appropriate form of therapy: (1) completely resectable, in which definitive surgery is indicated with possible adjuvant chemotherapy; (2) locally unresectable or incompletely resectable,

Table 29-1. TNM Staging of Gastric Cancer*

Ia	T1, N0, M0
Ib	T1, N1, M0
	T2, N0, M0
II	T1, N2, M0
	T2, N1, M0
	T3, N0, M0
IIIa	T2, N2, M0
	T3, N1, M0
	T4, N0, M0
IIIb	T3, N2, M0
	T4, N1, M0
IV	T4, N2, M0
	any T, any N, M1

T1	Tumor invades lamina propria or submucosa
T2	Tumor invades muscularis propria or subserosa
T3	Tumor penetrates serosa without invasion of adjacent structures
T4	Tumor invades adjacent structures
N1	Metastasis in perigastric lymph nodes within 3 cm of primary
N2	Metastasis in perigastric lymph nodes beyond 3 cm from primary or lymph nodes along left gastric, common hepatic, splenic, or celiac arteries
M1	Distant metastasis

*American Joint Committee on Cancer Staging and End Results Reporting, 1988

indicating appropriate use of radiation therapy (XRT); and (3) disseminated disease, in which systemic chemotherapy is most appropriate. Although this simple classification is of practical value, the TNM staging system is necessary for more precise comparisons of theraputic results.

After definitive surgical resection, patterns of failure have been analyzed by reoperation and autopsy series.[9] About 30% of those failing have loco-regional relapse only. If those with localized intraperitoneal spread are included in the loco-regional relapse group, then this increases to 54%. It was unusual for distant metastasis to be the only type of relapse occurring in 6% of cases. These results provide the impetus to develop more effective modalities for achieving local control.

Treatment

Surgery

Surgery remains the primary modality for treating gastric cancer. At present, the only hope for long-term survival is adequate resection of relatively early disease. Palliative gastrectomy is advised in all patients with resectable tumor even if complete resection is not possible or metastatic disease is present. This surgery decreases the chance of bleeding, perforation, or obstruction, and the debulking of tumor improves the chances for successful postoperative XRT and chemotherapy. For these reasons, the initial theraputic approach should be exploratory surgery with intent to resect unless the patient is a poor surgical risk or preoperative assessment unambiguously demonstrates that the tumor is unresectable. Fixation of the stomach on upper G.I. series, metastasis to vital organs with evidence of organ dysfunction, and ascites secondary to peritoneal carcinomatosis are the major contraindications to attempted resection of the primary tumor.

Factors influencing the type of operation chosen include location and size of the primary lesion, extent of intra-abdominal spread, prior gastric surgery, and whether definitive cure or palliation is the goal. Curative resection involves wide excision of the primary lesion with at least 5 cm margins and en bloc resection of regional lymph nodes and any other locally invaded tissue or organ. Lesions of the distal stomach require a radical distal subtotal gastrectomy in which 80–90% of the stomach is removed. Proximal lesions require a radical proximal gastrectomy that includes removal of the distal esophagus. A total gastrectomy is indicated for patients with linitis plastica or excessively large lesions. Large retrospective analyses of patients undergoing gastrectomy show the best survival occurring with radical subtotal gastrectomy (30–46% 5-yr survival).[10]

Chemotherapy

Treatment of advanced cancer, particularly in patients with metastatic disease, involves the use of chemotherapy. A number of single agents with partial response (PR) rates of >20% have been identified, including 5-

fluorouracil (5-FU), 21%; mitomycin-C (MIT), 30%; doxorubicin (ADR), 25%; and cisplatin (DDP), 25%. Other agents with response rates of 10–20% include hydroxyurea (HYD), carmustine (BCNU), chlorambucil (CLB), triazinate, dacarbazine (DTIC), and methotrexate (MTX). In general, most authors have concluded that combinations of agents result in improved response rates.[11,12] Several combinations have been identified that give PR rates of 30–50%. These include 5-FU + ADR + MIT (FAM, see Appendix), 5-FU + ADR + DDP (FAP), 5-FU + ADR + meCCNU (FAMe), and 5-FU with high-dose leucovorin (see Appendix). In a large phase 2 study, a combination of etoposide (ETO, VP-16), ADR, and DDP was reported to produce a response rate of 64% in 67 patients, with 21% complete responses (CRs).[13] The impact of combination chemotherapy on survival is less clear. Studies with FAM have shown that responding patients survive longer than nonresponding patients (13 mo vs. 3 mo). Randomized trials comparing different combinations have shown only modest differences in survival.[14] It is difficult to recommend one combination as a standard approach, although at this time, FAM is most widely used. It is a well-tolerated outpatient regimen, with the only significant toxicity being moderate myelosuppression.

Chemotherapy has been administered as an adjunct to surgery in an attempt to eradicate residual micrometastasis. The results of several prospective randomized studies evaluating postoperative adjuvant chemotherapy have been published. An initial study showing a survival advantage using 5-FU and meCCNU was not confirmed in 2 more recently reported trials.[15] Several trials using FAM as adjuvant therapy are in progress. The first completed and published study using adjuvant FAM did not show an overall benefit to treatment, although subset analysis suggested that survival might be improved in patients with more advanced disease at presentation.[16] Because of the high incidence of local relapse following complete surgical resection, a number of trials are in progress combining FAM or 5-FU and XRT as adjuvant therapy.[17] At present, postoperative adjuvant therapy cannot be recommended. Patients should be left untreated or entered on well-designed prospective, randomized trials.

Radiation therapy

The major role for XRT is in treatment of locally advanced disease. This includes initially unresectable cases, patients with residual disease following gastrectomy, and patients with local recurrence only. More recently, attempts have been made to incorporate XRT into the postoperative adjuvant therapy of completely resected gastric carcinoma. Although XRT alone can be curative in a small percentage of patients, its major benefit occurs when it is used in combination with chemotherapy. Several studies have demonstrated improved results from XRT + 5-FU compared to XRT alone. In a Mayo Clinic study, a 13-mo median survival was achieved using XRT + 5-FU (see Appendix) versus 6 mo with XRT alone.[18] The GITSG performed a study comparing XRT and chemotherapy alone (5-FU + meCCNU).[19] Although early survival favored the chemotherapy-only arm, 5-yr survival significantly favored the combined modality arm (16% vs. 7%). More recently, several groups have piloted the use of FAM in combination with XRT for locally advanced gastric carcinoma.[20,21] The XRT is generally sandwiched between several cycles of FAM (see Appendix). Preliminary results suggest a median survival of >13 mo with acceptable toxicity.

References

1. Mirvuish SS. The etiology of gastric cancer. J Natl Cancer Inst 1983; 71:631–47.
2. Moertel CG. The stomach. In: Holland JH, Frei E III, eds. Cancer medicine. Philadelphia: Lea & Febiger, 1973; 1527–41.
3. Kurtz RC, Sherlock P. The diagnosis of gastric cancer. Semin Oncol 1985; 12:11–18.
4. Wittenberg J. Computed tomography of the body. N Engl J Med 1983; 309:1223–30.
5. Douglass HO. Potentially curable cancer of the stomach. Cancer 1982; 50:2582–89.
6. Prolla JC, Kobayashi S, Kirsner JB, Arch Intern Med 1969; 124:238–46.
7. Kennedy BJ. The staging of gastric cancer. Semin Oncol 1985; 12:19–20.
8. Kennedy BJ. TNM classification for stomach cancer. Cancer 1970; 26:971–83.
9. Gunderson LL, Sosin H. Adenocarcinoma of the stomach—areas of failure in a reoperation series. Int J Radiat Oncol Biol Phys 1982; 8:1–11.
10. Dupont JB Jr, Cohn I Jr. Gastric adenocarcinoma. Curr Probl Cancer 1980; 4:1–46.
11. Macdonald JS, Schein PS, Woolley PV, et al. 5-fluorouracil, doxorubicin, and mitomycin (FAM) combination chemotherapy for advanced gastric cancer. Ann Intern Med 1980; 93:533–536.
12. Macdonald J, Gohmann J. Chemotherapy of advanced gastric cancer: present status, future prospects. Semin Oncol 1988; 15, suppl 4:42–49.
13. Preusser P, Wilke H, Achterrath W, et al. Phase 2 study with combination etoposide, doxorubicin, and cisplatin in advanced measurable gastric cancer. J Clin Oncol 1989; 7:1310–17.
14. Gastrointestinal Tumor Study Group. Triazinate and platinum efficacy in combination with 5-fluorouracil and doxorubicin: results of a three-arm randomized trial in metastatic gastric cancer. JNCI 1988; 80:1011–15.
15. Higgins GA, Amadeo JH, Smith DE, Humphrey EW, Keehn RJ. Efficiency of prolonged intermittent therapy with combined 5-FU and methyl-CCNU following resection for gastric carcinoma. Cancer 1983; 52:1105–12.
16. Coombes RC, Schein PS, Chilver CED et al. A randomized trial comparing adjuvant fluorouracil, doxorubicin, and mitomycin with no treatment in operable gastric cancer. J Clin Oncol 1990; 8:1362–1369.
17. Moertel CG, Childs DS, O'Fallon JR, Holbrook MA, Schutt AJ, Reitmeir RJ. Combined 5-fluorouracil and radiation therapy as a surgical adjuvant for poor prognosis in gastric carcinoma. J Clin Oncol 1984; 2:1249–54.
18. Childs DS, Moertel CG, Holbrook MA, Reitemeier RJ, Colby M. Treatment of unresectable adenocarcinoma of the stomach with a combination of 5-fluorouracil and radiation. Am J Roentgenol 1968; 102:541–44.
19. Gastrointestinal Tumor Study Group. A comparison of combination chemotherapy and combined modality therapy for locally advanced gastric carcinoma. Cancer 1982; 49:1771–77.
20. Le Chevalier T, Smith FP, Harter WK, Schein PS. Chemotherapy and combined modality therapy for locally advanced and metastatic gastric carcinoma. Semin Oncol 1985; 12:46–53.
21. Gunderson LL, Hoskins B, Cohen AM, Kaufman S, Wood WC, Carey RW. Combined modality treatment of gastric cancer. Int J Radiat Oncol Biol Phys 1983; 9:965–75.

30

APUDOMAS OF THE DIGESTIVE
SYSTEM

William B. Solomon, M.D.

WITHIN MOST ORGANS OF the human body are nests of cells capable of amine precursor (AP) uptake (U) and decarboxylation (D). These so-called APUD cells, which are related in function to cells descended from the neuroectoderm, are capable of synthesizing various regulators of the neuroendocrine system. Thus, amines and peptides such as serotonin, insulin, gastrin, and glucagon are synthesized and secreted by APUD cells.

APUD cells appear to be a uniform population of clear cells when viewed by light microscopy. Also classed as argentaffin cells, they are readily stained by silver-containing dyes. Using electron microscopy, characteristic secretory granules can be identified. The sine qua non of pathological identification of APUD cells is identification of a peptide within a cell by staining with antibodies, using an immunoperoxidase reaction, specific for each peptide.

APUD cells can become hyperplastic, form adenomas, undergo nesidioblastosis (formation of islets), exhibit carcinoid changes, or become frankly malignant carcinomas. Neoplastic disorders of APUD cells, generically termed apudomas, can occur within any organ system; however, they are found predominantly within organs of the G.I. tract/pancreas/adrenal medulla. The incidence of symptomatic apudomas is about 1/100,000 population; between 200 and 1,000 apudomas of the G.I. tract/pancreas are diagnosed each year in the United States.[1,2]

Apudomas produce their symptoms not because of location or tumor bulk but rather by secretion of peptides that regulate the functions of many organs. Although individual apudomas can actually secrete a variety of peptides, usually only one peptide causes symptoms. Indeed, peptides secreted by apudomas may produce dramatic symptomology such as profuse diarrhea (caused by the vasoactive intestinal peptide), head-to-toe flushing (due to serotonin), multiple G.I. ulcerations (caused by gastrin), or change in mental

572

status (produced by insulin excess). Because symptoms are nonspecific, there is often a long interval between the onset of symptoms and the diagnosis of an apudoma. Indeed, only one-third of insulinomas are diagnosed within a year of onset of symptoms, and as many as one-fifth of insulinomas are diagnosed after 5 yr of symptoms.

Diagnosis of an apudoma requires recognition that a symptom complex may be produced by a specific peptide. A radioimmunoassay (RIA) of the patient's serum for the peptide suspected of engendering the symptoms is then performed. If the RIA indicates that the level of peptide is inappropriately high, further diagnostic evaluation is warranted. Because the location of apudomas is generally restricted to specific sites within the G.I. tract or pancreas, abdominal CT scans, sonograms, or selective angiography can often yield information about the putative site of the apudoma. Once found, the putative apudoma can either be removed if solitary or biopsied if found to be multiple and unresectable. It is not possible to distinguish benign from malignant apudomas by pathological criteria. By light microscopy, all apudomas look alike; therefore, cells are stained with antibodies specific for the peptide that was found to be elevated in the serum. If the specimen does stain for the secreted peptide, this confirms that the specimen is a secretory apudoma. If the apudoma has been removed in its entirety, the level of the secreted peptide in the serum should return to normal.

Although apudomas are rare, a number of specific symptom complexes produced by secreted peptides have been identified. Most apudomas are sporadic in incidence, but a number of inherited syndromes involving multiple apudomas in multiple organs have been identified. Discussion of the major apudoma syndromes follows.

Carcinoid Apudomas

Carcinoid tumor capable of synthesizing and secreting the amine serotonin (5-hydroxytryptamine) is the most common apudoma, but it rarely causes symptoms. Although carcinoid tumors may be found in the bronchus, testes, ovaries, or bladder, they are most commonly found in 3 locations—appendix, rectum, and small intestine.

Most appendiceal carcinoid tumors are incidental findings at appendectomy. It is estimated that 1/250 appendectomies results in the finding of an appendiceal carcinoid. Because most appendiceal carcinoids are located at the tip of the appendix, they rarely obstruct the appendix and thus present as appendicitis. It is the rare appendiceal carcinoid tumor that is capable of metastasis to lymph nodes or liver: If the largest dimension of the appendiceal carcinoid is <2 cm, it never metastasizes, and nothing more than a simple appendectomy need be done. Appendiceal carcinoids >2 cm in their largest dimension have the potential for metastasis. Because the time to metastasis for larger appendiceal carcinoids is often >10 yr, only younger patients should undergo surgery more extensive than an appendectomy.[3]

At perhaps 1/2,500 proctoscopic examinations, at anywhere between 6 and 15 cm from the anal verge, a submucosal nodule will be found that has the pathological appearance of a carcinoid tumor. Because rectal carcinoids do not stain with antibodies to serotonin, they never cause carcinoid syndrome when metastatic. As with appendiceal carcinoids, size is the determinant of metastatic potential. Tumors <1 cm in size never metastasize and can be treated with local excision or fulguration; rectal carcinoids >2 cm in size frequently metastasize, indicating that a more extensive cancer removing operation is in order. As with appendiceal carcinoids, the time to onset of metastatic disease is measured in many years.

About 25% of small intestinal tumors are carcinoid tumors. Almost all small intestinal carcinoid tumors are located in the distal ileum and about 30% are multifocal in nature (see chapter 11, figures 11-32 and 11-33). Early in the course of their growth, they are asymptomatic. As the small intestinal carcinoid grows through the wall of the bowel, an intense desmoplastic reaction occurs, often resulting in painful small bowel obstruction. In addition, carcinoid tumors may occasionally encase the mesenteric artery, causing small bowel ischemia or infarction. Here, too, size of the primary lesion is the best prognostic indicator of metastatic potential. Lesions of <1 cm never metastasize, while those >2 cm almost always do. Because the symptoms of small intestinal carcinoids such as pain and bloating are nonspecific, diagnosis is often made when the tumor has already spread beyond the confines of the bowel wall. Even tumors that have spread to the local lymph nodes should be resected. Because small intestinal carcinoid tumors grow very slowly, local recurrences can occur even 15–20 yr after the initial resection. Once metastatic to the liver, they continue to grow slowly, and 5-yr survival with metastasis to the liver is not uncommon.

Serotonin secreted by G.I. carcinoid tumors into the portal vein is metabolized and rendered inactive in the liver. Thus, the carcinoid syndrome can occur only when G.I. carcinoid tumors are metastatic to the liver and serotonin entry is thus allowed into the systemic venous circulation. Carcinoid tumors that secrete serotonin directly into the systemic circulation (e.g., bronchial or bladder lesions) may induce the carcinoid syndrome in the absence of liver metastasis.

The Carcinoid Syndrome

When the mass of carcinoid tumor in the liver becomes sufficient to produce elevated levels in the urine of a metabolite of serotonin, 5-hydroxyindoleacetic acid (5-HIAA), a patient may suffer from the carcinoid syndrome. Patients may report paroxysmal flushing and sweating from head to toe that occasionally is accompanied by hypotension. Diarrhea is also frequently reported, and with longstanding carcinoid syndrome, carcinoid heart disease may develop. The endocardium of the heart becomes coated with a layer of smooth muscle causing valvular deformities, particularly tricuspid insufficiency or pulmonic stenosis. Treatment of the valvular heart disease is aimed at amelioration of congestive heart failure.

Gastrinomas (Zollinger-Ellison Syndrome)

Rarely, a patient will present with peptic ulcer disease in an unusual location or with multiple peptic ulcers. Thus, ulceration of the second or third portion of the duodenum or of the jejunum may be an indication of truly excessive gastric acid production secondary to increased secretion of gastrin. At times, patients will suffer recurrent ulcers or have ulcers accompanied by persistent diarrhea (not related to antacid use). These symptoms are also suggestive of increased gastrin production and consequential increased basal level of gastric acid production. In these cases, a serum gastrin level should be obtained. The level of gastrin secretion in patients with gastrinomas is frequently greater than 10 times normal. Other illnesses, such as pernicious anemia, are associated with elevated serum gastrin levels, but these illnesses usually are accompanied by the absence of gastric acid, not an increased basal level of gastric acid secretion. The combination of a 10-fold increase in serum gastrin level and an increase in basal level of gastric acid secretion accompanied by peptic ulcer disease is pathognomonic for gastrinoma.[4]

About 25% of patients with gastrinomas have apudomas involving multiple organs, especially the parathyroid gland and pituitary, a disorder known as Wermer's syndrome, or multiple endocrine adenomatosis [MEA] type 1. Patients with gastrinoma should be screened for MEA type 1 by obtaining serum calcium, phosphorus, and parathormone levels. Elevation of serum calcium or parathormone hormone levels is indicative of a parathyroid apudoma found in all MEA type 1 patients.

Fortunately, the treatment of gastrinoma has been made easy with the advent of histamine type 2 receptor antagonists, which inhibit the response of parietal cells to gastrin stimulation. Thus, the first step in the treatment of gastrinoma today is the initiation of therapy with cimetidine, ranitidine, or famotidine. Omeprazole, an inhibitor of the gastric parietal cell H^+-K^+ ATPase, may be used instead of histamine type 2 receptor antagonists. These agents surpress gastric acid secretion, allow ulcer healing, and abolish gastric acid-associated diarrhea. Once acid secretion is surpressed by H_2 receptor antagonists, the search for the site of the gastrinoma can be made. In general, most gastrinomas are found in the pancreas, although they may also be located in the wall of the duodenum or jejunum. CT scan or selective angiography may identify about 50% of gastrinomas, usually when they are >5 cm in diameter. Unfortunately, most gastrinomas are multiple and malignant, and extensive surgery such as partial or complete pancreatectomy results in cure of only a small portion (perhaps 20%) of gastrinomas.

Most gastrinomas and resultant peptic ulcer disease can be kept under control by drug therapy for a number of years; those patients who escape control may require removal of the end organ that responds to gastrin—that is to say, a total gastrectomy. The treatment of metastatic gastrinomas will be discussed in the section on treatment of metastatic apudomas.

Insulinomas

Insulin-producing apudomas of the pancreas are often difficult to diagnose because of their nonspecific symptoms. Frequently, patients have symptoms such as weakness, loss of consciousness, or personality changes for years prior to diagnosis. The initial diagnostic test is for blood sugar, which will be low. The hallmark of the disease is fasting hypoglycemia. Patients suspected of having insulinomas are subjected to a prolonged 24- 72-hr fast, and a blood glucose determination is made every 4 hr, or when the patient exhibits symptoms. A concomitant RIA for serum insulin levels is also obtained. Patients with insulinomas will demonstrate inappropriate elevations of serum insulin, with consequent hypoglycemia during the fast. Patients who surreptitiously administer insulin to themselves will present with symptoms similar to insulinoma. Here, RIA for the C peptide is invaluable. Patients with insulinoma have elevated levels of C peptide, which is a breakdown product of processed proinsulin. Patients who administer insulin to themselves will not have elevated levels of C peptide.

Once it is determined that the serum C peptide and insulin levels are elevated, the site of insulinoma must be determined. Almost all insulinomas are located in the pancreas. Some insulinomas can be diagnosed preoperatively by either CT scan or selective angiography; however, in most cases surgical exploration must be performed for localization. Fortunately, most insulinomas are benign and solitary, and surgical cure by removal of the insulinoma is achieved in about 90% of cases.

In patients with persistent hypoglycemia prior to surgery or patients unable to be cured by surgery, diazoxide, an antihypertensive toxic to B cells of the pancreas, may be given. Because diazoxide causes water retention, a diuretic must be given in addition.

Glucagonomas and Vipomas

Apudomas that secrete glucagon are relatively rare, but they do have a pathognomonic skin lesion-migratory necrolytic erythema. This rash, which is similar in appearance to toxic epidermal necrolysis, characteristically involves the perineal area and upper thighs. Most other symptoms are nonspecific, although most patients are mildly diabetic and have an increased incidence of phlebitis and pulmonary embolism. Most glucagonomas are found in the pancreas, and although they are solitary, most are malignant. Pancreatic resection should be tried in most cases, as debulking may decrease tumor mass enough to ameliorate symptoms.

Vasoactive intestinal polypeptide (VIP) is a hormone that produces profuse diarrhea. Prolonged diarrhea leads to dehydration and hypokalemia, causing malaise and muscle weakness. Many of these patients also have decreased gastric acid production. Again, the symptoms are nonspecific, and delay in diagnosis of this apudoma is often measured in years from time of symptom onset. In patients suspected of having a VIP-producing apudoma, a RIA for VIP is readily available. An increase in serum levels of VIP is highly suggestive of a vipoma, which is often localized to the pancreas.

Treatment of Unresectable or Metastatic Apudomas

Although drug therapy may control symptoms of gastrinoma, and diazoxide may be helpful in the treatment of insulinoma, these illnesses and other apudomas often become refractory to symptomatic management. Paradoxically, a peptide secreted by some apudomas may be useful in the symptomatic management of advanced apudoma.

Somatostatin is a peptide secreted in the CNS and in many other tissues. It is able to inhibit the secretion of many secreted peptides, including growth hormone, gastrin, vasoactive intestinal peptide, and insulin. A synthetic somatostatin analogue (trade name: Sandostatin) has been synthesized. Sandostatin has a much longer serum half-life than naturally occurring somatostatin and can be given subcutaneously by twice daily injection. It appears to be able to control the diarrhea caused by vipomas and carcinoid tumors as well as gastrin secretion by gastrinomas. It now appears to be the drug of choice in symptomatic apudomas refractory to other therapy.[5-7]

Because apudomas grow very slowly, surgical resection of metastatic disease is useful for debulking the tumor and may cause a dramatic decrease in symptoms.

For tumors not amenable to resection and not symptomatically controlled, cytotoxic chemotherapy may be of help. The most active combinations are streptozotocin (STZ) + 5-fluorouracil or STZ + Adriamycin (ADR) (see Appendix). Although many different treatment schedules are available, STZ 500 mg/m^2 is generally given as a short infusion by I.V. bolus on 5 consecutive days every 4 wk. ADR can be given by bolus 50 mg/m^2 q. 3 wk along with a STZ infusion. Response rates are about 30–40%. Many metastatic apudomas can be controlled for long periods with a combination of resection and cytotoxic chemotherapy.

Summary

Apudomas are rare tumors that manifest themselves by secreting peptides that produce often dramatic but nonspecific symptoms. Specific symptom complexes are produced by some of the secreted peptides. Measurement of an inappropriately high level of a peptide by serum RIA is the first step in diagnosis. Further diagnostic evaluation includes abdominal CT scan and/or selective angiography of these highly vascularized tumors.[8]

Surgical removal of solitary apudomas often results in cure; however, the distinction between benign and malignant apudomas cannot be made by light microscopy. Size of the apudoma is often an indicator of recurrent or malignant potential. For gastrinomas, histamine H_2 receptor antagonists are specific first-line treatment. For other apudomas, a variety of agents may control symptoms, and somatostatin analogues may be the mainstay of symptomatic therapy in the near future. Among treatment modalities also showing promise for the future is alpha interferon.[9]

Metastatic disease may be controlled for a long time with the judicious use of surgical resection and cytotoxic chemotherapy.[10-13]

References

1. Brennan MF, MacDonald JS. Cancer of the endocrine system. In: Devita VT, Hellman S, Rosenberg SA, eds. Cancer: principles & practices of oncology. 2nd ed. Philadelphia: Lippincott, 1985.

2. Moertel CG. An odyssey in the land of small tumors. J Clin Oncol 1987; 5:1503–22.

3. Moertel CG et al. Carcinoid tumor of the appendix: treatment and prognosis. N Engl J Med 1987; 317:1699–1701.

4. Wolfe MM, Jensen RT. Zollinger-Ellison syndrome: current concepts in diagnosis and management. N Engl J Med 1987; 317:1200–08.

5. Vinik AI et al. Somatostatin analogue (SMS201–995) in the management of gastroenteropancreatic tumors and diarrhea syndromes. Am J Med 1986; 81 suppl. 6B 23–39.

6. Deghenghi H et al. Somatostatin analogues in the treatment of carcinoid syndrome. Biomed Pharmacother 1988; 42:585–88.

7. Parmar H et al. Somatostatin and somatostatin analogues in oncology. Cancer Treat Rev 1989; 16:95–115.

8. Welbourn RB, Manolas KJ, Khan O, Galland RB. Tumors of the neuroendocrine system (APUD cells tumours-apudomas. Curr Prob Surg 1984; 21(8):1–73.

9. Smith DB et al. Phase 2 trial of rDNA alpha 2b interferon in patients with malignant carcinoid tumor. Cancer Treat Rep 1987; 71:1265–66.

10. Maton PN, Gardner JD, Jensen RT. Recent advances in the management of gastric acid hypersecretion in patients with Zollinger-Ellison syndrome. Gastroenterol Clin N Amer 1989; 18(4):847–63.

11. Vinayek R et al. Zollinger-Ellison syndrome. Recent advances in the management of the gastrinoma. Gastroenterol Clin N Amer 1990; 19(1):197–217.

12. Feldman JM. Carcinoid tumors and the carcinoid syndrome. Curr Probl Surg 1989; 26(12):829–918.

13. Mozell E et al. Functional endocrine tumors of the pancreas: clinical presentation, diagnosis, and treatment. Curr Probl Surg 1990; 27(6):301–386.

31

COLORECTAL AND ANAL CARCINOMA

C. Julian Rosenthal, M.D., F.A.C.P.

Incidence and Epidemiology

CARCINOMA OF THE COLON and rectum is one of the most common human malignancies, being second only to lung and breast cancer. In the United States, about 60,000 deaths per year are due to colorectal carcinoma. Several epidemiologic factors that account for variations in its distribution include:

Geographic distribution. Colorectal cancer is found with increasing incidence in industrially developed countries—in the urban regions in each country as well as in residents of countries with low incidence who move to countries with high incidence (e.g., Japanese in the United States, Indians in South Africa).

Sex. Colorectal cancer is equally distributed between the sexes in white and black Americans but has a heavy male predominance among Chinese in the United States and a heavy female predominance among blacks in Rhodesia and Uganda.

Age. The incidence of colorectal cancer peaks between the ages of 50 and 70.

Social class. It is significantly more common among those with very high incomes.

Diet. The major differences between diets of populations prone to colonic cancer and those not prone to it are an increase in calories by the doubling or more of intakes of sugar, protein, and fat and a decrease in intake of crude fiber contained in cereal foods, resulting in a considerable fall in the diet's bulk-forming capacity.

Bowel behavior. Factors that predispose to colon carcinoma include a decrease in the frequency of defecation (in the primitive populations in South Africa with a very low incidence of carcinoma, 2–3 bowel movements daily is the norm); and a decrease in the amount and the consistency of feces voided, which is directly related to the fiber content of the daily diet (when wholewheat bread [200–500 g/day] or bran [15–20 g/day] were eaten daily by Western populations, the incidence of colon cancer started to decline). However, studies are contradictory on the impact of transit time on the incidence of colon carcinoma. Davies' study in London (1918) showed that constipation was twice as common in colon cancer patients than in the general population, but in Hawaii, it was shown that a nonconstipated study group had the same incidence of colon cancer as a constipated group.[1]

Chemical and microbiologic composition of feces.[2] Feces of populations prone to colonic carcinoma as well as those of patients with ulcerative colitis contain a higher amount of bile acids, sterols, nitrogen, fat, and total solids. The concentration of bile acids, sterols, and fat can be lowered by halving the intake of fat and by increasing the fiber intake. In rats, lithocholic, taurodeoxycholic, and deoxycholic acids act as colon tumor promotors. Colonic tumors caused in rats by 1,2-dimethylhydrazine (DMH) were induced in a much higher incidence when rats were fed diets rich in corn oil and lard or beef fat than in those fed diets with a low content of these substances.

Chronic dietary deficiency of vitamin A and of dietary lipotropes (choline and methionine) also increased the carcinogenic action of dimethylhydrazine. Feces of populations prone to colonic carcinoma have a higher concentration of bacteroides bacteria, known to degrade bile acid cholate to potentially carcinogenic deoxycholate, and of clostridium bacteria, which are able to desaturate bile acids.

Precancerous Lesions and Pathogenesis

Precancerous lesions seen in patients with colon carcinoma are represented by colonic polyps (outgrowths of the mucosal surface). These polyps can be of 3 types:[3]

1. *Hyperplastic polyps* due to benign hyperplasia. In these polyps, the zone of cell division is expanded but remains restricted to the lower portion of the crypts of Lieberkuhn (like in normal mucosa). The differentiation into goblet and absorptive cells is maintained. In a few polyps, increased DNA labeling with titriated thymidine is found not only in the proliferative and transitional zones of the crypts but also in their mature zone. For this reason, it appears that the hyperplastic polyps may be precursors to adenomatous polyps. In a few cases studied, the Kirsten ras oncogene was found amplified in these polyps.[4]

2. *Adenomatous polyps, or pedunculated adenoma.* They are small (usually <2 cm in diameter), have a stalk with a well-vascularized fibrous core covered by fairly normal colon mucosa, and a head. Microscopically, the mucosa of these polyps varies from a normal glandular structure to the clinical picture of elongated hyperplastic glands, sometimes with budding and branching crypts and cells having increased mitotic activity, and finally to that of a mucosa with focal atypia. In a few cases, the glands can present focal or *in situ* cancers that can be cured by removal of the polyp if the stalk is not involved.

3. *Villous polyps, or sessile adenomas.* These are papillary lesions attached to the colonic mucosa by a broad base—usually single and quite large (≤ 15 cm

in diameter) and typically found in the sigmoid colon and rectum. Microscopically, they present fingerlike papillary villi that branch and secrete large quantities of mucus and potassium. Hybrids of villous and adenomatous polyps may also be encountered.

Rarely, polyps are hereditary; hereditary forms can have a higher incidence of malignant transformation than others. The following 5 forms of hereditary polyposis are most common:

- *Familial polyposis coli,* an autosomal dominant transmitted disorder diagnosed usually at 35 yr and rarely before 10 yr; characterized by hundreds of thousands of pedunculated polyps, most of them with the histologic structure of adenomatous polyps and a few with that of villous adenomas; untreated, the patient lives <50 yr
- *Gardner's syndrome,* which has autosomal dominant transmission; diagnosed before 32 yr and associated with other abnormalities of the skeleton and soft tissues: osteomas, cortical thickening of the long bones and ribs; abnormal dentition; desmoid tumors frequently in surgical scars; sebaceous cysts; and lipomas. In this disease, most polyps are adenomatous and pedunuclated; they are precancerous but their malignant transformation occurs late, usually after age 30.
- *Turcot syndrome,* an autosomal recessive disease associated with glial tumors
- *Peutz-Jeghers syndrome* (also has an autosomal dominant inheritance); consists of multiple polyps throughout the G.I. tract excluding the esophagus; usually nonmalignant, containing mucin-filled cysts (hamartomas); melanin spots on the bucal mucosa, lips, and fingers; occasional ovarian tumors accompany this syndrome
- *Juvenile polyposis coli,* a disorder with autosomally dominant inheritance; consists of multiple benign polyps containing mucin-filled cysts (hamartomas).

It is generally agreed that villous adenomas have significant potential for malignant transformation, especially if they measure ≥ 5 cm in diameter (30–40% become malignant).

Whether tubular (pedunculated) adenomatous polyps and hyperplastic polyps are premalignant is the basis of a major controversy. They were thought to be precancerous until 1958, when Spratt—and later, Castleman and Krickstein—noted that adenomatous polyps are rather evenly distributed throughout the colon, whereas cancers occur more frequently in the cecum, sigmoid colon, and rectum.[5,6] No adenomatous polyp was found in continuity with any of the adenocarcinomatous lesions. However, Marson[7] and Fenoglio and Lane[8] found that in 10% of pedunculated polyps with a diameter of >1.5 cm, continuity with invasive adenocarcinoma can be noted. This was confirmed by Lipkin in recent experimental studies on mice with colonic carcinoma induced by dimethylhydrazine.[9]

Active proliferation was expanded at the surface of the colonic crypts, possibly due to the fact that 2 enzymes (the thymidine kinase and thymidilate synthetase) that catalyze steps leading to DNA synthesis were not repressed in the upper third of the crypts, as occurs in normal mucosa. Also, 2 abnormal nuclear nonhistone proteins were detected after malignant transformation of colon mucosa by dimethylhydrazine. Studies by Kopolovich et al have also shown that predisposition to neoplasia of patients with hereditary adenomatosis of the colon and rectum (ACR) is associated with abnormalities of their skin fibroblasts, including loss of contact inhibition, decreased serum requirement for growth (from 15% to 1%), and a heightened susceptibility to transformation by the Kirstein strain of murine sarcoma virus.[10]

A recent study of 670 persons in 34 kindreds of patients with one adenomatous polyp and a cluster of relatives with colon cancer strongly supported the dominant inheritance of susceptibility to colorectal adenomas and cancers, with a gene frequency of 19 percent.[11] This study is supported by data concerning the significant consistency of genetic alterations in 172 colorectal tumor specimens at various stages of neoplastic development.[4] Ras gene mutations occurred in 58% of adenomas >1 cm in diameter and in 47% of carcinomas but in only 9% of adenomas <1 cm in size. A specific region of chromosome 18 frequently was deleted in carcinoma and in advanced adenomas and (rarely) early adenomas, whereas the chromosome 17p sequence was lost only in carcinomas. Sequences on chromosome 5 linked to the gene for familial adenomatous polyposis was lost in 29% and 35% of adenomas and carcinomas, respectively.

Based on all these data indicating the potential for malignant transformation of many polyps, a number of preventive measures are recommended:

1. Adenomatous (pedunculated) polyps are removed through sigmoidoscopy and, if necessary, colonoscopy (only 10% of all pedunculated polyps occur proximal to the sigmoid colon) if their diameter is >1 cm.

2. In cases of familial polyposis coli and Gardner's syndrome, due to the high incidence of villous polyps with advancing age, subtotal colectomy with ileoproctostomy and fulguration of polyps remaining in the rectal segment are recommended at time of diagnosis. If the number of rectal polyps is too great for removal or if the patient is not amenable to quarterly proctoscopic follow-up, the treatment of choice is total colectomy with abdominoperineal resection (APR) of the rectum and anus and the establishment of an ileostomy.

3. First-degree relatives of patients with colorectal cancer should be regularly screened for colonic tumors.

Anatomopathology and Staging Classification

There is a physiologic distinction between the 2 major halves of the colon: the right colon absorbs sodium through an active process, dependent upon aldosterone, with consequent passive reabsorption of water and loss of potassium, whereas the left colon and the rectum function primarily as a storage organ where the stool gains its normal consistency.[12]

Carcinoma of the right colon tends to be polypoid, whereas in the left colon the carcinoma tends more frequently to be infiltrative and constrictive (see chapter 11, figure 11-34), presenting as scirrhous, which is relatively uncommon, or as a sessile nodule, which commonly undergoes ulceration and necrosis.

Rectal carcinoma shows considerable diversity. Lesions can be soft, friable, hemorrhagic, mucinous or papillary, sessile or polypoid, with or without ulceration. It can be transmural, invading the bladder, ureters, or vaginal wall. Colonic and rectal malignant lesions extend from the mucosa through the muscularis to the serosa and the contiguous structures.

Within the framework of anatomic staging are various pathologic features of the disease that influence the prognosis: tumor size, extent of penetration through the bowel wall, venous invasion, and regional lymph node involvement. In relation to these factors, a pathologic staging system has existed since 1932, when Duke proposed the following classification of the rectal carcinomas:[13,14]

- *Stage A*. Tumor limited to the wall of the rectum
- *Stage B*. Spread by direct contiguity to extrarectal tissues
- *Stage C*. Involvement of regional lymph nodes (C_1, only paracolic nodes; C_2, involvement of the lymphovascular pedicle).

This classification was modified first by Kirklin, then by Astler and Coller, and finally by Turnbull.[15,16,17] The most commonly used current classification consists of 8 stages:

A	Involvement of the mucosa and submusoca only
B1	Involvement into but not through the muscularis
B2	Involvement into and through the muscularis to the serosa
B3	Involvement through the serosa in contiguous tissues or organs
C1	Involvement of regional lymph nodes with a B1 lesion of the intestinal wall
C2	Involvement of regional lymph nodes with a B2 lesion of the intestinal wall
C3	Involvement of regional lymph nodes with a B3 lesion of the intestinal wall
D	Adjacent organ invasion, peritoneal seeding, and distant metastases.

This classification has prognostic significance because colon cancer tends to penetrate perpendicularly through the bowel wall rather than by lateral intramural extension (usually, lateral extension is around 2 cm and no more than 4 cm). For this reason, surgeons leave a 5-cm margin between the tumor and the point of resection. The percentage of patients surviving 5 yr after surgery in these stages decreases significantly in the more advanced stages. Survival ranges between 70–100% for stage A, 60–70% for stage B, 40–60% for stage B2, and 4–40% for stage C. Patients in stage D at time of surgery do not generally survive 5 yr.[13]

Lymphatic invasion is present in > 50% of cases at time of surgery. It occurs in an orderly manner, first in the pericolic lymph nodes and then in the lymph nodes at the root of the mesentery, except in the distal 8 cm of rectum, where the lymphatic anatomy allows rapid lateral and distal spread. Prognosis depends on the number and location of lymph nodes. Five-year survival is 27% for 1 involved node; 9% for > 5 nodes; 41% for pericolic nodes exclusively; and 13% for nodes involved at the highest point of the mesenteric root. Venous invasion has a negative impact on 5-yr survival only in cases associated with lymph node involvement.

In rectal carcinoma, neoplastic dissemination has special characteristics due to specific anatomic conditions; the lack of serosal layer of the rectum permits easier involvement of extrarectal tissues, while the special lymphatic drainage of the rectum leads to dissemination—to the inferior mesenteric nodes from any point of the rectum, to the internal iliac nodes for lesions <8 cm from the anus, and to the inguinal nodes for lesions below the pectinate.

Clinical Manifestations

The symptoms vary for lesions at the 3 major sites of the large bowel (right colon, left colon, and rectum) due to specific morphologic and functional characteristics of these sites.[12]

The right colon has a large caliber and distensibility; its fecal material is liquid, and tumors have a tendency to occupy only a part of the circumference. For these reasons, obstruction is infrequent and major clinical manifestations are abdominal pain and anemia. The latter has features that cannot be explained by blood loss alone and is detected in only 30% of cases. It also has characteristics of anemia of chronic disease caused possibly by toxin reabsorption.

The left colon has semisolid fecal material and a lumen with a smaller caliber than the right colon; its tumors have a greater tendency toward annular spread. For these reasons, obstruction is frequent, with muscular hypertrophy above the stenosis. Other frequent manifestations are abdominal pain, bleeding (in 35–55% of cases), and changes in bowel habits.

The rectum, with the larger caliber of its ampulla, makes obstruction by cancer less frequent than in the left colon. Major clinical manifestations of rectal carcinoma include bleeding (present in 65–88% of cases), changes in bowel habits, increased frequency of stools and "morning diarrhea", tenesmus (sense of incomplete evacuation), pain, and a palpable mass. The last 2 symptoms occur late, being caused by extensive local fixation of the mass and by infiltration of nerve trunks, which causes dull sacral pain with or without radiation down the legs.

Natural History and Diagnostic Workup

The natural course of colorectal carcinoma was best studied through "second look" operations performed at the University of Minnesota on 75 patients who had initial APR for carcinoma of the rectum or sigmoid colon.[13] Of this group, 66% had recurrent disease. In 48% of these, there was only local or regional node recurrence. In 8%, only distant metastases were present, and in 44%, distant metastases accompanied local recurrence. The proportion of regional and distant metastases is somewhat different in cases of carcinoma of the right colon (fewer pelvic metastases but more liver metastases).

Distant metastases occur in the liver in 15–25% of cases at the time of initial surgery and in 65% at autopsy; in the lung in 15–20% of cases; and in bones, ovaries, and brain in <10% of cases.

Unresectable carcinoma of the colon has a rapid progression that results in short survival. Median survival from the time of proof of incurability is 7 mo (10% of patients reach 18 mo). Median survival for patients with recurrent disease is 5 mo, and median survival after diagnosis of liver metastases is only 4½ mo.

The workup for the early detection of metastatic and/or recurrent lesions in patients with resected colorectal carcinoma should include periodic screening for lesions at the more frequent sites of recurrence or metastasis.[18] The most useful procedures include flexible colonoscopy, which, repeated yearly, can detect local recurrence or a second primary lesion (seen in 5% of patients with adenocarcinoma of the colon); and CT scan of the pelvis, which, performed yearly up to 5 yr after tumor resection, detects regional recurrences. CT scan of the abdomen (see chapter 10, figures 10-31 and 10-32), also performed yearly, can detect liver metastases, lesions in the omentum, in other abdominal organs, and in the paraortic lymph nodes. An incidence of 15–20% false-positive lesions and 5–10% false-negative lesions occasionally can be picked up by a ^{99m}technetium scan of the liver or by liver sonogram. Currently, these tests are recommended only when the CT scan is equivocal or there are clinical reasons to suspect that it is falsely positive or negative. The ^{99m}technetium liver scan can, in its turn, be falsely negative in 24% of cases or falsely positive in 30% of cases. The liver sonogram is the best test capable of differentiating a cyst from a solid lesion. It appears that MRI scan of the liver is the most sensitive test for detecting early metastatic lesions.

Abnormal liver functions (SGOT, SGPT, GGT, LDH, alkaline phosphatase, 5′ nucleotidase) are generally late indicators of metastases or recurrent lesions. However, LDH and alkaline phosphatase elevation occur before abnormalities of the other tests and should be checked periodically after tumor resection (every 3–4 mo for 5 yr). LDH elevation at time of surgery also has been found to be a bad prognostic predictor of the course of disease. LDH values, like those of carcino-embryonic antigen, have been found to correlate with tumor size and can be used to monitor response to therapy.

Blind liver biopsies to confirm the presence of liver metastases are rarely necessary. They are recommended only in patients who develop liver metastases after >3 yr from the time tumor was resected primarily to differentiate metastatic lesions from a primary hepatocellular carcinoma. The blind liver biopsy yields positive results in 46–90% of cases. This yield can be improved by nearly 100% if biopsy is performed under CT scan guidance.

Chest x-ray and bone scan should also be done yearly for 5 yr in order to detect, at an early stage, possible metastases at the respective sites. CT scan of the head is not recommended for regular metastatic screening because it cannot detect lesions before neurologic deficit occurs.

Tumor markers of clinical significance in colorectal carcinoma are known to be represented by oncofetal antigens.[19] The first of these antigens, the alpha-fetoprotein, was discovered in 1963 by Abelev and was found to be an antigen common to a transplantable murine hepatoma and a component of newborn mouse serum.[20] In 1965, Gold and Freeman identified a serum antigen in patients with colon cancer that he called the carcino-embryonic antigen (CEA).[21] This antigen reacts with an antibody to an extract of colon cancer and cross-reacts with embryonal tissue. In order to be useful clinically, a tumor antigen should meet 4 criteria: (1) it must pass from the tumor into the body fluids, (2) it must be specific, (3) its level in the serum and urine must bear some relationship with the amount of tumor present, and (4) it must be detected by a reproducible assay.

CEA is currently detected by a radioimmunoassay; a level of ≤5 ng/ml is considered normal. Its determination is useful for 3 purposes in colorectal carcinoma:

- *As a prognostic test.* At a level >4 ng/ml at the time of surgery, 60% of cases developed recurrence within 14 mo; only 12% of those without recurrences after 14 mo had a level of >4 ng/ml.
- *For detection of recurrent lesions.* A rise in CEA level precedes clinical detectable recurrences in 40–60% of cases. A consistent rise in CEA level performed every 2 wk in 3 consecutive occasions is highly suggestive of recurrence.
- *For monitoring response to therapy.* Of patients whose CEA level decreased during 5-FU therapy, 30% were alive at 18 mo, whereas only 12% of those whose CEA level did not fall were alive at 18 mo.[19]

Determination of CEA level is not useful for mass screening of colorectal cancer because of >50% false-negative data in patients with confirmed cancer and frequent false-positive data in patients with benign diseases. For instance, CEA was found moderately elevated in patients with alcoholism, uremia, inflammatory bowel disease, peptic ulcer, and emphysema, as well as in 15% of heavy smokers.[19] At the same time, CEA was found elevated (>10 ng/ml) in patients with malignant diseases other than colonic carcinoma. These included pancreatic carcinoma (in 91% of cases), lung cancer (71%), gastric carcinoma (61%), and breast carcinoma (47%).

At present, the diagnostic techniques recommended for early detection of colorectal carcinoma include the following:[8]

- *Testing for fecal occult blood* with guaiac as a reagent. This test was found to give 30% false-positive results even on a restricted diet. However, when performed after 3 days of meat-free diet, it gave only 1% false-positive data. In the general asymptomatic population over 40 yr old, 1–5% tested positive; most significant causes included diverticulosis, ademonatous polyps, and colon carcinoma.
- *Sigmoidoscopy* can detect carcinoma of the rectum or sigmoid colon in 1/667 asymptomatic persons over 40. At the Strang Clinic, 58 cancers were detected among 26,000 individuals examined. Their survival at 15 yr after diagnosis was 90% versus the usual 40–50% survival for unselected cases of colorectal cancer.
- *Colonoscopy* has significantly improved the ability to detect early lesions in the ascending and transverse colon; 46% additional polyps were discovered by colonoscopy after barium enema, of which 25% were malignant.
- *Lavage and brush cytology* was found to increase the incidence of detectable malignant lesions.

Air-contrast barium enema was found too time-consuming and costly to serve as a screening test.

Current recommendations for screening colorectal cancer are tailored to the presence of symptoms and the appartenence of individuals to one of the high-risk groups for colorectal cancer. Recommendations are as follows:

- *In symptomatic patients.* Barium enema will visualize obvious lesions or suspicious areas of the bowel. Colonoscopy is then performed, even in cases highly suggestive of carcinoma; it is useful for obtaining the biopsy necessary for a definitive diagnosis and for demonstrating additional colonic lesions not seen on barium enema. In $\leq 20\%$ of cases, these have been proved to be carcinomas. In cases of diverticulosis detected on barium enema, colonoscopy is recommended because diverticuli often hide polyps or carcinomas; gentle colonoscopy or at least lavage cytology must be performed even in cases of acute diverticulitis.

- *In asymptomatic patients over 40.* Recommendations include an annual sigmoidoscopy or at least an initial sigmoidoscopy repeated every 3–4 yr and an annual slide test for occult blood. If this is positive, barium enema with air contrast followed by colonoscopy should be performed; an upper G.I. series is recommended if the above tests are negative. In asymptomatic patients with significant family history of single or primary colon carcinoma, multiple carcinomas in different anatomic sites (ovary, colon, breast, uterus) or polyposis syndromes, the same screening tests should be performed, starting at age 20.
- *In patients already known to have premalignant diseases of the colon.* As in ulcerative colitis, sigmoidoscopy with rectocolonic cytologic lavage should be performed every 6 mo. Once a year, these patients should have a complete colonoscopy with colonic lavage.
- *In patients with previous villous colon polyps or previous colon cancers.* In view of the fact that these patients are at high risk within 5 yr after removal of the initial lesion, with a 10–20% recurrence rate due largely to synchronous lesions, air contrast barium enema and colonoscopy should be performed 2 mo after removal of the lesion and every 2–3 yr thereafter. Slide testing for occult blood and sigmoidoscopy should be performed annually.

Treatment

The therapy of colorectal carcinoma involves all 3 modalities of antineoplastic treatment: surgery, irradiation (XRT), and chemotherapy; however, colorectal cancer can be effectively treated for cure only by surgical resection of early lesions.

Surgery

Surgery is the most effective therapy. Patients scheduled for colon or rectal resection should be adequately prepared. The mechanical cleansing of bowel should be properly performed in cases of nonobstructing tumors. The curative resection of colorectal carcinoma includes a wide excision of the cancer-bearing bowel segment and the widest feasible excision of the lymphatics draining the involved bowel segment. Cancer cell contamination and embolization should be held to a minimum.

The lymphatics from the cecum and ascending colon drain along the ileocolic and right colic systems to their origin from the superior mesenteric vessel. The transverse colon drains along the midcolic to the superior mesenteric trunk. The entire rectum drains along the superior hemorrhoidal plexus to the inferior mesenteric trunk. In addition, from the lower rectum (6–7 cm from the anal verge), lymphatics drain along the inferior hemorrhoidal plexus or laterally along the middle hemorrhoidal vessels. This lymphatic drainage explains the need for a right or left hemicolectomy even for small lesions located in the ascending, transverse, or descending colon.

For lesions in the upper rectum (6–11 cm from the anal verge), a sphincter-saving procedure is generally possible in 75% of cases, usually an anterior resection with restoration of bowel continuity by an end-to-end anastomosis; occasionally, a "pull-through" type of resection is necessary.

For infiltrating lesions in the distal rectum (up to 6 cm from the anal verge) an APR with colostomy is necessary. With these techniques, 5-yr survival has been reported in 81–85% of cases of stages A and B. In stage C, with regional involvement of lymph nodes, the 5-yr survival for colon carcinoma is 57.3% in males and 67.2% in females. For carcinoma of the rectum, it is 35.5% in males and 51.9% in females.[22]

Palliative limited procedures consisting of a local resection of the cancer without extensive hemicolectomy is recommended in cases with distant metastases (stage D) before obstructive symptoms develop. This leads to a mean survival of 14 mo; when only a diverting procedure is performed without resection of the primary tumor, the mean survival drops to 5.5 mo. With no procedure, mean survival is 6–8 wk. In cases of stage D carcinoma of the rectum, lysis of the lesions by laser therapy or by electrocoagulation can bring temporary reinstallment of the bowel transit and palliation of the destructive symptoms.

Radiotherapy

Radiotherapy is curative only for rectal carcinoma. In colon carcinoma, ongoing studies are attempting to reassess its effectiveness; old studies with orthovoltage therapy did not show any effect. XRT can be administered before surgery in clinically operable patients with carcinoma of the rectum with the purpose of preventing local and regional recurrences, reducing the possibility of distant metastases, eliminating disease in the lymph node drainage system, increasing tumor resectability by destroying extension of tumor to adjacent structures, and prolonging life.[23] Preoperative XRT in 1,276 patients with carcinoma of the rectum (Duke's C disease—positive lymph nodes in the operative specimen) led to 5-yr survival of 37% versus only 23% in a comparable group not receiving XRT.

Similar results were reported in 4 different studies that recorded improved 5-yr survival in patients with carcinoma of the rectum receiving preoperative irradiation.[24-27] However, in a more recent study by Siearus, this survival advantage was not confirmed; instead, a higher operative mortality rate (5.3%) was found in the group receiving preoperative XRT.

XRT can also be administered postoperatively in operable carcinoma of the rectum; in a small series by Gunderson, postoperative XRT reduced the recurrence rate at 5 yr to <5% and improved overall survival.[28] In patients with pelvic residual disease after surgery, postoperative XRT improves survival only in cases in which lymph nodes were free of disease.[28]

Finally, XRT can be administered with palliative intent to patients with primary inoperable and recurrent carcinoma of the rectum and colon. In operable cases, XRT can effectively control bleeding, pain, tenesmus, and mucous discharge in 70–90% of cases and can spare colostomy in 41% of cases of unresectable adenocarcinoma of the rectum.

Chemotherapy

Chemotherapy of colorectal carcinoma still gives poor results.[29] Clinical antitumor activity has been established for several agents, and combinations of antineoplastic agents have been found to increase the response rate. Despite this, chemotherapy of of colorectal carcinoma has not yet resulted in clear prolongation of survival.

The list of single effective agents includes 5-FU and its metabolite floxuridine (FUdR), the first agents with consistently demonstrable effectiveness (21% response rate in >2,000 cases); Mitomycin-C (MIT); methyl CCNU (MeCCNU) and carmustine (BCNU); streptozotocin; and melphalan (MEL).

Various combinations of agents with individual activity that have induced higher response rates in comparison with 5-FU alone but have not improved overall survival include:[29]

- *5-FU + MeCCNU* (led to partial remission in 30% of cases)[30]
- *5-FU + BCNU + vincristine (VCR) + dacarbazine (DTIC)* (induced partial remission in 43% of cases)[31]
- *5-FU + MeCCNU + VCR* (induced responses in 43% of cases).[32]

Although patients receiving these combinations did better than those receiving 5-FU alone (this group achieved PRs in only 14–22% of cases), the median duration of their remission was short (3.5–4.5 mo). However, all these data were generated by uncontrolled, nonrandomized studies. Other combinations (cyclophosphamide + 5-FU + methotrexate; cyclophosphamide + cytarabine + 5-FU) did not give better results than 5-FU alone.

The most reproducible and promising data have been obtained from a combination of 5-FU (370–400 mg/m^2/day) and high-dose leucovorin (200 mg/m^2/day) for 5 days every 3 wk (see Appendix); it induced a remission rate of 45% in untreated patients and 18% in patients previously treated with 5-FU alone.[33]

These data were confirmed by a phase 3 study in which after 4 mo of observation, 28.4% of patients receiving 500 mg/m^2 leucovorin (LCV) over a 2-hr infusion and 600 mg/m^2 5-FU by I.V. push every week × 6–8 wk achieved (and were still in) PR, whereas only 12.1% of patients receiving 5-FU alone (500 mg/m^2 I.V. bolus × 5 days q. 4 wk) achieved the same status (p < 0.01).[34] The PR rate increased to 44% in a study in which patients with advanced measurable colorectal carcinoma received 5-FU (370 mg/m^2/day) and concomitant C.I. leucovorin (500 mg/m^2/day) for 5 and 6 days, respectively, every 4 wk.[35] This compared favorably with the patients receiving only C.I. 5-FU alone for 5 days (13% response rate). A different schedule of C.I. 5-FU alone (300 mg/m^2/day) was also found to induce an increased rate of PRs (28%) when followed for >10 wk.[36] Finally, recombinant alpha 2a interferon was found[37] to modulate 5-FU on in vitro colon cancer cell lines as well as in a clinical study in which it was administered subcutaneously as a 9 MU dose 3 times/wk to 17 previously untreated patients; they received 5-FU I.V. in a loading course of 750 mg/m^2/day × 5, followed by weekly bolus I.V. therapy at 750 mg/m^2. Fourteen patients achieved PRs. In all these studies the mean duration of PR is still disappointing, varying between 6 and 16 mo.

Perfusion techniques for delivering 5-FU intra-arterially (I.A.) to the pelvis or liver or doxorubicin (ADR) to the liver were used with some success in patients with metastatic colorectal cancer. Hepatic perfusion of 5-FU or FUdR led to 35–60% response rate but without prolongation of the overall survival.

Adjuvant chemotherapy in colorectal carcinoma was extensively tested, using a variety of regimens. 5-FU alone administered by I.V. bolus for 5 days every 4 wk appeared to improve survival at 3 and 5 yr after surgery, especially in stage C patients, in at least 2 cooperative studies.[38,39] However, more significant results were presented in 2 recent reports of randomized studies[40,41] in which levamisole, an anthelmintic drug with immunostimulatory activity, was administered orally at a dose of 150 mg/day × 3 every 2 wk in combination with 5-FU at a dose of 450 mg/m^2/day weekly for 1 yr after an initial loading dose of 450 mg/m^2/day for 5 days (as an I.V. bolus). Among Duke's stage C patients, 3-yr disease-free survival of 61% and overall survival of 73% were significantly better than the same parameters determined in control patients who did not receive any postoperative treatment (49% and 65%, respectively).[41]

Immunotherapy is another antineoplastic treatment modality still in the experimental phase. To date, the only immunotherapy trial in colorectal carcinoma that demonstrated proven effectiveness in prolonging survival is the previously mentioned surgical adjuvant 5-FU–levamisole study.[17]

Different types of immunotherapy were attempted: nonspecific stimulation of the immune system with bacille Calmette-Guerin (BCG) by scarification, corynebacterium parvum I.V., or subcutaneously, and levamisole p.o.; active specific immunotherapy in which BCG was mixed with a tumor cell extract; specific adoptive immunotherapy with transfer factor and immune RNA; and immunotherapy combined with adjuvant chemotherapy.

Numerous ongoing trials are testing new biologic immune modifiers (interferon, tumor necrosifactor, etc.) as well as such new approaches as the use of monoclonal antibodies to specific antigents and to the carcino-embryonic antigen.

Carcinoma of the Anus

The anus, although it represents the direct continuation of the rectum (from which it is not separated by anatomic bounderies) has, in fact, histologic and functional features completely distinct from those of the rectum. For this reason, it is not surprising that the malignant tumors of the anal region have different characteristics and behavior from those of the colorectum.

Anatomopathology and Epidemiology

Tumors of the anal region are almost exclusively epidermoid carcinomas; they represent only 1–4% of all tumors of the alimentary tract. In relation to their location above or below the dentate line, these tumors are defined as anal canal neoplasms if originating above the dentate line and as anal margin tumors if they lie mainly or entirely below the dentate line down to an imaginary line located within a 5-cm radius from the anal verge. A so-called transitional zone begins just above the anal valves and merges with the squamous epithelium below the valves. The transitional zone is an area of significant epithelial instability from which most anal cancers originate.

Histologically, anal canal tumors produce little keratin, whereas squamous cell tumors of the anal margin are mostly keratinizing and have a better prognosis. The World Health Organization (WHO) classification of anal carcinoma recognizes 5 types: (1) squamous cell carcinoma, by far the most common anal tumor; (2) basaloid carcinoma, found exclusively in the anal canal, where it arises from the junctional zone above the dentate line (a type of squamous cell carcinoma, this tumor is also known as cloacogenic carcinoma); (3) mucoepidermoid carcinoma, which originates from the anal glands and has been frequently reported at the site of chronic anal fistulae; (4) adenocarcinoma, which has the same characteristics as type 3; and (5) undifferentiated small-cell carcinoma, an exceptionally rare tumor presumably of neuroendocrine origin.[42]

Epidemiologic studies indicate that anal carcinomas are seen with greater frequency in homosexual men,[43] in multiparous women and women with lower genital tract cancers, in patients with associated anorectal conditions causing chronic irritation (condylomas, fistulae, fissures, abscesses, hemorrhoids, leukoplakia),[44] and in patients who have had XRT for other malignancies.[45]

Patterns of Spread and Staging

In anal cancer patients, metastasis usually occurs via lymphatics in 3 directions: upward, with involvement of the pararectal area; in superior rectal and inferior mesenteric nodes; lateral along the inferior rectal vessels, with involvement of nodes along the levator muscles; and in the internal iliac nodes on the side wall of the pelvis. Tumors arising at the anal verge and the perianal skin usually metastasize by lymphatics in the inguinal nodes. Lateral extension may occur by direct invasion in the perianal tissues and longitudinally along the submucosa and above the sphincter muscles, from where the tumor may invade the prostate, urethra, bladder, and vagina.

Several staging systems for anal cancer have been proposed; the Roswell Park Memorial Institute classification recognizes 5 stages, starting with carcinoma *in situ* (stage 0), and progressing to stage I, with tumor confined to the anal epithelium and subepithelial connective tissue; stage II, with invasion of the sphincter anal muscles; stage III, with regional lymph node metastases (IIIa—in the perirectal nodes only; IIIb—in the inguinal nodes); and stage IV, with distant metastases.[46] A more detailed but somewhat cumbersome classification of anal carcinoma is used by WHO following the TNM system (table 31-1). A simplified classification recognizes only 3 stages: A, in which tumor is confined to the anal mucosa and submucosa; B, with tumor invading extra-anal tissues but not yet the regional lymph nodes; and C, with tumor metastasizing to the regional lymph nodes.[47] This classification is widely used, being predictive of survival. Additionally, prognosis is related to histology, as

Table 31-1. TNM Staging System for Primary Carcinomas of Anal Canal

T Primary	Tumor
Tis	Preinvasive tumor (carcinoma *in situ*)
T0	No evidence of primary tumor
T1	Tumor occupying not more than one-third of the circumference or length of the canal and not infiltrating the external sphincter muscle
T2	Tumor occupying more than one-third of the circumference or length of the canal and not infiltrating the external sphincter muscle
T3	Tumor with extension to rectum or skin but not to other neighboring structures
T4	Tumor with extensions to neighboring structures
TX	The minimum requirements to assess the primary tumor cannot be met
N	Regional lymph nodes
N0	No evidence of regional involvement
N1	Evidence of involvement of regional lymph nodes
NX	The minimum requirements to assess the regional lymph nodes cannot be met
M	Distant metastasis
M0	No evidence of distant metastasis
M1	Evidence of distant metastasis
MX	Minimum requirements to assess the presence of distant metastasis cannot be met.

proven by poorer survival rates in patients with nonkeratinizing squamous cell and basoloid type carcinoma than in those with low-grade keratinizing squamous cell carcinoma. In the latter group, about 70% of patients presented with tumor limited to the anal canal wall, 20% had regional lymph node involvement, and 2% had distant metastases.[48] In contrast, only 50% of patients with basaloid nonkeratinizing carcinoma presented with disease limited to the anal canal wall, whereas 30% had regional lymph node involvement and 20% presented with distant metastases.

Clinical Manifestations and Treatment

The most common presenting symptom of patients with anal carcinoma was bleeding (usually not severe enough to cause significant anemia), seen in 27–74% cases of various series.[49] Rectal pain or discomfort, the second most common complaint, was found in 21–39% of patients.[50] Other presenting symptoms included pressure, awareness of an anal mass, change in bowel habits, pruritus, anal discharge, and tenesmus. Because these symptoms are associated also with benign anorectal conditions, the diagnosis established by adequate biopsy is frequently delayed until the tumor reaches advanced stages.

Surgical resection is the treatment modality of choice for most cases with lesions of the anal margin and perianal skin as well as with superficial lesions (<2 cm in diameter) of the anal canal located under the dentate line.[49] More invasive lesions are treated surgically by APR but generally are better treated by XRT alone or in combination with chemotherapy, an approach that usually preserves the anal sphincter and permits a better quality of life.

Radiation therapy is effective because the epidermoid carcinoma of the anal canal and anal margin are generally radiosensitive. Radium implants and external beam radiation have been used alone or in combination for various sites of anal carcinoma. Complications, represented by strictures, infections, hemorrhage, necrosis, and severe postirradiation pain,[49] can generally be limited with more fractionated schemes and careful planning as recommended by Papillon.[50] Overall, complete remissions (CRs) are reported in various series in 75–100% of cases, of which 30–50% also have local surgical excision or APR (in a maximum of 20% of cases).[51]

Current recommendations for XRT include the following:

1. Small tumors of the anal margin can be treated by local excision or radium implant or external irradiation.

2. Large tumors of the anal margin may be treated with external irradiation combined with an interstitial implant, which is preferable to APR.

3. Small tumors of the anal canal should be treated with a radium implant alone, with careful fractionation; advanced tumors are suitable for either a fractionated radium implant or a combination of implant and external beam irradiation.[50] The latter is generally administered to the whole pelvis up to a total of 4,500–5,000 cGy, using the 4-field pelvic techniques associated with a perineal field.[51] This is followed by a boost to the tumor of 1,500–2,000 cGy.

Combined concomitant modality treatment (see Appendix) generally includes 5-FU, administered by C.I. infusion at a dose of 1,000 mg/m^2/day × 5 in the first and fourth week of irradiation; MIT, delivered as an I.V. bolus in the first day of this combined regimen; and XRT in 25 fractions over 5 wk to a total of 4,000–5,000 cGy to the perineum and pelvis plus a boost of 1,000 cGy in 100-cGy fractions to the tumor. Initially used by Nigro,[52] this regimen was then popularized by Sishy's large series[53] and by other recent studies,[54] and has become the preferred therapy for anal carcinoma. APR is performed only in patients with residual disease at biopsy performed 1 mo after combined modality treatment is completed. The toxicity of this treatment is generally limited to perineal erythema and desquamation, and radiation proctitis, all of which resolve after brief interruptions in treatment.

The treatment of recurrent epidermoid carcinoma of the anal region is successful only for lesions of the anal margin. These recurrent lesions, rarely accompanied by distant metastases, generally can be locally resected in 90% of cases; remaining lesions require APR or inguinal node dissection. For lesions of the anal canal, which generally are accompanied by distant metastases, APR or combination chemotherapy do not bring lasting CR; median survival of these patients is 8 mo.

Patients with metastatic anal carcinoma can be treated with combination chemotherapy. PRs were noted with MIT + 5-FU or a cisplatin and 5-FU combination regimen.[49] Unfortunately, prolongation of survival with these regimens is minimal. Overall, however, the treatment of anal carcinoma has made significant progress; it has become one of the few malignancies for which cure can be achieved even in cases with advanced locoregional disease, with preservation of the organ in most cases.

References

1. Walker AR, Burkitt D. Colon cancer: epidemiology. Semin Oncol 1976; 3:341–50.
2. Baserga R. Biochemical, molecular and pharmacologic approaches to large bowel cancer: an overview—Cancer 1980; suppl 45:1168–71.

3. Rawson RW. Colonic polyps: antecedent or associated lesions of large bowel cancer. Semin Oncol 1976; 3:361–68.

4. Vogelstein B, Pearson ER, Hamilton SR, et al. Genetic alterations during colo-rectal tumor development. N Engl J Med 1988; 319:525–32.

5. Spratt JS Jr, Ackerman LV, Moyer CA. Relationship of polyps of colon to colonic cancer. Ann Surg 1958; 148:682–96.

6. Castleman B, Kirkstein HI. Do adenomatous polyps of the colon become malignant? N Engl J Med 1962; 267:469–75.

7. Morson BC. Evolution of cancer of the colon and rectum. Cancer 1974; 34:845–49.

8. Fenoglio CM, Lane N. The anatomical precursor of colo-rectal carcinoma. Cancer 1974; 34:819–823.

9. Lipkin M. Phase 1 and phase 2 proliferative lesions of colonic epithelial cells in disease leading to colonic cancer. Cancer 1974; 34:878–88.

10. Kopolovich L, Pfeffer L, Lipkin M. Recent studies on the identification of proliferative abnormalities and of oncogenic potential of cutaneous cells in individuals at increased risk of colon cancer. Semin Oncol 1976; 3:369–72.

11. Cannon-Albright LA, Skolnick MH, Bishop T, et al. Common inheritance of susceptibility to colonic adenomatous polyps and associated colo-rectal cancer. N Engl J Med 1988; 319:533–37.

12. Wooley PV III. Clinical manifestations of cancer of the colon and rectum. Semin Oncol 1976; 3:373–76.

13. Hoth DF, Petrucci PE. Natural history and staging of colon cancer. Semin Oncol 1976; 3:331–36.

14. Dukes CE. The classification of cancer of the rectum. J Pathol Bacter 1932; 35:323–32.

15. Kirklin JW, Docherty MB, Waugh JM. The role of the peritoneal reflection in the prognosis of carcinoma of the rectum and sigmoid colon. Surg Gynecol Obst 1949; 88:326–31.

16. Astler UB, Coller FA. The prognostic significance of direct extension of carcinoma of the colon and rectum. Ann Surg 1954; 139:846–51.

17. Turnbull RB, Kyle K, Watson FR, Spratt J. Cancer of the colon; the influence of the nontouch isolation technique on survival rates. Ann Surg 1967; 160:420–25.

18. Winawer SJ, Sherlock P. Approach to screening and diagnosis in colo-rectal cancer. Semin Oncol 1976; 3:387–397.

19. Holyoke ED, Cooper EH. CEA and tumor markers. Semin Oncol 1976; 3:377–86.

20. Abelev GI, Porova SD, Khromkova NI, et al. Production of embryonal alphaglobulin by transplantable mouse hepatomas. Transpl Proc 1963; 1:174–80.

21. Gold P, Freeman SO. Demonstration of tumor-specific antigens in human colonic carcinomata by immunologic tolerance and absorption techniques. J Exp Med 1965; 121:439–43.

22. Stearns M Jr. Surgical aspects of colo-rectal carcinoma. Semin Oncol 1976; 3:399–406.

23. Kligerman MM. Radiation therapy for rectal carcinoma. Semin Oncol 1976; 3:407–14.

24. Fletcher WS, Allen CV, Dunphy JE. Preoperative irradiation for carcinoma of the colon and rectum. Am J Surg 1965; 109:76–83.

25. Kligerman MM, Urdaneta N, Knowlton A, et al. Preoperative irradiation of rectosigmoid carcinoma including its regional lymph nodes. Am J Roentgenol Radium Ther Nucl Med 1972; 114:498–503.

26. Higgins GA, Conn JH, Jordan PU, et al. Preoperative radiotherapy for colo-rectal cancer. Ann Surg 1975; 181:624–31.

27. Rider WD. The 1975 Gordon Richards memorial lecture: is the Miles operation really necessary for the treatment of rectal cancer? J Can Assoc Radiol 1975; 26:167–75.

28. Schild SE, Martenson JA Jr, Gunderson LL, Dozois RR. Long term survival and patterns of failure after postoperative radiation therapy for subtotally resected rectal adenocarcinoma. Int J Radiat Oncol Biol Phys 1989; 16:452–63.

29. Haller DG. Chemotherapy in gastro-intestinal malignancies. Semin Oncol 1988; 15 (suppl 4):50–64.

30. Baker LH, Matter R, Talley R, et al. 5 FU vs. 5 FU + MeCCNU in gastrointestinal cancer. Proc Amer Soc Clin Oncol 1975; (abstr) 16:229.

31. Falkson G, van Eden EG, Falkson HC. Fluorouracil, imidazole carboxomide dimethyltriazine, vincristine and bis-chloroethylnitrosourea in colon cancer. Cancer 1974; 33:1207–09.

32. Moertel CG, Schutt AJ, Hahn RG, et al. Therapy of advanced colo-rectal cancer with a combination of 5-fluorouracil methyl-1,3-cis (2-chloroethyl) -1-nitrosourea and vincristine. JNCI 1975; 54:69–72.

33. Macher D, Timus M, Schwartzenberg L, et al. Treatment of adjuvant colo-rectal and gastric adenocarcinomas with 5 fluorouracil combined with high dose calcium leucovorin. In: An update in the current status of 5 fluorouracil-leucovorin calcium combination 1984; 55–65.

34. Petrelli N, Douglas HO, Herrera L, et al. The modulation of fluorouracil with leucovorin in metastatic colorectal carcinoma. A prospective randomized phase III trial. J Clin Oncol 1989; 7:1419–26.

35. Doroshow JH, Multhauf P, Leong L, et al. Prospective randomized comparison of fluorouracil versus fluorouracil and high dose continuous infusion leucovorin calcium in the treatment of advanced measurable colo-rectal cancer in patients previously unexposed to chemotherapy. J Clin Oncol 1990; 8:491–501.

36. Lokich JJ, Ahlgren JD, Gullo JJ, et al. A prospective randomized comparison of continuous infusion fluorouracil with a conventional bolus schedule in metastatic colo-rectal cancer: a Midatlantic Oncology Program study. J Clin Oncol 1989; 7:425–29.

37. Wadler S, Schwartz EL, Goldman M, et al. Fluorouracil and recombinant alfa 2a-interferon: an active regimen against advanced colo-rectal cancer. J Clin Oncol 1989; 7:1769–75.

38. Fisher B, Wolmer CN, Rockette H, et al. Adjuvant chemotherapy of postoperative radiation for rectal cancer: 5 years results of NSABP R-01, Proc Am Soc Clin Oncol 1987; 6:92 (abstr 359).

39. Wolmark N, Fisher B, Rockette H, et al. Adjuvant therapy in carcinoma of the colon five year results of NSABP protocol C-01. Proc Am Soc Clin Oncol 1987; 6:92 (abstr 358).

40. Lourie JA, Moertel CG, Fleming T, et al. Surgical adjuvant therapy of large bowel carcinoma: an evaluation of levamisole and the combination of levamisole and fluorouracil. J Clin Oncol 1989; 7:1447–56.

41. Hamilton JM, Sznol M, Friedman MA. 5 fluorouracil plus levamisole: effective adjuvant treatment for colon cancer. In: DeVita VT Jr, Hellman S., Rosenberg SA, eds. Important advances in oncology 1990. Philadelphia: Lippincott, 1990; 115–30.

42. Morson BC, Sobin LH. Histologic typing of intestinal tumors. In: International histologic classification of malignant tumors. No. 45. Geneva: World Health Organization, 1976.

43. Daling JR, Weiss NS, Hoffenstein LI, et al. Correlates of homosexual behaviour and the incidence of anal carcinoma. JAMA 1982; 247:1988–90.

44. Brennan JT, Stewart CF. Epidermoid carcinoma of the anus. Am Surg 1972; 176:787–90.

45. Greenall MJ, Quan SH, Stearns MW, et al. Epidermoid cancer of the anal region. Pathologic features, treatment and clinical results. Am J Surg 1985; 149:95–101.

46. Paradis P, Douglass HO, Holyoke ED. The clinical implications of a staging system for carcinoma of the anus. Surg Gynecol Obstet 1975; 141:411–16.

47. Richards JC, Beahrs DH, Woolner LB. Squamous cell carcinoma of the anus and canal and rectum in 109 patients. Surg Gynecol Obstet 1962; 114:475–82.

48. Bomou BM, Moertel CG, O'Connell MJ, et al. Carcinoma of the anal canal. A clinical and pathologic study of 188 cases. Cancer 1984; 54:114–25.

49. Mitchell EP. Carcinoma of the anal region. Semin Oncol 1988; 15:146–53.

50. Papillon J. Radiation therapy in the management of epidermoid carcinoma of the anal region. Dis Colon Rectum 1974; 17:181–87.

51. Green JP, Schaupp WC, Cantril ST, et al. Anal carcinoma: current therapeutic concepts. Am J Surg 1980; 140:151–55.

52. Nigro ND, Vaitkevices VK, Considine G. Combined therapy for cancer of the anal canal. A preliminary report. Dis Colon Rectum 1974; 17:354–6.

53. Sishy B. The use of radiation therapy combined with chemotherapy in the management of squamous cell carcinoma of the anus and marginally resectable adenocarcinoma of the rectum. Int J Radiat Oncol Biol Phys 1985; 1587–93.

54. Knecht BH. Combined chemotherapy and radiotherapy for carcinoma of the anus. Am J Surg 1990; 159:518–21.

32

PANCREATIC CANCER

Howard Bruckner, M.D.

DESPITE RECENT ADVANCES REGISTERED in its earlier detection and in the understanding of its pathogenesis, pancreatic cancer has remained a disease difficult to diagnose, unsatisfactory to treat, rapidly debilitating to the patient, and difficult to study effectively. There is generally a sense of frustration in the medical community toward this malignancy, the incidence of which has climbed during the last decade to fourth place as a cause of death from cancer in the United States.[1]

Incidence and Epidemiology

Pancreatic cancer ranks ninth in frequency of nonskin cancers. It makes up only 3% of the newly diagnosed cancers but 5.5% of cancer deaths (about 20,000 per year in the United States).

In blacks, pancreatic cancer comprised 3.8% of incident cancers and 5.9% of lethal cancers. No significant variations with race have been seen except for American Indian men, who have a lower than average rate of carcinoma of the pancreas, and Jews and blacks, who show a tendency for higher than average risk. A slightly increased incidence of carcinoma of the pancreas is seen in the rural regions in comparison with urban areas.

In all races, pancreatic cancer is more frequently seen in men, with a sex ratio (men: women) of 1.7:1. However, special uncommon types of pancreatic cancer—squamous cell and intracystic papillary—are more common in women.

Islet cell carcinoma of the pancreas is more common in the young; median age at diagnosis for adenocarcinoma of the pancreas is 60–70.

Generally, there is a small coefficient of variation in the incidence of pancreatic cancer among various nations. Nonetheless, it has a higher incidence in the Western industrialized countries, and mortality rates among new immigrants from countries with low incidence (Africa, Japan) increase after a single generation.

Among specific risk factors that lead to an increased incidence of pancreatic cancer, tobacco has a premier role. Cigarette smokers of >2 packs/day have an increased risk of 2.75; among Japanese smokers, this risk increases 10-fold.

Diabetes mellitus represents a risk factor for pancreatic cancer, especially in women, among whom a 6-fold increased incidence is noted. Among diabetic men, no increase in the pancreatic cancer incidence has been noted if correction for recent onset diabetes mellitus is applied. Recent-onset diabetes is generally attributed to the destruction of pancreatic cells by the malignant tumors themselves.

Data are contradictory concerning the association of chronic alcoholism and chronic pancreatitis with pancreatic cancer and about the role high daily intake of coffee may play in increasing the risk for cancer of the pancreas, as may petrochemical, nuclear, industrial, and unspecified environmental exposure.[1]

Histopathology

Among all patients with nonendocrine cancer of the pancreas (endocrine islet cell carcinoma is discussed in the chapter of this book on apudoma), the most common histopathologic presentation is that of *duct cell adenocarcinoma* (see chapter 11, figure 11-41).[2] Accounting for ≤75% of all cancer of the pancreas, this tumor often resembles adenocarcinoma at other sites (intestinal tract, lung, uterus). Generally, large and small glands, poorly or well differentiated, are intermingled. The tumor glands are formed by tall columnar cells with mucin in the cytoplasm, but some are lined with cuboidal cells with scant cytoplasm. Nuclei vary in size, shape, polarity, and distribution of chromatin. The mucin is generally present in the apex of cancer cells or in the extracellular pools. Papillary and cystic features are occasionally present. In two-thirds of patients with this histologic type, the primary lesion is located in the head of the pancreas. Other less common histologic types include the following:

Giant cell pleomorphic carcinoma, a rare type (4% of cases), has a relatively higher distribution in the tail and body of the pancreas. It is made up of large polypoid, often bizarre mono- or multinucleated tumor giant cells and of malignant spindle cells. Necrosis and hemorrhages frequently occur, often leading to the impression that the tumor is made up of large hemorrhagic cysts.

A more differentiated variant of giant-cell carcinoma is the epulis type, a rare tumor in which, in addition to the bizarre giant cells and spindle cells seen in the common variety of giant cells, one can recognize numerous benign-appearing epulis-type cells (osteoclast-like cells). It resembles the benign giant cell tumor of the bone. Patients with this tumor survive longer than all other pancreatic cancer patients (average: 3–5 yr).

Adenosquamous cell carcinoma of the pancreas, or adenoacanthoma, is encountered in 4% of cases. It consists of a mixture of glandular and squamous cell carcinoma components that generally are moderately well differentiated. Of interest is the fact that this histologic type was found primarily in patients that either had another primary malignancy or received radiation therapy (XRT) to the abdomen. Early metastases to liver, lymph nodes, and/or peritoneum, and perineural invasion are common features of adenosquamous carcinoma of the pancreas.

Miroadenocarcinoma of the pancreas is another rare histologic type (3% of cases) that resembles the carcinoid tumors but does not stain with silver stains characteristic for carcinoid. Encountered more frequently in the body of the pancreas, it consists of small glands centered in sheets or solid foci of cells. This histologic type has an aggressive behavior, leading to death within days to months.

Mucinous adenocarcinoma (see chapter 11, figure 11-41), or colloid, gelatinous carcinoma of the pancreas is yet another rare tumor (2% of cases) found always in the head of the pancreas in male patients with history of chronic pancreatitis. It presents as large cystic spaces filled with mucin and lined by tall columnar cells or as lakes of mucin with floating nests of cells, some forming glandular patterns, many having "signet ring" morphology.

Cystadenocarcinoma (mucinous) of the pancreas is an extremely rare tumor seen only in women and only in the tail of the pancreas. It presents as a huge gray tumor with multiloculated cysts containing mucinosis fluid. These tumors generally are resectable. Patients with these tumors survive longer than those with common ductal carcinoma of the pancreas (12–16 mo).

Acinar cell carcinoma is another rare malignant tumor of the pancreas (1% of cases) encountered in patients younger than those with common ductal pancreatic cancer. These tumors present with areas of characteristic acinus formation (with large polyhedral cells) alternating with areas of necrosis or of sclerosis formation; sometimes these tumors can be confused with lymphomas.

Very rare types of pancreatic cancer include *pancreaticoblastoma,* with a predominant glandular arrangement of small cells with clear cytoplasm mixed with larger eosinophilic cells containing zymogengranules; and *papillary cystic carcinoma,* with sheets of cells surrounding thin-walled vessels or papillae containing red cells that have a low mitotic index and a more indolent course.

Finally, about 10% of all cases are defined as anaplastic carcinoma of the pancreas, which usually diffusely involves the pancreas and can present with 1 of the following 3 types of cells: large cells, small cells resembling lymphomas, and clear cells resembling renal cell carcinoma but staining positive for mucin.

Diagnosis and Clinical Features

Because the pancreas is located deep in the retroperitoneum, its lesions are generally detectable by physical examination only when far advanced. They are highly suspected at an early stage only when biliary obstruction or steatorrhea occurs due to a small lesion of the head of the pancreas.

During the past decade, the introduction of new imaging techniques, notably the CT scan and the MRI scan, together with the ability to obtain valuable cytologic material from the pancreas with the help of percutaneous fine-needle biopsy, has improved the frequency of accurate radiologic and cytologic diagnosis. Although performing multiple aspirations with a cytologist on site proves efficient, the most important differential diagnosis—particularly in the case of endocrine tumors and lymphomas—sometimes requires special supplementary tests.

The algorithm of a rational stepwise sequence of tests necessary to reach the diagnosis of pancreatic cancer is slightly different for patients in whom there is just a remote suspicion than for these with high-suspicion of pancreatic carcinoma.

The following relatively early clinical manifestations of carcinoma of the pancreas should raise our suspicion for a diagnosis of pancreatic cancer. These clinical manifestations are usually evidence of locally advanced unresectable or metastatic disease late in its clinical course.

Local G.I. symptomatology in the form of intermittent epigastric pain or periumbilical pain not related to meals and frequently radiating to the back accompanied by nausea and (rarely) vomiting is frequently associated with systemic manifestations that include anorexia and rapid weight loss. Frequently an unexplained reactive depression represents manifestation of this disease. There is also a high incidence of recurrent thromboembolic events often associated with an antithrombin III deficiency. This chronic, recurrent thromboembolic syndrome described by Trousseau requires heparin and is usually resistant to coumadin.

A high suspicion for pancreatic carcinoma is usually generated by the rapid development of obstructive jaundice in an otherwise asymptomatic patient.

A conventional barium study of the stomach and duodenum (upper G.I. study) has a relatively low accuracy in establishing the diagnosis of pancreatic carcinoma (50% of cases). A widened retrogastric space, together with mural and mucosal irregularities of the posterior gastric wall, are the main positive findings in carcinoma of the tail and body of the pancreas. Carcinoma of the head of the pancreas can cause deformity of the gastric antrum, its displacement, or the ulceration of its mucosa by tumor infiltration while the duodenal loop is widened. The upper G.I. series assists in deciding the individual necessity for double bypass surgery.

Hypotonic duodenography and selenomethionine ([75]SE) pancreatic scanning, which had low accuracy in establishing the diagnosis of pancreatic carcinoma, have been recently replaced by ultrasonography and CT scanning.

In a collaborative study in the diagnosis of pancreatic carcinoma, ultrasonography was found to be the best initial test for any patient suspected of carcinoma of the pancreas.[3] It has a failure rate of only 11% and a sensitivity of 82%; the predictive value of a positive test is 77% and that of a negative test, 88%. It has high patient acceptability and is relatively inexpensive and devoid of radiation hazards. However, these superior results can be achieved only by highly trained practitioners. The test is less effective in the obese or in those with bowel gas.

Being fully automated, *CT scanning* is less dependent on the radiologist's skills (see chapter 10, figures 10-10 to 10-12). It has a failure rate of 11%, a sensitivity of 77%, and a predictive value of 73% for a positive test and 85%

for a negative one.[3] A similar predictive value and sensitivity was found with longitudinal multiplane emission tomography. CT scans sometimes supplement sonography, which is technically unsatisfactory.[3]

Patients with abnormalities of the pancreas on ultrasonography or CT scan may be further evaluated with *endoscopic retrograde cannulation of the papilla (ERCP)*. This may be efficient when the same procedure allows placement of a biliary stent, which will obviate surgery. In the absence of biliary obstruction, percutaneous biopsy has a better yield than endoscopy. In establishing the visual diagnosis of pancreatic carcinoma, ERCP has a failure rate of 21%, specificity of 90%, and predictive values of 85% for a positive test and 91% for a negative test.[3] The success rate of ERCP depends on the skills of the endoscopist, but even the very skillful have a technical failure rate of 15%. Pancreatic duct cytology can be obtained with the help of ERCP through direct punch biopsy and by the analysis of the intraductal washing obtained by ERCP. If ERCP fails to establish the diagnosis, then curative surgery is indicated for cases that appear to be clinically resectable. Small, apparently inoperable (<3 cm) tumors also warrant attempts at surgery even if the percutaneous or endoscopic biopsy establishes the diagnosis. Some, however, believe that any biopsy decreases the chance of curative surgery.

For cases that appear unresectable or present with questionable masses on radiologic tests, a *percutaneous transperitoneal fine-needle biopsy* under sonographic or CT scan guidance is indicated; this procedure has a predictive positive value of 94%. The procedure has almost eliminated the need for exploratory laparotomy when a histologic diagnosis is needed. Perhaps the only contraindications to percutaneous biopsy other than the high risk of bleeding are planned curative surgery, in order to avoid tracking of cells, and mandatory bypass surgery, in order to avoid duplication. A highly unusual clinical or radiologic presentation—a reason to suspect a rare tumor—may also be a contraindication, depending on the skills of the available cytologist.

Finally, *celiac and superior mesenteric angiography* is available as a staging tool, primarily in patients thought to have a resectable pancreatic tumor. In these cases, it is essential to define the tumor vascularization as supportive evidence that the tumor is resectable and to help the surgeon to achieve hemostasis at the time of tumor resection as supporting evidence that the tumor is resectable. The angiogram can be used also for supplementary diagnostic purposes. An irregularity in the pancreatic artery or of one of its branches has a predictive value for a positive diagnosis of 63% and an 81% negative predictive value.[3] *Sonographic endoscopy* may also have a role in defining operability. It provides the best nonsurgical visualization of lymph nodes and sometimes tumor on vessels.

In addition to the above radiologic tests, a number of serologic tests have been studied for their possible diagnostic value for pancreatic carcinoma. However, none of the current serologic tests has specificity for this malignancy. Three serologic tests, the carcino-embryonic antigen (CEA), the pancreatic oncofetal antigen (POA), and the CA 19-9 appear to have primarily a prognostic value, for the reason that they are present at a high level in confirmed cases of pancreatic carcinoma. These tests also can be used to monitor patient response to treatment. More expensive radiologic tests can be used sparingly, but not omitted when the marker serves as the "screening" test. It has been found that levels of both CEA and POA often vary with changes of the tumor mass related to disease remission or relapse. When greater than 20 U, the POA can also have a positive predictive value for the diagnosis of pancreatic carcinoma (71%). POA elevation has a tendency to be associated with tumor differentiation. These tests and the CA 19-9 and CA 125 assays only supplement other evidence and cannot stand alone. Assays may rise with the degree of biliary and hepatic dysfunction, independent of tumor size. Abnormal assays are not evidence of metastatic disease and probably do not even contraindicate attempts at curative surgery.

Staging and Prognosis

Pancreatic carcinoma has a tendency to metastasize via the lymphatic channels, primarily to the peripancreatic, celiac, and paraortic lymph nodes, and hematogenously to liver, lung, bones, and adrenal glands.

Clinically, direct invasion with local obstruction of the bile duct or gastric outlet, painful invasion of retroperitoneal strictures, metastases with replacement of liver tissue, and peritoneal carcinomatosis represent the life-threatening modes of progression.

At time of diagnosis, 35–45% of patients have metastatic disease; however, >90% probably have clinically occult distant metastases and are technically inoperable due to local extension to blood vessels. Without regard to type of therapy, survival has varied with the site of the tumor in the pancreas (patients with tumors in the head have the longest survival) and the stage of the tumor. The latter is primarily related to the size and extension of the tumor and the presence of lymph node or distant metastases. The TNM classification applied to malignant tumors of the pancreas defining several categories is displayed in table 32-1.

Treatment

Treatment still has disappointing results, despite progress achieved in the earlier radiologic diagnosis of this disease. However, new therapies are slowly improving the abysmal results of standard treatment.

Pancreatic insufficiency frequently produces symptoms (indigestion and increased motility of the bowel) that can be partially alleviated with pancreatic enzymes. Infrequently, oral medium-chain triglycerides can provide fat. Parenteral hyperalimentation is useful only as an acute support for surgery, and providing fewer than usual calories may be ideal in order to avoid fluid overload and unexplained early deaths.

Pain is common and often accompanied by depression. Early use of methadone and antidepressants can be very helpful. These require concurrent

Table 32-1. TNM Staging Classification of Cancer of the Pancreas

Primary tumor (T)
TX	Primary tumor cannot be assessed
T0	No evidence of primary tumor
T1	Tumor limited to the pancreas
T1a	Tumor ≤ 2 cm in greatest dimension
T1b	Tumor >2 cm in greatest dimension
T2	Tumor extends directly to the duodenum, bile duct, or preipancreatic tissues Limited extension
T3	Tumor extends directly to the stomach, spleen, colon, or adjacent large vessels Contraindicates surgery

Regional lymph nodes (N)
NX	Regional lymph nodes cannot be assessed
N0	No regional lymph node metastasis
N1	Regional lymph node metastasis

Distant metastasis (M)
MX	Presence of distant metastasis cannot be assessed
M0	No distant metastasis
MI	Distant metastasis

Stage grouping

I	T1,N0,M0
	T2,N0,M0
II	T3,N0,M0
III	any T, N1, M0
IV	any T, any N, M1

use of prophylactic cathartics. Nerve block, sometimes effective for localized severe back pain, is best reserved for pain that is refractory to simple oral treatment or used as an alternative when narcotics produce excess sedation.

Historically, median survival rates for localized resected, regional unresected, and metastatic disease, respectively, are 12 mo (9% at 5 yr); 6 mo (5% at 2 yr, 1% at 5 yr); and 3 mo (10% at 1 yr, 1% at 5 yr). Best survival results in new trials for the same stages of disease are 22 mo (20% at 5 yr);[4] 11 mo (5% at 2 yr);[5] and 7-9 mo (40% at 1 yr).[6]

The overall survival of patients with early pancreatic carcinoma appears to be demonstrably influenced by therapy, and several regimens may produce modest rates of response, with benefit for "responding" patients (table 32-2). These new treatment options are relevant for the many patients who present or could be diagnosed while they are still in an early stage of disease and have good performance status and intact physiologic function. Nihilism is unwarranted. It only delays diagnosis and discourages both application and development of potentially effective treatments.

Improved survival in specific controlled trials appears to be due to novel treatments. It cannot be attributed either to early diagnosis or to improved supportive care because early diagnosis has no impact on the survival of "stage-adjusted" patients. Such new measures as percutaneous drainage or antibiotics, although they are beneficial for individual patients, as yet have had no impact on overall survival. In testing conventional treatments, collaborative studies have not found any improvements in stage-adjusted survival.

Table 32-2. Pancreatic Cancer: Development of Treatment

Stage	Trial status	Treatment	Trials
Perisurgical	Phase 2 early	XRT	XRT&5-FU,XRT + 5-FU + MIT, XRT + 5-FU + DDP + STZ
Adjuvant	Phase 3[a], 2	XRT + 5-FU[a]	
Regional	Phase 3[b]	XRT + 5-FU[b]	SMF + XRT + 5-FU + SMF**
	Phase 3	CMF–5-FU + MIT[b]	vs. SMF or FAM (S)
	Phase 2	FAP + XRT	
Metastatic			
Small	Phase 3	CMF–5-FU + MIT[b]	
Metastatic	Phase 3, 2	SMF[c]	LCV + 5-FU[c]
Large	Phase 2	FAM-S[c]	PALA + 5-FU[c]
Measurable	Phase 3	5-FU[uk]	

Key to abbreviations: a = possibly curative; b = clearly palliative; c = increases response rate and survival of patients with response; uk = efficacy unknown; XRT = radiation therapy; CMF = cyclophosphamide, methotrexate, 5-fluorouracil (5-FU); SMF = streptozotocin, mitomycin-C, 5-FU; FAM-S = 5-FU, doxorubicin, mitomycin-C, streptozotocin (STZ); LCV = leucovorin
**best preliminary finding

Surgery

All patients with localized tumors in the head or body—but not the tail—of the pancreas deserve exploration in order to attempt resection, intraoperative XRT, or isotope placement. Exploration is no longer warranted simply for diagnosis or staging. Biliary bypass is ideally coordinated with additional treatment.

Complete resection is the only treatment that offers any possibility of cure (seen in 9% of cases).[7] The chance of benefit is increased by the availability of intraoperative XRT and postoperative adjuvant therapy. Surgical morbidity (19%) is diminished by selection of physiologically young, nondiabetic, normal-performance-status patients. It is further lowered by relieving jaundice before surgery, restaging patients after any delay for ancillary treatment, intensively correcting physiologic status before surgery, and providing intensive intraoperative and postoperative care.[8] This type of surgery is evolving into a special center function.[9] Rushing to surgery adds nothing and is often harmful.

Surgery is especially feasible if patients have small (<4 cm) tumors. An angiogram can determine eligibility for resection (no vessel involved) and isotope implant (no venous thrombosis). Laparoscopy, performed as the first step, using the same anesthesia intended for exploration, may correct some errors in staging and avoid some laparotomies and the 7% mortality associated with exploration.

Patients with biliary obstruction benefit from bypass surgery only occasionally. The 10–15% morbidity of this procedure may indicate the need for both improved selection of patients for bypass surgery and the more frequent use of stents.[10] In these patients, 15% need relatively immediate gastroenterostomy and another 15% need gastroenterostomy within 3 mo. The need for gastroenterostomy is among the best indications for choosing biliary surgery in preference to the stent. Gastroenterostomy does not noticeably add to the morbidity of biliary bypass surgery.[10]

The conservative position is that bypass surgery is superior to resection, even for operable tumors.[11] Bypass surgery leads to a median survival of 12 mo, and is briefly palliative for patients with unresectable localized tumors (median survival: 4–6 mo) but is of questionable benefit for patients with metastatic disease (median survival: 12 wk). Bypass surgery should be coordinated with therapeutic investigations of adjuvant and regional therapy in order to give the patient 2 chances to benefit from surgery—e.g., IORT or perioperative treatment.[12]

Biliary stents are used (1) if bypass surgery fails, (2) to speed a slow improvement in serum bilirubin after bypass, (3) for postoperative cholangitis, and (4) for poor-risk surgical and survival patients (cardiacs, infected, poorly controlled diabetics, poor performance status, and physiologically elderly). It may also serve for perisurgical supportive care, preparation for surgery, and to allow time for investigational perisurgical adjuvant therapy. Stenting with endoscopy is preferred, especially in patients with ascites or poor coagulation function; percutaneous stents are reserved for patients with prior surgery, large tumors, or high bile duct obstruction distorting duodenal access.[13,14]

A bypass or stent is a prerequisite for chemotherapy of the severely jaundiced patient. In the presence of jaundice, complication-free time is inadequate, and altered biliary excretion adversely affects the safety of several drugs. Anecdotally, low-dose infusion of 5-fluorouracil (5-FU), full-dose streptozotocin (STZ), and simultaneous XRT can be beneficial as a last resort for the jaundiced patients. Some efforts center on combining STZ, cisplatin (DDP), and 5-FU infusion with XRT. The former attempts to take advantage of the acute response rate associated with STZ and its relative lack of bone marrow toxicity, and the latter attempts to use the synergism of 5-FU infusion, extrapolating from success against other G.I. tumors.[13]

Chemotherapy

The chemotherapeutic approach to carcinoma of the pancreas will be presented in relation to its use in patients at various disease stages.

ADJUVANT THERAPY

Adjuvant therapy may double median survival to 20 mo and may triple 5-yr survival to 20–30% of cases in comparison with resection alone for patients who recover rapidly and fully from surgery. These conclusions are based on an adjuvant controlled trial[4] and a confirmatory phase 2 trial.[5] Treatment consisted of bolus 5-FU and XRT. The adjuvant trial had few patients and took several years to accrue them; therefore, it is not widely accepted as a conclusive test. Nevertheless, the burden of proof now rests with those who choose the uniformly fatal practice of withholding potentially curative surgery.

All resected patients are candidates for the still investigational adjuvant therapy if they have both kidneys and if their hepatorenal function is normal.

Due to the controversy surrounding the risk and benefit of radical surgery, there is a body of theoretical constructs—and actual clinical experience— testing preoperative XRT[15,16] and periadjuvant combined modality therapy.[13,14] The CT scan remains the best restaging test to assess treatment. Radiologists often underestimate the degree of response and chance of operability. In particular, they fail to recognize sterilization of enlarged nodes in patients with apparent stable disease or minor response after combined modality therapy. Failure after resection surgery is both local and distant; adjuvant therapy has decreased local failure. Bile duct obstruction/cholangitis not due to cancer has been misdiagnosed as local failure after adjuvant therapy.

REGIONAL DISEASE

Combined modality therapy clearly increases the survival of patients with surgically staged inoperable cancer confined to the pancreas or adjacent regional nodes (8–11 mo median survival) compared to no treatment or XRT alone (4–6 mo median survival) (table 32-3). Chemotherapy alone appears to be nearly equal in efficacy (8–11 mo) to combined modality therapy (table 32-2). However, early studies of chemotherapy alone versus XRT + chemotherapy were, with one exception, uncontrolled.[17]

Table 32-3. Pancreatic Cancer: Regional Disease

| | | Median survival (mo) | | |
Investigator	No. pts.	5-FU + XRT	XRT	Comment
Moertel, 1969	64	10[a]	6[a]	6 mo[b] no treatment
GITSG, 1981	194	11,8	5	XRT, only 25 pts.
Dobelbower, 1979	44	15	12	Not randomized
Klaassen, 1985	47	8	—	8 mo; 5-FU alone
				5-FU more toxic

| | | Prognostic issues | | |
		CT	XRT	
Mallinson, 1980	14	11 MIT + 5-FU + CMF	—	3 mo b;no treatment
Smith, 1983	17	8 FAM	—	5-FU + XRT superior historically
	47	8 FAM	—	See above
Bruckner, 1989	9	9 HexMF	—	HexMF
Douglas, 1987		SMF	—	6 mo; XRT + 5-FU superior

Key to abbreviations: 5-FU = 5-fluorouracil; XRT = radiotherapy; CT = chemotherapy; a = mean survival; b = survival of a "no treatment" control group; HexMF = hexamethylmelamine, mitomycin-C, 5-FU (see also table 32-2 key)

A double-blind trial demonstrated an improvement in mean survival when bolus 5-FU in a 3-day schedule was added to XRT.[18] This was confirmed when 5-FU was given with XRT, either 4,000 or 6,000 cGy, compared to 6,000 cGy without chemotherapy.[5] Small, independent studies of combined modality therapy produced similar results.[12,19] The burden of proof rests with the advocates of XRT because there was no clear practical survival advantage with more XRT.[5] Also, sites of failure analyses did not find any evidence demonstrating the efficacy of XRT in controlling local tumor growth.[20]

XRT combined with 5-FU or doxorubicin (ADR) produces similar (8–11 mo) median survival results.[21] Treatment with 5-FU is the best tested and the least toxic. Nevertheless, many considerations favor priority for attempts to improve both XRT and chemotherapy within the context of combined modality programs. Its only failure is questionable. Single-agent 5-FU was equal to XRT + 5-FU in an Eastern Cooperative Oncology Group (ECOG) trial;[19] however, the trial was slow to accrue patients, marginally small-sized, marked by high ineligibility rates, and had many clearly identified—and therefore possibly confounding—poor prognostic variables.

In multivariate analyses, combined modality treatment using XRT + 5-FU was slightly superior (see above) to historical comparison with the FAM regimen (5-FU + ADR + mitomycin-C [MIT]). The Gastrointestinal Tumor Study Group (GITSG) found that XRT + 5-FU was statistically superior to SMF, but the small size of the trial and the small advantages are not enough to resolve the question.[22]

Some factors favor continued use and development of XRT: Local progression in at least 50% of cases is the first evidence of progression and is clinically important; XRT alone is sometimes palliative. Published reports on combined modality treatment programs are all suboptimum tests of XRT because of their use of low dosages, undesirable split courses, or poor field plans. There is clear direction for improvement in the application of XRT as part of a combined modality strategy. Based on the best results with high-technology particle therapy, XRT alone offers no advantages; results only approach those consistently reproducible with combined modality therapy or chemotherapy alone.

Nonsurgically staged patients with apparent localized disease may also do well with simultaneous XRT and chemotherapy because this combines the best leads derived from clinical trials against both localized and small metastatic pancreatic cancer. A simultaneous attempt at local control with XRT need not compromise systemic therapy for suspected "occult" metastatic disease.

Computer modeling and sites of failure analyses suggest reserving surgery for responders or unequivocally stable good-risk patients (Bruckner, unpublished). Percutaneous stents can be used initially and for nonresponders, thereby avoiding much surgical morbidity and many early surgical deaths. Three phase 2 trials have found substantial improvement in local control when combination chemotherapy is used with XRT, either sequential FAP[23] or concurrently with F-MIT or with FSP.[13]

OCCULT METASTASES

Patients with "early metastatic" pancreatic cancer, without clinical evidence of distant metastases or with nonmeasurable metastases, represent the best candidates for survival-oriented trials. Chemotherapy probably improves survival, although modestly. Chemotherapy may be effective against small tumors in spite of its failure against large, measurable tumors. Cyclophosphamide (CTX) + methotrexate (MTX) + 5-FU, followed by MIT + 5-FU (CMF-MMF) and 5-FU induction and maintenance immediately after staging surgery was superior to observation alone.[24] Median survival increased from 9 to 44 wk.

Chemotherapy also appeared to increase survival in other early stages of disease relevant to small or "occult" disseminated pancreatic cancer.[4,5,18] Mallinson's regimen[24] may be similar in efficacy to 5-FU + MIT (FAM), STZ + MIT + 5-FU (SMF), and HexMF (table 32-3). Even 5-FU alone appears to be the equal of FA or FAM[22] and therefore possibly of the Mallinson regimen. Nevertheless, although controversial, survival-associated response[26] and me-

Table 32-4. Pancreatic Cancer: Selected Phase 2 Combinations

Investigator	Regimen	Response (%)	Comment
Bukowski, 1982	FAF-S	48	S*
Wiggans, 1978;	SMF	43–34–32	S
Bukowski, 1980 & 1983			S
Seligman, 1977	SF	21	—
Bitran, 1979;	FAM	40–37	SY[†]
Smith, 1980			
Steinberg, 1984	MIFA III	14–21	SY
Lokich, 1972;	5-FU + BCNU	60–33	S
Kovach, 1974			
Bruckner, 1983 & 1989	HexMF	22–23	SY

*Responders survive longer than patients with stable disease or progressive disease.
[†]Responders' median survival is 1 yr or more.
Additional comments: Streptozotocin and 5-FU combinations are most consistent in producing best rates of response. Doxorubicin and 5-FU combinations tend to produce responses associated with best median survival.
BCNU = carmustine (see also keys to tables 32-2 and 32-3)

Table 32-5. Pancreatic Cancer: Selected Phase 3 Trials

Investigator	Regimen		Comment
Mallinson, 1980	CMF-F (MIT) > Control	S	44 wk vs. 9 wk
Moertel, 1969	5-FU + XRT > XRT	S	—
Moertel, 1981	5-FU + XRT > XRT	S	—
Bukowski, 1983	SMF > MF	T	Active, survival effect for responders
Moertel, 1986	SMF > FAM	T	Marginally active, 2°R Best survival not significant
Buroker, 1978	5-FU–MIT > 5-FU–CCNU	T	Active, 33% vs. 17%
Kovach, 1974	5-FU–BCNU > 5-FU > BCNU	T	Active, 33% vs. 16% vs. 0%
Cullinan, 1985	FAM-FA-F	—	Active 21–30%, no survival impact, MST 16 wk
Oster, 1982	SMF-FAM	—	Barely active, 4% vs. 9% No benefit
Moertel, 1977	SF-SC	—	Barely active, 12% Majority complete response Survival 9–13 wk, <10%, 1 yr

Trials demonstrate response (R) and survival advantage (S) or survival trends (T) among responders; 2°R SMF produces responses with apparent benefit after other chemotherapy fails; CCNU = lomustine (see also keys to tables 32-2 and 32-3)

dian survival of the best 5-FU historical studies appear to be inferior to the results of the historical trials of combination therapy (tables 32-4 and 32-5).

Occult metastatic disease may be a major target for comparative and developmental trials due to the patient's uniformly poor prognosis without therapy and the evidence of some benefit of treatment. Also, they are sufficiently intact to tolerate therapeutic trials, and the primary tumor and perhaps markers can now be used to assess response.

MEASURABLE METASTATIC DISEASE

Some tumors regress, even completely. Response is associated with prolongation of useful median survival beyond 1 yr. The FAM-S, FAM, and SMF regimens (see Appendix) produce the best rates of response, but they do not improve overall survival (table 32-4).[19,20,23-31] Adding STZ to a combination probably improves the rate of response (table 32-4) and possibly tends to improve survival. STZ-containing regimens appear most consistent and most active in producing high rates of response compared with 5-FU or possibly even FAM.[40] Some trials of STZ-containing regimens, however, have failed to find any evidence of benefit.[41,42] The most recent look at SMF found clinically and statistically insignificant trends favoring SMF over FAM.[43]

The CT scan only recently has been used to define measurable disease. CT scan evidence of primary (pancreatic mass) tumor shrinkage is associated with improved survival.[43] Because the CT scan can measure smaller tumors in normally unevaluable locations, these patients may have a better prognosis than historical patients. It will be necessary to know the site(s) and size(s) of measurable disease and the method of measurement in order to avoid confusion in comparing future reports.

The route and schedule of 5-FU administration are both important: The oral route failed entirely in a controlled trial.[44] Infusion is incompletely tested but may be less toxic than bolus loading.[37] Other "active" drugs include STZ and possibly MIT. The case for MIT has been severely damaged by new trials and increasing evidence of its toxicities.[25] Similarly, the anthracyclines have produced highly inconsistent results in phase 2–3 trials. Marginally active drugs include semustine, ICRF-159, B-2-deoxythioguanosine, hexamethylmelamine, vindesine, and chlorozotocin. Rarely, single agents produce complete remissions (CRs) of good duration. None of these marginally active drugs represent viable options for combination or single-drug therapy unless there is a preclinical rationale for testing the drug (advantage against early disease, drug synergism, inhibition of tumor angiogenesis, or potentiation of XRT). An excellent response or long period without progression is still reason to review the diagnosis.

Anecdotally active, incompletely tested drugs include chlorambucil, lomustine, CTX, mechlorethamine, and high-dose MTX. The alkylating agents are not likely to be of benefit. Ifosfamide, active in 3 small trials, is of current interest.[40]

Advanced pancreatic cancer is sometimes resistant to chemotherapy for reasons other than classic drug resistance. Clonogenic assay studies find that tumors from individual patients are sensitive to drugs that fail in the treatment of the same patients. Patients with advanced disease may not be suitable subjects for "conclusive" phase 2 or phase 3 trials. Drugs demonstrating antitumor activity in the in vitro assay may need to be tested against early disease.

5-FU + ADR + MIT + STZ (FAM-S) is the most active combination (48%, 12/25 patients) reported to date.[29] Realistically, adding active drugs to 5-FU may only produce 10–20% increments in response rates. Only 10–25%—or at best, 30%—of tumors respond to any form of single drug chemotherapy. Because these results can affect only the tail of the survival curve, it is almost unrealistic to compare regimens due to the small size of past trials and the severe debility, fragile physiology, and poor prognosis of many patients in these advanced disease trials. Clinical judgment remains critical in selecting drugs that are safe enough for the individual patient. It is unlikely that one can produce a statistically demonstrable impact on survival of patients with advanced disease by testing the addition of any of the current drugs to 5-FU. This may not be the case with regional disease.

Anecdotally, leucovorin (LCV) appears to increase the frequency and quality of response to 5-FU, sometimes after failure of SMF or FAM. Early results include 3 CRs and 1 partial response among 8 patients.[46] Similar findings of response in patients failing 5-FU have followed LCV + 5-FU treatment of patients with 5-FU–resistant colon cancer. In phase 2 trials, PALA, in another biochemical modulation therapy, also appears to increase response compared to 5-FU alone.[47]

Research Efforts

Research efforts are centered on new drugs, biochemical modulation and radiosensitizers, and integrating methods of intraoperative and external beam XRT into a total treatment plan. Tests of monoclonal antibodies seek to improve both staging and therapy. Endocrine measures, tamoxifen, LhRH and somatostatin-like drugs, although they are clinically problematic, have achieved preclinical successes.

Preoperative chemotherapy and XRT may identify or produce patients with slow disease and the best chance of benefiting from surgery and additional intraoperative combined modality treatment. Neoadjuvant therapy has created an additional role for the endoscopically placed prosthesis.[48] The safety of preoperative XRT has been demonstrated, including the ability to perform radical surgery after XRT.[13,15] Its efficacy probably will be improved by more complex drug therapy, as this is largely the experience in controlled trials of regional inoperable cancer.

References

1. Borg JW, Connelly RR. Updating the epidemiologic data on pancreatic cancer. Semin Oncol 1979; 6:275–83.
2. Cubilla AL, Fitzgerald P. Cancer of the pancreas (non-endocrine): a suggested morphologic classification. Semin Oncol 1979; 6:285–97.
3. Monassa AR, Levin B. Collaborative studies in the diagnosis of pancreatic cancer. Semin Oncol 1979; 6:298–308.
4. Gastrointestinal Tumor Study Group. Pancreatic cancer: adjuvant combined radiation and chemotherapy following curative resection. Arch Surg 1985; 120:899–903.
5. Douglass HO Jr, Stablein DM. Ten-year follow-up of first generation surgical adjuvant studies of the Gastrointestinal Tumor Study Group. In: Salmon SE, ed. Adjuvant therapy of cancer VI. Proc 6th Int Conf Adj Ther Cancer, Tucson Ariz March 1990. Philadelphia: Saunders, 1990; 405–15.
6. Bruckner HW, Storch JA, Brown JC, Goldberg J, Chamberlin K. Phase II trial of combination chemotherapy for pancreatic cancer with 5-fluorouracil, mitomycin-C, and hexamethylmelamine. Oncology 1983; 40:165–69.

7. Schein P, Levin B. Neoplasm of the pancreas: In: Calabresi P, Schein PS, Rosenberg SA, eds. Medical oncology. Basic principles and clinical management of cancer. New York: MacMillan, 1985; 828–50.

8. Andren-Sandberg A, Ihse I. Factors influencing survival after total pancreatectomy in patients with pancreatic cancer. Ann Surg 1983; 198:605–10.

9. Warshaw AL, Gu Z-y, Wittenberg J, Waltman AC. Preoperative staging and assessment of resectability of pancreatic cancer. Arch. Surg., 125:230–233, 1990.

10. Douglass HO Jr, and Holyoke ED. Pancreatic cancer: initial treatment as the determinant of survival. JAMA, 229:793–797, 1974.

11. Crile G Jr. The advantages of bypass operations over radical pancreatoduodenectomy in the treatment of pancreatic carcinoma. Surg Gynecol Obstet 1970; 13:1049–53.

12. Nori D, Hilaris BS. Intraoperative brachytherapy in pancreatic cancer. Cancer Invest 1988; 6:695–704.

13. Bruckner HW, Kalnicki S, Sung MW, et al. Combined modality therapy for stage II pancreatic cancer with simultaneous radiotherapy, 5-fluorouracil (FU) infusion, streptozotocin, and cisplatin with leucovorin and FU maintenance. Proc Am Assoc Cancer Res 1989; 30:1024.

14. Weese JL, Nussbaum ML, Paul AR, et al. Increased resectability of locally advanced pancreatic and periampullary carcinoma with neoadjuvant chemoradiotherapy. Int J Pancreatol 1991 (in press).

15. Pilepich MV, Miller HH. Preoperative irradiation in carcinoma of the pancreas. Cancer 1979; 46:1945–49.

16. Kopelson G. Curative surgery for adenocarcinoma of the pancreas/ampulla of vater: The role of adjuvant pre or postoperative radiation therapy. Int J Radiat Oncol Biol Phys 1983; 9:911–15.

17. Klaassen DJ, MacIntyre JM, Catton GE, Engstrom PF, Moertel CG. Treatment of locally unresectable cancer of the stomach and pancreas: a randomized comparison of 5-fluorouracil alone with radiation plus concurrent and maintenance 5-fluorouracil. An Eastern Cooperative Oncology Group study. J Clin Oncol 1985; 3(3):373–78.

18. Moertel CG, Childs DS, Reitemeier RJ, Colby MY, Holbrook MA. Combined 5-fluorouracil and supervoltage radiation therapy for locally unresectable gastrointetinal cancer. Lancet 1969; 2:865–67.

19. Dobelbower RR Jr. The radiotherapy of pancreatic cancer. Semin Oncol 1979; 6:378–89.

20. Bruckner HW, Stablein DM (for the Gastrointestinal Tumor Study Group). Sites of treatment failure: Gastrointestinal Tumor Study Group analyses of gastric, pancreatic, and colorectal trials. Cancer Treat Symp 1983; 2:199–210.

21. Douglass HO Jr, Thomas PRM, Stablein DM (for Gastrointestinal Tumor Study Group). Radiation therapy combined with Adriamycin or 5-fluorouracil for the treatment of locally unresectable pancreatic carcinoma. Cancer 1985; 56:2563–68.

22. Douglass HO Jr, Stablein D (for the Gastrointestinal Tumor Study Group). A randomized comparison of radiation plus streptozotocin + mitomycin + 5-fluorouracil (SMF) versus SMF alone for locally unresectable pancreatic carcinoma. Proc Am Soc Clin Oncol 1987; 6:76.

23. Wagener D, van Hoesel Q, Hoogenraad W, Strijk S, Wobbes T, Yap S. A phase II study of 5-FU, Adriamycin and cisplatin (FAP) followed by a split course irradiation in combination with 5-FU for locally advanced pancreatic cancer. Proc Am Soc Clin Oncol 1987; 6:77.

24. Mallinson CN, Rake MO, Cocking JB, et al. Chemotherapy in pancreatic cancer: results of a controlled prospective, randomized multicentre trial. Br Med J 1980; 281:1589–91.

25. Cullinan SA, Moertel CG, Fleming TR, et al (for the North Central Cancer Treatment Group). A comparison of three chemotherapeutic regimens in the treatment of advanced pancreatic and gastric carcinoma. Fluorouracil vs. fluorouracil and doxorubicin vs. fluorouracil, doxorubicin, and mitomycin. JAMA 1985; 253:2061–67.

26. Cullinan S, Moertel C, Wieand H. A phase III evaluation of drug combinations in the therapy of advanced pancreatic cancer. Proc Am Soc Clin Oncol 1989; 8:124.

27. Smith FP, Stablein D, Korsmeyer S, et al. Combination chemotherapy for locally advanced pancreatic cancer: Equivalence to external beam irradiation and implication for future management. J Clin Oncol 1983; 1(7):413–15.

28. Wiggans RG, Woolley PV III, Macdonald JS, Smythe T, Ueno W, Schein PS. Phase II trial of streptozotocin, mitomycin-C, and 5-fluorouracil (SMF) in the treatment of advanced pancreatic cancer. Cancer 1978; 41:387–91.

29. Bukowski RM, Schacter LP, Groppe CW, Hewlett JS, Weick JK, Livingston RB. Phase II trial of 5-fluorouracil, adrimaycin, mitomycin-C, and streptozotocin (FAM-S) in pancreatic carcinoma. Cancer 1982; 50:197–200.

30. Bukowski RM, Abderhalden RT, Hewlett JS, Weick JK, Groppe CW Jr. Phase II trial of streptozotocin, mitomycin-C, and 5-fluorouracil in adenocarcinoma of the pancreas. Cancer Clin Trials 1980; 3:321–24.

31. Seligman M, Bukowski RM, Groppe CW Jr, et al. Chemotherapy of metastatic gastrointestinal neoplasms with 5-fluorouracil and streptozotocin. Cancer Treat Rep 1977; 61:1375–77.

32. Bitran JD, Desser RK, Kozloff MF, Bilings AA, Shapiro CM. Treatment of metastatic pancreatic and gastric adenocarcinomas with 5-fluorouracil, Adriamycin and mitomycin-C (FAM). Cancer Treat Rep 1979; 63:2049–51.

33. Smith FP, Hoth DF, Levin BL, et al. 5-fluorouracil, Adriamycin and mitomycin-C (FAM) chemotherapy for advanced adenocarcinoma of the pancreas. Cancer 1980; 46:2014–18.

34. Sternberg CN, Magill GB, Sordillo PP, Cheng EW. MIFA III (mitomycin-C, 5-fluorouracil, and adriamycin) chemotherapy for advanced adenocarcinoma of the pancreas. Am J Clin Oncol 1984; 7(5):529–33.

35. Lokich J, Chawla PL, Brooks J, et al. Chemotherapy in pancreatic carcinoma: 5-fluorouracil (5-FU) and 1,3-Bis-(2-chlorethyl)-1-nitrosourea (BCNU). Ann Surg 1974; 179:450–53.

36. Kovach JS, Moertel CG, Schutt AJ, Hahn RG, Reitemeier RJ. A controlled study of 1,3 bis-(2-chlorethyl)-1-nitrosourea and 5-fluorouracil therapy for advanced gastric and pancreatic cancer. Cancer 1974; 33:563–67.

37. Bruckner HW, Kalman J, Gorbaty I, et al. Primary treatment of regional and disseminated pancreatic cancer with hexamethylmelamine, mitomycin-C and 5-fluorouracil infusion. Oncology 1989; 46:366–71.

38. Buroker T, Kim PN, Heilbrun L, Vaitkevicius V. 5-FU infusion with mitomycin-C (MMC) vs. 5-FU infusion with methyl-CCNU (Me) in the treatment of advanced upper gastrointestinal cancer. A phase III study. Proc Am Soc Clin Oncol 1978; 19:310.

39. Bukowski RM, Balcerzak SP, O'Bryan RM, Bonnett JD, Chen TT. Randomized trial of 5-fluorouracil and mitomycin-C with or without streptozotocin for advanced pancreatic cancer. A Southwest Oncology Group study. Cancer 1983; 52:1577–82.

40. Oster MW, Theologides A, Cooper MR, et al. Fluorouracil (f), Adriamycin (A), and mitomycin-C (M) (FAM) versus fluorouracil (F), streptozotocin (S), and mitomycin-C (M) (FSM) in advanced pancreatic cancer. Proc Am Soc Clin Oncol 1982; 1:90.

41. Moertel CG, Douglass HO Jr, Hanley J, et al. Treatment of advanced adenocarcinoma of the pancreas with combinations of streptozotocin plus 5-fluorouracil and streptozotocin plus cyclophosphamide. Cancer 1977; 40:605–08.

42. Moertel CG, Stablein DM (for the Gastrointestinal Tumor Study Group). Phase II studies of drug combinations in advanced pancreatic carcinoma: fluorouracil plus doxorubicin plus mitomycin C and two regimens of streptozotocin plus mitomycin C plus fluorouracil. J Clin Oncol 1986; 4:1794–98.

43. Barkin JS, Lindblad AS, Bruckner HW (for the Gastrointestinal Tumor Study Group). The evaluation of CT and sonographic pancreatic measurements in determining tumor response. Proc Am Soc Clin Oncol 1986; 5:22.

44. Stolinsky DC, Pugh RP, Batemena JR. 5-fluorouracil (NSC-19893) therapy for pancreatic carcinoma: comparison of oral and intravenous routes. Cancer Chemother Rep 1975; 59:1031–33.

45. Loehrer PJ Sr, Williams SD, Einhorn LH, Ansari R. Ifosfamide: An active drug in the treatment of adenocarcinoma of the pancreas. J Clin Oncol 1985; 3(3):367–72.

46. Bruckner HW, Crown J, McKenna A, Hart R. Leucovorin and 5-fluorouracil as a treatment for disseminated cancer of the pancreas and unknown primary tumors. Cancer Res 1988; 48:5570–72.

47. Schilder RJ, Paul AR, Walczak J, et al. Phase II trial of PALA/5-fluorouracil in pancreatic cancer. Proc Am Soc Clin Oncol 1990; 9:109.

48. Siegel JH, Snody H. The significance of endoscopically placed prostheses in the management of biliary obstruction due to carcinoma of the pancreas: results of nonoperative decompression in 277 patients. Am J Gastroenterol 1986; 81:634–41.

33

PRIMARY CARCINOMA OF THE LIVER AND BILIARY DUCTS

C. Julian Rosenthal, M.D., F.A.C.P.

PRIMARY CANCER OF THE liver and of the biliary tract are related diseases in that a major histologic type of liver cancer originates in the intrahepatic bile ducts, which have structure identical with that of the extrahepatic bile ducts and the gallbladder. Nonetheless, the epidemiology and clinical presentation of the gallbladder and extrahepatic biliary ducts carcinoma generally differ from those of the intrahepatic carcinoma; for these reasons, these 2 entities will be separately presented.

Primary Carcinoma of the Liver

Incidence and Histologic Classification

Primary cancer of the liver is a rare disease in the United States, representing <1% of all neoplastic diseases. It accounts for about 6,000 new cases of cancer yearly, almost all fatal, and 1% of all cancer deaths in this country and in Europe. The 2 principal histologic types of cancer of the liver are hepatocellular carcinoma (hepatoma), arising from hepatocytes, and cholangiocarcinoma, arising from the intrahepatic biliary system. Hepatocellular carcinoma predominates, with a ratio of 10–30:1; mixed forms can rarely occur. Other rare forms of primary liver cancer include (1) angiosarcoma, a fast-growing and always fatal malignancy whose etiology is related to exposure to the chemical agents thorotrast, vinyl chloride, and arsenic; (2) hepatoblastoma in children, particularly infants, usually a solitary tumor highly curable by surgical resection; and (3) a variety of sarcomas and lymphomas that can originate in the liver, although rarely. The following discussion will refer exclusively to the 2 most common forms of carcinoma of the liver— hepatocellular carcinoma and cholangiocarcinoma.

Epidemiology

Because hepatocellular carcinoma has unique geographic incidence rates throughout the world, it is thought to be caused by environmental factors. A high incidence is encountered in the eastern regions of China, Thailand, and northern Africa, where the disease may account for 30–40% of all cancer deaths. Nearly all patients (97%) have been exposed to the hepatitis B virus. In some areas with high incidence of hepatocellular carcinoma, especially in North Africa, aflatoxin (a mold toxin) was found in the canned food consumed by many patients who developed the disease.

Finally, cirrhosis of the liver following hepatitis B (macronodular), but more frequently caused by chronic ethanol drinking (micronodular), was found to be frequently associated with hepatocellular carcinoma. It has been roughly calculated that hepatocellular carcinoma may develop in 3–10% of patients with alcoholic cirrhosis, 10% of those with posthepatic cirrhosis, 20% of patients with hemochromatosis and cirrhosis, and in 40% of cases of cirrhosis caused by alpha 1 antitrypsin deficiency (cases in which a genetic susceptibility is evident).[2] There are also reports of clustering of hepatocellular carcinoma cases in a few families,[3] sometimes in association with adenomas.[2]

Another factor with a debatable role in the etiology of hepatocellular carcinoma is oral contraceptives taken regularly for >6 mo; however, the fact that there are only 100 cases of such an association raises the possibility that this is just a random phenomenon among the >10 million women taking oral contraceptives.[4] The case is much stronger for benign liver adenomas, which have been reported during the last decade as occurring almost exclusively in women taking oral contraceptives.

The only etiologic factor described with increased incidence among patients with cholangiocarcinoma in the Orient was the high incidence of infestation with the parasite *Opisthorchis sinensis.*[5]

Clinical Presentation

The clinical presentation of hepatocellular carcinoma and cholangiocarci- noma is frequently nonspecific; a few cases in all series are discovered only at surgery. The most common symptoms are vague epigastric pressure, discom- fort, and early satiety. A dull upper abdominal pain, abdominal distension, and a palpable abdominal mass are also frequently noted. In <30% of cases, patients present with fever, ascites, and acute abdominal pain. On rare occasions, patients present with signs of peritonitis due to rupture of the tumor mass into the peritoneum and massive intra-abdominal hemorrhage.

Because of the propensity of hepatocellular carcinoma to invade veins, symptoms of accelerated portal hypertension, ascites, and esophageal bleeding may herald development of cancer. Occasionally, the tumor may invade the inferior vena cava (see chapter 10, figures 10-1 to 10-3), the right heart, and even the pulmonary artery, with the respective symptoms caused by the vessel occlusion.

In 1–3% of cases, hepatocellular carcinomas are accompanied by paraneoplastic syndromes, including (1) hypoglycemia due to a proinsulin peptide secretion or due to the extensive involvement of the liver with consequent decreased glycogenolysis; (2) polycythemia due to the secretion of an erythropoietin-like peptide; and (3) fever due to a pyrogen secreted by the tumor.

Cholangiocarcinomas were not found to be associated with paraneoplastic syndromes. Their clinical presentation is similar to that of hepatocellular carcinoma, with the exception that they are more frequently solitary in the liver and less commonly associated with liver cirrhosis. They have no propensity for intravascular growth or rupture in the peritoneal cavity and have less propensity for diffuse intrahepatic growth than hepatocellular carcinoma.

Particularly in areas in which the disease is endemic, the cause of death in patients with hepatocellular carcinoma is hemorrhage in almost 50% of cases. Site of hemorrhage is equally divided between esophageal varices and the abdomen (from rupture of the tumor). Hepatic failure is usually the cause of death in the other 50% of cases.

In <20% of cases, patients may die from metastases; these were found in up to 32% of cases at autopsy but in only 8% of cases at diagnosis. Frequent sites of metastases are bone and lung.

Histopathology

The common histopathologic presentations of hepatocellular carcinoma are: a soft vascular lesion that can develop as a solitary mass; a primary large lesion with multiple surrounding satellite lesions; or diffuse nodules throughout the liver, suggesting a multifocal origin. Individual lesions may be pale or evenly stained by bile stain and are not fibrotic. Four grades of pathologic differentiation are recognized. The first grade is a well differentiated tumor with a papillary or trabecular pattern (see chapter 11, figure 11-35); the second grade has an alveolar pattern (see chapter 11, figure 11-36); the third grade presents as a so-called solid pattern; and the fourth grade is undifferentiated, with either a predominant small-cell component or a syncitial pattern.

The cholangiocarcinoma tends to be firm, fibrotic, and relatively avascular. (see chapter 11, figure 11-38). Unlike hepatocellular carcinomas, this tumor generally does not penetrate vessels. The usual growth of hepatocellular carcinoma is rapid, with a doubling time as short as 5–7 days. However, in ≤10% of cases, hepatocellular carcinomas can present as encapsulated tumors that are unifocal and may achieve large sizes without metastases; they have a distinctly lower growth rate and may progress over several years.

Prognosis and Treatment

Median survival duration for hepatocellular carcinoma is only 4–6 mo in most of the series. Occasionally, patients survive longer, but rarely beyond 2 yr from time of diagnosis. More differentiated histology (papillary, trabecular, or alveolar) is generally accompanied by longer survival.

Survival rates in a large series from Japan that included resected cases were 22% at 1 yr, 5% at 3 yr, and 2% at 5 yr. Only 6/22 patients surviving at 5 yr had their lesions resected, but 1 patient survived 10 yr without resection.[5] Survival generally correlates with the level and the rapidity of the rise of the level of alpha-fetoprotein (AFP).[5] It had a mean of 7.6 mo for AFP elevations >5000 U, 16 mo for lower AFP levels, and 34 mo with no AFP elevation. However, in patients with no AFP elevation were a few anaplastic hepatoma cases whose mean survival was only 3.8 mo. The overall survival for cholangiocarcinomas is also short: 20% at 1 yr, 3% at 3 yr, and 1% at 5 yr.[5]

Among the less common types of primary liver cancer, the angiosarcomas have a median survival of 5 mo (range: 2–22 mo). Hepatoblastomas seen in children can be resected and cured in 50% of cases; the remaining cases have an aggressive course, with a mean survival around 5 mo.

In primary cancer of the liver, resection currently represents the only possibility for cure. The significant capacity for regeneration and the ability of small fragments of liver to sustain function make possible the resection of even 70–80% of the organ. Unfortunately, only 5–20% of patients with primary liver cancer are acceptable candidates for surgical resection. They must have disease limited to 1 lobe, independent blood supply and biliary drainage for the portion of the liver left after resection (proven by angiography and cholecystography), normal liver function, no evidence of liver cirrhosis, no liver enzyme abnormalities, and no extrahepatic lesions. A current controversy concerns the resectability of multiple lesions in the same lobe. Niederhuber and Ensminger are advocates of resection of multiple lesions if at exploration the other lobe of the liver is free of disease.[6] Others believe that multiple lesions indicate the likely presence of microscopic lesions in the opposite lobe and consequently are a contraindication to resection, a fact supported by the very low 3-yr survival rate for patients with more than 1 hepatic primary lesion. One recommendation—not validated in controlled studies—is that surgical exploration be performed in all patients with primary liver cancer without extrahepatic metastases in order to insert at least a Silastic catheter in the hepatic artery for floxuridine (FUdR) administration in cases in which resection is not possible.[6] External beam irradiation with concomitant infusion chemotherapy may be equally effective in the same cases.[8]

Liver transplantation for primary cancer of the liver represents another surgical approach that has been tested primarily at the universities of Colorado and Cambridge.[6] Half of the 50 patients receiving transplants to date survived >3 mo, but 95% developed distant metastases and were dead within 1 yr. Thus, this is not yet a technique ready for broader clinical application.[20]

Chemotherapy has been tested extensively in hepatocellular carcinoma. Among numerous agents tested, doxorubicin (ADR) and 5-fluorouracil (5-FU) gave the best results by I.V. administration. ADR administered as an I.V. push at a dose of 60–100 mg/m^2/day q. 3 wk induced partial remission (PR) in 18–35% of cases in a number of studies.[7] The response rate to I.V. 5-FU 500 mg/m^2/day ×5 q. 4 wk was 15–25%. Combination chemotherapy did not lead to better results.

In all studies, patients responding to chemotherapy had a median survival duration of 7–9 mo—at least twice as long as patients who did not respond. Due to these relatively poor results of I.V. therapy, regional infusion chemotherapy in the intrahepatic artery through catheters attached to implantable pumps that can be refilled percutaneously has been extensively tested during the past 5 yr. ADR 2 mg/m^2/day for 3 wk or 12 mg/m^2/day × 5 q. 4–6 wk and FUdR 0.3 mg/m^2/day for 3 wk q. 5–6 wk to date have led to mixed results. The response rate was improved to 30–40% of all cases, but the median survival of the responders remained the same.[7] Recombinant alpha 2 interferon was also recently used in the treatment of inoperable hepatocellular carcinoma and was found to be superior to doxorubicin in a prospective, randomized trial.[21]

Another experimental method of delivering chemotherapy locally for protracted periods is the selective intrahepatic artery infusion of microcapsules (microbeads) containing mitomycin-C (MIT) or ADR, which is slowly released. This technique induced a 65% tumor reduction in a preliminary study.[8]

Radiation therapy (XRT) administered as external beam irradiation has only limited impact on primary cancer of the liver because of the poor tolerance of hepatic tissue for XRT alone. It tolerates a maximum total dose of 3,500 cGy, which does not have curative effect on hepatocellular carcinoma, but could be administered either for palliation of pain due to tumor infiltration of Glisson's capsule or for relief of intrahepatic or porta hepatis obstruction of the biliary tray due to enlarged lymph nodes. The efficacy of XRT appears to be enhanced by the concomitant administration of chemotherapy with ADR 12 mg/m^2/day × 5 q. 3 wk[9] or by its intralesional delivery as radioactive iodine labeled to an antibody to ferritin, found to have special affinity for hepatoma cells.[10] This delivery was accompanied by I.V. administration of ADR. In both of these experimental regimens, good PRs are seen in about 30% of cases with limited disease (≤ 3 lesions in the same lobe), with a mean duration of remission of 11–14 mo. No responses were seen among patients with multiple lesions.

Carcinoma of the Extrahepatic Biliary Tract and of the Gallbladder

Epidemiology

Carcinoma of the gallbladder (GB) and extrahepatic biliary ducts (EBD) ranks fifth in incidence among G.I. carcinomas, with 2.5–4.4 cases per 100,000 population in the United States each year.[11] It is diagnosed in 1–2% of all operations for biliary tract pathology.[11] Its peak incidence is in the sixth and seventh decades of life. Whereas GB carcinoma occurs 3 times more frequently in women than men, EBD carcinoma is seen just slightly more frequently among men.

The precise etiology of GB and EBD carcinoma is unknown, but significant epidemiologic associations have been established. In 74–92% of patients with GB carcinoma, gallstones were found at surgery, whereas only 30% of patients with EBD carcinoma have gallstones.[11] The relative risk for GB carcinoma increases with stone size—from 2.4 for patients with stones 2.0–2.9 cm in diameter to 10.1 for patients with stones >3.0 cm in diameter. In calcified GBs, carcinomas occur in 22% of cases.[11] Epithelial dysplasia, atypical hyperplasia, and carcinoma *in situ* are found in the gallbladder and biliary ducts in 83%, 13.5%, and 3.5%, respectively, of patients with gallstones, as well as in those with cholecystitis and chronic inflammation of the extrahepatic biliary ducts. This pattern represents the successive steps of mucosal transition toward carcinoma. Sclerosing cholangitis, chronic suppurative cholangitis, biliary parasites, and typhoid carrier's cholangitis were all reported as predisposing to carcinoma of the bile ducts due to local dysplastic events. Finally, a higher incidence of EBD carcinoma was found among patients with ulcerative colitis, in some cases occurring many years after bowel resection.[12]

Adenomatous polyps and metaplasia are thought to represent premalignant conditions. Smaller polyps (<12 mm in diameter) are less likely to harbor carcinomas than are larger polyps.[13] It was possible to trace histologically the transition from benign adenomas to carcinomas; foci of residual adenomas are found in 20% of patients with invasive GB carcinoma.[13]

Finally, mucosal metaplasia of the GB and EBD was also found in patients with chronic reflux of pancreatic fluid, due usually to an anomalous confluence of the distal pancreatic and bile ducts above the ductal sphincter. This aberration ultimately leads to an increased incidence of GB and EBD carcinoma in patients without stones.

Pathology and Staging

Most GB and EBD carcinomas are pure adenocarcinomas, 1–2% are anaplastic carcinomas, and 8–10% of GB carcinomas are adenoacanthomas. Morphologically, GB carcinomas are infiltrating and desmoplastic, although 15% may be purely papillary and 9% are predominantly mucinous.[13]

EBD carcinomas, along with tumors of the intrahepatic biliary ducts (which together are also called cholangiocarcinomas (see chapter 11, figure 11-38), can be divided morphologically in 3 categories: sclerosing (70% of cases), nodular (10%), and papillary (20%). Proximal cancers tend to be nodular, whereas distal cancers are frequently papillary and carry a relatively better prognosis. Half of EBD carcinomas occur proximally in the hepatic duct or at the duct confluence, 25% occur in the suprapancreatic common duct, and 20% in the intrapancreatic common bile duct. Multifocal lesions occur in <5% of patients.

Regardless of histology, the patterns of spread of GB and EBD carcinoma are similar. Advanced local and regional disease is the hallmark of this disease at presentation. The gallbladder fossa of the liver is invaded in 69–83% of patients with GB carcinoma. Direct invasion of the surrounding structures (liver, portal vein, pancreas) and extension into the bile ducts and frequently into the duodenum and transverse colon occur in ≤70% of cases, although direct microscopic invasion of the liver and peritoneal seeding by GB carcinoma have been found in <12% and 10% of cases, respectively, at time of diagnosis. Invasion or encasement of the portal vein or hepatic artery occurs in 15% of cases, and regional lymphatic metastases in the cystic, choledochal, and pancreaticoduodenal lymph nodes are seen in 40–70% of cases. Distant lymphatic metastases along the aorta and inferior vena cava are found in 25% of cases. During the course of disease, noncontiguous metastases to liver, lung, and bone are found in 66%, 24%, and 12%, respectively, of patients with GB carcinoma; 90% of these patients will have perineural invasion.

There is no uniform staging classification for GB and EBD cancer. Nevin has classified GB carcinoma as follows: stage I—intramucosal involvement only (*in situ*); stage II—involvement of the mucosa and muscularis; stage III—transmural involvement; stage IV—transmural and cystic lymph node involvement; and stage V—contiguous or metastatic liver involvement or distant metastases.[14] Only patients in stages I and II, representing <25% of all patients, survive a median of 5 yr.

Clinical Presentation and Diagnosis

Symptoms and signs of GB carcinoma are nonspecific and occur insidiously with advanced disease. Clinical findings associated with early carcinoma reflect concurrent biliary tract disease. Pain occurs in 75% of cases; jaundice due to obstruction of the neighboring extrahepatic biliary tree in 45%; nausea, vomiting, and anorexia in 40%; and weight loss in 37%. An abdominal mass, jaundice, and hepatomegaly are predominant physical signs that reflect advanced disease.

Virtually all patients with EBD carcinoma present with painless obstructive jaundice that is often insidious in onset. Half of patients have bilirubin 13 mg/100 ml. In rare occasions when only a single hepatic duct is obstructed, patients are not icteric, but they have increased alkaline phosphatase or gamma glutamyl transferase. Weight loss, pruritus, steatorrhea, and anemia symptoms are also frequently encountered. Jaundice and hepatomegaly are the most common physical findings of EBD carcinoma. A palpable distended gallbladder (Curvoisier's sign) is also frequently encountered unless the gallbladder wall has been thickened by previous unrelated attacks of cholecystitis and cholelithiasis. Following the onset of jaundice, clinical deterioration rapidly occurs, with intervening biliary sepsis and hepatocellular failure (spider nevi, ascites, palmar erythema), then increased ammonia level within a period of 6 mo.

Although EBD carcinoma is always suspected in cases of obstructive jaundice, the preoperative diagnosis of GB carcinoma is uncommon; still, recent advances in biliary tract imaging have provided alternatives for increasing the diagnostic yield.

Ultrasonography can diagnose early GB carcinoma if suspected; it is also the primary imaging modality in screening for biliary tract disease. Early tumors can be recognized as a polypoid mass projecting in the gallbladder lumen or as a focal thickening of the gallbladder wall. The newest ultrasound equipment can detect a mass as small as a 5 mm in diameter. Ultrasonography also can define the extent of the disease by detecting bile duct obstruction, regional lymphadenopathy, and hepatic metastases in conjunction with a mass in the gallbladder.

Ultrasonography is also the procedure of choice for detecting bile duct obstruction by cholangiocarcinoma, the main ultrasonographic features of which are proximal ductal dilatation, focal narrowing and thickening of the duct, persistent intraluminal soft-tissue echoes, and echogenic transluminal bands. Ultrasonography is accurate in 90% of cases of bile duct obstruction. As in GB carcinoma, it can also detect the extent of the disease and the presence of lymph node or liver metastases. CT imaging is helpful primarily in defining GB carcinoma but can also recognize the dilatation of bile ducts in an obstruction. The main CT scan findings (see chapter 10, figure 10-9) in cases of GB carcinoma are diffuse or focal gallbladder wall thickness of >0.5 mm and gallbladder wall contrast enhancement (95% of cases), an intraluminal mass (90%), direct invasion of the liver (85%), lymphadenopathy (65%), gallstones (50%), dilated bile ducts (50%), noncontiguous liver metastases (20%), G.I. tract invasion (8%), and intraluminal gallbladder gas (4%). Both CT and ultrasonography can be used for guidance of percutaneous needle biopsy performed to confirm the diagnosis of GB and EBD carcinoma.

Cholangiography has little diagnostic value in GB carcinoma, but is a prerequisite diagnostic procedure for defining the operability and resectability of EBD carcinoma. Percutaneous transhepatic cholangiography is preferred over endoscopic cholangiography because the intrahepatic ductal extension of the tumor and the intrahepatic ductal anatomy available for bilioenteric bypass is better defined. Tumors without bilateral involvement of the secondary intrahepatic ducts are potentially resectable; visceral angiography should subsequently be employed to verify or rule out resectability. Criteria for unresectability for carcinoma of the proximal bile ducts include (1) bilateral intrahepatic spread beyond second-order ducts on cholangiography or multifocal disease, (2) involvement of the main trunk of the portal vein, (3) bilateral involvement of hepatic artery or portal vein structures, and (4) vascular involvement of one side of the liver with contralateral extensive ductal involvement.

Prognosis and Treatment

The overall survival of patients with GB and EBD carcinoma is poor. Median survival at 5 yr is <5%, with the exception of patients with carcinoma of the distal intrapancreatic duct (Vater's ampulla), whose 5-yr survival reaches 40%.

The introduction of percutaneous and endoscopic intubation of the biliary tract in cases of biliary duct obstruction has provided new therapeutic options in the management of the patient with malignant obstructive jaundice. It is primarily used as a definitive palliative procedure for patients who are clearly beyond the possibility of a curative surgical resection. A preliminary trial comparing endoscopic endoprosthesis with surgical bypass in 37 patients has revealed a mortality of 5% for endoprosthesis and 21% for surgery.[16] The use of endoscopic endoprosthesis for preoperative drainage is not recommended because it did not decrease the operative mortality but, in fact, prolonged hospitalization because of its significant morbidity.[11]

SURGERY

About 15–25% of patients with GB carcinoma have tumors in stages I to III disease that appear grossly resectable for cure. Additionally, some patients with stage IV disease and a few with stage V who have only gross focal invasion of the liver are candidates for extensive surgical resection, including cholecystectomy, resection of the gallbladder fossa of the liver, regional lymphadenectomy, and focal resection of the liver. However, this type of radical surgery performed in cases with advanced disease results in only an occasional survivor at 5 yr. This target is reached after surgery by 12% of patients with stage III disease with intramural invasion and 70–80% of cases with stages I and II disease.

Limited results with surgery also are seen for patients with EBD carcinoma. Frequently, surgery has only the palliative intent of establishing a bilioenteric bypass. When it is performed with curative intent, the extent of resection is dependent on tumor location and may require en bloc resection of the head of the pancreas and of part of the duodenum, as in Whipple's procedure; radical pancreaticoduodenectomy, recommended for the carcinoma of the distal common duct; en bloc cholecystectomy and resection of the hepatic and supraduodenal common duct; lymphadenectomy of the cystic and choledochal nodes; or Y hepaticojejunostomy for carcinoma of the midduct. Resection of a tumor of the proximal bile duct incorporates the procedures used for midduct tumors and extends the resection proximally to include the confluence of the hepatic bile ducts and a segmental or lobar resection of the liver, if invaded. Although Whipple's procedure as performed in cases of distal EBD carcinoma has been demonstrated to lead to 5-yr survival in 16–68% of cases, with an average of 42% and perioperative mortality that has decreased to 3%,[11] 5-yr survival after radical resection of midduct or proximal duct tumors is only anecdotal. Combined results from 3 major hepatobiliary units indicate that proximal and midduct radical resections, including the adjacent portion of the liver, can be performed in <30% of cases, with 16.6% operative mortality and median survival of 30 mo.[11] Survival decreases to 20 mo in less specialized centers.

In cases treated palliatively, mean survival after tumor resection and decompression is 12–16 mo. Mean survival of patients who have undergone percutaneous or endoscopic decompression is 2–9 mo. Still, the difference is not statistically significant, and the operative procedure may not be indicated for most patients with poor performance status.

RADIOTHERAPY

GB and EBD tumors are generally radiosensitive; still, responses to radiation therapy (XRT) have been limited. External beam irradiation has led to objective responses, including palliation of pain and jaundice, in 80% of patients. However, median survival has not exceeded 11 mo.[11] Similarly, intraoperative XRT in patients with stage IV disease has led to objective responses, but their median survival was only 6 mo. Half of XRT failures occur locally or regionally.[17]

In patients with EBD carcinoma of the intrabile duct, boost transcatheter ^{192}iridium irradiation has been administered in conjunction with external beam radiation. This led to a mean survival of 11–12 mo and significant morbidity (bile duct stenosis, biliary sepsis, liver dysfunction). Concomitant XRT with continuous I.V. infusion of 5-FU as radiosensitizer seems to prolong median survival, but definitive results of a randomized study are not yet available. The role of adjuvant XRT following curative resection is unknown. In a nonrandomized study, a significant prolongation of survival after adjuvant radiotherapy was suggested.[22]

CHEMOTHERAPY

The role of chemotherapy in GB and EBD carcinoma has not been fully defined, primarily because of the poor performance status of patients referred for such therapy and the overall low incidence of these tumors. A few chemotherapeutic agents—5-FU MIT, ADR, and streptozotocin—used either alone or in combinations (see Appendix) have led to limited and rare objective responses (5–30% of cases). Median duration of response was 8.5–18 mo.[18] Hepatic arterial infusion of MIT with or without systemic 5-FU has led to increased survival over historical controls.[19] Adjuvant chemotherapy has not been investigated.

Overall, treatment of biliary tract neoplasms is still limited in scope, and results indicate that new therapeutic approaches are needed.

References

1. Underwood JCH, Huek P. Thorotrait-associated hepatic angiosarcoma with 36 years latency. Cancer 1978; 46:2610–12.
2. Cady B. Natural history of primary and secondary tumors of the liver. Semin Oncol 1983; 127–34.
3. Hagstrom RM, Ho YC. Family cancers among cases of primary liver cancer. Cancer 1972; 29:1264–67.
4. Shur SR, Kew MC. Oral contraceptives and hepatocellular carcinoma. Cancer 1982; 149:487–90.
5. Okuda K et al. Primary liver cancers in Japan. Cancer 1980; 45:2663–69.
6. Niederhuber JE, Ensminger WD. Surgical considerations in the management of hepatic neoplasia. Semin Oncol 1988; 15:102–07.
7. Ramming KP. Hepatic artery infusion for liver cancer. Semin Oncol 1983; 10:201–05.
8. Guo JY, Yen D, Huang ZZ, et al. Transcatheter arterial chemoembolization with anticancer drug in iodized oil for primary hepatic carcinoma. Cardiovasc Interv Radiol 1989; 12:181–187.
9. Rosenthal CJ, Rotman M. Pilot study of interaction of radiation therapy with doxorubicin by continuous infusion. Nat Cancer Inst monogr 1988; 6:285–89.
10. Order SE, Klein JL, Leichner PK, et al. Radiolabeled antibody in the treatment of primary and metastatic liver malignancies: recent results. Cancer Res 1986; 100:307–14.
11. Nagorney DM, McPherson GAD. Carcinoma of the gallbladder and extrahepatic bile ducts. Semin Oncol 1988; 15:108–15.
12. Akawri OE, van Heerden JA, Foulk WT, et al. Cancer of the bile ducts associated with ulcerative colitis. Ann Surg 1975; 181:303–09.
13. Aldridge MC, Bismuth H. Gallbladder cancer; the polyp-cancer sequence. Br J Surg 1990; 77:363–4.
14. Nevin JF, Moran TJ, Kay S, et al. Carcinoma of the gallbladder: staging treatment and prognosis. Cancer 1976; 37:141–48.
15. Thorsen MK, Quirez F, Lawson TL, et al. Primary biliary carcinoma: CT evaluation. Radiology 1984; 152:479–83.
16. Shepherd HA, Dibs A, Ross AP, et al. Endoscopic prosthesis in the palliation of malignant biliary tract obstruction: a randomized trial (abstr). Gut 1987; 27:A1284.
17. Buskirk SJ, Giunderson LL, Adson MA, et al. Analysis of failure following curative irradiation of gallbladder and extrahepatic bile duct carcinoma. Int J Radiat Oncol Biol Phys 1984; 10:2013–23.
18. Harvey JH, Smith FP, Schein PS. 5-Fluorouracil, mitomycin and doxorubicin (FAM) in carcinoma of the biliary tract. J Clin Oncol 1984; 2:1245–48.

19. Smith GW, Bukowski RM, Hewlett JS, et al. Hepatic artery infusion of 5-fluorouracil and mitomycin C in cholangiocarcinoma and gallbladder carcinoma. Cancer 1984; 54:1513–16.
20. Pishlymayr R, Ringe B, Wittekind C et al. Liver grafting for malignant liver tumors. Transplant Proc 1989; 21:2403–5.
21. Yeoh EC and Arnold M. Recombinant alpha 2 interferon is superior to doxorubicin for inoperable hepatocellular carcinoma: a prospective randomized trial. Brit J Cancer 1989; 60:928–33.
22. Basset JF, Mantion G, Gillet M et al. Primary carcinoma of the gallbladder. Adjuvant posoperative external irradiation. Cancer 1989; 64:1843–7.

34

CARCINOMA OF THE PROSTATE

Richard J. Macchia, M.D., Gobind B. Laungani, M.D., and C. Julian Rosenthal, M.D., F.A.C.P.

CARCINOMA OF THE PROSTATE is the most common urologic malignancy in the United States. In terms of appropriate treatment, it is also the most controversial. Several reasons exist for this. Because prostate cancer occurs in men of advanced age, illness and death from other causes are quite frequent. Of all men with prostate carcinoma, only about half die from it; the others die of some other disease. Thus, anyone contemplating a controlled study needs to have very large number of patients.

A second problem is the variable natural history of prostatic carcinoma. It is well-known that carcinoma of the prostate does not progress at a predictable rate. Among patients with early stage disease limited to the prostatic gland who for one reason or another have not received treatment, about 10% will not have progression of their disease. This characteristic of prostatic cancer contributes to uncertainty regarding the validity of all uncontrolled studies. It is also known that about 80% of autopsies performed on 80-yr-old men reveal carcinoma of the prostate *in situ* in those who did not have any clinical sign of prostatic cancer. This, however, is not an indication that prostate cancer is not a deadly disease.

Incidence and Epidemiology

About 32,000 males in the United States die each year of prostatic cancer.[1] This represents the second most common cause of cancer death in males (after lung cancer). The crude mortality rate of 23.2/100,000 males has slightly increased during the past 5 yr; incidence of the disease apparently has increased from 69/100,000 in 1982 to 98/100,000 in 1990, due largely to improved detection and reporting.

Significant racial differences exist in the distribution of prostate cancer. The incidence and mortality rate in American blacks is 1.5 times higher than in whites, but it is quite low in American Indians and American Orientals. This indication of a probable genetic predisposition for carcinoma of the prostate is supported also by a 3-fold increase in the incidence of prostatic cancer among blood relatives.[2] However, no significant association of prostatic cancer with any HLA antigen type or with any of the recently described cellular proto-oncogenes so far has been found.

Significant differences that can be seen in the age-adjusted mortality rates from country to country cannot be explained by the racial composition of the population but rather indicate the importance of environmental factors in the pathogenesis of prostate cancer. Thus, the mortality rates per 100,000 population varied in 1977 from 4 deaths in Japan to 14 deaths in Yugoslavia and Germany, 23 deaths in United States and Australia, and 30 deaths in Norway and Sweden.

Among Japanese migrating to Hawaii or to the continental United States, the incidence of prostate cancer changes from low to high after just one generation. These environmental influences could be related to occupational hazards or diet. It has been reported that exposure to automobile exhaust fumes and chemical fertilizers and to the environment found in rubber factories and printing shops is conducive to a slight increase in the incidence of prostatic carcinoma.[3] A high-fat diet, as well as the presence of retinoids and vitamin C in the diet, may lead to an increased incidence of carcinoma of the prostate.[4] A possible indirect relationship to infectious venereal agents is suggested by the increased incidence of prostatic cancer among males with multiple sex partners.

Epidemiologic studies have also pointed toward the androgen dependence of prostatic carcinogenesis. Thus, eunuchs were never found to have prostatic cancer; carcinoma of the prostate was found with decreased incidence among patients with hepatic cirrhosis, which is usually accompanied by an increase of serum estrogen level; and there is a slight but consistent increase in serum testosterone level in blacks as compared to whites.

Prostatic carcinoma is not familial. Although benign prostatic hypertrophy (BPH) and prostate cancer frequently coincide, there is no evidence that BPH predisposes to prostate cancer. In analogous fashion, the performance of a prostatectomy for benign disease does not diminish the possibility of subsequent development of prostate carcinoma. This is because prostatectomy, which is performed for benign disease, leaves a rim of prostate intact.

Histopathology

More than 95% of prostatic cancers are adenocarcinomas arising from the epithelium of prostatic acini, usually in the periphery of the prostatic gland. Four architectural patterns of distribution of prostatic carcinoma have been described: small acinar, large acinar, cribriform, and solid trabecular. Other rare forms of adenocarcinoma arising from the glandular acini include the papillary mucinous and adenoid cystic types.

Rarely, carcinomas can arise within the prostatic ductal system. These lesions may present as transitional cell carcinomas, adenocarcinomas, or squamous cell carcinomas. Although extremely rare, a carcinosarcoma containing malignant epithelial and mesenchymal elements has been described.

Malignant prostatic epithelial cells (see chapter 11, figures 11-53 and 11-54) generally exhibit pleomorphism, with an increased nuclear cytoplasmic ratio, and may have indistinct cell borders. Their nuclei are hyperchromatic, variable in size and shape, and have prominent, intensely eosinophilic nucleoli.

With colorimetric and immunohistochemical techniques, it is possible to detect acid phosphatase within secretory granules of prostatic epithelial cells. There is a general inverse correlation between the degree of anaplasia of the cancer cells and their acid phosphatase content. However, the presence of acid phosphatase in the cell is not exclusive for prostatic cancer and prostatic cells; for this reason, it does not have an absolute diagnostic value.

For prognostic purposes, various histologic grading systems have been developed (Gleason, Mostofi, Gaeta, and Mayo Clinic). One of the most commonly used systems is that of Gleason,[5] which recognizes 5 grades in relation to the degree of glandular differentiation of the tumor and its relationship to the prostatic stroma under low-power magnification, without consideration for the cellular anaplasia (table 34-1). Gleason improved his system by adding stage numbers to grade numbers, resulting in a sum that he called "categories." He found 75% 5-yr survival in patients in categories 3–7, 60% for categories 8–9, 20% for categories 10–12, and no survivors for categories 13–14.

Table 34-1. Gleason's Classification of 5 Patterns of Adenocarcinoma of the Prostate

Pattern	Description
1	*Very well differentiated.* Single, separate round to oval glands. Uniform size of glands, closely packed and well-defined areas of tumor involvement.
2	*Well differentiated.* Single, separate glands with more variation in size and shape. More stroma occurs between glands and tumor masses are not as well circumscribed.
3	*Moderately differentiated.* Single separate glands with variation in size. Glands may be irregular in shape, closely packed, or widely separated by stroma; larger glands may have papillary infoldings; tumors have indistinct borders or may appear as circumscribed masses of papillary or cribriform tumors.
4	*Poorly differentiated.* Irregular masses of fused glands that branch and coalesce and may appear as solid masses of epithelium containing multiple glandular lumina. Tumors appear to aggressively infiltrate the stroma. Tumors may also be composed of large cells with clear cytoplasm resembling hypernephroma.
5	*Very poorly differentiated.* Raggedly infiltrating masses of epithelial cells with minimal glandular differentiation, or sharply circumscribed broad cords and masses of compactly arranged epithelial cells with occasional tiny glandular lumina.

Adapted from Gleason DF (ref 5)

Clinical Presentation and Diagnosis

There are several common settings in which prostate carcinoma is suspected and diagnosed. About 10 percent of patients who undergo a prostatectomy for BPH are found to have occult carcinoma in the specimen. A second presentation is that of a patient with difficulty in urination caused by enlargement of the prostate gland. Third, a rectal examination done as part of a physical examination for other reasons can reveal a suspicious prostatic nodule. Finally, the patient may present with symptoms suggestive of metastatic disease. Very rarely, a patient with locally invasive prostatic carcinoma may present with hematuria or hematospermia.

The digital rectal examination is the best screening test for prostate cancer, although it actually is not very efficient. If one looks for the classic nodule of medical textbooks, many lesions could be missed. A solitary nodule of the prostate has about a 50% chance of being carcinoma. The differential diagnosis includes nodular BPH, granulomatous prostatitis, prostatic infarct, and prostatic calculi. In some cases, the prostate feels entirely normal despite other evidence of prostatic carcinoma, such as an elevated acid phosphatase or an abnormal bone scan. In other cases, the prostatic gland feels diffusely enlarged like BPH, and the tumor is detected only at the time of prostatectomy. Although many cases of BPH are asymmetric, one should be extra cautious with an asymmetrical gland, as the incidence of cancer is somewhat higher in these glands than in symmetrical glands. Indistinct borders of the gland should also alert the clinician to the possibility of malignancy. A diffusely nodular, rock-hard gland is another rare presentation of prostatic carcinoma that is easily identifiable.

The rectal examination should be carefully and slowly performed. An examination performed in a cursory manner will almost always miss all but the most obvious cases. The examination also provides a clue as to whether the disease is confined to within the prostate, has extended beyond the confines of the capsule laterally, or has progressed superiorly to invade the seminal vesicles.

A prostate cancer detection rate by digital rectal examination (DRE) of 1.4 percent was reported in several large screening series.[36] This number can be doubled (2.6 to 2.8%) when modern techniques of transrectal ultrasound (TRUS) are used.[37] The smaller size of the detected lesions by TRUS is similar to that detected by DRE: usually between 8–14 mm, never smaller than 4 mm. This is useful because lesions <5 mm in diameter are likely to be clinically insignificant. However, due to its cost and its evolving technology, TRUS is not yet ready for large-scale screening. Recent studies also have shown that results at par with those of TRUS can be obtained when the prostatic-specific antigen (PSA) serum level is used to complement DRE. PSA is a recently described tumor marker specific for the prostate tissue. When a PSA value of >4 ng/ml was considered positive, an increase detection rate of 34% was added to the DRE detection rate. DRE combined with PSA was capable of detecting 91% of all positive biopsy cases for cancer of prostate, whereas TRUS and DRE detected 94% of cases. This rate was increased to 97% when all 3 modalities were used.[38] PSA values were also found to correlate with the prostatic tumor mass;

values of >40 ng/ml have been associated with microscopic capsular penetration, seminal vesicle invasion, and microscopic invasion of pelvic nodes (stages C and D-1), whereas values of >100 ng/ml have been correlated with high incidence of distant metastases (stage D-2).[38] Unfortunately, PSA lacks specificity for cancer; values of <100 ng/ml can also be encountered in patients with benign prostatic hyperplasia and prostatitis.

Once suspected, the diagnosis of prostatic cancer is usually established by needle biopsy of the prostate, performed transrectally with a spring-driven Biopsy gun needle under ultrasound guidance; this permits outpatient acquisition of multiple prostate biopsy specimens with low morbidity and high patient acceptance. Complications represented by moderate bleeding and occasional sepsis can occur in 5 and 31% of cases, respectively.

Recently, fine-needle aspiration biopsy, using transrectal or percutaneous approaches, was also introduced in clinical practice. It has the advantage of being practically devoid of complications but has the disadvantage of obtaining specimens represented by isolated cells that require an experienced cytologist for interpretation. When biopsy reveals dysplasia defined as prostatic intraepithelial neoplasia (PIN) it should be repeated;[38] this is because PIN occurs in a high number of patients with prostatic cancer in areas adjacent to the cancer.

Staging and Pattern of Spread

Between 50 and 80% of patients have metastatic disease at time of diagnosis. Dissemination occurs at times only through lymphatics to the common iliac, inguinal, para-aortic, mediastinal, and supraclavicular nodes after escaping the groups of nodes surrounding the prostate. A high incidence (80%) of lymphatic involvement occurs in patients who present with seminal vesicle involvement. The rectal examination described above gives an indication as to the local extent of disease. Any palpable lymph nodes should undergo aspiration cytology or possible open biopsy. The most common pattern of dissemination is through the blood; the most common sites of hematogenous metastases are the bones (85% of cases), followed by lung, liver, and adrenal glands (10%). Chest x-ray, bone scan, and acid phosphatase determination are performed to detect these metastases. A CT scan of the abdomen and pelvis is recommended because it can reveal metastases to the liver and enlarged lymph nodes in the pelvis (see chapter 10, figure 10-21). It can also yield information regarding the local contiguous growth of the prostatic cancer.

The determination of serum prostatic acid phosphatase is a useful biologic marker for monitoring the course of the disease, but it is far from infallible. A negative acid phosphatase result does not indicate the absence of disease, nor does it indicate the absence of metastases. Only ≤80% of patients with metastatic disease have an elevated serum acid phosphatase. Most patients whose disease is limited to the prostate have a normal reading.

Determination of prostatic-specific antigen (PSA) in the serum can also be used to monitor tumor mass, being even more sensitive than acid phosphatase level.

Certain patterns that appear on the bone scan are pathognomonic for metastatic disease. However, a characteristic situation is an atypical pattern. It may be an isolated "hot spot" that should be confirmed by cone-down x-ray films of the area. However, in some cases, no abnormalities are seen on plain x-ray despite the increased uptake on bone scan; this is because the bone scan is more sensitive—but less specific—than the x-rays.

The most reliable method of determining the status of the lymph nodes is by a systematic extraperitoneal bilateral lymph node dissection. A less invasive method is CT-guided fine-needle aspiration cytology. False-negative results, however, are common, whereas false-positive data are uncommon in the hands of an experienced cytologist. Bipedal lymphangiography is not very useful in prostatic carcinoma patients because of its lack of sensitivity.

All radiologic and laboratory data mentioned above provide the information needed to stage each case of carcinoma of the prostate. Staging has a significant prognostic value and is important in choosing the most appropriate form of treatment.

Table 34-2. Staging Nomenclature: The Modified Whitmore-Jewett System

Stage	Description
A	Incidental pathologic findings
A-1	Focal
A-2	Diffuse (<5% of specimen and/or poorly differentiated grade)
B	Confined to the prostate
B-1	Confined to <1 lobe
B-2	Involving 1 lobe or more
C	Extension beyond prostate without distant metastases
C-1	Minimal extracapsular extension
C-2	Bulky tumor with outlet and/or ureteral obstruction
D	Distant metastases
D-1	Pelvic lymph node metastasis found by surgery or aspiration cytology
D-2	Clinical evidence of distant metastases
D-3	Relapse following endocrine therapy

The Whitmore-Jewett system is the most commonly used staging system for prostatic cancer.[32] It groups patients into 4 categories, A through D, and is based on both clinical and pathological information. Stages of the disease are described as follows (table 34-2):

Stage A includes tumors detectable only by histologic examination of prostatectomy specimens; 10–20% of samples obtained at prostatectomy of patients with BPH contain prostatic carcinoma. This stage is further divided into 2 classes: (1) substage A-1, for only focal involvement of the examined sample; and (2) A-2, indicating diffuse involvement defined by the presence of malignant cells in >4 chips or in >5% of a transurethral resection specimen. It was suggested that focal, poorly differentiated stage A-1 lesions should be classified as stage A-2 due to their more aggressive behavior. In studies reported by Catalona in 1984,[6] 37–53% of cancer of the prostate was detected in stage A, whereas in a 1967 Veterans Administration Cooperative Urological Research Group (VACURG) study, only 5% were in stage A.[7] In 12% of stage A cases, elevated acid phosphatase was detected by RIA. Two percent of patients with clinical stage A-1 and 23% of those with stage A-2 disease were found to have lymph node metastases on staging pelvic lymphadenectomy.

Stage B includes tumors that are evident on digital rectal examination and are confined to the gland. This stage has been subdivided into stage B-1 for tumors localized to just one lobe and B-2 for involvement of both lobes.

In recent series,[33] stage B patients accounted for 22–26% of patients, whereas in the old VACURG series they accounted for only for 8%.[7] In 30% of these patients, the serum acid phosphatase was elevated at the time of diagnosis. Lymph nodes were found involved at lymphadenectomy in 18% of patients with clinical stage B-1 and in 35% of those with stage B-2 disease.

Stage C includes tumors that extend beyond the prostatic capsule but have not produced distant metastases. They are subclassified as C-1 (when the palpable extracapsular extension is minimal and does not involve the seminal vescicles) and C-2 (when the extracapsular extension is bulky or invades the seminal vescicles or is causing bladder outlet or ureteral obstruction).

In the VACURG series, 48% of patients were in stage C but only 9–15% of cases in recent studies were in this stage.[7] In 45% of these cases, the acid phosphatase was elevated; lymph nodes were involved in 50% of patients with stage C-1 disease and in 80% of those with C-2 disease.

Stage D includes tumors that have metastasized distantly. They are further divided into 3 categories: (1) stage D-0—patients with clinically localized prostatic cancer and persistent elevation of the acid phosphatase after performance of prostatectomy; (2) stage D-1—patients found to have metastases only in the pelvic or other lymph nodes not contiguous with the primary prostatic lesion; and stage D-2—patients with clinical evidence of distant metastases in bones or other organs. Acid phosphatase elevation is detected in 90% of D-2 patients but in only 50% of D-1 patients.

In recent series,[33] 10–28% of patients were in stage D at diagnosis, whereas 38% were so classified in the old VACURG series.[7]

A more cumbersome staging classification (shown in table 34-3), the tumor-nodes-metastases (TNM) system,[33] is generally little used in the United States.

Treatment

As with all cancer, the basic information required to make a sound decision on therapy is an accurate estimate of the extent of disease and the ability to forecast the clinical behavior of the tumor. Unfortunately, in prostate cancer considerable uncertainty exists in both of these areas. Nevertheless, decisions must be made. There is no more controversial area in urologic oncology than the treatment of prostatic carcinoma.

This section will first review the indications and results of the 2 modalities of treatment—surgery and radiotherapy (XRT) used with curative intent in the treatment of patients with localized disease—then present a few problems posed by treatment of special groups of patients, and finally review therapy for

Table 34-3. Staging Nomenclature: Tumor-Nodes-Metastases (TNM) System

Stage	Description
TX	Minimum requirements to assess the primary tumor cannot be met
TU	No tumor present
T1a	No palpable tumor; on histologic sections no more than 3 high-power fields of carcinoma found
T1b	No palpable tumor; histologic sections revealing >3 high-power fields of prostatic carcinoma
T2a	Palpable nodule <1.5 cm in diameter with compressible, normal-feeling tissue on at least 3 sides
T2b	Palpable nodule >1.5 cm in diameter or nodule or induration in both lobes
T3	Palpable tumor extending into or beyond the prostatic capsule
T3a	Palpable tumor extending into the periprostatic tissues or involving one seminal vesicle
T3b	Palpable tumor extending into the periprostatic tissues, involving one or both seminal vesicles; tumor size >6 cm in diameter
T4	Tumor fixed or involving neighboring structures
NX	Minimum requirements to assess the regional nodes cannot be met
N0	No involvement of regional lymph nodes
N1	Involvement of contralateral, bilateral or multiple regional lymph nodes
N3	Fixed mass on the pelvic wall with a free space between it and the tumor
MX	Minimum requirements to assess the presence of distant metastasis cannot be met
M0	No (known) distant metastasis
M1	Distant metastasis present (specify)__________________

metastatic disease, with its 2 major components of hormonal therapy and chemotherapy.

Localized Prostatic Carcinoma

SURGERY

Surgery represented by radical prostatectomy is 1 of the 2 treatments of choice. It consists of the removal of the entire prostate and seminal vesicles with adequate margins, using either a retropubic or perineal approach.

Patients in stages A-2, B-1, and B-2 are appropriate candidates for definitive primary radical prostatectomy. Patients should have no combined disease and should have completed a negative staging evaluation for distant metastases.

Pelvic lymphadenectomy for staging should be performed simultaneously with a retropubic prostatectomy or preceding a perineal prostatectomy. Adequate information can be obtained with a limited node dissection that includes nodes within the boundaries of the external and internal iliac vessels and obturator fossa, this in order to minimize complications such as lymphedema and lymphocele.

Radical prostatectomy is associated with perioperative morbidity that can include urinary incontinence, urethral stricture, and impotence. The last possibility can be held to a minimum by using newer surgical techniques involving an anatomical dissection that preserves nerves necessary for erection.[34]

The results of radical prostatectomy are excellent, especially for patients with stage B-1 disease (limited to one lobe); their disease-free survival rates at 15 yr approaches the expected survival of men a comparable age group in in the general population.[8] However, this survival rate falls to 25–50% in patients with stage B-2 disease who have infiltration of the seminal vesicles and to 20% in patients with stage C disease.[9]

RADIATION THERAPY

XRT has been used in the treatment of prostatic cancer since 1914, when Pasteau and Degrais applied intraurethral radium.[10] Interstitial irradiation was especially popular among urologists: Whitmore[11] introduced interstitial applications of ^{125}iodine, and Carlton[12] used ^{198}gold seeds. External beam irradiation has been effectively used with curative intent since the introduction of megavoltage equipment, especially through the efforts of Bagshaw et al.[13] Currently, linear accelerators generating photons that have energy averaging 4 million electron volts (MeV) are preferred to the ^{60}cobalt machines emitting photons averaging 1.25 MeV. The former produce more sharply defined beams that can be focused more accurately; thus, smaller volumes of normal tissue are irradiated, reducing radiation morbidity. A 360° radiational technique usually is used to deliver 7,000 cGy to the prostate over a 6-wk period through a small portal (6×6 to 10×10 cm). In patients with clinical evidence or suspicion of lymph node metastases, 5,000–5,500 cGy are also delivered to the whole pelvis through 4 field parallel opposed portals and 5,500 cGy to the paraortic nodes through anterior and posterior fields. Higher energy equipment delivering 22 MeV (betatron) was recently used, requiring lower total doses (5,000 cGy to the prostate and only 2,000 cGy to the peripheral lymph nodes (a shrinking technique).[14]

In selected instances, interstitial irradiation with ^{125}iodine, ^{198}gold, or ^{192}irridium can be delivered with or without external beam irradiation when the disease is confined to the prostate gland (stages A and B-1). Although lower local control rates were reported with interstitial therapy, its results can be improved with careful attention to technique and dosimetry. Newer radiation modalities such as the use of heavy particles (neutrons, pi-mesons, and protons) are currently being tested; neutrons and pi-mesons are less dependent on tissue oxygenation and may be associated with less loss of efficacy with dose fractionation; on the other hand, protons are ideal for radiation boosts to the prostate. Candidates for definitive XRT must have a confirmed pathological diagnosis of cancer that is clinically confined to the prostate and/or surrounding tissues (stages A-2, B, C) and should have completed a negative staging evaluation for distant metastases.

Definitive XRT is associated with both acute and chronic effects on normal tissues, including proctitis, enteritis, and cystitis. These side effects are generally moderate and reversible; they may be chronic, but are rarely sufficiently severe to require corrective surgical intervention. Other complications include occasional urethral stricture formation in patients who have undergone a previous transurethral resection of the prostate. In most patients undergoing definitive irradiation of the prostate, potency is preserved but can diminish over time.

Assessment of local control is critical in evaluating the results of XRT. By clinical criteria alone, local control rates are higher than if postradiation positive needle biopsies are used as end results; the latter were reported to be positive in 20–67% of patients ≥ 1 yr after the completion of XRT.[15]

By clinical and radiologic criteria, local control after definitive XRT was reported in all patients with clinical stage A and B prostatic carcinoma, 94% of patients with clinical stage C-1, and 82% of those with C-2 lesions.[15] However, patients with a positive biopsy at 18 mo postradiation have an abysmal prognosis and require salvage prostatectomy and hormonal manipulations. For this reason, although the survival statistics for XRT and surgery are similar, we generally recommend total prostatectomy for patients under 70 with disease pathologically confined to the prostate, whereas XRT is preferred for those over 70 or medically debilitated.

XRT is also successfully used to palliate pain and to prevent possible fractures and spinal cord compression in patients with metastatic disease to the bones (stage D-2) refractory to hormonal manipulations. In stage D-1 disease with metastases to the iliac or paraortic lymph nodes, attempts to treat for cure with XRT did not lead to an improvement in 5-yr survival.

Disseminated Prostatic Carcinoma

When prostatic carcinoma spreads distantly from the prostate and its contiguous tissue, no therapeutic modality currently available is able to cure the disease. Due to the widespreaded distribution of metastases, surgery and XRT cannot play a major role in controlling stage D prostatic cancer. Chemotherapy or the systemic administration of hormones leading to ablation of androgen production are the 2 modalities most likely to succeed.

HORMONAL THERAPY

Hormonal therapy has been the mainstay for patients with advanced prostatic carcinoma for 40 years, ever since the Nobel-prize-winning observations of Huggins and Hodges[16] indicated that prostatic cancer is under the trophic influence of male hormones and that disease regression occurred with endocrine ablation. DES administered orally generally has been used as the drug of choice in inducing androgen ablation, based on initial good response of most patients, especially with respect to palliation of pain. The belief that estrogen therapy could have a major impact on survival was partly contraindicated by studies done by VACURG.[17] In the first of these studies, in which patients with stages C and D disease were entered, 4 regimens were compared: placebo, orchietomy plus placebo, DES (5 mg/day), and orchiectomy plus DES (5 mg/day). Among 992 patients with stage C disease, it was confirmed that in patients receiving hormonal therapy, survival was lower. Among 772 patients with stage D disease, a reduction of about 20% in mortality due to cancer of the prostate was noted after 5- and 10-yr observation in patients receiving DES. However, mortality due to cardiovascular or other causes was increased as compared with patients receiving only placebo.

In a second study, 3 different doses of DES (0.2 mg, 1 mg, and 5 mg/day) were compared within one group and with a group of patients with stage D disease receiving only placebo. A decrease in the death rate from 55% in patients with stage D disease receiving placebo or 0.2 mg DES to 24% and 22%, respectively, in patients receiving 1 mg and 5 mg DES per day was noted at 10 yr, indicating a clear benefit for DES. However, in view of an increase in the cardiovascular deaths in patients receiving 5 mg DES, it was concluded that the 1 mg/day DES dose was the best. This dose does not completely ablate the synthesis of testosterone, but usually inhibits it by about 90%. For this reason, the customary dose now used is 3 mg/day, which was found to induce complete inhibition of testosterone synthesis and a low incidence of cardiovascular and thrombogenic complications. Even so, this dose has not yet been tested in a large cooperative study. The VACURG studies also indicated that adequate estrogen therapy and orchiectomy are equivalent in the initial treatment of prostatic carcinoma and that there is little to gain from the use of both concomitantly. Orchiectomy should be the treatment of choice in patients at risk for cardiovascular and thrombogenic complications. In other patients, because of the relatively short-term benefit of orchiectomy (6–12 mo), DES should be the treatment of choice, in view also of the results of the Finnish National Prospective Prostatic Cancer Study.[18] This study showed a clear benefit at 2 yr for patients on DES as compared with those who had orchiectomy only, especially for patients with poorly differentiated tumors.

Over the past decade, a number of new hormonal therapies were introduced to improve the overall duration and quality of survival. Among them, agents that have had a major impact on the overall management of patients with metastatic prostatic carcinoma are the luteinizing hormone releasing hormone (LHRH) analogues or gonadotropin-releasing hormones (Gn-RH).[35] These substances are likely to replace DES in the primary hormonal management of stage D prostate cancer in all patients. They are currently the treatment of choice for patients with stage D disease who are at risk for development of thromboembolic events or who have had congestive heart failure or coronary insufficiency.

Under normal circumstances, LHRH is secreted in a pulsatile fashion by the hypothalamus. It appears that LHRH attaches to receptors at the level of the anterior pituitary gonadotroph that induces the redistribution of the calcium-binding protein calmodulin; this allows the release of "prepackaged" amounts of luteinizing hormone (LH) and follicular stimulating hormone (FSH). Consequently, the testis responds to the surge of gonadotropins by producing 3 products: (1) an androgen-binding protein (from the Sertoli's cells) involved in spermatogenesis; (2) inhibin, a peptide hormone produced by the Sertoli's cells that inhibits gonadotropin release; and (3) testosterone, produced by the Leydig cells. The increased secretion of the last 2 products has a negative feedback at the level of the hypothalamus and pituitary, leading ultimately to the inhibition of LH and FSH release.

Many agonistic-antagonistic analogues of LHRH have substitutions of D amino acids at the sixth position and some also at the ninth and tenth position, prolonging the biologic half-life of these agents from several minutes to many hours and sometimes days. After an initial transient increase in patients' symptoms—and possibly their tumor size—due to an increase in serum testosterone level lasting about 1 wk, these analogues in the long term cause a complete receptor down-regulation, producing castrate levels of testosterone and dihydrotestosterone, with consequent objective responses, in 40–50% of cases.

The prototype LHRH analogue leuprolide has been subjected to several clinical trials, including a prospective randomized multicenter trial comparing it to the use of DES.[19] This trial of 200 patients showed similar efficacy for 1 mg/day subcutaneous leuprolide as for oral DES 3 mg/day. However, there were significantly fewer side effects with leuprolide: Gynecomastia, nausea and vomiting, peripheral edema, and a tendency toward vascular complications (including phlebitis, pulmonary embolism, and congestive heart failure), which were encountered in a small but measurable fraction of patients on DES, were almost nonexistent in those receiving leuprolide. Only hot flushes were more commonly seen in the group taking leuprolide as compared with those taking DES. Long-acting Gn-RH analogue preparations requiring monthly parenteral administration have replaced the short-lasting ones requiring daily administration and are likely to become the primary hormonal treatment of choice in patients with stage D-2 prostatic cancer.

Use of the so-called primary hormonal therapy, represented by either estrogens (DES), LHRH analogues, or orchiectomy—which essentially lead to the absence of testosterone from the patients' serum—results in objective responses of tumor regression in 40–50% of cases. An additional 30% of these patients demonstrate improvement in subjective complaints. Duration of the hormonal responsiveness is about 10–24 mo, depending on the clinical situation at the time treatment is initiated. Patients who become clearly refractory to hormonal therapy in the presence of castrate levels of testosterone will, on occasion, demonstrate some subjective improvement with second-line therapies, although objective responses are rarely encountered, and the duration of subjective responses is limited to from 3 to 8–10 mo.

Second-line therapy includes some older derivatives of DES (estramustine and high-dose diethylstilbestrol diphosphate) as well as some of the more recent agents introduced into the therapy of prostatic carcinoma that have activity primarily at the level of the adrenal gland or in the prostatic neoplastic cell itself.

The function, survival, and proliferation of the neoplastic prostatic cells are under the influence not only of the hypothalomic-pituitary axis and the testis but also under that of androgens secreted by the adrenal gland (androstanedione and dehydroepiandrosterone). This gland is stimulated by adrenocorticotrophic-releasing factor (CRF) from the hypothalamus as well being under the influence of the metabolic events to which testosterone and other androgens are subjected in the prostatic cells. Testosterone, as well as other adrenal androgens, diffuses passively through the prostatic cell membrane into the cytoplasm only if unbound from the testosterone-estrogen binding globulin or albumin, the 2 proteins that keep 97% of the circulating testosterone bound.

In the prostatic cell cytoplasm as well as in that of neoplastic prostatic cells, androgen-dependent testosterone and the adrenal gland-derived androgens are readily converted to dihydrotestosterone (DHT) by 5-alpha reductase (figure 34-1). DHT then binds to a specific cytoplasmic receptor protein, forming a complex that is then translocated into the nucleus of the prostatic cell, where it binds to acceptor sites on the DNA of nuclear chromatin. This leads to the production of messenger RNA, which codes for proteins important to the metabolic functions of the prostatic cells and of the androgen-dependent prostatic carcinoma cells. These proteins are not produced in the absence of androgens; consequently, the growth of androgen-dependent prostatic carcinoma cells is inhibited and the prostate itself becomes atrophic.

Worth noting is the fact that androstanedione and dehydroepiandrosterone, the androgens secreted by the adrenal gland even though they are 3–6 times less potent than testosterone, are produced in larger daily quantities (1.4 and 29 mg, respectively, vs. 6.6 mg of testosterone). Thus, the adrenal gland androgens secreted daily represent about one-third of the relative total androgen effect present in the serum. Therefore, the adrenal androgens can still a stimulate prostatic carcinoma cell growth after the complete suppression of testosterone by orchiectomy, or by administration of DES or LHRH analogues. It was also reported that one-fourth to one-fifth of patients who relapsed with prostatic cancer following orchiectomy had DHT levels of 2 ng/g, significantly higher than nonandrogen target tissues from their body, which averaged 0.9 ng/g.[20]

For these reasons, some of the new hormonal therapies used at present as second-line treatment are directed primarily at the inhibition of the androgen production (corticosteroids that inhibit ACTH released by the pituitary gland) and at the synthesis (aminoglutethimide, spironolactone, ketoconazole) of androgens from the adrenal gland. Also, these therapies aim at competing with DHT receptors or with testosterone for 5-alpha reductase at the level of prostatic neoplastic cells, which are androgen dependent.

Following are some of the newer hormonal therapies that are being used as second-level therapies but have the potential of being used as first-line therapies, especially in combination with some of the current first-line agents aiming at a total androgenic blockade.

Estramustine phosphate sodium (Emcyt) is a combination of the estrogen estradiol and a nitrogen mustard. The extent to which each of these contributes to the antitumor activity is not clear, but it is believed that this agent has primarily an enhanced estrogenic activity. About 20% of patients with advanced prostatic carcinoma refractory to DES responded subjectively to treatment with estramustine.[21] In a double-blind prospective trial comparing estramustine with DES in 153 patients not previously treated with hormones, the 2 drugs were comparable in effectiveness and side effects.

Diethylstilbestrol diphosphate (Stilphostrol), administered in high doses (500–2,000 mg in 5% dextrose over 1–4 hr), is thought to have a cytotoxic effect due to its binding to DNA. It was reported to induce subjective responses in 75% of patients who have relapsed after primary endocrine therapy.[22] Acid phosphatase decreased in 30% of patients and the prostate decreased in size in 11%. Favorable immediate responses were also reported in paraplegic and paraparetic patients.[23]

Progestational agents. Megestrol acetate (Megace) and cyproterone acetate, with or without associated estrogen, may induce subjective and objective responses in patients with prostatic cancer refractory to DES. Megesterol acetate and other progestational agents induce a decrease of LH release at the level of the pituitary gland and exhibit antiandrogenic action directly at the prostatic cell site, competing with DHT receptors and with testosterone for 5-alpha reductase. Megesterol acetate 80 mg/day was found to induce 90% inhibition of testosterone synthesis; for this reason, it was shown to produce remissions when used also as primary hormonal therapy.[24] Adding a small dose of DES (0.1 mg) to megesterol acetate (80 mg/day) can suppress all sources of DHT more effectively than use of megesterol acetate alone. With this combination, it was found that 81% of patients with prostatic carcinoma who relapsed after the primary hormonal therapy became objectively stable for an average time interval of 7 mo.[24] In previously untreated patients, the same combination stabilized the disease for a mean of 22 mo, comparing favorably (although statistically insignificantly) with the mean of 16 mo for patients who underwent prostatectomy or received DES.[24]

Antiandrogens. These agents interfere with cytoplasmic receptor binding of DHT and nuclear translocation of the DHT-receptor complex. Among them, cyproterone acetate and megestrol acetate inhibit also the gonadotropin released from the anterior pituitary, whereas flutamide has exclusive activity in the prostatic cell. Flutamide was extensively tested and found to induce some side effects, including diarrhea, flushing, and gynecomastia. However, patients maintain potency—the testosterone level is actually increased—and are not exposed to an increased risk of the thromboembolic or cardiovascular side effects seen with administration of DES. As second-line therapy, flutamide (250 mg p.o. t.i.d.) induced favorable responses in 23% of patients who failed prior therapy[25] and in 90% of those not previously treated, with a mean duration of response of 10.5 mo.

Aminoglutethimide is a derivative of glutethimide, which induces the blockage of several cytochrome P-450 hydroxylation-dependent steps involved in the conversion of cholesterol to pregnenolone and in the aromatization of androgens to estrogens; thus, it inhibits the adrenal production of steroids, androgens, and estrogens. It should be administered at a dose of 250 mg p.o. q.i.d. concomitantly with hydrocortisone 10 mg p.o. b.i.d. in order to prevent the reflex rises in ACTH that would override the metabolic inhibitory capabilities of aminoglutethimide. Subjective responses were reported with this regimen in 20–40% of prostatic cancer patients who had relapsed after primary hormonal therapy.[26]

Ketoconazole, an antifungal agent that inhibits a variety of cytochrome P-450-dependent enzymes, also was found capable of lowering serum testosterone to castrate levels when administered in high doses (400 mg q. 8–12 hr) to 15 patients with advanced prostatic carcinoma.[27] The agent also relieved their pain for an average of 5–6 mo. However, it can cause rare episodes of hepatotoxicity, nausea, vomiting, anaphylaxis, and xerostomia.

Tamoxifen citrate, an antiestrogen, has also produced 13% objective remissions in 38 patients who failed to respond to first-line hormonal therapy.[28]

The concept of combining various hormonal agents in order to achieve total blockade of androgen production was advanced by Labrie et al,[29] who combined leuprolide, a Gn-RH agonist, with flutamide in 1 study and with orchiectomy in another. They reported that only 26% of patients progressed at 17 mo average follow-up, in marked contrast with historical controls, in which progression was reported in average of 70% of cases. A recent multicenter randomized trial comparing leuprolide with placebo to the combination of leuprolide and flutamide in >500 patients with stage D-2 prostatic cancer indicated a trend toward a superior disease-free interval (16.9 vs. 13.9 mo) and overall survival (35.6 vs. 28.3 mo) for the flutamide-leuprolide combination;[39] however, this was statistically significant only in patients with minimal metastatic disease, which suggests that this treatment should be started before patient becomes symptomatic.

In discussing hormonal therapy for prostatic carcinoma patients, a legitimate question refers to the optimal timing for initiating the hormonal therapy. Based on VACURG studies, the early institution of hormonal therapy did not prolong overall survival; indeed, for certain patients with stage C disease, survival was shortened. For this reason, stage D patients should receive hormonal therapy when symptoms develop; this will also preserve their sexual activity. Excepted from this recommendation are patients with bilateral hydronephrosis secondary to para-aortic lymphadenopathy and those with extensive vertebral disease with early epidural extension that may not yet have caused symptoms or objective findings. In view of the gravity of the potential complications these patients may have, they should receive hormonal therapy even when free of symptoms.

CHEMOTHERAPY

About 25% of patients with metastatic prostatic cancer do not respond to hormonal therapy. Median survival for these patients and for the large group who relapse within 3 yr of achieving hormone-induced remission is about 12 mo; as mentioned above, only a few of them have a second short-lived remission. In these nonresponsive or relapsing patients, chemotherapy has been administered for the past 2 decades. Before 1973, very few studies of chemotherapy were carried out in advanced prostatic cancer because of the dramatic response to hormonal therapy, the debilitated status of patients who relapsed from hormone-induced remissions, and the difficulties in quantifying tumor response. To date, chemotherapy has demonstrated limited benefits. A recent review of about 1,500 patients participating in 17 chemotherapeutic trials showed that only 4.5% achieved a partial or complete remission (PR or CR) and another 20% had stable disease at 12 wk.[30] Despite these generally disappointing results, several single agents have been found to be active in inducing responses defined by PR (reduction of tumor mass by $\leq 50\%$) or stabilization of disease. Cyclophosphamide (CTX) induced responses in 26–53% of cases in various trials,[31] dacarbazine (DTIC) in 28% of cases, and doxorubicin (ADR) in 22–28% of cases. ADR was found effective when administered on a weekly schedule at a relatively low dose of 25 mg/m^2, which has low toxicity. Some response was seen in 83% of patients; 19% had a decrease in acid phosphatase level by more than half, and 58% had an equivalent decrease of alkaline phosphatase. 5-Fluorouracil (5-FU) was also found to induce PRs in a limited number of cases (12–20%); methotrexate (MTX) induced a few responses, but at a price of significant toxicity. Cisplatin (DDP) was found successful as single agent, primarily at Roswell Park Memorial Institute.

Combination chemotherapy was developed in an effort to improve the results of single agents.[31] To date, 2 regimens—CTX + 5-FU + ADR and ADR + MIT + 5-FU (see Appendix) have led to results superior to those given by single agents alone (PRs in 30–50%). With the second regimen, better responses were obtained in patients with visceral metastases than in those with osseous metastases.

Overall, chemotherapy of advanced carcinoma of the prostate is still limited in scope, having primarily a palliative intent. On the other side, in view of the generally advanced age of prostatic carcinoma patients, the goal of achieving a relatively sustained, even if incomplete, remission would likely suffice, as they could live out their normal life span without distressing symptoms.

References

1. Boring CC, Squires TS, Tong T. Cancer statistics 1991. CA 1991; 1:19–36.
2. Schuman IM, Mandel J, Blackard C, et al. Epidemiologic study of prostatic cancer: preliminary report. Cancer Treat 1977; 61:181–86.
3. Winkelstein W Jr, Sacks ST, Ernster VL, Selvin S. Correlation and incidence rates for selected cancers in the nine areas of the third National Cancer Survey. Am J Epidemiol 1977; 105:407–19.
4. Blair A, Fraumeni JF. Geographic patterns of prostatic cancer in the United States. JNCI 1978; 61:1379–84.
5. Gleason DF. Classification of prostatic carcinomas. Cancer Chemother Rep 1966; 50:125–128.
6. Catalona WJ. Prostate cancer staging in prostate cancer. New York: Grune and Stratton, 1984; 57–83.
7. Veterans Administration Cooperative Urological Research Group. Treatment and survival of patients with cancer of prostate. Surg. Gynecol Obstet 1967; 124:1011–17.
8. Cochran JS, Kadevsky MC. Private practice experience with radical surgery treatment of cancer of prostate. Urology 1981; 17:547–49.
9. Schroeder FH, Bolt E. Carcinoma of the prostate. A study of 213 patients with stage C tumors treated with total perineal prostatectomy. J Urol 1975; 114:257–60.
10. Pasteau O, Degrais P. The radium treatment of cancer of the prostate. Arch Roentgen Ray 1914; 18:396–410.
11. Whitmore WT Jr, Hilaris B, Grabstald H. Retropubic implantation of iodine 125 in the treatment of prostatic cancer. J Urol 1972; 108:918–20.
12. Carlton CE Jr, Dawoud F, Hudgins P, Scott R Jr. Irradiation treatment of carcinoma of the prostate: a preliminary report based on 8 years of experience. J Urol 1972; 108:924–27.
13. Bagshaw MA. Definitive radiotherapy in carcinoma of the prostate. JAMA 1969; 210:326–27.
14. Perez CA, Bauer W, Garzia R, Royce RK. Radiation therapy in the definitive treatment of localized carcinoma of the prostate. Cancer 1977; 40:1425–33.
15. Neglia WJ, Hussey DH, Johusson DE. Megavoltage radiation therapy for carcinoma of the prostate. Int J Radiat. Oncol Biol Phys 1977; 2:873–82.
16. Huggins C, Hodges CV. Studies on prostatic cancer. The effect of castration, of estrogen and of androgen injection on serum phosphatases in metastatic carcinoma of the prostate. Cancer Res 1941; 1:293–97.
17. Byar DP. VACURG studies on prostate cancer and treatment. In: Tannenbaum M, ed. Urologic pathology: the prostate. Philadelphia: Lea and Febiger, 1977; 241–67.
18. Haapiainen R, Rannikko S, Alfthan O. Comparison of primary orchiectomy with oestrogen therapy in advanced prostatic cancer. Br J Urol 1986; 58:528–33.
19. The Leuprolide Study Group: leuprolide versus diethylstilbestrol for metastatic prostatic cancer. N Engl J Med 1984; 311:1284–86.
20. Geller J, Albert JD, Nachtschein DA, et al. Comparison of prostate cancer tissue, dihydrotestosterone levels at the time of relapse following orchiectomy or estrogen therapy. J Urol 1984; 132:693–96.
21. Benson RC, Loear JB, Gill GM. Treatment of stage D hormone resistant carcinoma of the prostate with estramustine phosphate. J Urol 1979; 121:452–54.

22. Rohlf PI, Flocks RH. Stilphosterol therapy in 100 cases of prostatic carcinoma. J Iowa Med Soc 1969; 59:1096–98.
23. Hawtrey CE, Welch MJ Jr, Schmidt JD, et al. Paraplegia and paraparesis due to prostatic cancer. Urology 1974; 4:431–34.
24. Geller J, Albert J, Vik A. Advantages of total androgen blockade in the treatment of advanced prostatic cancer. Semin Oncol 1988; 15 (suppl) 53–61.
25. Sogani PC, Ray B, Whitmore WF Jr. Advanced prostatic carcinoma. Flutamide therapy after conventional endocrine treatment. Urology 1975; 6:164–66.
26. Block M, Trump D, Rose DP, et al. Evaluation of aminogluthetamide in stage D prostatic cancer. An assessment of efficacy and toxicity in patients with tumor refractory to hormonal therapy. Cancer Treat Rep 1984; 68:719–22.
27. Tachtenberg J, Pont A. Ketoconasole therapy for advanced prostatic carcinoma. Lancet 1985; 2:433–35.
28. Glik JH, Wein A, Padavic K, et al. Phase II trial of tamoxifen in metastatic carcinoma of the prostate. Cancer 1982; 49:1367–72.
29. Labrie F, Dupont A, Belanger A, et al. Treatment of prostate cancer with gonadotropin releasing hormone agonists. Endocr Rev 1986; 7:67–74.
30. Eisenberg MA, Simon R, O'Dwyer PV, et al. A reevaluation of nonhormonal cytotoxic chemotherapy in the treatment of prostatic carcinoma. J Clin Oncol 1985; 3:824–41.
31. Torti FM. Approaches to chemotherapy of prostate cancer. Adv Oncol 1988; 4:18–24.
32. Whitmore WF Jr. Natural history and staging of prostate cancer. Urol Clin N Am 1984; 11:205–08.
33. Paulson DF. The natural history of prostate cancer. Adv Oncol 1988; 4:10–17.
34. Walsh PC. Nerve sparing radical prostatectomy. Semin Oncol 1988; 4:351–58.
35. Waxman J. Gonadotrophin-releasing hormone analogues for prostatic cancer: an overview. Semin Oncol 1988; 4:366–70.
36. Chodack GW, Wald V, Parmer E, et al. Comparison of digital examination and transrectal ultrasonography for the diagnosis of prostate cancer. J Urol 1986; 135:951–54.
37. Lee F, Littrup PJ, Torp-Pedersen ST, et al. Prostate cancer: comparison of transrectal US and digital rectal examination for screening. Radiology 1988; 168:389–94.
38. Drago JR, Badaloment R. The role of new modalities in the early detection and diagnosis of prostate cancer. CA 1989; 39:325–35.
39. Crawford ED, et al. A controlled clinical trial of leuprolide with and without flutamide in prostatic carcinoma. N Engl J Med 1989; 321:419–24.

35

RENAL CELL CARCINOMA

Thomas J. Forlenza, M.D., F.A.C.P.

RENAL CELL CARCINOMA OCCURS principally in the fifth decade of life and has a male predominance. Because of the protean manifestations of hematuria, abdominal mass, pain, fever, and weight loss, it poses an intriguing differential diagnosis and has been called the internist's tumor;[1] renal cell carcinoma occasionally has been associated with systemic amyloidosis, which at times can be a very confounding problem.[2] Tobacco and tobacco products, ionizing radiation, and hormonal manipulation (in animals) have been associated with an increased incidence of renal cell carcinoma. A specific cause has not been isolated.

Pathology and Diagnosis

Three histologic types of tumor are distinguished by their microscopic appearance: clear cell (see chapter 11, figures 11-42A & B), granular cell, and sarcomatoid. They are graded by the histologic atypia. It is important to distinguish among these, as the sarcomatoid type behaves much more aggressively as compared to the other types.[3] The most common sites of metastases are lung, lymph node, liver, and bone, with >50% of tumors being metastatic at time of presentation. A curious hepatic dysfunction and hypertension have been reported;[4,5] these disappear when the tumor is resected. Thyroid and vaginal metastases also have been reported.[6]

The patient's chief complaint will indicate where diagnostic testing should start. Usually, the patient will have an abdominal mass, pain, or hematuria as

640

a presenting symptom. The classic triad of gross hematuria, abdominal mass, and pain was reported in only 29/309 patients (9%) in Skinner's series.[1]

The CT scan (see chapter 10, figures 10-26 through 10-29) can be very helpful in the evaluation of an abdominal mass and does not appear to raise the cost of a hospital stay.[31] In a survey of British practitioners, when renal carcinoma was suspected, ultrasound was preferred by 93% of respondents as a routine investigation versus 16% of respondents who preferred abdominal CT scanning.[7] The vast majority of renal lesions will be cysts and not tumors. Lang reports that 70% of lesions identified by nephrotomogram will be benign renal cysts with only 5.5% incidence of malignancy.[8] Malignant lesions are vascular by angiographic study and have a worse prognosis than avascular tumors.[9] Blath relates that 19/72 patients in his series had avascular tumors with papillary adenocarcinoma predominating. These patients had a lower incidence of vein and capsule invasion and an increased survival rate.

An interesting entity, xanthogranulomatous pyelonephritis, is mentioned because it is indistinguishable from renal cell carcinoma diagnostically, and nephrectomy is required to make the distinction.[10] It has been reported in conjunction with renal cell carcinoma.[11]

Staging and Treatment

As with most tumors, the more advanced, the worse the prognosis. The local extent of the tumor is an important indicator of survival in the nonmetastatic group of patients. Capsular invasion, lymphoid involvement, and the presence of distant metastases are important prognostic factors. Renal vein involvement does not appear to influence survival.[1] Lymph node involvement implies systemic disease and has a 5–10% 5-yr survival rate.[12] Various classifications have been used to categorize renal cell carcinoma. The TNM classification is an acceptable grouping of clinical and pathologic findings (table 35-1); the extent of tumor at the time of surgery is the best predictor of survival.[13]

The cornerstone of treatment is surgery at as early a stage as possible.[14] Renal cell tumors are usually large and bulky abdominal masses. They can be uncomfortable, painful, and a potential source of fever, infection, and blood loss. For these reasons, nephrectomy, even in the presence of metastatic disease, is usually recommended even though this may not increase survival time.[15] The extent of resection will be determined by the preoperative evaluation. Partial nephrectomy may be indicated in the presence of solitary or bilateral renal carcinoma.[16] Only 2.5% of patients will present with an apparently solitary metastasis. If the solitary metastasis presents after nephrectomy, the prognosis is somewhat better. In O'Dea's series, the average time to presentation of a metastatic lesion was 2 yr 7 mo, with a 5-yr survival rate of 33%.[17] Therefore, removal of a solitary metastasis, despite location, should be attempted.[19]

Extension of tumor into the inferior vena cava is not necessarily a contraindication to resection. This occurs in 4–10% of patients, and surgery is indicated.[19] Cumulative data in the literature show a 50% survival with follow-up ranging from 3–30 mo.[20,21]

Table 35-1. Renal Cell Carcinoma: TNM Classifications

Primary tumor (T)

TX	Minimum requirements cannot be met
T0	No evidence of primary tumor
T1	Small tumor, minimal renal and calyceal distortion or deformity; circumscribed neovasculature surrounded by normal parenchyma
T2	Large tumor with deformity or enlargement of kidney or collecting system
T3a	Tumor involving perinephric tissues
T3b	Tumor involving renal vein
T3c	Tumor involving renal vein and infradiaphragmatic vena cava
	Note: Under T3, tumor may extend into perinephric tissues, into renal vein, and into vena cava as shown on cavography. In these instances, the T classification may be shown as T3a, b, and c, or some appropriate combination, depending on extension. For example, T3a & b is tumor in perinephric fat and extending into renal vein.
T4a	Tumor invasion of neighboring structures (e.g., muscle, bowel)
T4b	Tumor involving supradiaphragmatic vena cava

Nodal involvement (N)

	The regional lymph nodes are the para-aortic and paracaval nodes. The juxtaregional lymph nodes are the pelvic nodes and the mediastinal nodes.
NX	Minimum requirements cannot be met
N0	No evidence of involvement of regional nodes
N1	Single homolateral regional nodal involvement
N2	Involvement of multiple regional or contralateral or bilateral nodes
N3	Fixed regional nodes (assessable only at surgical exploration)
N4	Involvement of juxtaregional nodes

Distant metastasis (M)

MX	Not assessed
M0	No (known) distant metastasis
M1	Distant metastasis present

Arterial embolization preoperatively may be indicated to reduce bleeding at nephrectomy,[22] but in general it does not enhance survival[23] and may be associated with distant embolization,[24] flank pain, fever, and nausea and vomiting. Therefore, this procedure should be used—if it is used at all—only after thorough consideration has been given to other treatment modalities. It may reduce bleeding when resecting metastases,[25] and it has been used to reduce pain.[26]

Radiation has a small role in the management of renal cell carcinoma. It may decrease pain, hematuria, or bleeding from metastases, but it does not seem to increase 5-yr survival.[15] Again, this treatment modality must be tailored to the patient and should not be viewed as a routine form of treatment.

Chemotherapy has had a minimal effect on renal cell carcinoma, with responses ranging from 5–16%. Stolback reported hematologic toxicity from hydroxyurea, with a 5% response rate, and an ichthyosis-like skin rash from nafoxidine, with a 16% response rate.[27]

Vinblastine was found to give somewhat better results, with a response rate in the 10–15% range.

Hormonal manipulations also have been tried. Estrogen and/or progesterone receptors were found in 83% of renal cell carcinoma specimens tested;[29] however, only a few patients had significant titers. Animal studies have shown that renal cell carcinoma can be induced by estrogen and inhibited by testosterone, cortisone, and provera or by adrenalectomy and orchiectomy.[29] Bloom and other investigators have administered large doses of progesterone derivatives or testosterone to patients with advanced renal cell carcinoma, with only limited results.[30] Objective response rates in various series were only 16% for progestinic agents (e.g., megestrol acetate) and only 9% for androgen therapy, with a range of 7–25%; generally, a higher response rate was seen in males than in females,[39] and the effect was greater on lung metastases than on bone lesions.[29] All responses to hormonal therapy were, however, short lasting (3–7 mo). Immunologic therapies were also extensively tested due to the rarely reported regressions of the tumor attributed to a process of immunologic regression of a highly antigenic tumor. Through the years, short-lasting partial or complete remissions (PRs or CRs) were reported in 10% of renal cell carcinoma patients treated with bacille Calmette-Guerin, 5% of those receiving "immune RNA," and 21% of those receiving autologous tumor cell suspensions.[31] Recently, alpha interferon, in doses of 3–50 MU I.M. or subcutaneous daily or every other day, was reported to induce responses in 22–46% of cases. However, when translated to standard responses using the accepted criteria defining PRs and CRs, these were only 11–28% responses, with a mean duration of 3–6 mo.[31] The most recent biologic modifier treatment, applied with some success to patients with advanced renal cell carcinoma, has been the administration of interleukin-2 activated autologous killer lymphocytes. CRs and PRs were reported in 19 to 33% of cases.[32]

Newer agents such as echinomycin, a cyclic peptide isolated from *Streptomyces echinatus,* and trimetrexate, a potent inhibitor of dihydrofolate reductase not requiring polyglutamination, are being tested in various cooperative trials.

In summary, although the main modality of treatment of renal cell carcinoma is surgery, the long natural history of the disease allows many palliative modalities to be used. Renal cell carcinoma, therefore, poses a great challenge to the oncology team. Supportive measures and a humanistic approach will help the patient with this disease to live out his life with as much freedom from pain as possible.

References

1. Skinner DG, Colvin RB, Vermillion CD, Pfister RC, Leadbetter WF. Diagnosis and management of renal cell carcinoma. Cancer 1971; 28(5):1165–77.
2. Hind CR, Tennent GA, Evans DJ, Pepys MB. Demonstration of amyloid A (AA) protein and amyloid P component (AP) in deposits of systemic amyloidosis associated with renal adenocarcinoma. J Pathol 1983; 139(2):159–66.
3. Tomera KM, Farrow GM, Lieber MM. Sarcomatoid renal carcinoma. J Urol 1983; 130(4):657–9.
4. Ramon CU. Hepiatic dysfunction in renal cell carcinoma. Cancer 1972; 20:1287–89.
5. Leckie B, Brown JJ, Fraser R, et al. A renal carcinoma secreting inactive renin. Clin Sci Mol Med 1978; 55(suppl 4):159s–61s.
6. Jonsson K, Hellsten S, Lindholm CE, Bondestam S. Angiographic work-up in a patient with late vaginal metastasis from a renal carcinoma. Scand J Urol Nephrol 1980; 14(1):122–4.
7. Ritchie AWS, Chisholm GD. Management of renal cell carcinoma—a questionnaire survey. Br J Urol 1983; 55:591–94.

8. Lang FK. Roentgenographic assessment of asymptomatic renal lesions. Radiology 1973; 109:257–69.

9. Watson RC, Flemming RJ, Evans JA. Arteriography in the diagnosis of renal carcinoma: review of 100 cases. Radiology 1968; 91:888.

10. Lorentzen M, Nielsen HO. Xanthogranulomatous pyelonephritis. Scand J Urol Nephrol 1980; 14(2):193–200.

11. Schoborg TW, Saffos RO, Urdaneta L, Lewis CE. Xanthogranulomatous pyelonephritis associated with renal carcinoma. J Urol 1980; 124(1):125–27.

12. De Kernion JB, Berry D. The diagnosis and treatment of renal cell carcinoma. Cancer 1980; 45:1947–51.

13. Selli C, Hinshow WM, Woodard BH, Paulson DF. Stratification of risk factors in renal cell carcinoma. Cancer 1983; 52:899–903.

14. Jonas D, Weber W, Beckert H, et al. Surgery of the primary tumor of metastasizing renal carcinoma. Urol Int 1984; 39(2):110–3.

15. Rafla S. Renal cell carcinoma—natural history and results of treatment. Cancer 1970; 24:26–60.

16. Palmer JM. Role of partial nephrectomy in solitary or bilateral renal tumors. JAMA 1983; 249(17):2357–61.

17. O'Dea MJ, Zincke H, Utz DC, Bernatz PE. The treatment of renal cell carcinoma with solitary metastasis. J Urol 1978; 120:540–546.

18. Hubmer G, Gnad H, Vilits P. Renal carcinoma with solitary distant metastasis. Urol Int 1984; 39:46–8.

19. Skinner DG, Pfister RR, Colvin R. Extension of renal cell carcinoma into the vena cava—the rationale for aggressive surgical management. J Urol 1972; 107:711–15.

20. Kearney GP, Waters WB, Klein LA, Richie JP, Gittes RF. Results of inferior vena cava resection for renal cell carcinoma. J Urol 1980; 125:769.

21. Clayman RV, Gonzalez R, Fraley EE. Renal cell cancer invading the inferior vena cava—clinical review and anatomical approach. J Urol 1980; 123:157–160.

22. Christensen K, Dyreborg U, Andersen JF, Nissen HM. The value of transvascular embolization in the treatment of renal carcinoma. J Urol 1985; 133(2):191–3.

23. Gottesman JE, Crawford ED, Grossman HB, Scardino P, MacCracken JD. Infarction-nephrectomy for metastatic renal carcinoma. Urology 1985; 25(3):248–50.

24. Milewski JB, Malewski AW, Malanowska S, Borkowski A, Skowronski IA, Tomankiewicz Z, Sawicka E. Spinal cord damage as a complication of renal artery embolization in patients with renal carcinoma. Int Urol Nephrol 1981; 13(3):221–9.

25. Bowers TA, Murray JA, Charnsangavej C, Soo CS, Chuang VP, Wallace S. Bone metastases from renal carcinoma. The preoperative use of transcatheter arterial occlusion. J Bone Joint Surg (Am) 1982; 64(5):749–54.

26. Chuang VP, Wallace S, Swanson D, et al. Arterial occlusion in the management of pain from metastatic renal carcinoma. Radiology 1980; 133(3 pt 1):611–4.

27. Stolbach LL, Begg CB, Hall T, Horton J. Treatment of renal carcinoma: a phase III randomized trial of oral medroxyprogesterone (Provera), hydroxyurea, and nafoxidine. Cancer Treat Rep 1981; 65(7–8):689–92.

28. Concolino G, Marocchi A, Conti C, et al. Human renal cell carcinoma as a hormone dependent tumor. Cancer Res 1978; 38:4340.

29. Harris DT. Hormonal therapy and chemotherapy of renal cell carcinoma. Semin Oncol 1983; 10:422–430.

30. Bloom HJG. Medroxy progesterone acetate (Provera) in treatment of metastatic renal cell carcinoma. Br J Cancer 1971; 25:250.

31. Quesada JR. Biologic response modifiers in the therapy of metastatic renal cell carcinoma. Semin Oncol 1988; 15:396–407.

32. Rosenberg SA. Immunotherapy of patients with advanced cancer using interleukin-2 alone or in combination with lymphokine activated killer cells. In: Important advances in oncology. Philadelphia: Lippincott 1988; 217–57.

36

MALIGNANT TUMORS OF THE UROTHELIUM

Richard J. Macchia, M.D., Mark Horowitz, M.D., and Gobind B. Laungani, M.D.

THE UROTHELIUM IS THE epithelial lining of the lumenal surface of the urinary tract, extending from the tips of the calices of the kidney to the distal urethral meatus. Thus, it involves the lumenal surfaces of the kidney (calices, infundibulas, and pelvis), the ureter, the urinary bladder, and the urethra. Histologically, it is transitional cell epithelium throughout its entire length with the exception of the distal few centimeters of the urethra, which is squamous cell tissue. It is important that the urothelium be regarded as a single organ. Any cancer that appears in one portion of the urothelium has a high propensity to occur either simultaneously or consecutively in another.

Recent research into urothelial cancer has led to a much greater understanding of the basic pathophysiology of the disease process. Clinical research has led to dramatic changes in the management of both superficial and invasive carcinoma of the urinary bladder. This field of endeavor is a constantly changing and rapidly expanding one in which controversy abounds. Unless otherwise noted, the rest of this chapter is devoted to carcinoma of the urinary bladder.

Incidence and Epidemiologic Risk Factors

It is estimated that 50,200 cases of bladder cancer are diagnosed in the United States each year and that 9,500 deaths from the disease occur each year.[1] Bladder cancer is the fifth most common cancer in men in Western society and is the second most common urologic malignancy. The disease has its highest prevalence among those 60–70 yr old; fewer than 1% of bladder cancers are seen in patients under 40. The overall incidence in persons over 40 is 20/100,000 population. Men outnumber women by a ratio of 2.5:1. Bladder cancer occurs twice as frequently among white males as among black males. The geographic distribution of bladder cancer in the United States follows the general pattern of higher incidence of all kinds in the urban areas, especially along the East Coast.

Because bladder cancer follows the general geographic distribution of cancer, environmental factors are presumably significant. The major known causes in industrialized areas are cigarette smoking and certain occupational exposures. There is a 2.5 increased incidence rate of the disease for those who have smoked >100 cigarettes in their lifetime (a relatively small number) as compared with a rate of 1 for those who have not.[2] Tobacco abuse is also the most easily preventable risk factor for carcinoma of the bladder.

Workers exposed to a small group of aromatic hydrocarbon dyestuff intermediates have a risk 30 times that of nonexposed individuals.[2] Less than 1% of the work force has exposure to these chemicals. However, a larger group of workers in 5 occupational categories—dyestuffs, rubber, leather, painting, and use of other organic chemicals—was found to have 1.8 times elevated risk of transitional cell carcinoma of the bladder, as compared with those unexposed. Occupational exposure defined in this way accounts for about one-fifth of all cases.

Among many other suspected risk factors are coffee drinking, artificial sweetener ingestion, exposure to certain chemotherapeutic agents (especially cyclophosphamide, whose metabolites are active cytotoxic substances that can irritate the bladder mucosa if diuresis is not increased at the time of drug administration), pelvic irradiation, and any kind of prolonged irritation of the bladder mucosa.

Many years ago, when indwelling urethral catheters were used for such benign conditions as neurogenic bladder associated with paraplegia, the development of urinary bladder cancer after 20 yr of irritation was a well-known phenomenon. A unique form of chronic irritation is found in regions endemically infested with schistosomiasis. Distribution of histologic types of cancer in these countries shows a shift toward squamous cell types. Another unusual risk factor is the emergence of adenocarcinoma in persons who originally had exstrophy and whose bladders were reconstructed. Any person who has undergone extensive pelvic radiation should be considered in the high-risk category.

Anatomy and Histology

The dome of the bladder is derived from the urachus. Embryologically, the trigone consists of 2 layers. The trigone is triangular in shape and is situated on the posterior wall or floor of the bladder, with its apex exiting through the internal meatus of the urethra, i.e., the bladder neck. The ureteral orifices empty into the bladder at the lateral apices of the trigone. The bladder itself is a hollow muscle lined with mucosa. For the purposes of our discussion, the bladder can be regarded as having 2 layers—mucosal and muscular (or detrusor).

The important anatomic relationships of the bladder are as follows: In the male, its junction with the prostate gland is the so-called bladder neck. The urothelium continues from the bladder and lines the prostate; at its superior border are the seminal vesicles, which, after they extend cephalad of the prostate, abut directly against the posterior wall of the trigone. Laterally, the prostate is bordered by the extraperitoneal structures, including muscles, nerves, and blood vessels. Posteriorly and extraperitoneally is the rectum. The superior and posterior aspects of the bladder are covered with peritoneum. The bowel, especially the sigmoid colon and the ileum, frequently lie upon the peritonealized surface of the bladder.

In the female, the cervix sits immediately subjacent to the trigone and is situated between the ureters immediately prior to their entrance into the bladder wall. The fundus of the uterus is posterior to the bladder and can frequently be seen as an indentation when the bladder is filled with irrigating fluid at cystoscopy.

The 3 most frequent types of bladder carcinoma are transitional cell, squamous cell, and adenocarcinoma. Ninety percent of bladder cancers are transitional cell carcinomas (see chapter 11, figures 11-45A, B, C), either in isolation or distributed with elements of squamous metaplasia, glandular differentiation, squamous cell carcinoma, or adenocarcinoma. Squamous cell carcinoma accounts for 7–9% of bladder cancers and adenocarcinoma for 1–2%. The incidence, risk factors, gender distribution, worldwide distribution, age incidence, stage at diagnosis, natural history, treatment, and prognosis frequently differ across the 3 types.

As already noted, squamous cell carcinoma is primarily reported in regions in which schistosomiasis is endemic, whereas adenocarcinoma (see chapter 11, figure 11-46) is more frequently seen in persons who were born with bladder exstrophy. Both these rare types occur at an earlier mean age—32 for adenocarcinoma, 45 for squamous cell carcinoma—as compared with the mean age of 64 at the time of diagnosis of transitional cell carcinoma. At variance with the latter common histologic type, among patients with adeno-carcinoma and squamous cell carcinoma there is no gender difference. The prognosis is generally more favorable for the transitional cell carcinoma than for the other 2 rare histologic types.

Patients present with either superficial or invasive tumors. More than 70% of bladder cancers occur in the superficial form, of which about 70% will recur, with worsening of the histological grade in 20% and development of invasion in 10%. Initial therapy for these superficial tumors should be directed at eliminating existing disease and preventing recurrence and progression to locally invasive and metastatic disease. Most patients with muscle-invasive disease exhibit the invasive quality at initial presentation; these patients have a worse prognosis, with a higher incidence of metastases.

Grading tumor histologic presentation at time of diagnosis was found to have prognostic significance in view of the fact that most bladder tumors had not begun to invade when diagnosis was made.[4] Most bladder tumors have a luminal surface configuration that is papillary, and because cells forming the papillae may represent various degrees of departure from the morphological appearance of normal transitional cells, they are graded on this basis. Grade I papillary carcinoma is almost indistinguishible from benign papillomas. Grading II and III papillary carcinoma differs from normal papillae in relation to the nuclear cytoplasm ratio, degree of chromatin concentration, etc. Highly undifferentiated tumors are graded IV.[4] Numerous studies present a good correlation of grade with survival. Among a large group of cases with follow-up of at least 8 yr, the mortality from bladder cancer was zero for papillomas, negligible for grade I papillary carcinoma but increased abruptly to 50% for grade II and to 90% and 100% for grades III and IV, respectively.[5] There is certain correlation between pathologic grading and clinical staging because low pathologic grade correlates well at the time of diagnosis with low clinical stage.

Among other biologic factors, chromosomal abnormalities were shown to be of certain significance that is not yet completely defined. In 2 of the most extensive studies, it was found that in more invasive tumors that generally recurred there was an increased number of chromosomes (up to triploidy) and of marker chromosomes; in patients with tumors without marker chromosomes, only 0.5% recur.[6] Recently, alteration of chromosome 3 was found in 30% of karyotypes of patients with transitional cell carcinoma of the bladder whose karyotype was analyzed.[7] Also, it was found that p21 protein, a product of the cellular oncogene ras, has an increased expression in bladder carcinoma with higher grade histology.[8]

Clinical Manifestations

Gross or microscopic hematuria is present in 85% of cases and is by far the most common presenting symptom. The amount of hematuria does not correlate with the severity of the tumor. In adults, hematuria means tumor until proven otherwise, and a diagnostic evaluation should be undertaken to attempt to define its precise cause. Large series have shown that even with a thorough workup a definitive cause for microscopic hematuria can be identified in only 50% of patients. Fortunately, long-term follow-up of patients whose thorough workup was negative does not disclose an incidence of subsequent benign or malignant disease that exceeds their age- and sex-related cohorts. The percentage of patients who will have a malignancy with hematuria varies greatly—1–20%, depending on a variety of circumstances.

Diagnostic pitfalls abound. Hematuria must not be ascribed to excess anticoagulation unless evidence exists for that premise. Hematuria in the presence of a urinary tract infection may be safely ascribed to the urinary tract infection in a sexually active female. However, because bladder cancer and urinary tract infections frequently coexist, bladder cancer must be suspected in the older patient even in the presence of a urinary tract infection. Intermittency of hematuria, or the fact that it is microscopic rather than gross, cannot be used as an argument against the existence of bladder or other urologic cancer.

Although it is the most common symptom or sign, hematuria is not invariably present. One of the causes of the lower tract irritability (LTI) syndrome is carcinoma of the bladder. The patient complains of symptoms suggestive of an infection, such as urinary frequency, dysuria and urgency. Incidental microhematuria, found on routine examination, is not an unusual presentation.

Staging

An important fact is that, in contradistinction to prostate cancer, most cases of bladder cancer are localized to the bladder at time of diagnosis. Only about 10% of patients have demonstrable metastatic lesions at time of diagnosis. It

Table 36-1. TNM Staging Classification of Carcinoma of the Bladder

Primary tumor (T)
    Note: The suffix *m* should be added to the appropriate T category to indicate multiple tumors. The suffix *is* may be added to any T to indicate the presence of associated carcinoma *in situ*

TX	Primary tumor cannot be assessed
T0	No evidence of primary tumor
Tis	Carcinoma *in situ:* "flat tumor"
	Ta Noninvasive papillary carcinoma
T1	Tumor invades subepithelial connective tissue
T2	Tumor invades superficial muscle (inner half)
T3	Tumor invades deep muscle or perivesical fat
	T3a Tumor invades deep muscle (outer half).
	T3b Tumor invades perivesical fat
T4	Tumor invades any of the following: prostate, uterus, vagina, pelvic wall, abdominal wall

Regional lymph nodes (N)
    Note: Regional lymph nodes are those within the true pelvis; all others are distant nodes

NX	Regional lymph nodes cannot be assessed
N0	No regional lymph node metastasis
N1	Metastasis in a single lymph node, ≤ 2 cm in greatest dimension
N2	Metastasis in a single lymph node, >2 cm but not >5 cm in greatest dimension, or multiple lymph nodes, none >5 cm in greatest dimension
N3	Metastasis in a lymph node >5 cm in greatest dimension

Distant metastasis (M)

MX	Presence of distant metastasis cannot be assessed
M0	No distant metastasis
M1	Distant metastasis

Stage grouping

0	Tis, N0, M0
	Ta, N0, M0
I	T1, N0, M0
II	T2, N0, M0
III	T3a, N0, M0
	T3b, N0, M0
IV	T4, N0, M0
	Any T, N1, N2, N3, M0
	Any T, any N, M1

Table 36-2. Comparison of Local Extent of Tumor According to Jewett-Strong-Marshall and TNM Classifications

Jewett-Strong-Marshall	TNM
0 Epithelial	Tis, Ta—Papillary carcinoma confined to mucosa
A Lamina propria	T1
B Superficial muscle	T2
B Deep muscle	T3a
C Perivesical fat	T3b
D Adjacent organs	T4—Adjacent organs
Lymph nodes	N + —Pelvic lymph node metastases
	M + —Metastatic lesions other than lymph nodes

must be remembered, however, that even with the most sophisticated of imaging techniques available today, a lesion of about 1 cm in diameter must be present before it is detectable. If an evaluation for metastatic lesions is "negative," the patient and his family should be educated about the possible existence of micrometastases, which justifies adjuvant therapy. This is especially important in patients who have tumors invasive of the detrusor muscle and who frequently undergo a total cystoprostatectomy as definitive therapy. Despite the extensive nature of the surgical procedure, 50% of these patients die from metastatic disease.

Staging Classification

The most widely used staging system in the world is the TNM system (table 36-1); however, American urologists in general only recently have begun to use this system rather than the older system outlined by Jewett, Strong, and Marshall. Table 36-2 compares the Jewett-Strong-Marshall classification with now more widely used TNM system. Several points about the TNM system merit special attention. The 3 basic divisions are tumors limited to the mucosa, tumors infiltrating the detrusor muscle, and finally, metastatic disease. The likelihood of metastases being present—even though undetectable—with disease infiltrative of the detrusor muscle is extremely high, as evidenced by the above statement about patients subjected to cystoprostatectomy. Although the TNM system is undoubtedly useful, it has significant limitations. For example, it provides no method for quantifying the amount of disease present. The patient with a solitary small T lesion in the bladder is placed in the same classification as a patient whose entire bladder is covered with T lesions. Yet we know from examination of surgically removed bladders that such a diffusely involved bladder most likely has a more penetrating lesion that is simply not detected due to the limitations of biopsy techniques.

Staging procedures

Bladder cancer is generally staged in the following manner: A cystoscopy is performed, and if a lesion is noted, it is excised as completely as possible, using the transurethral resectoscope. The procedure is known as *transurethral resection of the bladder tumor (TUR-BT)*. The cystoscopy and TUR-BT provide a great deal of information. Visually, the urothelium of the bladder and urethra can be inspected to detect multicentricity of visible lesions as well as erythematous areas that may indicate concomitant carcinoma *in situ* (CIS). The location of the lesions has been correlated with prognosis. Lesions in or near the trigone and the bladder neck have the worst prognosis, and multiple lesions carry a worse prognosis than solitary lesions. Given the same grade and stage of tumor, large lesions carry a worse prognosis than small lesions. Cystoscopic visualization allows one to determine whether or not the ureteral orifices are obstructed by tumor. The physical appearance of the tumor also gives an idea of the seriousness of the disease. A cauliflower-shaped exophytic lesion is usually less ominous than a sessile one.

In addition to the excision of a visible lesion by the resectoscope, one ordinarily would perform a procedure known as *bladder mapping*. This consists of using a different instrument, a cold-punch biopsy forceps, to take samples from other portions of the bladder. It is well known that there is a high incidence of concomitant carcinoma *in situ* when a visible bladder lesion is detected. Any lesion carries a more ominous prognosis with it in the presence of concomitant CIS. Patients who demonstrate carcinoma *in situ* in association with a visible bladder lesion have a reported recurrence rate of >80%, with about 60–70% of patients developing infiltrating cancers.

The TUR-BT is performed in a way that attempts to remove the entire tumor if this is technically possible. The procedure removes not only the superficial portions of the tumor, but every effort is made to remove the involved underlying detrusor muscle. Pathologic examination then determines the histologic nature of the tumor. The grade of tumor is estimated. A specific statement should be made on the pathology report as to whether or not muscle is present in the specimen. If so, there should be an indication as to whether or not there is any infiltration of the muscle layer by the tumor.

One must be alert to the fact that urethral involvement is not uncommon; for this reason, transurethral biopsy of the prostatic urethra usually is necessary.

The TUR-BT is routinely performed under general or spinal anesthesia. Upon introducing the instrument, urine is taken for cytologic evaluation. At the conclusion of the procedure, a rectal and bimanual examination is performed to determine any abnormalities in the bladder and in the pelvis, such as a frozen pelvis or a palpable mass. This is also the best time to conduct a thorough examination of the abdomen.

The search for metastatic disease consists of a chest x-ray, radionuclear bone scan, and CT scan of the abdomen and pelvis (see chapter 10, figure 10-25). A simple chest x-ray is most commonly used, although some institutions advocate a chest CT scan. Bone lesions are uncommon in the early phase of bladder cancer. Although the CT scan of the abdomen can be performed at any time, the pelvic CT scan is best performed after the initial cystoscopy but before the TUR-BT. The reason for this is that the TUR-BT frequently leads to inflammation, making interpretation of the CT scan difficult. The CT scan is also useful for detecting enlarged lymph nodes. Percutaneous fine-needle aspiration biopsy of these lymph nodes can easily be accomplished.

An excretory urogram (ExU) is performed to detect urothelial carcinoma of the renal calices and pelvis and ureter. This is ordinarily performed before the

TUR-BT. If a lesion suspicious for cancer is detected, the following manipulations can be undertaken: Selective cytology can be obtained from the ureter on the involved side. If the quality of the ExU leaves something to be desired, a retrograde ureteropyelogram can be performed to better delineate the lesion. A flexible or rigid ureteropyeloscopy can also be performed in order to directly visualize the lesion and obtain a biopsy. On rare occasions, the retrograde passage of an instrument is technically impossible. In these situations, we have performed the selective cytology and biopsy of upper tract lesions by the percutaneous transrenal antegrade route.

Prostatic involvement by transitional cell carcinoma has an impact on the treatment, so it is important to identify all patients with bladder cancer involving the prostate. Of patients with bladder carcinoma, 10–42% demonstrate extension into the prostatic urethra.[17,18] This number increases to 46–68% in patients with carcinoma *in situ*.[19]

Whether the MRI scan will improve clinical staging beyond that obtained by CT scanning remains to be seen. Sonography has been used via the abdominal transrectal and transurethral approaches, and although it occasionally produces interesting images, it has not been adopted for routine use by most medical schools and cancer centers.

Treatment

In discussing treatment modalities, it is convenient to divide patients into 3 categories. The first category is for superficial disease limited to the mucosa and/or submucosa. It includes carcinoma *in situ* as well as visible lesions that do not invade the bladder muscle. In the second category, the disease has infiltrated the bladder muscle. The third category is metastatic disease.

Superficial Disease Therapy

The TUR-BT used in diagnosis is frequently the definitive therapy. If the lesion is superficial, low-grade, and solitary, it is usually the only therapy,[9] and the patient is then subjected to the follow-up routine described at the end of this section. However, the TUR-BT is not sufficient if the lesions are multiple and widespread (or high-grade despite their being superficial) or if CIS is present. The reason is that the recurrence rate after TUR-BT alone in these cases is 50–80%.

Because not all patients will benefit from intravesical therapy, patients who are at higher risk for tumor recurrence and progression must be identified. This high-risk group includes patients with T1 papillary tumors (especially if multiple), multifocal papillary Ta tumors (grade II or III), multifocal and/or symptomatic Tis, persistently positive urine cytology after transurethral resection, and papillary tumors not amenable to resection. In these cases, it seems appropriate to administer intravesical therapy prophylactically to prevent recurrences of superficial bladder tumors as well as progression to deeper bladder wall invasion noted in 15% of Ta cases and 29% of T1 tumors.[11] Half of these patients will die of bladder cancer. Besides the prophylactic intent, intravesical therapy was used with curative intent as definitive therapy for the treatment of disease that cannot be resected surgically. This method of treatment permits the contact of high concentration of cytotoxic agents with tumor-bearing mucosa with limited systemic absorption, thus minimizing toxicity.

Among the agents used for intravesical therapy, 4 were used in a sufficient number of cases to permit an overall assessment of results: thio-tepa, doxorubicin (ADR), mitomycin-C (MIT), and bacille Calmette-Guerin (BCG).[10] Composite data of multiple studies indicate the following rates of complete remission (CR), defined by lack of evidence of disease after therapy-cystoscopy and by biopsy and urine cytology; and partial remission (PR), defined by a 50% reduction in the number of tumors or of the involved bladder surface area or in the size of overt lesions and—in the case of Tis—by a negative biopsy but a positive urine cytology.[10] Among 231 patients treated intravesically with thio-tepa, 38% CRs and 24% PRs were noted. This result was similar to the 33% CR and 31% PR rates seen after ADR intravesical therapy in 366 patients. Among 236 patients given MIT, 48% achieved CRs and 34% PRs. In 401 patients receiving BCG, a 71% CR rate was reported. BCG appears to give consistently better results, which, when stratified for carcinoma in situ (Tis) and papillary tumor (T1), resulted in a CR rate of 82% and 58%, respectively.

In 10 controlled studies in which the above-mentioned drugs were used with prophylactic intent, BCG again gave best results, with a net benefit in treated patients of 42%. This result compared favorably with the 16% benefit after MIT, 13% after ADR therapy, and 6% after thio-tepa. This benefit was defined by the decrease seen in the rate of recurrences at 1 yr in the treated group of patients as compared with the control group. Currently, the 2 most common agents used, based on previous studies, are MIT and BCG.

The protocol currently used by the authors is to instill MIT 40 mg dissolved in 60cc sterile water into the bladder 1 wk after the TUR-BT. The patient then gets weekly treatment for 7 additional weeks at the same dosage. The patient then undergoes cystoscopy and urine cytology 3 mo after the original TUR-BT. If the followup cystoscopy and urine cytology are not clear, the protocol is repeated. If the patient fails again, alternative therapy must be used (e.g., crossover to BCG or total cystectomy).

Besides being effective, BCG has the advantage of being relatively inexpensive. Three different strains were used: Tice, Connaught, and Pasteur.

The efficacy of intravesical BCG for the treatment and prophylaxis of recurrent superficial bladder cancer has been documented by numerous studies[20,21,22] since the initial report by Morales et al in 1976.[23] Martinez-Piniero et al compared the prophylactic effect of ADR, thio-tepa, and BCG against recurrences and progression of superficial transitional cell bladder cancer in 202 patients.[24] The number of patients with recurrences was significantly lower in the BCG arm (9/67) compared to the ADR (23/53) and thio-tepa (20/56) arms. BCG was also superior in preventing recurrences and progression of high-risk tumors. The dosage of BCG used by most authors is 120 mg/50 ml/wk for 6 wk.

The added efficacy of maintenance versus nonmaintenance BCG is still open to discussion. Kavoussi et al reported a success rate of 36% in patients treated after 6 wk of therapy; this increased to 65% after 12 wk of therapy.[25] Badalament et al compared patients receiving BCG weekly for 6 wk with patients receiving the 6 weekly doses plus monthly BCG for 2 yr.[26] Patients receiving maintenance and nonmaintenance therapy had similar tumor recurrence and progression rates. The group concluded that monthly BCG does not prevent, delay, or reduce tumor recurrence or progression observed with the 6-wk regimen.

Catalona et al reported that 58% of the patients who had recurrence after 1 course of BCG were rendered free of tumor by a subsequent course.[27] Bretton et al treated 28 patients with 2 courses of BCG in an effort to identify patients who might benefit from a second course.[28] Their data showed that the usefulness of a second course of BCG is related to the duration of response to the first course. They concluded that patients with a long-lasting response to the initial course of BCG ($\geq$ 21 mo) are likely to benefit from another course.

Side effects of intravesical therapy are relatively modest. Myelosuppression is the chief side effect of thio-tepa and ADR because of their systemic absorption (greater for thio-tepa because its molecule is smaller than that of ADR). Because MIT is not absorbed from the bladder, myelosuppression does not occur; instead, chemical cystitis is seen in 15% of cases and contact dermatitis in the perineal area in 5–10%.

In most patients, BCG produces an intense local inflammatory reaction manifested by dysuria, urgency, frequency, and passing shreds of tissue lasting from 6–24 hr after instillation. The local effects of BCG can be ameliorated with the systemic administration of isomiazed BCG, which has a cumulative effect. Serious complications are extremely rare. Among 1,287 patients treated with BCG, fever of > 103° F was seen in 3.9% of cases, pneumonitis and hepatitis in 0.9%, arthritis in 0.5%, skin rash in 0.4%, ureteral obstruction in 0.3%, and bladder contraction and epididymo-orchitis in 0.2%.[10] Relative contraindications to BCG administration are represented by active tuberculosis and AIDS.

Failure to respond to intravesical therapy should be assessed at 6 mo after treatment. In a multivariate analysis of 221 patients treated with BCG, Herr et al reported that 32% with positive biopsies at 3 mo were free of disease at 6 mo without additional therapy, suggesting a delayed therapeutic effect of BCG.[29] Follow-up should consist of cystoscopy, mapping of recurrent bladder tumors on standardized diagrams, cytological evaluation, and TUR/fulguration, with biopsy of any suspicious areas.

Muscle-Invasive Disease

This has been an area of considerable change over the past few years. In the 1970s, preoperative radiation (XRT) with 2,000 cGy given over the course of 1 wk followed by immediate total cystoprostatectomy was the therapy of choice. This was usually accompanied by the performance of a bilateral systematic pelvic node dissection and urinary diversion by means of an ilial conduit. All these elements are currently undergoing reevaluation.

CYSTOPROSTATECTOMY

Cystoprostatectomy remains the most widely used therapy, but in spite of its extensive and mutilating nature, it yields only a 50% cure rate. Almost all people who die after cystoprostatectomy die of distant metastases, despite the fact that the metastatic evaluation was negative. Incorporation of XRT into the overall therapy was begun in the early 1970s, and it was felt that, based on historic controls only, the addition of preoperative XRT led to a considerable improvement in survival rate and the virtual elimination of recurrent disease in the pelvis. However, there is little evidence based on controlled, randomized studies that indicates a survival advantage in the use of preoperative XRT..

In 1984, Skinner et al compared 100 patients receiving preoperative XRT with 97 treated by surgery alone; they found no significant difference in survival or pelvic recurrence rates.[30]

The role of pelvic lymph node dissection continues to be controversial. About 20–35% of patients thought to have locally invasive but nonmetastatic disease will have metastases to the pelvic lymph nodes. The most critical factors associated with nodal metastases are muscle invasion and penetration into the perivesical fat. Dretler et al showed that in patients followed without adjuvant therapy, up to 33% of those with only 1 or 2 positive lymph nodes achieved long-term cure with surgery alone.[31] Findings of macroscopic nodal disease at time of surgery usually indicated systemic disease and a poor long-term prognosis.

Urinary diversion for patients undergoing cystectomy can be accomplished in 1 of 3 ways: ileal conduit, continent urinary pouch, or neobladder creation. Since 1950, the ileal conduit has been the most widely used form of diversion.[32] Concern needs to be given to the status of the ileum in patients receiving preoperative radiation. Segments of ileum that demonstrate radiation damage should be avoided at all cost. The jejunum should be used only in the patient for whom no other alternative exists. Up to 40% of patients with a jejunal conduit demonstrate electrolyte disturbances characterized by hyperkalemia, acidosis, azotemia, hypovolemia, and hyponatremia. Use of the sigmoid colon has the advantage of providing a means to create a larger cutaneous stoma with fewer complications. The use of the ileocecal diversion offers a stoma that seldom develops stenosis; an antireflux mechanism can be provided by enhancing the ileocecal valve.

Urinary diversion via a continent ileal reservoir was first introduced in the United States in 1982 by Kock and associates.[33] However, this technique has largely been replaced by the creation of a continent urinary pouch using ileal and cecal segments.[34] In highly selected patients, an alternative approach is to create a neobladder from intestinal segments and connect it to the natural urethra.[35]

The ileo neobladder came out of the search for a true bladder substitute that could avoid an external stoma and nocturnal enuresis.[35] It is the only completely detubularized low-pressure reservoir without any valves constructed from ileum. Contraindications against the neobladder are tumor infiltration of the prostatic urethra and impaired kidney function.

Another recent surgical development is the application to cystoprostatectomy of the technique of potency-sparing radical prostatectomy. The potency-sparing total prostatectomy preserves the neurovascular bundles that run posteriolateral to the prostate. Preservation of this bundle may maintain potency in $\leq 80\%$ of patients.

RADIATION THERAPY

Even though radical cystoprostatectomy has been the preferred method of treatment in the United States for patients with invasive bladder cancer, XRT as definitive treatment has been used in a significant proportion of patients who are older, medically inoperable, or who refuse radical cystectomy. With this largely negative selection of patients, definitive external beam XRT to 5,500 cGy led to a 5-yr survival rate of 20–39% for patients presenting with clinical stage T2 and T3 bladder tumors.[12,13] Bladder function was preserved in only 30–50% of cases.

The 5-yr survival in responders to XRT varied in different studies between 72 and 79%, whereas the 5-yr survival in nonresponders was 11–17%.[14] The addition of concomitant chemotherapy (cisplatin[39] or 5-fluorouracil[40] by I.V. infusion) to the XRT has led to an improved local control rate in some patients with clinically advanced (T3 and T4) bladder tumors, causing only a few transient side effects.

CHEMOTHERAPY

Chemotherapy alone has been was used in treating invasive bladder carcinoma in a few institutions. The response rates (preoperatively estimated), counting only patients who achieved CRs, ranged from 6–7% for cisplatin (DDP) alone or in combination with cyclophosphamide (CTX), to 9% for intermediate high-dose methotrexate (MTX) with folinic acid rescue, to 25–45% for a combination of DDP + CTX + ADR (CISCA) (see Appendix), and to 28–55% for the combination regimen M-VAC (MTX + vinblastine (VLB) + ADR + CTX) (see Appendix). The last regimen, developed at the Memorial Sloan-Kettering Cancer Center, proved also to give best results in patients with advanced metastatic disease.[14]

When chemotherapy was combined with XRT, an initial randomized study in which a combination of ADR and 5-fluorouracil (5-FU) was administered following definitive XRT to 110 patients with T3 NX M0 carcinoma of the bladder, no improvement in survival or disease-free interval was found to result from the postirradiation chemotherapy. However, in a prospective study by the National Bladder Cancer Group, patients with muscle-invading bladder cancer stages II to IV who were not candidates for cystectomy received definitive XRT and weekly DDP. A CR rate of 77% was noted among the 57 patients entered in the study (88% for patients with T2 disease, 84% for those with T3, and 50% for T4 lesions). Similar results were obtained at the University of Innsbruck. The CR rates for DDP + XRT seem to be higher than those for XRT alone (43–51%) or for XRT + ADR or 5-FU (50%). At the Health Science Center at Brooklyn, XRT administered with concomitant 5-FU infusion led to a CR rate of 66% in locally advanced bladder carcinoma cases.

The failure rate of 50–70% seen in patients with muscle-invasive disease treated by cystectomy is considered a result of failure to eradicate micrometastatic tumor deposits. Neoadjuvant chemotherapy is an attempt to debulk or downstage the tumor and eradicate the micrometastases by combining radical cystectomy with preoperative systemic chemotherapy. McCullough et al, who studied 17 patients with stages T2 to T4, NX, M0 disease, found that 53% exhibited pathological downstaging after receiving neoadjuvant CISCA.[37] All were clinically free of disease at a median follow-up of 19 mo. At Memorial Sloan-Kettering Cancer Center, where the use of M-VAC was evaluated, significant downstaging occurred in 68% of patients, with 57% achieving T0 and 11% Tis.[38] Further prospective studies are under way at this time.

Salvage cystectomy following combined chemotherapy and full-dose XRT for local recurrences is likely to be more difficult and risky than for recurrence following irradiation alone. For this reason, current studies are focusing on defining criteria for selecting patients who are more likely to respond to definitive XRT and combination chemotherapy, whereas the other cases with locally advanced bladder carcinoma may receive preoperative chemotherapy followed by cystoprostatectomy.

Metastatic Bladder Carcinoma

Due to its tendency to spread hematogenously to many sites, primarily to lung, bone, and liver, the only possible way to approach the therapy of metastatic carcinoma of the bladder is by administering systemic chemotherapy.

Initial trials with single agents showed that DDP, ADR, MTX, and VLB were capable of inducing CRs in 20–35% of cases; unfortunately, the remissions could not be maintained longer than a mean of 2.5–4 mo.[14] For these reasons, a number of combination regimens using drugs that were found active as single agents were tested in small phase 2 trials (without comparison control arms). Among them, the M-VAC regimen, in which 2 drugs (MTX and VLB) were given weekly and all 4 every 5 wk, has generated some enthusiasm in view of a 37% CR rate and 32% PR rate, which are superior to any other regimen. Duration of remission to date averages 8 mo, with a broad range (6–22 mo).[16] It is conceivable that this regimen may represent the first truely curative chemotherapy, at least for some cases of advanced metastatic carcinoma of the bladder.

References

1. Boring CC, Squires TS, Tong T. Cancer statistics 1991. CA 1991; 41:19–36.
2. Cole P. A population based study of bladder cancer. In: Doll R, Vedopija I, eds. Host environmental interactions in the etiology of cancer in man—implementations in research. Lyon: Int Agency for Research in Cancer, 1973; 83–87.
3. Morrison AS. Public health value of using epidemiologic information to identify high risk groups for bladder cancer screening. Semin Oncol 1979; 6:184–88.
4. Farrow GM. Pathologist's role in bladder cancer. Semin Oncol 1979; 6:198–206.
5. Bergkoust A, Lyiengquist A, Mobercer G. Classification of bladder tumors based on the cellular pattern. Preliminary report of a clinical pathological study of 300 cases with a minimal follow-up of eight years. Aeta Chir Scand 1965; 130:371–78.

6. Sandberg AA. Chromosome markers and progression in bladder cancer. Cancer Res 1977; 37:2950–56.

7. Helm S, Mittelman F. Cancer cytogenetics. New York: Alan R. Liss, 1987.

8. Viola MV, Fromowitz F, Orovez S, Deb S, Schlom J. Ras oncogene p21 expression is increased in premalignant lesions and high grade bladder carcinoma J Exp Med 1985; 161:1213–68.

9. Whitmor WF Jr. Surgical management of low stage bladder cancer. Semin Oncol 1979; 6:207–16.

10. Herr HW, Landone VP. Intravesical therapy for superficial bladder cancer. In: Cancer updates. Philadelphia: Lippincott, 1988; 2:1–10.

11. Malmstrom PO, Busch C, Norlen BJ. Recurrence, progression and survival in bladder cancer. Scand J Urol Neph 1987; 21:185–91.

12. Cummings KB, Shipley WU, Einstein AB, Cutler SJ. Current concepts in the management of patients with deeply invasive bladder carcinoma. Semin Oncol 1979; 6:220–27.

13. Shipley WU, Rose MA, Perrone TL, et al. Full dose irradiation for patients with invasive bladder carcinoma: clinical and histological factors prognostic of improved survival. J Urol 1985; 134:679–83.

14. Shipley WU, Kaufman SD, Pront GR Jr. The role of radiation therapy and chemotherapy in the treatment of invasive carcinoma of the urinary bladder.

15. Sternberg I, Yagoda A, Scher HI, et al. Preliminary results of M-VAC (methotrexate, vinblastine, doxorubicin and cisplatin) for transitional cell carcinoma of the urothelium. J Urol 1985; 133:403–07.

16. Yagoda A. Chemotherapy of urothelial tract cancer: Memorial Sloan-Kettering Cancer Center experience. In: Hellman S, Rosenberg SA eds. Important advances in oncology. Philadelphia: Lippincott, 1988; 143–59.

17. Schellhammer PF, Bean MA, Whitmore WF Jr. Prostatic involvement by transitional cell carcinoma: pathogenesis, patterns and prognosis. J Urol 1977; 118:399.

18. Wood DP Jr, Montie JE, Pontes JE, Vanderbrug Medendorp S, Levin HS. Transitional cell carcinoma of the prostate in cystoprostatectomy specimens removed for bladder cancer. J Urol 1989; 141:346.

19. Prout GR Jr, Griffin PP, Daly JJ, Heney NM. Carcinoma in situ of the urinary bladder with and without associated neoplasms. Cancer 1983; 52:524.

20. Lamm DL, Thor DE, Harris SC, Reyna JA, Stogdill VD, Radwin HM. Bacillus Calmette-Guerin immunotherapy of superficial bladder cancer. J Urol 1980; 124:38.

21. Camacho F, Pinsky C, Kerr W, Oettgen H. Treatment of superficial bladder cancer with intravesical BCG. Proc Am Cancer Res Am Soc Clin Oncol 1980; 21:359 (abstract c-160).

22. Brosman SA. Experience with bacillus Calmette-Guerin in patients with superficial bladder cancer. J Urol 1982; 128:27.

23. Morales A, Eidinger D, Bruce AW. Intracavitary bacillus Calmette-Guerin in the treatment of superficial bladder tumors. J Urol 1976; 116:180.

24. Martinez-Pineiro JA, Leon JJ, Martinez-Pineiro L, et al. Bacillus Calmette-Guerin versus doxorubicin versus thio-tepa: a randomized prospective study in 202 patients with superficial bladder cancer. J Urol 1990; 143:502.

25. Kavoussi LR, Torrence RJ, Gillen DP, et al. Results of 6 weekly intravesical bacillus Calmette-Guerin instillations on the treatment of superficial bladder tumors. J Urol 1988; 139:935.

26. Badalament RA, Herr HW, Wong GY, et al. A prospective randomized trial of maintenance versus nonmaintenance intravesical bacillus Calmette-Guerin therapy of superficial bladder cancer. J Clin Oncol 1987; 5:441.

27. Catalona WJ, Hudson MA, Gillen DP, Andriole GL, Ratliff TL. Risks and benefits of repeated courses of intravesical bacillus Calmette-Guerin therapy for superficial bladder cancer. J Urol 1987; 137:220.

28. Bretton PR, Herr HW, Kimmel M, et al. The response of patients with superficial bladder cancer to a second course of intravesical bacillus Calmette-Guerin. J Urol 1990; 143:710.

29. Herr HW, Badalament RA, Amato DA, Laudone VP, Fair WR, Whitmore WF Jr. Superficial bladder cancer treated with bacillus Calmette-Guerin: multivariate analysis of factors affecting tumor progression. J Urol 1989; 141:22.

30. Skinner DG, Lieskovsky G. Contemporary cystectomy with pelvic node dissection compared to preoperative radiation therapy plus cystectomy in management of invasive bladder cancer. J Urol 1984; 131:1069.

31. Dretler SP, Ragsdale BD, Leadbetter WF. The value of pelvic lymphadenectomy in the surgical treatment of bladder cancer. J Urol 1973; 109:414.

32. Bricker EM. Substitution for the urinary bladder by the use of isolated ileal segments. Surg Clin North Am 1956; 36:1117–21.

33. Kock NG, Nilssen AE, Nilssen LD, et al. Urinary diversion via a continent ileal reservoir; clinical results in 12 patients. J Urol 1982; 728:469–75.

34. Comey M. Bladder replacement by ileal cystoplasty following radical cystectomy. World J Urol 1985; 3:161–64.

35. Hautmann RE, Egghart G, Frohneberg D. The ileal neobladder. J Urol 1988; 133:39–44.

36. Walsh PC, Lepor H, Egghaston GC, et al. Radical prostatectomy with preservation of sexual function: anatomical pathological considerations. Prostate 1983; 4:473–78.

37. McCullough DL, Cooper RM, Yeaman LD, et al. Neoadjuvant treatment of stages T2 to T4 bladder cancer with cis-platinum, cyclophosphamide and doxorubicin. J Urol 1989; 141:849.

38. Scher HI, Yagoda A, Herr HW. M-VAC effect on the primary bladder lesion. J Urol 1988; 139:470.

39. Shipley WU, Prout GR, Einstein AB, et al. Treatment of invasive bladder cancer by cisplatinum and radiation in patients unsuited for surgery. JAMA 1987; 258:931–35.

40. Rotman M, Macchia R, Silverstein M, et al. Treatment of advanced bladder carcinoma of the bladder with irradiation and concomitant 5-fluorouracil infusion. Cancer 1987; 59:710–14.

37

TESTICULAR CANCER

Seymour Ritter, M.D.

Incidence and Histologic Classifications

TESTICULAR CANCER ACCOUNTS FOR only about half of 1% of all new cancer cases in the United States per year (about 5,000 cases), and a tenth of 1% of all deaths. Of these tumors, 95% are of germinal origin. Other tumors are of sarcomatous origin, adrenal rest tumors, or mestastic tumors. Because the testicle also appears to be a protected area for leukemic cells, it is occasionally—together with the central nervous system—an area of recurrence. Germinal cell tumors may also arise from the mediastinum or other midline rest areas, where residual germ cells may remain after the descent of testis and ovary sharing the embryonal life. In females, most germinal cell tumors are benign; in the male, most are malignant.

Most germ cell tumors have a typical chromosomal abnormality, an i(12p) (figure 37-1).[18] The normal cells of the patient do not have this, but an increased number of genetic abnormalities is seen in patients with germ cell tumors. Klinefelter's syndrome is associated with primary mediastinal germ cell tumors. Down's syndrome and Marfan's syndrome seem to be associated with testes primaries.[19]

Several classifications for testicular tumors have been suggested.[1,17] The World Health Organization classification of germinal tumors is as follows:
* Tumors of 1 histological type
  — Seminoma with its variant spermatocystic seminoma (see chapter 11, figure 11-48)
  — Embryonal carcinoma with its variant polyembryoma (see chapter 11, figure 11-49)

— Teratoma that could be mature or immature with or without malignant transformation (see chapter 11, figure 11-52)
— Yolk sac tumor or endodermal sinus tumor (see chapter 11, figure 11-50 A & B)
— Choriocarcinoma (see chapter 11, figure 11-51)
* Tumors of more than 1 histological type
  — Embryonal carcinoma with teratoma with or without seminoma
  — Embryonal carcinoma and yolk sac tumor with or without seminoma
  — Yolk sac tumor and teratoma with or without seminoma
  — Choriocarcinoma with any other type
  — Other combinations.

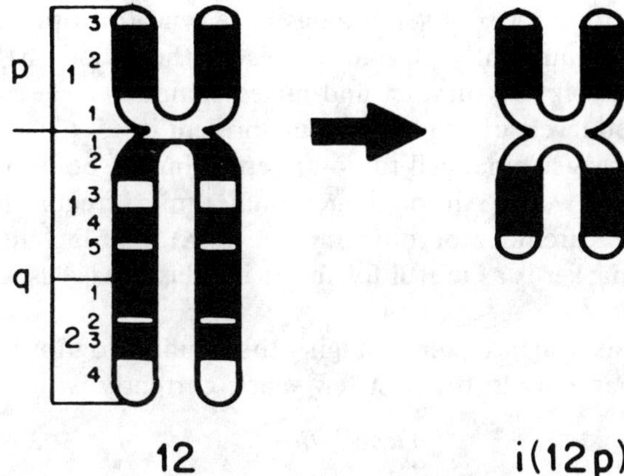

Figure 37-1. Schematic presentation of i(12p), seen in the preponderant number of germ cell tumors of the testis, showing loss of the whole long (q) arm. Whether the i(12p) is dicentric or not remains to be determined. (Source: Castedo SM et al, ref 18)

The treatment approach depends on whether the tumor is pure seminoma or not, and on the stage of the tumor. This classification is of some prognostic significance, although not the primary prognostic factor. The histologic differentiation between pure seminoma and nonseminomatous testicular tumors is the most significant determinant in early stage tumors of the testes.

Patterns of Spread; Diagnosis and Staging

Testicular germinal neoplasms spread primarily via the lymphatic system, the anatomy of which follows that of the vascular system deriving from the genital ridge.[2] Arteries to the testes originate from the aorta just below the renal arteries. The vein from the right testis drains to the vena cava several centimeters below the right renal vein; that of the left testicle drains into the left renal vein. The lymphatics follow the same pathways, draining to the high lumbar nodes, which are connected to the thoracic duct and the left supraclavicular nodes. Primary therapy for testicular neoplasms depends on staging and a knowledge of basic anatomy.

Initial diagnosis depends on finding a testicular mass. At time of diagnosis, 93% of patients with testicular tumors have a palpable intrascrotal mass, 35% have para-aortic node spread revealed by an abnormal I.V. pyelogram or lymphangiogram, and 16% have pulmonary metastases seen on chest x-ray. Testicular scans and sonograms occasionally play a role, but diagnosis hinges on testicular biopsy, which should always be done through an inguinal approach to preserve the lymphatic patterns described above and to prevent abnormal drainage toward inguinal nodes. Tumor markers, alpha-fetoprotein (AFP), and the beta subunit of human chorionic gonadotropin (HCG) must be obtained prior to the biopsy of a testicular mass.[3] HCG is produced by all choriocarcinoma cells, whether or not they are in pure or mixed germinal tumors. In addition, 7.5% of seminomas have syncytiotrophoblastic cells that relapse HCG at significantly elevated levels in the blood. AFP is present in embryonal cells, yolk sac tumors, and mixed tumors.

Elevated blood levels of AFP or HCG are present in 45–65% of patients with nonseminomatous germinal cell tumors, depending on body burden of tumor and cells secreting AFP. Although germinal tumors regularly secrete other markers, such as carcinoembryonic antigen (CEA), and lactate dehydrogenase (LDH), neither marker is as useful for following the disease as AFP and the beta subunit of HCG.

After diagnosis, the next step is staging the tumor. Prognosis by stage, which has improved markedly in the past few years, currently is:

Stage	Description	Prognosis
I	Local	>95%
II	Regional	>95%
III	Distant	75%
		>90%

The American Joint Committee on Cancer has designated staging by TNM classification, as shown in table 37-1.[14]

Because initial spread is via the lymphatics to the thoracic duct and thence to the subclavian vein in the left supraclavicular fossa, investigation is so directed prior to the next step. Chest x-ray and CT scans or tomograms of the chest are the only important radiologic tests needed outside the abdomen. Bone and brain involvement tends to be late. For the determination of stage II, defined by the presence of retroperitoneal nodes, lymphangiography or pelvic and abdomen CT scan are used.[13] At present, the latter permits the most accurate detection of para-aortic lymph node enlargement (see chapter 10, figure 10-19). If markers (AFP and/or HCG) were positive prior to removal of the testicle and negative afterward, this would be good evidence for negative nodes. Chemotherapy is now so effective in curing metastatic disease that efforts have been made to define stage I patients who do not require exploration even though they have nonseminomatous germ cell tumors.[15] Factors that are associated with a worse prognosis (in the case of a stage I

Table 37-1. TNM Classifications Applied to Testicular Cancer

Primary tumor (T)
The extent of primary tumor is classified after radical orchiectomy

TX	Primary tumor cannot be assessed (in the absence of radical orchiectomy, TX is used)
T0	Histologic scar or no evidence of primary tumor
Tis	Intratubular tumor: preinvasive cancer
T1	Tumor limited to testis, including rete testis
T2	Tumor invades beyond tunica albuginea or into epididymis
T3	Tumor invades spermatic cord
T4	Tumor invades scrotum

Regional lymph nodes (N)

NX	Regional lymph nodes cannot be assessed
N0	No regional lymph node metastases
N1	Metastasis in a single lymph node, 2 cm or less in greatest dimension
N2	Metastasis in a single lymph node, more than 2 cm but not more than 5 cm in greatest dimension, or multiple lymph nodes, none more than 5 cm in greatest dimension
N3	Metastasis in a lymph node more than 5 cm in greatest dimension

Distant metastasis (M)

MX	Presence of distant metastasis cannot be assessed
M0	No distant metastasis
M1	Distant metastasis

Stage Groupings

0	Tis, N0, M0
I	T1, N0, M0
	T2, N0, M0
II	T3, N0, M0
	T4, N0, M0
III	Any T, N1, M0
IV	Any T, N2 or N3
	Any T, any N, M1

tumor this would be the likelihood of positive retroperitoneal nodes) would be vascular invasion in the primary tumor, and absence of teratomatous elements. The latter results in a patient with absence of AFP, which is produced in the yolk sac elements of malignant teratomas and embryonal cell carcinomas.[16]

The reason for the attempt to avoid prophylactic chemotherapy concerns the problem of long-term toxicity of these regimens.[20] Cisplatin (DDP) certainly produces a reduction in glomerular filtration rate, and although most recover, long-term reduction has been reported. Several reports have been published on the development of hypertension in young men after DDP-containing chemotherapy. Bosl et al reported increased serum renin and aldosterone levels in nonhypertensive men 9–54 mo after therapy.[20] This suggests that more renovascular problems may arise as time goes on. Other long-term toxicities of these regimens include an effect on sterility, with decreased spermatogenesis and decreased Leydig cell function. Some of this may predate the chemotherapy. No convincing evidence has yet been seen of increased numbers of secondary malignancies from modern treatment of nonseminomatous germ cell tumors, but this may appear in the future. Vascular toxicity has been reported, primarily Raynaud's phenomenon, but myocardial and cerebral episodes have been rarely suspected as secondary to platinum-based chemotherapy. Neurological toxicity, primarily paresthesias, may persist for years after therapy. Ototoxicity is a complication of DDP therapy, but is not a major complaint in young men who do not have audiometry. In nonseminomatous germinal tumors, exploration and retroperitoneal node dissection may be indicated in cases in which lymph node enlargement has been shown by radiologic imaging. The surgery can be nerve sparing, since chemotherapy is so effective. One complication of retroperitoneal node dissection is retrograde ejaculation; preserving the nerve chain can prevent this.

In summary, then, workup becomes a logical progression. In seminoma, once biopsy is done, a CT scan of the abdomen (which may show the presence of massive nodes), a chest x-ray, and liver chemistries usually will be all the workup needed, because if all are negative, the patient has clinical stage I or IIa disease (occult involvement of lymph nodes). If bulky nodes are present in the pelvic or retroperitoneal regions, the patient has IIb disease, and if mediastinal or cervical nodes are involved, patient is stage III, which in some classifications[5] includes also distant organ involvement, while in others[4] the latter represents stage IV disease (table 37-1).

In nonseminomatous germinal tumors, if markers are positive and turn negative after orchiectomy, the patient is in stage I. Further x-rays and CT scans are usually done to confirm this. In marker-negative disease, CT scan of the retroperitoneal nodes and chest x-ray are again the most cost-efficient method of determining if stage III disease is present.[6] Node dissection is needed unless there is bulky retroperitoneal disease or disease outside of the abdomen.[7]

Treatment

Pure seminoma is a very radiosensitive tumor, and because a dose of only 3,000 cGy constitutes a curative dose, standard therapy is radiation of the retroperitoneal and possibly mediastinal and left supraclavicular areas. Because the cure of stages I and II seminoma is >90%, a search for retroperitoneal nodes is not usually done. Chemotherapy with one of the current regimens used for nonseminomatous tumors is generally reserved for seminomas that relapse after irradiation.

Advanced nonseminomatous testicular tumors have been treated successfully since the 1950s, when Li et al used a combination of actinomycin-D (ACT), chlorambucil (CLB), and methotrexate (MTX) to get a 12% complete response (CR) rate and a 39% total response rate.[8]

A variety of other single agents and combinations were used with no better results until Samuels in 1975 reported that a combination of vinblastine (VLB) and bleomycin (BLM) produced a 35% CR rate and a 61% total response rate.[8] The Memorial group (Citkovik et al) introduced the VAB-3 (VLB + doxorubicin [ADR] + BLM + cisplatin [DDP]) protocal in 1977, at about the same time that Einhorn introduced the PVB[9] (DDP + VLB + BLM) (see Appendix). Both produced a CR rate of about 70% in advanced disease.

Subsequent work in both places showed that maintenance therapy with low doses did not add to previous results. It was found that short, intensive courses produced fewer relapses than more widely spaced intensive courses. Patients who recurred on these regimens were treated with rescue regimens using etoposide (ETO, VP-16) and DDP. Because ETO appears to be more active than VLB, it recently replaced the latter in the initial treatment. The BEP (BLM + ETO + DDP) regimen has become the preferred upfront chemotherapy.[10]

Response rate and recurrence rate vary primarily with the bulk and extent of disease. After completion of the chemotherapy course, the patient is evaluated for residual markers or residual masses. Residual markers almost invariably mean residual tumor, but residual masses are represented by fibrosis or benign germ cell tissue in 75% of cases; for this reason, residual masses in patients with negative markers must be surgically removed for identification and salvage cure. In terms of response to therapy of metastatic disease, a regimen such as BEP produces close to 100% CRs in patients with minimal pulmonary or abdominal disease, whereas most of the incomplete responses are converted to CRs with surgical debulking of residual disease. With bulky disease, the CR rate is about 75%.

Adjuvant therapy is used in primary treatment only with poor prognostic factors. The 3 most important independent variables predicating poor prognosis were found to be the levels of LDH and HCG and the total number of metastatic sites.[11] Because minimal recurrent disease has an excellent prognosis and 90% of recurrences will be in the first 2 yr, patients with good surgical chances of cure need not be treated unless and until they recur. Patients with presumed stage I disease, i.e., marker-positive prior to orchiectomy and marker-negative afterward, or patients with no retroperitoneal nodes on exploration do not need to be given adjuvant therapy. In patients with only microscopically positive nodes that are grossly negative, or patients with <5 positive nodes, none of them larger than 2 cm, the surgical cure rate has been estimated at >80%. Because the 20% due to recur can be cured if recurrence is found early, treating the 80% who will never need therapy may be poor strategy. In patients with >6 positive nodes, any node of >2 cm, or extension into adjacent tissue, chemotherapy is used as adjuvant to prevent recurrence. The PEB regimen or a modified VAB-6 regimen can be administered.

Although most patients with germ cell tumors will achieve a CR with the above chemotherapy, poor-risk patients—those likely not to achieve CRs—can be identified. Patients with an estragonadal primary germ cell tumor have a poor prognosis. Only 3 other variables were found to be independent predictors of prognosis. These are actual level of LDH, actual level of HCG, and total number of sites of metastasis. For the latter, size or bulk was not a factor, and the markers were considered as continuous variables rather than using a cutoff level.[11]

Extragonadal Germ Cell Tumors

Germ cell tumors arise from areas other than the testicle; indeed, they can arise from any area along the embryonal germinal ridge. Primary germ cell tumors can arise from the pineal gland to the retroperitoneal area. The second most common primary site after the testicle is the mediastinum.[12] Treatment for extragonadal germ cell tumors usually has been chemotherapy (same regimens as for testicular tumors), but response rates are inferior to rates of testicular germ cell tumors of the same tumor bulk (i.e., between 40–65% CRs in bulky disease).

Recently, suggestions have been made that any undifferentiated tumor of unknown primary origin be treated as a germinal cell primary, and in this series the cure rate of these tumors was 23%. Some had alpha-fetoprotein present on immunoperoxidase staining of the bioptic material, and most were midline tumors.

References

1. Hajdu SI. Pathology of germ cell tumors of the testes. Semin Oncol 1979; 6:14–25.
2. Watson CR. Lymphography of testicular carcinoma. Semin Oncol 1979; 6:31–36.
3. Rowland RG. Serum markers in testicular germ-cell neoplasms. Hematol/Oncol Clin N Am Sept 1988; 2 (3):485–9.
4. Smithers DW, Wallace ENK. Radiotherapy in the treatment of patients with seminomas and teratomas of the testicle. Br J Urol 1962; 34:422–35.
5. Mostofi FK. Comparison of various clinical and pathological classification of tumors of testes. Semin Oncol 1979; 6:26–30.
6. Barzell WE, Whitmore WF. Clinical significance of biologic markers: Memorial Hospital experience. Semin Oncol 1979; 6:48–52.
7. Whitmore WF Jr. Surgical treatment of adult germinal testes tumors. Semin Oncol 1979; 6:55–68.
8. Jacobs EM, Muggia FM, Rozencweig M. Chemotherapy of testicular cancer: from palliation to curative adjuvant therapy. Semin Oncol 1979; 6:3–13.
9. Einhorn LH, Donohue JP. Cis-diamminedichloroplatinum, vinblastine and bleomycin combination chemotherapy in disseminated testicular cancer. Ann Intern Med 1977; 87:293–98.
10. Peckham MJ, Barrett A, Liew KH, et al. The treatment of metastatic germ cell testicular tumors with bleomycin, etoposide and cisplatin (BEP). Br J Cancer 1983; 47:613–19.
11. Bossl GJ, Geller NL, Bajorin D. Identification and management of poor risk patients with germ cell tumors: the Memorial Sloan-Kettering Cancer Center experience. Semin Oncol 1988; 15:339–44.
12. Reynolds TF, Yagoda A, Vugriu D, Golbey R. Chemotherapy of mediastinal germ cell tumors. Semin Oncol 1979; 6:113–15.
13. Pectasides D, Vonorta P, Tsialta-Salihou A, Pateniotis K, et al. Immunoscintigraphy with ^{131}I-labeled H17E2 monoclonal antibody compared with conventional lymphangiography and computed tomography in the detection of metastases in patients with testicular germ cell tumours. Br J Cancer Suppl Jul 1990; 10:74–7.
14. Manual for Staging of Cancer (American Joint Committee on Cancer). 3rd ed. Pt II—Staging of cancer at specific anatomic sites. Philadelphia: Lippincott 1988; 183–87.
15. Williams SD, Stablein DM, Einhorn LH, et al. Immediate adjuvant chemotherapy versus observation with treatment at relapse in pathological stage II testicular cancer. N Engl J Med 1987; 317(23):1433–38.
16. Klepp O, Olsson AM, Henrikson H, et al. Prognostic factors in clinical stage I nonseminomatous germ cell tumors of the testis: multivariate analysis of a prospective multicenter study. J Clin Oncol 1990; 8(3):509–18.
17. Mostofi FK, Sesterhenn IA, Davis CJ. Developments in histopathology of testicular germ cell tumors. Semin Urol 1988; 6(3):171–88.

18. Castedo SM, de Jong B, Oosterhuis JW, et al. Chromosomal changes in human primary testicular nonseminomatous germ cell tumors. Cancer Res 1989; 49(20):5696–701.
19. Dexeus FH, Logothetis CJ, Chong C, Sella A, Ogden S. Genetic abnormalities in men with germ cell tumors. J Urol 1988; 140(1):80–4.
20. Roth BJ, Einhorn LH, Greist A. Long-term complications of cisplatin-based chemotherapy for testis cancer. Semin Oncol 1988; 15(4):345–50.
21. Increased plasma renin and aldosterone in patients treated with cisplatin-based chemotherapy for metastatic germ-cell tumors. J Clin Oncol 1986; 4(11):1684–9.

38

MALIGNANCIES OF THE UTERINE CORPUS

Alexander Sedlis, M.D.

MALIGNANT TUMORS OF THE uterine corpus may arise either from the endometrial lining (adenocarcinoma of endometrium) or from the uterine wall muscle (uterine sarcoma). Of the 2, adenocarcinoma of the endometrium is by far the most frequent. Endometrial adenocarcinoma occurs predominantly in older, postmenopausal women, whereas the sarcoma has no age predilection.

Adenocarcinoma of the Endometrium: Pathology and Natural History

Endometrial adenocarcinoma is the most common malignancy affecting female genital organs. About 38,000 new cases of this tumor appear each year in the United States,[1] >80% among postmenopausal women. In addition to age, risk factors for endometrial carcinoma include obesity, hypertension, diabetes, low parity, and history of ovulatory disorders. Women who develop adenocarcinomas of the endometrium before menopause very frequently suffer from dysfunctional uterine bleeding in association with anovulation.

Adenocarcinoma arising from the uterine mucosa forms polypoid growths, usually multiple, that initially fill the endometrial cavity. Grossly, the malignancy may resemble endometrial hyperplasia or polyp. The uterus does not become enlarged in women with endometrial carcinoma because its cavity is not easily distended and the wall becomes invaded by the tumor only in later stages. Microscopically, adenocarcinoma is composed of glands that, in some respects, resemble normal endometrial glands during proliferative phase (see chapter 11, figure 11-55). Unlike the normal endometrium, however, the malignant glands have distorted shape, intraluminal or stromal invaginations, and multilayered epithelial lining. Epithelial cells also tend to be larger, lighter in color than benign cells, and have larger nuclei, prominent nucleoli, and multiple mitotic figures. Malignant glands grow at the expense of the stroma, forming a "back to back" growth pattern with very little stroma between the glandular walls.

Endometrial tumors are graded according to the histological degree of differentiation. Grade 1 tumors are well differentiated and most closely resemble the normal proliferative phase endometrium. They are composed of glands without solid tumor growth pattern. Grade 2 tumors exhibit areas of solid, poorly differentiated tumor alongside glands. In addition to solid pattern, a cribriform pattern may be also noted that is characterized by intraglandular bridges that divide the glands into small compartments. In Grade 3 tumors, the poorly differentiated solid growth pattern predominates. In some endometrial cancers, regardless of grade, benign squamous epithelium may be noted. Tumors with areas of squamous epithelium are termed adenocarcinoma with squamous differentiation, or adenoacanthoma. Although in most instances squamous differentiation is associated with grade I tumors, the mere presence or absence of squamous epithelium does not change the natural history or prognosis of endometrial cancer.

In addition to the most common "endometroid" tumor (also known as common endometrial), there are special types of endometrial cancer that generally have a poorer prognosis. One such rare type, papillary serous carcinoma (see chapter 11, figure 11-56), histologically resembles the serous papillary tumor of the ovary, showing complex papillations and psammoma bodies. Papillary tumors are very aggressive, rapidly infiltrating the myometrium, penetrating into the lymphatic system, and widely metastasizing into the cervix and peritoneum of pelvic and abdominal organs.[2] Another rare type of endometrial cancer is clear cell carcinoma, histologically characterized by clear cells with abundant transparent cytoplasms and hyperchromatic nuclei that form glands and solid areas. Clear cell carcinoma, sometimes found in association with papillary tumors, is also very virulent. Adeno-squamous carcinoma shows on microscopic examination a combination of adenocarcinoma and squamous cell cancer. The squamous cell component in this tumor has malignant appearance on histologic examination as opposed to the benign squamous cells seen in the so-called adenoacanthoma. Adeno-squamous carcinoma also tends to be clinically more aggressive than the endometroid tumor.

Endometrial cancer expands from its initial site in the lining of the uterus into the underlying uterine wall. Initially, tumor penetration into the uterine wall is slow, especially if the tumor is of the common endometroid variety. Consequently, when first diagnosed, most endometrial tumors are found in the most superficial portions of the uterine wall. It is possible that the initially slow growth of endometrial tumor may be due to the relative resistance of the thick muscular structure of the uterine wall. As the tumor advances through the uterine wall, it enters the lymphatic channels, which become more numerous in the deeper portions of the myometrium. Consequently, the risk of lymphatic involvement rises with the depth of penetration. From the lymphatic channels in the uterine wall, tumor may be carried to the regional lymph nodes draining the uterus that are located either in the pelvis or in the para-aortic region. In further expansion, the tumor may reach the cervix or, in the opposite direction, the ovaries and pelvic structures. The tumor may also spread by hematogenous route to lung, which is a common site for distant metastases of endometrial cancer. The most frequent site of recurrence, however, is the upper vagina, where tumor may be carried through the pelvic lymph channels.

Clinical Manifestations

Abnormal uterine bleeding is the most important symptom of endometrial cancer. Because most endometrial cancers occur in postmenopausal women, the bleeding is of the postmenopausal type. By definition, any bleeding that is 12 mo after the most recent normal period in the menopausal age is abnormal. About one-third of postmenopausal bleeding episodes are caused by endometrial cancer. Other causes of postmenopausal bleeding may be benign endometrial or endocervical polyps, endometrial hyperplasia, abnormal estrogenic stimulation from exogenous medication, ovarian tumors, or other nonspecific sources. Bleeding may also be due to cervical cancer or inflammatory diseases of the cervix or vagina.

Abnormal bleeding caused by the endometrial cancer may also occur in the perimenopausal period, not necessarily preceded by ≥ 12 mo of amenorrhea. In premenopausal women, bleeding caused by endometrial cancer is of the intermenstrual or metrorrhagia type. Bleeding from endometrial cancer is rarely accompanied by other manifestations such as pain or systemic disorders. Physical examination reveals no abnormal findings other than bleeding from the cervical os. The uterus is usually of normal size unless it is enlarged from other causes, such as benign fibroids or from an advanced stage of endometrial cancer.

Diagnosis and Staging

The index of suspicion of endometrial cancer must be high when dealing with patients with postmenopausal, perimenopausal bleeding, or any type of abnormal bleeding after 40. Diagnostic measures must be directed toward detection of endometrial cancer in all these women if no obvious cause of bleeding is found on examination of the cervix or vagina. Diagnosis of endometrial cancer is confirmed by histologic examination of an endometrial tissue sample. The sampling must be obtained regardless of whether or not bleeding is active at the time of examination if the patient reports a history of postmenopausal bleeding. Endometrial tissue may be obtained by dilatation and curettage, a procedure that usually requires use of an operating room and anesthesia. Currently, endometrial sampling is often carried out in an ambu-

Table 38-1. International Federation of Gyncologists and Obstetricians (FIGO) Staging of Corpus Cancer

Stage and grades	Description
Ia—G 1,2,3	Tumor limited to endometrium
Ib—G 1,2,3,	Invasion to $<1/2$ myometrium
Ic—G 1,2,3	Invasion to $>1/2$ myometrium
IIa—G 1,2,3	Endocervical glandular involvement only
IIb—G 1,2,3	Cervical stromal invasion
IIIa—G 1,2,3	Tumor invades serosa and/or adnexae and/or positive peritoneal cytology
IIIb—G 1,2,3	Vaginal metastases
IIIc—G 1,2,3	Metastases to pelvic and/or para-aortic lymph nodes
IVa—G 1,2,3	Tumor invades bladder and/or bowel mucosa
IVb	Distant metases including intra-abdominal and/or inguinal lymph node

latory setting using vacuum aspiration methods or endometrial biopsy. Endometrial biopsy through a specially constructed thin (4 ml in diameter) cannula does not require cervical dilatation; consequently, it can be done without anesthesia or with a local paracervical block.

The revised FIGO staging of corpus cancer is shown in table 38-1. Corpus cancer is now surgically staged. Stage I tumor confined to the uterine corpus is further divided into Ia (tumor limited to the endometrium), Ib (invasion to $<1/2$ myometrium), and Ic (invasion to $>1/2$ myometrium). Stage II involves the cervix in addition to the uterine corpus. A stage III tumor invades peritoneal serosa (positive peritoneal cytology), vagina, adnexae, and pelvic and para-aortic lymph nodes. The stage IV tumor invades bladder and bowel mucosa and/or distant metastatic sites. In addition, each stage is further classified as G 1, 2, or 3, according to histologic grade.

Treatment

Treatment of adenocarcinoma of endometrium depends on the stage. The great majority of patients with endometrial cancer have stage I disease when first diagnosed. The tumor in most of these patients is localized to the uterus, with no (or minimal) lymphatic spread outside the uterus. Therefore, the main objective of treatment in this early stage is to remove the affected organ by simple hysterectomy and bilateral salpingo-oophorectomy. In patients with grade 2 or 3 tumor or special aggressive types (e.g., papillary or clear-cell), in addition to hysterectomy, pelvic and para-aortic lymph nodes are sampled and peritoneal washings are obtained for cytological examination.

The pathological specimen is then examined for prognostic risk factors, such as the tumor grade, depth of penetration into the uterine wall, lymph node metastases, and malignant cells in peritoneal washings. For good prognosis, in tumors that are histologically grade 1 (having only superficial or no myometrial penetration), the postoperative adjuvant treatment consists of local application of radium to the vagina. If the tumor is grade 2 or 3 and it extends to the middle or outer third of the uterine wall, the risk of recurrence is increased; therefore, external radiotherapy (XRT) to the entire pelvis is required. Lymph node metastases and positive peritoneal cytology may require chemotherapy or abdominal XRT in addition to pelvic XRT. At present, the significance of peritoneal cytology is not completely clear-cut. It is possible that some malignant cells in peritoneal washings are from tumor metastases, but some might have been propelled through the fallopian tube into the peritoneal cavity during diagnostic procedures. For this reason, no consensus has yet been reached on what additional treatment, if any, is required for a patient with positive peritoneal cytology.

In stage II endometrial cancer, the cervix is involved; it is therefore assumed that the natural history of the disease will be similar to primary cervical cancer. For this reason, treatment strategy aims at the potential routes of spread of cervical cancer in addition to the cancer in the corpus: pelvic XRT from external radiation source and intracavitary radionuclide applications for stage II cancer, followed or preceded by a total hysterectomy. The value of radical hysterectomy as an alternative treatment of stage II disease has not been established.[3]

Treatment of stage III or IV disease is not governed by any set rules. Treatment may vary according to exact location of extrauterine tumor. A combination of surgery, XRT, and chemotherapy is usually required. Progestational agents are often used for systemic treatment of advanced or recurrent endometrial cancer. The rationale for use of these agents is their known ability to inhibit estrogen-induced epithelial proliferation in endometrial cancer as well as the normal endometrium. For progestational therapy to be effective, tumor cells must have estrogen and progesterone receptors.[4] Testing for receptors is recommended prior to initiating the therapy, although it may be difficult because the endometrial tissue sample is small, especially from metastatic sites. The immunohistochemical method for *in situ* receptor testing should overcome this difficulty because it can be performed on a histological slide. Progestational therapy is tried first because of its minimal toxicity. Prolonged remissions of advanced endometrial cancer have been achieved with progestational agents in about 30% of patients.[4] For women in whom progestational therapy failed, chemotherapy is given, using either doxorubicin (ADR) or cisplatin (DDP) (see Appendix). So far, no significantly favorable results have been obtained with these compounds.

Prognosis and Pathogenesis

The 5-yr survival rate for endometrial cancer patients of all stages is 67%.[5] This relatively favorable survival figure reflects the high preponderance of early-stage disease among the total number of patients and the generally slow rate of progression of this tumor. The positive prognostic factors are histologic grade 1 and no or superficial endometrial penetration.[6] Generally, "good prognosis tumors" are estrogen-dependent cancers, e.g., those associated with postmenopausal estrogen replacement therapy or polycystic ovarian syndrome and other anovulatory disorders producing unopposed estrogen stimulation. The most important unfavorable prognostic indicators are grade 3 tumor and greater than one-third myometrial thickness penetration (see table 38-2).[6] Other poor prognostic factors include special cell types, e.g., papillary and clear-cell tumors, and positive lymph nodes.

Table 38-2. Frequency of Pelvic Node Metastasis Versus Grade and Myometrial Invasion

| Histological grade | None n (%) | Muscle invasion | | |
		Inner 1/3 n (%)	Mid 1/3 n (%)	Outer 1/3 n (%)
1	1/77 (1)	2/85 (2)	1/20 (5)	3/15 (20)
2	1/19 (5)	5/91 (5)	7/15 (14)	11/53 (21)
3	0/11 —	4/35 (11)	3/18 (7)	21/53 (23)

Source: Creasman et al (ref 6)

There is strong evidence that estrogen promotes the growth or even initiation of most endometrial cancers. Prolonged estrogen activity unopposed by progesterone increases the risk of endometrial cancer. For example, rates of endometrial cancer are high in women with estrogen-producing ovarian granulosa theca cell tumors and with chronic anovulatory states (e.g., polycystic ovary syndrome). Obese women, who often have excess estrogen from aromatization of adrenal androstenedione into estrone also show increased rates of endometrial cancer. Clinicians have been long aware of frequent association of endometrial cancer with obesity, hypertension, and diabetes. It is now clear that the obesity is primarily responsible for increased estrogen and increased endometrial cancer risk, whereas hypertension and diabetes are consequences of obesity. Another evidence supporting the role of estrogen in endometrial cancer is the reported increased rate of endometrial adenocarcinoma in postmenopausal women undergoing estrogen replacement therapy.

Early Detection and Prevention

Most cases of endometrial cancer are detected relatively early because the initial manifestation of abnormal vaginal bleeding usually brings on medical attention and endometrial sampling. However, a small proportion of endometrial cancers are asymptomatic. That asymptomatic endometrial cancer exists has been shown by the occasional discovery of cancer on pathological examination of uteri removed for benign indications in asymptomatic patients. Unfortunately, no practical and reliable clinical detection test for asymptomatic endometrial cancer exists. The cervical vaginal cytologic smear (Pap test) is of little value because false-negative results have been observed in 50% of Pap smears from women with endometrial cancer. The accuracy of cytological tests may be improved if the specimen is obtained directly from the endometrial cavity by means of a special aspiration cannula or a scraper. The use of this method, however, is hampered by discomfort to the patient and difficulty in interpreting the cytological material. As a means of cancer prevention, the endometrium should be protected form any prolonged unopposed estrogen. When giving estrogen replacement therapy to postmenopausal women, it is recommended that estrogen should be combined with progestational agents for at least 10 days of the 20-day cycle. Women diagnosed with persistent anovulation (e.g., polycystic ovary syndrome) should be treated with cyclic progestational therapy, such as oral contraceptive pills. Postmenopausal women at higher risk for endometrial cancer (obese, hypertensive and diabetic, or receiving estrogen replacement) should be carefully observed for any vaginal bleeding. Periodic endometrial biopsies have been recommended for screening these women.

Uterine Sarcoma: Pathology and Natural History

Uterine sarcoma originates from the mesenchymal portion of the uterine corpus, myometrium, and endometrial stroma. These tumors are much less frequent then adenocarcinoma but have a more aggressive clinical course and poor prognosis.

Classification of uterine sarcoma is shown in table 38-3. Leiomyosarcoma, one of the most common types, arises from the smooth muscle of the uterine wall and on histological examination presents a pattern similar to normal smooth muscle. It is composed of spindle-shaped small muscle cells arranged parallel in cords and solid sheets (see chapter 11, figure 11-56B). Individual cells show bizarre shapes, nuclear pleomorphism, and an increased number of mitotic figures. Presence of mitoses and their numbers are important diagnostic and prognostic features of leiomyosarcoma. Five or fewer mitotic figures/10 high-power field indicate a benign character of the tumor. Counts of 5–10 mitoses per high-power field are found in an intermediate type of sarcoma that may or may not recur but rarely metastasizes. Sarcomas with counts of >10 mitotic figures per high-power field frequently recur, metastasize, and carry a poor prognosis.[7]

Endometrial stroma sarcoma is histologically a fibrosarcoma. Similarly to leiomyosarcoma, the mitotic count in this tumor is an important prognostic factor. The lymphatic stromal myosis, a variant of endometrial stromal

Table 38-3. Common Types of Uterine Sarcoma

Leiomyosarcoma

Endometrial stromal sarcoma
  (including endolymphatic stromal myosis)

Malignant mixed mullerian tumor

  A. Homologous (carcinosarcoma)

  B. Heterologous

---

sarcoma, has low malignant potential but may extend into the lymphatic spaces of the uterine wall and the parametria.

Malignant mixed mullerian tumors present a combination of 2 or more cell types on histological examination. Homologous malignant mixed mullerian tumors, also known as carcinosarcoma, contain sarcomatous and adenocarcinoma elements. Heterologous malignant mixed mullerian tumors contain elements not usually found in normal uteri, e.g., malignant cartilage, striated muscle, or bone. The striated muscle elements in these tumors are often in immature form and are known as rhabdomyoblasts or "strap cells" characterized by deep eosinophilic cytoplasm and multiple nuclei with occasional striation detected with special stains. Other types of uterine sarcoma include liposarcoma and pure rhabdomyosarcoma.

Clinical Manifestations

Leiomyosarcoma usually presents as a tumor mass replacing the uterus. On palpation, the tumor resembles the benign leiomyoma in that it is firm and multinodular. However, unlike the benign leiomyoma, leiomyosarcoma tends to grow rapidly. Abnormal bleeding may occur in leiomyosarcoma if the tumor extends into the endometrial cavity and erodes the endometrial lining. Leiomyosarcoma should be suspected in cases of rapidly expanding uterine tumors. Preoperative diagnosis of leiomyosarcoma is rarely made because the diagnostic curettage or sampling of endometrial cavity may miss the tissue from a sarcoma unless the tumor is present in the endometrial cavity. For this reason, the diagnosis is made in most instances upon pathological examination of the excised uterus. Leiomyosarcoma occurs at all ages. In young women, sarcoma may be present in a preexisting benign leiomyoma. If myomectomy is performed instead of hysterectomy, the tumor is detected on examination of the myomectomy specimen.

Endometrial stromal sarcoma is found mainly in older women. Like endometrial adenocarcinoma, it causes uterine bleeding and is usually diagnosed on curettage or endometrial biopsy.

The malignant mixed mullerian tumor is seen almost exclusively in postmenopausal women. Clinical manifestations include postmenopausal bleeding or presence of a polypoid mass protruding through the cervical os. The diagnosis is made either by biopsying the mass or by curettage.

Regardless of cell type, sarcomas grow locally and metastasize through the vascular system into the abdominal cavity or the lung. The prognosis is generally poor, especially if the mitotic count is high and the tumor extends outside the uterine body.

Treatment

Surgery, XRT, and chemotherapy singly or in combination have been tried with limited success in treatment of uterine sarcoma. Surgery, the initial step, accomplishes local control of the primary disease. It is usually limited to total hysterectomy, bilateral salpingo-oophorectomy, and excision of visible tumor; radical surgery does not improve the results. Adjuvant chemotherapy with ADR has been disappointing in that the results were as poor in patients treated with chemotherapy as those without.[8] XRT has only a limited indication for treatment of uterine sarcoma because the tumor spreads by hematogenous route and is relatively radioresistant. Recently, however, XRT has been used with limited success for local control of advanced malignant mixed mullerian tumors.[9]

In uterine sarcomas, as in other soft-tissue sarcomas, combination chemotherapy based primarily on the concomitant use of ADR and dacarbazine (DTIC) led to a response rate of 30–42%, with a mean duration of 10 mo. This appeared superior to the response rate of 17–20% with single agents that led to a mean response duration of only 6 mo.[10] However, no improvement of the long-term survival was seen with the combined drugs. The addition of vincristine, cyclophosphamide (CTX) or actinomycin-D did not improve the response rate or survival.[11] Recently, ifosfamide, a CTX analogue activated by hepatic microsomes, was introduced in the treatment of advanced soft-tissue sarcomas with the concomitant administration of MESNA, which prevented the severe hemorrhagic cystitis caused by ifosfamide alone. It lacks cross-resistance with CTX and can be used in combination with etoposide as a salvage regimen.[12] Uterine sarcomas were recently treated with a combination of ifosfamide with MESNA, ADR, and DDP with favorable results.[13,14] Three of 4 patients with measurable disease achieved complete remission; just 1/7 patients relapsed.[13] This phase 2 study, too limited to permit any conclusion, leads to the hope of seeing improved results in ongoing phase 3 trials in which ifosfamide is used in 1 of the regimens.[14]

References

1. Silverberg E, Lubera JA. Cancer statistics. CA 1988; 38:14.
2. Chambers JT, Merino M, Kohorn EI, et al. Uterine papillary serous carcinoma. Obstet Gynecol 1987; 69:109–13.
3. Lewis GC, Bundy B. Surgery for endometrial cancer. Cancer 1981; 48:568.
4. Creasman WT, Soper GT, McCarty KS Jr, et al. Influence of cytoplastic steroid receptors content on prognosis of early stage endometrial carcinoma. Am J Obstet Gynecol 1985; 151:922.
5. Kottmeier HL, ed. Annual report of the results of treatment in gynecologic cancer. Stochholm: Int Federation of Gynecology and Obstetrics. vol. 17, 1979.
6. Creasman WT, Morrow CP, Bundy B. Surgical pathologic spread patterns of endometrial cancer. Cancer 1987; 60:2035.
7. Bartes JF, Smith EB, Szpak CA. Leiomyosarcoma of the uterus: clinical pathologic study. Gynecol Oncol 1984; 21:320.
8. Omura GA, Blessing JA, Major FJ, et al. A randomized clinical trial of adjuvant Adriamycin in uterine sarcomas: a Gynecologic Oncology Group Study. J Clinical Oncol 1985; 3:1240.
9. Hornback NB, Omura G, Major FJ. Observations on the use of adjuvant radiation therapy in patients with stage I and II uterine sarcoma. Int J Radiat Oncol Biol Phys 1986; 12:2127.
10. Gottleib JA, Benjamin RS, Baker LH, et al. The role of DTIC (NSC-45388) in the chemotherapy of sarcomas. Cancer Treat Rep 1976; 60:199–203.

11. Baker LH, Frank J, Fine G, et al. Combination chemotherapy using Adriamycin, DTIC, cyclophosphamide and Actinomycin D for advanced soft tissue sarcomas. A randomized comparative trial. A phase III Southwest Oncology Group study (7613). J Clin Oncol 1987; 5:851–61.
12. Miser JS, Kinsella TJ, Triche TJ, et al. Ifosfamide with MESNA uroprotection and etoposide: an effective regimen in the treatment of recurrent sarcomas and other tumors in children and young adults. J Clin Oncol 1987; 5:1191–98.
13. Nishida T, Nagasue N, Kishi N, et al. A preliminary study of a combination chemotherapy with ifosfamide, Adriamycin and cisplatin for endometrial carcinoma. Acta Obstetr Gynecol Jpn 1988; 490:1883–88.
14. Thigpen T, Lambuth BW, Vance RB. Ifosfamide in the management of gynecologic cancers. Semin Oncol 1990; 17:11–18.

39

CANCER OF THE CERVIX

Jean Claude Remy, M.D.

ALTHOUGH CERVICAL CANCER IS a preventable disease in the United States through early detection and treatment of its precursors, it remains a major problem. It is the most common gynecologic malignancy and is the leading cause of cancer deaths in young women in Third World countries. In this country, cervical cancer is most common in women of low socioeconomic status and in immigrants who have not had adequate screening and health education.[1] One can hope that with better health education and worldwide socioeconomic assistance, cancer of the cervix would one day disappear as a world threat. Cervical cancer starts as an intraepithelial lesion of the squamo-columnar junction in a gradual and reversible onset and progresses to invasive cancer. This process is very slow, perhaps lasting 8–12 yr.

Incidence, Epidemiology, and Histopathology

Invasive cervical cancer occurs at an average age of 48, with peak incidence at age 45–55—10 yr older than the average age for carcinoma *in situ* of the cervix. Recently, however, carcinoma *in situ* and invasive cancer have been found in women in their late teens and early 20s. Cervical intraepithelial neoplasia has almost no symptoms; usually the only manifestation is an abnormal Pap smear that requires a colposcopic examination.

In 1980, the American Cancer Society issued a general guideline suggesting 2 annual Pap tests at the age 20 (or earlier if sexually active), followed by cytologic smears at least every 3 yr.[1] This recommendation was revised after criticism from the American College of Obstetrics and Gynecology and the

Society of Gynecologic Oncologists. Current guidelines are for 3–4 negative annual smears, with the frequency of subsequent tests at the physician's discretion, taking in consideration the degree of risk.

It is well established that squamous cell carcinoma of cervix is a sexually transmitted disease.[1] Menstrual and family histories are not significant risk factors. Early marriage and divorce have been correlated with an increased incidence of cervical cancer. Some studies indicate that Catholic nuns and unmarried women have a low incidence of cervical cancer. It appears that squamous cell carcinoma is related to sexual contact and depends on low socioeconomic status, early sexual activity, and multiple sexual partners. Some recent reports suggest an increased incidence in cigarette smokers.

An etiology involving a sexually transmitted virus has received much attention. At one time herpes type 2 virus was thought to be a strong causative agent of cervical carcinoma; recent data have not supported that role, but some investigations are still under way.[2]

Human papillomaviruses (HPV) are closely related to cervical cancer, but they cause only local manifestations.[2] Although HPV cannot be grown in cell culture, by using recent advances in molecular biology, HPV have been classified into up to 45 different types. Types 6, 11, 16, 18, 31, 33, and 35 are found in genital neoplasia. HPV type 6 and 11, which contain koilocytotic cells, are associated with genital warts, whereas types 16 and 18 show a lesser degree of koilocytosis and high atypia are found in cervical intraepithelial neoplasia II and III. Recently, HPV 31 and 33 have been isolated, the first associated with cervical dysplasia and the second with cervical carcinoma.

The incidence of the human papilloma has increased tremendously in recent years, making it one of the most common sexually transmitted diseases in the United States. Evidence that human papillomavirus is involved in cervical cancer is based on the following facts: Papillomas can progress to carcinomas, koilocytotic atypia of the cervix is induced by HPV, koilocytotic atypia can progress to carcinomas, HVP DNA is detected in a large percentage of dysplasias

Table 39-1. Histologic Classification of Carcinoma of the Cervix

I.   Squamous Cell Carcinoma
   a.   Keratinizing
   b.   Large-cell nonkeratinizing
   c.   Small-cell nonkeratinizing
   d.   Verrucous
II.   Adenocarcinoma
III. Mixed carcinoma
   a.   Adenosquamous
   b.   Mucoepidermoid
   c.   Glassy cell
   d.   Adenocystic
IV.   Undifferentiated carcinoma
V.   Carcinoid tumor
VI.   Malignant melanoma
VII. Malignant nonepithelial tumors
   a.   Sarcoma
   b.   Lymphoma

and cervical cancer, and dysplastic changes occur in human tissues after a laboratory infection with HPV type 2.

More than 85–90% of malignant cervical tumors are squamous in origin, ranging from well differentiated to poorly differentiated (see table 39-1). Squamous cell carcinomas are classified into large-cell keratinizing (epithelial pearls), large-cell nonkeratinizing, and small-cell (possibly neuroendocrine tumors). The gross appearance of the tumor varies with the site and extent of the cancer involvement. Endophytic and exophytic are the 2 major modes of presentation. The former is subdivided into ulceroinfiltrative and nodular infiltrative and the latter into polypoid and papillary forms, with bulky, friable masses protruding into the vagina.

Dissemination of Squamous Cell Carcinoma and Staging

Cancer of cervix spreads by direct extension to adjacent tissues (parametria, uterosarcral ligaments, bony pelvis, bladder, rectum), by lymphatic drainage, and (less commonly) by the blood vessels.[3] The primary nodes involved are those in the parametrial and paravaginal tissues draining to the external iliac, the internal iliac, and the obturator and presacral nodes.[4,17] Disease may spread cephalad though the common iliac nodes to para-aortic nodes and thence to mediastinal and left supraclavicular nodes.[5,18] Retrograde spread to inguinal nodes sometimes occurs. The incidence of pelvic node metastases is about 15% in stage I, 25% in stage II, 36–50% in stage III, and >50% in stage IV.[16] The staging classification initially adopted by the International Federation of Gynecologic Oncologists took into account the patterns of spread of this malignancy (table 39-2).

Table 39-2. Revised International Federation of Gynecologists and Obstetricians (FIGO) Staging Classification for Cancer of Cervix (with 1985 Modifications)

Stage	Description
0	Carcinoma *in situ,* intraepithelial carcinoma (cases of stage 0 should not be included in any therapeutics statistics for invasive cancer)
I	Carcinoma strictly confined to cervix (extension to corpus should be disregarded)
Ia	Preclinical carcinomas of the cervix (i.e., those diagnosed only by microscopy
Ia1	Minimal microscopically evident stromal invasion
Ia2	Lesions detected microscopically that can be measured; upper limits of measurement should not show a depth of invasion of >5 mm taken from the base of the epithelium, either surface or glandular, from which it originates; a second dimension, the horizontal spread, must not exceed 7 mm. Larger lesions should be staged as Ib.
Ib	Lesions of greater dimensions than stage Ia2
II	Carcinoma extending beyond the cervix but not onto the pelvic wall
IIa	Extension to upper two-thirds of vagina; no obvious parametrial involvement
IIb	Obvious parametrial involvement
III	Involvement of the lower third of the vagina or extension to the pelvic sidewall
IIIa	Involvement of the lower third of the vagina; no extension to the pelvic sidewall
IIIb	Extension onto the pelvic sidewall and/or hydronephrosis or nonfunctioning kidney
IV	Carcinoma extending beyond the true pelvis
IVa	Involvement of the mucosa of bladder and rectum
IVb	Distant metastases

Symptomatology and Diagnosis

In the preinvasive phase, cervical neoplasia causes no symptoms; its only manifestation may be an abnormal Pap test during a routine pelvic examination or an examination for vaginitis. The few symptoms of early invasive cancer may include postcoital bleeding, postdouche staining or bleeding, or blood-tinged vaginal discharge. When the lesion becomes more obvious, frank bleeding secondary to ulceration, necrosis, or sloughing of the tumor occurs, and it can be described as menometrorrhagia. Pain occurs when tumor extends to the pelvic sidewall and to the sacrum, with involvement of nerve trunks and the sacral plexus. Late symptoms such as leg edema and swelling are due to lymphatic obstruction by tumor or to venous compression by enlarged lymph nodes. In patients with bladder or rectal involvement, fistulae may be present; hydronephrosis with renal pain and uremia indicates extension of cancer to the parametrium with ureteral obstruction.

Pelvic examination reveals an apparently normal cervix or a cervical ulceration with a granular base and hard nodular edge, or a fungate, friable mass (cauliflower shape) that bleeds easily on touch or instrumentation.

A rectovaginal examination is necessary to assess the extent of the cancer to parametria and utero sacrals. The diagnosis is finally made by a punch biopsy. The clinical evaluation of the tumor is completed with a metastatic workup that includes a CBC with differential, electrolytes, liver chemistries, serology for syphilis, prothrombin time, chest x-ray (PA lat), cystoscopy, partial thromboplastin time, proctosigmoidoscopy, barium enema, and a CT scan of the pelvis and abdomen (see chapter 10, figure 10-22). If an enlarged node is found in the para-aortic area, a fine-needle biopsy should be performed under fluoroscopy (see chapter 10, figure 10-23). If the fine-needle biopsy is negative, the patient should undergo an exploratory laparotomy and an intraperitoneal or extraperitoneal para-aortic node biopsy.

Treatment

Intraepithelian Neoplasia

Surgery is the treatment of choice for carcinoma of the cervix *in situ.* Surgical treatment includes excisional biopsy, cone biopsy, and hysterectomy.[7] A focal or single lesion can be treated by excisional biopsy; however, when several quadrants of the cervix are involved, cone biopsy or hysterectomy are the surgical procedures of choice. Of patients treated with cone biopsy, 3.5% develop recurrence, whereas with hysterectomy the recurrence rate is 0.5–2%. The rates of invasive carcinoma following conization or hysterectomy are 0.5% and 0.3%, respectively, based on collected series.

Other means also are used in the therapy of intraepithelial carcinoma of the cervix. Many physicians and patients favor cryosurgery or laser therapy over electrocautery because less pain and discomfort is associated with it. The criteria for laser vaporization are similar to those used for cryosurgery, and the cure rates are the same (96–98%). However, with laser therapy, tissue destruction is well controlled, tissue reaction is less, and the overall morbidity is minimal.

Microinvasive Cancer

When the lesion is < 1 mm no metastases to pelvic nodes have been found, and the treatment of choice is simple hysterectomy.[8] In patients who desire more children, a provisional treatment may be a cone biopsy with close follow-up, but only if the cone margins and endocervical curettage are negative. If the lesion is 1–3 mm, a modified radical hysterectomy or a radical hysterectomy with pelvic node dissection is indicated.

Frank Invasion

For patients with stages Ib and IIa disease, therapy is either radical hysterectomy and pelvic node dissection or radiotherapy (XRT).[9,15,17] Surgical management is indicated when the size of the lesion is ≤4 cm and when the patient is young, in order to preserve the vaginal and ovarian functions. In all patients who are poor surgical risks or who have cervical lesions of >4 cm, XRT is indicated. Urologic complications related to radical surgery are minimal and, with careful surgery, manageable. The incidence of ureterovaginal fistula has decreased from 1.4% per 1,000 population in 1973 to 0% in 1978.[10] Patients with positive nodes after radical hysterectomy should be treated with adjunctive XRT or chemotherapy.[11]

Patients with stages IIb, III, and IV disease are treated by XRT with or without systemic chemotherapy. The XRT is given in the form of intracavitary radium or cesium (brachytherapy), 8,000 mg/hr, to the main tumor, external radiation (teletherapy), 4,500–5,000 cGy,[12] to the pelvis, and a booster dose of 800–1,000 cGy to the involved side. An extended radiation field is used if there are metastases to the para-aortic node region.[12] Use of the extended field leads to an increased incidence of G.I. (diarrhea, abdominal cramps) and urologic (dysuria, contracted bladder) complications.[13,16] Chemotherapeutic drugs used in combination with XRT are cisplatin (DDP), 5-fluorouracil (5-FU), bleomycin (BLM), and hydroxyurea (HYD) as single-drug or multidrug regimens. If there is evidence of para-aortic node metastases by fine-needle biopsy under CT scan or sonogram or by intra- or extraperitoneal node biopsy, extended field radiation is the appropriate therapy, followed perhaps by chemotherapy. The XRT dose to the para-aortic area is 4,500 cGy.

Special Treatment Categories

Special therapeutic problems are raised by tumor of the cervix with unusual presentation. About 8–10% of stage I and II cancers are bulky endocervical lesions, for which local failure is high when treated with XRT alone because of anoxia at the central core of the tumor. In such cases, most gynecologic oncologists favor XRT followed by extrafascial hysterectomy. The radiation is

Table 39-3. Stages and 5-Yr Survival Rates in Cancer of the Cervix Following Optimal Therapy

Stage	5-Yr survival rate (%)
0	100
Ia	98+
Ib	80–90
IIa	75–80
IIb	55–65
IIIa	40–50
IIIb	30–40
IVa	10–15
IVb	None

given in the form of 4,000 cGy to the whole pelvis, followed by over 72-hr intracavitary radium or cesium application.

Invasive cervical cancer may be found in the surgical specimen when a hysterectomy is performed for benign disease. The prognosis correlates well with the extent of disease. Adjunctive therapy may consist of a combination of vaginal ovoids and external pelvic XRT, which delivers an adequate dose to upper vagina, parametrial tissue, and lymph nodes. A surgical alternative is radical excision of upper vagina with pelvic lymphadenectomy.

Squamous cell carcinoma may develop in the cervical stump of patients who have undergone hysterectomy for nonmalignant conditions. Therapy for cervical stump carcinoma varies with the stage; Stages Ib and IIa can be managed by radical cervicectomy and pelvic node dissection if the patient is a good surgical candidate. If the patient is a poor surgical risk, for stages IIb, III, and IV the therapy of choice is radiation. However, a high rate of small bowel complications should be expected.

Patients with recurrent or persistent cervical cancer after XRT are best managed by pelvic exenteration if the disease is resectable. In patients with widespread metastatic disease, chemotherapy (see Appendix) can be tried. Some of the best results, consisting of 45% partial remission with a mean duration of 11 mo in patients with lung, bone, or liver metastases, were obtained with a combination chemotherapy regimen including BLM, DDP, vincristine, and methotrexate.[14,16] Research is under way in advanced stages using multidrug regimens before XRT in order to reduce the size of the tumor. Such patients can then be treated by radical hysterectomy or XRT, depending on the response to chemotherapy.

The prognosis for patients with carcinoma of the cervix, although it has significantly improved during the past 3 decades, is dependent on the stage of the disease at the time of diagnosis (table 39-3).[15]

References

1. Berek JS, Hacker NF, Fu Y-S et al. Adenocarcinoma of the uteri cervix: histologic variables associated with lymph node metastasis and survival. Obstet Gynecol 1985; 65:46.

2. Kurman RJ, Jenson AB, Lancaster WD. Papilloma virus infection of the cervix. Relationship to intraepithelial neoplasia based on the presence of specific viral structural proteins. Am J Surg Pathol 1983; 7:39.
3. Boyce JG, Fruchter RG, Nicastri AD, et al. Vascular invasion in stage I carcinoma of the cervix. Cancer 1984; 53:1175.
4. Boronow RC. Stage I cervix cancer and pelvic node metastasis. Am J Obstet Gynecol 1977; 127:135.
5. Buchsbaum HJ. Extropelvic lymph node metastases in cervical carcinoma. Am J Obstet Gynecol 1979; 133:814.
6. Averette HE, Dudan RC, Ford JH Jr. Exploratory celiotomy for surgical staging of cervical cancer. Am J Obstet Gynecol 1972; 113:1090.
7. DiSaia PJ. Surgical aspects of cervical carcinoma. Cancer 1981; 48:548.
8. Seski JD, Abell MR, Morley GW. Microinvasive squamous carcinoma of the cervix. Obstet Gynecol 1977; 50:410.
9. Averette HE, Mikuta JJ, Park RC, Wharton JT. Surgery or irradiation? Selecting the best treatment for cervical cancer. Contemp OB/Gyn 1979; 13:80.
10. Remy JC, Fruchter RG, Choi K, Rotman M, Boyce JG. Complications of combined radical hysterectomy and pelvic radiation. Gynecol Oncol 1986; 24, 317–26.
11. Morrow CP, Shingleton HM, Austin JM, et al. Is pelvic radiation beneficial in the post-operative management of stage IB squamous cell carcinoma of the cervix with pelvic node metastases treated by radical hysterectomy and pelvic lymphadenectomy? Gynecol Oncol 1980; 10:105.
12. Fletcher GH, Rutledge FN. Extended field technique in the management of the cancers of the uterine cervix. Am J Roentgenol 1972; 114:116.
13. Delgado G, Caglar H, Walker P. Survival and complications in cervical cancer treated by pelvic and extended field radiation after para-aortic lymphadenectomy. Am J Roentgenol 1978; 130:41.
14. Rosenthal CJ, Khulpateea N, Boyce J, Mehrotra S. Effective chemotherapy for advanced recurrent and metastatic carcinoma of the cervix with bleomycin, cisplatin, vincristine and methotrexate. Cancer 1983; 52:2025–30.
15. Burke TW, Hos-Kins WJ, Heller PB et al. Prognostic factors associated with radical hysterectomy failure, Gynecol Oncol 1987; 26:153.
16. Morrow CP, Townsend DE. Synopsis of gynecologic oncology. 3rd ed. New York: Wiley, 1987; 103–58.
17. Larson DM, Copland LJ, Stringer CA, Gershenson DM, Malone JM Jr, Edwards CL. Recurrent cervical carcinoma after radical hysterectomy, Gynecol Oncol 1988; 30:381–87.
18. Downey GO, Potish RA, Adcock LL, Perm KA, Twiggs LB. Pretreatment surgical staging in cervical carcinoma: therapeutic efficacy of pelvic lymph node resection. Am J Obstet Gynecol 1989; 160:1055–61.

40

INVASIVE CANCER OF THE VAGINA

Jean Claude Remy, M.D.

MALIGNANCIES OF THE VAGINA are uncommon, accounting for only about 2% of all gynecologic cancers.[1] The most common histologic type (95%) is squamous cell carcinoma. Other malignancies include adenocarcinoma, verrucous carcinoma, dethylstilbestrol (DES)-associated clear cell adenocarcinoma, melanoma, sarcoma, and (in children) rhabdomyosarcoma and endodermal sinus tumor.[2]

Squamous Cell Carcinoma: Incidence, Symptoms, and Clinical Appearance

Squamous cell carcinoma of the vagina has the highest incidence in the sixth and seventh decades of life. Chronic irritation associated with uterine prolapse and pessaries, genital viruses, and previous radiation to the vagina have been incriminated as etiologic factors.[1] Before the diagnosis is made, one should eliminate the possibility of cervical carcinoma or vulvar carcinoma with vaginal involvement by means of meticulous examinations of cervix and vulva and by appropriate biopsies. Vaginal bleeding and discharge are the most common presenting symptoms. Sometimes, in advanced stages, a patient may have pain. Urinary symptoms occur in anterior vaginal lesions and G.I. symptoms in posterior lesions.[3] The lesion may appear exophytic, ulcerative, or (rarely) infiltrative. Secondary involvement must be suspected when the lesion is submucosal.

Location, Diagnosis, and Staging

Lesions of the upper third of vagina are the most common, followed by lesions in the middle third and lower third.[2] The posterior wall of the vagina is involved more often than the anterior and lateral walls. Location of the lesion determines the pattern of spread, which takes place by direct invasion and via the lymphatics.[4] Anterior lesions of the upper two-thirds of the vagina metastasize to internal and external iliac nodes; posterior lesions metastasize to the obturator, pararectal, and para-aortic nodes. The lymphatic drainage of the distal vagina, similarly to that of the anus and vulva, is primarily to the inguinal nodes. Diagnosis ordinarily is made by punch biopsy, but immunohistochemical studies sometimes are necessary to make a totally accurate diagnosis.[2,3] The next step in patient management is the metastatic workup, including biopsy of cervix, endometrium and vulva; hematologic studies; blood chemistries; cystourethroscopy; proctosigmoidoscopy; CT scan of pelvic and abdomen; and chest x-ray. At the end of the workup, the stage of vaginal carcinoma can be determined using the criteria of the International Federation of Gynecologists and Obstetricians (FIGO) classification (table 40-1).

Table 40-1. Staging of Primary Vaginal Carcinoma (FIGO Classification)

Stage	Description
0	Carcinoma *in situ,* intraepithelial carcinoma
I	Carcinoma limited to vaginal wall
II	Carcinoma involving the subvaginal tissue but not extending onto the pelvic wall
III	Carcinoma extending onto the pelvic wall
IV	Carcinoma extending beyond the true pelvis or involving the mucosa of the bladder or rectum (bulious edema, as such, does not permit a case to be allotted to stage IV)
IVa	Spread to adjacent organs
IVb	Spread to distant organs

Treatment

Therapy for invasive squamous cell carcinoma depends on the age of the patient, location and extent of the tumor, and the desire for preservation of a functional vagina.[5] Because of the proximity of the bladder and rectum, treatment complications must be expected. Radiotherapy (XRT) remains the preferred treatment for squamous cell carcinoma of the vagina. It is given in the form of external radiation, 4,500–5,000 cGy, followed by interstitial or intracavitary implant. If the lower third of the vagina is involved, 5,000 cGy should be added to both groins.

In some patients with stage I carcinoma, radical hysterectomy, pelvic node dissection, and vaginectomy with split-thickness skin graft can be done successfully.

Patients with recurrent or persistent squamous cell carcinoma are treated the same way as patients with cervical cancer. Exenteration can be attempted for patients in good medical condition with localized central disease. In patients with disseminated disease or unresectable disease, a systemic chemotherapy regimen with cisplatin (DDP) can be tried.[6]

Table 40-2. 5-Yr Survival in Squamous Cell and Clear Cell Carcinoma of the Vagina

Stage	5-Yr survival (%)
Squamous cell carcinoma	
I	55–60
II	35
III	25–30
IV	8
Clear cell carcinoma	
I	87
II	76
III	37
IV	None

Prognosis of carcinoma of the vagina is favorable for patients with stage I disease but poor for patients whose disease is diagnosed in higher stages (see data on their 5-yr survival in table 40-2).

Clear Cell Carcinoma: Etiology and Incidence

In 1971, an association between maternal DES use and clear cell adenocarcinoma in the adolescent offspring was found; since then, more than 550 cases have been identified and entered in a special registry.[7] From 1946–71, an estimated 2–3 million pregnant women were given DES to improve pregnancy outcome because they had signs of threatened abortion or a history of habitual spontaneous abortion. About two thirds of patients with clear cell adenocarcinoma had a history of intrauterine exposure to DES. The risk of developing clear cell carcinoma in the exposed female offspring is about 1:1,000 to 1:10,000. It is even higher if DES was taken before the twelfth week of pregnancy. The youngest child to develop clear cell adenocarcinoma was 7 and the oldest 33, with a peak at age 19. Benign cervicovaginal structural changes can occur, including transverse ridges, cervical hoods and collars, cockscombs and septa, cervical incompetence, and (sometimes) cervical stenosis. DES-exposed women should undergo annual inspection and palpation of the vagina and cervix, cytological examination of vaginal epithelial cells, and iodine staining of vagina and cervix. Colposcopy and biopsy should be performed when any of the previous examinations is abnormal.

Location, Symptoms, Diagnosis, and Treatment

Clear-cell adenocarcinoma arises with almost equal frequency in the vagina and cervix; however, some investigators report a predominance (68%) in the vagina. It originates in the upper third of the vagina along the anterior wall and sometimes in the posterior and lateral walls; it is rarely found in the lower vagina. Early spread to regional pelvic nodes may occur. The pelvic nodes are positive in 16% of stage I lesions and in about 50% of stage II and more advanced stages.

Clear cell adenocarcinoma may be asymptomatic, discovered only on routine pelvic examination in a patient with or without history of DES exposure. In most instances, the symptoms range from heavy vaginal discharge to frank bleeding. The diagnosis is made by colposcopically directed biopsy or by punch biopsy of an obvious lesion. When the diagnosis is made, a metastatic workup should be done to determine the extent of disease. The same staging for squamous cell carcinoma of cervix and vagina is used for clear cell adenocarcinoma.

The therapy for clear cell adenocarcinoma should be individualized. Tumor size and location, extent of disease, and patient age must be considered. In stage I and early stage II, the treatment of choice is radical hysterectomy, pelvic node dissection, and partial or complete vaginectomy with reconstruction. The ovaries are preserved to prevent early menopause. Primary XRT is reserved for advanced stages. The overall survival for all stages is about 78%; the 5-yr survival for each of the stages is similar to that of patients with vaginal squamous cell carcinoma, with the exception of patients with stage II clear cell carcinoma, who have a much better prognosis than those with squamous cell disease (table 40-2).

Recurrent or persistent disease is treated by exenteration when indicated, or by XRT, chemotherapy (see Appendix), or various combinations of these modalities similar to those used for squamous cell carcinoma of the cervix and vagina.

References

1. Blaustein A, Sedlis A. Diseases of the vagina. In: Blaustein A, ed. Pathology of the female genital tract. 2nd ed. New York: Springer-Verlag, 1982; 59.
2. Herbst AL, Green TH, Ulfelder H. Primary carcinoma of the vagina. An analysis of 68 cases. Am J Obstet Gynecol 1970; 106:210.
3. Rutledge F. Cancer of the vagina. Am J Obstet Gynecol 1967; 97:635.
4. Wharton JT, Fletcher GH, Delcos L. Invasive tumors of the vagina: clinical features and management. In: Coppleson M, ed. Gynecologic oncology—principles and clinical practice. New York: Churchill Livingstone, 1981; 345.
5. Annual report on the results of treatment in gynecological cancer. vol 19 FIGO, Radiumhemmet Stockholm, 1985.
6. Rubin SC, Young J, Mikuta JJ. Squamous carcinoma of the vagina: treatment complications and long term follow-up. Gynecol Oncol 1985; 20:346.
7. Herbst AL, Anderson S, Hubby MM, et al. Risk Factors for the development of diethylstilbestrol associated clear cell adenocarcinomas—a case control study. Am J Obstet Gynecol 1986; 154–814.

41

CARCINOMA OF THE OVARY

Alexander Sedlis, M.D.

OVARIAN TUMORS ARE CLASSIFIED into 3 types according to their origin from 1 of the 3 components of the embryonal ovary: (1) common epithelial tumors arising from the celomic lining of the ovary; (2) germ cell tumors from the embryonal germ cell; and (3) sex cord mesenchymal tumors deriving from the ovarian stroma in the region of the embryonal cords. The 3 tumor types will be discussed separately because each category has its distinct symptoms, natural history, prognosis, and response to therapy, in addition to a different embryogenesis.

Common Epithelial Tumors: Terminology and Staging

The common epithelial tumor is the most frequent type of ovarian malignancy, comprising nearly 85% of all cases. Occurring most often in women over 40, its frequency rises with age. These tumors develop from the single layer mesothelial lining of the ovary and its extension into the "germinal inclusion cysts."[1] Ovarian mesothelial cells are capable of transforming into mullerian-like tissues; the tumors that derive from them often resemble endosalpinx, endocervix, or endometrium tissue.

Common epithelial tumors are classified according to (1) cell type, (2) tumor architecture, and (3) malignant behavior (table 41-1). The most common cell types of epithelial tumors of the ovary are serous, mucinous, and endometroid. The less common types are clear-cell tumor and the malignant variety of the Brenner tumor.

Table 41-1. Classification of Common Epithelial Ovarian Tumors

Cell type	Tumor architecture	Malignant behavior
Serous	Cystic	Benign
Mucinous	Papillary	Low malignant potential
Endometrioid	Adenomatous	Carcinoma
Clear cell	Fibrous	
Brenner		

Table 41-2. Histologic Criteria of Benign, Low Malignant Potential (LMP), and Malignant Common Epithelial Ovarian Tumors

	Benign	LMP	Malignant
Multilayering	0	+	+
Atypia	0	+	+
Detachment	0	+	+
Mitoses	0	+	+
Stromal invasion	0	0	+

The serous tumors (see chapter 11, figures 11-58A & B) are composed of cuboidal, sometimes cilliated, cells that resemble the endosalpinx and often show papillary projections and psammoma bodies—round, laminated calcium crystals. The mucinous tumors (see chapter 11, figure 11-59) are made up of columnar, mucin-producing cells that resemble either the endocervix or the goblet cell of intestinal mucosa. The endometroid tumor is characterized by glandlike spaces lined by stratified cuboidal epithelium reproducing the pattern of endometrial mucosa. Clear cell tumors feature solid groups of cells with clear cytoplasm and prominent hyperchromatic nuclei and glandlike spaces lined by "hobnail cells." The malignant Brenner tumors show solid sheets of squamous or transitional-like cells.

The tumor architecture may be either (1) cystic, characterized by fluid-filled spaces; (2) papillary, with fingerlike projections; or (3) adenoid, with glandlike structures.

The malignant behavior of an ovarian tumor may be absent, as in a benign type; predominant, as in a clearly malignant type; or only occasional, as in low malignant potential (LMP) tumor. Histological appearance of a tumor accurately predicts its clinical behavior. Microscopic features of malignancy shared by clearly malignant and LMP tumors are (1) complex papillations, slender branching papillae composed of malignant epithelial cells with thin or absent fibrous stalks; (2) "detachment" of the papillary tips; (3) increased mitotic activity; and (4) cellular pleomorphism or variation in size, shape, and staining characteristics. The feature that distinguishes the clearly malignant tumors from the LMP tumors is the invasion of the tumor into the ovarian stroma, present in malignant but absent in LMP tumors (table 41-2). The diagnostic

Table 41-3. International Federation of Gynecologists and Obstetricians (FIGO) Ovarian Cancer Staging

Stage	
I	Growth limited to the ovaries
Ia	Growth limited to 1 ovary, no ascites 1. No tumor on the external surface; capsule intact 2. Tumor present on the external surface, or capsule(s) ruptured, or both
Ib	Growth limited to both ovaries; no ascites 1. No tumor on external surface; capsule intact 2. Tumor present on external surface, or capsule(s) ruptured, or both
Ic	Tumor either stage 1a or stage 1b, but with ascites present or with positive peritoneal washings
II	Growth involving 1 or both ovaries with pelvic extension
IIa	Extension and/or metastases to uterus and/or tubes
IIb	Extension to other pelvic tissues
IIc	Tumor either stage IIa or stage IIb, but with ascites present or with positive peritoneal washings or with capsule(s) ruptured
III	Tumor involving 1 or both ovaries, with peritoneal implants outside the pelvis and/or positive retroperitoneal or inguinal nodes; superficial liver metastasis qualifies as stage III
IIIa	Tumor grossly limited to the true pelvis, with negative nodes but with histologically confirmed microscopic seeding of abdominal peritoneal surfaces
IIIb	Tumor of 1 or both ovaries with histologically confirmed implants of abdominal peritoneal surfaces, none exceeding 2 cm in diameter; nodes negative
IIIc	Abdominal implants >2 cm in diameter and/or positive retroperitoneal or inguinal nodes
IV	Growth involving 1 or both ovaries with distant metastases. If pleural effusion is present, there must be positive cytology to allot a case to stage IV. Parenchymal liver metastases equals stage IV
Special category	Unexplored cases thought to be ovarian carcinoma

term applied to any given common epithelial tumor is a composite of all 3 characteristics: cell type, tumor architecture, and malignant behavior.

The staging system for ovarian tumor developed by the International Federation of Gynecologists and Obstetricians is shown is table 41-3. Stage I tumors are confined to one (Ia) or both ovaries (Ib). Tumors confined to 1 or 2 ovaries with capsule ruptured, ascites, or malignant cells in peritoneal fluid are classified Ic. Stage II tumors are confined to the pelvis; IIa tumors are limited to the genital organs, fallopian tubes or uterus; IIb tumors also involve the bladder, cul-de-sac and the rectosigmoid; and the classification IIc is used when ascites with or without malignant cells is present. Stage III tumors involve the organs of the peritoneal cavity above the pelvic brim, including the omentum, the bowel serosa, parietal peritoneum, surface of the liver, serosa of the hemidiaphragm, and/or positive retroperitoneal or inguinal lymph nodes. Stages IIIa, b, c are described in the table. Stage IV tumors extend outside the peritoneal cavity to the pleura or distant foci. The stage of ovarian cancer is determined at surgery and radiological survey for metastases.

Clinical Presentation

Advanced Tumors

In nearly two-thirds of patients with malignant common epithelial ovarian tumors, diagnosis is made first in an already advanced stage. The reasons for the delayed diagnosis are absence of symptoms in early disease and rapid progression of peritoneal metastases. The initial symptoms often reflect the involvement of the G.I. tract with tumor. These symptoms are usually vague and nonspecific—for example, "indigestion," postprandial discomfort, nausea, "gas pains," or constipation. Not infrequently, the first symptom is tightness of clothing from increased abdominal girth due to ascites. Some patients may present with symptoms of intestinal obstruction, nausea, vomiting, constipation, and colicky abdominal pains.

On physical examination, the predominant finding may be distended abdomen due to multiple abdominal masses representing primary and metastatic tumor and ascites with shifting dullness and fluid wave. Tumor masses that are characteristically fixed are also felt in the adnexa and the cul-de-sac. Hydrothorax may be found in cases with pleural metastases.

Women with ovarian cancer frequently present in a state of malnutrition (e.g., dehydration, emaciation, and muscle wastage) due to (1) shift of water, electrolytes, and proteins to the ascitic fluid; (2) "parasitic" affinity of tumor cells to circulating amino acids and glucose; (3) inefficient anaerobic carbohydrate cycle in the tumor tissue; (4) compensatory mobilization of glucose from the liver and amino acids from the skeletal muscles; or (5) inadequate food intake because of anorexia and diminished intestinal absorption brought on by impaired peristalsis following blockage of myoenteric plexuses by tumor implants and by ascites.

Early Disease

Early ovarian cancers usually produce no symptoms; a palpable adnexal mass is often the only manifestation of disease. Pain may occur in exceptional instances of tumor torsion, hemorrhage, or rupture. Metrorrhagia, which may occur infrequently, is probably caused by unopposed estrogen produced in the stroma stimulated by the tumor.

Diagnosis

Advanced ovarian malignancy should be suspected in women with vague G.I. symptoms, weight loss, ascites, and pelvic masses. Malignancy of G.I. tract tumors or metastatic tumors from other sites may be differentiated from primary ovarian tumor on colonoscopy, small intestine series, barium enema, and other imaging techniques, including CT scans, sonography and MRI.

Cytologic examination of ascitic fluid aspirated by paracentesis is of little diagnostic help because the cytology is often negative even in presence of obvious malignancy, and the origin of tumor cannot always be ascertained by cytological examination.

Laparoscopy is not useful for the diagnosis of advanced ovarian cancer because the procedure may be technically difficult in the presence of abdominal masses, the findings are not specific, and biopsy through the laparoscope is impractical. Laparotomy is a procedure of choice for definitive diagnosis, staging, and initial therapy of advanced ovarian cancer.

Early ovarian malignancy must be considered as a differential diagnosis in all instances of palpable pelvic masses, especially in adnexal location. Most adnexal masses require laparotomy for final diagnosis because no noninvasive test can reliably rule out ovarian malignancy. Expectant management of an adnexal mass may be justified only if there is (1) clinical evidence of inflammatory disease by history or physical findings, (2) endometriosis, or (3) a small 5–6 cm cystic, freely movable unilateral adnexal mass suggesting a functional ovarian enlargement (e.g., corpus luteum in a young woman). A woman with such findings should be reexamined during the next cycle; if her mass fails to shrink as expected with corpus luteum, she must be surgically explored. In all other instances, mere observation of adnexal masses for a prolonged period of time is inexcusable, because in an event of ovarian malignancy early intervention offers improved prognosis. Prior to surgery, evaluation with sonography, colonoscopy, and barium enema examination should be done to ascertain that the palpable masses do not originate from the G.I. or G.U. tract (e.g., diverticulosis or pelvic kidney).

Although it is impossible to predict with certainty whether adnexal tumor is malignant or benign, certain clinical findings, including large tumor size, lack of mobility, solid consistency, sonographic evidence of irregular contour and inner echos, and presence of ascites in a woman over 40, may favor malignancy. Patients in whom the suspicion for malignancy is high must have preoperative colonoscopy or barium enema and a bowel prep, inasmuch as malignancy increases the risk of entering the bowel lumen (e.g., accidental injury or need for resection). Also, the surgeon who plans to operate on such patients must have the necessary knowledge and skill to perform the required extensive procedure.

The role of the tumor marker, Ca-125, measured by radioimmunoassay (RIA) and found elevated in 80% of the sera of patients with epithelial ovarian cancer, is still debated.[2] However, it is useful in monitoring tumor response to therapy and tumor progression.[2]

Treatment

Patients with ovarian malignancy usually require all 3 modalities of oncologic treatment: surgery, chemotherapy, and radiotherapy (XRT). The initial step is surgery, followed in most patients by adjunctive chemotherapy or XRT for residual tumor. Re-operation, or second-look laparotomy, is also required to evaluate the results of adjunctive therapy.

Surgery

Operative intervention in patients with ovarian malignancy serves 3 purposes: diagnosis, staging, and tumor resection. The abdominal incision for this type of surgery is midline in location, extending from the symphysis to above the umbilicus. The diagnosis of malignancy may be established if findings are grossly obvious (e.g., tumor masses with irregular surface, papillations, hemorrhages and adhesions in ovarian and other intra-abdominal locations). If malignancy is not grossly obvious, a frozen section examination should be done.

For proper tumor staging, the following steps are required:[3]

1. Peritoneal fluid is sampled for cytological examination. Ascitic fluid, if present, is aspirated or, in absence of ascites, peritoneal washings are obtained with 200 ml of saline mixed with 1,000 units of heparin that is poured in and reaspirated from the peritoneal cavity.

2. The entire abdominal cavity is explored by palpation and inspection in search for visible tumor implants.

3. In the absence of any gross tumor implants, multiple biopsies are taken for occult metastases from the peritoneum of the cul-de-sac, paracolic gutters, rectosigmoid, the bladder dome, and the undersurface of the right hemidiaphragm.

4. Omentum is removed below the transverse colon and para-aortic and pelvic nodes are sampled.

Any gross tumor is removed from the primary and metastastic sites together with the ovaries and tubes, in an attempt to "debulk," even in cases in which the entire tumor cannot be resected without sacrificing adhering organs. The purpose of "debulking," or cytoreductive surgery, is to facilitate chemotherapy both by reducing the number of target cells and by stimulating the inactive G-0 phase cells to enter an active cell cycle that is susceptible to chemotherapy. The less residual tumor left after cytoreductive surgery, the better the prognosis. Patients with <1 cm residual tumor are considered in the optimal category and those with >1 cm tumor in the suboptimal category.[4]

Conservative surgery consisting of only unilateral oophorectomy may be done instead of hysterectomy in young women desiring continuation of reproductive function whose tumor is stage Ia, unilateral, with no evidence of spread beyond the ovary and of well differentiated histologic grade. However, even with conservative surgery, the standard staging procedure is required, including cytology samples and omentectomy as well as peritoneal and lymph node biopsies.

Chemotherapy

Because surgery alone cannot eradicate all gross and microscopic tumor, all patients with advanced ovarian cancer require adjuvant therapy. Currently, chemotherapy (see Appendix) is the preferred mode of adjuvant treatment for ovarian cancer because of its systemic effect capable of reaching local and distant metastases. The standard chemotherapy regimen for ovarian cancer is a cisplatin (DDP) and cyclophosphamide (CTX) combination.[15] Hexamethymelamine (HMM) plus doxorubicin (ADR) also produces a response. The multiagent combination has a documented advantage over the single alkylating agent therapy used in the past.[5] Of the 3 agents, DDP achieves the most consistent tumor response. Chemotherapy is usually given at 3-wk intervals for 8–10 treatments. Prolonging chemotherapy beyond this point is not practical because of acquired resistance to the drugs and because of serious drug side effects, including cardiotoxicity (ADR), nephro- and neurotoxicity (DDP), and bladder toxicity (CTX).

Recently, carboplatin, a DDP analogue, was found to be equally effective with DDP in first-line chemotherapy of advanced ovarian cancer. It lacks DDP's renal and G.I. toxicities, and the myelosuppression it induces is tolerable and reversible at a dose of 400 mg/m^2 as single agent and 200–300 mg/m^2 in combination with other alkylating agents or ADR.[16] Ifosfamide (IFX), a CTX analogue, is another new drug currently under investigation. It induced 19–25% partial or complete responses (CRs) in patients with epithelial ovarian cancer that became resistant to DDP-based chemotherapy and to other alkylating agents.[17,18] The intraperitoneal (I.P.) route for chemotherapy is still experimental. Drugs tested so far include melphalan (MEL), ADR, 5-fluorouracil (5-FU), mitomycin (MIT), and DDP. The theoretical advantage of I.P. chemotherapy is that it achieves much higher drug concentration in the peritoneal cavity but a lower concentration in the systemic circulation as compared with the I.V. route. This way, the direct drug effect on peritoneal tumor is enhanced and systemic toxicity is lessened. For I.P. treatment, the chemotherapeutic agent is injected via a Tenthoff catheter implanted in the peritoneal cavity. About 2,000 ml of fluid containing the chemotherapeutic agent is injected, left in the peritoneal cavity for 4 hr, then drained. The instillation is repeated several times during the course of treatment. However, in the case of DDP, which does not induce significant irritation of the peritoneal lining, drainage of the fluid and repetition of the instillation are unnecessary;[19] for this reason, DDP has become the agent of choice for I.P. administration. Adequate fluid distribution is assessed by ultrasound, CT scan, or radiopaque medium. The complications of I.P. chemotherapy include peritonitis and ileus. Extensive I.P. adhesions may interfere with equal distribution of the agent in the peritoneal cavity. The effectiveness of I.P. chemotherapy has not yet been adequately evaluated.

Radiotherapy

External beam radiation has been used less frequently for adjunctive therapy for ovarian cancer than has chemotherapy. Considering the pattern of spread of ovarian carcinoma to the entire peritoneal cavity, XRT must be delivered to the entire peritoneum by total abdominal irradiation in order to match the effectiveness of chemotherapy. The ability to deliver an adequate dose of radiation to the abdominal cavity is limited by potential harm to normal organs, including liver, kidneys, and intestines. It is estimated that to treat a residual tumor of < 5 mm, the XRT dosage should be between 4,500–5,000 cGy. On the other hand, 2,500 cGy may be sufficient for the treatment of peritoneal metastases < 1 mm in size. Irradiation of the abdomen is accomplished either by whole abdominal and pelvic open field technique, the moving strip technique, and abdominal irradiation with the pelvic boost. The best results have been achieved with 2,250 cGy abdominal irradiation plus pelvic boost in patients with early ovarian malignancy who have been initially treated by surgery with complete resection of the malignancy.[7]

Radioactive substances have been used for postoperative instillation into the abdomen. Good results have been reported with radioactive phosphorus (^{32}P), which is a beta emitter with superficial range of action.[8] Currently, the use of ^{32}P is being reevaluated because of reported late complications (intestinal obstruction and injury).

Second-Look Operation

An exploratory laparotomy to assess the results of treatment is performed on patients who have completed adjuvant therapy and show no clinical signs of residual or recurrent tumor. The second-look procedure, similar to the initial staging laparotomy, consists of careful exploration, palpation and inspection of all peritoneal surfaces, peritoneal washings, and multiple peritoneal biopsies. The residual tumor, if encountered, is excised. Results of the second-look operation are used for planning of further management—that is, whether to continue chemotherapy using the same or different agent, change therapeutic modality, or discontinue therapy. More than 50% of patients either have no residual disease or only microscopic disease on the "second-look" and have a 25% chance of survival.

Results of Treatment

The mortality from epithelial cancer of the ovary is 60%, higher than in other common gynecologic cancers (cervix 40%, uterine corpus 20%). One reason for high mortality is delayed diagnosis: Most patients are first diagnosed with advanced stage III or IV disease. Survival is much better in patients with early disease stages I and II: 55–90% in stage I and 20–55% in stage II. It must be noted, however, that the survival figures for early disease are probably inaccurate because (1) only a few patients with early disease are on record and (2) the staging laparotomy is not always according to the accepted standards, so that some patients might have been understaged. Other than the stage, the residual disease and histological grade also influence survival. The cell type (serous, mucinous, or endometroid) is of no prognostic significance.

Overall survival of patients with epithelial ovarian cancer has not improved significantly since the advent of modern chemotherapy, although response is being achieved in 50–88% of patients, of whom 23–44% have a complete response. The median survival of patients is 13–23 mo. Experimental use of immunotherapy so far has not resulted in improved survival.

Tumors of Low Malignant Potential

These tumors, also known as borderline tumors, share many histologic features with well differentiated ovarian cancers but lack stromal invasion.[9]

LMP tumors are much less aggressive than truly invasive ovarian carcinoma, affect younger women, are mostly confined to a single ovary, and in 70% of cases are first diagnosed as stage I or II (in contrast to only 35% in cases of clearly malignant tumor). The 5-yr survival of women with LMP is >90% and at 10 yr is 80%, compared to 40% 5-yr survival with frankly malignant tumors.

The diagnosis of LMP tumors is determined strictly by histologic criteria, namely the absence of stromal invasion. Neither size nor spread outside the ovary influences the diagnosis as long as there is no evidence of stromal invasion in extraovarian locations.

Management of LMP tumors is similar to management of frank ovarian malignancy. The first step is staging laparotomy, including peritoneal washings, search for implants, peritoneal and lymph node biopsies, and omentectomy. Hysterectomy and bilateral salpingo-oophorectomy is the treatment of choice, but young, nulliparous women may be managed conservatively by unilateral oophoretomy only, provided that stromal invasion is definitely ruled out on pathologic examination of multiple sections of the tumor.

The role of adjuvant therapy for women with LMP tumors has not been established, because the high 5- and 10-yr survivals of women with LMP were been reported before the chemotherapy era. Currently, investigational trials are being conducted to assess the value of the single-agent versus multiagent chemotherapy or no therapy in various stages of LMP tumors.

Epidemiology

The frequency of common epithelial malignant tumors of the ovary increases with age; very few have been reported in prepubertal girls. The incidence remains low until the 40s, when it begins to rise progressively with age. Other than age, few risk factors have been identified for epithelial tumors of the ovary. Heredity plays some role, as there are several families with exceptionally high frequencies of these tumors. Obesity, high-unsaturated-fat diet, and previous breast, endometrial, or colon cancer have been named as risk factors. Use of oral contraceptive drugs lowers the risk of ovarian cancer.[10] Theoretically, it is possible that the contraceptive pills diminish the risk of cancer by inhibiting ovulation, thus reducing the scarring of the surface of the ovary that leads to an ingrowth of celomic epithelium into the stroma and formation of germinal inclusion cysts.

Germ Cell Tumors

Although germ cell tumors comprise only 10% of all ovarian tumors, they are the most frequent type of ovarian malignancy in children and adolescents. These tumors derive from the embryonal germ cell that migrates into the gonadal ridge or the future ovary from its original site at the caudal end near the yolk sac during the fifth week of embryonal life. The route of the germ cell

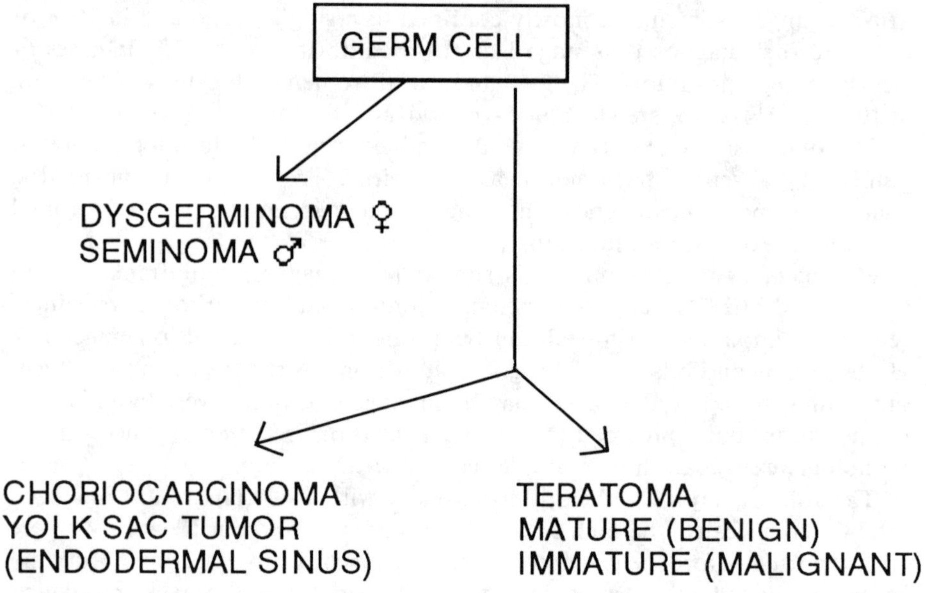

Figure 41-1. Classification of ovarian germ tumor.

migrating in the midline along the mesentery explains why some germ cell tumors develop in the presacral area, the mediastinum, or the pineal gland (see figure 41-1).

Germ cell tumors may reproduce either the undifferentiated germ cell (e.g., ovarian dysgerminoma and testicular seminoma) or in the tissues of the conceptus—as placenta in choriocarcinoma, yolk sac in the yolk sac tumor, and the embryo in teratoma. The mixed germ cell tumor may contain any combination of principal types of tumor.

Dysgerminoma occurs most frequently around the age of 20. At particular risk are individuals with gonadal dysgenesis (xy and xx/xy) and "streak ovaries," which often contain gonadalblastoma, a dysgerminoma precursor. For this reason, streak ovaries should be prophylactically removed. Dysgerminoma, like most ovarian tumors, is usually asymptomatic; its first clinical manifestation may be abdominal or pelvic tumor. Tumor markers are absent in the blood of most patients with dysgerminoma, although human chorionic gonadotropin (HCG) and alpha-fetoprotein (AFP) may be detectable if dysgerminoma contains foci of choriocarcinoma or if endodermal sinus tumor is present.

The tumor is bilateral in $< 10\%$ of cases, and on pathological examination it is solid, with a yellowish-gray cut section surface. Microscopic examination reveals solid sheets of uniformly large cells with round vesicular nuclei and prominent nucleoli. The cell cytoplasm stains positively with para-aminosalicylic acid (PAS), as does the embryonal germ cell. Interspersed between sheets of tumor cells are strands of fibrous connective tissue, diffusely infiltrated with lymphocytes.

Management of dysgerminoma begins with a standard staging laparotomy. The tumor is removed together with the affected ovary. In stage Ia disease, conservative surgery consisting of only unilateral oophorectomy is often warranted to preserve the reproductive function because recurrence and metastases are relatively infrequent. The opposite ovary, if preserved, must be carefully inspected and palpated for presence of tumor. Biopsy of the preserved ovary has been advocated by some and opposed by others on grounds that it may cause adhesions and infertility. For adjuvant therapy in dysgerminoma, XRT has been a method of choice because the tumor is highly radiosensitive— 2,500 cGy eliminates the tumor in the primary and metastatic sites. XRT has been used not only for residual disease after hysterectomy and bilateral salpingo-oophorectomy but also after unilateral oophorectomy. In these patients, reproductive function may be preserved by shielding the uterus and the unaffected ovary while delivering adequate radiation to the residual tumor. Recently, good results and preservation of fertility have been reported with chemotherapy using vincristine (VCR), actinomycin-D (ACT), and chlorambucil (CLB).

The prognosis of patients with dysgerminoma is generally good; 10-yr survival is 90%. The tumor's relatively low malignant potential diagnosis at early stage and susceptibility to radiation and chemotherapy all contribute to high survival figures.

Immature teratoma (formerly malignant teratoma) occurs primarily in children and young adults and is extremely rare after 35. Bilateral involvement is found in only 2% of cases. On histological examination, a mixture of immature tissues and organs resembling embryonal tissues is seen. The degree of maturity of various components determines the histologic grade of tumor. As a rule, immature neuroepithelial elements denote a high degree of immaturity, so that the percentage of neuroepithelial tissue is used as an index of histologic grade of immature teratoma. Neuroepithelial elements can be recognized on histological sections as nests of closely packed elongated cells arranged around a central cleft.

Similarly to common epithelial tumors, immature teratoma spreads to the serosa of the abdominal cavity, and the risk of metastases spread correlates with tumor's histological grade. In some cases, the tumor is more mature in metastatic sites than in the primary site. Histologic tumor grade in metastatic sites correlates with the prognosis for recurrence and survival; if the metastatic tumor is completely mature (e.g., neuroglia), the prognosis for survival is usually excellent.

The surgical procedure for patients with immature teratoma consists of staging laparotomy and removal of the tumor from the primary and metastatic sites. The uterus and contralateral ovary may be preserved because the tumor is rarely bilateral and there is no evidence that the additional surgery improves the prognosis.

Patients with stage I, grade I, completely resected tumor do not require any additional therapy. For grades II and III teratomas, or for tumors with extraovarian spread, adjuvant chemotherapy is indicated, using a VAC combination (VCR + ACT + CTX or CLB). CLB has an advantage over CTX in that it causes less damage to the normal ova. Vinblastine (VLB) + bleomycin (BLM) + DDP also achieves good results, but is reserved for second-line therapy because of its serious side effects. Either combination is administered in 3 or 4 courses (see Appendix).

A second-look operative procedure is indicated for patients with pure teratoma with no measurable tumor markers. In recent years, use of chemotherapy has greatly improved the outcome for patients with high-grade and extensive stages of immature teratoma. Many patients treated with modern combination chemotherapy are now in prolonged remission and free of recurrence.

Yolk sac tumor (also known as endodermal sinus tumor), choriocarcinoma, and embryonal carcinoma are rare types of malignant germ cell tumors. A large proportion of these tumors are of mixed type, containing 2 or more malignant germ cell elements. Endodermal sinus tumor (yolk sac tumor) is composed of loosely arranged interlacing thin tubules. The Schiller-Duval body, a glomeruloid structure with a central tuftlike projection, is the second component found on histological examination. Eosinophilic colloid droplets containing AFP are identifiable by immunocytochemistry.

These tumors, which occur mainly in children and young adults, are usually asymptomatic until a pelvic or abdominal tumor becomes evident. In rare instances, choriocarcinoma may cause hemoperitoneum and acute abdominal pain that simulate ectopic pregnancy. The false impression of ectopic pregnancy may be reinforced by the positive HCG produced by the tumor. HCG and AFP produced by endodermal sinus tumor are important tumor markers that can be measured in the blood for diagnosis and for monitoring treatment results. For this reason, it is advisable to routinely determine the baseline HCG and AFP titers preoperatively on young women with a solid ovarian tumor. Endodermal sinus tumor, choriocarcinoma, and embryonal carcinoma are extremely aggressive tumors that spread so rapidly from the onset that they are often diagnosed in advanced stage. Surgical treatment consists of staging procedure and resection of all visible tumor. The uterus and other ovary may be preserved, because there is no evidence that their removal improves survival.

Although until recently these tumors were universally fatal and caused death within several months after diagnosis, modern chemotherapy has dramatically improved the outcome.[11] As in immature teratomas, many patients are now in prolonged remission after chemotherapy. The choice of chemotherapeutic regimen is the same as for immature teratoma: either VAC or VLB + BLM + DDP. Second-look laparotomy is not always necessary because the HCG and AFP are reliable indexes of tumor recurrence or persistence.[12]

Sex Cord Mesenchymal Tumors

Approximately 5% of ovarian malignancies belong to the sex cord mesenchymal tumor group. These tumors derive from the gonadal mesenchymal cells that in the developing embryo are arranged into cordlike structures and later develop either into the follicular wall of the ovary or the spermatic tubules in the testicles. Theca granulosa tumor reproduces the components of the ovarian follicle and the Sertoli-Leydig cell tumors those of the testicle. The common characteristic of mesenchymal tumors is their ability to produce steroid hermones, either estrogenic or androgenic, and their relatively low malignant potential.

Theca granulosa tumors are more common than Sertoli-Leydig cell tumors, are mostly solid or contain cystic cavities, and are rarely bilateral. Microscopically, they present solid sheets of uniformly sized, mostly round, occasionally elongated cells with rare mitotic figures that resemble the follicular cells of normal ovary. The granulosa cells are interspersed with areas of thecalike cells of elongated shape and arranged into parallel bundles. The common microscopic patterns of granulosa theca cell tumors are: (1) microfollicular, featuring Call-Exner bodies—small follicle-like spaces that contain eosinophilic material; (2) macrofollicular, with large cystic spaces; (3) trabecular, with cells arranged into wavelike cords; and (4) sarcomatoid, a solid tumor. The last-named variety may sometimes be confused with an undifferentiated common epithelial cancer, and may require special techniques such as electron-microscopy or immunocytochemistry for differential diagnosis.

Theca granulosa tumors may be found in all age groups, including children. These tumors secrete estrogen, affecting the endometrium and other targets and producing symptoms. In women of reproductive age, the symptom of unopposed estrogen is metrorrhagia from endometrial hyperplasia. In postmenopausal women, the tumors cause postmenopausal bleeding, and in prepubertal girls, bring forth a pseudoprecocious puberty characterized by vaginal bleeding and telarche. Abnormal vaginal bleeding that accompanies these tumors leads to early diagnosis, in contrast with common epithelial tumors, which are usually asymptomatic. Diagnosis of these tumors is confirmed by finding a palpable or sonographically evident pelvic tumor.

The risk of metastases in granulosa cell tumor is low, and recurrences are seen in only 10–20% of patients, usually after an interval of 10–20 yr.[13] Because the malignant potential of these tumors is relatively low, they are managed more conservatively than are the highly virulent epithelial tumors. The recommended treatment of granulosa cell tumor is staging laparotomy and a unilateral oophorectomy for stage I disease. Adjuvant therapy with VAC chemotherapy has been used only for extensive disease and residual tumor after surgery.

Because testosterone-producing Sertoli-Leydig cell tumors are very rare, their natural history and response to therapy has not been adequately investigated. These tumors usually do not attain a large size, perhaps because of early diagnosis based on pronounced signs of virilization. On miscroscopic examination, the dark-staining, elongated Sertoli cells are found arranged in ductlike formation. The testosterone-producing Leydig cells are large, have abundant, dense eosinophilic cytoplasm, and appear in clusters scattered among Sertoli cells. Symptoms produced by these tumors include amenorrhea, hirsutism, baldness, clitoral hypertrophy, and deepening of the voice. High levels of testosterone may be detected in the blood. Sertoli-Leydig cell tumors of the ovary must be differentiated from adrenal tumors or hyperplasia, which also may cause virilization. The differential diagnosis may be complicated because the usually small ovarian tumor may be missed on palpation or even sonography.

Sertoli-Leydig cell tumors are known to metastasize and recur, but exact figures on mortality are not available. Patients with these tumors are managed similarly to those with other tumors of low malignant potential, namely, by staging laparotomy and unilateral oophorectomy for stage Ia tumor and more extensive surgery if extraovarian spread is noted. The role of adjuvant therapy for these tumors has not been well investigated, but response to VAC and other chemotherapeutic agents has been reported.

Ovarian Cancer Control

Ovarian cancer control through early detection has not been successful mostly because the tumor is asymptomatic in the early stages and the because usual warning symptoms of gynecological cancers (e.g., bleeding or pain) are absent. No screening techniques are available, and Pap smears are rarely positive and then usually only with disseminated disease when the malignant cells spread outside of the ovary into the fallopian tubes, the uterine cavity, and the cervix.

The few options for ovarian cancer prevention are as follows: Periodic pelvic examination is recommended for women over 40, in whom the frequency of ovarian cancer is increased. Women with palpable adnexal tumors must be carefully evaluated for possible ovarian malignancy. Laparotomy is advisable for any adnexal mass that is larger than 6 cm and persistent unless nonneoplastic etiology can be firmly established (e.g., infection or endometriosis). Women of postmenopausal age should be considered for surgical exploration, even with lesser degree of ovarian enlargement. Surgery has been recommended for the so-called postmenopausal palpable ovary syndrome. According to one view, any palpable ovary in postmenopausal women should be considered suspicious because normal postmenopausal ovaries are too small to be discernable on pelvic examination. Periodic screening of all women over 40 by pelvic sonogram also has been advocated. Potential usefulness of newly developed ovarian tumor markers for screening purposes is being investigated.[14]

References

1. Gondos B. Surface epithelium of the developing ovary. Possible correlation with ovarian neoplasia. Am J Pathol 1975; 81:303.
2. Niloff JM. The role of CA 125 assay in the management of ovarian cancer. Oncology 1988; 2:67–72.
3. Wharton JT, Herson J. Surgery for common epithelial tumors of the ovary. Cancer 1981; 48:582.
4. Griffiths CT, Parker LM, Fuller AF. Role of cytoreductive surgical treatment in the management of advanced ovarian dancer. Cancer Treat Rep 1979; 63:235.
5. Thigpen T, Blessing JA. Current therapy of ovarian carcinoma: an overview. Semin Oncol 1984; 12:47–52.
6. Piver MS, Lele SB, Marchetti DL, et al. Surgically documented response to intraperitoneal cisplatin, cytarabine and bleomycin after intravenous cisplatin-based chemotherapy in advanced ovarian adenocarcinoma. J Clin Oncol 1988; 6:679–84.

7. Dembo AJ, Bush RS. Radiation therapy of ovarian carcinoma. In: Griffith CT, Fuller AF, eds. Gynecological oncology. Boston: Martinus Nijhoft, 1983; 263–298.

8. Hilaris BS, Clar GC. The value of post-operative intraperitoneal injection of radiocolloids in early cancer of the ovary. Am J Roentgenol Rad Ther Nucl Med 1971; 112:749.

9. Colgan TJ, Norris HJ. Ovarian epithelial tumors of low malignant potential: a review. Int J Gynecol Pathol 1983; 1:367.

10. Stadel BV. The etiology and prevention of ovarian cancer. Am J Obstet Gynecol 1975; 123:772.

11. Slayton RE, Park RC, Silverberg SG, et al. Vincristine, actinomycin and cyclophosphamide in the treatment of malignant germ cell tumors of the ovary. A Gynecologic Oncology Group study (final report) Cancer 1985; 56:243.

12. Gershenson DM, Copeland LJ, DelJunco G, et al. Second-look laparotomy in the management of malignant germ cell tumors of the ovary. Obstet Gynecol 1986; 67:789.

13. Bjozkholm E, Silfversward C. Prognostic factors in granulosa-cell tumors. Gynecol Oncol 1981; 11:261.

14. Klug TL, Bast RC, Niloff JM, et al. Monoclonal antibody immunoradiometric assay for an antigenic determinant (CA125) associated with human epithelial ovarian carcinoma. Cancer Res 1984; 44:1048.

15. Omura GA, Bundy BN, Berek JS, et al. Randomized trial of cyclophosphamide plus cisplatin with or without doxorubicin in ovarian carcinomas. A Gynecology Oncology Group study. J Clin Oncol 1989; 7:457–69.

16. Alberts DS, Canetta R, Mason-hiddil N. Carboplatin in the first line chemotherapy of ovarian cancer. Semin Oncol 1990; 17:54–60.

17. Sutton GP, Blessing JA, Photopoulos G, et al. Phase II experience with iphosphamide/MESNA in gynecologic malignancies. Preliminary report of Gynecologic Oncology Group studies. Semin Oncol 1989; 16:68–72 (suppl 3).

18. Thigpen T, Lambuth BW, Vance RB. Ifosfamide in the management of gynecologic cancers. Semin Oncol 1990; 17:11–18 (suppl 4).

19. Marksman M. Intraperitoneal cisplatin chemotherapy in the management of ovarian carcinoma. Semin Oncol 1989; 16:79–82 (suppl 6).

42

CARCINOMA OF THE BREAST

*Joseph Aisner, M.D., F.A.C.P., Jeffrey S. Abrams, M.D.,
and N. Simon Tchekmedyian, M.D., F.A.C.P.*

CANCER OF THE BREAST is a common and important problem for women and for society in general. Known since ancient times, breast cancer has recently received considerable attention with changes in treatment approaches. The oncologist's role in the management of patients with breast cancer, which has expanded in recent years, now includes not only the treatment of recurrent and metastatic cancer but also participation in the initial therapy of many patients. The approach to this disease has become a multidisciplinary undertaking. To achieve optimal interactions, surgeons, radiation oncologists, medical oncologists, and other specialists need to understand the natural history of breast cancer and the role of each treatment modality according to stage. This chapter will focus on treatment by stage. As with the rest of this book, when chemotherapy programs are mentioned, their doses, schedules, and routes of administration and dose adjustment are described in the Appendix.

Epidemiology

Incidence and Mortality

The incidence of invasive female breast cancer has increased slightly in recent years and was estimated at about 150,000 new cases in the United States for 1990.[1,2] Data from the National Cancer Institute's Surveillance, Epidemiology and End Results (SEER) program indicate that breast cancer accounts for 26% of all female cancer and is responsible for 18% of female cancer deaths in this country.[2] The probability at birth of eventually developing breast cancer is 10.2% for white females and 7.5% for black females. The mortality from breast cancer has remained mostly unchanged since 1930 and is estimated at 44,000 deaths for 1990, indicating that overall, 2 of 5 patients who develop breast cancer will die of it. Breast cancer remains the most common invasive malignancy in females, second only to lung cancer as a cause of female cancer death. There are also about 900 cases of male breast cancer each year that lead to 300 male breast cancer deaths.[1]

Etiology and Risk Factors

The cause of breast cancer is unknown. Both hereditary and environmental factors seem to be important.[3] A positive family history is probably the most important risk factor, increasing the risk of breast cancer several fold. Women with diets high in fat content and total calories have an increased incidence of breast cancer, leading some to postulate a causal relationship.[3-5] There is growing literature suggesting that environmental factors such as diet, social habits, and viral exposure may have at least a partial etiologic role in the development of breast cancer. Studies in the Japanese female population illustrate this very well. Japanese women in Japan have a very low incidence of breast cancer, whereas second- or third-generation Japanese women in the United States have a breast cancer incidence approaching that of the U.S. Caucasian population.[6] Japanese women in Hawaii have an intermediate incidence. These epidemiologic findings, together with demonstrations of differences in urinary excreted estrogens that parallel the shift in incidence, suggest that some factors external to the genetic composition are at work.

The risk of breast cancer increases progressively with age. Although uncommon, the disease is not rare between the ages of 15 and 34. The major risk factors are (1) prior breast cancer, invasive or *in situ;* (2) family history of breast cancer, especially in a first-degree female relative, the risk being highest when either the relative developed premenopausal bilateral breast cancer or both mother and sister developed breast cancer;[7-9] and (3) no pregnancies, or first pregnancy after age 18. Benign proliferative breast disease, i.e., atypical hyperplasia and fibroadenoma, has also been suggested by some to have prognostic significance.[10] Interpretation of data on benign breast disease is made difficult by the variability of pathologic interpretation, but atypical hyperplasia is an important factor.[11,12] The relationship, if any, between "fibrocystic disease" and breast cancer is unclear, and the definition of "fibrocystic disease" is clearly not uniform.[13]

Other statistically subordinate but associated risk factors include early menarche and late menopause.

A history of ovarian and uterine cancer has also been associated with breast cancer. In addition, an excess of breast cancer (as compared to expected) has been identified in women previously exposed to ionizing irradiation. Increased incidence of breast cancer has been observed in women treated with irradiation for postpartum mastitis or with fluoroscopic chest examinations as part of tuberculosis treatment, as well as in Japanese women who survived exposure from atomic bomb irradiation.[14] Certain mammographic parenchymal breast patterns identified on mammography have been claimed to be associated with an increase in breast cancer risk, but the value of this pattern in predicting breast cancer remains unconfirmed.[10,14a,16] Other factors such as duration of menses, body size, number of pregnancies, breast feeding, and socioeconomic status have been associated with breast cancer, but statistical analysis shows them to be dependent factors when corrections for the major risk factors are considered.

The identification of risk factors may help determine when and how often breast examinations and mammograms should be used as screening for early breast cancer detection. Certainly, high-risk populations should be screened at an earlier age and more often than the general population.

Prevention

The role of dietary prevention is currently being investigated,[16a] but at present no dietary preventive is known. Other potential preventives are being discussed, such as medical intervention with antiestrogens and retinoids.[14a] Currently, however, the only effective preventive measure is bilateral mastectomy. This approach and all of its social implications may be indicated when the risk of breast cancer is unacceptably high to the patient and her physician (tables 42-1 and 42-2). In practice, such an approach is offered infrequently, usually only to patients with 2 or more first-degree relatives with breast cancer or occasionally to patients with 1 first-degree relative with bilateral premenopausal breast cancer. Patients with a strong family history of breast cancer and large breasts that are difficult to examine may desire bilateral mastectomies when they cannot accept emotionally the relative uncertainty of the presence of breast cancer as assessed by mammography and breast examination. This option may also be reasonable if biopsy of a suspicious lesion reveals atypical hyperplasia or *in situ* carcinoma.[16b] The refinements in modern breast reconstruction techniques have made mastectomies potentially more acceptable as a preventive measure. Bilateral mastectomy has also been offered to some patients with premalignant diseases such as lobular carcinoma *in situ*.[16b] However, more conservative treatment with close clinical follow-up and mammography have been advocated for compliant patients.[17] Bilateral subcu-

Table 42-1. Increased Risk of Breast Cancer in Relatives of Patients with Breast Cancer

Nature of disease in proband	Increased risk in relatives*	Calculated lifetime risk (%)[†]
Premenopausal	x 3.1	28
Postmenopausal	x 1.5	14
Bilateral	x 5.4	49
Premenopausal	x 8.8	79
Postmenopausal	x 4.0	36

*Ratio of incidence of breast cancer in relatives of described patient/incidence of breast cancer in relatives of controls who do not have breast cancer
[†]Increased risk multiplied by average lifetime risk for American women
Source: Pertrakis (in part), 1977 (ref 8)

Table 42-2. Benign Breast Disease: Histologic Types and Interactions with Family History in Determining Relative Risk of Breast Cancer

Histology	Fam history	No. patients	Relative risk*	P
All histologic types	—	3,308	1.5	0.0001
Nonproliferative	—	1,378	0.89	0.51
Proliferative	—	1,925	1.9	0.0001
All histologic types	N	2,934	1.4	0.007
	Y	309	2.5	0.0001
"Proliferative" no atypia	N	149	1.5	0.002
	Y	195	2.1	0.009
Atypical hyperplasia	N	193	3.5	0.001
	Y	39	8.9	0.0001

*Relative to an age-matched reference population in Atlanta from the 3rd National Cancer Survey
Source: Dupont and Page, 1985 (ref 12)

taneous mastectomies have also been suggested, but they have the major disadvantage of leaving residual glandular tissue, and the nipples are denervated. Therefore, subcutaneous mastectomy does not have a major benefit over simple mastectomy.

Pathology

Histopathology

Histopathologic classification is very important, inasmuch as some breast carcinoma subtypes require only very limited therapy. Thus a diagnosis of "adenocarcinoma" but not otherwise specified is inadequate, and such pathology readings should be reviewed to allow more specific information if possible. For clinical purposes, the histopathology of breast cancer can be classified as follows:

Infiltrating ductal and lobular adenocarcinomas (see chapter 11, figures 11-77 to 11-80) are the most common forms of breast cancer, with several subtypes that account for nearly 90% of all breast cancers. These are generally aggressive cancers characterized by early invasion through basement membranes into surrounding breast fat and lymphatics with hematogenous spread to distant organs. In some instances, the subtypes of breast cancer cannot be specified because the tumor is very poorly differentiated. These latter tumors are very aggressive, commonly lack hormone receptor proteins, and carry a very poor prognosis.

Medullary carcinomas. Medullary carcinomas (see chapter 11, figure 11-82) tend to grow slowly and are usually found as a large, locally invasive, circumscribed and hemorrhagic breast mass. When metastases to lymph nodes occur, however, the clinical behavior then closely parallels the infiltrating ductal pattern with frequent hematogenous dissemination. When this occurs, it is clinically indistinguishable from all the other infiltrating forms.

Papillary carcinoma (see chapter 11, figure 11-83), another unusual variant of infiltrating carcinoma that occurs predonominantly in older women, has a somewhat more favorable prognosis, with slower growth than infiltrating ductal carcinoma. Lymph node metastases are unusual. However, when lymph node metastases do occur, the prognosis becomes indistinguishable from infiltrating ductal carcinoma.

Mucinous carcinoma (colloid carcinoma) is a rare form with slow growth and more favorable prognosis. Nontheless, when the lymph nodes are involved, this overrides the prognostic significance of the histology.

Tubular carcinomas. Tubular carcinomas are uncommon, generally slowly growing tumors that behave less aggressively than the other invasive forms (see chapter 11, figures 11-81 and 11-86). This histology has a lesser tendency to involve the axillary lymph nodes or to spread hematogenously.[18] These carcinomas generally have a better prognosis with an excellent chance of cure with only local therapy, and many surgeons advocate a simple mastectomy without lymph node dissection.

Lobular carcinoma in situ (LCIS) is considered by many as either a premalignant condition or as a marker for the eventual occurrence of invasive cancer. Between 10 and 25% of such patients will develop invasive carcinoma within 20 yr of diagnosis; the invasive cancer can occur in either breast with equal frequency.[17-19] In most cases, the invasive malignancy is infiltrating ductal adenocarcinoma. Conservative management of LCIS is usually advocated.

Intraductal carcinoma is also an *in situ* malignancy, but it should not be confused with LCIS. The natural history of intraductal carcinoma and its management are different. First, intraductal carcinomas are frequently multi-centric and occasionally palpable.[20] Second, subsequent invasive carcinomas develop in ≤50% of patients treated with biopsy alone. The invasive tumors are primarily ductal, localized to the ipsilateral breast and, in general, to the quadrant initially affected. These data argue for adequate local therapy initially, and this is the subject of ongoing investigations.

Paget's disease of the breast is a rare disorder characterized by subacute or chronic eczematoid changes of the nipple and areola with itching and bleeding. This entity presents with an underlying ductal carcinoma in two-thirds of cases. Management and prognosis under these circumstances do not differ from the common approach to ductal carcinomas. In one-third of cases, the disease seems limited to skin infiltration, with large cells having pale cytoplasm; wide excision, without further treatment, may suffice, since it may be considered as an *in situ* process. Careful evaluation for an underlying mass is critical, however.

Other forms include metaplastic carcinoma, apocrine carcinoma, adenoid cystic carcinoma, squamous carcinoma, and carcinosarcoma. These account for a very small percentage of all breast cancers. They are generally aggressive forms and need to be considered clinically as invasive cancers.

Malignant cystosarcoma phyllodes is a rare soft-tissue tumor of the breast that seldom affects the axillary lymph nodes (see chapter 11, figure 11-88). Mastectomy without axillary dissection is thus the recommended therapy. A benign form, cystosarcoma phyllodes benigna, should not be confused with the malignant form.

Metastatic carcinoma, lymphoma and a variety of nonepithelial tumors such as sarcomas do occasionally occur in the breast. They are best managed with treatment appropriate for the site of origin and the histopathologic grade of the lesion.

Inflammatory breast cancer is a clinicopathologic entity characterized clinically by inflammation (swelling, erythema, and heat) of the breast mimicking infection, or pathologically identified by diffuse infiltration of the intradermal lymphatics with malignant breast cancer cells (see chapter 11, figure 11-84). Inflammatory carcinoma most often presents with both clinical and histopathological criteria, but the clinical findings are sufficient for diagnosis once infectious mastitis is excluded. The disease, usually disseminated at diagnosis, is considered as advanced and unresectable disease even when metastases are not identified. This disease has a high systemic and local recurrence risk and portends a poor prognosis. Recently, aggressive combined modality treatment with chemotherapy, surgery, and radiotherapy (XRT) has yielded promising results, with about 20% of patients alive and free of cancer at 5 yr in some series.[21,22a]

Biologic Predictors of Breast Cancer Behavior

HORMONE RECEPTORS

Jensen et al demonstrated that some breast cancers contained proteins in the cell cytoplasm that bound estrogens.[23] These proteins, called *estrogen receptors,* were found to provide important prognostic information regarding disease behavior and response to hormone treatments. Subsequently, progesterone receptor proteins were also identified.[24a] The presence of estrogen or progesterone receptor proteins or both in a tumor specimen is generally associated with a better prognosis as determined by a longer disease free interval after primary treatment and a better survival after recurrence.[24]

In order to obtain a biochemical (quantitative) assay for the presence of these proteins in the tumor, about 500 mg of tumor is required (about 1 c.c.). These proteins are labile at room temperature, making careful tissue handling crucial. The tumor sample must be placed in iced saline immediately and frozen at $\leq -70°C$ until processed. The results of the assay are expressed in fentimols (of receptor protein) per milligram (fmol/mg) of cytosol protein. Depending on the standards of the various laboratories, estrogen receptor (ER) and progesterone receptor (PR) values are usually considered "positive" if they are ≥ 6–10 fmol/mg cytosol protein. The assays are well standardized with good quality control so that they are reliable. Recently, the technique of immunocytochemistry has been applied to estrogen receptor analysis allowing determinations (qualitative) upon smaller tissue samples and even on cytology specimens.[24b] In addition, immunohistochemistry upon paraffin-embedded material is also possible, thus raising the possibility of prospectively tracing such information on prior tissue specimens. If this approach is confirmed, then small samples for diagnosis need not be divided to obtain ER/PR information.

Because of the prognostic information and the impact on the treatment at all stages, ER and PR proteins should be measured in new tumor specimens from the breast and in all biopsy specimens. Usually, the receptor status remains unchanged when the tumor recurs, as assessed by subsequent biopsies. Liver metastases, however, may be more often receptor negative. In addition to predicting the course of the disease, the receptor analysis helps to predict response to hormone treatments. A positive result for ER or PR or both correlates well with responsiveness to hormonal treatment. Seventy percent or more of receptor-positive tumors in soft tissue respond to first-line hormonal therapy, whereas < 10% of receptor-negative tumors respond to hormonal therapy. Thus, negative receptors are most predictive. The data also show that the higher the absolute level of ER and PR positivity, the more likely the response to hormones.[25] Borderline values may represent "false positives." However, because negative receptor results are most accurately predictive (poorer prognosis and lack of response to hormonal treatments) and tend to preclude hormone treatments, false negatives are the more important consideration.

False negatives may result from: (1) inadequate preservation before processing, leading to protein denaturation; (2) dilution of tumor tissue with large amounts of receptor-negative stroma; or (3) competitive binding of the receptor sites by endogenous or replacement hormones or antihormones (e.g., tamoxifen). Usually, patients should be off tamoxifen for 4–6 wk before a reliable receptor assay is performed. Careful attention to hormonal therapies before biopsy is thus important in assessing receptor analysis data.

TUMOR DIFFERENTIATION, LYMPHATIC OR VASCULAR INVASION, AND PROLIFERATION INDEXES

Some investigators have suggested that less-differentiated tumors, as assessed by light microscopy, have a worse prognosis than well-differentiated tumors. There is a rough correlation between the degree of differentiation (poorly, moderately, and well differentiated) and the level of receptor protein. In contrast with histologic gradings, nuclear grading has been proposed as a more objective method for predicting outcome on histologic review.[26] Most of the claims for this approach have not yet been confirmed, however. In contrast, lymphatic and vascular invasion have been associated in several reports with a high recurrence rate and a relatively short disease-free interval.[27,28] This finding, however, correlates closely with axillary lymph node involvement. A high labeling index, in vitro high S phase on flow cytometry, and aneuploidy of the tumor (also assessed on flow cytometry) have also been associated with a shorter disease-free interval and an increased risk of recurrence.[29] These parameters are in vitro correlates of the adverse biology of the tumor and can be assessed by flow cytometry of dissagregated fixed tissue.[29a,29b] In addition, recent reports suggest that increased expression of the HER-2/neu oncogene may impart prognostic information for recurrence-free survival.[29c] These biologic parameters are being used with increasing frequency to determine post-operative treatment options.

Natural History

A number of clinical characteristics predict for local and distant disease recurrence, disease-free survival, and overall survival.[30] These factors, which are the basis of the staging classification of breast carcinoma, include: local characteristics, tumor size, and involvement of the axillary lymph nodes. The so-called grave local signs, such as large bulky disease, inflammation, peau-d'orange, diffuse skin edema, skin ulceration, and fixation of mass or nodes to the chest wall, are all indicators of extensive local disease and predict for disease recurrence in the vast majority of women despite surgery, XRT, or both. Even at the earliest point of detection where the primary tumor is ≤1 cm and the axillary lymph nodes are found to be free of disease on histopathology, only 70% of the women will remain disease-free at 10 yr despite surgery, XRT, or both. These extremes of presentation of the local disease stress the point that most breast cancer is not strictly a loco-regional disease, but rather a systemic process whose biologic virulence can be predicted in part by the current in vitro assessments. Because it probably takes many years, on average, for a breast cancer to grow into a 1 cm mass (limits of palpation), there has been a long opportunity for the entire body to become seeded through hematogenous spread during the preclinical period. The various prognostic factors thus give indications of how well the host has been able to confine this spread. Perhaps the greatest advance in breast cancer management in recent years has been the conceptual recognition that breast cancer disseminates early and via hematogenous routes; spread does not occur centrifugally from the breast through lymphatics into the blood stream.

Tumor Size

It has been known for many years that the size of the primary tumor plays an important role in all aspects of treatment planning, such as the technical resectability, the irradiation portals, and the probability of local and distant disease recurrence as a manifestation of treatment failure. As can be seen in figure 42-1, the 5-yr survival is affected by the size of the primary tumor.[31] The prognostic importance of tumor size has been recognized by its impact upon the staging systems, as will be discussed.

Despite the well-recognized effect of size upon outcome, some patients with large (and even very large) tumors but uninvolved axillary lymph nodes have a better prognosis than patients with smaller primary tumors and involved (histologically positive) axillary lymph nodes (figure 42-1). This suggests that axillary node involvement may be a more powerful predictor of natural history than tumor size. Careful analysis of many prospective trials, especially those conducted by the National Surgical Adjuvant Breast Project (NSABP), have confirmed the priority of these 2 prognostic factors, i.e., size of tumor is an independent prognostic variable but subordinate to the involvement of the axillary lymph nodes.[31-33] The location of the primary tumor in the breast, however, has no prognostic significance.[34]

Axillary Lymph Node Involvement

Data derived from trials of surgical therapies and postoperative manipulations such as radical or modified radical mastectomies and postoperative adjuvant XRT have clearly established the prognostic impact of assessing the

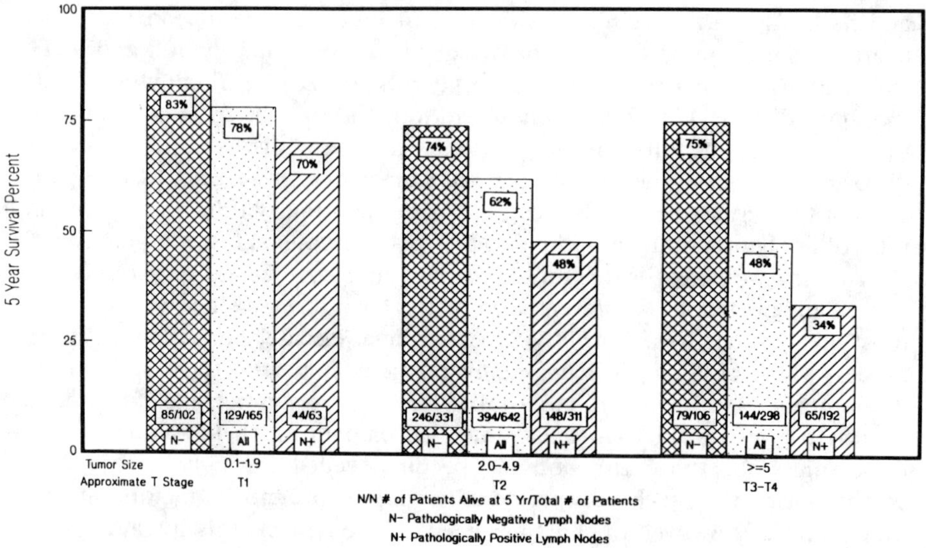

Figure 1. Comparison of tumor size (T), nodal status (N), and percentage of patients surviving 5 yr. Note that tumor size predicts for survival at 5 N + has consistently worse survival than N − disease. Furthermore, N + disease is consistently worse than N − disease, even when T size is greater. For example, compare T, N + with T3, T4, N − . (Data derived in part from Fisher et al, ref 31.)

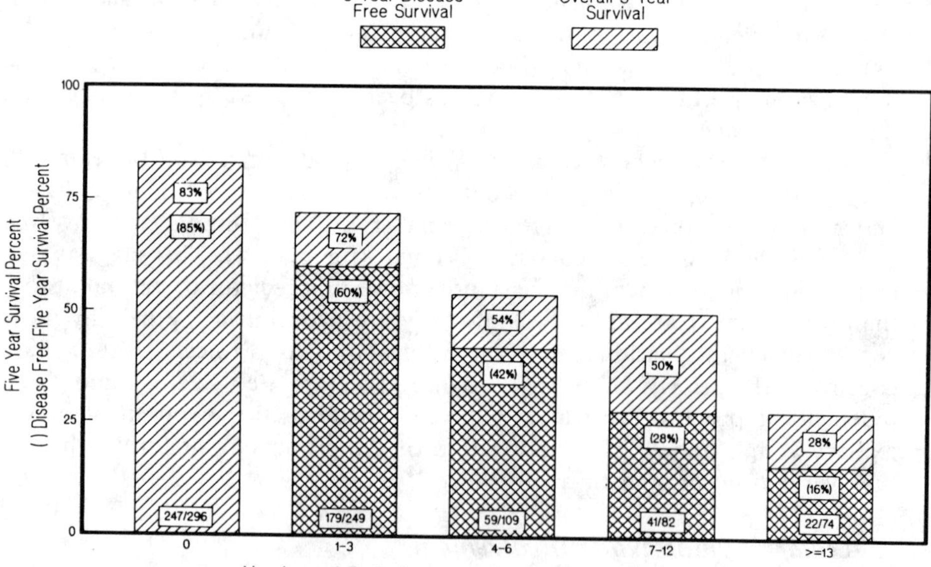

Figure 2. Comparison of the number of pathologically involved nodes (in an adequate axillary sampling—see text) and the 5- and 10-yr survival. Note the direct (linear) relationship between the number of pathologically involved nodes and the survival. (Data derived from Fisher et al, ref 32.)

axillary nodes for tumor involvement.[32,33] Furthermore, there is a direct correlation between the number of nodes involved and the 5- and 10-yr survival.[32,33]

As demonstrated in figure 42-2, 10-yr survivals are clearly lower than 5-yr survivals. The difference is mainly due to breast cancer deaths. Most (>80%) cancer recurrences, however, occur by 5 yr, suggesting that the 5-yr disease-free survival is an important indicator of the efficacy of adjuvant systemic treatment modalities.[33]

In order to accurately assess lymph node involvement, which has important implications for treatment options, it is necessary that there be an adequate axillary sampling, i.e., as many nodes should be removed as technically feasible. Generally, 20 or more nodes is considered to be an adequate sampling. Furthermore, most surgical series now suggest that the axillary dissection can be carried out through a separate incision and not necessarily at the same time as the breast biopsy.

A clinical assessment of the axillary nodes is not adequate to determine whether the nodes are involved. Nearly one-third of clinically palpable lymph nodes will not contain tumor on histology, and about one-third of the clinically negative nodes will be found to contain gross or microscopic disease. Large mated or fixed lymph nodes are usually involved with tumor and are associated with the subsequent development of distant metastases and poor survival.

Sites of Metastases and Recurrence

Even in patients with early stage disease, there seems to be a lifetime risk of breast cancer recurrence, suggesting that the term "cure" should be used with caution for patients with invasive breast cancer.[35]

The incidence of local, loco-regional, and distant metastases after primary therapy for loco-regional (stages I and II) disease are summarized in table 42-3,[34a] and the sites of recurrence are shown in table 42-4.[36] The recurrence

Table 42-3. Incidence and Location of Recurrences After Primary Therapy for Breast Carcinoma

First site of recurrence	Clinically negative axillary nodes	Clinically positive axillary nodes
	Percent (N = 1,079)	Percent (N = 586)
Local[a]	5	5
Regional[b]	3	9
Distant[c]	30	39
Combinations[d]	3	7
Total recurrence rate at 12 yr	41	60

After Fisher et al (ref 34a)
[a]Includes chest wall, scar, or both
[b]Includes axillary, supraclavicular, internal mammary, or subclavicular lymph nodes
[c]Includes all major organ systems and opposite breast
[d]Includes patients with loco-regional, local or regional and distant, and widespread presentations

Table 42-4. Analysis of the Locations of Distant Metastases When Detected as First Site of Recurrence in 532 Patients

Location of metastases	Percent (N = 554)
Skeletal system	30
Respiratory	22
More than 1 site	16
Opposite breast[a]	14
Digestive system	8
Hemopoietic and lymphatic system	6
Other	4

[a]Includes second primary breast tumors
Source: after Fisher et al (ref 34a)

rates are considerably higher for regionally advanced disease (stages IIIa and IIIb).[37] As can be seen in this table, alterations in loco-regional therapies have little impact on disease recurrence elsewhere, giving further testimony to the concept that breast cancer is a systemic disease even in its earliest presentation.

Within the broad spectrum of disseminated (stage IV, M1) disease, there is a wide prognostic variation according to several factors such as the number and sites of metastases. Patients with skin, lymph node, or subcutaneous (soft-tissue) metastases and no other site of involvement have higher response rates to hormonal and chemotherapy and a longer survival than patients with metastases to other sites. Patients with liver metastases, lymphangitic lung spread, symptomatic (low blood counts) bone marrow involvement, and multiple brain metastases have a poor prognosis, with a median survival of <6 mo. Patients with malignant pleural effusions or nodular metastases in the lungs have a prognosis similar to that of patients with soft-tissue disease. Patients with involvement of bone, including those whose disease extends into the bone marrow but does not affect blood counts, have an intermediate prognosis. Patients with metastases limited to bone can have a protracted course characterized by a relatively slow progression for long periods (months to years) until they are progressively debilitated and die of visceral metastases, hypercalcemia, or various medical complications. The range of survival is, however, very wide for each subgroup, and prediction of behavior in an individual case is virtually impossible. The range of survival of patients after developing metastases varies from a few months to >25 yr, but the median is 15–18 mo. With rare exceptions, "local" recurrences (that is, recurrences limited initially to the ipsilateral chest wall) are usually soon followed by disseminated metastases. Therefore, local recurrences should be considered as metastatic implants, i.e., the local manifestations of a systemic disease. This concept is supported by the near-uniform development of systemic disease despite adequate "local" therapy. The therapeutic approach to local recurrence will be discussed below.

There are several other important factors: The number of affected sites, the duration of the disease-free interval (time from diagnosis to first disease recurrence), and the location of metastases are of important prognostic value in determining survival after recurrence. These factors are shown in table

Table 42-5. Median Survivals According to Disease-free Interval and Number of Sites Involved

No. sites	DFI*			
	0–1 yr	1–2 yr	2–5 yr	5+ yr
1	(50)[†] / 11	(57) / 16	(92) / 20	(50) / 40
2	(43) / 7	(38) / 13	(73) / 14	(46) / 22
3	(28) / 5	(31) / 7	(29) / 12	(26) / 14
4+	(14) / 5	(16) / 6	(14) / 5	(7) / 21

*Disease-free interval
[†]( ) = number of patients
  N = median survival (in months)
After Cutler et al (ref 38)

42-5.[38,29] In general, the shorter the disease-free interval and the greater the number of affected sites, the shorter the survival.

Staging

Two basic staging systems are in wide use nationally and internationally: (1) a numerical staging system using 4 distinct staging levels (I–IV) and (2) the TNM (tumor, node, and metastases) staging system (tables 42-6 and 42-7). The TNM system can easily be converted to the numerical system, but the reverse is not easily accomplished; therefore, the TNM system is preferred by most investigators, especially those dealing with early-stage disease. Familiarity with both staging systems is important so that practitioners can speak a common language.

Some important aspects of these 2 systems should be highlighted:

1. Stage IV is defined by the presence of distant metastases (M1).

Table 42-6. Numerical Staging of Breast Cancer

Stage	Description
I	Breast tumor <2 cm in greatest dimension and no involvement of axillary nodes
II	Breast tumor <5 cm in greatest dimension or movable axillary nodes involved
IIIa*	Breast tumor >5 cm in greatest dimension with or without movable axillary involvement (technically resectable)
IIIb	Any inflammatory breast cancer or any tumor with direct extension to chest wall or skin (edema, peau d'orange, ulcers, or satellite lesions) or involvement of fixed axillary nodes or supraclavicular or infraclavicular nodes
IV	Any tumor with distant metastases other than regional nodes

*Stage III is arbitrarily divided into *a* and *b* on the basis of technical resectability (b = nonresectable)

Table 42-7. TNM Classification of Breast Cancer

Primary Tumor (T)

TX	Minimum requirements to assess the primary tumor cannot be met
T0	No evidence of primary tumor
Tis	Carcinoma *in situ*
T1	Tumor ≤ 2 cm in greatest dimension
T2	Tumor >2 cm but not >5 cm in greatest dimension
T3	Tumor >5 cm in greatest dimension
T4	Tumor of any size with direct extension to chest wall or skin (chest wall includes ribs, intercostal muscles, and serratur anterior muscle, but not pectoral muscle)

       T4a—Fixation to chest wall

       T4b—Edema (including peau d'orange), ulceration of the skin of the breast, or satellite skin nodules confined to the same breast

       T4c—Both of the above

       T4d—Inflammatory carcinoma

Note: Dimpling of the skin, nipple retraction, or any other skin changes except those in T4b may occur in T1, T2, or T3 without affecting the classification.

Lymph nodes (N)

Definition for clinical-diagnostic stage

NX	Minimum requirements to assess the regional nodes cannot be met (e.g., previously removed)
N0	Homolateral axillary lymph nodes not considered to contain growth
N1	Movable homolateral axillary nodes considered to contain growth
N2	Homolateral axillary nodes considered to contain growth and fixed to one another or to other structures
N3	Homolateral internal mammary lymph nodes

Definitions for surgical-evaluative and postsurgical resection—pathologic stages (pN)

pNX	Minimum requirements to assess the presence of distant metastases cannot be met
pN0	No evidence of homolateral axillary lymph nodes metastasis
pN1	Metastasis to movable homolateral axillary nodes not fixed to one another or to other structures
pN2	Metastases to homolateral axillary lymph nodes fixed to one another or to other structures
pN3	Metastasis to homolateral internal mammary lymph nodes

Distant metastasis (M)

MX	Not assessed
M0	No (known) distant metastasis
M1	Distant metastasis present

Stage Grouping

Stages	
0	Tis, N0, M0
I	T, N0, M0
II	T0, N1, M0
	T1, N1, M0
	T2, N0, M0
IIb	T2, N1, M0
	T3, N0, M0
IIIa	T0, N2, M0
	T1, N2, M0
	T3, N1, M0
	T3, N2, M0
IIIb	Any T, N3, M0
	T4, any N, M0
IV	Any T, any N, M1

2. T4 (stage IIIb) is defined by tumor extension to the chest wall or skin as evidenced by fixation to chest wall, skin ulceration, or diffuse skin edema (peau-d'orange).

3. Inflammatory breast cancer (without distant metastases; M0), a clinical or histopathologic diagnosis, also falls into the T4 (stage IIIb) category.

In general, the staging system carries the most important prognostic information. Staging is usually based on clinical evaluation, but in recent years staging has been modified for the operative and histopathologic findings, including involvement of underlying structures, lymph nodes, and vascular or lymphatic invasion. Survival according to numerical stage is shown in figure 42-3.[39]

Screening and Early Detection

Because advanced stage correlates with decreased survival, it follows that earlier diagnosis might lead to intervention at an earlier stage and improved survival. This concept has led to various attempts at earlier diagnosis, including public education, self-examination programs, and mass screening. Whereas the impact of education and self-examination programs is felt to be positive,[40,41] there is clear-cut evidence that mass screening with the use of

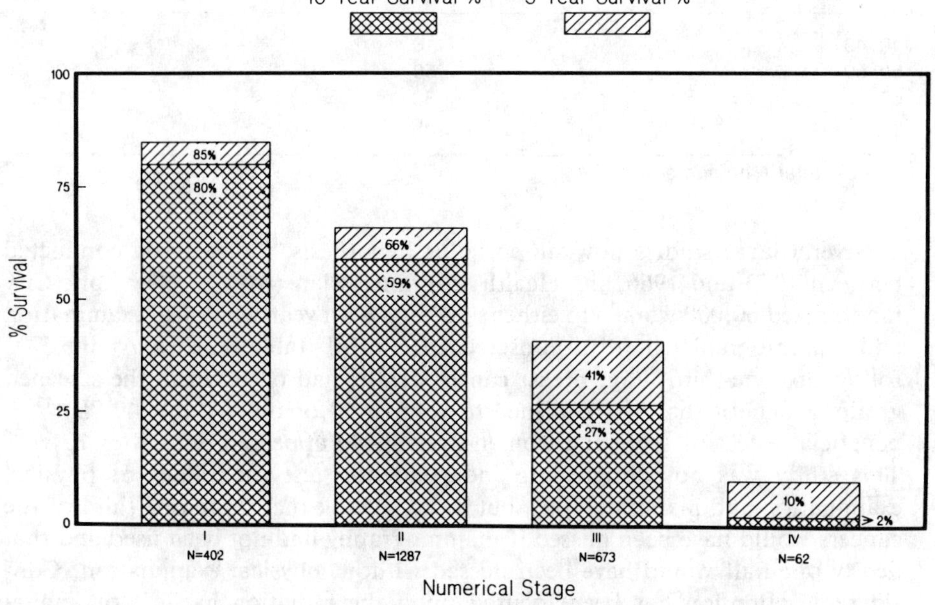

Figure 3. Five and 10-yr survival according to clinical numerical stage at initial presentation of breast cancer. Except for stage IV disease, data are based primarily on local therapy. (Data derived from Cutler et al, ref 39.)

breast mammography has made an impact on both early diagnosis and survival. Pioneering efforts in the 1950s[42] led to the well-established role of mammography as an adjuvant to the clinical evaluation of breast pathology.[43] With further improvements of technique and equipment, mammography evolved into a tool that currently enables the physician to increase the rate of detection of nonpalpable tumors. Its main value is to identify a previously unnoticed or unsuspected lesion, leading to earlier diagnosis and improved survival.

Table 42-8A. Health Insurance Plan (HIP) Study of Cumulative Breast Cancer Deaths (Cancer Diagnosed in First 5 Yr)

| Yr from | No. breast cancer deaths | | Difference |
entry onto study	Study group	Control group	(%)
N	306	300	—
5	39	63	38.1
7	71	106	33.0
10	95	133	28.6
14	118	153	22.9

Source: after Shapiro et al (ref 44)

Table 42-8B. Health Insurance Plan (HIP) Study of Breast Cancer Deaths After 7 Yr of Evaluation

| | No. dying of disease | |
Age at death (yr)	Control group	Study group
40–49	16	17
50–59	59	32
60 +	33	21
Totals	108	70

Source: after Morrison et al (ref 43)

Several large studies now support this hypothesis.[43] In a study conducted between 1963 and 1966, the Health Insurance Plan (HIP) of New York City randomized 60,000 women to either screening with yearly physical examination and mammography or to a nonscreened control (table 42-8A). At the 7-yr follow-up, one-third fewer breast cancer deaths had occurred in the screened group, a benefit that was confined to women 50 or older (table 42-8B).[43] A beneficial effect of screening women ages 40–49 appeared only after 10 yr.[44] This study was not designed to independently test the values of physical examination and mammography, but it did suggest that up to one-third of the cancers would have been missed if mammography had not been used and that nearly one-half would have been missed without physical examination. Considerable attention has been focused upon the radiation hazards of annual screening mammography, based upon a finding of increased incidence of breast cancer in women exposed to ionizing radiation.[14] Virtually all investigators have concluded that the benefits of mammography far exceed any risks.

Further development in mammographic techniques with decreased radiation exposure and higher imaging resolution have further improved the risk/benefit ratio.

In an attempt to confirm and expand the HIP study, the National Cancer Institute (NCI) and the American Cancer Society (ACS) funded the Breast Cancer Detection and Demonstration Project (BCDDP). This project of annual screening, breast examination, breast self-examination training, and mammography was not a randomized study. Thus, although the BCDDP study was not designed to test the efficacy of screening, it did generate important data about the contributions of mammography to early breast cancer detection.[43,45] More than 280,000 women were enrolled in the program starting in 1973. Screening was completed in 1981. After 1977, routine mammography was restricted towomen age 50 or over based on the early results of the HIP study; women younger than 50 had mammography only if they belonged to a high-risk group for breast cancer or if they had abnormal physical findings.[43] Data generated by the BCDDP further established the value of mammography in early breast cancer detection; 35% of breast carcinomas detected in women ages 40–50 and 42% of breast cancer found in women ages 50–59 were found by mammography alone. Overall, more than 4,400 breast cancers were recorded for the entire population followed; of these, 80% were first detected at the BCDDP centers. Of the more than 3,500 breast carcinomas detected by the project centers, <20% had positive nodes at surgery. One-third of the cancers were either noninvasive or <1 cm in size. Although there was no control group, these data suggest that most cancers detected in this program were localized to the breast according to surgical-pathologic staging. The relative contribution of mammography to early detection seemed higher in the BCDDP project than in the HIP study; this was likely due to better mammographic technique. When considered together, the HIP and the BCDDP studies provide a strong rationale for a yearly screening program for women over age 50 and is highly suggestive for women ages 40–49. Recently, a joint recommendation for screening mammography was published as a consensus of multiple organizations including NCI, ACS, and various medical specialty societies.[45a] These recommendations include annual screening for women over 50 and screening every 1–2 yr of women 40–50. In addition, the ACS recommends a baseline at age 35–40. It is generally agreed that women in high-risk groups require regular screening annually beginning at age 35, and even earlier in selected cases.

The current state of the art technique of film mammography provides superior imaging with minimal (as little as 0.1 cGy per procedure) exposure to radiation. This low level of radiation, less than that of a chest x-ray, is considered relatively "safe."

Routine screening mammography is not recommended under age 35 because the density of normal breast tissue precludes adequate imaging. Diagnostic mammography in patients with palpable abnormalities may be indicated at any age. Although diagnostic mammography is both specific and sensitive, it is less reliable when considered "negative" (i.e., no identifiable suspicious area) in the presence of a palpable mass. Therefore, any persistent (longer than 1–2 mo) distinct palpable mass should be biopsied regardless of whether there is mammographic evidence of its presence. In young women, a mass waxing and waning with the menses may be managed more conservatively with frequent (1–3 monthly) examinations before embarking on a course of repeated biopsies for "fibrocystic" disease.

Diagnostic and Pretreatment Staging Workup

Detection

More than two-thirds of women consult their physician on finding a lump in a breast. Thus, most breast tumors are found first by the patient herself. A small, yet fortunate minority are found to have a small tumor on routine physical examination or mammography. Unfortunately, too many women, nearly one-third of all cases, present with locally advanced breast tumors or with evidence of metastases. When a breast mass is found and the clinical diagnosis of its nature is uncertain, subsequent evaluation is important. A number of possible approaches can be followed, depending in large measure on the nature and consistency of the mass as well as clinical and historical findings. For example, in women with a strong family history there should be a low threshold for biopsy. If the mass has a cystic consistency, sonography might distinguish solid and cystic structures. Mammography is a very important diagnostic tool in these settings, although there is a greater confidence in a "positive" reading than a "negative" one. If a cyst is encountered, it can be aspirated and the fluid sent for cytologic examination. If the initial impression is one of a benign mass, frequent (1–2 monthly) follow-up examinations and follow-up mammography are then performed. If the patient has a persistent or distinct solid mass, a biopsy would be indicated. If a mammogram is suspicious or shows a possible carcinoma, even in the absence of a palpable mass, then a biopsy should be obtained. Localization under mammographic guidance can be used when a mass is not palpable. In this setting, mammography of the pathologic specimen obtained at surgery is sometimes used to confirm resection of affected tissue. A negative mammogram does not rule out malignancy, and a palpable mass should not be ignored because the mammograms are "normal."

Once it has been decided that a tissue biopsy is necessary, careful planning becomes critical in order to assure proper handling of tissue. In addition to histopathologic examination, a portion of the biopsy specimen should be reserved for estrogen and progesterone receptor protein determination. Thus, a frozen section of the biopsy specimen may guide the pathologist and surgeon in obtaining an adequate specimen for hormone receptor determinations. The frozen section should have less of a role, however, in determining the exact diagnosis; also, it should not be used to determine the need for an immediate mastectomy. There is no evidence that a delay of several days before definitive therapy makes any difference in either local control or eventual outcome. Considering the multiple options available today for primary treatment, this time period is important for the patient to understand and consider the various alternatives so that she can make an informed and educated choice.

Pretreatment staging is intended to develop clinical and laboratory information that will guide treatment, provide prognostic information, and allow the clinician to anticipate disease developments. The extent of the pretreatment evaluation depends upon the clinical circumstances, the findings, the anticipated interventions, and available resources. For example, if a woman had a small, questionable lesion to be biopsied, then a minimal diagnostic workup such as history and physical examination, alkaline phosphatase, liver function studies, and chest x-ray may be adequate. When the patient is asymptomatic, except for the loco-regional process in the breast, and the initial staging evaluation is unrevealing, further laboratory tests usually carry little benefit. CT scans of the abdomen, radionuclide liver and bone scans, and survey roentgenograms are discouraged in this setting; they seldom provide useful information. On the other hand, a woman with obvious breast cancer and adverse prognostic features would most likely benefit from a thorough and careful search for metastatic disease. A reasonable evaluation for metastatic disease would include complete history and physical examination, chest x-ray posteroanterior and lateral views, CBC with platelet count and differential, serum chemistries including blood urea nitrogen (BUN) or creatinine, bilirubin, aspartate aminotransferase (SGOT), lactic dehydrogenase (LDH), and alkaline phosphatase (Alk P). Isotopic scans of the liver or bone are usually performed if the serum chemistries are abnormal. Positive areas on the bone scan should be examined roentgenographically, especially in weight-bearing bones, because large lytic, unstable lesions may be relatively asymptomatic and may become manifest only at the time of a pathologic fracture. Other imaging techniques or invasive procedures are required at times when unusual metastatic sites are suspected, such as marrow aspiration and biopsy in patients with an leuko-erythroblastic picture in the peripheral blood smear and a myelogram in patients with suspected spinal cord compression. Patients with meningeal involvement may complain of irritability, headaches, cranial nerve palsies, or other focal changes. This complication is uncommon and may be difficult to diagnose because the cerebrospinal fluid is often paucicellular. Sequential spinal taps for cytology may thus be required. Although brain metastases are seen in breast cancer with considerable frequency, they usually are symptomatic. A CT scan of the brain is thus indicated when neurological signs and symptoms occur.

Treatment

The primary treatment of breast cancer depends on several variables, the most important of which are clinicopathologic stage, hormone receptor content of the tumor, biologic activity of the tumor, age, and menopausal status. In the subset of patients with stage IV (M1) breast cancer, location, extent, type (diffuse vs. discrete) and number of metastases are also important for treatment planning.

For practical purposes, treatment can also be divided into 3 components: (1) management of loco-regional disease (breast tumor, axillary metastases, skin and soft-tissue involvement in breast and axillary region); (2) treatment of systemic micrometastasis; and (3) management of macroscopic distant metastases (any site outside the loco-regional area). Supraclavicular and cervical involvement of breast cancer should be considered as distant sites because they are virtually always associated with distant metastases and have the same outcome statistics as soft-tissue metastases in other distant sites.

The 3 major therapeutic options are surgery, XRT, and systemic therapies. Systemic treatment currently includes hormonal and chemotherapeutic agents. Surgery plays a major role in establishing the diagnosis and is the cornerstone of therapy for local control. The application of surgery thus predominantly influences early stage disease. Surgery is also a modality for endocrine manipulation (oophorectomy) and may have a role in debulking advanced disease. Likewise, XRT is a treatment having application to regional areas, since it affects the area targeted within the radiation field. Because recent studies have shown that XRT after complete excisional biopsy is as effective as total mastectomy, breast radiation has become part of the primary treatment approach. XRT is thus an important component of local control both at the primary site and for various specific metastatic foci such as CNS, unstable bones, or painful sites. It can be an ideal therapy for a regional recurrence. Large-field irradiation (hemibody) may have some palliative role in pain control as well.

Originally applied for advanced and recurrent disease, systemic therapies have now been successfully applied as an adjuvant to local therapy for control of micrometastasis. This approach was derived from the recognition of breast cancer as a systemic disease. It has long been appreciated that breast cancer can recur despite adequate local treatment. Inasmuch as the primary tumor was removed and the disease recurred in other sites, it was clear that these metastases occurred before removal of the primary tumor. These sites were micrometastases at the time of the original surgery. Chemotherapy to treat these micrometastases for some patients with high probability of disease recurrence has improved both the disease-free and overall survival. For advanced disease, systemic therapy is chosen according to patient and tumor prognostic factors such as sites of metastases and tumor hormone receptors. In general, hormonal treatment is less toxic and easier to administer; therefore, it is used first when appropriate. Chemotherapy is given in multiple drug combinations after hormonal therapy is no longer feasible.

Due to the evolutions in treatment approaches for each modality alone and together for breast cancer, the roles of surgery, XRT, and systemic therapy are less meaningful individually but acquire more significance when they are placed in the perspective of an organized, planned, and comprehensive attack on the disease. Initial chemotherapy is already being used in locally advanced breast cancer to reduce or "debulk" the mass. Radioactively labeled antibody may make XRT a systemic treatment. Thus, the distinction between domains for different modalities is becoming arbitrary.

The application of the various modalities is best considered according to stage at the time of treatment. Although some of the options presented didactically suggest a standard approach to various stages, it is the firm belief of the authors and others that ongoing clinical research is needed to refine and improve upon these suggestions. All clinicians should participate in such ongoing clinical trials, which have become widely available to physicians. The evolving rationale for a logical approach to therapy is presented, but the recommendations are not intended to be construed as formulas or recipes for treatment.

Management of Minimal Breast Cancer

MANAGEMENT OF STAGE I

As shown in tables 42-6 and 42-7, stage I disease is small-volume disease confined to the breast. Survival figures for local therapy are excellent (figure 42-3), indicating that many patients will be able to contain their disease process with local treatment (only to the breast). The cornerstone of therapy is therefore surgery, with attention paid to local control. In the past, adequate local control was defined by radical mastectomy (with or without postoperative irradiation). This approach was derived from the anecdotal experiences with the treatment of advanced local disease and was based on the concept that breast cancer spread centrifugally from the point of origin into the lymph nodes (which acted as a barrier to distal spread), and then into the circulation for distant hematogenous spread. Radical mastectomy was advocated by Halsted, meaning that the radix or root of the problem was removed in its entirety, including adjacent lymph nodes in the axilla together with the pectoralis muscles. Some surgeons even advocated a "super-radical" procedure that included the removal of supraclavicular and internal mammary nodes. These procedures were obviously deforming and there was considerable doubt raised about their impact in early disease. Many investigators suggested that less deforming surgery such as a simple mastectomy was adequate and led to equivalent results.

In recent years, many reports have shown that a modified radical mastectomy (the entire pectoralis muscle is left intact) is equivalent to either a radical or super-radical mastectomy but considerably less deforming. Modified radical mastectomy then became the standard to which all other therapies have been compared. The recognition of the systemic nature of breast cancer indicated that local therapies affected local control but not overall survival. Thus, in early-stage disease, less deforming procedures would likely do as well for overall outcome. After considerable anecdotal experience, several prospectively randomized, controlled studies in England, the United States, and elsewhere have shown that "quadrantectomy" or "lumpectomy" (wide excisional biopsy) plus breast radiation is equivalent to mastectomy.[34,46] Axillary dissection is still necessary in order to adequately stage the disease. For example, a 3-arm, prospectively randomized study by the National Surgical Adjuvant Breast and Bowel Project (NSABP protocol B-06)[34] tested 3 alternatives for local therapy: (1) total mastectomy and axillary dissection (modified radical mastectomy); (2) segmental mastectomy (mass excised with a 2-cm rim of normal tissue) and axillary dissection; and (3) segmental mastectomy, axillary dissection, and breast radiation. This study, which accrued patients 1976–84, with >5 yr of median follow-up, so far has shown no significant difference in either local control or survival between mastectomy and the segmental mastectomy plus breast radiation groups. Women who received a segmental mastectomy alone had a higher rate of disease recurrence in the affected breast than the irradiated patients or those undergoing modified radical mastectomy; in most cases, however, a subsequent mastectomy provided adequate local control. Thus, there are no significant differences in survival for any of the 3 groups.

Most investigators have accepted these findings as showing that there are no differences in survival outcome according to local control maneuvers for early-stage disease. These findings also argue that XRT after modified radical mastectomy to the chest wall and lymph nodes (axillary, supraclavicular, and internal mammary) is not necessary.

Not all women with early-stage (I or II) breast cancer are appropriate candidates for breast-sparing surgery and breast radiation (5,000 cGy to the breast by tangential fields plus, in some series, a boost to the tumor bed with either iridium implants or electron beam). In some instances when the breast is very small, excision of the mass will result either in so much breast deformity or the radiation fields will be so difficult that mastectomy would be preferable. Patients requiring mastectomy may still maintain or even have an improvement in body image with available breast reconstruction techniques. This approach should be discussed with the patient initially when breast-sparing surgery is not feasible, as it may alter the initial approach technically. The timing for reconstruction is controversial; it is best planned with the patient by the general and plastic surgeons.[47] Reconstruction has been performed at the time of initial surgery; some surgeons advise a minimum period of several months (usually 4–6) after mastectomy and before reconstruction to allow for good local healing and revascularization.

Analysis of hormone receptor data has shown that women whose tumors have positive hormone receptors have a better prognosis than women whose tumors are negative for these proteins.[29,30] In addition, there is evolving statistical evidence that biologic markers of tumor activity also confer prognostic significance.[29] In 1990, data from several studies were reported at the NCI consensus meeting on breast cancer.[47a] These studies indicate that adjuvant systemic therapy has resulted in significant improvement in disease-free survival in breast cancer patients who are node negative, although the median follow-up to date is still short. In 1 study, node-negative patients with negative estrogen receptors (NSABP protocol B-13) received methotrexate (MTX), 5-fluorouracil (5-FU), and calcium leucovorin (LCV) given after surgery; 80% of 368 patients were free of disease at 4 yr, versus only 71% in the control group. The second study (NSABP protocol B-14) for ER-positive, node-negative patients used tamoxifen postoperatively. The treatment group has an 82% (1,218 patients) disease-free survival at 4 yr, whereas only 77% of the control group (1,326 patients), who received placebo, were free of disease at 4 yr (p <0.00001). The third study (Intergroup-0011) included all node-negative, ER-negative patients and a subgroup of node-negative, ER-positive patients with >3 cm tumors. Patients were randomized after surgery to the "standard" CMFP (cyclophosphamide [CTX] + MTX + 5-FU + prednisone) regimen for 6 cycles versus observation alone. This study showed that regardless of their ER status, the 406 patients who received chemotherapy had a 3-yr median disease-free survival of 84% compared to only 69% for the control group (p <0.0001). These data, corroborated with other studies from Europe, show that adjuvant hormonal or cytotoxic chemotherapy can have a meaningful impact on the natural history of node-negative breast cancer patients. Currently, premenopausal women with stage I breast cancer are offered chemotherapy if their tumor is >1 cm, is estrogen receptor negative, has high labeling index (or high S phase fraction), or is aneuploid. Postmenopausal women with ER-positive stage I disease are usually offered tamoxifen. The approach for premenopausal women with stage

I ER+ tumors and postmenopausal women with ER-negative stage I tumors remains controversial; these women should also be included in national studies.

MANAGEMENT OF STAGE II

For practical purposes, the loco-regional management of stage II disease is identical to that for stage I, with the same alternatives and considerations applying for local control, including mastectomy or breast-sparing surgery plus irradiation. In stage II disease, however, there is an increased probability of local and distant recurrence, and these data have led to the application and testing of postoperative (or postlocal control) adjuvant therapies. Postoperative radiation to the chest wall and loco-regional lymph nodes following mastectomy has been advocated for many years as a means of improving outcome for patients with stage II disease. It has been shown that postoperative XRT will decrease the incidence of chest wall (local) recurrences, but that distal recurrence rates (and sites) and overall survival are unaffected by such radiation.[48] This should not, however, be confused with breast irradiation as part of primary local therapy. Postoperative adjuvant XRT increases morbidity (e.g., lymphedema and radiation pulmonary fibrosis) and can potentially interfere with either timing or dose of chemotherapy. Because it does not improve survival, can increase morbidity, and might potentially interfere with other adjuvant therapies, postoperative adjuvant XRT to the chest wall and regional nodes is not recommended. Furthermore, because this irradiation can only modify local control, it is best saved for the relatively small percentage of patients whose disease recurs in that area (table 42-3); excellent local control can be achieved at that time.

Hormonal manipulations have been shown to be effective in advanced disease (see below) and were therefore logically tested as adjuvant therapy for breast cancer. One of the first of these studies was the adjuvant oophorectomy trial conducted by the NSABP and others.[49] Most of these studies, conducted in groups of patients with unknown receptor status, showed that there was a prolongation of disease-free interval but not overall survival for patients undergoing oophorectomy. Because of a loss of information about the subsequent hormonal management of patients, this modality was not recommended for adjuvant treatment. Most of these studies were conducted before the era of hormone receptor analysis; therefore, only a small subgroup (about one-third of premenopausal patients having tumors with positive receptors) may have benefited from this treatment, and the benefit could have been obscured by the larger, nonresponsive population. Adjuvant chemotherapy has since proven beneficial to premenopausal patients, making it difficult to repeat these studies.

In the postmenopausal group, however, hormonal therapies appear to have an important role. For the approximately one third of postmenopausal women with estrogen-negative tumors, hormonal therapies have no established role. For the remaining postmenopausal women with estrogen receptor-positive tumors, there is a small but consistent advantage for both disease-free and overall survival in favor of the use of the antiestrogen tamoxifen as adjuvant therapy.[50-52] This conclusion, however, is based on a compilation of randomized studies, a statistical tool needed because of the relatively small advantage.[51,52] Because the differences between treated and untreated groups is small, patients should be entered onto ongoing studies of adjuvant treatments. Such studies offer the "state-of-the-art" therapies with the intent of improving outcome and accumulating valuable prospective data. Where such studies are not available or acceptable to the postmenopausal patients, adjuvant tamoxifen may be given because of its minimal side effects.

Another approach to adjuvant treatment is chemotherapy. Chemotherapy with cytotoxic agents is known to have antitumor activity in advanced disease, and multiple animal model experiments have shown that postoperative adjuvant chemotherapy can cure an animal, whereas neither surgery alone nor chemotherapy is curative after the metastases become apparent.[53] This treatment approach was tested in stage II breast cancer. Initial reports of some of these studies demonstrated a significant impact upon both disease-free and overall survival, but subsequent analysis has shown that outcome varied with menopausal status and number of affected nodes.[54-58] Furthermore, a number of studies with apparently conflicting results have led to considerable confusion about the application of chemotherapy with respect to dose, timing, chemotherapy regimen to be used, and to which subgroup the chemotherapy should be given.[58] An overview of these issues is difficult, requiring an understanding of the principles of chemotherapy and an appreciation of both the animal data and the various reported studies. For example, dose is a critical factor in chemotherapy. Animal studies clearly show a dose-related effect on the cure rate,[59] and studies in advanced disease in women have also suggested a dose-dependent response frequency.[60,61] None of the adjuvant studies has shown that a lower dose is equivalent to a "standard" dose. Low-dose, so-called "nontoxic" therapy therefore cannot be currently justified outside a study setting. At least one current study (by the Cancer and Leukemia Group B (CALGB)) addresses the issue of dose.

The timing of adjuvant chemotherapy has also been considered important. In animals, a delay in adjuvant chemotherapy has a detrimental impact on the cure rate.[62] In women, the data in most studies were derived from the application of chemotherapy within the first 4–6 wk after surgery. Furthermore, several studies have suggested that earlier (intraoperative or immediately postoperative) chemotherapy may produce enhanced beneficial results.[63] At least one review (by Cooper et al) has suggested that a delay of chemotherapy to allow adjuvant chest irradiation was detrimental to survival.[64] These pieces of information would suggest that adjuvant chemotherapy, when used, should be given as early as possible—perhaps intraoperatively or in the recovery room. In addressing this issue, the Ludwig Breast Cancer Study Group failed to show a time of chemotherapy effect; immediate and intraoperative chemotherapy was not significantly better than chemotherapy delayed 6 wk after surgery.[64a] At present, delay of chemotherapy beyond 6 wk would not be justified. Therefore, some consideration of the timing of chemotherapy and primary breast radiation needs to be made. It has been our practice—and the approach of CALGB—to administer the adjuvant chemotherapy, where appropriate, for up to 6 courses before the breast is given definitive irradiation.

Which subgroups of patients should receive adjuvant chemotherapy is a more difficult matter, however. Nearly all studies have shown an advantage for chemotherapy in the premenopausal patients, and a compilation of randomized studies has led to the recognition that such patients should receive adjuvant combination chemotherapy, preferably on one of the cooperative group studies. Premenopausal women with 10 or more nodes have such a dire prognosis that many investigators have taken a more radical approach to chemotherapy, such as high-dose chemotherapy and autologous bone marrow transplantation. The results in postmenopausal patients, however, are less clear. Although many studies do not show an advantage for chemotherapy over no treatment in the postmenopausal group, several studies show a consistent advantage in favor of chemotherapy.[54,56-58,65] These studies used treatment principles of drug combinations given uniformly and at adequate dose. A compilation of adjuvant chemotherapy data that includes treatments with single agents and lower doses therefore might be suboptimal and might miss a beneficial effect. Obviously, the issue of dose and treatment is not settled for the postmenopausal group, and further studies are needed. At present, such patients should be given the opportunity to participate in cooperative group studies. Because of the lack of convincing benefit, toxic chemotherapy probably should be given to the postmenopausal patients only within the confines of a study.

MANAGEMENT OF STAGE III

Stage III breast cancer identifies a heterogeneous group of patients who present with large (>5 cm) primary lesions, fixed masses or fixed lymph nodes, skin edema or ulceration, and inflammatory disease. This group is further divided into IIIa and IIIb (table 42-6). In general, patients with stage IIIa disease have loco-regional disease that can be adequately resected by a modified radical or radical mastectomy. Patients with stage IIIb disease have such an advanced loco-regional process that surgery as a primary modality is not a reasonable option because even a very extensive "super-radical" resection would not offer adequate local control. Subgroups according to TNM staging are given in table 42-7. Most patients with stage III disease have micrometastasis and eventual—often early—disease progression or recurrence.[66] Although no clear consensus has been reached on the approach to stage III disease, there is growing realization that systemic treatment is an important component of therapy. Multiple uncontrolled studies have shown that combined modality approaches, including systemic therapies, are superior to loco-regional treatments alone.[21,22] Also, several pilot studies have indicated that initial chemotherapy may improve both local and systemic disease control.[21,22,67] First, such an approach usually produced tumor regression and made the disease technically more resectable or more easily contained within a port of irradiation or both. Second, systemic therapy may also provide initial control of micrometastasis, which grows unchecked during the course of loco-regional therapy. An alternative approach might be to use hormonal therapies as the systemic treatment for receptor-positive tumors, but recent studies of this approach are lacking.

Although patients with stage IIIa disease often have technically resectable tumors, both the local failure rate and the high frequency of systemic failure dictate the need for additional therapies. Initial XRT to such lesions requires high dosages and large volumes of radiation, leading to severe local morbidity. This is especially important because the XRT dose necessary to sterilize a tumor increases exponentially as the tumor volume increases. Despite high doses of 6,000–8,000 cGy, there is a high local failure rate, and often subsequent mastectomy is required even in the face of the complications of such a combined approach.[66] Initial mastectomy followed by chest irradiation improves local control but offers no advantage for micrometastasis, thus having no impact on distant recurrence or survival.

Loco-regional therapy (either surgery or XRT followed by chemotherapy or chemotherapy followed by loco-regional therapy) is preferred.[22] The latter approach has some advantages. Typically, a woman with a large mass will have an incisional or needle biopsy to confirm histology. Initial chemotherapy would produce tumor regression in most cases, meaning that surgery could be done more easily and completely. Excision of the mass, if chosen by the woman, would offer less deformity in this situation. Based on pilot studies at the University of Maryland Cancer Center[22] and at Mount Sinai Hospital in New York,[67] as well as on data from the Cancer and Leukemia Group B,[68] our approach has been to offer initial combination chemotherapy with CAF or CMFVP for 3 courses.[22] This is followed by mastectomy or complete excision, depending on the choice of the patient and surgeon. Chemotherapy is then continued for an additional 3 courses, after which the patient is offered breast radiation if the breast is not removed. Obviously, multiple timing permutations are possible. The local complications of concurrent doxorubicin (ADR) and breast radiation, however, suggest the described sequence with XRT after chemotherapy. In stage IIIa disease, there is no suggestion that both mastectomy and chest wall radiation are necessary. One study by the CALGB using chemotherapy initially suggested that surgery and XRT as local control measures are not significantly different, thus either approach is justified.[68] Such combined modality approaches have resulted in nearly 50% disease-free survival at 5 yr for this subgroup, suggesting that a similar approach to unresectable disease is appropriate.

A number of clinical features such as fixation to chest wall, edema of skin, or inflammatory disease suggest that a tumor is initially not resectable (table 42-6). Adequate local control is frequently not achieved, and widespread metastases occur in the vast majority. In this subgroup, systemic therapy, i.e., chemotherapy, has become a cornerstone of treatment. One goal of treatment is to control the primary lesion, because the morbidity of uncontrolled local cancer in the chest wall produces ulceration, infection, foul smell, bleeding, and pain. Chemotherapy can initially reduce the size of the primary lesion or eliminate its inflammatory component in nearly 80% of cases.[22,22a,67,68] Chemotherapy with CAF or CMFVP is continued for at least 3 courses or until the surgeon feels that the lesion has become resectable. A "hygienic" mastectomy is then performed and chemotherapy is resumed, but could be interrupted after 3 more courses for chest wall radiation. Initial disease progression or no response after 2 or 3 courses of chemotherapy indicates the need for aggressive XRT, followed, if feasible, by surgery for local control. The duration of chemotherapy after loco-regional therapy is not established, but has ranged from 8–24 mo. The timing of XRT is somewhat arbitrary; a reasonable approach is to add chest radiation after 6 mo of chemotherapy. Again, many permutations of the timing of each modality are possible, and the best approach is not known. Nevertheless, data from the University of Texas M.D.

Anderson Cancer Center and elsewhere suggest that such combined modality treatments are important and effective.[21,22] Five-year survival of about 30% has been reported with aggressive combination modality treatment.

MANAGEMENT OF STAGE IV

Stage IV disease is defined by the occurrence of metastases beyond the regional area initially or the recurrence of breast cancer anywhere after adequate local therapy. The therapeutic options for stage IV are relatively limited. Surgery is useful primarily to confirm disease presence and to obtain tissue for hormone receptor analysis. XRT, the treatment of choice for CNS metastases, can produce local palliation such as stabilization of weight-bearing bone, control of pain, or reduction of a local mass. Neither modality, however, can be expected to have much impact on survival or overall palliation, making systemic treatments necessary. Few patients remain free of disease, and the goal of treatment for stage IV disease is maximal palliation. In other words, patients should have treatment applied in a manner that maximizes the benefits of therapy for symptom-free survival to enhance their quality of life. The physician should apply the various modalities in a manner that maximizes potential benefit. A treatment flow that we have used at the University of Maryland Cancer Center is shown in figure 42-4.

LOCAL RECURRENCE

A *local recurrence* (recurrence on the chest wall at the site of mastectomy and without regional lymph node involvement or systemic metastases) after mastectomy is usually accompanied or followed by distant failure within months. The disease-free survival at 10 yr after local failure is <5%, making local failure almost synonymous with systemic cancer.[69] The fact that occasional patients do survive free of disease for many years after local therapy does, however, suggest that true local recurrence does occur rarely. For all practical purposes, local failure is a marker of systemic relapse that may explain why postsurgical XRT to prevent local failure does not improve survival. The most common presentation is multiple skin nodules along the surgical scar. Metastases, however, may have a predilection for scar tissue at any site. When a local recurrence is easily resected, it should be removed, because an occasional patient will be disease-free for prolonged periods with no other therapy. XRT to the chest wall can be added after resection to prevent further local recurrence or may be delayed until there is further local recurrence. When the local recurrence is not resectable, it should be managed with XRT if this can be given in adequate dosage. Newer modalities of local therapy are also being investigated, including phototherapy using light-activated dyes such as porphyrin derivatives.[70] Such approaches are potentially useful to palliate or control local problems. Systemic therapy, however, may be needed when local treatment cannot be given. Hormonal therapy should be considered first (as outlined in Figure 42-4); chemotherapy is indicated in patients with negative hormone receptor status or visceral crises (see below).

Loco-regional recurrence refers to recurrence in ipsilateral supraclavicular, infraclavicular, or ipsilateral axillary nodes with or without local lesions in the chest wall and in the absence of distant metastases. Development of distant

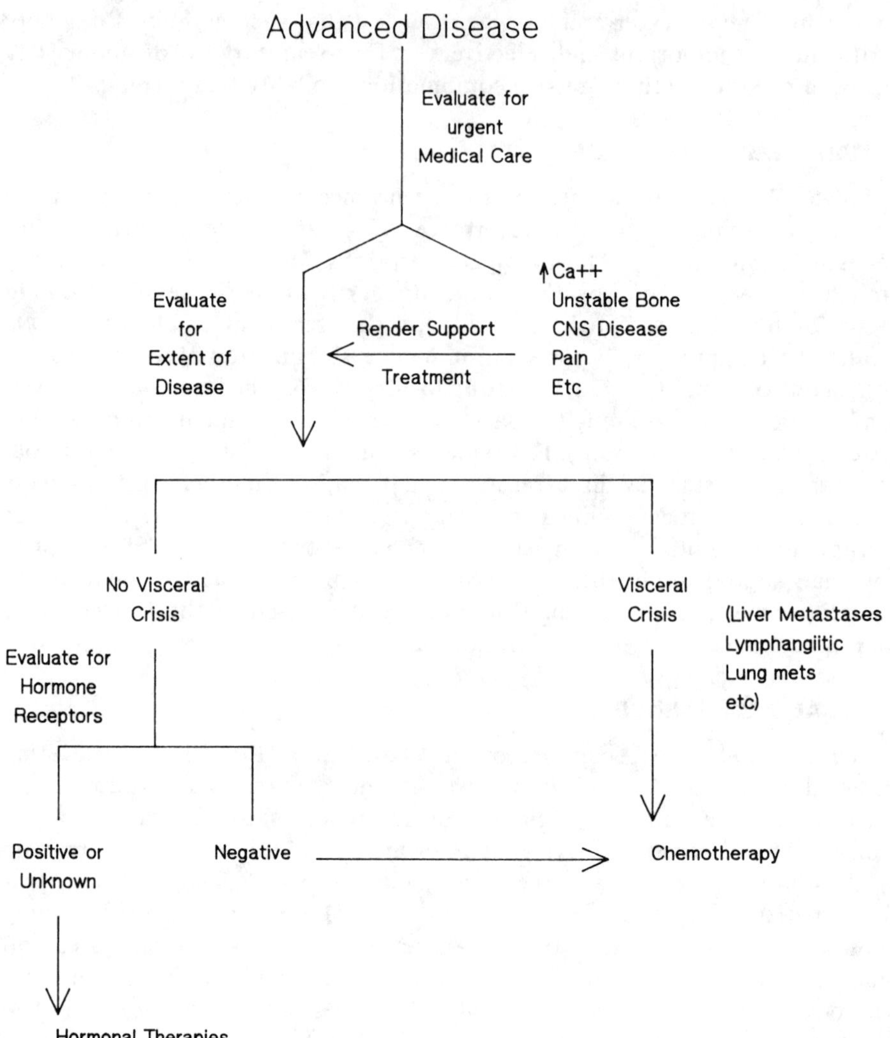

Figure 4. Flow diagram for treatment approach to advanced (metastatic) disease. Patients are first evaluated for any life-threatening problems that require immediate intervention. Subsequent workup focuses on defining extent of disease (site involved). Patients requiring a rapid tumor response, i.e., these with visceral crisis (see text) and those with estrogen receptor-negative tumors are placed on chemotherapy. Patients without visceral crisis having either positive or unknown hormone receptors in their tumor are placed on hormonal treatments.

metastases in a short interval is the rule. Vigorous attempts to resect recurrent disease in these areas (e.g., deep-seated supraclavicular nodes) are not warranted. If concomitant chest wall lesions are present, XRT would be indicated, and electron beam therapy might have some advantages. In the absence of chest wall metastases, the need for XRT is less compelling, because axillary and supraclavicular nodes often can be managed with systemic chemotherapy or hormonal therapy; XRT, adequate for these recurrences, often involves a large radiation port. If the disease becomes worse regionally during systemic therapy, then XRT is very useful for symptom control. Whether hormonal therapy or chemotherapy is chosen depends on hormone receptor status and sites of disease (figure 42-4).

Occasionally, patients will have clinically evident disease recurrence at only one site (e.g., brain, lung, skin, bone) and an extensive staging evaluation fails to reveal any additional sites of disease involvement. Furthermore, biopsy of such sites will frequently render the patient without evidence of disease (NED). Because it is nearly certain that such patients will have further disease recurrence, there is often a tendency use systemic therapy. Whereas it is highly desirable to render the patients NED by removal of any disease where possible and add appropriate local therapy as needed, the addition of systemic therapy is currently not recommended. Several studies attempting to augment survival in such circumstances have failed to show an impact on survival, and such treatments (either hormonal or chemotherapy) are likely to confuse the treatment when the patient has further disease progression. In addition, it is entirely possible that by adding potentially toxic therapy, the patient's asymptomatic period of NED is consumed with treatment toxicity. For this reason, such therapy should not be considered outside of a formal study setting.

Treatment Flow for Metastatic Disease

When patients first present with recurrent or metastatic disease, it is very important that they be assessed and staged in order to define the sites of disease and determine which treatment option is best for each (figure 42-4). The need for urgent or emergent therapies can be determined, and the basis for subsequent evaluations can be established. The initial evaluation should provide the clinician with an assessment of disease sites of involvement.

Certain sites and problems should take precedence before systemic treatment choices are made. For example, brain metastases should be treated promptly with steroids and XRT; hypercalcemia should be controlled with appropriate hydration and medical management; unstable bone lesions should receive appropriate stabilization or XRT or both; pain should be managed with analgesics or appropriate radiation to painful sites; and symptomatic effusions should be drained. One particularly difficult and frustrating problem is the management of back pain and the assessment of the risks of epidural spinal cord compression, including the indications of myelography. Severe and progressive back pain associated with bone scan or radiologic evidence of spinal bone metastases are both highly suggestive of epidural cord compression, which is frequent in this setting even when neurological findings are totally absent.[71] The indication for myelography (or MRI scanning) is based on the need for an accurate definition of the anatomic extension of the epidural invasion so that precise radiation ports can be planned. Roentgenograms are crucial to assess the stability of the spine, particularly of the cervical region.

When lytic lesions threaten stability, immobilization and surgical evaluations are mandatory.

Once the assessment shows that the patient is not in need of urgent/emergent therapy or such appropriate therapy has been instituted, a decision between the various systemic treatment options is appropriate. Hormonal therapy is a preferred first treatment whenever possible or feasible, because it is both less toxic and much easier to manage. Because response to hormonal therapy may take 8–12 wk to become manifest, it is important to first determine if the patient has any potentially life-threatening organ involvement—a so-called visceral crisis. For example, patients with lymphangitic lung metastases, extensive liver metastases, or a leukoerythroblastic peripheral blood picture due to bone marrow involvement are considered to have visceral crisis, and progression of disease may be lethal. Therefore, the more immediate response of chemotherapy is highly desirable. Conversely, patients without visceral crisis can be considered to have a more stable clinical picture and could potentially be evaluated over a longer period for response to hormonal therapy. Patients with known estrogen receptor-negative tumors should also proceed to chemotherapy, because the response frequency to hormones in this setting is very low. However, patients with hormone receptor-positive tumors and those with unknown (and unobtainable) hormone receptor status should undergo hormonal therapy.

Hormonal Therapy

The mechanism of action of hormonal manipulations in breast cancer is not well understood, but is a subject of intensive research. For clinical purposes, the main concept is that a sudden change in the hormonal microenvironment of the cancer cell may change its growth kinetics. An organized approach to hormonal therapies is shown in figure 42-5. Oophorectomy in premenopausal patients removes the source of estrogen; estrogen at physiologic levels binds to estrogen receptors located in the nucleus of the cell, where it is thought to promote the synthesis of m RNA, which in turn induces protein synthesis and cell growth. Antiestrogens such as tamoxifen are thought to alter this process, thus inhibiting cell growth. These mechanisms also trigger the release of potent growth factors and inhibiting substances that can alter the expression of the receptor proteins themselves.

Oophorectomy

Oophorectomy is often the initial treatment for premenopausal women. An oophorectomy adds another level of hormonal manipulation for the premenopausal patient and, at least for the responding patient, offers the possibility of both more and longer hormonal control. During the perimenopausal and postmenopausal periods, estrogens can be produced in fat cells by aromatase enzymes that transform androgens of adrenal origin into estrogens. For this reason, oophorectomy is useless after menopause. Serum gonadotropin levels and a vaginal cytology smear to assess for estrogen effect may be helpful when the menopausal status is uncertain. Oophorectomy is best obtained by surgery, although in some countries XRT (1,000–2,000 cGy to the ovaries) has been

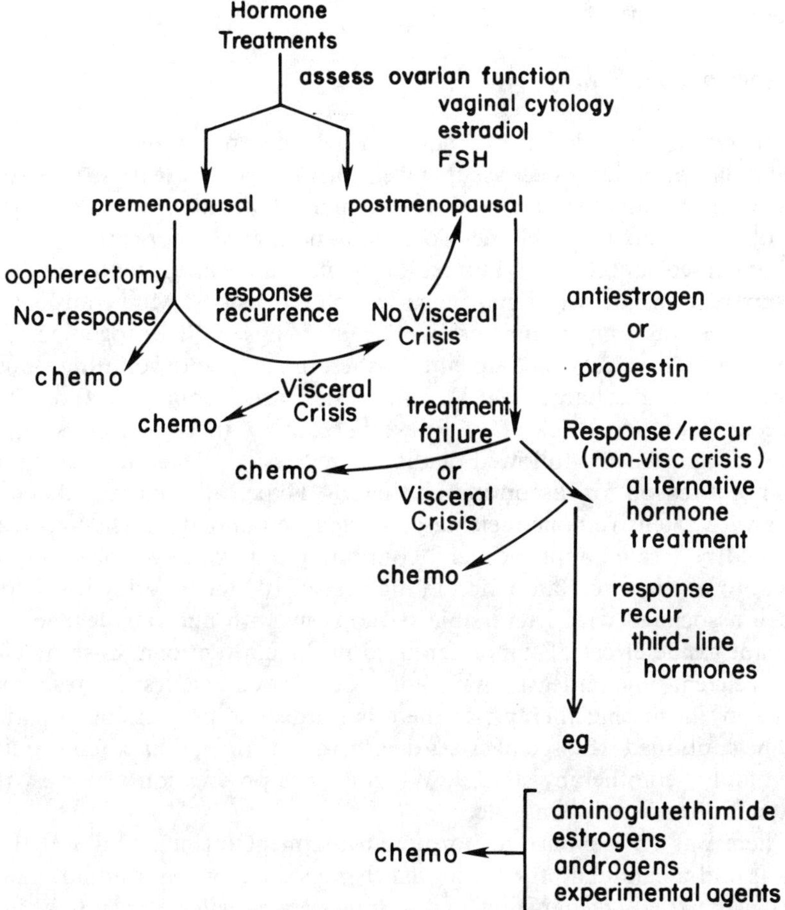

Figure 5. Flow diagram for hormonal treatments of breast cancer (patients without visceral crisis). Choice depends upon menopausal status. Serum gonadotropins and vaginal cytology estrogen effect can help differentiate pre- and postmenopausal status for the intermenopausal group. For premenopausal women, the first choice is usually oophorectomy, which can add a level of hormone therapy. Subsequent hormonal management, if indicated, is identical to that for the postmenopausal group. Primary failure (no response to treatment) should lead to chemotherapy. Response followed by progression or recurrence should lead to subsequent hormonal treatments unless visceral crisis occurs. For postmenopausal patients, the initial treatment is usually an antiestrogen (tamoxifen). Subsequent therapy, if indicated by response then progression, is usually a progestin (megestrol acetate). Alternatively, the sequence can be reversed (tamoxifen second). Multiple subsequent therapies (and permutations in the order of the therapies) are potentially possible with response/progression, provided visceral crisis does not ensue. Chemotherapy is used when there is primary treatment failure to a modality, visceral crisis ensues, or hormonal options are exhausted.

used. Suppression of estrogen production by XRT takes longer to occur and is usually less complete. For oophorectomy in general, patients with ER-PR-positive tumors can have a response rate up to 60–70% and a median duration of response of nearly 1 yr.

Antiestrogen Therapy

Tamoxifen is considered by many to be the treatment of choice for postmenopausal patients because it is well tolerated and at least as effective as other currently available hormonal treatments.[73] Tamoxifen is administered in a dose of 10 mg p.o. b.i.d. Higher doses have not proven more effective except in unconfirmed anecdotes. Tamoxifen is not associated with significant myelosuppression nor with renal, hepatic, or CNS toxicity. Mild transient falls in platelet counts may occur rarely. The drug has mild estrogenic effects. Uncommon side effects include hot flashes, nausea and vomiting, vaginal bleeding, vaginal discharge, and skin rash. Increasing bone pain (bone flare) may occur early (first few days to weeks) during therapy and is a good prognostic sign, usually followed by disease regression. Thus, increasing bone pain is not a reason for discontinuing therapy. Hypercalcemia may develop in patients with extensive bone metastases started on tamoxifen. The hypercalcemia should be treated appropriately; continuing tamoxifen whenever possible may lead to a response. Tamoxifen in high dose (100 mg/m^2/day for >6 mo) has been associated with irreversible retinopathy with macular degeneration. This is not a side effect of tamoxifen used in the conventional dose of 10 mg b.i.d. Sufficient time (at least 8 wk) should be allowed to assess for response to this and any hormonal therapy. If there is no disease progression, treatment should be continued. If visceral crises develop at any time, tamoxifen should be stopped and chemotherapy started. When disease progression develops, there are often 2 different circumstances:

1. There was no response to hormonal treatment (primary failure). If the patient is still a candidate for hormonal therapy, a second hormonal manipulation can be tried, recognizing that response rates will be very low, in the proximity of 10%.

2. There was disease stabilization or a response to treatment. Responding patients should be observed for several weeks after the drug is discontinued to see if there was stabilization or even improvement in the disease.

This "withdrawal" stabilization or response (seen occasionally with additive hormonal treatments) is uncommon with antagonist therapy, but it may provide a few months of stable disease. Once it is recognized that the disease is worsening, a second-line hormonal treatment is administered (figure 42-5).

Progesterone Compounds

Progestins are another class of compounds active in the hormonal treatment of breast cancer. Megestrol acetate (MA) is the commercially available oral agent with the widest use and applicability. MA is as effective as tamoxifen as first-line therapy, and either drug can be used in sequence with the other. At the conventional dose of 160 mg/day, MA is also relatively devoid of side effects or toxicity except for some mild weight gain and possible fluid retention, perhaps making it a better choice for underweight patients because it increases appetite. If tamoxifen is administered first, MA is the most reasonable second choice at a dose of 160 mg/day (40 mg p.o. q.i.d.). Preliminary evidence suggests a dose/response curve for the progestins in general for breast cancer. Pilot studies at the University of Maryland Cancer Center also suggest a dose/response curve for MA (with some patients responding to high dose even after primary failure of tamoxifen or conventional dose MA).[74] Higher doses result in considerable weight gain, however. Further studies are needed to define the optimal dose of MA.

Aromatase Inhibitors

Aminoglutethimide in a dose of 250 mg p.o. q.i.d. administered together with hydrocortisone, 25 mg p.o. b.i.d., persistently blocks adrenal steroidogenesis in >90% of patients.[75] Hydrocortisone is added to suppress ACTH hypersecretion, which could otherwise override aminoglutethimide-induced adrenal suppression. Aminoglutethimide has 2 potential mechanisms of action: (1) it blocks adrenal function and (2) inhibits aromatization of androgens to estrogens in peripheral tissues, mainly fat, by blocking the aromatase enzyme system. The latter effect is probably more effective in suppressing adrenal function as measured by plasma dihydroepiandosterone levels, which should fall below 25 mg/dl by 3 wk. Plasma dihydroepiandosterone levels are not measured routinely but this could be done if there were concern about inadequate adrenal suppression with the 1 g/day dose. Skin rash occurs in over one third of patients, but often fades without intervention with continuation of therapy. Mental changes, mainly somnolence, lethargy, and ataxia, are common. Thyroid dysfunction occasionally develops with chronic use. Side effects frequently lead to discontinuation of the drug because patients may find them unacceptable, and reassurance is usually very important. Patients stopping aminoglutethimide should have their adrenal function monitored to determine if normal function returns. Recently, newer aromatase inhibitors have been introduced into clinical trials. These new substances have the advantage of significantly fewer side effects, perhaps making them more desirable as part of initial hormone therapy.

Estrogens

Estrogens can also have important antitumor activity in the postmenopausal patient. Diethylstilbestrol (DES) in a dose of 5 mg p.o. t.i.d. has been effective in about 30% of patients unselected for hormone receptor status and previously untreated with hormonal therapy. The response frequency is higher in patients with predominately soft-tissue disease and with "positive" receptor tumors. There are several suggestions of a dose/response curve, and dose is usually escalated to tolerance.[76] Because side effects are more severe than with antiestrogens or MA, DES is seldom used initially despite its lower cost. Toxicity includes thromboembolic complications, endometrial hyperplasia and bleeding, salt and water retention, and (especially) nausea and vomiting. Patients with hypertension and heart failure may have severe decompensation unless aggressively treated with cardiotonics, diuretics, and antihypertensives. Again, bone flare or hypercalcemia is not always evidence of disease progression; some patients may benefit from symptomatic treatment and supportive care continuation of estrogens.

Androgens

Androgens have also been used, but because they are probably less effective than estrogens or any of the drugs discussed above, they are less preferred than estrogens. They also produce the undesirable side effect of masculinization. They may be preferable, however, in elderly women who cannot tolerate the fluid retention associated with estrogens. Fluoxymesterone, 10 mg p.o. t.i.d., or testosterone propionate, 100 mg I.M. t.i.w., have been used. Virilization is universal and may be unacceptable to many women; cholestatic jaundice is also a possible side effect, occurring in 10–20% of patients.

Glucocorticoids

Glucocorticoids are considered to have antitumor activity, but most of the benefit is a subjective improvement with little evidence for objective tumor regression. They can have marked side effects (Cushing's syndrome). They are used most often for control of brain edema associated with metastases, cord compression, for the control of hypercalcemia, and for symptomatic relief in some instances where other therapies are not effective.

Chemotherapy

Chemotherapy is indicated in patients with distant metastases when hormonal therapy is not a reasonable initial option (figure 42-4) or fails to control the disease. Because chemotherapy of overt metastatic breast cancer is a palliative intervention, morbidity and complications should be balanced with the benefit obtained. Palliation signifies improvement in the quality of life and prolongation of survival when definitive cure is not possible.

Virtually all currently available chemotherapeutic drugs used in breast cancer have been tested alone or as part of a combination for the treatment of advanced disease. Single agents that produce responses in ≥20% of treated patients when used alone are considered active (table 42-9).[77] Response frequencies with single agents in patients with advanced breast cancer who have not received prior chemotherapy range between 20–40%;[77] doxorubicin (ADR), CTX, 5-FU, mitoxantrone, MTX, thio-tepa, and mitomycin-C (MIT) are among the most active drugs. The activity of these single agents in patients given prior chemotherapy is consistently lower. In both previously treated and untreated patients, responses to single-agent chemotherapy are rarely complete and are usually relatively short. As is true for several malignancies, combination chemotherapy has proven more effective than single-agent therapy both in terms of response frequency and duration of response.[78] Chemotherapeutic agents can have different mechanisms of actions and can affect cell growth and division at different points of the cell cycle; often, toxicities are also different, allowing for the drugs to be combined at nearly full dose with acceptable side effects. Additive and sometimes synergistic combinations may be obtained.

Combination chemotherapy thus can increase response rates and prolong disease control and survival. The use of combinations of active single agents has resulted in cures of certain advanced malignancies such as testicular cancer, Hodgkin's disease, and diffuse histiocytic lymphoma.[78] Combination chemotherapy for breast cancer has not yet produced cures in advanced disease, but its application to earlier disease as an adjuvant has had a significant impact upon the cure rate. Thus, further study of advanced disease is likely to have 2 important benefits: (1) improved survival for patients with advanced disease and (2) development of new adjuvant therapies to improve the surgical cure rate.

First-line Chemotherapy for Advanced Disease

Selection of first-line chemotherapy depends on institutional preference, physician experience, and patient risk factors for toxicity. Several drug combinations have nearly similar response rates and fairly similar side effects (table 42-10). Responses to combination chemotherapy average 10–12 mo. The most popular multiagent chemotherapy programs, including their response rates, percentages of complete response (CR), and duration of response are outlined in table 42-10.[29,79-93] Combination chemotherapy clearly improves the duration and quality of survival for most patients.

Response rates and durations of response have a wide range because of the heterogeneity of metastatic breast cancer. Soft-tissue disease responds better than visceral disease, and bone disease is very difficult to evaluate. Patients with a longer disease-free interval (>1 yr) respond better than those with a short disease-free interval. This heterogeneity has led to some confusion in the

Table 42-9. Single-agent Chemotherapy in Breast Cancer

Agent	Approximate objective response rate (%)
Doxorubicin (Adriamycin) (A)	35
Cyclophosphamide (C)	35
Nitrogen mustard	35
Mitoxantrone	30
Thio-tepa (T)	30
Phenylalanine mustard	25
Chlorambucil	20
5-Fluorouracil (F)	25
Methotrexate (M)	35
Vincristine (V)	20
Vinblastine (Vbl)	20
Vindesine	20
Mitomycin-C (MIT)	40
Carmustine (BCNU)	20
Hexamethylmelamine (Hx)	30
Dibromodulcitol (D)	30

Objective response: complete or partial response (i.e., 50% decrease in cross-perpendicular dimensions)
Source: after Carater (ref 77)

Table 42-10. Popular Initial Combination Chemotherapies for Advanced Breast Cancer

Combination	Percentage range of total response rate (CR + PR)	Percentage range of complete response rate	Range of duration of response (mo)
TMF	75	—	7
CMP	44	4	7
CMV	33	7	8
CMF	40–70	8–15	6–10
CMF ± V ± P	30–80	7–25	6–14
CAF ± VP	40–80	8–15	8–16
CAMFVP	46	11	9
CAFM	50	10	11
CA	41–78	2–22	10–12
CAV	56,72	16,28	12,22
AV	52,53	8,—	7,8
Others (VFP, CFP, CFP-V, CFV)	42–63	2–6	6–10

Abbreviations: T = thio-tepa, M = methotrexate, F = fluorouracil, C = cyclophosphamide, P = prednisone, V = vincristine, A = Adriamycin (refs. 30,77,79–95)

comparison of chemotherapy regimens. In order to compare various chemotherapy combinations, large prospectively randomized trials with stratification for the various prognostic factors are needed. Combination chemotherapy for breast cancer was initiated by Greenspan et al, with a combination of thio-tepa, 5-FU, and MTX.[79] Subsequently, Cooper introduced a 5-drug regimen of CTX, MTX, 5-FU, vincristine (VCR), and prednisone.[80] Since then there have been multiple permutations of these drugs with substitution of ADR for MTX and/or the addition/substitution of other agents as well. An overview of such available trials would suggest that CMF[88,89,93] is the basic constituent of CMFVP; the V and P add little to the 3-drug regimen.[89,91] CAF is superior to CMF and is the usually preferred first-line regimen. The use of CAF, however, must be balanced against all patient factors. For example, women with significant cardiovascular disease may be more appropriately treated with CMFVP (or derivative) regimens. VATH is an effective second-line regimen after CMF or CMFVP,[90,94,103] and, in an ongoing CALGB study, appears to be about equivalent to CAF as a first-line therapy. The differences between the options are small, however, and further investigations are needed to improve the chemotherapy regimens. New approaches include further permutations of available drugs, but the best opportunities lie in the identification of new agents or the identification of newer treatment modalities derived from our understanding of the biology of these tumors. Although they are manageable, toxicities of the available chemotherapy can be considerable, generally consisting of mild nausea and vomiting, hair loss, and blood count suppression. The last effect is usually the dose-limiting toxicity, although the use of colony stimulating factors may alter the dosing capabilities. Other toxicities that are related to specific drugs include mucositis, stomatitis, diarrhea, constipation, paresthesia, muscle weakness, hematuria, heart damage, and liver function changes.

The optimal duration of chemotherapy is not well defined. Usually, therapy is continued until there is evidence of disease progression or recurrence, but it is unclear whether the chemotherapy is needed on a continuous basis; further studies are needed to define the optimal use of chemotherapy. In the small percentage (about 10%) of women who achieve a CR, there is no information or standardized approach on how long to continue treatment. Our practice has been to continue chemotherapy for 2 yr before considering discontinuance. Most women, however, have disease progression before there is an option for treatment discontinuation.

Salvage Chemotherapy

Eventually, the initially chosen combination chemotherapy regimen becomes ineffective by virtue of disease progression or recurrence. At that time, a second-line or "salvage" regimen is usually started. There are a number of second-line regimens[90,94,107] (see Appendix) with variable effectiveness (table 42-11), making the use of experimental agents highly desirable from both an ethical and a scientific viewpoint in these patients. The choice of which second-line regimen should be used depends upon the prior regimen. There is little rationale for choosing as a second-line combination a regimen with only minor changes (e.g., CAF after CMF). Furthermore, ADR as a single agent has <25% activity in salvage, and the combination of ADR and VCR offers little apparent advantage over ADR alone. On the other hand, VATH is a highly active salvage regimen after CMF or CMFVP and vice versa.[90,94,103] In general, patients are placed on regimens containing agents to which the tumor was not exposed in the prior combination. With a large fraction of the women with breast cancer receiving adjuvant chemotherapy, a common problem occurs when a patient has recurrent disease after such therapy is completed. Ongoing trials demonstrate that patients who develop recurrent disease within a year of finishing adjuvant chemotherapy rarely respond to the same regimen. Conversely, patients whose treatment fails >1 yr after adjuvant therapy may respond to the same regimen with response frequencies only slightly lower than those of previously untreated patients.

Table 42-11. Second-Line (Salvage) Combination Chemotherapies for Disseminated Breast Cancer

Combination	Approximate objective total response rate (%)
AV	25
AMit	40
FAVMit	54
VblMit	7,40
VAMit	17,73
VblATH	49,52
VAPt	42
VACMCf	78
HxVM	45

Abbreviations: A = Adriamycin, V = vincristine, Mit = mitomycin, F = fluorouracil, Vbl = vinblastine, T = tamoxifen, H = halotestin, Pt = cisplatinum, Cf = citrovorum factor, C = cyclophosphamide, M = methotrexate, V = vincristine Hx = hexamethylmelamine (refs. 90,94,96–107)

Male Breast Cancer

The primary surgical treatment for male breast cancer is modified radical mastectomy with axillary dissection. Because of the small size of the male breast, "lumpectomy" is not usually advocated. Although no data are available on adjuvant therapy, it seems reasonable to follow the same guidelines as for female breast cancer. Hormonal therapies, however, may be very important. Fro advanced disease, hormonal manipulations are indicated first in most patients, since 70% of tumors have positive hormone receptors. Orchiectomy is offered first because it removes the main source of estrogen (via aromatization of androgen). Tamoxifen has been effective and is a reasonable first- or second-line regimen.[108,109] Other hormonal treatments and chemotherapies are similar to those described for female breast cancer.

References

1. Cancer Facts and Figures 1990. New York: American Cancer Society, 1990.
2. Silverberg E, Boring CC, Squires TS. Cancer statistics 1990. CA 1990; 40:9–26.
3. Special report: the epidemiology and etiology of breast cancer. N Engl J Med 1980; 30:1246–48.
4. Gray GE, Pike MC, Henderson BE. Breast cancer incidence and mortality rates in different countries in relation to known risk factors and dietary practices. Br J Cancer 1979; 39:1–7.
5. Miller AB, Kelly A, Choi NW, et al. A study of diet and breast cancer. Am J Epidemiol 1978; 107:499–509.
6. Buell P. Changing incidence of breast cancer in Japanese-American women. JNCI 1973; 51:1479–83.
7. Anderson DE. A genetic study of human breast cancer. JNCI 1972; 48:1029–34.
8. Pertrakis NL. Genetic factors in the etiology of breast cancer. Cancer 1977; 39:2709–15.
9. Sattin RW, Rubin GL, Webster LA, Huezo CM, Wingo PA, Dry HW, Layde PM. Family history and the risk of breast cancer. JAMA 1985; 253:1908–13.
10. Moskowitz M, Gartside P, McLaughlin C. Mammographic patterns as markers for high-risk benign breast disease and incident cancers. Radiology 1980; 134:293–95.
11. Moskowitz M, Gartside P, Wirman JA, McLaughlin C. Proliferative disorders of the breast as risk factors for breast cancer in a self-selected screened population: pathologic markers. Radiology 1980; 134:289–91.
12. Dupont WD, Page DL. Risk factors for breast cancer in women with proliferative breast disease. N Engl J Med 1985; 3:146–51.
13. Love SM, Gelonam RS, Sileu W. Sounding board—fibrocystic "disease" of the breast: a non-disease? N Engl J Med 1982; 307:1010–14.
14. McGregor DH, Land CE, Choi K, Tokuoka S, Liu PI, Wakabayashi T, Beebe GW. Breast cancer incidence among atomic bomb survivors, Hiroshima and Nagasaki 1950–1969. JNCI 1977; 59:799–811.
14a. Muggia FM, Greenspan EM, Aisner J, et al. Workshop on chemoprevention of breast cancer. Cancer Res 1984; 44:3151–54.
15. Wolfe JN. Risk for breast cancer development determined by mammographic parenchymal pattern. Cancer 1976; 37:2486–92.
16. Ernster VL, Sacks ST, Peterson CA, Schweitzer RJ. Mammographic parenchymal patterns and risk factors for breast cancer. Radiology 1980; 134:617–20.
16a. Howe GR, Hirohata T, Hislop JM, et al. Dietary factors and risk of breast cancer: Combined analysis of 12 case controlled studies. JNCI 1990; 82:561–69.

16b. Beuhler PK. Patient selection for prophylactic mastectomy: who is at high risk? Plast Reconstr Surg 1983; 72:324-34.

17. McDivitt RW, Hutter RV, Foote FW Jr., Stewart FW. In situ lobular carcinoma. JAMA 1967; 201:96-100.

18. McDivitt RW, Stewart FW, Berg JW. Armed Forces Institute of Pathology. Atlas of tumor pathology. Fascicle 2, 2nd series. Carcinoma of mammary lobules, Washington, D.C.: The Institute, 1968; 63-86.

19. Rosen PP, Lieberman PH, Braun DH, et al. Lobular carcinoma *in situ* of the breast: Detailed analysis of 99 patients with an average follow-up of 24 years. Am J Surg Pathol 1978; 2:225.

20. Fisher ER, Gregorio RM, Fisher B, et al. The pathology of invasive breast cancer: a syllabus derived from findings of the National Surgical Adjuvant Breast Project (protocol 4). Cancer 1974; 36:1-85.

21. Fastenberg NA, Martin RG, Buzdar AU, et al. Management of inflammatory carcinoma of the breast: a combined modality approach. Am J Clin Oncol 1985; 8:134-41.

22. Aisner J, Morris D, Elias EG, Wiernik PH. Mastectomy as an adjuvant to chemotherapy for locally advanced or metastatic breast cancer. Arch Surg 1982; 117:882-87.

22a. Abrams JS, Aisner J. The evolving approach to stage III breast cancer. In: Kennedy BJ, ed. Breast cancer. New York: AR Liss, 1982; 143-62.

23. Jensen EV, Block GE, Smith S, Kyser KA, DeSombre ER. Estrogen receptors and breast cancer response to adrenalectomy. NCI monograph 1971; 34:55-70.

24. McGuire WL, Horowitz KB. Progesterone receptors in breast cancer. In: McGuire WL, ed. Hormones, receptors and breast cancer. New York: Raven Press, 1978; 31-42.

24a. McGuire WL, Clark GM, Dressler LG, Owens MA. Role of steroid hormone receptors as prognostic factors in primary breast cancer. NCI monogr 1986; 1:19-23.

24b. Mirecki DM, Jordan VC. Steroid hormone receptors and human breast cancer. Lab Med 1985; 16:287-94.

25. Fisher B, Redmond C, Brown A, et al. Influence of tumor estrogen and progesterone receptor levels on the response to tamoxifen and chemotherapy in primary breast cancer. J Clin Oncol 1983; 1:227-41.

26. Rosen PP, Kinne Lesser M, Hellman S. Are prognostic factors for local control of breast cancer treated by primary radiotherapy significant for patients treated by mastectomy? Cancer 1986; 57:1415-20.

27. Sampat MB, Sirsat MV, Gangadharan P. Prognostic significance of blood vessel invasion in carcinoma of the breast in women. J Surg Oncol 1977; 9:523-32.

28. Ketterhagen JP, Quackenbush SR, Haushalter RA. Tumor histology as a prognostic determinant in carcinoma of the breast. Surg Gyn Obstet 1984; 158:120-23.

29. Silvestini R, Daidone MG, Fronzo G, et al. Prognostic implication of labelling versus estrogen receptors and tumor size in node negative breast cancer. Breast Cancer Treat Res 1986; 7:161-69.

29a. Meyer JS, Coplin MD. Thymidine labelling index, flow cytometric S phase measurement and DNA index in human tumors. Am J Clin Pathol 1988; 89:586-95

29b. Kallioniemi OP, Blanco G, Alavaikko M, et al. Improving the prognostic value of DNA flow cytometry in breast cancer by combining DNA index and S phase fraction. Cancer 1988; 62:2183-90.

29c. Slamon DJ, Clark GM, Wong SG, et al. Correlation of relapse and survival with amplification of the HER-2/neu oncogene. Science 1987; 235;177-82.

30. Harris JR, Henderson IC. Natural history and staging of breast cancer. In: Hellman S, Henderson IC, Kinne DW, eds. Breast diseases. J.B. New York: Lippincott, 1987; 233-58.

31. Fisher B, Slack NH, Bross IDJ, et al. Cancer of the breast: size of neoplasm and prognosis. Cancer 1969; 24:1071-80.

32. Fisher B, Bauer M, Wickerham DL, et al. Relation of number of positive axillary nodes to the prognosis of patients with primary breast cancer—an NSABP update. Cancer 1983; 52:1551-57.

33. Fisher B, Slack N, Katrych D, Wolmark N. Ten year follow-up results of patients with carcinoma of the breast in a cooperative clinical trial evaluating surgical adjuvant chemotherapy. Surg Gyn Obstet 1975; 140:528-34.

34. Fisher B, Bauer M, Margolese R, et al. Five year results of a randomized clinical trial comparing total mastectomy and segmental mastectomy with or without radiation in the treatment of breast cancer. N Engl J Med 1985; 312;665–73.

34a. Fisher B, Redmond C, Fisher ER, et al. Ten-year results of a randomized clinical trial comparing radical mastectomy and total mastectomy with or without radiation. N Engl J Med 1985; 312:674–81.

35. Langlands AO, Pocock SJ, Kerr GR, Gore SM. Longterm survival of patients with breast cancer: a study of the curability of the disease. Br Med J Nov 1979; 17:1247–51.

36. Valagussa P, Bonadonna G, Veronesi V. Patterns of relapse and survival following radical mastectomy. Analysis of 716 consecutive patients. Cancer 1978; 41:1170–78.

37. Donegan WL, Skibba JL. Patterns of survival and disease recurrence after mastectomy for carcinoma of the breast. Cancer Treat Symp 1983; 2:107–31.

38. Cutler SJ, Asire AJ, Taylor SG. Classification of patients with disseminated cancer of the breast. Cancer 1969; 24:861–69.

39. Cutler SJ. Classification of extent of disease in breast cancer. Semin Oncol 1974; 1:91–96.

40. McGinnis LS. The importance of clinical breast examination. Cancer 1989; 64:2657–63.

41. Greenwald P, Nassa PC, Laurence CE, et al. Estimated effect of breast self-examination and routine physician examinations of breast-cancer mortality. N Engl J Med 1978; 299:271–73.

42. Leborgne R. Diagnosis of tumors of the breast by simple roentgenography. Calcifications in Carcinomas 1951; 65:1–22.

43. Morrison AS. Review of the evidence on the early detection and treatment of breast cancer. Cancer 1989; 64:2651–56.

44. Shapiro S, Venet W, Strax P, Venet L, Roeser R. Ten to fourteen-year effect of screening on breast cancer mortality. JNCI 1982; 69:349–55.

45. Morrison AS, Brisson J, Khahid N. Breast cancer incidence and mortality in the Breast Cancer Detection Demonstration Project. JNCI 1988; 80:1540–47.

45a. Bassett LW, Marijikian V, Gold RH. Mammography and breast cancer screening. Surg Clin North Am 1990; 70(4):775–800.

46. Veronesi V, Sacconzzi R, DelVechio M, et al. Comparing radical mastectomy with quadrantectomy, axillary dissection and radiotherapy in patients with small cancers of the breast. N Engl J Med 1981; 305:6–11.

47. Dowden RV, Horton CE, Rosato FE, McCraw JB. Reconstruction of the breast after mastectomy for cancer. Surg Gyn Obstet 1979; 149:109–15.

47a. Early stage breast cancer: NIH consensus development conference. Program and abstracts, NIH, June 18–21, 1990.

48. Fisher B. Breast cancer management: alternative to radical mastectomy. N Engl J Med 1979; 301:326–28.

49. Ravdin RG, Lewison EF, Stack NH, et al. Results of a clinical trial concerning the worth of prophylactic oophorectomy for breast carcinoma. Surg Gyn Obstet 1970; 131:1055–64.

50. Nolvadex Adjuvant Trial Organization. Controlled trial of tamoxifen as a single adjuvant agent in management of early breast cancer. Analysis at six years. Lancet Apr 1985; 13:836–840.

51. Peto R. Overview of mortality by allocated treatment in randomized comparisons of early breast cancer. Presented at Overview on Adjuvant Chemotherapy for Breast Cancer, Bethesda, Md., Sept 7–9, 1985.

52. NIH consensus development conference statement: adjuvant chemotherapy for breast cancer. CA 1986; 36:42–47.

53. Burchenal JH. Adjuvant therapy—theory, practice and potential. Cancer 1976; 37:46.

54. Bonadonna G, Valagussa P, Taneini G, et al. Current status of Milan adjuvant chemotherapy trials for node positive and node negative breast cancer. NCI monogr 1986; 1:45–50.

55. Fisher B, Redmond C, Fisher ER, Wolmark N. Systemic adjuvant therapy in treatment of primary operable breast cancer. National Surgical Adjuvant Breast and Bowel Project experiences. NCI monogr 1986; 1:35–44.

56. Goldhirsch A, Gelber R. Adjuvant treatment for early breast cancer. Ludwig Group studies. NCI Monogr 1986; 1:55–70.

57. Tormey DC, Gray R, Taylor SG, Knuman M, Olson JE, Cummings FJ. Postoperative chemotherapy and chemohormonal therapy in women with node positive breast cancer. NCI monogr 1986; 1:75–80.

58. Lippman ME, Chabner BA. NIH consensus development conference on adjuvant chemotherapy and endocrine therapy for breast cancer: editorial overview. NCI Monographs 1986; 1:5–10.

59. Skipper HE, Schabel FM, Lloyd HH. Dose-response and tumor cell repopulation rate in chemotherapeutic trials. In: Rosowsky A, ed. Advances in cancer chemotherapy. New York: Marcel Decker, 1979; 297.

60. Jones RB, Norton L, Bhadivaj S, Muss T, Holland JF. Single agent Adriamycin for metastatic breast cancer. A steep dose response relationship. Proc Am Soc Clin Oncol 1983; 2:C419.

61. Hyniuk WM, Levine MN, Levin L. Analysis of dose intensity for chemotherapy in early (stage II) and advanced breast cancer. NCI monogr 1986; 1:87–94.

62. Skipper HE, Schabel FM Jr. Quantitative and cytokinetic studies in experimental tumor models. In: J.F. Holland, E. Frei, eds. Cancer medicine. Philadelphia: Leu and Febiger, 1974; 624–50.

63. Nissen-Meyer R, Kjellgren K, Malmis K, Manson B, Norin T. Surgical adjuvant chemotherapy: Results of one short course with cyclophosphamide after mastectomy for breast cancer. Cancer 1978; 41:2088–98.

64. Cooper RG, Holland JF, Glidewell D. Adjuvant chemotherapy of breast cancer. Cancer 1979; 44:793–98.

64a. Goldhirsch A, Gelber RD. Randomized perioperative therapy in operable breast cancer: The Ludwig Study V. 3rd Int Conf on Adjuvant Therapy of Primary Breast Cancer. March 2–5, 1988; 8.

65. Osborne CK, Rivkin SE, McDivitt RW, et al. Adjuvant therapy of breast cancer: Southwest Oncology Group studies. NCI monogr 1986; 1:71–74.

66. Zucali R, Uslenghi C, Kenda R, Bonadonna G. Natural history and survival of inoperable breast cancer treated with radiotherapy followed by radical mastectomy. Cancer 1976; 37:1422–31.

67. Perloff M, Lesnick GJ. Chemotherapy before and after mastectomy in stage III breast cancer. Arch Surg 1982; 117:879–81.

68. Perloff M, Korzun A, Chu F, Lesnick GJ for CALGB. Combination chemotherapy (CT) with surgery (S) and radiotherapy (RT) for stage III breast carcinoma. Proc Am Soc Clin Oncol 1985; 4:60.

69. Chu FC, Lin FJ, Kim JH, Huh SH, Garmatis CJ. Locally recurrent carcinoma of the breast: results of radiation therapy. Cancer 1976; 37:2677–81.

70. Daughterty TJ, Wershaupt KR. Newer methods of cancer treatment: photo dynamic sensitizers. In: V.T. DeVita Jr., S. Hellman, S.A. Rosenberg, eds. Principles and practice of oncology. 2nd ed. Philadelphia: Lippincott, 1985; 2272–99.

71. Rodinchok LD, Harper GR, Ruckdeschel JC, Price A, Roberson G, Barron KD, Horton J. Early diagnosis of spinal epidural metastases. Am J Med 1981; 70:1181–88.

72. Lippman M, Bolan G, Huff K. The effects of estrogens and antiestrogens on hormone responsive human breast cancer in long-term tissue culture. Cancer Res 1976; 36:4595–4601.

73. Legha SS, Davis HL, Muggia FM. Hormonal therapy of breast cancer: new approaches and concepts. Ann Intern Med 1978; 88:69–77.

74. Tchekmedyian NS, Tait N, Aisner J. High dose megestrol acetate in the treatment of postmenopausal women with breast cancer. Semin Oncol 1986; 13 suppl 4:20–25.

75. Santeu RJ, Worgul TJ, Lipton A, et al. Aminoglutethimide as treatment of postmenopausal women with advanced breast carcinoma. Ann Intern Med 1982; 96:94–101.

76. Carter AC, Sedransk N, Kelley RM, et al. Diethylstilbestrol: recommended dosages for different categories of breast cancer patients. JAMA 1972; 237:2079–85.

77. Carter SK. Integration of chemotherapy into combined modality treatment of solid tumors. VII: Adenocarcinoma of the breast. Cancer Treat Rev 1976; 3:141–74.

78. DeVita VT, Schein PS. The use of drugs in combination for the treatment of cancer. N Engl J Med 1973; 288:998–1006.

79. Greenspan EM. Combination cytotoxic chemotherapy in advanced disseminated breast cancer. Mt. Sinai J Med, New York, 1966; 33:1–27.
80. Cooper R. Combination chemotherapy in hormone resistant breast cancer. Proc Am Assoc Cancer Res 1969; 10:15.
81. Carter SK. The chemical therapy of breast cancer. Semin Oncol 1974; 1:131–44.
82. Leone LA, Rege V. Treatment of metastatic, recurrent or inoperable carcinoma of the breast with VCR/Pred/5-FU/MTX/cyclo (Reg I) vs. VCR/Pred/5-FU (Reg II). Proc Am Assoc Cancer Res 1973; 55:183–87.
83. Ansfield FJ, Ramierz G, Korbitz BC, et al. Five drug therapy for advanced breast cancer—a phase I study. Cancer Chemother Rep 1971; 55:183–87.
84. Spigel SC, Coltman CA, Costanzi JJ. Disseminated breast carcinoma. Arch Intern Med 1973; 132:575–77.
85. David JH, Ramierz G, Ellerby RA, et al. Five-drug therapy in advanced breast cancer. Cancer 1974; 34:239–45.
86. Kaufmann S, Goldstein M. Combination chemotherapy in disseminated carcinoma of the breast. Surg Gynecol Obstet 1973; 137:83–86.
87. Ahman DL, Bisel HF, Hahn RG, et al. An analysis of a multiple-drug program in the treatment of patients with advanced breast cancer utilizing 5-fluorouracil, cyclophosphamide, and prednisone with or without vincristine. Cancer 197; 36:1925–35.
88. Otis PT, Arementrout SA. Combination chemotherapy in metastatic carcinoma of the breast: Results with a three drug combination. Cancer 1975; 36:311–17.
89. Aisner J, Weinberg V, Perloff M, et al. Chemoimmunotherapy for advanced breast cancer: a randomized comparison of six combinations (CMF, CAF, vs. CAFVP) each with or without MER immunotherapy. A CALGB study. Proc Am Soc Clin Oncol 1981; 22:443.
90. Hart RD, Perloff M, Holland JF. One day VATH (vinblastine, adriamycin, thiotepa and halotestin) therapy for advanced breast cancer refractory to chemotherapy. Cancer 1981; 48:1522–27.
91. Bull J, Tormey D, Li SH, Carbone PP, Falkson G, Blom J, Perlin E, Simon R. A randomized comparative trial of Adriamycin versus methotrexate in combination drug therapy. Cancer 1978; 41:1649–57.
92. Gutterman JU, Cardenas JO, Blumenstein GR, et al. Chemoimmunotherapy of advanced breast cancer: prolongation of remission and survival with BCG. Br Med J 1976; II:1222–25.
93. Canellos GP, Pocock SJ, Taylor SG, III, Sears ME, Klaasen DJ, Band PR. Combination chemotherapy for metastatic breast carcinoma. A prospective comparison of multiple drug therapy with L-phenylalanine mustard. Cancer 1976; 38:1882–86.
94. Perloff M, Hart RD, Holland JF. Vinblastine, Adriamycin, thio-tepa and halotestin (VATH): Therapy for advanced breast cancer refractory to prior chemotherapy. Cancer 1978; 42:2534.
95. DeLena M, Brambilla C, Morabito A, Bonadonna G. Adriamycin plus vincristine compared to and combined with cyclophosphamide, methotrexate and 5-fluorouracil for advanced breast cancer. Cancer 1975; 35:1108.
96. Brambilla C, DeLena M, Rossi A, Valasussa P, Bonadonna G. Response and survival in advanced breast cancer after two non-cross resistant combinations. Br Med J 1976; 1:801.
97. DeLena M, Brambilla C, Marabito A, Bonadonna G. Adriamycin plus vincristine compared to and combined with cyclophosphamide, methotrexate and 5-fluorouracil for advanced breast cancer. Cancer 1975; 35:1108.
98. Morgan LR. Adriamycin and mitomycin-C in advanced breast cancer. In: Carter SK, Crooke ST, eds. Mitomycin-C. New York: Academic, 1979.
99. DeLena M, Jirillo A, Villa S, Volonterio A, Villani F, Brambilla C, Bonadonna G. Preliminary results with Adriamycin plus mitomycin combination in metastatic breast cancer. Proc Am Soc Clin Oncol 1981; 22:400.
100. Denafrio JM, East DR, Troner MB, Vosel CL. Phase II study of mitomycin-C and vinblastine in women with advanced breast cancer refractory to standard cytotoxic therapy. Cancer Treat Rep 1978; 62:2113.

101. Konits, PH, Aisner J, Van Echo DA, Lichtenfeld K, Wiernik PH. Mitomycin-C and vinblastine chemotherapy for advanced breast cancer. Cancer 1981; 48:1295.
102. Shipp SK, Westrich MA, Muss HB, et al. Vincristine, doxorubicin and mitomycin-C in patients with metastatic breast cancer failing prior cyclophosphamide (C), methotrexate (M) and fluorouracil (F). Proc Am Soc Clin Oncol 1981; 22:381.
103. Oster MW, Park Y, Grossbard L. Vincristine, Adriamycin and mitomycin therapy for previously treated breast cancer. Proc Am Soc Clin Oncol 1981; 22:428.
104. Marcus FS, Friedman MA, Resser KJ, Cassidy MJ, Carter SK. 5-FU + Oncovin + Adriamycin + mitomycin-C (FOAM): An effective therapy for metastatic breast cancer in patients that have failed prior chemotherapy. Proc Am Soc Clin Oncol 1980; 21:412.
105. Trump DL, Ettinger DS, Abeloff MD. Doxorubicin, vincristine and cisdiaminedichloroplatinum (II) therapy in patients with advanced breast cancer. Med Pediatr Oncol 1981; 9:1.
106. Mattson W, Arwidi A, Von Eyben F, Lindholm CE. Phase II study of combined vincristine, Adriamycin, cyclophosphamide, and methotrexate with citrovorum factor rescue in metastatic breast cancer. Cancer Treat Rep 1977; 61:527.
107. Longacre D, Donavan M, Paladine W, Cunninsham T, Sponzo R. Hexamethylmelamine, vincristine and methotrexate chemotherapy in advanced neoplasms. Cancer Treat Rep 1977; 61:919.
108. Aisner J, Ross DD, Wiernik PH. Tamoxifen in advanced male breast cancer. Arch Intern Med 1979; 139:480–81.
109. Patterson JS, Battersby LA, Bach BK. Use of tamoxifen in advanced male breast cancer. Cancer Treat Rep 1980; 64:801–04.

43

ENDOCRINE MALIGNANT TUMORS

Anne C. Carter, M.D., and Jose R. Marti, M.D.

ENDOCRINE MALIGNANT TUMORS ARE relatively rare. It is estimated that in 1990 there were 13,600 new cases, of which 12,000 were thyroid cancers. Parathyroid, adrenocortical, and pheochromocytoma carcinomas are usually associated with endocrinopathies, whereas most thyroid cancers are not.

Pituitary Carcinomas

Adenohypophysial or pituitary carcinomas are very rare, occurring in < 1% of all pituitary tumors. The pathogenesis is unknown. About 10% of pituitary adenomas are invasive of bone and venous sinuses and should be called *invasive adenomas* rather than malignant pituitary adenomas. There are no adequate criteria indicating that these are malignant tumors.[1]

Pituitary carcinomas may be divided into 2 groups: those with cerebrospinal metastasis via the cerebrospinal fluid (CSF) and those with extracranial metastasis.[1] Cerebrospinal metastases may have implantation at the base of the brain, over the spinal cord, the cauda equina, and (rarely) within the ventricular system. Of reported cases, the average age was 41, with no sex prediliction. Radiographic studies showed sellar expansion with bony erosion and extrasellar extension. Most cases demonstrated no endocrine hyperfunction, although 2 cases with Cushing's syndrome were reported.[2] Spinal fluid cytology may be positive, and radioimmunoassay (RIA) of pituitary hormones may be helpful.

Extracranial metastases have been reported to lymph nodes, bone, liver, kidney, ovary, heart, and lung. There may also be cerebrospinal metastasis.

Seven of 16 patients had Cushing's syndrome and/or hyperpigmentation.[3] No clinical evidence of pituitary hypersecretion was seen in 9 cases. Radiographically, the tumors tend to have no sella enlargement but do have erosion and destruction of the sella floor. Cellular pleomorphism, atypia, and variable mitotic activity were noted in most. Survival ranged from 9 days to 4.8 yr, with a mean survival of 1.4 yr, excluding 1 patient, who is still alive 9 yr from time of original diagnosis.[3] Therapy of these rare tumors has been glucocorticoid suppression of increased ACTH secretion if present. Radiation therapy (XRT) also has been used.

Pituitary metastases from systemic cancer, although rare, must be recognized.[4] Usually, metastases to the pituitary present as diabetes insipidus and less commonly with occulomotor palsies. Symptoms usually occur after age 50. Breast cancer is the most common tumor to metastasize to the pituitary. Radiologic studies of the pituitary sella are not helpful. Transphenoidal removal of the tumor and XRT might be considered in the presence of symptoms from such metastases (headache, visual field impairment) provided there is no diabetes insipidus or other cranial nerve dysfunction.

Adrenal Carcinoma

Adrenocortical Carcinoma

The incidence is approximately 0.5 to 2 cases per million population per year in the United States.[48] Syndromes associated with these tumors are Cushing's syndrome (50%), virilization (20%), combination of Cushing's syndrome and virilization (4%), feminization (12%), and hyperaldosteronism (4%). About two-thirds of adrenocortical carcinomas occur in females.[6] The age range for their occurrence is 6 mo to 72 yr, with an average age of 36.7. In Cushing's syndrome, adrenocortical carcinomas are more frequent in children than in

Table 43-1. Criteria and Staging of Adrenocortical Carcinoma

Criteria	
T1	tumor ≤5 cm, invasion absent
T2	tumor >5 cm, invasion absent
T3	tumor outside adrenal in fat
T4	tumor invading adjacent organs
N0	no positive lymph nodes
N1	positive lymph nodes
M0	no distant metastases
M1	distant metastases

Staging	
Stage I	T1, N0, M0
Stage II	T2, N0, M0
Stage III	T1 or T2,N1,M0, T3,N0,M0
Stage IV	Any T, any NM1, T3,T4,N1

Source: Norton et al (ref 5)

adults—46% and 9%, respectively. They are larger than adrenal adenomas, usually >100 g. There are no absolute pathologic criteria for adrenocortical carcinomas, although they tend to have prominent nuclei with pleomorphism, a high nuclear/cytoplasmic ratio, and enlarged vesicular nuclei, with 1 or more prominent nucloeli.[7] Staging of adrenocortical carcinoma is shown in table 43-1.[5]

The signs and symptoms of adrenocortical carcinoma depend on whether there is an increased secretion of cortisol and corticosterone leading to Cushing's syndrome, increased secretion of aldosterone resulting in Conn's syndrome, or increased secretion of 11-hydroxyandrostenedione producing precocious puberty or virilization. The signs and symptoms of these syndromes have been well described.[8,49] Patients with Cushing's syndrome due to adrenocortical carcinoma usually have more virilization than with Cushing's disease due to adrenocortical hyperplasia.

Adrenal cortical excess can be determined by the following tests: (1) diurnal levels of cortisol, (2) morning level of cortisol after 1 mg dexamethasone at 11 p.m., (3) low-dose dexamethasone (DEX) (0.5 mg every 6 hr for 48 hr) with measurement of urine 17-hydroxycorticosteroids (17-OHCS) and/or cortisol, and (4) urine free cortisol.

The differential diagnosis of Cushing's syndrome includes Cushing's disease of anterior pituitary origin, adrenocortical adenoma, adrenocortical carcinoma, or ectopic ACTH-producing tumors. Tests necessary to differentiate the etiology of Cushing's syndrome are: (1) high-dose DEX (2 mg every 6 hr for 48 hr) with measurement of 17-OHCS and/or urine cortisol, (2) metyrapone test (750 mg every 4 hr for 48 hr with measurement of urine 17-OHCS and plasma 11-deoxycortisol, and (3) plasma ACTH. Urinary 17-ketosteroids and plasma testosterone should also be measured.[8]

Conn's syndrome, rarely caused by adrenocortical carcinoma, is diagnosed if there is hypertension, hypokalemia, high levels of plasma aldosterone in the presence of low or hyporesponsive levels of plasma renin.

The localization of adrenal tumors is done by CT and MRI scanning. Selective arteriography and retrograde venography are usually not needed. Selective venous sampling may be required. Radionuclide scanning with ^{131}I-19-iodocholesterol or ^{131}I-6 β-iodomethyl-19-norcholesterol (NP-59) may be useful to localize tumors.[5]

The treatment of adrenocortical carcinoma is en bloc resection through an abdominal incision that can be extended into the thoracic cavity. The patient must be treated with corticosteroids preoperatively, intraoperatively, and postoperatively.

Metastatic adrenocortical carcinoma with glucocorticoid excess may be treated with antihormonal agents to reduce the production of cortisol excess, namely metyrapone, an inhibitor of 11-β-hydroxylation or aminoglutethimide, which inhibits the enzymatic conversion of cholesterol to 5-pregnenolone. The usual dosage is 1–2 g/day. Aminoglutethimide is associated with toxicity.

Treatment with mitotane (o,p'DDD), an adrenolytic drug, inhibits steroid secretion and produces tumor regression.[5,9,10,50] Levels of cortisol must be measured and glucocorticoids administered. The dosage required is 8–10 g/day. Toxicity, particularly G.I., including anorexia, nausea, vomiting, and diarrhea, as well as neuromuscular disturbances, may be severe. Objective tumor regression ranges from 34 to 61%. Antitumor response is not seen for about 6 wk, and mean duration of response is about 10 mo. The effectiveness of ketoconazole in the treatment of adrenocortical carcinoma has been reported.[11] Cytotoxic chemotherapy has produced poor results to date.[5] Suramin may be beneficial.[51] Radiation therapy (XRT) is not beneficial except for palliation of bone pain.[52] The prognosis for adrenocortical carcinomas is poor.

Malignant Pheochromocytoma

The incidence rate of pheochromocytoma is 0.95 per 100,000 person years in the United States.[53] Ten to 14% of pheochromocytomas are malignant. About 0.1 percent of all hypertensive patients have pheochromocytomas. The incidence of malignant pheochromocytomas is about the same for sporadic and familial pheochromocytomas. Pheochromocytomas are bilateral in 5% of cases and extra-adrenal in 10%. The most common familial syndrome associated with pheochromocytomas is multiple endocrine neoplasia (MEN) (see section on medullary thyroid carcinoma, below). Pheochromocytomas in MEN are usually bilateral.[5,53]

Pathologically, pheochromocytomas show marked variability of cell and nuclear size and cell arrangement. It is not possible to distinguish histologically whether or not a pheochromocytoma is benign or malignant.[5,12] Recently, neuropeptide Y expression was reported to distinguish malignant from benign pheochromocytomas.[54]

The most common symptoms of pheochromocytomas, benign or malignant, are sweating, episodic attacks, palpitations, anxiety, and headache.[5,13,53] The physical findings may include hypertension, orthostatic hypotension, fever, weight loss, abdominal mass, and signs of neuroectodermal disease.

The diagnosis of pheochromocytoma depends on biochemical measurement of urinary catecholamines, total and free, and their metabolites vanillylmandelic acid (VMA), metanephrine, and normetanephrine. VMA levels may be decreased by monoamine oxidase inhibitors and alpha methyl dopa and increased by ingestion of bananas, citrus fruits, vanilla, coffee, nuts, and chocolate. Metanephrine levels are increased by monoamine oxidase inhibitors, alpha methyl dopa, and by vasopressin agents. The clonidine suppression test measuring plasma epinephrine, norepinephrine, and catecholamines is currently the test of choice.[5] Pharmacologic tests, adrenolytic or provocative, are rarely used today. Localization of the tumor is the same as for adrenocortical carcinoma. Vena cava catheterization with determination of plasma catecholamine levels at various locations is sometimes required for localization. Before localization studies, treatment with the alpha blocker phenoxybenzamine should be instituted, and sometimes a beta blocker such as propranolol is required for tachycardia. ^{131}I-metaiodobenzylguanidine (^{131}I-MIBG) scintigraphy appears to be useful for localizing tumors, particularly recurrent and metastatic lesions.[5,14,53]

Definitive treatment for pheochromocytoma is surgical. Patients must be well prepared preoperatively with phenoxybenzamine 10–100 mg b.i.d. Metyrosine, a tyrosine hydroxylase inhibitor, may be administered 250–500 mg q.i.d.

to reduce catecholamine biosynthesis. Intraoperatively, either phentolamine or sodium nitroprusside are used for hypertensive crisis. I.V. propranolol is sometimes indicated for cardiac arrhythmias.[5,53]

Metastatic pheochromocytomas are best treated with metyrosine. The tumors respond poorly to cytotoxic chemotherapy such as cyclophosphamide (CTX), vincristine (VCR), carmustine (BCNU), doxorubicin (ADR), and streptozotocin (STZ). The combined therapy of CTX, VCR, and dacarbazine (DTIC) has given the best results.[5] XRT may be useful to relieve osseous pain.

Prognosis in general is poor, although some patients have long survival. Adrenal malignant pheochromocytoma patients had a mean survival of 6.6 yr (range 2 mo to 16 yr) and 43% 5-yr survival compared to patients with extra-adrenal malignant pheochromocytomas, where mean survival was 1.2 yr and there were no 5-yr survivors.

Parathyroid Carcinoma

Hyperparathyroidism due to parathyroid carcinoma is rare, with a reported incidence of 0.5–4%.[15-17] Parathyroid carcinoma occurs with equal frequency in men and women and at a younger age than primary hyperparathyroidism. The histopathology of parathyroid carcinoma (see chapter 11, figure 11-96) as described by Schantz and Castleman[18] generally presents several elements, including pleomorphic chief cells, acellular trabeculation, and mitotic cells with capsular or vascular invasion. As with other endocrine carcinomas, the histopathology may be indistinguishable from that of benign tumors. DNA aneuploidy determined by flow cytometric analysis has diagnostic and prognostic value in parathyroid carcinoma.[55]

Symptoms of hypercalcemia, namely polyuria and polydipsia, generalized weakness and fatigue, anorexia, nausea, vomiting, weight loss, dyspepsia, vague abdominal pains, and constipation, were present in 98% of patients with parathyroid carcinoma. A palpable mass in the neck was found in 48% of cases of parathyroid carcinoma—a much higher percentage than in patients with primary hyperparathyroidism.[15]

Mean levels of serum calcium are much higher in patients with parathyroid carcinoma—15.5–15.9 mg/dl—compared to primary hyperparathyroidism (10.8–11.7 mg/dl), and mean levels of serum phosphorus are lower.[15,16] Levels of parathormone are 2–3 times normal. Renal involvement, including impaired renal function, renal calculi, and renal calcinosis, is far more common in parathyroid carcinoma (32–60% of cases) than in primary hyperparathyroidism. Incidence of skeletal involvement, including osteitis fibrosa cystica is high (55–73% of cases). Concomitant renal and skeletal involvement, which is rare in primary hyperparathyroidism, is not uncommon in parathyroid carcinoma.[15] Anemia is also common. Recently, elevated levels of plasma hCG have been reported in parathyroid carcinoma.[15] The differential diagnosis is between primary hyperparathyroidism and ectopic production of parathormone.

Neither preoperative localization of parathyroid carcinoma by selective venous sampling for parathormome nor selective arteriography is indicated when exploration of the neck is being performed for the first time. In patients who have had a previous neck dissection, this procedure may be justified. Localization with noninvasive imaging techniques (CT scan or high-resolution ultrasound) should be done first.[19]

Therapy for parathyroid carcinoma depends on meticulous en bloc resection of the parathyroid tumor and all adjacent invaded tissue, avoiding capsular violation or tumor spillage.[17] Radical neck dissection should be performed only when node involvement is clinically obvious. With recurrent disease, palliation can be achieved with repeated resections of local and distant metastases. Metastatic tumors are not responsive to XRT or combination chemotherapy. Control of persistent hypercalcemia is difficult, as most agents must be given parenterally and only act transiently, i.e., calcitonin with or without prednisone, disodium etidronate, mithramycin. Oral phosphates are associated with toxicity. Dichloromethylene diphosphonate (Cl_2 MDP, clodronate) was withdrawn from clinical investigation. Aminohydroxypropylidene diphosphonate (ADP) and gallium nitrate are investigational.[56]

Parathyroid carcinoma is a slowly progressive tumor. Disease-free survival may be as long as 17 yr. Five-year survival is around 55–60%, and 50% of patients who had recurrence survive 5 yr. Metastases occur locally in the neck, and the most common distant metastases are to lung, liver, bone, and pancreas.[15,17]

Thyroid Carcinoma

Thyroid carcinoma is an uncommon malignancy, even though it is the most common endocrine malignancy. It is estimated that in 1990 there were 12,100 new cases of thyroid carcinoma and 1,025 deaths in the United States.[65] This tumor occurs more frequently in women than men (ratio 2.6:1). The overall incidence of thyroid cancer for both sexes has increased from 3.8 to 4.4 per 100,000 between 1973–74 and 1985–86.[57] The prevalence of thyroid cancer at autopsy in patients dying of other diseases has been reported to be as high as 5.7%, and the absolute prevalence of thyroid cancer in nodular goiters is 10–15%.

The most common classification of the different types of thyroid cancers and their estimated frequency is shown in table 43-2.[20,21]

The TNM staging of thyroid cancer depends on size of the tumors (T), the presence or absence of regional lymph nodes (N), and the presence or absence of distant metastases (M). Staging groups take into account the age of the patient and tumor pathology (table 43-3).[22]

Papillary and Follicular Adenocarcinoma

The etiology of differentiated thyroid cancers remains unknown. Animal experiments have shown evidence that benign adenomas as well as malignant nodules can be induced by iodine-deficient diets, feeding of thiouracil or subtotal thyroidectomy. It has been suggested that thyroid carcinoma is mediated through increased pituitary thyroid-stimulating hormone (TSH) secretion.[20] However, there is no evidence that excess TSH induces thyroid

Table 43-2. Classification and Estimated Frequency of Thyroid Cancers

| | Frequency | |
Cancer type	Range (%)	Mean (%)
Carcinoma		
Papillary adenocarcinoma	57–73	60
Pure papillary carcinoma		
Mixed papillary and follicular carcinoma		
Follicular adenocarcinoma	18–25	21
Pure follicular carcinoma		
Clear cell carcinoma	rare	rare
Oxyphil cell (Hürthle) carcinoma	rare	rare
Medullary carcinoma	2–6	4
Undifferentiated (anaplastic) carcinoma	5–17	15
Small-cell carcinoma		
Giant-cell carcinoma		
Epidermoid carcinoma	rare	rare
Other malignant tumors		
Sarcoma		
Lymphoma		
Malignant teratoma		
Metastatic tumors		

Adapted from Bantle and Sommers (refs 20 and 21)

tumors in man, although there is evidence that established thyroid cancers in man regress with TSH suppression produced by administration of thyroid hormone.[20] Low-dose radiation exposure to the head and neck in infancy and childhood for benign conditions such as acne, thymic abnormalities, or hypertrophied tonsils or adenoids increases the risk of differentiated thyroid carcinoma.[23-25] The risk is increased with radiation doses of 180–1,500 cGy, and the younger the subject, the greater the risk. The risk for radiation-induced thyroid carcinoma, higher in women than in men, may appear up to 30 yr after radiation exposure. In one large series of 1,056 subjects irradiated, 27% had palpable thyroid abnormalities and 33% of 60 operated patients had thyroid carcinoma. There is some evidence that adults exposed to high-dose radiation for Hodgkin's disease and non-Hodgkin's lymphomas are at risk for thyroid cancer.[58] There is no significant increased incidence of thyroid carcinoma after the administration of ^{131}I for treatment of hyperthyroidism, although average follow-up was only 8 yr.[27]

Papillary adenocarcinomas are more common than follicular adenocarcinomas. They are usually subclassified as pure papillary carcinomas and the more common mixed papillary and follicular carcinomas. The latter behave like pure papillary carcinomas. They are usually small tumors, 0.5–4.0 cm in diameter, and are slow growing. The larger tumors may contain cystic areas. Microscopically, they contain well-differentiated epithelial areas arranged in fibrovascular stalks (see chapter 11, figure 11-92). Mitoses in nucleoli are seldom seen. About 50% of papillary carcinomas contain laminated calcified spherules (psammoma bodies) that are pathognomonic of papillary thyroid carcinoma. More than one-third are multicentric, presumably due to lymphatic spread; they tend to metastasize to cervical lymph nodes via regional lymphatics.[21,28] At time of

Table 43-3. Thyroid Cancer Stage Grouping

Cancer stage	Papillary or follicular	
	under 45 yr	45 yr and older
I	Any T, Any N, M0	T1, N0, M0
II	Any T, Any N, M1	T2, N0, M0
		T3, N0, M0
III		T4, N0, M0
		Any T, N1, M0
IV		Any T, Any N, M1
	Medullary	
I	T1 N0 M0	
II	T2 N0 M0	
	T3 N0 M0	
	T4 N0 M0	
III	Any T N1 M0	
IV	Any T Any N M1	
	Undifferentiated	
Stage IV*	Any T Any N Any M	

T1 = ≤ 1 cm
T2 = > 1 cm—≤ 4 cm
T3 = > 4 cm, limited to thyroid
T4 = Any size extending beyond thyroid capsule
*all cases are stage IV
Source: ref 22

surgery, 39–46% of patients have lymph node metastases.[29-31] Blood vessel invasion is uncommon, and most do not metastasize through the blood stream. Distant metastases occur in around 10% of patients.[21,28]

Follicular adenocarcinomas tend to be larger than papillary carcinomas.[21,28] Histologically, there may be many well-developed follicles that are indistinguishable from normal thyroid tissue or benign follicular adenomas from normal thyroid tissue, or they may be solid without any follicles (see chapter 11, figure 11-93). Mitoses and pleomorphism are uncommon. It may be difficult to distinguish between follicular adenoma and follicular carcinoma unless capsular or blood vessel invasion has occurred. Hematogenous dissemination is common, with metastasis to lung and bone.[21] Lymph node metastases are less frequent than with papillary thyroid carcinoma. A variant of follicular carcinoma is Hürthle cell carcinoma, which is characterized by oxyphilic follicular cells. These tumors behave like follicular carcinomas but are more aggressive.

Papillary and follicular thyroid adenocarinomas usually present as a "lump in the neck" representing a solitary thyroid nodule noted either by the patient or the physician. Papillary carcinomas typically occur between the ages of 20–60, although they also are seen in children.[29,30] These tumors are 2 times more frequent in women as in men, and (rarely) may present with an enlarged cervical or lymph node away from the midline and usually in the anterior cervical triangle. Hoarseness, dysphagia, or difficulty in breathing are less common presenting symptoms. Follicular carcinomas occur most commonly between the ages of 30–70, are uncommon in children, and are 3 times more frequent in women than in men.[29,32] Rarely, follicular carcinoma may present with metastatic disease in the lung and (very rarely) with symptoms of hyperthyroidism.

The presence of a thyroid nodule, a common finding, does not necessarily mean the existence of a thyroid cancer. Only 1 out of 4 "cold" (hypoactive) nodules removed surgically are malignant.[33] Therefore, the differential diagnosis between a benign nodule and a malignant thyroid neoplasm is a frequent challenge. High-risk patients for thyroid cancer are those with:

- A true single solitary cold thyroid nodule
- History of previous low-dose radiation to the neck
- Presence of a thyroid mass with associated cervical adenopathy
- Hoarseness
- Family history of thyroid cancer
- A cold nodule in males
- A cold nodule in very young or in older patients.

Baseline thyroid function tests should be obtained. Thyroid imaging is helpful in distinguishing cold thyroid nodules from "hot" (hyperfunctioning) nodules. The incidence of thyroid cancer in a cold nodule is estimated to be 12–16%.[33] Thyroid imaging with sodium pertechnetate has the advantage of lower radiation absorption than radioactive iodine, either ^{131}I or ^{123}I. However, some papillary carcinomas will concentrate ^{99m}Tc but not ^{131}I or ^{123}I.[34] The value of discerning multinodular goiters from true solitary nodules by this modality is questionable. Only 30–70% of solitary nodules clinically prove to be so at the time of surgery.

Fine-needle aspiration of clinically solitary cold thyroid nodules has proved to be a very valuable procedure that is safe and can be performed in the office. Adequate material for cytology can be obtained in >90% of aspirations. There is a high degree of specificity, false positives are rare, and false negatives occur in 5–10% of aspirations.[5,35,36] It may be difficult to distinguish follicular adenoma and follicular carcinoma by fine-needle aspiration. Core-needle biopsy is more difficult, has a higher morbidity, and is no more accurate than fine-needle biopsy. Thyroid imaging need not precede needle aspiration, which can be done on the initial visit.[37]

Ultrasonography of the thyroid can determine whether or not a nodule is solid or cystic. Cysts <4 cm in diameter are usually benign.[33] Thyroid carcinomas usually are solid but may be mixed solid and cystic lesions. Benign thyroid nodules may also be solid or mixed solid cystic lesions. Some believe that combined ultrasound and needle aspiration is the best diagnostic combination.[38]

The treatment of differentiated thyroid cancer is controversial. The greatest differences of opinion center on the extent of the primary thyroid surgery and the role of ablative radioactive iodine treatment. No prospective studies have been done, but there are many retrospective studies.[5,30-32,39,40,59] Authors who advocate a total thyroidectomy contend that most thyroid tumors are multicentric and that a total thyroidectomy adheres to traditional surgical principles. Most authors advocating a subtotal thyroidectomy respond that thyroid cancer can be controlled locally for long periods and that the morbidity associated with injury to the parathyroids or to the recurrent laryngeal nerves increases with the magnitude of the operation. Based on retrospective studies in the literature, most clinicians today would agree that for tumors situated near the isthmus and larger than 1.5 cm, a near-total thyroidectomy should be performed, preserving the posterior capsule of the thyroid in order to preserve parathyroid function. The procedure should be followed by postoperative radioactive iodine and suppressive thyroid hormone therapy. Smaller tumors and those away from the isthmus may be treated with hemithyroidectomy and postoperative thyroid hormone suppression. In patients with cervical node involvement, local excision of cervical lymph node metastases or, preferably, an ipsilateral modified neck dissection preserving the vital neck structures should be performed rather than radical neck dissection.

Postoperatively, it is recommended that the patients be treated with triiodothyronine 25 μg t.i.d. for 4 wk.[20] At that time, it should be discontinued, and 2 wk later TSH levels should be obtained and a total body scan with ^{131}I performed. Any remaining thyroid tissue is then ablated with 75 mCi [131]I. Three days after the ablative procedure, 100–150 μg L-thyroxine should be taken daily. The adequacy of thyroxine in achieving suppression can be monitored with a thyrotropin-releasing hormone (TRH) test or by measurement of serum TSH with a highly sensitive assay. If TSH is not suppressed, the thyroxine dose should be increased by 25 μg increments. About 6 mo after ^{131}I ablation, a ^{131}I scan to determine whether or not there is any remaining functioning thyroid tissue should be obtained; this is done only after thyroxine is discontinued and triiodothyronine 25 μg t.i.d. has been taken for 3 wk, because the half-life of thyroxine is much longer than that of triiodothyronine. Two weeks later, a serum TSH and ^{131}I scan should be carried out. If there is functioning thyroid tissue, the patient should be treated with 150 mCi ^{131}I, and 3 days later the thyroxine should be resumed. Serial measurements of serum thyroglobulin may be helpful for follow-up to determine whether or not thyroid tissue is present.[41,60]

The prognosis for papillary thyroid carcinoma is good. Recurrence rate is higher if thyroid carcinoma was diagnosed before age 30; however, the mortality rate is higher in patients over 40.[39] Overall mortality at 30 yr is 29%. Tumor size is an important prognosticator. No mortality was observed 3–32 yr after surgery in tumors 1.5 cm in diameter.[20,29] The presence of lymph nodes does not have an adverse effect on mortality;[30,40] indeed, mortality is lower in patients with lymph node metastases.[39] Survival with follicular carcinoma is somewhat inferior to that of papillary carcinoma. The mortality at 20 yr is 39%.[32] Prognosis is poor in patients whose diagnosis is made after age 40; however, tumor size does not influence prognosis. Follicular carcinoma with marked invasion of capsule and blood vessels has a high mortality (>50%).[29] Multifactorial analytic methods applied to thyroid cancer have permitted the development of prognostic scoring systems applicable to specific histologic cell types.[61]

Anaplastic Thyroid Carcinoma

No specific risk factors for anaplastic thyroid carcinoma (ATC) have been identified. These tumors usually occur in patients over 60. Pathologically, there are no papillary or follicular elements and no amyloid is present. ATC is classified as small-cell and large-cell types (see chapter 11, figure 11-95). In the former, mitoses are frequent and the stroma often fibrous. In the large-cell type, also known as *giant cell* or *spindle cell* carcinoma, the cells are large with pleomorphism, perhaps resembling fibrosarcoma. Frequent atypical mitoses are seen with giant cells.[28] Diagnostic procedures are similar to those described for differentiated thyroid carcinoma.

Therapy of ATC is frequently disappointing. In the rare instances in which a tumor is resectable, surgery should be very aggressive. The minimal procedure should be radical total thyroidectomy even if the parathyroids and recurrent laryngeal nerves are sacrificed.[42,62] If the tumor is not resectable, a case can be made for salvage procedures such as thyroidectomy with en bloc laryngectomy and radical neck dissection. With the small-cell type, external XRT should be given, as the tumor may be a lymphoma. With all inoperable cases, external XRT should be administered. Cytotoxic chemotherapy (see Appendix) has been disappointing. In a randomized trial of ADR alone or in combination with cisplatin (DDP), the latter produced 33% complete and partial remissions (CRs and PRs) compared to 5% with ADR. No statistical difference in survival was seen.[43] Combinations of ADR with DDP or with bleomycin (BLM), VCR, and melphalen or with VCR and BLM produced 9–64% response rates.[5]

The prognosis for ATC is poor, and the tumors progress rapidly, with local invasion and metastases. Due to lack of local control, the patient frequently expires with upper airway obstruction. Death frequently occurs in <6 mo. Five-year survival has been reported between 0 and 24%,[5] but it has been questioned whether those with long survival actually had true anaplastic tumors.

Medullary Thyroid Carcinoma

Medullary thyroid carcinoma (MTC) accounts for about 7% of all thyroid cancers. Of the 4 types of MTC, 3 are familial:[44]
- Nonfamilial—sporadic
- Familial
  —As a manifestation of the multiple endocrine neoplasia (MEN) type IIa: MTC plus pheochromocytomas and/or hyperparathyroidism
  —As a manifestation of the multiple endocrine neoplasia (MEN) type IIb: MTC plus pheochromocytomas, ganglioneuromatosis, multiple mucosal neuromas, and characteristic marfanoid phenotype
  —Medullary thyroid carcinoma non-MEN without extrathyroidal manifestations of MEN.

The familial types are inherited by autosomal dominant transmission. Some MEN IIb may present as a genetic mutation.[45]

Macroscopically, MTC is usually well demarcated from surrounding tissue, commonly occupying the superior portion of the thyroid lobe. The familial types are frequently bilateral, firm, gray, yellow, or tan. Microscopically, they are composed of epithelial cells, C cells, fibrous tissue, amyloid and varying amounts of calcium deposition (see chapter 11, figures 11-94A&B). Cells may be variable in size. C cell hyperplasia is thought to be a precursor of MTC, ranging from isolated hypertrophied cells to large unencapsulated aggregates or large accumulations of cells with a partial fibrous capsule.[46] Extrathyroidal extension has been reported in $\leq 64\%$ of cases (especially in sporadic cases and in patients with MEN IIb). The tumors could be aggressive.

The average age for patients with MEN IIa is 34; for MEN IIb, 19; and for the sporadic type, 50. Clinically, patients present with a thyroid nodule, cervical lymphadenopathy, or goiter.[63] MTC may be suspected because of the presence of MEN IIb syndrome, with marfanoid characteristics; ganglioneuromas, which may involve the tarsal plates of the eyes; nodules studding the tip and anterior third of the tongue; and nodules within the lip. The gangliomas may produce G.I. or neuromuscular symptoms. Skeletal abnormalities include abnormalities of the feet, chronic hip disorders, and kyphoscoliosis or lordosis.[45]

The definitive diagnosis of MTC is made by measuring calcitonin (iCT), the biological marker for this tumor. Levels of iCT may be elevated at the time of presentation and tend to be higher in patients with sporadic disease. Patients with familial MTC may have iCT in the normal range, and provocative tests must be used. Screening of family members of patients with a history of MTC must also be done with provocative tests.[64] The 2 stimulatory tests used are a calcium infusion test or I.V. injection of pentagastrin performed simultaneously or sequentially with measurement of iCT.[44] Stimulation with combined calcium and pentagastrin gives a higher level of iCT than either alone. Levels of iCT may be elevated with other malignancies, chronic renal failure, some G.I. disorders, and in children—although levels are not as high as in MTC. Patients with MTC must be screened for pheochromocytoma and hyperparathyroidism by methods discussed above.

MTC should be treated aggressively with total thyroidectomy, as bilateral disease is found in MEN IIa and IIb.[44] In the sporadic cases, there is frequently disease in the contralateral lobe. A modified "prophylactic" neck dissection of the central compartment of the neck from the hyoid bone to the thoracic inlet and anterior mediastinum should be performed. The internal jugular veins, spinal accessory nerves, and sternocleidomastoid muscles are usually preserved. Lymph nodes in the lateral compartments should be sampled and, if positive, removed. After surgery, the patient should receive thyroid replacement therapy while the iCT levels are monitored. Stimulatory tests should be performed periodically. If iCT is elevated, metastases should be sought. These occur primarily in the lymph nodes of neck and mediastinum, lung, liver, and bone. Cytotoxic chemotherapy and XRT in general have been ineffective.

Prognosis is related to preoperative iCT levels, with patients who show the higher levels having a poorer prognosis.[44] Patients with sporadic neoplasms had a less favorable survival rate than the familial MTC patients,[47] but if matched for tumor size and age the prognosis is the same.[63,64] Patients over 50 have a poorer survival rate than those under 50.

References

1. Scheithauer BW. Surgical pathology of the pituitary: the adenomas. Part II. In: Sommers SC, Rosen PO, eds. Pathology annual 1984. P2, 19. Norwalk: Appleton-Century-Crofts, 1984; 269–329.

2. Doniach I. Histopathology of the pituitary. In: Besser GM, Rees LH, eds. Clinics Endocrinol Metabol 1985; 14:765–89.

3. Kaiser FE, Orth DN, Mukai K, Oppenheimer JH. A pituitary parasellar tumor with extracranial metastases and high, partially suppressible levels of adrenocorticotropin and related peptides. J Clin Endocrinol Metab 1983; 57:649–53.

4. Max MB, Deck DF, Rottenberg DA. Pituitary metastasis: incidence in cancer patients and clinical differentiation from pituitary adenoma. Neurology 1981; 31:998–1002.

5. Norton JA, Doppman JL, Jensen T. Cancer of the endocrine system. In: DeVita VT Jr, Hellman S, Rosenberg SA, eds. Cancer principles and practice of oncology, 3rd ed. Philadelphia: Lippincott, 1989; 1269–1344.

6. Hutter AM, Kayhoe DE. Adrenal cortical carcinoma: clinical features in 138 patients. Am J Med 1966; 41:572–80.

7. Neville AM, O'Hare MJ. Histopathology of the human adrenal cortex. Clinics Endocrinol Metabol 1985; 14:791–820.

8. Bondy, PK. Disorders of the adrenal cortex. In: Wilson JD, Foster DW, eds. Williams' textbook of endocrinology. 7th ed. Philadelphia: Saunders, 1985; 816–90.

9. Hutter AM, Kayhoe DE. Adrenalcortical carcinoma: results of treatment with o,p'DDD in 138 patients. Am J Med 1966; 41:581–92.

10. Lubitz JA, Freeman L, Okun R. Mitotane use in inoperable adrenal cortical carcinoma. JAMA 1973; 223:1109–12.

11. Contreras P, Rojas A, Biagini L, Gonzales P, Massardo T. Regression of metastatic adrenal carcinoma during palliative ketoconazole treatment (letr to ed). Lancet 1985; 1:151–52.

12. Manger WM, Gifford RW Jr. Pheochromocytoma. New York: Springer-Verlag, 1977.

13. Landsberg L, Young JB. Catecholamines and the adrenal medulla. In: Wilson JD, Foster DW, eds. Williams' textbook of endocrinology. 7th ed. Philadelphia: Saunders, 1985; 891–965.

14. Swenson SJ, Brown ML, Sheps SG, et al. Use of ^{131}I-MIBG scintigraphy in the evaluation of suspected pheochromocytoma. Mayo Clinic Proc 1985; 60:299–304.

15. Shane E, Bilezikian JP. Parathyroid carcinoma: a review of 62 patients. Endocr Rev 1982; 3:218–26.

16. Holmes EC, Morton DL, Ketcham AS. Parathyroid carcinoma: collective review. Ann Surg 1969; 169:631–40.

17. Wang C, Gaz RD. Natural history of parathyroid carcinoma. Diagnosis, treatment and results. Am J Surg 1985; 149:522–27.

18. Schantz A, Castleman B. Parathyroid carcinoma. A study of 70 cases. Cancer 1973; 31:600–05.

19. Rossi RL, ReMine SG, Clerkin EP. Hyperparathyroidism. Surg Clin N Am 1985; 65:2,187–209.

20. Bantle JP, Oppenheimer JH. Differentiated thyroid carcinoma. In: Hollander VP, ed. Hormonally responsive tumors. Orlando: Academic Press, 1985; 529–40.

21. Sommers SC. Thyroid gland. In: Anderson WAD, Kissane JM, eds. Pathology. 7th ed. vol. 2. St. Louis: Mosby, 1977; 1641–45.

22. American Joint Committee on Cancer. Manual for staging of cancer. 3rd ed. Beahrs OH, Henson DE, Hutter RVP, Myers MH, eds. Philadelphia: Lippincott, 1988; 57–59.

23. Duffy, BJ, Fitzgerald PJ. Carcinoma of the thyroid in children. Cancer 1950; 3:1018–32.

24. DeGroot LJ, Paloyan E. Thyroid carcinoma and radiation. A Chicago endemic. JAMA 1973; 225:487–91.

25. Refetoff S, Harrison J, Karanfilski BT, Kaplan EL, DeGroot LJ, Bekerman C. Continuing occurrence of thyroid carcinoma after irradiation to the neck in infancy and childhood. N Engl J Med 1975; 292:171–75.

26. Carr RF, LiVolsi VA. Morphologic changes in the thyroid after irradiation for Hodgkin's and non-Hodgkin's lymphoma. Cancer 1989; 64:825–29.

27. Dobyns BM, Sheline GE, Workman JB, Tompkins EA, McConahey WM, Becker DB. Malignant and benign neoplasms of the thyroid in patients treated for hyperthyroidism: a report of the thyrotoxicosis therapy follow-up study. J Clin Endocrinol 1974; 38:976–98.

28. Oertel JE, LiVolsi VA. Pathology of thyroid diseases. In: Ingbar SI, Braverman LE, eds. Werner's the thyroid: a fundamental and clinical text. 5th ed. Philadelphia: Lippincott, 1986; 651–86.

29. Woolner LB, Beahrs OH, Black BM, McConahey WM, Keating FR. Classification and prognosis of thyroid carcinoma. A study of 885 cases observed in a 30-year period. Am J Surg 1961; 102:354-87.
30. Mazzaferri EL, Young RL, Oertel JE, Kemmerer WT, Page CP. Papillary thyroid carcinoma: the impact of therapy in 576 patients. Medicine 1977; 56:171-96.
31. Mazzaferri EL, Young RL. Papillary thyroid carcinoma: A 10 year followup report of the impact of therapy in 576 patients. Am J Med 1981; 70:511-18.
32. Young RL, Mazzaferri EL, Rahe AJ, Dorfman SG. Pure follicular thyroid carcinoma: impact of therapy in 214 patients. J Nucl Med 1980; 21:733-39.
33. Van Herle AJ, Rich P, Ljung BME, Ashcraft MW, Solomon DH, Keeler EB. The thyroid nodule. Ann Intern Med 1982; 96:221-32.
34. Shambaugh GE, Quinn JL, Oyasu R, Freinkel N. Disparate thyroid imaging. Combined studies with sodium pertechnetate Tc 99m and radioactive iodine. JAMA 1974; 228:866-69.
35. Gershengorn MC, McClung MR, Chu EW, Hanson TAS, Weintraub BD, Robbins J. Fine-needle aspiration cytology in the preoperative diagnosis of thyroid nodules. Ann Intern Med 1977; 87:265-69.
36. Wang CA, Vickery AL Jr, Maloof F. Needle biopsy of the thyroid. Surg Gynecol Obstet 1976; 143:365-68.
37. Silverman JF, West RL, Larkin EW, et al. The role of fine-needle aspiration biopsy in the rapid diagnosis and management of thyroid neoplasm. Cancer 1986; 57:1164-70.
38. Walfish PG, Hazani E, Strawbridge HTG, Miskin M, Rosen IB. Combined ultrasound and needle aspiration cytology in the assessment and management of hypofunctioning thyroid nodule. Ann Intern Med 1977; 87:270-74.
39. Cady B, Sedgwick CE, Meissner WA, Bookwalter JR, Romagosa V, Werber J. Changing clinical, pathologic, therapeutic, and survival patterns in differential thyroid carcinoma. Ann Surg 1976; 184:541-52.
40. Samaan NA, Maheshwari YK, Nader S, et al. Impact of therapy for differentiated carcinoma of the thyroid: an analysis of 706 cases. J Clin Endocrinol Metab 1983; 56:1131-38.
41. Pacini F, Lari R, Mazzeo S, Grasso L, Taddel D, Pinchera A. Diagnostic value of a single serum thyroglobulin determination on and off thyroid suppressive therapy in the follow-up of patients with differentiated thyroid cancer. Clin Endocrinol 1985; 23:405-11.
42. Nel CJC, VanHeeden JA, Goellner JR, et al. Anaplastic carcinoma of the thyroid: a clinicopathologic study of 82 cases. Mayo Clin Proc 1985; 60:51-58.
43. Shimanoka K, Schoenfeld DA, DeWys WD, Creech RH, DeConti R. A randomized trial of doxorubicin versus doxorubicin plus cisplatin in patients with advanced thyroid carcinoma. Cancer 1985; 56:2155-60.
44. Wells SA, Dilley WG, Fardon JA, Leight GS, Baylin SB. Early diagnosis and treatment of medullary thyroid carcinoma. Arch Intern Med 1985; 145:1248-52.
45. Carney JA, Sizemore GW, Hayles AB. Multiple endocrine neoplasia, type 2b. In: Iochim HL, ed. Pathobiology ann. vol. 8. New York: Raven Press, 1978; 105-53.
46. Sizemore GW. Medullary carcinoma of the thyroid gland. In: Oppenheimer JH, ed. Thyroid today. Deerfield, Ill.: Travenol Laboratories 1982; 5 (no. 3) 1-6.
47. Kakudo K, Carney JA, Sizemore GW. Medullary carcinoma of thyroid: biological behavior of the sporadic and familial neoplasm. Cancer 1985; 55:2818-21.
48. Lutton JP, Cerdas S, Billaud L, et al. Clinical features of adrenocortical carcinoma, prognostic factors and the effect of mitotane therapy. New Engl J Med 1990; 322:1195-1201.
49. Ribeiro RC, Neto RS, Schell MJ, Lacerda L, Sambaio GA, Cat I. Adrenocortical carcinoma in children: A study of 40 cases. J Clin Oncol 1990; 8:67-74.
50. Venkatesh S, Hickey RC, Sellin RV, Fernandez JF, Samaan NA. Adrenal cortical carcinoma. Cancer 1989; 64:765-769.
51. LaRocca RV, Stein CA, Danesi R, Jamis-Dow CA, Weiss GH, Myers CE. Suramin in adrenal cancer: Modulation of steroid hormone production, cytotoxicity in vitro, and clinical antitumor effect. J Clin Endocrinol Metab 1990; 7:497-504.
52. Soffen EM, Solin LJ, Rubenstein JH, Hanks GE. Palliative radiotherapy for symptomatic adrenal metastases. Cancer 1990; 65:1318-20.

53. Samaan NA, Hickey RC, Shutts PE. Diagnosis, localization, and management of pheochromocytoma. Pitfalls and follow-up in 41 patients. Cancer 1988; 62:2451–60.
54. Hellman LJ, Cohen PS, Averbach SD, Cooper MJ, Keiser HR, Israel MA. Neuropeptide Y expression distinguishes malignant from benign pheochromocytoma. J Clin Oncol 1989; 7:1720–25.
55. Obara T, Fujimoto Y, Hirayama A, Kanaji Y, Ito Y, Kodama T, Ogata T. Flow cytometric DNA analysis of parathyroid tumors with special reference to its diagnostic and prognostic value in parathyroid carcinoma. Cancer 1990; 65:1789–93.
56. Warrell RP Jr, Bockman, RS. Metabolic emergencies. In: VT DeVita Jr, S Hellman, SA Rosenburg, eds. Cancer principles and practice of oncology, 3rd ed. pp. 1986–2003, Philadelphia: J.B. Lippincott Co. 1989.
57. Cancer Statistics Review 1973–86. Including a report on the status of cancer control May 1989. U.S. Department of Health and Human Services NIH Publication No. 89–2789. Table III–1, 1989.
58. DeGroot LJ, Kaplan EL, McCormick M, Straus FH. Natural history, treatment, and course of papillary thyroid carcinoma. J Clin Endocrinol Metab 1990; 71:414–424.
59. Aiello DP, Manni A. Thyroglobulin measurement vs iodine[131] total-body scan for follow-up of well-differentiated thyroid cancer. Arch Intern Med 1990; 150:437–39.
60. Hay ID. Prognostic factors in thyroid carcinoma. In JH Oppenheimer, ed. Thyroid Today 12 (No 1, Jan./Feb.) pp. 1–9. Lincolnshire, IL. Boots-Flint, Inc. 1989.
61. Venkatesh YSS, Ordonez NG, Schultz PN, Hickey RC, Goepfert H, Samaan NA. Anaplastic carcinoma of the thyroid: A clinicopathologic study of 121 cases. Cancer 1990; 66:321–30.
62. Bergholm U, Adami H-O, Bergström R, Johansson H, Lundell G, Telenius-Berg M, Akerström G. Clinical characteristics in sporadic and familial medullary thyroid carcinoma: A nationwide study of 249 patients in Sweden from 1959 through 1981. Cancer 1989; 63:1196–1204.
63. Gagel RF, Tashjian AH Jr, Cummings T. Papathanasopoulos N, Kaplan MM, DeLellis RA, Wolfe HJ, Reichlin S. The clinical outcome of prospective screening for multiple endocrine neoplasia type 2a. N Engl J Med 1988; 318:478–84.
64. Samaan NA, Schultz PN, Hickey RC. Medullary thyroid carcinoma: prognosis of familial versus nonfamilial disease and the role of radiotherapy. J Hormone and Metab Res 1989; 21:21–25.
65. Silverberg E, Boring CC, Squires TS. Cancer statistics, 1990. CA 1990; 40:9–26.

44

OSTEOSARCOMAS

Engracio P. Cortes, M.D.

OSTEOSARCOMA IS DEFINED AS a spindle cell tumor that produces malignant osteoid.[1] It can have osteoblastic, chondroblastic, or fibroblastic components. This differentiation does not affect the prognosis of the disease.

Incidence

Osteosarcoma is the most common of all primary malignant bone tumors. Dahlin reported 28% of such tumors in his 6,221 cases.[2] In the United States, about 900 new cases occur each year.[3] Its peak incidence occurs in the 10- 25-yr age group, decreasing gradually with advancing age. Males are affected 1½–2 times more often than females. When it occurs in patients over 40, it is usually associated with a preexisting disease, (e.g., Paget's disease), irradiated bones, multiple hereditary exostoses, or polyostotic fibrous dysplasia.[1,2] The primary tumor usually is located at anatomical sites associated with maximum growth rate—the distal femur, the proximal tibia, and the proximal humerus.[4] Primary osteosarcoma of the axial skeleton, including the skull, jaw, vertebra, orbit, and pelvis, account for < 10% of tumors,[3] except for patients over 30, where the preponderance of axial skeleton location has been reported by Jenkins.[5]

Histopathology and Etiology

The pathological variants of osteosarcoma are many (see chapter 11, figure 11-75), including less aggressive parosteal, periosteal, and low-grade intraosseous osteosarcomas that are histologically and radiologically distinct lesions from the classical central, medullary osteosarcomas that are the primary focus of this review. The cause of osteosarcoma is unknown. Occurring throughout the animal kingdom, the tumor can be induced experimentally by chemicals, radiation, and DNA and RNA viruses. Osteosarcoma is transmissible by an RNA virus in newborn rats, mice, hamsters, and chickens.[6] Some relation to increased osteoblastic activity is indicated by the correlation between the period of maximum growth and the age of most patients and the location of most tumors. Johnson suggested that the tumors were quantitatively related to the amount of cell activity in the bone and that the risk of osteosarcoma is increased in diseases with excessive cellularity (e.g., benign fibrous lesions, Paget's disease, organizing bone infarcts, osteomyelitic scars, and unresolved callus).[7]

The only exogenous agent known to induce osteosarcoma is ionizing radiation. In a series of 600 osteosarcomas seen at the Mayo Clinic from 1909–64, 23 (3.8%) arose in previously irradiated bone.[1] Radiation-induced osteosarcoma may occur 3-4 yr after therapeutic or industrial exposure. Thorotrast, formerly used in radioactive scanning as a bone-seeking material, has been associated with osteosarcoma.[8] Osteosarcomas also complicate radiation osteitis in persons with residual body burdens of bone-seeking radionuclides such as "radium" watch dial painters (from tipping their brushes with the lips) and radium chemists.[9]

Goorin et noted the role of genetic factors in osteosarcoma.[10] Sixteen sets of siblings with the disease have been identified. Among patients with hereditary retinoblastoma, the incidence is increased to 500 times above the incidence in other groups. Deletion on the long arm of chromosome 13, which can occur in patients with retinoblastoma, has been found in some osteosarcoma tumors.

Clinical Manifestations

Pain, tenderness, and swelling are the usual presenting complaints. They have existed for about 3 mo when the average patient is first seen.[11] A blow or some other minor injury is usually related by the patient as an inciting or even causative factor. It is, however, much more likely that the injury drew the patient's attention to an already existing neoplasm. Ewing referred to this occurrence as "traumatic determinism." Trauma reveals more malignant growths than it produces.[12] Incidence of pathological fracture is <1%;[13] systemic symptoms are rare. Serum alkaline phosphatase is an important biologic marker of tumor activity in osteosarcoma patients.[14-16] In a review of 155 patients by Francis of his 2-yr survivors, 85% had normal alkaline phosphatase compared to only 12% of those who died of the disease.[17] Scranton and co-workers had similar findings.[18] Plasma carcinoembryonic antigen (CEA) was found to be elevated in 17/21 osteosarcoma patients with gross disease and normal in all 9 patients with no gross cancer after amputation of the involved extremity.[19] A rising CEA level coincided with clinical progression of disease in all 9 cases.

Diagnostic Procedures

Most osteosarcoma patients can be diagnosed with a reasonable degree of confidence from the appearance of the lesion on plain x-ray.[20,21] Typical findings are increased intramedullary radiodensity (due to tumor bone or calcified cartilage), an area of radiolucency (due to nonossified tumor), a pattern of permeative destruction with poorly defined borders, cortical destruction, periosteal elevation, and extraosseous extension with soft-tissue ossification.

In a correlative histologic and roentgenographic study of 245 patients with osteosarcoma of the extremities, Von Ronnen reported some distinct radiographic patterns.[23] Most frequent was the mixed pattern of radiologic bone formation and bone destruction with a poorly defined, irregular border and periosteal spicule or Codman's triangle (135 patients). The purely cystic, lytic, and periosteal variants were relatively uncommon. The predominant osteosclerotic type was slightly more common and present in a fairly large number of cases. No distinctive characteristics could be observed. Codman's triangle is a manifestation of extreme periosteal elevation forming an acute angle with the cortex. The periosteal new bone formation is a reactive response to the lifting of the periosteum; it is not specific for osteogenic sarcoma, since it can also be seen in Ewing's sarcoma. At Memorial Sloan-Kettering Cancer Center, New York, Wilner classified 600 radiographs of osteosarcoma into 3 broad categories: sclerotic (32%), osteolytic (22%), and mixed (46%).[24] No statistical difference in overall survival rates among these 3 types was noted.

Radioactive bone scans often reveal a greater degree of bone involvement than was suspected from review of regular films. The activity reflects both the gross (intraosseous) extent of the tumor as well as the reactive bone around it. Bone scan cannot detect microscopic, radiologically occult, intramedullary extensive of "skip" metastases with any degree of reliability.[24] The scan additionally acts as a screening technique for other osseous lesions unless they are easily seen on plain x-ray.[24]

Arteriographic evaluation of the primary osteosarcoma defines the extraosseous component of the tumor and identifies the venous drainage.[25] The highly vascular portion of an osteosarcoma is often seen to extend further than would be expected from plain x-ray. The most reliable sign of malignancy is the irregular, pathologic vessels of the tumor, which are filled with contrast medium at an early arterial phase; or an early venous filling, suggestive of arteriovenous shunting.[26] These findings are not specific for osteosarcoma, although occasionally the findings can distinguish benign from malignant tumors. Adequate angiography is quite accurate in delineating the extent of the soft-tissue component of a primary lesion and is very useful in planning both biopsy and definitive surgery.[27] Conversely, the arteriogram confirms the suggestion on plain x-ray that a lesion is completely intraosseous and offers the surgeon additional confidence that the tumor can be considered for radical resection with an adequate margin.[25,28]

Staging and Treatment

The surgical staging system for osteosarcomas adopted by the Musculoskeletal Tumor Society is based on the fact that mesenchymal sarcomas of bones behave alike, irrespective of histogenic type. The system is based on the GTM* classification (table 44-1) that defines for each tumor (1) its grade (G) as low (G1) or high (G2) in function of histology and other clinical data; (2) its location (T) as T1 (intracompartmental), defined as an anatomic structure or space bounded by natural barriers of tumor extension, or T2 (extracompartmental); and (3) its dissemination or lack of dissemination to lymph nodes or other organs and tissues (defined as metastases–M).

Table 44-1. GTM* Surgical Staging of Bone Sarcomas

Stage	Grade	Site
Ia	Low (G)	Intracompartmental (T1)
Ib	Low (G1)	Extracompartmental (T2)
IIa	High (G2)	Intracompartmental (T1)
IIb	High (G2)	Extracompartmental (T2)
III	Any G	Any T
	Regional or distant metastases (M)	

*G = histologic grade; T = anatomical site; M = lymph nodes and metastases

This staging classification has proven to have prognostic significance concerning patients' 5-yr survival.[29] In a study by Enneking et al, it was found to be 100% for stage Ia, 95% for Ib, 62% for IIa, 40% for IIb; no patient with stage III disease was alive at 5 yr.[29]

The selection and sequence of therapeutic modalities in the management of osteosarcomas is related to the presence or absence of metastases and the location of the primary lesion.

Therapy of localized disease

Surgery is the main modality of treatment for osteosarcomas localized to extremities. The traditional procedure has been amputation of the limb one joint above the tumor-containing bone or (occasionally) transmedullary amputation.

Within the past decade, parallel development of sophisticated imaging techniques permitting accurate anatomical determination of tumor location, of total joint replacement technique, and of effective chemotherapeutic regimens have made possible a nonamputative procedure represented by the resection en bloc of the tumor and surrounding tissues and their replacement by custom-made implants in selected cases.[28] Limb-sparing procedures are possible for osteosarcomas located in the proximal humerus proximal and distal femurus and only occasionally for the proximal tibia and fibula.

---

*G = histologic grade; T = anatomical site; M = lymph nodes and metastases

Many factors must be considered in the decision to perform limb-sparing surgery rather than amputation for an osteosarcoma. They include the risk of local recurrence (generally it is similar for the 2 procedures), the function of the limb, the procedure morbidity, and the duration of rehabilitation after surgery.[30] In 7 analyzed series, the local recurrence rate after a limb-sparing procedure was 3.4–16%.

Chemotherapy has been used in the treatment of primary osteosarcomas as adjuvant treatment in the pre- and postoperative procedure. Many single chemotherapeutic agents were tested, but only a few were found as effective as single agents in inducing partial or complete remissions (PRs and CRs) in advanced measurable disease. They included doxorubicin (ADR), methotrexate (MTX) in high doses with leucovorin (LCV) rescue, cisplatin (DDP), and to a lesser degree, bleomycin (BLM), cyclophosphamide (CTX), and actinomycin D (ACT). A steep response curve was found only for ADR and high-dose MTX.[31,32] These 2 drugs were introduced in the postsurgical treatment of resected osteosarcomas.[31,32] The disease-free survival rates in a multitude of studies carried out with the 2 drugs as adjuvant chemotherapy were 40–60%, an improvement by at least 20% in comparison with historical controls. However, the significance of this improvement should be viewed in the light of reports showing that with better surgical techniques combined with excellent postoperative care, the 5-yr disease-free survival has increased during the last decade to about 40% in patients who did not receive adjuvant chemotherapy.[33] A few studies performed during the past decade suggest that adjuvant chemotherapy may produce a more favorable outcome with early disease-free survival of >50%, which at 5 yr usually decreases to a level of 30–60%.[39] These results were similar when the dose intensity was increased or high-dose MTX was combined with ADR as well as other drugs (5-fluourouracil, CTX, etc.) (see Appendix). Better results, consisting of disease-free survival at 52 mo in 82% and at 24 mo in 90% of patients, were reported only by Rosen et al on the outcome of 2 studies.[34] The most obvious feature of these studies was the administration of preoperative chemotherapy with high-dose MTX with LCV rescue in 4 consecutive weeks before surgery and the administration of the same plus ADR, BLM, CTX, and dacarbazine (DTIC) every 11 wk or of ADR + DDP + BLM + CTX + ACT (see Appendix) every 9–10 wk in patients who had a poor response to high-dose MTX preoperatively. These data are being reevaluated in a phase 3 cooperative study group carried out by the Pediatric Oncology Group.

Radiation therapy (XRT) is used in the primary treatment of osteosarcomas in patients with tumors arising in surgically inaccessible sites. It is required in combination with limited surgery for osteosarcomas that arise in the maxilla, other sinuses, and mandible, which had a high failure rate when treated with surgery alone. In uncontrolled studies, results appeared better when irradiation (with either interstitial techniques or external beam) was administered preoperatively rather than postoperatively, when there generally is a long waiting time for wound healing. High-dose XRT followed immediately by surgery led to an 80% disease-free survival at 3 yr in 33 cases of osteosarcoma of the mandible.[35]

XRT is also recommended for patients with osteosarcomas in the pelvis, vertebral bodies, ribs, and other sites that are not amenable to extensive radical surgery. In these cases, XRT frequently can be combined with intra-arterial[36] or I.V. delivery[37] of chemotherapy (using DDP or ADR), which occasionally can shrink the tumor so that it becomes surgically resectable.

Management of Patients with Metastatic Osteosarcomas

The most common site of metastasis in patients with osteosarcomas is in the lung. Lung metastases can be synchronous with the primary site or may represent the first site of disease relapse.

In cases of osteosarcoma localized to 1 extremity with synchronous lung metastasis, treatment can still have a curative goal in patients whose lung metastases are amenable to complete surgical resection. There are 2 approaches. The first consists of surgical ablation of the primary tumor followed by thoracotomy and removal of lung metastases. Adjuvant chemotherapy is then administered for about 1 yr. In the second approach, chemotherapy is given first, permitting evaluation of response to the drugs; next, the primary lesion is resected along with the lung metastases, which frequently have become easier to remove.

In patients presenting only with lung metastases, the general recommendation is to attempt curative resection only for those with a single metastatic lesion or a few lesions located in the same lobe that developed >1 yr after adjuvant chemotherapy was completed.

Patients who relapsed while on chemotherapy or during the first year after completion of the adjuvant chemotherapy, along with all other patients with osteosarcoma that has already metastasized to various unresectable sites or to more than 1 site, should receive only chemotherapy,[38] using agents different from those initially used with only a goal of palliation (see Appendix). Radiation therapy can also be used for the same purpose.

Overall, the treatment of osteosarcomas has significantly improved during the last 2 decades, permitting the achievement of cures in 40–60% of cases with primary resectable lesions as well as in a smaller number of patients with single metastases.

References

1. Dahlin DC, Coventry MB. Osteogenic sarcoma: a study of six hundred cases. J Bone Joint Surg (Am) 1967; 49:101–10.
2. Dahlin DC. Bone tumors: general aspects and data on 6,221 cases. Springfield, Ill.: Thomas, 1978.
3. Dahlin DC. Osteosarcoma of bone and consideration of prognostic variables. Cancer Treat Rep 1978; 62:189–92.
4. Huvos AG. Bone tumors: diagnosis, treatment and prognosis. Philadelphia: Saunders, 1979.
5. Jenkin RDT. The management of osteosarcoma and Ewing's sarcoma. Bone-certain aspects of neoplasia. Colston papers no. 24. London: Butterworth, 1973; 229–39.
6. Owen LN. Bone tumours in man and animals. London: Butterworth, 1969.
7. Johnson LC. A general theory of bone tumors. Bull NY Acad Med 1953; 29:164–71.
8. Harris TJ, Schiller AL, Treistad RL, et al. Thorotrast-associated sarcoma of bone: a case report and review of the literature. Cancer 1979; 44:603–10.

9. Report of the United Nations Scientific Committee on the Effect of Atomic Radiation. General Assembly: 19th session, 1964; suppl 14 (A15814), 94–95.

10. Goorin A, Abelson H, Frei E. Osteosarcoma: Fifteen years later. N Engl J Med 1985; 313:1637–43.

11. Sweetnam R. Osteosarcoma. Ann R Coll Surg 1969; 44:38.

12. Ewing J. Modern attitude toward traumatic cancer. Arch Pathol 1935; 19:590–728.

13. Madewell JE, Ragsdale BD, Sweet DE. Radiographic and pathologic analysis of solitary bone lesions, Radiol Clin North Am 1981; 19:715–814.

14. Thorpe WP, Reilly JJ, Rosenberg SA. Prognostic significance of alkaline phosphatase measurements in patients with osteogenic sarcoma receiving chemotherapy. Cancer 1979; 43:2178–81.

15. Levine AM, Rosenberg SA. Alkaline phosphatase levels in osteosarcoma tissue are related to prognosis. Cancer 1979; 44:2291–93.

16. Cortes EP, Holland JF, Glidewell O. Adjuvant therapy of operable primary osteosarcoma—a Cancer and Leukemia Group B experience. Recent Results Cancer Res 1979; 16–24.

17. Francis KC, Kohn H, Malawer MM. Osteogenic sarcoma. J Bone Joint Surg 1976; 55:754.

18. Scranton PE Jr, DeCicco FA, Totten RS, et al. Prognostic factors in osteosarcoma: a review of 20 years experience at the University of Pittsburgh Health Center Hospital. Cancer 1975; 36:2179–91.

19. Cortes EP, Chu TM, Wang JJ, et al. Carcinoembryonic antigen in osteosarcoma. J Surg Oncol 1977; 9:257–65.

20. Von Ronnen JR. Histological and radiographical classification of osteosarcoma in relation to therapy. A review of 245 cases located in the extremities. J Belge Radiol 1968; 51:215–21.

21. Jaffe HL. Tumors and tumurous conditions of the bones and joints. Philadelphia: Len and Febiger, 1958; 256–78.

22. Lindbom A, Sondenberg G, Spjut AJ. Osteogenic sarcoma: a review of 96 cases. Acta Radiol 1961; 56:1–19.

23. Wilner D. Osteogenic sarcoma (osteosarcoma). In: Wilner D, ed. Radiology of bone tumors and allied disorders. Philadelphia: Saunders, 1982; 1897–2095.

24. Enneking W, Dempsey S. Osteosarcoma. Orthop Clin North Am 1977; 8:785–803.

25. Hudson T et al. Angiography in the management of musculo-skeletal tumors. Surg Gynecol Obstet 1975; 141:11–21.

26. Halpern M, Freiberge R. Arteriography in orthopedics. Am J Roentgenol Radium Ther Nucl Med 1965; 94:194–206.

27. Allan C, Soule E. Osteogenic sarcoma of the somatic soft tissues. Cancer 1971; 27:1121–33.

28. Marcove RC, Lewis M, Huvos A. En bloc upper humeral interscapular-thoracic resection. The Tikhoff-Linberg procedure. Clin Orthop 1977; 124:219–28.

29. Enneking WF, Spanies SS, Goodman MA. A system for the surgical staging of musculoskeletal sarcoma. Clin Orthop 1980; 153:106–20.

30. Mindoll ER. Long term results concerning function and quality of life. Chao EYS, Irins J, eds. Design and application of tumor prosthesis for bone and joint reconstruction. New York: Thieme-Stratton, 1983.

31. Cortes EP, Holland JF, Wang JJ, et al. Amputation and Adriamycin in primary osteosarcomas. N Engl J Med 1974; 291:998–1000.

32. Jaffe N, Frei E III, Traggis D, et al. Adjuvant methotrexate and citrovorum factor treatment of osteogenic sarcoma. New Engl J Med 1974; 291:994–97.

33. Taylor WF, Ivins JC, Dahlin DC, et al. Trends and variability in survival from osteosarcomas. Mayo Clin Proc 1978; 53:695–700.

34. Rosen G, Caparros B, Huvos AC, et al. Preoperative chemotherapy for osteogenic sarcoma. Selection of postoperative adjuvant chemotherapy based upon the response of the primary tumor to preoperative chemotherapy. Cancer 1982; 49:1221–30.

35. Chambers RG, Mahoney DE. Osteogenic sarcoma of the mandible. Current management. Am J Surg 1970; 36:463–68.

36. Benjamin R. Regional chemotherapy for osteosarcoma. Semin Oncol 1989; 16:323–27.

37. Rosenthal CJ, Rotman M. Pilot study of interaction of radiation therapy with doxorubicin by continuous infusion. NCI monogr 1988; 6:285–290.
38. Kane MJ. Chemotherapy of advanced soft tissue sarcomas and osteosarcomas. Semin Oncol 1989; 16:297–304.
39. Eilber FR, Rosen G. Adjuvant chemotherapy for osteosarcoma. Semin Oncol 1989; 16:312–23.

45

SOFT-TISSUE SARCOMA

Seymour D. Ritter, M.D.

SOFT-TISSUE SARCOMAS ACCOUNT for only 0.7% of all cancers, and there are only about 4,500 new cases per year in United States, with 1,600 deaths. The incidence rate is 2 per 100,000 population. In adults, the peak incidence is in the fourth and fifth decades of life. Childhood soft-tissue sarcomas, which are discussed elsewhere in this book, behave and respond differently.

Etiologically, genetics plays a small role.[12] Rare families have associated sarcomas, and some are associated with genetic diseases. Neurofibromatosis occasionally undergoes sarcomatous degeneration, and Gardner's syndrome is associated with malignant desmoid tumors. Chemicals such as methylcholanthrene and chlorophenols have been implicated as the cause of some sarcomas.[11] Ionizing radiation in children produces chondrosarcomas and osteogenic sarcomas years later. Mesothelioma is associated with asbestos as an etiological agent; the mechanism of action here appears to be the physical shape of the crystal. Kaposi's sarcoma is often associated with a virally mediated acquired immune deficiency. Trauma is a frequently cited etiology but is rarely proven; chronic infection and edema may be a cause in some cases of lymphangiosarcoma and fibrosarcoma. Because the tumors are of such diverse histology, the variety of etiologies should not be surprising.

Histopathology and Staging

Soft-tissue sarcomas are of mesenchymal origin and are usually classified and named by tissue of origin.

769

Table 45-1. Histologic Classification of Soft-Tissue Sarcomas

Tumors of clearly recognizable cell type
  Tumors of fibrous tissue: fibrosarcoma (chapter 11, figure 11-61)
  Tumors of adipose tissue: liposarcoma (chapter 11, figures 11-63A & B)
    Well-differentiated
    Myxoid
    Round-cell
    Pleomorphic
  Tumors of striated muscle: rhabdomyosarcoma (chapter 11, figures 11-66A & B)
    Pleomorphic
    Alveolar
    Embryonal
    Mixed
  Tumors of smooth muscle: leiomyosarcoma (chapter 11, figure 11-64)
  Tumors of vascular origin: angiosarcoma (chapter 11, figure 11-72)
    Lymphangiosarcoma
    Malignant hemangiopericytoma
  Tumors of synovial tissue: synovial sarcoma (chapter 11, figure 11-67)
    Tumors of mesothelium: malignant mesothelioma
    Tumors of neurogenic (nerve sheath) origin:
      Neurogenic sarcoma
      Malignant schwannoma (chapter 11, figure 11-68)
    Tumors of histiocytic origin: malignant fibrous histiocytoma (chapter 11, figure 11-62)
      Giant cell tumor of soft parts
  Tumors of cartilagenous origin: chondrosarcoma (chapter 11, figure 11-76)

Tumors of Debatable Origin
  Kaposi's sarcoma (probably endothelial) (chapter 11, figure 11-73)
  Alveolar soft parts sarcoma (probably myogenic)
  Epitheliod sarcoma (probably synovial)
  Extraskeletal Ewing's sarcoma (chapter 11, figure 11-70)

Tumors that cannot be further classified
  Undifferentiated sarcoma

One useful classification system is shown in table 45-1.[1] This classification is scarcely comprehensive, however. Synonyms for neurogenic tumors alone could cover a page. Developments in immunohistological, biochemical staining, and electron microscopic techniques have enabled better identification of tissue of origin over time. For example, S-100 protein is found primarily in neurogenic tumors and in melanomas of neural crest origin; factor VIII-related antigen is found in endothelially derived tumors. Over the years, these techniques have clarified diagnosis but have changed concepts. As early as 1961, Kaufman and Stout showed the histiocyte to be a facultative fibroblast.[3] They described tumors derived from histiocytes, naming them malignant fibrous histiocytomas, and were able to reclassify tumors that had been known as liposarcomas, fibrosarcomas, and rhabdomyosarcomas (without striations) to this classification. This sarcoma can have a storiform, pleomorphic, myxoid, giant cell, xanthomatous, or angiomatoid appearance, and several elements may be present in the same tumor. The cell of origin is a facultative fibroblast, capable of phagocytosis, and may be the same as the bone marrow histiocyte, a more primitive cell, or one that can become a macrophage or a fibroblast. Rosenberg et al, in a table summarizing the change in histological diagnosis of soft-tissue sarcomas over the years, showed no incidence of malignant fibrous histiocytomas (MFH) before 1972 and 22.8% of all soft-tissue sarcomas to be MFH in a 1984 review.[5] It is currently the most frequently reported type of soft-tissue sarcoma, with pathologists diagnosing many fewer fibrosarcomas.

There is a certain age association of different histologic types of soft-tissue sarcomas. Thus, in the neonatal period one sees more frequent fibrosarcomas; rhabdomyosarcomas of the embryonal or botryoid type are more frequently encountered in early childhood, whereas in late childhood and adulthood an increased incidence of alveolar rhabdomyosarcomas, fibrosarcomas, clear-cell sarcomas, synovial sarcomas, hemangiopericytomas, neurogenic sarcomas, and malignant fibrous histiocytomas is seen. Kaposi's sarcoma, giant-cell sarcoma of the soft parts, and angiosarcoma of the skin are associated more frequently with old age.

Some soft-tissue sarcomas have a certain prediliction for specific anatomic sites, as shown in table 45-2. The biologic behavior of different types of soft-tissue sarcomas varies considerably. Certain histologic types rarely metastasize (e.g., dermatofibrosarcoma protuberans).

Table 45-2. Association of Soft-Tissue Sarcomas by Site

Head and neck	Rhabdomyosarcoma (child)
	Angiosarcoma (elderly)
Thigh	Malignant fibrous histiocytoma
	Liposarcoma
	Synovial sarcoma
	Rhabdomyosarcoma (adult)
Retroperitoneum and mesentery	Leiomyosarcoma
	Liposarcoma
	Malignant fibrous histiocytoma
Distal lower extremity	Synovial sarcoma
	Clear cell sarcoma
	Kaposi's sarcoma (elderly)
Distal upper extremity	Epithelioid sarcoma
Genitourinary	Rhabdomyosarcoma (child)
	Leiomyosarcoma (adult)
Skin	Angiosarcoma and lymphangiosarcoma
	Epitheloid sarcoma

Although most soft-tissue sarcomas have primarily hematogenous spread, about 10% metastasize to lymph nodes. Some that do so are rhabdomyosarcoma, hemangiocytoma, malignant fibrous histiocytoma, synovial sarcoma, epithelioid sarcoma, and clear-cell sarcoma.[2]

Finally, among various histologic types one can identify some with good 5-yr survival: well-differentiated fibrosarcoma, infantile fibrosarcoma, well-differentiated and myxoid liposarcoma, malignant fibrous histiocytoma, and superficial epithelioid sarcoma.[2] In general, nuclear grade is of more importance than histological type.

With such a diffuse group of diseases, the histologic classification is somewhat less predictive of prognosis than in other diseases. A better predictor

Table 45-3. TNM Staging Classification of Soft-Tissue Sarcomas*

Primary tumor (T)
TX	Minimum requirements to assess primary tumor cannot be met
T0	No demonstrable tumor
T1	Tumor ≤5 cm in diameter
T2	Tumor >5 cm in diameter

Tumor grade (G)
G1	Well differentiated
G2	Moderately well differentiated
G3-4	Poorly differentiated; undifferentiated

Nodal involvement (N)
NX	Minimum requirements to assess the regional nodes cannot be met
N0	No lymph node metastasis
N1	Regional lymph node metastasis

Distant metastasis (M)
MX	Minimum requirements to assess the presence of distant metastasis cannot be met
M0	No distant metastasis
M1	Distant metastasis present

*This classification apples to the following tumors:

alveolar soft-part sarcoma	malignant hemangiopericytoma
angiosarcoma	malignant mesenchymoma
epithelioid sarcoma	malignant schwannoma
extraskeletal chondrosarcoma	malignant peripheral nerve sheath tumor
extraskeletal osteosarcoma	rhabdomyosarcoma
fibrosarcoma	synovial sarcoma
leiomyosarcoma	sarcoma, unclassified
liposarcoma	sarcoma, other
malignant fibrous histiocytoma	

is the stage of the disease as defined by the TNM classification (table 45-3).[1] More important than TNM in sarcomas is grading based both on nuclear characteristics and the number of mitoses per 10 high-powered fields (HPF).[13] In general, <3 mitoses per 10 HPF is benign and >10 is malignant. Pathologists use grades I, II, III for increasing malignancy in sarcomas. A classification was developed using both criteria (table 45-4). This staging system, devised by the American Joint Committee on Cancer, was based on a review of 1,215 cases from 13 institutions.[5]

Diagnosis and Treatment

Most soft-tissue sarcomas present as a mass. In adults, 80% occur in the extremities, but if children are included, 12% are in the head and neck, 30% in the trunk, 12% are retroperitoneal, and the rest are in the extremities. Diagnosis is usually made by palpation of the lesion. A mass may be felt subcutaneously. The skin is usually smooth over the mass, although some sarcomas do involve and discolor the skin—e.g., Kaposi's sarcoma presents frequently as a small, bluish mass, and angiosarcomas are red and purple. Lymphangiosarcomas and dermatofibrosarcoma protruberans also involve the skin. The latter rarely metastasizes, but unless it is completely removed, it will continue to recur locally and cause death. Most sarcomas are firm to hard on palpation. Pain is a late symptom, usually because the mass enlarges and presses on a nerve or bone. Swelling may cause limitation of motion if the tumor extends over a joint.

Biopsy, except of an extremely small lesion, should be incisional rather than excisional in nature.[6] Excision attempts usually result in a rim of tissue being left behind. This false capsule is usually tumor, and landmarks are no longer present, resulting in a final more extensive surgical procedure.

Because only about 10% of soft-tissue sarcomas metastasize to lymph nodes, nodal resection is less important. Preoperative workup therefore need include only chest films and diagnostic procedures for the primary tumor, e.g., CT scans (see chapter 10, figures 10-44 and 10-45) of the tumor area for extent of disease. Recurrences are either local or pulmonary in the vast majority of cases.

Surgical treatment involves removal of the tumor with wide margins.[6] Wide local excision for small tumors may be adequate if the tumors are low grade. More properly, a radical soft parts resection is done with a 2-cm margin around the tumor. Where narrower margins are needed, postoperative radiation may decrease the incidence of local recurrence. Because many tumors occur in the extremities, amputation may be needed to achieve local control. However, preoperative radiation therapy (XRT) and chemotherapy have made limb-sparing surgery more practical.[14] Adjuvant XRT in high-grade lesions can reduce local recurrence from 25–35% to 7–12%.[7]

Retroperitoneal sarcomas present a formidable problem for the surgeon. When discovered, they are usually large and are frequently wrapped around major vessels and nerves. Resections are often incomplete, and the recurrence

Table 45-4. American Joint Committee on Cancer (AJCC) Stage Grouping of Soft-Tissue Sarcomas

Stage	Grade	Description
Ia	G1, T1, N0, M0	Well-differentiated tumor ≤5 cm in diameter; no regional lymph nodal or distant metastases
Ib	G1, T2, N0, M0	Well-differentiated tumor >5 cm in diameter; no regional lymph nodal or distant metastases
IIa	G2, T1, M0S, M0	Moderately differentiated tumor ≤5 cm in diameter; no regional lymph nodal or distant metastases
IIb	G2, T2, N0, M0	Moderately differentiated tumor >5 cm in diameter; no regional lymph nodal or distant metastases
IIIa	G3, T1, N0, M0	Poorly differentiated tumor ≤5 cm in diameter; no regional lymph nodal or distant metastases
IIIb	G3, T2, N0, M0	Poorly differentiated tumor >5 cm in diameter; no regional lymph nodal or distant metastases
IIIc	Any G, T1, T2; N1, M0	Tumor of any differentiation, any size; regional lymph nodal metastases but no distant metastases
IVa	Any G, T3, any N, M0	Tumor of any differentiation of malignancy demonstrating clear radiographic evidence of destruction of cortical bone (with invasion) and histopathologic confirmation of invasion of major artery or nerve, with or without regional lymph nodal metastases but without distant metastases
IVb	Any G, any T, any N, M1	Tumor with distant metastases

rate is 80%. Head and neck sarcomas present some of the same problems of resection with adequate margins. Heavy particle beam therapy can be curative of localized sarcomas in otherwise inoperable locations.

Prognosis in extremity sarcoma worsens with more proximal location independent of grade. Nodal dissection is rarely if ever indicated, the incidence of positive nodes being only 2.6% in 1 study with no improvement of survival with node dissection. Adjuvant chemotherapy is controversial.[8] The problem is the variety of locations, histologies, grades, and tumor sizes, combined with the small number of tumors. This has resulted in equivocal outcomes. At least 1 study by Rosenberg at the National Cancer Institute using cyclophosphamide (CTX), doxorubicin (ADR), and methotrexate (MTX) showed a significant increase in survival for patients treated with chemotherapy. Other regimens with higher response rates have been suggested.[15]

Treatment of recurrence and metastases. Recurrent tumor is most common either locally or in the lungs. Additional local resection for recurrence plus radiation, i.e., amputation of extremity lesion or resection of a retroperitoneal lesion, is occasionally successful—5–10% of the time as opposed to about a 50% cure rate for primarily resected tumors. Single lesions in the lung have been resected, and there are rare 5-yr survivors after multiple lung metastases have been resected.[15] Chemotherapy for soft-tissue sarcomas is usually based on ADR-containing regimens (see Appendix).[10,16] The combination of CTX, ADR, dacarbazine (DTIC), and vincristine (VCR) pioneered by Gottlieb is an effective regimen, giving about 12% complete responses and 45% total responses in variety of tumors.[9] ADR alone, in higher doses of 30 mg/m^2/day $\times$ 3, ADR and DTIC with or without CTX, and all variations have response rates that may be better than ADR alone, but not convincingly so.[10] Cisplatin (DDP) and high-dose MTX with leucovorin rescue can induce occasional favorable responses in patients relapsing after an ADR-induced response. Actinomycin-D, CTX, and VCR are frequently used in pediatric tumors.

Finally, recently ifosfamide with MESNA protection for the bladder, administered in combination with VCR or etoposide and DTIC has led to improved results in a few preliminary studies.[17]

References

1. Manual for Staging of Cancer (American Joint Committee on Cancer). 3rd ed, Pt II—Staging of cancer at specific anatomic sites. Philadelphia: Lippincott, 1988; 25–282; 123–144; 127–31.
2. Enterline, HT. Histopathology of sarcomas. Semin Oncol Jun 1981; 8(2):133.
3. Kauffman, SL, Stout AP. Histiocytic tumors (fibrous xanthoma and histiocytoma) in children. Cancer 1961; 14:468–482.
4. Rosenberg SA, Suit HD, Baker LH. Sarcomas of soft tissue. In: De Vita VT, Hellman S, Rosenberg S, eds. Cancer—Principles and practice of oncology. Philadelphia: Lippincott, 1985.
5. Russell WA, Cohen J, Edmonsom JH, et al. Staging system for soft tissue sarcomas. Semin Oncol 1981; 8:156–59.
6. Yang JC, Rosenberg S. Surgery for adult patients with soft tissue sarcomas. Semin Oncol 1989; 16:289–296.
7. Tepper JE, Suit H. Radiation therapy of soft tissue sarcomas. Cancer 1985; 55:2273–77.

8. Elias AD, Antman KH. Adjuvant chemotherapy for soft tissue sarcoma: an approach in search of an effective regimen. Semin Oncol 1989; 16:305–12.
9. Gottlieb JA, Baker LH, O'Bryan RM, et al. Adriamycin used alone and in combination for soft tissue and bone sarcoma. Cancer Chemother Rep (Pt 3) 1975; 6:271–82.
10. Kane MJ. Chemotherapy of advanced soft tissue and osteosarcomas. Semin Oncol 1989; 16:297–306.
11. Johnson ES. Association between soft tissue sarcomas, malignant lymphomas, and phenoxy herbicides/chlorophenols: evidence from occupational cohort studies. Fundam Appl Toxicol 1990; 14(2):219–34.
12. McClay EF. Epidemiology of bone and soft tissue sarcomas. Semin Oncol 1989; 16(4):264–72.
13. Mandard AM, Petiot JF, Marnay J, et al. Prognostic factors in soft tissue sarcomas. A multivariate analysis of 109 cases. Cancer 1989; 63(7):1437–51.
14. Walker MJ, Wood DK, Briele HA, et al. Soft tissue sarcomas of the distal extremities. Surgery 1986; 99(4):392–98.
15. Jablons D, Steinberg SM, Roth J, Pittaluga S, Rosenberg SA, Pass HI. Metastasectomy for soft tissue sarcoma. Further evidence for efficacy and prognostic indicators. Thorac Cardiovasc Surg 1989; 97(5):695–705.
16. Chang AE, Kinsella T, Glatstein E, et al. Adjuvant chemotherapy for patients with high-grade soft-tissue sarcomas of the extremity. J Clin Oncol 1988; 6(9):1491–1500.
17. Elias A, Ryan L, Sulkes A, et al. Response to mesna, doxorubicin, ifosfamide, and dacarbazine in 108 patients with metastatic or unresectable sarcoma and no prior chemotherapy. J Clin Oncol 1989; 7(9):1208–16.

46

CUTANEOUS MALIGNANCIES

Neil I. Brody, M.D., Ph.D.

IN THIS CHAPTER, CANCERS of the skin are grouped according to their cell of origin. The skin is composed of a group of cells that are permanent residents, including epidermal cells, melanocytes, fibroblasts, vascular- and nervous system-associated cells, and fat cells. Also present are transient cells, primarily of immune system origin, such as Langerhans cells, lymphocytes, and monocytes. Although all cells of the skin are subject to malignant degeneration, only the more common cutaneous malignancies are considered in this discussion. The intent is to familiarize the oncology specialist with the variety of malignancies that confront the dermatologist in daily practice. The intent of this approach is to facilitate the recognition of cutaneous cancers and bring about an appropriate disposition of the patient being examined by the nondermatologist practitioner.

In describing these tumors, the following approach has been used: First, because all individuals relate to descriptive terms such as *flat* and *red,* these terms are used to describe cutaneous malignancies. Second, the fact that adequate and accurate skin examination requires both visual and tactile approaches is emphasized. The skin of the fingertips is uniquely capable of discerning alterations in texture and substance that are not visible, and the cutaneous sensory cortex is nearly as large as the visual. Third, the histologic descriptions are of specimens stained with hematoxylin and eosin, the most commonly used preparation.

Beyond teaching recognition, an attempt has been made to distill the essences of causation, prevention, and therapy. Many of the concepts presented can be extended to malignancies other than those of the skin. Where possible, the framework of discussing the projected etiology of cutaneous malignancies is interjected, as it is believed that it is fundamental to the teaching of cancer prevention regardless of the primary discipline of the examining physician. Counseling, prevention, and patient education are mandatory to enhance early detection, which still is the most powerful tool available to the practitioner aiming to reduce the morbidity and mortality of malignancy.

The skin is a unique window into the world of oncology. It allows recognition of numerous principles that apply throughout the specialty. Observation of the skin suggests that there is an early stage in cancer that dermatologists refer to as premalignant. Tumors in this category become malignant unless there is either medical intervention or an immunological response. Even when malignant, some tumors are well defended against by the host. These tumors progress slowly and are easily cured even when an inappropriate delay precedes their care. Other tumors—such as malignant melanoma—that are less readily checked by the host defense systems clearly demonstrate that early recognition results in cure. Even deadly tumors, typified by melanoma, often are present for long periods—perhaps years—before they are brought to the attention of a physician. Understanding that even deadly cancers have a long window of vulnerability to medical intervention requires that our current anticancer armamentarium intensify its interest in early methods of detection and diagnosis. Finally, the skin has served as a model demonstrating that common environmental agents induce, enhance, and predispose to malignancy.

Etiology

Chemicals

Arsenic is the archetype agent for chemical induction of malignancy. Our knowledge about its role in the induction of cancer comes primarily from epidemiological data. Individuals internalize arsenic from numerous sources. Arsenic was once used for medicinal purposes as diverse as the treatment of asthma (Fowler's solution), syphilis, and even as a "tonic to build the blood." Arsenic is present in the soil and well water at isolated distribution points around the world. Many industries have depended upon arsenic. In agriculture, it is used as a pesticide and herbicide. As recently as the 1960s, American cigarettes were tainted with arsenic.

Arsenic is a low inducer of both cutaneous and extracutaneous malignancies. In Taiwan, where certain provinces have contaminated well water, it has been shown that 5 yr of exposure results in the pigmentary alteration of arsenism, 15 yr induces keratoses, and 20 yr results in skin cancer. The interdependence of genetics and the carcinogen is demonstrated by the fact that no individuals in endemic Taiwanese villages get internal malignancies, whereas in other areas of the world where arsenic is part of the food and water supply, all forms of internal malignancies have been reported. Such factors as the rate of dose accumulation and the route of administration may affect the latency period and the type of malignancy induced. For example, where industrial exposure occurs by inhalation, the incidence of lung cancer increases. The mechanism of arsenic-induced malignancy is not known. As with other carcinogens, arsenic is capable of altering the genetic material, as is shown by an increased incidence of sister chromatid exchanges. Arsenic also interferes with the enzyme systems responsible for phosphorylation. Because DNA repair requires the energy that is a by-product of the phosphorylation pathways, the bipronged attack of inducing DNA changes and decreasing the rate of repair may be responsible for the generation of malignancy. Although these forms of alterations of cellular metabolism and genetic material may account for the generation of malignancy on the cellular level, they shed no light on the observation that there is a long hiatus between the initial insult and the recognition of malignancy.

Electromagnetic Energy

Ultraviolet light (UV) and X rays are 2 distinct spectrums of electromagnetic energy capable of inducing malignancy. Both agents are capable of altering DNA. Although everyone knows to avoid unnecessary x-ray examinations, informed avoidance of unnecessary UV exposure, as in sunbathing, seems not yet to be practiced knowledge. Much of the malignancy discussed in this chapter is etiologically associated with sun exposure. The actinic keratosis, a premalignant lesion, derives its name from its sun-induced heritage. Basal cell and squamous cell carcinomas occur primarily on sun-exposed skin. In fact, for basal cell carcinomas, the frequency of occurrence in a particular location on the skin surface is directly related to the level of sun exposure of that cutaneous locale.

For UV-induced malignancy, much is known about the role of this agent beyond its simply changing the phenotype of the cells from benign to malignant. UV light also alters the host's level of resistance to the malignancies it induces. In a mouse model in which UV-induced malignancy has been studied, daily exposure to the UVB (2,900–3,200 A) spectrum of sunlight for 20 wk results in numerous malignancies in the mouse's skin. These malignancies can be surgically removed and grown in vitro, or transferred to another mouse of the same strain. When transplanted, these sun-induced malignancies display 2 disparate characteristics. Some malignancies do not grow and are rejected; these are referred to as the regressor phenotype. Other malignancies grow and kill the mouse; these are referred to as the progressor phenotype.[1]

It is assumed that whether a tumor grows or doesn't grow is determined by the host's ability to reject the tumor. Evidence for this hypothesis comes from the fact that tumors of the regressor phenotype transplanted to a mouse that has been irradiated with UVB for only 5 or 6 wk can grow and kill the mouse. Other forms of immunologic alteration of the host—for example, by antilymphocyte serum cytotoxic agents and X-irradiation—also reduce the host's defense mechanisms sufficiently to allow tumors of the regressor phenotype to grow and kill the mouse. The most interesting aspect of this model stems from the fact that a specific suppressor T lymphocyte is responsible for allowing regressor tumors to prosper.[2] These suppressor T lymphocytes can be obtained from the spleen of a mouse that has been irradiated with UVB for 6 wk. Upon transfer to an unirradiated mouse, these cells confer susceptibility to the growth of UV regressor tumors. These suppressor T cells are specific for UV-induced tumors, as they do not alter the host's resistance to chemically induced malignancies or to other immunologic phenomena (such as response to myriad tested antigens). Commerically available nonprescription sun screens provide protection against both the development of malignancy and immunological alterations.

Genetics of DNA Repair

In the course of their existence, many cells accumulate alterations of their DNA that require repair to allow proper cell function and division and to avoid malignant degeneration. A large number of enzymes are involved in the DNA repair process. In 2 diseases, DNA repair mechanisms are deficient: Bloom's syndrome and xeroderma pigmentosum. In the latter, the cumulative effects of sun damage are devastating. Individuals with xeroderma pigmentosum develop vast numbers of basal and squamous cell carcinomas, as well as melanoma. Eventually they succumb to 1 of these cancers, most within the first 30 yr of life.

Basal Cell Carcinoma

Basal cell carcinomas are the most common of all skin cancers. They occur predominantly in areas of most solar exposure. Individuals with a history of sunburn have the highest incidence of basal cell carcinomas. Obviously, this depends upon skin coloration: type 1 individuals with blue or green eyes, blond or red hair and freckles are the most prone, whereas this tumor rarely if ever occurs in types 5 and 6 dark-skinned or black persons. Other factors that predispose to basal cell carcinomas include arsenic ingestion, X-irradiation, basal cell nevus syndrome, and diseases with faulty DNA repair such as xeroderma pigmentosum.

Types and Appearances

The nodular form of basal cell carcinoma is the most common. This lesion is raised and has a pink, translucent character that is most easily discernible at its borders. Frequently an increase in the vascularity of these tumors is seen that is recognizable by the telangiectasia coursing through and slightly beyond the discernible mass. The central area in larger lesions may be a crust, secondary to ulceration. Left untreated, this and other basal cell carcinomas continue to expand in a 3-dimensional fashion. In their progression, they will invade and erode nerves, blood vessels, and even bone; at this point, they are frequently referred to as rodent ulcers. Although locally aggressive, however, these and other basal cell carcinomas rarely metastasize.

The pigmented basal cell carcinoma is the melanized twin of the nodular carcinoma. Because its pigment is melanin, it is rarely found in lightly pigmented individuals, especially those with blue or green eyes. Most basal cell carcinomas cause some hypertrophy of the fibrous stroma in which they are embedded. The sclerosing basal cell carcinoma augments its imbedding milieu to such an extent that biopsy specimens are frequently mistaken for morphea. Because of the vast increase in stroma and the sparse distribution of malignant cells, the borders of this form of basal cell carcinoma are difficult to determine. An easily missed clinical appearance, it is difficult to treat and is frequently associated with a history fraught with recurrences. Basal cell carcinoma appears clinically as an area of hardened skin with an obliterated surface and none of the usual pink, "pearl-like" and telangiectatic character descriptive of the nodular basal cell carcinoma. Superficial basal cell carcinomas occur most frequently on the trunk as nonhealing, pink, slightly raised, and occasionally scaly lesions. Their borders are well defined but generally irregular. These lesions may masquerade as an eczematous dermatitis; however, they do not respond to treatments used for eczemas.

Histology

Microscopically, the proliferating cell in the basal cell carcinoma lives on the basement membrane of the dermoepidermal junction (see chapter 11, figure 11-89). The nodular, superficial, and pigmented types have clumps of these cells all attached at some point to the central surface lesion. In the sclerosing type, a vast quantity of collagen with dark blue basal cells can be seen scattered in groups in the vast array of dense, pink-staining collagen.

Treatment

A number of treatment modalities are available for the removal of basal cell carcinomas. The most common is referred to as curettage and electrodesiccation. In trained hands, the nodular, pigmented, and superficial basal cell carcinomas may be cured >95% of the time using this modality. The resulting scar is a flat, ivory-colored patch. Where the borders of basal cell carcinomas are easily discerned, excision and suture closure offers a rapidly healed, cosmetically improved mode of removal. For larger and more complicated lesions, Mohs (a surgeon) developed a technique in which tangential (salami-like) sections are cut and examined under the microscope.[3] Sections are sequentially cut until there is no residual microscopic evidence of tumor. The accuracy of this modality depends on the contiguous nature of the spread of this class of tumor. Because every strand is thought to be attached at some point to the initial central tumor, one is able to map the strands by continued sectioning. In difficult to treat and recurrent tumors, this is the method of choice.

Three other treatment approaches deserve mention. The first, *cyrosurgery,* uses liquid nitrogen to freeze the tumor to an arbitrarily accepted border selected because statistically it ought to be beyond the cancer. The technique is technically simple and applicable in contaminated individuals and certain areas that are anatomically difficult to treat. *X-irradiation* is much like cryosurgery in that a statistically determined border of clinically normal tissue is irradiated. It is most applicable where one does not want to use a cold steel surgical technique because the anatomical locale makes the procedure difficult or impossible (e.g., certain eyelid lesions). The x-ray modality should be used in the head and neck only in individuals 60 yr old or older. Finally, *laser surgery* offers many of the same benefits as cryosurgery and irradiation. Because it is a fairly new technique, no firm guidelines are yet available for its application.

Squamous Cell Carcinoma

Squamous cell carcinoma is the second most common form of skin cancer. A number of agents have been implicated in furthering the induction of this malignancy. Among these agents are UV light such as might be obtained by sun exposure, UV light that is part of the PUVA regimen (P = psoralens; UVA = UV light 320–400 nm, a common treatment modality for psoriasis); arsenic, as found in antiquated medications, insecticides, and some well water; tar pitches, to which chimney sweeps were exposed; x-ray therapy, such as that received for treatment of acne, other dermatoses, or even other skin cancers; burn scars; lupus vulgaris; and chronic granulomas. The other major predisposing factor is heredity. Individuals with fair skin who readily burn on sun exposure are more susceptible than darker individuals. Persons who have inherited the disease xeroderma pigmentosum are also more susceptible. In keeping with sunlight as a predisposing factor, men get this tumor more frequently than women, and those with higher doses of sun exposure (e.g., farmers and sailors) are at increased risk. Populations living closer to the equator have a higher incidence, and when the cancer occurs, it is most frequently present on exposed areas of the skin surface.

Types and Appearances

Because squamous cell carcinomas are derived from the keratinizing cells of the epidermis, many have differentiated to the point at which they are producing excess horn. This production of keratin accounts for the clinical appearance of 2 forms of this tumor. The first, known as a cutaneous horn, is a fingerlike projection of keratinous material. The second, verrucous carcinoma, takes on the appearance of a wart; it is found in the anogenital region in association with condyloma, in the mouth in association with florid oral papillomatosis, or on the foot. These associations with wartlike tumors are more likely due to the fact that certain papilloma viruses have recently been found in association with malignant degeneration. In adjacent sections of the same tumor, the DNA of the papilloma virus can be found in the nuclei of cells that were initially responsible for the wartlike growth, whereas cells that display malignant degeneration generally do not have detectable fragments of wart virus.

Other forms of squamous cell carcinoma initially look like basal cell carcinomas. As these tumors grow, they become large exophytic masses. Descriptively, squamous cell carcinomas begin as small, red, slightly scaly patches, grow into raised lesions of similar coloration whose surface generally displays increased vascularity, and eventually become large, warty growths or red masses with blood-tinged surfaces.

Histology and Treatment

As the clinical appearance varies, so does the histology. The early tumor shows masses of pink-staining cells—some of which are producing keratin—

expanding initially within the epidermis, then progressing beyond the dermoepidermal junction. The presence of keratin-containing areas within the tumor is helpful diagnostically, but they may not be present. As these tumors enlarge, individual cells may become more undifferentiated. Some forms of squamous cell carcinomas have a cell type indistinguishable from cells of other spindle cell tumors such as malignant melanoma and fibrosarcomas.

Many of the same treatment modalities appropriate for basal cell carcinomas are used in the treatment of squamous cell carcinomas. A rule of thumb frequently followed by the dermatologist states that malignancies arising on sun-damaged skin have a slower growing, less metastasizing phenotype than those arising on unexposed skin. It is important to recognize that part of the workup of squamous cell carcinomas includes inspection of regional lymph node chains for signs of metastases. Early recognition and elimination of the precursors of malignant transformation are always the stepping stone of ideal care. Depending on the size and location of the tumor, curettage and electrodesiccation, excision and primary closure, Mohs surgery, cryosurgery, X ray, and laser surgery are all appropriate modalities.

Bowen's Disease

Bowen's disease is a specific clinical and histological presentation of squamous cell carcinoma *in situ*. The malignant cells are contained entirely within the epidermis (e.g., above the basement membrane). Most patients do not report any predisposing conditions that account for the presence of Bowen's disease, but there is an association between Bowen's disease and arsenic ingestion. Because of this association and the increased incidence of internal malignancies with arsenic ingestion, intense cross-examination to elicit this history is warranted. In one large series, about 5% of patients with Bowen's disease were found to have an additional underlying malignancy.

The lesion of Bowen's disease is round or oval with an irregular border. It is either flat or slightly raised from the surrounding surface, may be covered with varying amounts of scale, and is pinker than the surrounding skin. Although its pinkness and sharply defined border help demarcate it from its normal surrounds, these lesions expand centrifugally with time and can easily be 5–7 cm in diameter. Left unattended, about 5% of these lesions become squamous cell carcinomas. In this event, the squamous cell carcinomas that they breed tend to be more aggressive than those occurring on sun-exposed skin.

The histopathology of Bowen's disease is characteristic. Within the epidermis and never descending below the basement membrane, cellular atypia and complete disorganization of the normal maturation process from the basal cell zone to the horny layer are seen.

Treatment of Bowen's disease is the same as that for basal cell and squamous cell carcinomas. Their *in situ* nature should not be misconstrued as indicating that they are more easily eradicated than equivalently sized squamous cell or basal cell carcinomas. Treatment with topical anticancer agents such as 5-fluorouracil (5-FU) is only occasionally successful.

Erythroplasia of Queyrat

It is most convenient to think of erythroplasia of Queyrat as Bowen's disease of a semimucous or mucous membrane. This lesion is found on the glans penis, especially in the uncircumcised male, and on the vulva of the female. It occurs with increasing frequency after age 50. It differs in 2 substantial ways from Bowen's disease: It more frequently degenerates into squamous cell carcinoma, and it is not associated with underlying malignancy.

Clinically, this is a red, velvety and flat lesion with an irregular but sharply defined border. Because of its location in moist areas, its surface is frequently glistening. In past years, this precancerous lesion was excised by radical surgery. Today, topical 5-FU or ablation with the carbon dioxide laser and careful follow-up seem more appropriate and certainly adequate. The period of treatment with 5-FU is frequently very uncomfortable.

Paget's Disease

Paget's disease is an intraepidermal malignancy occurring in areas of the body where there are apocrine glands. Most commonly, Paget's disease occurs on the nipple of women. However, it can also be found in the urogenital and perirectal area, where it is referred to as extramammary Paget's disease. When this lesion occurs on the nipple, it is frequently associated with an underlying adenocarcinoma of mammary ducts. Extramammary Paget's disease is also associated with an increased incidence of underlying malignancies. In extramammary Paget's disease, the malignancies may not be contiguous with the overlying *in situ* Paget's disease.

Paget's disease of the nipple frequently masquerades as an eczematous dermatitis. Suspicion should be aroused in situations of asymmetry, when one nipple is involved with a red, scaly lesion for any substantial period of time. Individual lesions are red, slightly scaly, irregularly bordered, and sometimes eroded. Usually, only a portion of the areola is involved with extension beyond the normal areola border. Lesions of extramammary Paget's disease are generally red, slightly eroded, crusted, and oozing. They may or may not be elevated above the surrounding skin.

Histologically, large round cells are seen, with a nearly clear, pale staining, and abundant cytoplasm. These pagetoid cells, found within all layers of the epidermis, contain mucin. Special staining to demonstrate the mucin helps differentiate Paget's disease from similar-appearing cells that are found in malignant melanoma or Bowen's disease.

Paget's disease is treated by excisional surgery. In the case of breast disease, mastectomy is frequently indicated. For extramammary Paget's disease, wide local excision is the treatment of choice. Needless to say, a workup for underlying malignancies is warranted. Mohs surgery has been used for extramammary Paget's and may be tissue sparing.

Keratoacanthoma

Keratoacanthomas are rapidly growing tumors that closely resemble squamous cell carcinomas clinically and histologically. Their etiology is not known, but many suspect that they have a viral pathogenesis. Some keratoacanthoma lesions regress spontaneously; however, because they may become large and destructive before they regress, many advocate treating them when first recognized. Keratoacanthomas have been known to occur both as solitary lesions and as a more aggressive multiple form. In both forms, the lesions have the same clinical appearance, although when they appear in multiples they are frequently smaller in size. Immunosuppression, environmental factors such as sun and tar exposure, and x-ray and PUVA therapy may predispose to the occurrence of keratoacanthomas. There is a predilection for these tumors to occur in males, but no hereditary pattern has emerged.

Histologically, this tumor cannot be reliably differentiated from squamous cell carcinoma. An optimal biopsy specimen includes a lateral margin; the configuration of this margin with its arboreal pattern confirms the diagnosis. However, frequently this border is not well defined or is not obtained in the surgical biopsy specimen. The cells within the specimen and their patterns are identical to those described for squamous cell carcinoma. At the borders of this lesion, the well-defined basement membrane may be absent. Therefore, most pathologists hesitate to unequivocally diagnose keratoacanthomas.

Clinically, the keratoacanthoma is a rapidly enlarging red and dome-shaped lesion with a central umbilicated core of yellowish keratinous material. The border of the lesion is ill defined as it gradually ascends to elevation above the skin surface.

The most reasonable treatment of keratoacanthoma is local excision of the earliest lesion. The linear scar of a simple excision is cosmetically superior to the eroded pockmarked area left after spontaneous resolution of this tumor. This is especially true for solitary tumors diagnosed while they are still small. Multiple keratoacanthomas occur infrequently, and no consensus exists for their therapy. Some cases have been treated with antimetabolites such as methotrexate (MTX). Both solitary and multiple keratoacanthomas may be treated with injections of 5-FU.

Precursors of Nonmelanoma Skin Cancer

Arsenical Keratoses

Arsenical keratoses are lesions that arise after many years of exposure to arsenic. These lesions may occur anywhere on the skin surface, but seem to have a predilection for the palms and soles. In this location, they are heaped-up masses of keratin that appear as small horns. Individual lesions do not commonly degenerate into squamous cell carcinomas. Their major importance lies in the recognition that the patient has been exposed to toxic quantities of arsenic and should be examined for underlying malignancies.

Actinic Keratoses

Actinic keratoses are sun-induced premalignant lesions. As the name implies, these lesions occur exclusively on areas exposed to solar radiation and exist for extended periods without degenerating into frank malignancy. However, because of their propensity to become squamous cell carcinomas, treatment during an early phase is warranted. Individual lesions of actinic keratoses are rough-textured, red, slightly scaly, and flat. Having a sandpaper texture, they are usually more discernible to the touch than to visualization.

Numerous modalities are available for the treatment of actinic keratoses, but the 2 most commonly used are topical 5-FU and surgical curettage. A new modality for the treatment of these lesions is on the horizon: topical and systemic derivatives of vitamin A may aid in maintaining the proper differentiation state of squamous epithelium. In this case, treatment with these agents may cause them to remit, prevent them from occurring, or prevent additional malignant degeneration.

Actinic Cheilitis

Actinic cheilitis, best thought of as actinic keratosis of the semimucous membrane of the lip, is a precursor to squamous cell carcinoma of the lip. It occurs exclusively in individuals who have had heavy solar exposure. Because solar radiation is from above, the lower lip is involved more often than the upper.

Clinically, actinic cheilitis presents as a slightly red, enlarged, scaly, fissured lower lip. The border between the lip and the glabrous skin is frequently white, denoting an abnormal production of keratin. When erosions and ulcerations are present, one should think more seriously of squamous cell carcinoma. The histology of actinic cheilitis is identical to that of actinic keratoses. Solar degeneration of the supporting tissues in the papillary dermis is present, and within the epidermis are seen disorder of the keratinizing cells, anaplasia of nuclei, and areas of keratinization not commonly present in the vermilion surface. More careful scrutiny, including step-sectioning of these lesions, is warranted because the prognosis of squamous cell carcinoma of the lip is worse than that for squamous cell carcinoma in other sun-induced areas. This lesion is ideally managed by carbon dioxide laser ablation. The procedure is well tolerated and the cosmetic results are superb.

Leukoplakia

Leukoplakia is a white patch occurring on a mucous membrane. On biopsy, this white patch displays epidermal hypertrophy. The white area demonstrates that the mucous membrane in this area is producing keratin, a product it does not normally produce. Keratin, when saturated with water, increases in volume and becomes opalescent. Beyond this clinical and histologic description, leukoplakia represents a cutaneous response to a number of exogenous stimuli. It may represent a benign, premalignant, or malignant lesion. Friction-producing habits such as cheek biting produce a benign form of leukoplakia, whereas tobacco use produces a premalignant form. In the vagina, senile atrophy with alteration in the volume of friction-fighting fluids can induce leukoplakia.

Despite its existence as a clinical entity, it would be convenient to limit the term leukoplakia to lesions in which histological observation reveals the generation of atypical epidermal cells. Using this limited, not yet accepted definition, about 6–13% of leukoplakic areas become malignant. As with actinic cheilitis, malignancy in this area is more aggressive than malignancy occurring on solar-damaged glabrous skin.

Cutaneous Horn

Cutaneous horn is a clinical diagnosis. It represents an accretion of keratinous material above a keratin-producing lesion. Four common keratin-producing lesions may be found at the base of a cutaneous horn: actinic keratosis, squamous cell carcinoma, verruca vulgaris, and seborrheic keratosis. From this list, it is apparent that both benign and malignant lesions may produce enough horn to develop the same clinical characteristics. It is therefore mandatory and cosmetically enhancing to remove and biopsy all cutaneous horns. After histological identification of the parental pathogenic process, appropriate additional therapy can be undertaken.

Melanoma

Melanoma is a malignancy of pigment-producing cells distributed in the skin, mucous membranes, retina, and meninges. Although this lesion accounts for only a small percentage of total skin cancer, it is responsible for nearly all the deaths from skin cancer and an undue proportion of all cancers. About 25% of all patients diagnosed with melanoma will die of their disease. The rate of increase of malignant melanoma in our society is nearly as great as that for lung cancer. If this progression is unchecked, nearly 1 in 100 people will acquire melanoma by the year 2000.[4,5] Despite this gloom, >95% of all melanomas that are detected early can be cured. It is of paramount importance to disseminate to physicians and to the population at large the diagnostic parameters required for early recognition.

Etiology, Types, and Appearance

Epidemiological evidence has accrued indicating that sun exposure plays a significant role in the generation of melanoma. First of all, there is an increased incidence of melanoma as a susceptible population moves closer to the equator. By definition, a susceptible population has fairer skin and is therefore more susceptible to sunburn. This includes individuals with type 1 or 2 skin and excludes individuals with type 5 or 6 skin. In keeping with the skin type, patients with melanoma frequently report incidents of severe blistering sunburn as children. The severity of sunburn is enhanced by the solar phenomenon referred to as the sunspot. Following sunspots, an increased amount of UV radiation reaches the earth's surface; 2 to 4 yr after a sunspot, the incidence of melanoma reaches a peak. Melanoma occurs more frequently on sun-exposed or partially sun-exposed areas of the skin. Only areas that are covered with a double layer of clothing (e.g., swimming/sunbathing attire) have sufficiently less solar damage to decrease the frequency with which melanoma occurs in these areas. The incidence of melanoma increases as mankind exposes more of his cutaneous anatomy to the ravages of sunlight. In coastal regions, where leisure activity typically involves such exposure, the incidence of melanoma is higher than in inland areas.

It is assumed that the mechanism by which sunlight induces malignant changes of the melanocyte is similar to that producing other sun-induced tumors. The probability that a malignant hit of UV radiation will occur on a melanocyte is probably inversely proportional to the frequency with which that cell coats its nucleus with a large number of fully developed UV-absorbing melanosomes. With lighter skin types, the pigment barrier surrounding the nucleus is more transparent. Clinical signs of sunburn are indicators that UV exposure has exceeded the skin's potential to develop a melanosome barrier. It is a bizarre indicator of man's failure to understand his future that as individuals we value the cosmetic effect of today's tan over the avoidance of tomorrow's cutaneous malignancy.

Melanoma is a pigmented lesion (a rare unpigmented variety is referred to as amelanotic melanoma). Its color range includes brown, dark brown, black, blue, red, and white. Very frequently, more than a single color is present within the lesion. Although these lesions may begin with the same external dimension as the average nevus, they are frequently larger when initially recognized. Rarely are they smaller than 4–5 mm in diameter in their initial size, but they grow to be large, extending to 4–5 cm. Close scrutiny of the surface of the melanoma frequently reveals that normal skin markings have been effaced. With progression, it is common that small hills and valleys demark the surface topography. With time, both tumors and erosions occur. It is difficult to assess the exact border of a melanoma as it oozes its malignancy into surrounding normal skin. It is rarely regular in shape, demonstrating a penchant for an angular, irregular edge. Patients frequently will report some symptomatology associated with early melanomas—e.g., itching or some nondescript sensation that draws attention. Additionally, the patient may report that the lesion grew or appeared in a short time. Despite this rapidity of appearance, lesions may linger at 1 stage or another of this slow and relentless growth for years.

Three forms of melanoma can be described by clinical appearance: superficial spreading melanoma, nodular melanoma, and lentigo maligna. Superficial spreading melanoma is a lesion in which the radial growth phase of malignant cells exceeds the vertical growth rate. In this situation, cells from the tumor migrate laterally to increase the diameter of the lesion before they have the ability to descend deeper into the dermis. It is believed that for some melanomas, clones of malignant cells arise that have enhanced ability to penetrate the dermis. Before appreciable lateral spread takes place, these tumors increase in thickness. Clinically, they are referred to as nodular melanomas. Lentigo maligna melanoma occurs on sun-damaged skin. It begins life as a lentigo maligna, a premalignant lesion in which all of the transformed cells are maintained within the epidermis and above the basement membrane. This melanoma may arise as the result of direct carcinogenic effects of sunlight. The lesion becomes melanoma when it demonstrates the capacity of individual cells to penetrate the basement membrane, one of the hallmarks of malignant cells that normally live within the epidermis (see chapter 11, figure 11-91).

Prognosis and Staging

Once melanoma is found, there are defined guidelines for predicting prognosis of the host/tumor interaction. The 6 widely accepted indicators are: thickness of the primary tumor, location, presence of ulceration, mitotic rate, presence of a lymphocytic response, and the clinical or microscopic presence of metastases to regional lymph nodes. Survival from melanoma can be stratified most readily by the single prognostic indicator, thickness of the primary tumor.[6] Thickness is determined by measuring distance from the granular zone of the epidermis to the deepest malignant cell. For lesions <0.76 mm in thickness, the survival rate after simple excision is 85–98%. By contrast, lesions that measure >3 mm have a survival rate of <50%. Adding the location of the lesion also influences stratification for lesions of comparable thickness. Lesions on the head and neck have the worst prognosis, and those on the limbs have a better prognosis than those on the trunk. Lesions that are ulcerated or have high mitotic indexes also have a poor prognosis. Both of these are indicators of rapid-growth tumor cells. Lesions that have an increased lymphocytic response tend to do better than those without one. When regional metastases to lymph nodes are present, regardless of the thickness of the primary lesion, survival rates are very poor. Only about 30% of patients with regional lymph node metastasis survive 5 yr, and <10% reach the 10-yr mark.[7] For this reason, clinical staging at time of diagnosis is important in melanoma patients. Staging workup should include a careful examination of the patient's skin over the whole body for other primary sites or the presence of satellite lesions. In 12% of cases, white areas on the skin can be recognized in the vicinity of the melanoma lesions; they are indicative of spontaneous regression.[8] All sites of possible lymph node enlargement should be carefully examined, and the following procedures should be performed: chest radiogram completed by a CT scan of the chest in case of suspicious lesions; blood chemistry profiles and a gallium-67 citrate scan, which could detect occult metastases in sites other than brain or bones;[9] CT scan of the pelvis and abdomen and bi-pedal lymphangiogram, which can detect para-aortic lymph node enlargement.

Based on data so assembled, patients can be staged according to a relatively simple clinical staging system that recognizes 3 stages. Stage I, with local disease, has only 4 substages: A—when only the primary lesion is present; B—when there is a primary and a satellite lesion within a 5-cm radius from the primary; C—when there is local recurrence within a 5-cm radius from a resected primary; and D—when skin metastases are located >5 cm from the primary site but within the primary lymphatic drainage area. Stage II is defined by the presence of regional lymph node metastases, and stage III indicates the presence of distant metastases, including those in lymph nodes beyond the regional drainage.

Table 46-1. TNM Classification of Malignant Melanoma

Primary tumor (PT)

pTX	Primary tumor cannot be assessed
pT0	No evidence of primary tumor
pTis	Melanoma *in situ* (atypical melanocytic hyperplasia, severe malanocytic dysplasia), not an invasive lesion (Clark's level I)
pT1	Tumor 0.75 mm or less in thickness; invades the papillary dermis (Clark's level II)
pT2	Tumor >0.75 mm but not >1.5 mm in thickness and/or invades to papillary-reticular dermal interface (Clark's level III)
pT3	Tumor >1.5 mm but not >4 mm in thickness and/or invades the reticular dermis (Clark's level IV)
pT3a	Tumor >1.5 mm but not >3 mm in thickness
pT3b	Tumor >3 mm in thickness but not >4 mm in thickness
pT4	Tumor >4 mm in thickness and/or invades the subcutaneous tissue (Clark's level V) and/or satellite(s) within 2 cm of the primary tumor
pT4a	Tumor >4 mm in thickness and/or invades the subcutaneous tissue
pT4b	Satellite(s) within 2 cm on the primary tumor

Regional lymph nodes (N)

NX	Regional lymph nodes cannot be assessed
N0	No regional lymph node metastasis
N1	Metastasis >3 cm in greatest dimension in any regional lymph node(s) and/or in-transit metastasis
N2a	Metastasis >3 cm in greatest dimension in any regional lymph node(s)
N2b	In-transit metastasis
N2c	Both N2a and N2b

Distant metastasis (M)

MX	Presence of distant metastasis cannot be assessed
M0	No distant metastasis
M1	Distant metastasis
M1a	Metastasis in skin or subcutaneous tissue or lymph node(s) beyond the regional lymph nodes
M1b	Visceral metastasis

Stage Grouping	
I	pT1, N0, M0
	pT2, N0, M0
II	pT3, N0, M0
III	pT4, N0, M0
	Any pT, N1, N2, M0
IV	Any pT, Any N, M1

A cumbersome TNM pathologic staging system was also developed (table 41-1), but is generally not used for practical purposes. The clinical staging helps design the appropriate therapeutic plan.

Treatment

Only the early surgical treatment of the primary lesion (stage I disease) is generally curative. After an initial biopsy has established the diagnosis, a wide excision followed by split-thickness skin grafting is the recommended procedure. According to the thickness of the primary lesion, various sizes of borders beyond the clinically apparent tumor have been proposed. These borders grow smaller each year, and through the years have changed according to the regional anatomical distribution. These data indicate that small lesions do well even with borders as small as 3–5 mm, whereas larger lesions do poorly regardless of how much skin the surgeon is able to excise.[20]

Radiation therapy (XRT) was found in a few studies to be occasionally effective in the treatment of primary lesions located at unresectable anatomic sites. However, only in patients with stage I lentigo maligna was XRT found to give results similar to surgery and prove satisfactory as an alternative treatment.[10]

In patients with stage II disease, lymph node dissection is the recommended procedure in addition to the wide excision of the primary lesion. It leads to cure in a small fraction of stage II patients (13–39% 5-yr survival). For patients who are not cured, lymphadenectomy of the involved chains prevents later complications (pain, ulceration, functional disability) due to the rapid growth of the involved nodes.

The role of lymph node dissection for stage I disease is still being debated.[20] The controversy arises from the diversity of results among studies comparing the outcome of wide excision plus regional lymph node dissection with that of wide local excision only. Results vary from a 50% increase in survival at 5 yr to a 19% decrease in survival for patients who had lymph node dissection. Two recently performed prospective studies seem also to confirm the lack of benefit derived from the lymph node dissection in stage I disease.[11]

Adjuvant therapy represented by systemic bacille Calmette-Guérin (BCG) or chemotherapy with dacarbazine (DTIC) (see below) was found ineffective for patients with stage I or II disease after being brought to a disease-free status by surgery. BCG was found effective only when injected intralesionally in patients with stage Ib or Ic disease (satellite or recurrent lesions within a 5-cm radius from the primary).[12]

Regional perfusion with alkylating agents (melphalan (MEL), thio-tepa, or mechlorethamine), applying the technique of isolation perfusion of the involved limb, was found beneficial only for patients with multiple cutaneous metastases in an extremity otherwise not amenable to surgery in patients with stage Id disease.[20]

No curative treatment has been found for patients with stage III (disseminated) disease. Surgery can be used with a palliative role to resect lesions that have a tendency to bleed or to obstruct the bowel or airways only if the disease is not widely disseminated.

Palliative XRT was administered with mixed results to soft-tissue, osseous, visceral, and CNS metastases as well as to bulky lymph node metastases. Melanoma is generally a radioresistant tumor, with a response rate averaging 57% when conventional radiation fractionation with total doses of ≤4,000 cGy were used. Large individual fractions with doses of >400 cGy per fraction up to the same total were found to improve the response rate up to 80% in cases of skin lesions and visceral lesions; however, no improvement was seen for osseous metastases, which generally benefited from a higher total dose of radiation.[13]

Systemic chemotherapy was found only modestly effective as palliative treatment in patients with stage III melanoma.[21] DTIC is the most active single agent for the treatment of metastatic melanoma. At a dose of 150–250 mg/m^2/day $\times$ 5 every 3–4 wk, DTIC has induced an overall response rate of 21%, with a mean response duration approaching 1 yr.

Synthetic nitrosoureas (carmustine, lomustine) and MEL were also found to induce occasional responses. Combination chemotherapy, also including other drugs (vinblastine, cisplatin), did not fare better than DTIC alone. The best and most consistent results have been achieved with the 3-drug regimen of carmustine, hydroxyurea, and dacarbazine (see Appendix), which led to an overall response rate of almost 30% and an average duration of 6 mo.[21]

Biologic modifiers have been continuously tested in this disease because of occasional reports indicating spontaneous disappearance of melanoma lesions due likely to the rejection of the cells by the patient's immune system. However, BCG was not found effective in stage III disease. Alpha interferon was reported to give modest results (6–15% objective responses) of short duration (3–6 mo). Recently, the use of interleukin-2 (IL-2) activated killer lymphocytes (LAK) has led to a 19% response rate (partial and complete remissions) of relatively short duration.[14] This treatment, which causes many side effects, is in the course of being improved. IL-2 alone can also induce partial remissions without as much toxicity.[21]

Overall, therapy for stage III melanoma is poorly effective, with mean survival ranging from 3½ to 5 mo in nonresponders and 9–14 mo in responders.

Precursors of Melanoma

The question of whether melanoma arises anew from any melanocyte or preferentially arises from particular pigmented lesions is of paramount importance. As we now realize that melanoma is curable when recognized at its earliest stages, it stands to reason that recognition at a premalignant level, if such a stage exists, is most beneficial. Three pigmented lesions have been identified as having an increased frequency of degenerating into melanoma: dysplastic nevi, congenital nevi, and lentigo maligna.

Dysplastic Nevus

Dysplastic nevi were originally described by Clark et al as the B-K mole syndrome, referring to the 2 families in which the initial observations were made.[15] Dysplastic nevi can be recognized clinically by their variation in color, irregular shape, increase in size to >5 or even 10 mm, and increase in number and distribution as compared to normal nevi. Typically, whereas a normal nevus is uniform in color, the dysplastic nevus is various shades of brown. The border of a normal nevus is sharply demarcated and either round or oval in shape, but the dysplastic nevus has an irregular border that is not sharply demarcated. Most normal nevi are <5 mm in diameter. Rarely does an individual have more than 40 normal nevi. However, individuals with the dysplastic nevus syndrome frequently have 100 or more nevi. Dysplastic nevi occur most commonly on the back, but are also found on the scalp, breast, and buttocks; normal nevi rarely involve the scalp, breast, and buttocks, but occur most frequently on sun-exposed skin. Individuals with the familial form of the dysplastic nevus syndrome have an increased frequency of melanoma. Individuals with the familial form of dysplastic nevus syndrome and a first-degree relative with malignant melanoma have a lifetime risk of developing melanoma of nearly 100%. The dysplastic nevus syndrome does not always occur in the familial setting, and sporadic cases can occur. In addition, individual nevi on patients whose remaining nevi are of normal appearance and number are now recognized as dysplastic by their microscopic appearance.

Because the risk of developing melanoma in individuals with the familial dysplastic nevus syndrome and even the sporadic form was high, a pattern for evaluating lesions in these individuals was codified. When suspected, an individual lesion should be biopsied in order to establish the diagnosis in the appropriate clinical setting. All members of the family of an individual with the dysplastic nevus syndrome must be examined. It is convenient and appropriate to photograph the entire skin surface in a standard fashion in order to follow the evolution of individual lesions. It has been recommended that the body be divided into 24 sections and be photographed with a 55 mm macro lens at a distance of 2½ ft. Patients should be reexamined every 3–6 mo and any lesion that has changed by comparison with the prior set of photographs should be biopsied. These individuals should pay particular attention to avoiding excessive sunlight, as there is some evidence that UV light plays a role in inducing or facilitating the growth of melanoma. It is not yet clear whether ocular melanoma will occur in greater frequency in these patients, but it seems prudent to have them obtain a routine ophthalmologic examination. Finally, it is of crucial importance to teach these individuals what to look for in examining their own skin surfaces. Weekly examination using a mirror is recommended.

Congenital Nevus

Controversy exists as to whether pigmented lesions present at birth have an increased incidence of evolving into melanoma. These pigmented lesions are present in about 1 in 100 births, and it is estimated that the lifetime risk for malignant evolution is about 6%, as compared with the <1% risk for the population at large. The magnitude of the risk seems to increase with the size of the congenital nevus. Unfortunately, the larger lesions frequently referred to as bathing trunk nevi (because they may cover large portions of the skin surface) are less susceptible to surgical removal.

It is important to recognize that the statistics quoted represent a skewed sample of individuals who return to the physician's office for medical care. A prospective study that follows a population of adequate size is required to determine the real risk of melanoma development in congenital nevi. Most dermatologists today feel comfortable excising congenital nevi whenever possible.

Lentigo Maligna

By definition, a lentigo maligna is a pigmented lesion composed of atypical melanocytes occurring on sun-damaged skin. It represents sun-induced melanoma *in situ*. In this situation, a typical biopsy reveals melanocytes at all levels of the epidermis but not descending below the basement membrane. As previously noted, this lesion supports the concept that sunlight plays a role in the development of malignant melanoma.

Cutaneous T Cell Lymphomas

Lymphocytes normally traffic through the skin. It is appropriate to consider the skin as an immune-associated organ—the abbreviation SALT is used to refer to "skin-associated lymphoid tissue." When malignant degeneration occurs in the pool of lymphocytes that normally recirculate through the skin, the term *cutaneous T cell lymphoma* applies. Several clinical variations of cutaneous T cell lymphomas have been described, including mycosis fungoides, Sézary syndrome, D'emblee variant, and adult T cell lymphoma (ATL). Although these clinical entities are lumped together as cutaneous T cell lymphoma (CTCL), they need not be clinical variations of the same disease. Evidence is now accruing that mycosis fungoides and ATL are distinguishable.[16]

Mycosis fungoides is an arcane descriptive term that refers to the end-stage clinical appearance of this disease, in which large fungating tumors occur. Etiologically, this term (coined by Alibert) is a misnomer because it has no relationship to fungal organisms. However, the term is useful for the practicing clinician in that it depicts an indolent lymphoma in which the malignant cell, a T lymphocyte, accumulates in the skin and, as it divides, changes the surface of the skin from a red patch to a large fungating tumor. Although these malignant helper T cells multiply in the skin, they are present in the circulation at the earliest stage; for this reason, the disease must be considered systemic at its onset. The earliest lesion of mycosis fungoides is atrophic, flat, and pink, with a surface resembling cigarette paper. Scale and crust may be present. Lesions in this stage are referred to as large-patch parapsoriasis or poikiloderma vasculare atrophicans. These lesions are asymptomatic, frequently escaping detection, and are treated as nonspecific eczematous dermatoses that do not respond. With time, the number of malignant cells increases and the lesion begins to elevate, going through a plaque stage to eventually become a tumor. Mycosis fungoides is manageable by the application of nitrogen mustard or by electron beam therapy. It is not yet clear whether either of these modalities cures or even extends the survival of patients with this indolent malignancy. The average lifespan from time of diagnosis varies with the stage at which the diagnosis is made: From the patch stage to the tumor stage, 7 or more years may elapse.

The appellations D'emblee variant and Sézary syndrome refer to clinical presentations of cutaneous T cell lymphomas. For the D'emblee variant, the patient presents without or with a very brief past history of a cutaneous T cell lymphoma in which there suddenly and rapidly appear fungating tumors of the same form found in the end stages of mycosis fungoides. Because this presentation is rare—and the science of understanding and discerning the variants of cutaneous lymphoma is new—the etiology and the proper place of classification of this disease are not yet clear. The Sézary syndrome is the clinical presentation in which a patient with a cutaneous T cell lymphoma presents for the first time or at some stage during his lymphoma with red skin of a generalized nature (erythroderma) and a circulating leukemia of T cells. The etiology of Sézary syndrome is unknown, but it consists of the triad of erythroderma, leukemia, and large peripheral lymph nodes. The leukemic cell is a large, mononuclear cell with a convoluted nucleus. By electron microscopy, this cell is identical to the cell found in infiltrates of patients with mycosis fungoides. Inasmuch as mycosis fungoides patients frequently have a leukemic phase during the end stage of the disease, it was proposed that mycosis fungoides and Sézary syndrome were different poles of the same disease.

In 1981, a new type C retrovirus referred to as the human T cell leukemia virus (HTLV) was isolated from patients who had "Sézary cell leukemia."[17] Because the clinical presentation was consistent with the picture of Sézary syndrome, it became a simple step of logic to assume that all of these cutaneous T cell lymphomas—whether they presented as D'emblee variant, mycosis fungoides, or Sézary syndrome—were all a virus-induced malignancy. This simplistic view has not been borne out by the data. To date, all patients who have been HTLV positive present with a picture that looks like Sézary syndrome, but not all patients with Sézary syndrome turn out to be HTLV positive. No patients with classical forms of mycosis fungoides, with its slow clinical evolution, have been shown to be HTLV positive.[18,19] Therefore, the virus-induced malignancy is now considered a distinct and separate entity and is referred to as adult T cell lymphoma. It is fair to conclude that until the etiology and the initiating pathological event(s) for mycosis fungoides, Sézary syndrome, and D'emblee variant are as well described as for ATL, maintaining these clinical syndromes as separate diseases under the heading of CTCL is appropriate and rational. (ATL is described in detail in another chapter of this book.)

Kaposi's Sarcoma

Kaposi's sarcoma (KS), initially described in 1872 by Moritz Kaposi, is a multicentric malignancy of a cell associated with the vascular system. The malignant cell is thought to be a pericyte, but final proof of this is lacking. Three forms of KS are delineated by the clinical presentation: the classical form, the endemic aggressive form encountered in Central Africa, and the rapidly progressing form seen in some patients with AIDS.

In the classical form of KS, elderly people in a well-defined geographic area are primarily involved. This geographic area extends in its southern pole to the tip of Italy, east to the Turkish border, and north through Russia and Poland to the North Sea, involving all the nationalities that now live in these areas. These include central European Jews, Poles, Russians, and Italians. In these individuals, the onset of the disease begins as subtle purplish patches on the lower extremities. In indolent, slow progression, these lesions extend proximally at all depths from the papillary dermis to the deep fascia, with only the most cutaneous aspects visible. With proliferation, the patches become plaques and the plaques become nodules. These nodules may be friable, bleeding on mild trauma. While the disease is progressing in the lower extremities, it also begins to involve the upper extremities and the entire G.I. tract. Heavily involved lower extremities present with a woody, nonpitting edema that initially may be unilateral but eventually becomes bilateral. Progressive G.I. tract involvement can lead to abdominal pain, bowel obstruction, and bleeding. One cause of death in patients with advanced disease is uncontrollable bleeding from multiple foci in the G.I. tract.

The near-term prognosis in the classical KS is generally good. Patients easily survive for 10 yr and many for much longer. Frequently, elderly persons afflicted with this tumor die from some other cause. If the pace of appearance of new lesions changes and becomes more rapid, then the disease has taken an unfavorable course and the prognosis is more guarded. Death from KS is from progressive pulmonary involvement, G.I. bleeding, or involvement of other viscera, including the spleen and liver. Patients younger than 45 yr at the onset of the disease frequently have a more rapid and fulminant course.

No excellent therapies for KS have been developed. Perhaps the indolent nature, favorable prognosis, and rareness of its occurrence in this classical form have impeded progress in its treatment. Currently favored modalities include low doses of vincristine and/or vinblastine as well as electron beam therapy. Although the tumor is radiosensitive, forms of treatment other than electron beam therapy are doomed to failure because of the multifocal nature of the disease and lack of definable borders. For this disease, whole-body therapy such as chemotherapy or perhaps electron beam are required.

Another endemic area for KS is in Central Africa, particularly the Congo. In this area, at least 13% of all registered cancers are KS. It appears that the Bantus are affected and that interbreeding with the white population effectively eliminates the disease. In Africa, the disease is not limited to the elderly, and even children are afflicted. There is a significant preponderance of males over females, perhaps as many as 10 to 1. Other differences from the classical form of the disease include the high frequency of lymphadenopathy and hepatosplenomegaly and a particularly fulminant course with rapidly fatal outcome. In Africans, particularly in children, cutaneous involvement need not occur.

KS as described in Africa is clinically akin to the disease as it presents in AIDS victims. Recognized as early as 1981 was the clustering of clinically atypical but histopathologically consistent KS in homosexuals. In addition to KS, these homosexual men also had numerous opportunistic infections, including pneumocystis carinii, candidiasis, cryptococcosis, toxoplasmosis, viral hepatitis, and cytomegalic virus infection (CMV). The disease in these individuals is rapidly progressive and fatal. It presents with a few cutaneous lesions occurring most frequently on the trunk, head, or neck, but rarely on the extremities. The cutaneous lesions in these individuals begin as pink macules of irregular but elongated configuration rather than as the violaceous lesions of the lower extremities that are associated with the classic presentation in the elderly. Although cutaneous lesions are few, there is frequently hepatosplenomegaly and always lymphadenopathy in these individuals. High-dose (10–25 million U/m^2 subcutaneously 3 times/wk) alpha interferon (INF-α) was found to be the only agent inducing objective responses in $\leq 40\%$ of patients with epidemic KS. This regimen is generally well tolerated; it induces a flulike syndrome and moderate myelosuppression, but these side effects are transient and rapidly reversible.[22]

The clustering of KS among homosexuals as well as its spread along with other sexually transmitted diseases gives credence to the concept that the disease may be infectious in nature. Its potential spread by an infectious agent is also consistent with its distribution in Africa. Moreover, its genetic localization within particular ethnic groups, including the Bantus, Italians, and Central European Jews supports the concept that this infectious agent is more readily transmissible in a particular genetic background. Studies looking at the histocompatibility (HLA) phenotype of individuals with KS indicate that there is a preponderance of the Dr5 gene allotype in patients with AIDS-associated KS and in the elderly with classic KS. Numerous etiologic agents are being considered as predisposing factors to KS. A viral agent seems the most likely culprit. In this regard, nearly all individuals with KS and AIDS have high titers of CMV. Unfortunately, these data are tainted because nearly all homosexuals have signs of CMV infection. On the other hand, it is true that a high percentage of individuals with the classic KS also have CMV virus. Moreover, in several studies, CMV virus has been isolated from tissue cultures of KS lesions. Unfortunately, these latter experiments are not readily reproducible. Some role for the CMV virus, along with a helper virus, seems reasonable in view of the current data.

Recent studies suggest that the human immunodeficiency virus (HIV) itself may play a direct role in the development of KS.[22] It was found that 15% of the male mice in whom the "tat" gene of HIV was successfully implanted into their germ line developed, at age 12–18 mo, skin tumors similar to those of human KS.[23] It was also noted that established long-term cultures of spindlelike cells derived from patients with epidemic KS were nonspecifically stimulated by lymphokines released from lymphocytes infected by a variety of retroviruses.[24] This would suggest that KS is a polyclonal tumor proliferation in response to paracrine angiogenic signals.[22]

Despite the diversity of clinical presentations, the histopathological picture for lesions of all KS presentations is the same. Initially, these lesions begin as clusters of dilated blood vessels of diverse and bizarre shapes that leak or extravasate red blood cells. Surrounding these incontinent vascular channels are plump, spindle-shaped cells and a mononuclear cell infiltrate. With progression, the vascular channels may disappear; in its end stages, the disease is indistinguishable from other spindle-shaped tumors.

It seems likely that the new onslaught and increasing prevalence of this disease will lead to more rapid progress both in determining its etiology as well as improving therapeutic modalities. Numerous new modalities of therapeutic regimens are currently being tried.

References

1. Kripke ML, Fisher MS. Immunologic parameters of ultraviolet carcinogenesis. JNCI 1976; 57:211–15.
2. Daynes RA, Spellman CW. Evidence for the generation of suppressor cells by UV radiation. Cell Immun 1977; 31:182–87.
3. Mohs FE. Chemosurgery: microscopically controlled surgery for skin cancer. Boston: Charles C. Thomas, 1978.

4. Silverberg E. Cancer statistics, 1985. 1985; CA 35:19–35.
5. Kopf AW, Rigel DS, Friedman RJ. The rising incidence and mortality rate of malignant melanoma. J Dermatol Surg Oncol 1982; 8:706–761.
6. Breslow A. Thickness, cross-sectional areas, and depth of invasion in the prognosis of cutaneous melanoma. Ann Surg 1970; 172:902–08.
7. Balch CM, Soong SJ, Murad TM, et al. A multifactorial analysis of melanoma III. Prognostic factors in melanoma patients with lymph node metastases (stage II). Ann Surg 1981; 193:377–88.
8. McGovern. Spontaneous regression of melanoma. Pathology 1975; 7:91–99.
9. Kirkwood JM, Myers JE, Vlock DR, et al. Tomographic gallium 67 citrate scanning: useful new surveillance for metastatic melanoma. Ann Intern Med 1982; 97:694–99.
10. Storck H. Treatment of melanotic freckles by radiotherapy. J Dermatol Surg Oncol 1977; 3:293–94.
11. Veronesi U, Adamus J, Bandiera DC, et al. Delayed regional lymph node dissection in stage I melanoma of the skin of the lower extremities. Cancer 1982; 49:2420–30.
12. Rosenberg SA, Rapp H, Terry W, et al. Intralesional BCG therapy of patients with primary stage I melanoma. In: Terry WD, Rosenberg SA, eds. Immunotherapy of human cancer. New York: Elsevier, 1982; 289–91.
13. Habermalz HJ, Fisher JJ. Radiation therapy of malignant melanoma. Experience with high individual treatment doses. Cancer 1976; 38:2258–62.
14. Rosenberg SA. Immunotherapy of patients with advanced cancer using interleukin-2 alone or in combination with lymphokine activated killer cells. In: DeVita H, Rosenberg SA, eds. Important advances in oncology. Philadelphia: Lippincott, 1988; 217–57.
15. Clark WH Jr, Reimer RR, Greene M, et al. Origin of familial malignant melanomas from heritable melanocytic lesions. "The B-K mole syndrome." Arch Dermatol 1978; 114:732–38.
16. Brody N. Mycosis fungoides. Curr Concepts Dermatol 1986.
17. Poiesz B, Ruscetti FW, Gadzar AF, et al. Isolation of type C retrovirus particles from cultured and fresh lymphocytes of a patient with cutaneous T cell lymphoma. Proc Natl Acad Sci USA 1980; 77:7415–19.
18. Broder S, Bunn PA, Jaffe ES, et al. NIH conference: T cell lymphoproliferative syndrome associated with human T cell leukemia/lymphoma virus. Ann Intern Med 1984; 100:543–47.
19. Waldmann TA, Greene WC, Sarin PS, et al. Functional and phenotypic comparison of human T cell leukemia/lymphoma virus positive adult T cell leukemia and their distinction using anti-Tac. J Clin Invest 1984; 73:1711–18.
20. Boddie AW. Three unresolved issues in the surgical treatment of melanoma. Oncology 1988; 2:39–44.
21. Legha SS. Current therapy for malignant melanoma. Semin Oncol 1989; 16:34–44 (suppl 1).
22. Kriegel RL, Friedman-Kien AE. Epidemic Kaposi's sarcoma. Semin Oncol 1990; 17:350–60.
23. Vogel J, Hinrichs SH, Reynolds RK, et al. The HIV tat gene induces dermal lesions resembling Kaposi's sarcoma in transgenic mice. Nature 1988; 335:606–611.
24. Nakamura S, Salahuddin SZ, Biberfield P, et al. Kaposi's sarcoma cells: long-term cultures with growth factor from retrovirus infection DD4-T cells. Science 1988; 242:426–30.

47

CANCER OF UNKNOWN ORIGIN

Vladimir Benisovich, M.D.

Cancer of unknown origin (CUO) is a biopsy-proven metastatic tumor without an apparent primary site. CUO and poorly differentiated neoplasms are usually discussed together. Poorly differentiated tumors often are not only of undetermined primary site but could also be of uncertain tissue origin (e.g., adenocarcinoma, squamous cell carcinoma, lymphoma, sarcoma). Cancer of any organ or tissue may present as CUO. Patients with this diagnosis represent an extremely heterogeneous group who often pose problems in terms of workup and treatment.[1]

Pathogenesis and Incidence

Casciato et al proposed several hypothetical mechanisms that could explain the existence of occult primary neoplasms: "(1) unrecognized primary lesions (e.g., on the skin or endometrium) may have been destroyed or removed years before the appearance of metastatic lesions; (2) the primary cancer may have undergone spontaneous regression; (3) the primary cancer may be too small to be detected, even at postmortem examination; and (4) finally, the site or origin might be obscured by the extensiveness of metastases or by the nonspecific pattern of dissemination."[2] It is not clear which mechanism is most common. It appears, however, that the main distinctive features of CUO are: (1) ability to metastasize very early (at a size too small to be detected), and (2) atypical pattern of metastatic spread.

Table 47-1 shows data resulting when Nystrom et al[3] compared metastatic patterns of their patients with eventually discovered primary sites to those of patients with obvious primaries at presentation from a review by Gilbert and

Table 47-1. Percent of Metastatic Involvement: Cancer of Unknown Origin (A) Versus Obvious Primary sites (B)

Primary Site	Bone		Lung		Liver		Brain	
	A	B	A	B	A	B	A	B
Lung	4	30–50	90	34	36	30–50	21	15–30
Breast	33	50–85	66	60	60	45–60	33	15–25
Thyroid	0	39	100	65	50	60	0	1
Pancreas	28	5–10	31	25–40	72	50–70	3	1–4
Liver	31	8	19	20	100	—	6	0
Colorectal	13	5–10	40	25–40	87	71	0	1
Gastric	9	5–10	18	20–30	36	35–50	9	1–4
Renal	66	30–50	77	50–75	33	35–40	0	7–8
Ovary	0	2–6	25	10	25	10–15	0	1
Prostate	25	50–75	75	13–53	50	13	25	2

Metastatic sites (column group header spanning Bone, Lung, Liver, Brain)

Source: Nystrom et al (ref 3)

Kagan.[4] Among patients with CUO who were later proven to have lung cancer, only 4% had bone metastases at the time of diagnosis and 11% at autopsy, whereas 50% of patients with obvious lung cancer had bone metastases at autopsy. In contrast, patients with cancers of the pancreas or liver as the cause of CUO had a much higher incidence of bone involvement (30%) than patients with apparent primary tumors of these organs (10%). When presenting as CUO versus a known primary site, carcinoma of the prostate has a higher incidence of metastases to the liver (50% vs. 13%) and to the brain (25% vs. 2%), but less common bone involvement (25% vs. 50–75%). A random somatic mutation changing the metastatic properties of the tumor could partially explain atypical behavior of CUO. It is unclear, however, whether unknown primary tumors grow more slowly than cancers in general, and if so, why their growth rate is retarded. Primary tumors often remain silent for long periods and apparently proliferate more slowly than metastases.

Clinical and statistical data on CUO are scarce and controversial. Most studies have been retrospective, and criteria for diagnosis vary significantly from study to study.

CUO is not an uncommon problem. According to the tumor registry of the Charity Hospital at New Orleans, its incidence is 13.8 per 100,000 population, and it is the eighth most common cancer.[5] CUO patients account for 0.5–10% of all malignant solid tumors.[5-9] In cancer statistics, about 7% of patients had the diagnosis of CUO, making it more common than hypernephroma, ovarian cancer, or pancreatic cancer.[9]

Males and females are affected equally. Very few patients are younger than 20, and <10% of all patients are 20–39. A sharp increase in incidence occurs after 40 and peaks between ages 60 and 79. The median age is 60—somewhat older than in the general population of patients with cancer.[6,10]

The most common histological types are adenocarcinoma (>40%) and undifferentiated carcinoma (>30%).[5,10] Together, these tumors comprise 74–81% of all cases of CUO and until recently, because it was believed that they had similar natural histories, prognosis, and poor responsiveness to therapy, they were usually grouped and discussed together. During the past decade, it became apparent that undifferentiated cancers represent a different entity and require a different approach[38] (see discussion below). Squamous cell carcinoma accounts for most of the remaining cases (14%). Melanomas comprise up to 5%. Sarcomas, lymphomas, and even leukemias may occasionally present as undifferentiated cancers.

Prognosis

Median survival varies in different reports from 2 to 7 mo, depending at least partially on arbitrary decisions of the authors to record survival from the date of diagnosis versus the date of entry into the study or the date of referral. No difference was seen in survival between patients in whom the primary tumor site was identified while alive and those in whom the primary site was not determined.[6,41] However, patients who presented with metastases to lymph nodes survived longer than patients with metastases to visceral organs.[6,11]

Table 47-2 shows data gathered by Nystrom et al in comparing the distribution of primary cancer sites of patients who presented with CUO and eventually had their primary sites identified with distribution among patients

Table 47-2. Distribution of Primary Cancer Sites: Comparison with Literature and End Results

Primary site	Present N	Series %	Literature %	End results %
Above diaphragm				
Lung	28	18	17	10
Breast	3	2	3	26
Thyroid	2	1	5	1
Parotid	1	< 1	—	< 1
Subtotal	34			
Below diaphragm				
Pancreas	30	20	21	2
Liver	16	11	10	1.5
Colorectal	15	10	7	14
Gastric	12	8	10	5
Renal	9	6	3	2
Ovary	4	3	2	5
Prostate	4	3	3	17
Adrenal	1	< 1	2	—
Subtotal	91			
Other	4	2	—	—
No PCS found at necropsy	23	15	15	—
Total	152			

Source: Newman et al (ref 8)

Table 47-3. Role of Systemic Treatment in Certain Tumors

Curative potential	Lymphomas (non-Hodgkin's and Hodgkin's disease)
	Germ cell tumors
	Acute leukemia
	Ovarian carcinoma
	Small-cell carcinoma of the lung
	Pediatric sarcomas
Effective palliative potential	Breast*
	Prostate*
	Stomach
	Endometrium*
	Medullary carcinoma of the thyroid
	Islet cell tumors
	Head and neck tumors
	Sarcomas

*Treatment solely with hormonal therapy can be very effective.
Source: Robert et al (ref 12)

who presented with obvious primary sites (as indicated in "end results" statistics).[8] The distribution of primary cancer sites in Nystrom's series is very similar to that of the literature on CUO but differs markedly from the "end results." Organs that are readily accessible for physical examination (e.g., breast, prostate) rarely are the source of metastases of unknown primary sites: 2% CUO versus 26% known primary site for breast, and 3% versus 17% for prostate. On the other hand, cancers of the lung, liver, and (particularly) pancreas are much more common among patients presenting with CUO. Colorectal (15%), gastric (12%), and renal (9%) cancers are also quite common among patients with eventually identified primary sites. More than 80% of patients presenting with CUO have tumors that respond poorly to chemotherapy; therefore, most of these patients have a dismal prognosis whether the primary site is found or not. In other words, most patients with CUO are unlikely to benefit from extensive search for the primary site. Despite extensive clinical investigations, primary sites are found in only 11–34% of patients during life; in about 20% of patients, the primary site cannot be located even at autopsy.[3,10,11] However, 10–20% of patients presenting with CUO may have cancers that are curable or responsive to chemotherapy or even nontoxic hormonal treatment. Because the tumors noted in table 47-3[12] can potentially be cured or palliated, their diagnosis should not be missed; in certain circumstances, empirical therapy may be warranted.

Histopathology

Biopsy materials should be reviewed with an experienced pathologist. Depending on clinical presentation, additional pathological and clinical studies can be suggested. At times, certain histological findings may provide additional clues for narrowing the diagnostic possibilities. For example, psammoma bodies are characteristic of carcinoma of the ovary, thyroid, or breast.

Poorly differentiated cancers often can be identified by electron microscopy as squamous cell carcinoma, adenocarcinoma, small-cell carcinoma, melanoma, and so on. In some instances, electron microscopy can further define tumors. For example, lamellar surfactant bodies are pathognomonic for bronchoalveolar carcinoma of the lung and apical terminal webs for adenocarcinomas originating in the gut.[13]

Diagnosis

Electron microscopy and immunohistochemical studies of poorly differentiated specimens often may not only clarify the origin of the tumor but—more important—may also identify treatable or even curable subsets of patients. Antibodies against kappa or lambda light chains and common leukocyte antigen may help in differentiation of lymphomas from other poorly differentiated neoplasms. Positive immunohistochemical stains for alpha-fetoprotein (AFP) or beta subunit of human chorionic gonadotropin (B-HCG) suggest extragonadal germ cell cancer (EGCC).[14,42] The presence of dense core granules, identified either by electron microscopy or immunoperoxidase staining, establishes neuroendocrine differentiation of the tumor. In the near future, panels of monoclonal antibodies may become a useful tool in identifying the primary site or origin of the tumor. Mottolese et al analyzed cytospins of 60 malignant effusions of unknown origin, using a panel of monoclonal antibodies to tumor-associated antigens, and determined the origin of the primary tumor in 87% of the cases.[45] Patients with well- or moderately well-differentiated adenocarcinomas of unknown origin are less likely to benefit from chemotherapy, and electron microscopy, along with immunoperoxidase staining, is less useful.[38] As stated earlier, although adenocarcinomas of the prostate and breast rarely present as CUO, it is worthwhile to consider these sites in differential diagnosis because relatively nontoxic hormonal treatment is available for both malignancies. Metastatic breast carcinoma is also responsive to combination chemotherapy. Serum acid phosphatase[15] and particularly an immunologic marker in the biopsy specimen known as prostatic-specific antigen (PSA)[16] are very useful in the evaluation of males with CUO. Similarly, females with CUO should have their biopsy specimens checked for estrogen and progesterone receptors. Selected currently available tumor markers are listed in table 47-4.[17]

Most serum markers are not specific and may be elevated in many types of malignancies and benign conditions. Only the prostatic fraction of acid phosphatase, prostatic-specific antigen, AFP and β-HCG may occasionally be useful in establishing the origin of the tumor. Carcinoembryonic antigen (CEA) can be elevated in a variety of cancers and nonmalignant conditions. Even when positive, this serum marker does not suggest the primary site nor does it identify treatable cancers. For this reason, this test is not indicated in diagnostic evaluation of patients with CUO. Histochemical staining of tumor tissues for CEA, however, is reported to be useful in differentiation of anaplastic carcinoma of the stomach from lymphoma and poorly differentiated lung

Table 47-4. Selected Tumor Markers

Tissue marker	Diagnostic application
ENZYMES	
Acid phosphatase	Identification of metastatic carcinomas of prostate
Muramidase (hysozyme)	Differentiation of true histiocytic lymphoma. Myelomonocytic leukemias
Histaminase	Medullary thyroid carcinoma. Undifferentiated small (oat) cell carcinoma of the lung
Alkaline phosphatase (Regan lysozyme)	Ovarian carcinoma, other tumors
HORMONES	
Anterior pituitary hormones (ACTH, prolactin, TSH, LH, etc.)	Functional classification of pituitary tumors. Differentiation of pituitary tumors from poorly differentiated neoplasms originating from the ethmoidal and sphenoidal sinuses
Calcitonin	Medullary carcinoma of thyroid. C cell hyperplasia
Thyroglobulin, T3, T4	Metastatic thyroid carcinoma
Pancreatic islet cell and gastrointestinal hormones (insulin, glucagon, gastrin, etc.)	Functional classification of pancreatic islet cell and carcinoid tumors
HCG	Identification of trophoblastic elements in gonadal germ cell tumors. Other neoplasms
Testosterone	Sertoli-Leydig tumors
Estradiol	Granulosa and theca cell tumors
ONCOFETAL ANTIGENS	
α-Fetoprotein	Differential diagnosis and classification of gonadal and extragonadal germ cell tumors. Hepatocellular carcinoma, other tumors
Carcinoembryonic antigen (CEA)	Adenocarcinoma of colon, other tumors
SERUM PROTEINS	
Immunoglobulins	Differentiation of large (B) cell lymphomas from poorly differentiated carcinomas. Differentiation of atypical lymphocytic proliferations from lymphomas. Characterization of multiple myeloma
α-1-Antitrypsin	Hepatocellular carcinoma, gonadal and extragonadal germ cell tumors, other neoplasms
OTHER PRODUCTS	
α-Lactalbumin, casein	Metastatic breast carcinoma. Differentiation of extramammary Paget's disease from other tumors
Myoglobin	Tumors derived from skeletal muscle
Actin, myosin	Tumors derived from smooth and skeletal muscle, other neoplasms
Factor VIII-related antigen	Tumors derived from endothelial cells
Mesothelioma antigen	Differentiation of mesothelioma from other tumors
Glial fibrillary acidic protein	Differentiation of gliomas from other tumors
Keratin	Classification of poorly differentiated squamous carcinomas

Source: Mackay and Ordonez (ref 17)

cancer from mesothelioma.[18,19] Lymphomas and mesotheliomas are always negative for CEA.

In the past, patients without obvious primary sites automatically underwent extensive radiographic investigations, including upper G.I. series, barium

Table 47-5. Results of Contrast Roentgenography

	Upper gastrointestinal tract contrast roentgenograms	Full-column barium enema examination	Intravenous pyelogram	Total
No. cases	218	198	187	603
No. roentgenograms positive for carcinoma	14	17	16	47
No. true-positive	8	9	5	22
No. false-positive	6	8	11	25
No. false-negative	4	6	4	14

Roentgenographically positive study results include all examinations thought to be positive by the radiologist for a primary cancer site. True-positive studies were confirmed by a second procedure or necropsy. False-positive and false-negative results were verified by necropsy. Source: Neumann and Nystrom (ref 8)

enema, and I.V. pyelograms (IVP). However, when ordered without specific indications, contrast radiographs have a very low and misleading yield. This point was very well illustrated by Neumann and Nystrom (table 47-5).[8] In the series they report, only 36/129 patients with eventually proven primaries had an intra-abdominal primary cancer potentially demonstrable by upper G.I. series, barium enema, or IVP. Of these 36 patients, 22 were diagnosed by corresponding contrast studies. The remaining 14 patients had false-negative studies. Furthermore, false-positive results (25 cases), determined postmortem, were as common as true positive results (22 cases). In summary, only a small number of patients have primary tumors capable of detection by contrast radiologic studies. About one-third of these tumors will be missed, and any positive result will have a 50% chance of being false-positive.

Gaber et al found that only the bone scan had a high diagnostic yield in asymptomatic patients (almost 50%) (see figure 47-1).[20] Contrast studies were very useful in the presence of organ-specific symptoms but not in asymptomatic patients. Liver scans revealed abnormalities consistent with metastatic cancer in 20/22 patients (91%) with enlarged liver and elevated serum alkaline phosphatase, in 62.5% of patients with elevated enzyme level but normal physical examination, and in only 5.4% (2/37) patients with normal alkaline phosphatase, regardless of physical examination. In the absence of specific clinical findings, gallium scans, mammograms, and thyroid scans were of no value in locating the primary site.

Presently, most authors believe that a diagnosis of CUO should be made after initial evaluation, including history, thorough physical evaluation, routine laboratory tests, and chest x-ray, rather than after extensive search for the primary site. Diagnostic clues, such as the presence of blood in the stool or urine, may suggest further investigations.

The role of CT body scanning remains controversial. McMillan et al and Karsel et al found that with the introduction of CT scanning, the detection rate of primary sites increased to at least 30%, versus <10% in the pre-CT scan era.[21,22] According to these data, it seems reasonable to perform extensive CT scans on all patients with CUO because of their greater diagnostic yield and

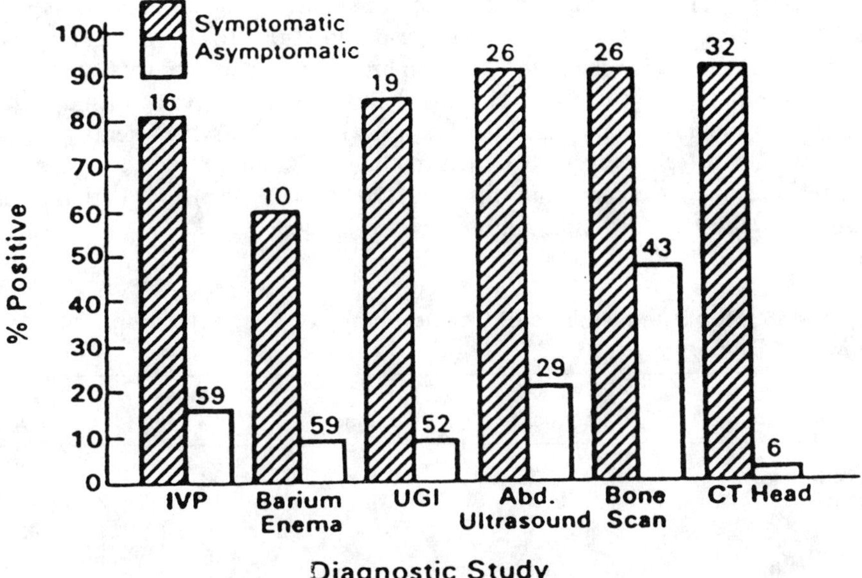

Figure 47-1. Results of multiple diagnostic studies in patients with metastatic carcinoma from an unknown primary tumor. IVP = intravenous pyelogram; UGI = upper gastrointestinal series; CT = computerized tomography. (Source: Gaber et al, ref 20)

expediency. However, others have not found that CT scans increase the diagnostic yield in searching for unknown primary sites.[23,24] Sonography is usually found to be inferior to CT scans in evaluation of patients with CUO.[21,25] At present, the use and extent of CT scans and sonography should be determined on a case-by-case basis.

Treatment

Because CUO by definition is metastatic disease at presentation, chemotherapy is the primary modality of treatment in most cases. A few attempts have been made to create effective regimens combining the drugs with broad therapeutic activity and encompassing as many tumors as possible. Woods et al, in a randomized study, compared a combination of doxorubicin (ADR) and mitomycin-C (MIT) (DM) with cyclophosphamide (CTX) + methotrexate (MTX) + 5-fluorouracil (5-FU) (CMF).[26] They found the DM combination was more effective than CMF, with a response rate of 36% versus 5%. Melliken et al found a similar response rate of 39% to a mitomycin and Adriamycin combination.[47] However, in series reported by Eagan et al, a response rate to this combination was only 7.1% and median survival in all reported groups did not exceed 6 mo.[46]

Bedikian et al reported a response rate of 29% with sequential use of tegafur and a combination of CTX, ADR, and cisplatin (DDP) (CAP).[27] Tegafur is an antimetabolite closely related to 5-FU with broad-spectrum activity, particularly against tumors of the G.I. tract. The CAP combination is active against a variety of cancers, including cancers of the lung, ovary, and breast. Patients who did not respond to tegafur were switched to the CAP combination. The response rate to other reported combinations was ≤20% (table 47-6).[27,28] Patients with a good baseline performance status survived longer.

Table 47-6. Published Results of Chemotherapy of Adenocarcinoma of Unknown Primary Site

Author/reference	Treatment	No. pts.	Response (%)	Overall survival
McKeen	FAM	28	22	?
Woods	AM	25	36	18 wk
	CMF	22	5	7 wk
Moertel	F	88	16	
	F + BCNU	11	18	
	M	9	22	4 mo
	FM	7	0	
Valentine	CAF	14	14	7 + mo
Rudnick	FAM	14	?	100 days
	Control	14	—	90 days
Bedikian	Tegafur CAP	21	29	18 wk
Fiore[28]	VnA	38	16	8 + mo
Eagan[46]	MA	28	7.1	5.5 mo
	MAP	27	18.5	4.6 mo
Milliken[47]	MA	51	39	4.5 mo
	PVB	50	30	6.2 mo

F = 5-FU; A = Adriamycin; M = mitomycin; C = cyclophosphamide; P = cisplatin; Vn = vindesine; B = bleomycin; V = vinblastine
Source: modified from Bedikian et al (ref 27)

In none of these studies was a treated group randomized against a nontreated control group. Because cancers of unknown primary sites are most likely to be cancers of the lung, pancreas, G.I. tract, or kidney, it is unlikely to expect improvement in chemotherapy results unless new effective agents are developed. Until then, it seems reasonable to approach a patient with CUO from the point of view of which responsive tumor he or she may have and to manage the patient accordingly.[12,39] Certain clinical syndromes should be recognizable even without documented primary sites.

About 75% of patients presenting with squamous cell carcinoma in a high cervical lymph node will have primary tumors located in the head and neck area. These patients should have a meticulous ENT examination and multiple directed and/or blind biopsies. CT or MRI scanning of the head and neck may identify submucosal tumor when endoscopy is negative.[1,29] Even if the primary tumor site is not found, radical surgery and/or radiation therapy (XRT) should be considered. The 3-yr survival after local and regional therapy in this group of patients is 35–59%.[30,31,40,43]

About 50% of females presenting with isolated axillary metastases from unknown primary sites were eventually found to have breast carcinoma.[32] A repeat biopsy for estrogen and progesterone receptors may be warranted. These patients should be treated as if they have breast cancer even if mammogram, estrogen and progesterone receptors, and histological examination of resected upper-outer quadrant of the breast are all negative. XRT should be given to the axilla and, if breast cancer is proven, a mastectomy and/or XRT to the breast should also be considered.[1,33]

In a female with malignant ascites of unknown origin, even without a detectable pelvic mass, an ovarian primary site should be suspected, and the approach of laparotomy by a skilled gynecologic surgeon followed by DDP-based chemotherapy is suggested.[37]

In a male under 50 with metastatic undifferentiated cancer involving midline structures, an extragonadal germ cell tumor would represent a treatable condition. Serum and biopsy material should be evaluated for AFP and β-HCG. In a series reported by Richardson et al, all of 12 patients responded to therapy, with complete remissions in 7.[34] In subsequent reports, Greco et al and Hainsworth at al came to a conclusion that not all patients with poorly differentiated cancers of unknown primary site who responded to DDP-based chemotherapy had germ cell tumors.[36,38,44] Other types of poorly differentiated carcinomas, including adenocarcinoma, might also be responsive and even cured with this treatment. The authors recommend that for purposes of treatment planning, patients with poorly differentiated adenocarcinoma should be grouped with the poorly differentiated carcinoma patients rather than with patients with well-differentiated adenocarcinomas of unknown primary site.[38] Patients with poorly differentiated neuroendocrine carcinoma identified either by electron microscopy or immunoperoxidase staining were reported to be responsive to chemotherapy. Major responses were seen in 18/25 patients; 6 patients achieved a complete response. Three patients remained disease-free >24 mo after completing therapy.[44]

In a patient with undifferentiated tumor involving multiple lymph nodes but without demonstrable disease outside the lymphatic system, tumor tissue should be evaluated for the presence of lymphocyte markers, and treatment protocol should include agents active against lymphomas.[12]

Although pathologists often use the term "poorly differentiated lung cancer," neither of the 2 currently available classifications of lung cancer (WHO and WP-L) includes this entity. Poorly differentiated lung cancer is a malignant pulmonary neoplasm that lacks distinctive light microscopic features and represents an unrecognized histological type of lung cancer, including small-cell carcinoma. Because chemotherapy is crucial in the management of small-cell lung cancer, combination chemotherapy active against this disease should be included in the treatment plan.[35]

In conclusion, CUO is a common and challenging problem. Life expectancy of patients is short, and even an extensive search for the primary site usually is unrewarding. In most cases, chemotherapeutic agents have no significant impact on the course of the disease. Maximum information should be obtained from biopsy specimens. A search for the primary tumor should be limited, prudent, expeditious, and directed mainly at identifying tumors with treatable or palliative potential. In certain clinical situations, empiric therapeutic trials for potentially responsive tumors are warranted.

References

1. Ultmann JE, Phillips TL. Cancer of unknown primary site. In: DeVita VT, Helman S, Rosenberg SA, eds. Cancer: Principles and practice of oncology. 3rd ed. Philadelphia: Lippincott, 1989; 1941–52.
2. Casciato DA, Tabbarah HJ, Rice DH. Metastases of unknown origin. In: Haskell CM, ed. Cancer treatment. 2nd ed. Philadelphia: Saunders, 1985; 225–43.
3. Nystrom JS, Weiner JM, Heffelfinger-Juttner J, et al. Metastatic and histologic presentations in unknown primary cancer. Semin Oncol 1977; 4:53–58.
4. Gilbert HA, Kagan AR. Metastases: Incidence, detection and evaluation without histologic confirmation. In: Weiss L, ed. Fundamental aspects of metastasis. New York: American Elsevier, 1976; 385–405.
5. Krementz ET, Cerise EJ. Metastatic lesions of undetermined source. Hosp Med 1970; 6:91–112.
6. Stewart JF, Tattersal MH, Woods RL, et al. Unknown primary adenocarcinoma: incidence of over investigation and natural history. Br Med J 1979; 1:1530–33.
7. Holmes FF, Fouts TL. Metastatic cancer of unknown primary site. Cancer 1970; 26:816–20.
8. Neumann KH, Nystrom JS. Metastatic cancer of unknown origin: nonsquamous cell type. Semin Oncol 1982; 9:427–34.
9. Silverberg E. Cancer statistics, 1982. CA 1982; 32:15–31.
10. Didolkar FN, Elias FG, Moore RH. Metastatic carcinomas from occult primary tumors: a study of 254 patients. Ann Surg 1977; 186:625–30.
11. Moertel CG. Adenocarcinoma of unknown origin. Ann Intern Med 1979; 91:646–47.
12. Robert NJ, Garnick MB, Frei E III. Cancers of unknown origin: current approaches and future perspectives. Semin Oncol 1982; 9:526–31.
13. Dvorak AM, Monahan RA. Metastatic adenocarcinoma of unknown primary site. Arch Pathol Lab Med 1982; 106:21–24.
14. Greco FA, Oldham RK, Fer MF. The extragonadal germ cell cancer syndrome. Semin Oncol 1982; 9:448–55.
15. Watson RA, Tang DB. The predictive value of prostatic acid phosphatase as a screening test for prostatic cancer. N Engl J Med 1980; 303:497–99.
16. Nadji M, Tabei SZ, Castro A, et al. Prostatic specific antigen: an immunohistologic marker for prostatic neoplasms. Cancer 1981; 48:1229–32.
17. Mackay B, Ordonez NG. The role of the pathologist in the evaluation of poorly differentiated tumors. Semin Oncol 1982; 9:396–415.
18. Ejeckam GC, Huang SN, McCaughey WTE, et al. Immunohistopathologic study on carcinoembryonic antigen (CEA)-like material and immunoglobulin A in gastric malignancies. Cancer 1979; 44:1606–14.
19. Wang, NS, Huang SN, Gold P. Absence of carcinoembryonic antigen-like material in mesothelioma: an immunohistochemical differentiation from other lung cancers. Cancer 1979; 44:937–43.
20. Gaber AO, Rice P, Eaton C, et al. Metastatic malignant disease of unknown origin. Am J Surg 1983; 145:493–97.
21. McMillan JH, Levine E, Stephens RH. Computed tomography in the evaluation of metastatic adenocarcinoma from an unknown primary site. A retrospective study. Radiology 1982; 143:143–46.
22. Karsell PR, Sheedy PF, O'Connell J. Computed tomography in search of cancer of unknown origin. JAMA 1982; 248:340–43.
23. Schildt RA, Kennedy PS, Chen TT, et al. Management of patients with metastatic adenocarcinoma of unknown origin: a Southwest Oncology Group study. Cancer Treat Rep 1983; 67:77–79.
24. Vannetzel J, Aymard A, Colbert N, et al. Scanographie abdominale dans les adenocarcinomes metastases de siege primitif inconnu. Results d'une etude prospective. La Presse Medicale 1985; 14:1612.
25. Kamin PD, Bernadino ME, Wallace S, et al. Comparison of ultrasound and CT in detection of pancreatic malignancy. Cancer 1980; 46:2410–12.

26. Woods RL, Fox RM, Tattersall MHN, et al. Metastatic adenocarcinoma of unknown primary site: a randomized study of two combination chemotherapy regimens. N Engl J Med 1980; 303:87–89.

27. Bedikian AY, Bodey GP, Valdivieso M, Burgess MA. Sequential chemotherapy for adenocarcinoma of unknown primary. Am J Clin Oncol (CCT) 1983; 6:219–24.

28. Fiore JJ, Kelsen DP, Gralla RJ, Casper ES, et al. Adenocarcinoma of unknown primary origin: treatment with vindesine and doxorubicin. Cancer Treat 1985; 69:591–94.

29. Muraki AS, Mancuso AA, Harnsberger HR. Metastatic cervical adenopathy from tumors of unknown origin: the role of computed tomography. Radiology 1984; 152:749–53.

30. Coker DD, Casterline PF, Chamber RG, et al. Metastases to lymph nodes of the head and neck from an unknown primary site. Am J Surg 1977; 134:517–22.

31. Fitzpatrick PJ, Kotalik JF. Cervical metastases from an unknown primary tumor. Radiology 1974; 110:659–63.

32. Copeland EM, McBride CM. Axillary metastases from unknown primary sites. Ann Surg 1973; 178:25–27.

33. Feigenberg Z, Zer M, Dintsman M. Axillary metastases from an unknown primary source: a diagnostic and therapeutic approach. Isr J Med Sci 1976; 12:1153–58.

34. Richardson RL, Schonmacher RA, Fer MF, et al. Unrecognized extragonadal germ cell cancer syndrome. Ann Intern Med 1981; 94:181–86.

35. Fer MF, Sherwin SA, Oldham RK, Greco FA, Matthews MJ. Poorly differentiated lung cancer. Semin Oncol 1982; 9:456–66.

36. Greco FA, Vaughn WK, Hainsworth JD. Advanced poorly differentiated carcinoma of unknown primary site: recognition of a treatable syndrome. Ann Intern Med 1986; 104:547–53.

37. Strnad MC, Grosh WW, Baxter J, Burnett LS, et al. Peritoneal carcinomatosis of unknown primary site in women. A distinctive subset of adenocarcinoma. Ann Intern Med 1989; 111:213–17.

38. Greco FA, Hainsworth JD. The management of patients with adenocarcinoma and poorly differentiated carcinoma of unknown primary site. Semin Oncol 1989; 16:116–22.

39. Sporn JR, Greenberg BR. Empiric chemotherapy in patients with carcinoma of unknown primary site. Am J Med 1990; 88:49–55.

40. Bataini JP, Rodriguez J, Jaulerry C, et al. Treatment of metastatic neck nodes secondary to an occult epidermoid carcinoma of the head and neck. Laryngoscope 1987; 97:1080–84.

41. Le Chevalier T, Cvitkovic E, Caille P, et al. Early metastatic cancer of unknown primary origin at presentation. A clinical study of 302 consecutive autopsied patients. Arch Intern Med 1988; 148:2035–39.

42. Kirsten F, Chi CH, Leary JA, et al. Metastatic adeno or undifferentiated carcinoma from an unknown primary site—natural history and guidelines for identification of treatable subsets. Q J Med 1987; 62:143–61.

43. De Braud F, Heilbrun LK, Ahmed K, et al. Metastatic squamous cell carcinoma of an unknown primary localized to the neck. Advantages of an aggressive treatment. Cancer 1989; 64:510–15.

44. Hainsworth JD, Johnson DH, Greco AF. Poorly differentiated neuroendocrine carcinoma of unknown primary site. A newly recognized clinicopathologic entity. Ann Intern Med 1988; 109:364–71.

45. Mottolese M, Venturo I, Donnorso RP, et al. Use of selected combinations of monoclonal antibodies to tumor associated antigens in the diagnosis of neoplastic effusions of unknown origin. Eur J Cancer Clin Oncol 1988; 24:1277–84.

46. Eagan RT, Therneau TM, Rubin J, et al. Lack of value for cisplatin added to mitomycin-doxorubicin combination chemotherapy for carcinoma of unknown primary site. Am J Clin Oncol 1987; 10:82–85.

47. Milliken ST, Tattersall NHM, Woods RL, et al. Metastatic adenocarcinoma of unknown primary site. A randomized study of two combination chemotherapy regimens. Eur J Cancer Clin Oncol 1987; 23:1645–48.

48

PEDIATRIC MALIGNANCIES

Sreedhar P. RAO, M.D.

MALIGNANT DISORDERS ARE SECOND only to trauma as a cause of death in children over the age of 1 yr.[1] The types of cancer seen in children differ markedly from those seen in adults. Whereas carcinomas comprise the bulk of adult cancer, leukemias, lymphomas, and embryonal sarcomas account for most cancer in children. Significant advances made in the field of pediatric oncology during the past 2 decades have resulted in a greatly improved prognosis for several forms of childhood cancer, most notably Wilms' tumor, acute lymphoblastic leukemia, rhabdomyosarcoma, Hodgkin's disease, and

Table 48-1. Major Malignancies (as a Percent of Total) in Children Under 15 by Site and Race, SEER Program 1973–76

Type and site of cancer	White (%)	Black (%)
Leukemia	30.9	24.1
Central nervous system	18.3	21.6
Lymphoma	13.8	11.3
Neuroblastoma	7.8	7.2
Soft-tissue	6.2	8.6
Kidney	5.8	9.0
Bone	4.7	3.6
Retinoblastoma	2.5	4.1
Germ cell	2.0	3.6
Liver	1.3	
Melanoma	1.0	0.05
Miscellaneous	5.7	6.4

Source: Young et al (ref 2)

non-Hodgkin's lymphomas. Improvements in the outcome of childhood cancer have come from the application of a multidisciplinary team approach that uses the skills of the pediatrician, pediatric oncologist, pediatric surgeon, diagnostic radiologist, pathologist, and the radiation oncologist. Tumors discussed in this chapter are CNS tumors, neuroblastoma, Wilms' tumor, rhabdomyosarcoma, Ewing's sarcoma, retinoblastoma, acute lymphoblastic leukemia, and non-Hodgkin's lymphomas.

Epidemiology of Childhood Cancer

The incidence of childhood cancer varies with sex, race, and geography. Table 48-1 shows the relative incidence of major malignancies in white and black children in the United States.[2]

Variations by Age and Sex

Most cases of acute lymphoblastic leukemia, neuroblastoma, Wilms' tumor, retinoblastoma, and hepatoma occur in children under 5. Hodgkin's disease, non-Hodgkin's lymphomas, and tumors of testis and bone frequently affect children over 10. CNS tumors are seen predominently in 5- 10-yr-old children.

The annual incidence of cancer in the United States is about 12.4 per 100,000 white children and 9.8 per 100,000 black children.[2] Ewing's sarcoma is very rare in blacks. The incidence of childhood cancer is the highest in Israel and the lowest in India. Primary malignancy of the liver is more common in the Far East.

Table 48-2. Environmental Factors as a Cause of Childhood Malignancy

Time of exposure	Carcinogen	Tumor
Prenatal	Diethylstilbestrol	Adenocarcinoma of vagina
	Ionizing radiation	Leukemia
	Benzene	Leukemia
	Alkylating agents	Leukemia
Childhood	Ionizing radiation	Leukemia
	Therapeutic radiation	Leukemia; osteosarcoma; fibrosarcoma; skin, breast, and thyroid cancer
	Asbestos	Mesothelioma (much later in life)
	Cytotoxic agents	Leukemia
	Anabolic steroids	Hepatocellular carcinoma
	Immunosuppressive agents	Non-Hodgkin's lymphoma
	Polyvinyl chloride	Squamous cell carcinoma
	Epstein-Barr virus	Burkitt's lymphoma (Africa) Nasopharyngeal cancer
	Human T cell lymphotrophic	T cell lymphoma and leukemia in adults
	Schistosoma haematobium	Urinary bladder cancer (Egypt)

Source: Miller (ref 3)

Environmental Factors

Several environmental agents have been implicated in the causation of childhood cancer. The latent period can vary considerably. In some cases, exposure to a carcinogen during the prenatal period or early childhood can manifest during adulthood. Table 48-2 lists the known association between various carcinogens and the nature of the tumor.[3]

Several types of chromosomal abnormalities (aneuploidy, deletion, translocation, and increased chromosomal fragility) are associated with an increased incidence of cancer (table 48-3).

Immunodeficiency syndromes, both congenital and acquired, are known also to have an increased incidence of malignancy (table 48-4).[4] Some sporadic congenital anomalies are associated with specific types of malignant tumors (table 48-5).[5]

Recent data have indicated that overall death rates in children fell 50% for leukemia and bone cancer, 80% for Hodgkin's disease, 32% for non-Hodgkin's lymphomas, and 31% for all other cancers between 1965 and 1979 compared with the previous 15 yr. This significant reduction in mortality is attributed primarily to improved therapy and, to a lesser extent, to a decrease in incidence of certain cancers (e.g., leukemia).[6]

Central Nervous System Tumors

Primary malignant tumors of the brain, the second most common form of cancer in children, constitute the largest group of solid tumors in children. Each year, nearly 1,200 new cases are diagnosed in the United States, and the annual incidence is about 24 per million in children under 15.[2] Most childhood brain tumors arise from glial cells and rarely metastasize preoperatively.

PATHOGENESIS AND HISTOLOGY

Although the etiology of these tumors is unclear, genetic factors seem to play an important role. Evidence for this is based on an association of certain brain tumors with autosomal dominant neurocutaneous disorders (neurofibro-

Table 48-3. Chromosomal Abnormalities and Cancer in Childhood

Abnormality	Cancer
Down's syndrome	Acute leukemia
Klinefelter's syndrome	Breast carcinoma
13 q –	Retinoblastoma
11 p –	Wilms' tumor
Translocation 3,8	Renal cell carcinoma
Translocation 4q –	Osteosarcoma
Fanconi's anemia	Acute myelomonocytic leukemia
Bloom's syndrome	Acute leukemia
Ataxia/telangiectasia	Lymphoma

Table 48-4. Association Between Immunodeficiency and Cancer

Abnormality	Cancer
Wiskott-Aldrich syndrome	Lymphoma
Common variable immunodeficiency	Lymphoma
Ataxia/telangiectasia	Lymphoma
Chédiak-Higashi syndrome	Lymphoma
Bruton's agammaglobulinemia	Acute lymphoblastic leukemia
Immunodeficiency post-transplantation	Lymphoma
	Epithelial tumor
AIDS	Kaposi's sarcoma
	B cell lymphoma

Table 48-5. Sporadic Congenital Abnormalities and Cancer

Abnormality	Cancer
Aniridia, sporadic	Wilms' tumor
Hemihypertrophy and Beckwith's syndrome	Wilms' tumor
	Hepatoma
	Adrenocortical carcinoma
Genitourinary abnormalities	Wilms' tumor
Poland syndrome	Acute leukemia
Cryptorchidism	Testicular cancer
Enchondromatosis	Chondrosarcoma

Source: Miller (ref 5)

Table 48-6. Common Primary Central Nervous System Tumors in Children

Tumor type	Percentage
Medulloblastoma	25
Cerebellar astrocytoma	13
Cerebral astrocytoma (low-grade)	23
Astrocytoma (high-grade)	11
Ependymoma	9
Brain stem glioma	10
Others	9

matosis and tuberous sclerosis), a male preponderence in medulloblastoma, and the frequent deletion of chromosome 22 in meningiomas. Patients with basal cell nevus syndrome have an increased incidence of medulloblastoma. Other disorders with an increased incidence of CNS tumors have also been found in association with other primary tumors: adrenocortical tumors, acute leukemia, adenocarcinoma of the colon, hepatoma, and the rhabdoid form of Wilms' tumor.

Tumors in children usually arise in the posterior fossa and in the midline.[7] About two-thirds of tumors in children under 15 are infratentorial, whereas most tumors in the first year of life are supratentorial. The commonest infratentorial tumors are cerebellar astrocytomas, medulloblastomas, and brainstem gliomas. Supratentorial tumors in children include astrocytomas, ependymomas, malignant gliomas, and craniopharyngiomas (table 48-6).

CLINICAL MANIFESTATIONS

Symptoms and signs are related to the location and rate of tumor growth. Slow-growing tumors tend to be very large and fast-growing tumors relatively small at time of presentation. The most common symptoms and signs are related to increased intracranial pressure and/or focal neurological deficit. Clinical manifestations of increased intracranial pressure are headache and vomiting, especially in the morning; rapid head enlargement in infants; sixth cranial nerve palsy; papilledema in children over 2 yr, and nonspecific personality changes (irritability and lethargy). Focal neurological manifestations include seizures, visual and speech problems, and motor weakness.

Physical examination may reveal a large head with bulging fontanelle in infants. In older children, there may be evidence of papilledema and sixth cranial nerve palsy. Prolonged increased intracranial pressure may lead to optic atrophy. Atonia, impaired motor coordination, hemiparesis, and multiple cranial nerve palsies may also be found in patients with cerebellar or brainstem tumors.

DIAGNOSTIC EVALUATION

Development of CT scanning has greatly improved diagnostic accuracy in patients with suspected CNS tumor. This noninvasive procedure is very accurate and is safe. It may demonstrate cyst or hemorrhage within the tumor or metastasis to other parts of the brain. Postcontrast CT scan may also help predict the histological features of the tumor. Slow-growing tumors generally produce minimal contrast enhancement, whereas rapidly growing tumors show greater enhancement due to disruption of the blood/brain barrier.

Cerebrospinal fluid (CSF) cytology may identify tumor cells and serve as a guide to effectiveness of therapy. Lumbar puncture is hazardous in a patient with a posterior fossa tumor and increased intracranial pressure. CSF should be obtained at the time of ventriculoperitoneal shunt or definitive surgery.

A myelogram is recommended for all patients with suspected spinal cord tumor and in all patients with medulloblastoma, even in the absence of neurological abnormalities suggestive of a spinal cord lesion. Nearly a third of patients with medulloblastoma have myelographic evidence of spinal metastasis at the time of initial diagnosis.[8]

Cerebral angiography, EEG, echoencephalogram, and pneumoencephalography are done very infrequently or not done at all.

Medulloblastoma

Medulloblastoma is the most common malignant brain tumor in children, accounting for 25% of cases (see chapter 11, figure 11-5). It arises from the roof of the fourth ventricle and causes early hydrocephalus, resulting in headache, vomiting, lethargy, and ataxia. Males are affected more often than females, and most cases manifest symptoms before the age of 8. The proximity of the tumor to the ventricle leads to metastasis to all areas of the CNS. The most common appearance of the tumor on CT scan consists of a solid, contrast-enhancing midline mass in the posterior fossa associated with obstructive hydrocephalus.

MANAGEMENT

Surgery. The main objectives of surgery are to relieve obstruction to the CSF flow and to remove as much tumor as possible. The extent of tumor resection is judged by the neurosurgeon and findings on CT scan done on the fourth or fifth postoperative day. A myelogram with CSF cytology and bone marrow biopsy and aspiration complete the metastatic workup. Patients may then be staged by T and M criteria (table 48-7).[9]

Table 48-7. Staging of Medulloblastoma by the 'T' and 'M' Criteria

T1-2	Relatively small and noninvasive tumors
T2-4	Tumors >3 cm in diameter with extension into adjacent structures
M0	CSF negative for malignant cells
M1	CSF cytology is positive
M2	Intracranial subarachnoid spread
M3	Spinal subarachnoid spread
M4	Disseminated extracranial metastasis

Radiation therapy. Because of the tendency to spread through CSF pathways, the entire craniospinal axis is irradiated.[10] The usual dose is 5,000 cGy to the posterior fossa and 3,600 cGy to the craniospinal axis. Generally, the dose is decreased by 500 cGy in children under 3 yr. The 5- and 10-yr survival rates are 40–55% and 30–40%, respectively. A Connecticut survey has shown that patients treated at a university cancer center have a better prognosis than those treated in community hospitals.

Chemotherapy. Medulloblastomas are highly chemosensitive due to rapid growth and high mitotic index. The tumor is responsive to vincristine (VCR), methotrexate (MTX), cyclophosphamide (CTX), procarbazine (PCZ), nitrogen mustard, the nitrosoureas, and cisplatin (DDP). The Children's Cancer Study Group (CCSG) and International Society of Pediatric Oncology (SIOP) have completed similar protocols in which patients were randomized to receive standard radiotherapy (XRT) with or without chemotherapy represented by a combination of VCR, lomustine (CCNU), and prednisone in the CCSG study and VCR + CCNU in the SIOP study.[11,12]

Disease-free survival (DFS) was the end point in both studies. Nearly one third of the patients in both studies were T1 or T2. Although no significant difference was noted in DFS between T1-2 and T3-4 groups in the CCSG study, patients with small tumors (T1-2) did significantly better in SIOP study. Patients with normal CSF cytology (M0) had higher DFS compared to those with abnormal CSF cytology or intracranial or spinal subarachnoid disease. The overall DFS was as shown in table 48-8.

Based on the above studies, chemotherapy may not be indicated in all patients with medulloblastoma. Patients with a poor prognosis—children under 4 yr, children with locally invasive tumors (T3-4), and children with positive CSF cytology with or without radiographic evidence of subarachnoid metastasis—should be treated with combined XRT and chemotherapy. A more intensive chemotherapy regimen known as "8 drugs in 1 day" has been used in patients with recurrent medulloblastoma.[13] Nearly 50% of patients showed objective response.

High-Grade Astrocytomas

Astrocytoma usually refers to low-grade tumors that grow very slowly and have low infiltrative potential. The most common location for such tumors is the cerebellum. Surgical resection is the mainstay of treatment for patients with this disease. If not resectable, the eventual outcome is poor because of infiltration into adjacent structures, i.e., the brain stem, diencephalon, and optic chiasm.

High-grade astrocytomas, malignant astrocytoma, and glioblastoma multiforme commonly arise above the tentorium, occasionally in the brain stem, but rarely in the cerebellum (see chapter 11, figures 11-1 and 11-2). Patients may present with focal neurological deficits or symptoms and signs of elevated intracranial pressure.

Until recently, the management of these lesions consisted of surgical resection and XRT. Although XRT produced remission, the recurrence rate was very high, with a 5-yr survival of <20%. In view of the poor prognosis, the CCSG conducted a randomized, chemotherapeutic clinical trial.[14] Following maximal resection of the tumor, XRT to the tumor was delivered (dose 4,500–5,200 cGy, depending on age of patient). Half the patients received the same chemotherapy used in patients with medulloblastoma. At 30 mo, the DFS was 43.8% for the chemotherapy group and 21.3% for the XRT group, demonstrating that adjuvant chemotherapy was superior in the treatment of children with high-grade cerebral astrocytoma. Currently, the CCSG is conducting a study in which intensive chemotherapy ("8 drugs in 1 day") will be compared with a standard chemotherapy arm using VCR + CCNU + prednisone.

Brain Stem Glioma

Brain stem gliomas comprise 10–15% of primary brain tumors in children. Despite their relatively small size, these tumors produce severe morbidity and early death. Although most patients have low-grade astrocytoma at biopsy, most are histologically high grade at autopsy.[15]

The diagnosis of brain stem glioma is entertained in patients presenting with multiple cranial nerve dysfunction, abnormal gait, and cerebellar and pyramidal tract signs.[16] A CT or MRI scan reveals an intrinsic brain stem lesion. Although surgical confirmation of the diagnosis is not always required, it is considered strongly in patients with exophytic or cystic lesions. Brain stem encephalitis, abscess, or arteriovenous malformations are included in the differential diagnosis. At some institutions, all patients suspected of brain stem glioma undergo biopsy. Although the small piece of tissue obtained at biopsy may not be representative of the entire tumor, children with biopsy-proven low-grade tumor have a better prognosis than those with high-grade tumor.

Conventional management consists of corticosteroids, followed by radiation to the posterior fossa. The usual dose is 5,000–5,500 cGy delivered over a 6-wk period. Despite initial response in over half the patients, recurrence is very common. Adjuvant chemotherapy has been tried in a randomized 2-arm study by the CCSG.[16] XRT alone was compared with XRT plus chemotherapy (VCR + prednisone + CCNU). No significant difference was noted in survival between the 2 treatment modalities; the 2-yr survival rates were 22% for XRT and 29% for XRT plus chemotherapy. In another study, administration of preradiation chemotherapy (5-flourouracil [5-FU] and CCNU) followed by XRT with hydroxyurea (HYD) and misonidazole did not improve survival. Currently, studies using hyperfractionation XRT (6,400–7,200 cGy) are in progress. Preliminary findings suggest better response to this form of XRT than to conventional radiotherapy.

Neuroblastoma

Neuroblastoma is a unique tumor that may regress spontaneously. Adrenal neuroblastoma was first described by Virchow in 1964. Cushing and Wolback reported the transformation of malignant neuroblastoma into a benign ganglioneuroma with spontaneous regression of the tumor.[18]

Epidemiology and Etiology

The etiology of neuroblastoma is not known. It occurs in about 9.6 white children and 7 black children per million in the United States each year.[2] Nearly half of the cases are diagnosed during the first 2 yr of life and over two-thirds are diagnosed in children under 5. Neuroblastoma has been associated with fetal hydantoin syndrome, fetal alcohol syndrome, neurofibromatosis, and Hirschsprung's disease. Some cases are thought to be inherited in autosomal fashion.

Although chromosomal localization for a neuroblastoma gene has not been found, nearly 80% of neuroblastomas studied by modern banding techniques have shown chromosomal abnormalities. The most frequently detected abnormality has been deletion or rearrangement of part of the short arm of chromosome 1.

Pathology

Neuroblastoma is a very primitive tumor of the sympathetic nervous system. On microscopic examination, the tumor is shown to have small round cells with minimal cytoplasm (see chapter 11, figure 11-69). There may be rosettelike structures. In some cases, it is extremely difficult to differentiate neuroblastoma from other small round-cell malignant tumors such as embryonal rhabdomyosarcoma, non-Hodgkin's lymphoma, and Ewing's sarcoma. Also, it may be difficult to distinguish metastatic neuroblastoma from acute leukemia. Electron microscopy, culture of tumor cells, and monoclonal antibodies may be helpful in the differential diagnosis. A recently proposed histologic grading system may be helpful in predicting prognosis.[19] Ganglioneuroma is the benign counterpart of neuroblastoma, and the prognosis is excellent. Ganglioneuroblastoma has an intermediate degree of cellular differentiation and variable prognosis.

Clinical Manifestations

The clinical manifestations of neuroblastoma depend upon the age of the patient and the extent of tumor spread at time of diagnosis. The tumor may arise at any location in the sympathetic nervous system and has a tendency for rapid dissemination. Nearly two thirds of patients have evidence of widespread disease at time of diagnosis. The commonest sites of distant metastasis are bone, bone marrow, liver, lymph nodes, and subcutaneous tissue.

Approximately two-thirds of these tumors arise in the abdomen, the commonest intra-abdominal site being the adrenal medulla. Affected children may present with an abdominal mass. In addition, there may be symptoms of fever, poor appetite, weight loss, and bone and joint pain, all indicative of disseminated tumor. Neuroblastoma originating from the paravertebral region may produce symptoms and signs of spinal cord compression if epidural extension has occurred. Early recognition and prompt surgery or XRT are crucial in reducing the risk of permanent paralysis. Tumor arising from the thoracic paravertebral region may produce symptoms of cough or respiratory difficulty or be completely asymptomatic. Usually, the tumor is seen on chest x-ray done to rule out pneumonia. Neuroblastoma arising from the cervical sympathetic chain may produce Horner's syndrome, which consists of miosis, anhydrosis, enophthalmos, and ptosis. Rarely, affected children may present with opsoclonus-myoclonus syndrome or chronic diarrhea. Newborn infants with neuroblastoma may present with rapidly enlarging liver or subcutaneous nodules from metastasis. Metastasis to the retro-orbital area is quite typical in older children, who present with proptosis and characteristic echymoses of the upper and lower eyelids. Pulmonary metastasis is rare in neuroblastoma.

Diagnostic evaluation

Diagnostic evaluation includes the following tests:
* Complete blood count, which may reveal no abnormalities in early stages. However, anemia, thrombocytosis, and disseminated intravascular coagulation with thrombocytopenia have been well described.
* Levels of catecholamines and their metabolites in the urine (elevated in >90% of children with neuroblastoma). Most frequently, VMA (vanillylmandelic acid) and HVA (homovanillic acid) are measured. Serial measurements are helpful to determine response of the tumor to treatment and to detect recurrence.
* In cases of adrenal neuroblastoma, the typical findings on I.V. urogram (IVU) are inferior and lateral displacement of the kidney, with no distortion of the calyceal system (see chapter 10, figure 10-54). Calcifications are often present.
* Abdominal CT scan may be helpful in the evaluation of the para-aortic nodes and liver for metastatic disease.
* Skeletal survey and ^{99m}Tc MDP bone scan detect skeletal metastasis (see chapter 10, figure 10-54). Both should be performed.
* If bone marrow biopsy and aspiration reveal extensive marrow replacement by tumor, it may be difficult to distinguish from acute leukemia.

Urinary catecholamines, electron microscopy, and testing the bone marrow with monoclonal antibodies against neuroblastoma may be useful in the differential diagnosis.

- Elevated levels of serum ferritin, lactate dehydrogenase (LDH), and neuron-specific enolase (NSE) are associated with poor prognosis.

Staging

The following staging system, proposed by Evans et al, is widely used:[20]

Stage I Tumor confined to the organ or structure or origin

Stage II Tumor extending beyond the organ or structure of origin but not crossing the midline. Ipsilateral lymph nodes may be involved.

Stage III Tumor crossing the midline. Regional lymph nodes may be involved bilaterally.

Stage IV Remote disease with involvement of bones, bone marrow, liver, or distant lymph node regions.

Stage IV-S Generally, stage I or stage II disease with metastasis to 1 or more of the following: liver, bone marrow, or skin, but without radiographic evidence of bone metastasis. Majority of patients in this group are under 1 yr old.

Prognosis

Of the several factors identified as having prognostic significance, patient age and extent of the disease at diagnosis are the 2 most important.[21] Generally, patients with stage I or II disease have a very good prognosis, whereas those with stage III or IV disease have a poor prognosis. Patients with stage IV-S disease have an excellent prognosis and may not require antineoplastic therapy. Important among other prognostic factors are site of the primary tumor (thoracic, cervical, and pelvic tumors have better prognosis than abdominal tumors), histopathology of the tumor, serum ferritin levels, and the number of copies of N-myc oncogenes.[22] Ganglioneuroma or ganglioneuroma with few areas of neuroblastoma, normal serum ferritin, and <3 copies of N-myc oncogenes are associated with better prognosis. Spontaneous tumor regression with eventual long-term survival may occur in 7% of all children with neuroblastoma, mostly young infants with stage I, II, or IV-S disease.

Treatment

Surgery. Patients with localized disease should undergo surgical resection of the tumor. Biopsy of regional lymph nodes should be done to accurately determine the stage. Despite microscopic residual tumor in patients with stage II tumor, probably no additional therapy is necessary. The precise role of surgery in patients with stage III or IV disease is not clear. Although debulking of the tumor in stage III patients has been widely recommended in the past, there is no concrete evidence that outcome is any different from that in patients who had only biopsy. An inoperable tumor may become operable after chemotherapy, XRT, or both.

Table 48-8. Disease-Free Survival at 54 Months in Meduloblastoma Studies

Study group	Treatment regimen	Survival (mo)
Children's Cancer Study Group	XRT	49.4
	XRT + chemotherapy	59.5
International Society of Pediatric Oncology	XRT	43.4
	XRT + chemotherapy	56.3

Radiation therapy. Although neuroblastoma is a radiosensitive tumor, the exact role of XRT is not well defined. XRT has not improved outcome in patients with stage II disease even if macroscopic or microsopic residual tumor is present. Despite routine XRT in stage III patients, there is no convincing evidence for improvement in survival. In patients with stage IV disease, XRT is primarily used for palliation.

Chemotherapy. Despite the availability of various chemotherapeutic regimens that have produced excellent tumor response rates, long-term survival has not significantly improved during the past 2 decades. CTX, VCR, doxorubicin (ADR), DDP, dacarbazine (DTIC), and teniposide (VM-26) are all effective drugs with at least a 20% response rate when used as single agents. Several drug combinations have been used (see Appendix). The regimen CTX + VCR + DTIC has produced an overall response rate of 80% in studies conducted by the CCSG (table 48-9).[23] Despite the high response rate, 5-yr survival is still very poor.

A chemotherapeutic regimen based on cell kinetics, developed at St. Jude's Children's Research Hospital, Memphis, Tenn., produced a 70% response rate in patients with stage III or IV disease.[24] The drug regimen consisted of CTX + ADR.

Patients with stage IV-S disease need to be treated cautiously.[21] These tumors tend to regress spontaneously, especially in very young infants. A tissue diagnosis alone may be adequate in the absence of serious complications. Some investigators recommend surgical resection of the primary tumor. These patients should be closely monitored. In the event of symptoms of compression by the tumor (i.e., rapidly enlarging liver), small doses of radiation are recommended.

Patients who present with evidence of spinal cord compression have an excellent survival rate. Emergency laminectomy or XRT is required to prevent neurological sequelae. XRT alone appears to be as effective as surgery.

Because of poor survival rates for patients with stage III or IV neuroblastoma who receive conventional chemotherapy or XRT, several experimental treatment modalities are being investigated. These consist of allogeneic or autologous bone marrow transplantation preceded by XRT and intensive chemotherapy. Monoclonal antibodies have been used to purge the bone marrow of tumor cells.

Sequelae

Neuroblastoma arising from the neck may lead to permanent neurological deficit (Horner's syndrome). The patient with opsoclonus often has residual

Table 48-9. Three-Year Disease-Free Survival in Children with Neuroblastoma

Stage	DFS (%)
I	95–100
II	90
III	50–70
IV	10–20
IV-S	70–75

Table 48-10. Congenital Abnormalities Observed in Patients with Wilms' Tumor

Anomaly	Incidence (%)
Hemihypertrophy or Beckwith-Wiedemann syndrome	3.0
Genitourinary abnormalities	4.9
Nonfamilial aniridia	1.0

neurological abnormalities after the resolution of neuroblastoma. Children with stage IV-S neuroblastoma have minimal or no residual effects. Patients with stage IV disease who survive may have evidence of permanent damage due to tumor, i.e., pathological fracture.

Treatment-related sequelae are a decrease in height and scoliosis due to a combination of surgery and XRT. The immediate short-term toxicity consists of bone marrow depression due to chemotherapy and associated infections and bleeding complications. The use of alkylating agents may also impair gonadal function.

Wilms' Tumor

Wilms' tumor is the commonest malignant neoplasm of the genitourinary tract in children. Among children under 15, it occurs in the United States at a rate of 7.5 cases per million white children and 7.8 cases per million black children.[2] Most cases are diagnosed between the ages of 1 and 5. Occasional cases have been described in adolescents and even in adults.

Associated Congenital Abnormalities

Several congenital abnormalities are associated with an increased incidence of Wilms' tumor.[5] The incidence of congenital abnormalities observed in 547 children with Wilms' tumor enrolled in the first National Wilms' Tumor Study (NWTS-1) are shown in table 48-10.

Several primary tumors are also described in association with Wilms' tumor, notably fibrosarcoma, retinoblastoma, and neurofibromatosis. Deletion of the short arm of the chromosome 11 (11-P) has been reported in several children with Wilms' tumor. When malformations with a known increased incidence of Wilms' tumor are detected, the affected child should be carefully followed until the age of 15. This should include physical examination every 3–6 mo and abdominal ultrasound every 6 mo until the age of 7, then less frequently until the age of 15.

Pathology and Microscopic Features

Wilms' tumor may attain a very large size before becoming symptomatic. Often the tumor tends to grow into the renal vein and inferior vena cava. The commonest sites of metastasis are regional lymph nodes, lungs, and liver; bone and brain are sites of metastases in a few cases.

There is usually an admixture of 3 cellular components: epithelial, blastematous, and stromal (see chapter 11, figure 11-43). These components may demonstrate different degrees of differentiation. Based on a review of a large number of specimens from the NWTS pathology center, 2 distinct subtypes of Wilms' tumor are described: tumor of favorable histology (FH) and of unfavorable histology (UH).[25] Patients with FH Wilms' tumor have an excellent prognosis but those with UH have a poor prognosis. The UH was further classified into (1) anaplastic type, focal or diffuse, (2) clear-cell sarcoma, and (3) rhabdoid tumor of kidney. Clear-cell sarcoma patients have a predilection for bone and CNS metastasis, whereas those with rhabdoid features have a higher incidence of CNS metastasis as well as primary CNS tumors.

Clinical Findings and Diagnostic Evaluation

Most patients present with symptoms of enlarging abdomen or an abdominal mass, usually detected by a family member. Pain in the abdomen is another frequent symptom; microscopic hematuria or hypertension are found in about 25% of patients. Generally, patients with Wilms' tumor appear to be in good health at the time of initial presentation.

Physical examination should include careful examination of the abdomen to determine the nature of the mass and a search for commonly associated congenital abnormalities. The following conditions must be considered in the differential diagnosis: suprarenal neuroblastoma, intrarenal neuroblastoma, mesoblastic nephroma (also known as renal hamartoma), renal cell carcinoma, and cystic kidney disease.

The diagnosis is usually made by excretory urography. The intrinsic structure of the kidney is distorted and the calyceal system splayed (see chapter 11, figure 11-55). Abdominal ultrasound is very useful to determine whether a renal mass is solid or cystic when the kidney is nonvisualized on excretory urography; a solid mass favors Wilms' tumor. Patency of the inferior vena cava can also be determined by ultrasound. In doubtful cases, inferior vena cavography is recommended to confirm or rule out the presence of tumor in the inferior vena cava. Plain chest x-rays and chest and abdominal CT scans are useful in looking for metastasis in lung or liver (see chapter 11, figure 11-56). A skeletal survey, bone scan, and CT scan of the head are indicated if the histology of the tumor warrants such an evaluation.

Table 48-11. National Wilms' Tumor Study Staging System

Group	Description
I	Tumor limited to kidney and completely removed Renal capsule intact No tumor rupture during removal No residual tumor apparent beyond margins of resection
II	Tumor extended beyond kidney but completely resected Renal vessels outside the kidney have tumor Biopsy or local spillage of tumor may have occurred Lymph nodes are not involved
III	Residual nonhematogenous tumor confined to abdomen Lymph nodes at any level are involved Gross tumor spillage Implants found on peritoneal surface Tumor not completely resected because of local infiltration into vital structures
IV	Hematogenous metastasis to lung, liver, bone, or brain
V	Bilateral renal involvement at diagnosis

Staging

Staging is based on operative and pathological findings. The most widely used staging was developed by the NWTS (table 48-11).

Bilateral Wilms' tumor is considered to represent 2 primary tumors and not a metastatic disease. The prognosis for bilateral Wilms' tumor at diagnosis is excellent, with 87% survival in contrast to 50–60% survival in patients with widespread metastases or metachronous bilateral Wilms' tumor. It is extremely important to identify even small tumor in the opposite kidney at the time of initial surgery.

Treatment

Surgery. The first major step in the treatment of a child with Wilms' tumor is abdominal exploration and removal of the affected kidney. A transabdominal route is used. The opposite kidney should be inspected and palpated. Any suspicious lesion, including in lymph nodes, is biopsied. Extreme care should be taken not to rupture the tumor when the affected kidney is being removed.

Radiation therapy. Several critical questions were asked in the NWTS studies pertaining to indications for XRT and the minimal dose required for optimal local control.[26-28] It has been shown that routine postoperative XRT is not necessary for patients with stage I tumor who receive chemotherapy with actinomycin D (ACT) and VCR. Some early evidence suggests that XRT may not be required for stage II patients and that 1,000 cGy is adequate for patients with stage III disease if accompanied by appropriate chemotherapy. However, XRT is recommended in all patients with UH tumors because of a high incidence of local relapse. The field of irradiation includes the original tumor bed as seen on the preoperative excretory urogram. Entire vertebral bodies are irradiated to minimize post-XRT scoliosis.

Chemotherapy. The most effective chemotherapeutic agents are ACT, VCR, and ADR. A combination of ACT and VCR was shown to be more effective than either agent alone. Also, addition of ADR to the above regimen was shown to be better than the 2-drug combination. Current guidelines for chemotherapy of FH tumors are as follows: stage I—VCR and ACT for 6 mo; stage II—intensive combination chemotherapy with VCR and ACT for 15 mo; stages III & IV—VCR, ACT, and ADR for 15 mo. Chemotherapy details are shown in the Appendix, and results of treatment in 1 of the studies are shown in table 48-12.

More effective treatment is needed for patients with UH tumors. Currently, all patients with UH tumors are treated with VCR, ACT, and ADR with or without CTX.

Treatment of Patients with Metastasis

Pulmonary metastasis at diagnosis is not an indication that nephrectomy should be delayed. Postoperative XRT is given to both lungs regardless of the location or the number of pulmonary lesions. A dose of 1,000–1,200 cGy is used. Patients with liver metastasis may undergo resection if feasible, followed by chemotherapy. Those with unresectable tumor should receive XRT and chemotherapy in an effort to achieve resectability.

Renal Cell Carcinoma

Renal cell carcinoma is a rare tumor in children. The tumor is indistinguishable from that seen in adults. Patients present with hematuria, abdominal mass, or pain. Excretory urogram findings are those of an intrinsic renal tumor. Most common sites of metastasis are lung, liver, regional lymph nodes, and bone. Nephrectomy is the only recommended therapy for patients with localized and well encapsulated tumors. XRT is recommended in patients who have residual disease. The role of chemotherapy is unclear.

Rhabdomyosarcoma

Rhabdomyosarcoma is the commonest soft-tissue sarcoma in children and adolescents. Fibrosarcoma, synovial sarcoma, liposarcoma, neurofibrosarcoma, and hemangiosarcoma are the other soft-tissue sarcomas seen in children, with an annual incidence in the United States of 4.5 per million in white children and 1.3 per million in black children.

Epidemiology and Pathology

Rhabdomyosarcoma has 2 age peaks, the first in children aged 2–6 and the second during adolescence. In young children, common sites are the head and neck and genitourinary tract. In adolescents, the male genitourinary tract, the retroperitoneal region, the trunk, and extremities are common sites. Rhabdomyosarcoma has been described in association with neurofibromatosis and

Table 48-12. Results of Therapy in Second National Wilms' Tumor Study

Group	Regimen	No. patients	3-yr RFS (%)	3-yr survival (%)
I	E—6 mo ACT, VCR	106	96	97
I	F—15 mo ACT, VCR	109	90	91
II,III,IV	C—15 mo ACT, VCR	159	65	74
II,III,IV	D—15 mo ACT, VCR + ADR	155	79	84

ACT = actinomycin-D; VCR = vincristine; ADR = Adriamycin; RFS = relapse-free survival

basal cell nevus syndrome. An excess incidence of rhabdomyosarcoma is described in siblings of children with brain tumors and adrenocortical carcinoma.

Three major histological types are described: embryonal, alveolar, and pleomorphic.[29] Embryonal is the commonest type, accounting for nearly 60% of tumors. It is characterized by large numbers of primitive round and spindle-shaped cells with little myoblastic differentiation (see chapter 11, figure 11-66A). Sarcoma botryoides, distinguished by its polypoid appearance, is histologically similar to embryonal rhabdomyosarcoma. Alveolar rhabdomyosarcoma resembles the pattern of pulmonary alveoli, in which tumor cells and multinucleated giant cells line septa and protrude into open alveolar spaces. This subtype carries a worse prognosis than embryonal rhabdomyosarcoma. The pleomorphic subtype is only rarely seen in children (see chapter 11, figure 11-66B).

Recently, a new pathologic classification has been proposed by the Intergroup Rhabdomyosarcoma Study (IRS) in which tumors are classified into favorable and unfavorable types based on cytologic features.[30] Two unfavorable types have been identified: anaplastic and monomorphous round-cell. Nearly 80% of the tumors belong to the "favorable" category.

Clinical Manifestations

The relative frequency of primary tumor sites is shown in table 48-13. Most children present with a mass in the head and neck region or in the genitourinary tract. Orbital rhabdomyosarcoma presents with proptosis and rarely extends into the CNS. Tumors of the middle ear present with ear pain, symptoms of chronic otitis media, discharge from the middle ear, or signs of intracranial extension (e.g., increased intracranial pressure and cranial nerve palsies). Nasopharyngeal rhabdomyosarcoma presents with nasal obstruction, epistaxis, or symptoms of sinusitis. These tumors may also spread to the CNS. Tumor arising from the prostate or urinary bladder may present with urinary obstruction, hematuria, or abdominal mass. Uterine or vaginal tumors present with vaginal bleeding or a polypoid mass extruding through the vaginal opening.

The commonest sites of rhabdomyosarcoma in adolescents are paratesticular, extremity, or trunk, presenting with a painless mass or scrotal swelling. The latter may be mistaken for scrotal abscess, hydrocele, or testicular torsion. Nearly half the patients with a paratesticular primary lesion will have intra-abdominal lymph node metastasis. A retroperitoneal rhabdomyosarcoma usually presents with an abdominal mass.

Table 48-13. Primary Sites of Rhabdomyosarcoma

Site	Incidence (%)
Head and neck	38
Genitourinary tract	21
Extremity	18
Trunk	7
Retroperitoneum	5

Table 48-14. Clinical Grouping System of Intergroup Rhabdomyosarcoma Studies

Group	Description
I	Localized disease, completely resected; regional nodes not involved Confined to muscle or organ of origin Contiguous involvement, infiltration outside the muscle or organ of origin, as through fascial planes
II	Regional disease, grossly resected tumor with microscopic residual disease; no evidence of gross residual disease; no clinical or microscopic evidence of regional node involvement Regional disease, completely resected (regional nodes involved and completely resected with no microscopic residual)
III	Incomplete resection or biopsy with gross residual disease
IV	Metastatic disease present at onset

The tumor spreads via lymphatics and the blood stream. Paratesticular, genitourinary, extremity, and perineal tumors have a much higher incidence of lymphatic spread than orbital tumors. The common sites of hematogenous metastasis are lung, bone, bone marrow, and liver. Nearly 40% of patients with parameningeal primary develop meningeal spread unless given prophylactic therapy. Evaluation should consist of chest x-ray, CT scan of the chest, bone survey, bone scan, and bone marrow aspiration and biopsy. In addition, head CT scan and CSF cytology should be obtained in patients with parameningeal primaries.

The clinical grouping system adopted by the IRS is displayed in table 48-14.[31]

Treatment

Treatment strategy depends on the site of the primary tumor and extent of tumor spread (clinical group). In general, certain primary sites (e.g., orbit and middle ear) are managed with biopsy, XRT, and chemotherapy. Primary tumors of the trunk, extremity, and the paratesticular regions are managed by gross resection of the tumor followed by multiagent chemotherapy.

Surgery. Historically, despite intensive and frequently disabling surgery, local recurrence rates were very high, leading to a low cure rate. Complete surgical excision is now indicated only when it leads to no major functional disabilities. In cases of locally invasive tumor, even radical surgery may not lead to greatly improved survival. If the tumor cannot be resected completely, a biopsy followed by trial chemotherapy and XRT may make the tumor resectable. Lymph node biopsy is recommended for tumors of the paratesticular region, genitourinary tract, extremity, and perineum.

Radiation therapy. Based on the results of IRS-1, XRT is not necessary for patients with group I tumors (total excision without microscopic residual).[32] In more advanced disease, the recommended dose of radiation for microscopic residual is 4,500–5,000 cGy, and for gross residual tumor, 5,000–5,500 cGy.

Chemotherapy. The 4 most effective drugs in the treatment of rhabdomyosarcoma are VCR, ACT, CTX, and ADR. The most commonly used regimens consist of combinations of VCR, ACT, and CTX (standard VAC and pulse VAC) (see Appendix).

Significant refinements have been made in the chemotherapy of rhabdomyosarcoma from the IRS-1 and IRS-2 studies.[33,34] Among relevant conclusions of the above studies: XRT was unnecessary in group I patients if they received VAC chemotherapy; ACT and VCR were as effective as 3-drug (VAC) therapy in group II patients; adding ADR to the pulse VAC regimen did not improve the outcome in patients with group III or IV disease; and intrathecal prophylaxis improved survival in children with parameningeal tumors.[29,31,32]

The relapse-free survival rates at 3 yr were >80% for group I and 63–72% for group II patients. In contrast, 3-yr survival was 54–61% for group III patients and 17–23% for group IV patients. Long-term survival in relapsed patients is extremely poor.

Ewing's Sarcoma

Ewing's sarcoma is the second most common primary malignant tumor of bone in children and adolescents; 75% of these tumors occur before the age of 20. Males are affected more frequently than females (1.6:1). The tumor is rare in blacks. The most frequent primary sites are femur, tibia, humerus, rib, vertebra, fibula, scapula, and sacrum. In extremity lesions, the diaphysis is usually affected.

The patient may present with pain, swelling, tenderness, warmth over the tumor, and fever, or with pathologic fracture following minor trauma. Advanced disease patients may present with pulmonary metastases. Metastases occur in other bones and bone marrow. Nearly a third of patients have evidence of metastatic disease at diagnosis.

Radiology and Pathology

The radiographic findings may appear as roughening of the periosteum, mimicking osteomyelitis. In advanced cases, the entire shaft of a long bone may be involved. Periosteal thickening, associated with laminar deposit and subperiosteal new bone formation, produces an "onionskin" appearance. This particular abnormality is not specific for Ewing's sarcoma. In this tumor, in contrast to osteosarcoma, no ossification occurs. CT scan of the lesion may provide additional details as to extent of bone and soft tissue involvement.

Histological examination reveals an area of necrosis, hemorrhage, and calcification (see chapter 11, figure 11-70). The tumor cells, polyhedral-shaped, are arranged in monotonous sheets. The cytoplasm is scanty and lightly stained. The cells have small nuclei and fine nucleoli. About 10% of patients may show a rosettelike pattern similar to that seen in metastatic neuroblastoma. The cytoplasm of cells of patients with Ewing's sarcoma often has PAS-positive glycogen granules—a very useful feature in differential diagnosis, which includes chronic osteomyelitis, metastatic neuroblastoma, rhabdomyosarcoma, and lymphoma.

Treatment

Once the diagnosis is established after a biopsy, the following studies should be done to define the extent of the disease:
- Complete blood count
- CT scan of the lesion and chest
- Bone scan and bone survey
- Bone marrow aspiration and biopsy
- Tests of hepatic and renal function to monitor effects of therapy.

Surgery. The major role of surgery is to obtain a biopsy for diagnostic purposes. Only lesions of expendable bones are surgically resected for local control (e.g., lesions of ribs or fibula).[35] Patients in whom radio- and chemotherapy have failed to control the local tumor are also candidates for surgical resection.

Radiation therapy. XRT is still considered a major mode of treatment for control of the primary tumor. Megavoltage equipment is used to deliver 5,500–6,000 cGy to the entire bone. Recently, the need for irradiation of the entire bone has been questioned, especially if the patient will receive systemic chemotherapy. There is some evidence that limited field irradiation and concurrent chemotherapy have produced excellent local control.[36] The major contributing factors in satisfactory local tumor control are dose, location of tumor, age of the patient, and treatment method. Prophylactic pulmonary XRT should not be routinely given.

Local tumor control can be achieved in about 90% of patients with a radiation dose of 5,000-5,500 cGy and chemotherapy. Generally, tumors of femur are frequently associated with poor post-XRT functional results as compared to other tumor sites. Pathologic fractures related to a large tumor, large biopsy, excessive weight bearing, or asymmetrical muscle atrophy may occur.

Functional results are less favorable in children under 15, mostly manifested by discrepancy in leg length due to epiphyseal irradiation. The major delayed complications of XRT are joint deformity, fracture, soft tissue and muscle atrophy, and second malignant neoplasms.

Chemotherapy. The major chemotherapeutic agents used in Ewing's sarcoma are VCR, ACT, CTX, and ADR.[37,38] These agents are ususally given concurrently with XRT. Because ACT, ADR, and (to a lesser extent) CTX have a radiomimetic effect, care must be used while administering combined modality therapy. The 2 most commonly used regimens are VAC (VCR + ACT + CTX) and VACA (above 3 drugs plus ADR).

Recently, efforts have been made to avoid XRT in the treatment of patients with this tumor. The strategy consists of presurgical chemotherapy to obtain tumor-free margins at the time of resection. If that is accomplished, the patient will not receive radiation but will continue chemotherapy. However, if the tumor cannot be completely resected, XRT is then administered at a lower dose because of reduction in tumor size.[36]

Despite some controversy, most authorities still consider radiotherapy and chemotherapy as the major treatment modalities for patients with Ewing's sarcoma.

Prognosis

Patients with pelvic primary tumor have the least favorable outcome, followed by patients with primaries of proximal bones. Although rib lesions have been considered to carry a poor prognosis, recent studies have shown >50% disease-free survival. Overall, the 5-yr survival rate for patients with primary tumor limited to the bone and without distant metastasis is about 85%. However, soft-tissue extension or distant metastasis carries a poorer prognosis. In Intergroup Ewing's Sarcoma Study 1, patients who received only VAC without pulmonary irradiation had a higher incidence of pulmonary metastasis. The addition of ADR to VAC decreased the incidence of pulmonary metastasis in nonirradiated patients.

Retinoblastoma

Retinoblastoma is the most common intraocular tumor of childhood, accounting for nearly 3% of all childhood cancer.

Incidence and Genetic Factors

The incidence of retinoblastoma is estimated to be 11 per million children under age 5; about 200–300 new cases are diagnosed each year in the United States.[39] There is no significant difference in its incidence between whites and blacks or boys and girls. More than 90% of the cases are diagnosed in children under 5.

Despite a strong genetic implication for developing retinoblastoma, nearly 90% of affected patients do not have a positive family history for the tumor.[40] These cases probably represent the first mutation within a family. About 20–25% of genetically inherited tumors are associated with a deletion in the q14 band of chromosome 13.[41] Whereas the deletion is seen in all the cells in genetic retinoblastoma patients, it is seen only in tumor cells of nongenetic retinoblastoma. Half of the offspring of patients with genetic retinoblastoma are affected. The gene for retinoblastoma, located in the region of 13q14 of chromosome 13, is closely linked to the genetic locus for esterase D. Genetic linkage analysis is being done to attempt the prenatal diagnosis and presymptomatic diagnosis.

Clinical features

The most common symptoms and signs are leukokoria (white pupil), strabismus, glaucoma, and impaired vision. Occasionally, children present with orbital cellulitis, unilateral dilated pupil, hyphema, and nystagmus. A distinct clinical syndrome has been described consisting of microcephaly, broad nasal bridge, microphthalmia, hypertelorism, epicanthal folds, ptosis, micrognathia, low-set ears, and thumb abnormalities in association with retinoblastoma and deletion of the long arm of chromosome 13. The tumor may spread locally to the orbit and extraorbital structures. Sites of distant metastases include bone, bone marrow, and other organs.

The patient with metastatic disease presents with an orbital mass or proptosis, failure to thrive, anorexia, vomiting, and neurologic defects. Children are diagnosed at an early age when they have a family history of retinoblastoma. These children present more often with strabismus than leukokoria; the latter represents a more advanced local tumor.

Diagnosis requires careful examination of both eyes (under general anesthesia) by indirect ophthalmoscopy after the pupils are dilated. Documentation of the tumor is done with photography and drawings. Occasionally, the tumor may not be visualized adequately because of vitreous hemorrhage or retinal detachment. In these circumstances, ultrasonography and a constrast CT scan are very helpful. The CT scan not only will show the tumor, frequently with calcification, but may also demonstrate intracranial extension. The diagnosis is confirmed by histopathological examination of the tumor after enucleation. Once the diagnosis is confirmed, patients are evaluated for metastases. The following studies are recommended: Skeletal survey, bone scan, bone marrow biopsy and aspiration, chest roentgenogram, and CSF examination. The most commonly used classification for intraocular retinoblastoma is that of Reese-Ellsworth (table 48-15).

Differential diagnosis. In patients who present with retinal detachment, persistent hyperplastic primary vitreous and retinopathy of prematurity are considered in the differential diagnosis. Astrocytic hamartoma and toxacara granuloma are important considerations in patients presenting with a retinal mass.

Treatment

The major objectives of treatment are preservation of life, perservation of the eye, retention of vision, and favorable cosmetic results. Every attempt

Table 48-15. Reese-Ellsworth Classification of Intraocular Retinoblastoma

Group I: very favorable prognosis
  (a)   Solitary tumor, <4 disc diameters in size, at or behind the equator
  (b)   Multiple tumors, none over 4 disc diameters in size, all at or behind the equator
Group II: favorable prognosis
  (a)   Solitary tumor, 4–10 disc diameters in size, at or behind the equator
Group III: doubtful prognosis
  (a)   Any lesion anterior to the equator
  (b)   Solitary tumors >10 disc diameters behind the equator
Group IV: unfavorable prognosis
  (a)   Multiple tumors, some >10 disc diameters
  (b)   Any lesion extending anteriorly to the ora serrata
Group V: very unfavorable prognosis
  (a)   Massive tumors involving over half the retina
  (b)   Vitreous seeding

should be made to improve the chances of survival.

Enucleation. The indications for enucleation are (1) unilateral group V disease, (2) blind eye with active tumor, (3) eye with glaucoma from tumor invasion, (4) eye that did not respond to other forms of therapy, (5) most bilateral group V disease, and (6) some patients who are not available for further follow-up.[42] Extreme care should be taken to remove the affected eye by proper marking of the eye as well as examination of the eye before enucleation. Effort is made to remove a long stump of optic nerve because leaving a portion of optic nerve infiltrated by the tumor may seed the orbit.

External beam radiation. Retinoblastoma is a very radiosensitive tumor. For tumors at the posterior pole, either a single temporal portal or both temporal and frontal portals may be used. The patients are treated 4–5 times a week in 200-cGy fractions to a total dose of 3,500–4,500 cGy.[43] All tumors will show tumor response, and in some it will be complete. If only a temporal portal is used, the incidence of cataract is about 5%. Other adverse effects of XRT consist of erythema of the skin and underdevelopment of the bones in the radiation field.

Cryotherapy. Cryotherapy, generally used for very small tumors, has an overall success rate of 70%. It is easily applied to tumors anterior to the equator. Cryotherapy may also be used to treat new tumors that appear after external beam radiation or tumors that respond poorly to radiation.

Photocoagulation. The objective is to obliterate blood supply to the retina. The indications are similar to those for cryotherapy. When tumors are very small (< 1 disk diameter, DD), more than 90% are cured. The cure rate is about 50% when tumors are 3–4 DD in size.

Chemotherapy. Although objective responses have been observed in patients following administration of VCR, CTX, and ADR, the exact role of chemotherapy is not well defined in this tumor.[44] Adjuvant chemotherapy following enucleation, using VCR + CTX in unilateral group V patients, showed no improvement in survival over enucleation alone. Grabowski et al recently reported sustained remission in 10/12 children with extraocular retinoblastoma using systemic and intrathecal chemotherapy as well as irradiation.[45]

Bilateral retinoblastoma. Enucleation of the most affected eye is recommended only in markedly asymmetric cases in which 1 eye belongs to group V and the other to group I or II. Otherwise, XRT is employed to treat both eyes. Guidelines for the treatment of unilateral retinoblastoma are followed in those who undergo enucleation of the severely affected eye. The incidence of metastasis is identical in patients with unilateral or bilateral retinoblastoma.

Second tumors. Patients with the hereditary form of retinoblastoma are at greatest risk for second malignant tumors. Thus, all patients with bilateral retinoblastoma and about 15% of unilaterally affected patients are at risk. Tumors appear both inside and outside the radiation field and also in those who have not received XRT. The most common second malignant tumor has been osteogenic sarcoma; other tumors include fibrosarcoma and other soft-tissue sarcomas. Osteogenic sarcoma of the skull is estimated to be 2,000–5,000 times more common in survivors of bilateral retinoblastoma than in the general population. The average interval between the treatment for retinoblastoma and the appearance of a second malignancy is 11 yr.

Acute Lymphoblastic Leukemia of Childhood

Acute lymphoblastic leukemia (ALL) is the commonest form of cancer in children. About 1,800 new cases are diagnosed annually in children under 15 in the United States.[2] It is slightly more common in boys than in girls and also is more common in whites than in nonwhites. The peak age incidence for ALL in white children is 3–5 yr, but it is seen almost uniformly in all age groups in black children.

The cause of leukemia is not known. It is considered a clonal disease resulting from malignant transformation of a single cell.[46] Increased incidence of leukemia is seen in patients with the following disorders: Down's syndrome, Bloom's syndrome, Fanconi's aplastic anemia, Wiskott-Aldrich syndrome, and ataxia telangiectasia. Whereas a slightly increased incidence of ALL is seen in a sibling of an affected child, the incidence is 25% for an identical twin of a child with the disease.

Clinical Presentation and Diagnosis

The symptoms and signs are related to bone marrow failure secondary to uncontrolled growth of malignant lymphoid cells. Patients may present with 1 or more of the following: fever, pallor, bleeding manifestations, bone or joint pain, lymphadenopathy, and hepatosplenomegaly. Sometimes, patients may present with a variety of nonspecific symptoms such as anorexia, malaise, irritability, and persistent fever.

Most patients have evidence of anemia and thrombocytopenia. Nearly a third of the patients may have a platelet count of >100,000 /cmm. The leukocyte count is >10,000/cmm in over half of patients. About 20% of patients have a leukocyte count of >50,000/cmm. Although lymphoblasts may be seen on peripheral blood smear in some children, a bone marrow examination is essential to establish the diagnosis of leukemia. If aspirate is difficult to obtain, a bone marrow biopsy is required to distinguish between ALL and aplastic anemia. Clinical disorders that may be confused with leukemia are infectious mononucleosis, acute infectious lymphocytosis, pertussis, aplastic anemia, juvenile rheumatoid arthritis, and malignant tumor with metastasis to the bone marrow (e.g., neuroblastoma, rhabdomyosarcoma and non-Hodgkin's lymphoma).

Definitive diagnosis of leukemia type requires special stains (Wright stain, Sudan black B stain, nonspecific esterase, PAS stain of bone marrow smear), immunophenotyping, and chromosome analysis.

Elevated serum levels of LDH, uric acid, potassium, and phosphate may be seen in some patients at diagnosis. Serum immunoglobulin levels are decreased in nearly a third of patients at diagnosis. About 5% of children with ALL have evidence of CNS leukemia at diagnosis as evidenced by CSF pleocytosis and presence of leukemia cells in the CSF.[47]

Morphologic and Immunologic Classification

ALL is classified into 3 morphologic categories (L-1, L-2, L-3) according to the French-American-British (FAB) classification.[48] The classification takes into account the following features of lymphoblasts: cell size, cytoplasmic nuclear ratio, nucleus shape, and nucleoli. Nearly 85% of the ALL lymphoblasts are of L-1 type, about 15% L-2, and <1% L-3. Although no correlation can be made between L-1, L-2 morphology and immunophenotype, L-3 lymphoblasts usually demonstrate surface immunoglobulin and other B cell properties.[49]

About 15–20% of cases have T cell lymphoblast properties and 1–2% have B cell lymphoblast features as demonstrated by the presence of surface immunoglobulin. Most cases (about 80%) have no detectable surface markers and are considered to have non-T, non-B cell leukemia. About 80% of these patients are positive for common ALL antigen (CALLA positive).[50] Recent studies using monoclonal antibodies for the classification of ALL have shown that most cases of non-T, non-B ALL are indeed of B cell origin. More recently, molecular biologic studies of lymphoblasts have demonstrated immunoglobulin gene rearrangement in B cell precursor ALL. This parallels the different stages of normal B cell maturation.

Using modern cytogenic technology, cytogenetic abnormalities in leukemia cells are demonstrated in nearly 90% of ALL patients.[51] The abnormalities involve the number of chromosomes per cell and the presence of translocation. Patients with hyperdiploidy and a chromosome number above 50 have a better prognosis than those with pseudodiploidy.

Prognosis

Several factors have recently emerged that predict the prognosis in children with ALL.[52,53] The 2 most important factors are the level of the WBC and age of the child. Children between 2 and 10 with a WBC of <10,000/cmm have the best prognosis. Infants under 1 yr and patients with a WBC of >50,000/cmm regardless of age have poor prognosis. Patients 2 to 10 having a WBC of 10,000–50,000/cmm have an intermediate prognosis. Factors that suggest adverse prognosis are M-3 bone marrow on day 14 (an indication of slow response), FAB morphology L-2 or L-3, sex (males), bulk disease (large spleen and liver), surface markers (B, pre-B or T cell), race (nonwhites), chromosomal abnormalities (pseudodiploidy, Philadelphia chromosome), immunoglobulin deficiency, higher hemoglobin (>10 gm/dl) and platelet count (<100,000/cmm).

For nearly a decade, cooperative study groups have been refining the therapy based on front-end prognostic factors. Patients with good prognosis features are treated less intensively to minimize acute and long-term toxicity. In contrast, patients with poor prognostic factors are treated with more intensive therapy in order to improve their long-term DFS. Indeed, these principles of therapy have produced substantial improvement in the outcome of children with poor prognosis ALL.

Treatment

Therapy of ALL consists of supportive measures as well as specific antileukemia therapy. I.V. fluids at the rate of twice maintenance, alkalization of urine, allopurinol to prevent hyperuricemia, blood product transfusion, and antibiotics form the mainstay of supportive therapy. Remission-induction therapy consists of VCR, prednisone, and L-asparaginase, a regimen that yields a remission rate of >95% in children with good-risk ALL.[54] Intrathecal MTX during induction, consolidation, and maintenance therapy consistitutes adequate CNS prophylaxis in these children. Maintenance therapy consists of daily 6-mercaptopurine and weekly MTX (both orally), with monthly pulses of VCR and prednisone. With the above therapy, 85% of low-risk ALL patients are expected to have long-term DFS.[55]

The prognosis for patients with poor-risk ALL (WBC >50,000/cmm) has improved dramatically with use of multidrug, aggressive chemotherapy. One of the regimens, Berlin-Frankfurt-Munster (BFM), used intensive induction, consolidation, delayed intensification, and standard maintenance.[56] Another aggressive regimen, developed at Memorial Sloan-Kettering Cancer Center, New York, consists of intensive induction followed by intensive maintenance therapy with drugs in rapid rotation.[57] Both regimens employ cranial irradiation (1,800 cGy) for CNS prophylaxis. The 4-yr event-free survival rate for high-risk ALL patients has gone from <40% to nearly 70% with use of 1 of above aggressive therapies. The outcome in infants with leukemia is still poor, even through their event-free survival has doubled (from 20% to 40%) with aggressive chemotherapy. The optimal duration of therapy for patients with ALL is not known. Maintenance therapy for 2 yr appears to be adequate for girls, whereas boys seem to require somewhat more (2½–3 yr). However, when intensive therapies are used, 2 yr of maintenance may be adequate. About 20% of children with ALL relapse when therapy is discontinued, with most relapses occurring within 12 mo thereafter.

Patients who relapse while on chemotherapy or within 6 mo after the end of chemotherapy have a poor prognosis. Although a second remission can be achieved in most patients, long-term DFS is only about 10%. If the patient has an HLA (human leukocyte antigens)-compatible, MLC (mixed lymphocyte culture) nonreactive sibling, bone marrow transplantation early in the second remission is the treatment of choice. Other options include autologous bone marrow transplantation or marrow transplantation from an unrelated matched donor.

In summary, the long-term DFS for children with ALL has gone from 1% to 60% in the past 2 decades. This has been possible with (1) use of intensive multiagent induction therapy, (2) prevention of extramedullary disease, (3) better supportive care, and (4) therapy designed to prevent the risk of relapse based on front-end prognostic factors.

Non-Hodgkin's Lymphomas*

Incidence

The lymphomas (non-Hodgkin's and Hodgkin's) are the third most common malignancy in childhood and account for 13.8% of all childhood cancers in the

---

*This brief presentation will review only those features of lymphomas that are primarily encountered in childhood. Details of the pathogenesis, clinical presentation, and management of the lymphoproliferative disorders are extensively reviewed in another chapter of this book. For the same reason, no comments will be made on Hodgkin's disease, whose characteristics in childhood are identical with those seen in adults.

United States. About 450 cases of non-Hodgkin's lymphomas (NHL) and 375 cases of Hodgkin's disease are diagnosed each year in children in the United States. There are 2 age peaks for NHL—3–6 yr and adolescence. The disease has a marked preponderance for male children, with a male-to-female ratio of about 3:1. Etiology, epidemiology, and classification of NHL in childhood are similar to those of the disease in adults.

Nearly 95% of NHL in children are diffuse and histologically high-grade tumors. The correlation between morphology, immunologic subtype, and clinical behavior is fairly good. About 40% of childhood NHL is T cell-derived and 40% B cell-derived; the remaining cases are non-T, non-B. T cell NHLs often arise in the mediastinum, thymus, or peripheral nodal tissue and have diffuse lymphoblastic histology. Prior to effective therapy, transformation or progression to ALL occurred in nearly 50% of cases. B cell lymphomas arise in the G.I. tract, peripheral nodes, or bone marrow. Histologically, B cell tumors have an undifferentiated or large-cell (histiocytic) appearance.

Clinical Manifestations and Diagnosis

Clinical manifestations depend on the site of lymph node involvement. These tumors progress very rapidly, and patients present with a brief duration of symptoms. The most common primary sites are the abdomen, mediastinum, head and neck, and peripheral nodal region.

The abdomen is the primary site in 30–40% of children with NHL, with nearly one-third in the intestine (see chapter 10, figures 10-14 through 10-18).[58,59] Other intra-abdominal sites are colon, ovary, kidney, stomach, liver, and spleen. Initial symptoms and signs include abdominal pain, vomiting, fever, and an abdominal mass. Symptoms are frequently due to intussusception. After the first year of life, NHL must be ruled out in any child who presents with intussusception, even if it is reduced by barium enema. Most children with abdominal lymphoma present with large unresectable tumors often associated with metabolic abnormalities such as hyperuricemia, hyperphosphatemia, and hyperkalemia.

The mediastinum is the next most common site of primary involvement (see chapter 10, figures 10-36A & B). The usual symptoms are fever, cough, malaise, and progressive dyspnea. Many of these patients have supraclavicular cervical adenopathy and pleural effusion. A few patients may present with superior vena cava (SVC) syndrome. Symptoms and signs of SVC syndrome are dyspnea, cough, orthopnea, swelling of the face and upper trunk, distension of neck veins, facial plethora, and cyanosis. The SVC syndrome is a medical emergency requiring prompt diagnosis and appropriate therapy.

Some patients present with rapidly enlarging lymph nodes in the neck, axilla, and (less frequently) the inguinal region. About 15% of children with T cell NHL have bone marrow involvement at diagnosis. T cell NHL with marrow involvement and T cell ALL have many clinical and immunological features in common, making it difficult to distinguish one from the other, and therapy is similar. Burkitt's lymphoma is a B cell malignancy endemic to Central Africa. It is often of multifocal origin and very aggressive. It often involves extranodal sites, including abdominal and pelvic viscera, facial bones (mandible and maxilla), salivary glands, bone marrow, and the CNS.[60]

The diagnosis of NHL should be considered in any child with adenopathy, a mediastinal mass, or intestinal obstruction. Biopsy should be performed at a major treatment center with fresh tissue submitted for light- as well as electron microscopy. The latter will be useful in differentiating NHL from neuroblastoma, rhabdomyosarcoma, and Ewing's sarcoma. In addition, studies to determine cell surface and biochemical markers, chromosomes, and cytochemistry should also be performed.

The site of biopsy should be carefully chosen; the least invasive procedure should be used for diagnosis. Children who present with a large mediastinal mass and respiratory difficulty have an increased risk of respiratory arrest, even after endotracheal intubation.[61] Before considering biopsy of a large mediastinal mass, a bone marrow examination should be done even if the CBC is normal; the bone marrow aspirate may obviate the need for more invasive procedures. Another potential means of diagnosis is thoracentesis with cytocentrifuge examination of the pleural fluid. Cervical lymph nodes are frequently enlarged in patients presenting with an anterior mediastinal mass. In such patients, lymph node biopsy should be performed under local anesthesia if possible. If biopsy of a mediastinal mass is required, extreme care must be taken. Corticosteroid therapy for 1–2 days may be necessary to shrink the tumor mass in order to prevent serious respiratory complications during anesthesia; radiation has also been used to shrink the tumor mass prior to biopsy. It is possibile that either treatment may confuse the histological diagnosis.

Staging

Due to rapid progression of NHL and associated serious complications, staging studies should be completed very quickly. These studies include thorough physical examination, CBC, bone marrow aspiration and biopsy, and lumbar puncture to examine the CFS for abnormal cells. Serum LDH, uric acid, electrocytes, BUN, creatinine, calcium, and phosphate levels should be determined in all patients.

Imaging studies consist of chest x-ray, bone scan, and bone survey. Patients with mediastinal or abdominal presentation should have a CT scan. Ultrasound, myelography, and tomograms are less useful.

A number of staging procedures have been suggested for childhood NHL but none is widely used because the progression of NHL in children does not follow a predictable course. Even what appears to be a well-localized mediastinal NHL can spread very rapidly to the bone marrow and the CNS. Children with NHL fall into 2 broad groups: those with localized disease and those with disseminated disease. Nearly two thirds of patients with NHL have disseminated disease at diagnosis. Localized disease is defined as a tumor limited anatomically either to a single extranodal site with or without regional lymph node involvement or to tumor in 1 or 2 adjacent lymph node regions. Only patients in whom the abdominal disease is completely resected are considered to have localized disease. All patients with mediastinal NHL are considered to have disseminated disease.

Treatment

Although optimal therapy for childhood NHL patients has not been defined, the prognosis for these children has dramatically improved during the past decade.

Because of the similarities between NHL and ALL, several investigators have used multiagent chemotherapy even in patients with localized NHL, along with XRT to bulk disease. This leads to a dramatic improvement in outcome. Chemotherapy with agents effective against childhood ALL has thus become the standard therapy for NHL in children. More aggressive multiagent chemotherapy is being used, with improved results, in patients with disseminated NHL.

The Children's Cancer Study Group (CCSG) compared the effectiveness of 4-agent chemotherapy (COMP) with that of 10-drug therapy (LSA_2-L_2) in childhood NHL[62] (see Appendix). Histopathology of the tumor was grouped into 2 broad categories: lymphoblastic and nonlymphoblastic. COMP was as effective as LSA_2-L_2 in patients with localized NHL regardless of the histology. Six months of therapy may be adequate for such patients. However, LSA_2-L_2 was far more effective in disseminated lymphoblastic NHL than was the COMP regimen. At the same time, COMP was more effective in disseminated nonlymphoblastic NHL than the LSA_2-L_2 regimen. Because NHL is very sensitive to chemotherapy and many patients may present with bulky and disseminated disease, supportive treatment is extremely important in these patients prior to and during specific antilymphoma therapy. Special attention should be paid to the problems of airway and vascular compromise and acute tumor lysis syndrome.

With modern induction therapy, at least 90% of patients with NHL achieve remission.[59,62] All children should receive CNS prophylaxis. It appears that intrathecal chemotherapy alone is not as effective as cranial irradiation plus intrathecal chemotherapy in preventing CNS disease. Some investigators have suggested that children with localized NHL involving the G.I. tract need not receive CNS prophylaxis because of a low risk of CNS disease.

The precise role of XRT in childhood NHL is not clear. Its role in children with localized NHL is under investigation by the CCSG. Currently, some children with NHL do receive XRT to the areas of bulky disease at the time of presentation. If XRT is given, the usual dose is 1,500 cGy.

Recent studies have shown that nearly 60–80% of children with advanced lymphoblastic lymphoma can be cured. However, children with advanced abdominal NHL (usually of undifferentiated histology) have a less favorable outcome. Relapse is uncommon in children who are in complete remission for 12 mo after institution of therapy. Based on this, current studies are exploring the role of intensive chemotherapy for 1 yr or less in patients with abdominal NHL.

Recurrence of the tumor generally carries a very poor prognosis, especially if relapse occurs while a patient is on therapy. Bone marrow transplantation (usually allogeneic) after intensive chemotherapy offers some hope for cure for children with recurrent NHL.

Complications of Treatment

The acute complications of chemotherapy are nausea, vomiting, neuropathy, pancytopenia, and alopecia. XRT produces erythematous skin changes in the treatment field. The major long-term complications of chemotherapy are sterility, particularly in males; underdevelopment of soft tissues and bones in the radiation field; and chemical hypothyroidism. There is general agreement that sitting height is diminished in children treated with radiation prior to age 13 compared to minimal or no effect in children treated after age 13.

The incidence of morbidity and mortality from postsplenectomy sepsis is considerably decreased following institution of pneumococcal vaccine and antibiotic prophylaxis. Herpes zoster, very common in patients receiving combined radiation and chemotherapy, may be quite debilitating. A major concern to all physicians treating patients with Hodgkin's disease is the risk of second malignancy. In a recent study, the incidence of second malignancy was 2.3%. Second malignancies seen in order of frequency are ANLL, non-Hodgkin's lymphoma, and solid tumors. The risk is greatest in patients who received XRT therapy and chemotherapy, least (nonexistent) in those treated with XRT alone, and intermediate in those given chemotherapy.

References

1. Vital Statistics of the United States, 1976. vol 2. Mortality, Pt A. Hyattsville, Md.: U.S. Dept of Health and Human Services, 1980.
2. Young JL Jr, Ries LG, Silverberg E, et al. Cancer incidence, survival and mortality for children younger than 15 years. Cancer 1986; 58:598–602.
3. Miller RW. Environmental causes of cancer in children. Adv Pediatr 1978; 25:97–119.
4. Filipovich AH, Spector BD, Kersey J. Immunodeficiency in humans as a risk factor in the development of malignancy. Prev Med 1980; 9:252–59.
5. Miller RW. Relation between cancer and congential defects in man. N Engl J Med 1966; 75:87–93.
6. Miller RW, McKay FW. Decline in US childhood cancer mortality, 1950 through 1980. JAMA 1984; 251:2567–70.
7. Finlay JT, Croins SC, Uteg R, Griese W. Progress in the management of childhood brain tumors. Hematology/Oncology Clinics of North America 1987; 1 (4):753–76.
8. Deutsch M, Laurent JP, Cohen ME. Myelography for staging medulloblastoma. Cancer 1985; 56:1763.
9. Harisiadis L, and Chang C. Medulloblastoma in children: a correlation between staging and results of treatment. Int J Radiat Oncol Biol Phys 1977; 2:833–41.
10. Berry M, Jenkins D, Keen C, et al. Radiation therapy for medulloblastoma. Cancer 1981; 48:2296–2309.
11. The treatment of medulloblastoma: results of a prospective randomized trial of radiation therapy with and without CCNU, vincristine and prednisone. J Neurosurg 1990; 72:572–82.
12. Bloom H, Thornton-Jones J. Adjuvant chemotherapy for medulloblastoma. The multicenter controlled trial of the International Society of Pediatric Oncology (SIOP), from Proc 13th Int Cong Chemother 1983.
13. Pendergrass TW, Milstein JM, Geyer JR, et al. Eight drugs in one day chemotherapy for brain tumors. Experience in 107 children and rationale for preradiation chemotherapy. J Clin Oncol 1987; 5(8):1221–1231.

14. Sposto R, Ertel IJ, Jenkin RD, et al. The effectiveness of chemotherapy for treatment of high grade astrocytoma in children: results of a randomized study. A report from the Childrens Cancer Study Group. J Neuro-oncol 1989; 7:165–177.
15. Montravadi R, Phatak R, Bellus S, et al. Brainstem gliomas: An autopsy study of 25 cases. Cancer 1982; 49:1294–96.
16. Allen JC. Newly diagnosed and recurrent brain tumors. Pediat Clin North Am 1985; 32(3):633–49.
17. Wara WM, Edwards MSB, Levin VA, et al. A new treatment regimen for brainstem glioma. A pilot study of the Brain Tumor Research Center and Children's Cancer Study Group. Int J Radiat Oncol Biol Phys 1986; 12 (Suppl 1):143.
18. Cushing H, Wolbach BB. The transformation of a malignant paravertebral sympathicoblastoma into a benign ganglioneuroma. Am J Pathol 1927; 3:203–15.
19. Shimada H, Chatten J, Newton WA, et al. Histopathologic prognostic factors in neuroblastic tumors: definition of subtypes of ganlioneuroblastoma and an age linked classification of neuroblastomas. JNCI 1984; 73:405–16.
20. Evans AE. Staging and treatment of neuroblastoma. Cancer 1980; 65:1799.
21. Evans AE. Neuroblastoma: diagnosis and management. Curr Concepts Oncol 1982; 4(2):10–20.
22. Finkelstein JZ. Neuroblastoma: the challenge and frustration. Hematol/Oncol Clin North Am 1987; 1(4):675–694.
23. Finkelstein JZ, Klemperer MR, Evans AE, et al. Multiagent chemotherapy for children with metastatic neuroblastoma: A report from Children's Cancer Study Group. Med Pediatr Oncol 1979; 6:179–88.
24. Green AA, Hayes FA, Hsistu HO. Sequential cyclophosphamide and doxorubicin for induction of complete remission in children with disseminated neuroblastoma. Cancer 1981; 48:2310–17.
25. Beckwith JB, Palmer NF. Histopathology and prognosis of Wilms' tumor. Cancer 1978; 41:1937–48.
26. D'Angio GJ, Beckwith JB, Breslow NE, et al. Wilm's tumor: an update. Cancer 1980; 45:1791–98.
27. D'Angio GJ, Evans A, Breslow NE, et al. The treatment of Wilms' tumor: results of the second National Wilms' Tumor Study. Cancer 1981; 47:2302–11.
28. D'Angio GJ, Breslow N, Beckwith JB. Treatment of Wilms' tumor: results of the third National Wilms' Tumor Study. Cancer 1989; 64:349–60.
29. Horn RC, Enterline HT. Rhabdomyosarcoma: a clinicopathological study and classification of 39 cases. Cancer 1958; 11:181–99.
30. Palmer N, Foulkes M. Histopathology and prognosis in the second intergroup rhabdomyosarcoma study (IRS-III) (Abstr) Proc Am Soc Clin Oncol 1983; 2:229.
31. Maurer HM, Moon T, Donaldson M, et al. The intergroup rhabdomyosarcoma study: a preliminary report. Cancer 1977; 40:2015–26.
32. Maurer HM. The intergroup rhabdomyosarcoma study: update, Nov 1978. NCI monogr 1981; 56:61–68.
33. Crist WM, Garnsey L, Beltangady MS, et al. Prognosis in children with rhabdomyosarcoma. A report of the intergroup rhabdomyosarcoma studies I and II. J Clin Oncol 1990; 8(3):443–52.
34. Miser JS, Pizzo PA. Soft tissue sarcomas in childhood. Pediat Clin North Am 1985; 32(3):779–800.
35. Pritchard DJ. Indications for surgical treatment of localized Ewing's sarcoma of bone. Clin Orthop 1980; 153:39–43.
36. Razek A, Perez CA, et al. Intergroup Ewing's sarcoma study: local control related to radiation dose, volume and site of primary lesion in Ewing's sarcoma. Cancer 1980; 46:516.
37. Nesbit ME, Perez CA, Teft M, et al. Multimodal therapy for the management of primary nonmetastatic Ewing's sarcoma of bone: an intergroup study. NCI monogr 1981; 56:255–262.
38. Rosen G, Caparros B, Nirenberg A, et al. Ewing's sarcoma: ten years experience with adjuvant chemotherapy. Cancer 1981; 47:2204–13.
39. Abramson DH. Retinoblastoma: diagnosis and management. CA 1982; 32:130–140.
40. Abramson DH, Ellsworth RM, Grumbach N, et al. Retinoblastoma: survival, age at detection and comparison 1914–1958, 1958–1983. J Pediatr Ophthalmol Strab 1985; 22:246–250.
41. Potluri VR, Helson L, Ellsworth RM, et al. Chromosome abnormalities in human retinoblastoma. Cancer 1986; 58:663–671.

42. Abramson DH, Ellsworth RM. The surgical management of retinoblastoma. Ophthalmic Surg 1980; 11:596.

43. Abramson DH, Ellsworth RM, Jereb B. External beam radiation for retinoblastoma. Bull NY Acad Med 1981; 57:787.

44. White L. The role of chemotherapy in the treatment of retinoblastoma. Retina 1983; 3:194.

45. Grabowski EF, Ellsworth RE, Mccormick B, et al. Extraocular retinoblastoma: substained remission in 10 of 12 children treated with irradiation and combination chemotherapy. Pediatr Res 1987; 21:299a.

46. Dow LW, Martin P, Moohr J, et al. Evidence of clonal development of childhood acute lymphoblastic leukemia. Blood 1985; 66:902–07.

47. Bleyer WA, Poplack DG. Prophylaxis and treatment of leukemia in the central nervous system and other sanctuaries. Semin Oncol 1985; 12(2):131–48.

48. Bennett JM, Catovsky D, Daniel MT, et al. French-American-British (FAB) Cooperative Group. The morphological classification of acute leukemias—concordance among observers and clinical correlation. Br J Haematol 1981; 47:553–61.

49. Miller DR, Leikin S, Albo V, et al. Prognostic importance of morphology (FAB classification) in childhood acute lymphoblastic leukemia. Br J Haematol 1981; 48:199–206.

50. Greaves MF, Janossy G, Peto J, et al. Immunologically defined subclasses of acute lymphoblastic leukemia in children: their relationship to presentation features and prognosis. Br J Haematol 1981; 48:179–97.

51. Williams DL, Raimondi S, Rivera G, et al. Presence of clonal chromosome abnormalities in virtually all cases of acute lymphoblastic leukemia. N Engl J Med 1985; 10:640–41.

52. Robison L, Sather H, Coccia P, et al. Assessment of the interrelationship of prognostic factors in childhood acute lymphoblastic leukemia. Am J Pediatr Hematol Oncol 1980; 2(1):3–5.

53. Miller DR, Krailo M, Bleyer WA, et al. Prognostic implication of blast cell morphology in childhood acute lymphoblastic leukemia. A report from the Children's Cancer Study Group. Cancer Treat Rep 1985; 69:1211–21.

54. Ortega JA, Nesbit ME Jr, Donaldson MH, et al. L-asparaginase, vincristine and prednisone for induction of first remission in acute lymphocytic leukemia. Cancer Res 1977; 37:535–40.

55. Bleyer A, Nickerson J, Coccia P, et al. Monthly pulses of vincristine and prednisone prevent marrow and testicular relapse in childhood acute lymphoblastic leukemia. One conclusion of the CCG-161 study of good prognosis ALL. Proc Am Soc Clin Oncol 1985; 4:160.

56. Riehm H, Langermann HJ, Gadner H, et al. The Berlin childhood acute lymphoblastic leukemia therapy study, 1976–79. Am J Pediatr Hematol Oncol 1980; 2:299–306.

57. Steinherz PG, Gaynon P, Miller DR, et al. Improved disease free survival of children with acute lymphoblstic leukemia with high risk for early replase with the "New York" regimen. A new intensive therapy protocol: a report from the Children's Cancer Study Group. J Clin Oncol 1986; 4:744–52.

58. Wollner N, Burchenal JH, Lieberman PH, et al. Non-Hodgkin's lymphoma in children. A comparative study of two modalities of therapy. Cancer 1976; 37:123–34.

59. Murphy SB. Management of childhood non-Hodgkin's lymphoma. Cancer Treat Rep 1977; 61:1161–73.

60. Ziegler JL. Burkitt's lymphoma. N Engl J Med 1981; 305:735–45.

61. Halpern S, Chatten J, Meadows AT, et al. Anterior mediastinal masses: anesthesia hazards and other problems. J Pediatr 1983; 102:407–10.

62. Anderson JR, Wilson JF, Jenkin DT, et al. Childhood Non-Hodgkin's lymphoma. The results of a randomized therapeutic trial comparing a four-drug regimen (COMP) with a ten-drug regimen (LSA1-2L2) N Engl J Med 1983; 308:559–65.

APPENDIX

COMBINATION CHEMOTHERAPY AND SUPPORTIVE THERAPY IN NEOPLASTIC DISEASES

A Compendium of Regimens and Schedules of Administration

Contents

Introduction

The chief objective of this appendix is to present, over the span of a few pages, a listing of combination chemotherapy regimens currently used in the treatment of malignant diseases (abbreviations used herein are shown in table A-1).

These regimens include, with sufficient details, drug dosages, their route, and frequency of administration (dose adjustments related to the common side effects these drugs produce are listed in a table at the end). This compendium includes the more frequently used chemotherapeutic cytotoxotic agents and the reductions that must be applied to their calculated dose in relation to some of the side effects they induce on various organs and systems.

This appendix does not contain an exhaustive presentation of all of the side effects that can possibly be caused by the recommended drugs, nor the details of therapeutic measures that can counteract or control these side effects. Also, full details on administration of these drugs are not included. It is the belief of the editor that such details cannot be entirely reduced to writing; some can be acquired only through clinical experience. For this reason, administration of the combination chemotherapy regimens presented in this appendix should be directed and carried out only by specialized physicians, medical oncologists, hematologists, or gynecologic oncologists with adequate training and experience in the field of therapy of malignant neoplasms. This appendix is intended primarily to serve these specialists as well as the trainees in the respective specialties as a useful reference for the exact dosage and sequence of administration of drugs included in relatively complex combination regimens.

The editor as well as the publisher of this book would like to caution physicians who lack adequate training in this field not to administer the regimens listed in this appendix without adequate supervision of qualified physicians. Although every effort was made to check the accuracy of the drug regimens published herein, the editor and publisher cannot take responsibility for any error that could occur in the way in which these drugs are administered resulting from their use under the direction of inexperienced physicians.

The choice of the combination chemotherapy regimens presented here followed several criteria. For malignant neoplasms in which drug regimens with curative intent exist (e.g., acute leukemias, lymphomas, germ cell tumors), as well as for advanced neoplasms in which significant prolongation of survival can be achieved by chemotherapy (e.g., breast cancer, small-cell lung cancer), all combination regimens known to have led to successful outcomes have been listed.

Conversely, for other advanced malignant tumors representing the approximately 70% of all neoplasms for which no chemotherapy that could meaningfully prolong survival has been clearly identified, the choice of combination chemotherapy regimens was somewhat arbitrary. The regimens given include some of those most commonly used as well as some that, in the opinion of the editor, are among the most effective currently (November 1990) available and have tolerable side effects.

The appendix also includes, in a section on supportive therapy, the exact formulations for antiemetic and analgesic drugs widely used in the palliation of symptoms in patients with advanced neoplasms.

This appendix does not represent an exhaustive compendium of all combination chemotherapy regimens that have ever led to favorable results in patients with advanced malignancies; rather, it includes concise listings of the most commonly used drug regimens in clinical practice that could help the practicing oncologist to prescribe a detailed and complex regimen without needing to consult the original reference.

It is hoped that this compendium of chemotherapy regimens will be useful in the daily practice of clinical oncology.

Hematologic Malignancies

Acute Myelocytic Leukemia

Regimen	Drugs	Dose/admin. rte.	Days of treatment	Frequency/ comments
Remission Induction Regimens				
DA	Daunorubicin	45 mg/m^2/d I.V. bolus	1,2,3	q. 3–4 wk
	Cytosine arabinoside (ara-C)	100 mg/m^2/d I.V.C.I.	1–7	1–3 times until CR
DAT	Daunorubicin	45 mg/m^2/d I.V. bolus	1,2,3	q. 3–4 wk × 1–3 cyc
	Cytosine arabinoside	100 mg/m^2/d I.V.C.I.	1–7	until CR
	Thioguanine	100 mg/m^2 p.o. q. 12 h	1–7	
MA	Mitoxantrone	12 mg/m^2/d I.V. bolus	1,2,3,17,18	
	Cytosine arabinoside (ara-C)	100 mg/m^2/d I.V.C.I.	1–7 & 17–21	
NOVE	Mitoxantrone (Novantrone)	10 mg/m^2/d I.V. bolus	1–5	q. 3–4 wk × 2–3 cyc until CR
	Etoposide	100 mg/m^{2}d I.V.Sh.I.	1–5	
IDAC	Idarubicin	12 mg/m^2/d I.V. bolus	1–3	q. 3–4 wk × 2–3 cyc
	Cytosine arabinoside	100 mg/m^2/d I.V.C.I.	1–7	until CR
L-10 MSKCC	Vincristine	1.5 mg/m^2 (max 2 mg) I.V. bolus	1,8,15,22,29	
(VDPM-	Prednisone	60 mg/m^2/d p.o.	1–29, then D/C on d 36	
CTACy)	Doxorubicin	20 mg/m^2 I.V. bolus	17,18,19	
	Methotrexate	15 mg/m^2 I.V. bolus	42–46; 78–82; 114–118	
		6.25 mg/m^2 i. thec, or Omaya reserv	2,5,16,19,30,33, 55,58,88,92,95	
	Cytosine arabinoside (ara-c)	30 mg/kg I.V. 3-h inf q. 12 h	56–63;92–98; 128–134	
	Thioguanine	2.5 mg/kg p.o. q. 12 h	56–63;92–98; 128–134	
	Asparaginase	200 IU/kg I.V. 1-h inf	135–144	
	Cyclophosphamide	1,200 mg/m^2 2-h inf	146	
Consolidation Regimens				
HiC-D	Cytosine arabinoside (high-dose)	3 gm/m^2 q. 12 h I.V. 3-h inf	1–6	Admin c̄ antiemetics, steroid ophthalmic drops, KCL
	Daunorubicin	30 mg/m^2 I.V. bolus	7,8	
HiC-AMSA	Cytosine arabinoside	3 gm/m^2 q. 12 h I.V. 3-h inf	1–5	This and previous regimen can also be used for reinduction of remissions after DA or DAT regimen
	M-AMSA	100 mg/m^2 I.V.Sh.I.	1–5	
D/DA	Doxorubicin (Adriamycin) *or*	45 mg/m^2/d I.V. bolus	1	q. 4 wk × 2
	Daunorubicin	55 mg/m^2/d I.V. bolus	1	
	Cytosine arabinoside	200 mg/m^2/d I.V.C.I.	1–5	
Maintenance Regimens				
CT	Cytosine arabinoside	100 mg/m^2 s.c. q. 12 h	1–5	q. 4 wk × 12
	Thioguanine	50 mg/m^2 p.o. q. 12 h	1–5	
TC	Thioguanine	40 mg/m^2 p.o. q. 12 h	1–4	q. wk × 26
	Cytosine arabinoside	60 mg/m^2 s.c.	5	

Acute Lymphocytic Leukemia

Regimen	Drugs/ procedures	Dose & admin. rte.	Days of treatment	Frequency & comments
Induction Regimens				
1. For Favorable Childhood ALL (L-1)				
PVD (M-CRT)	Prednisone	40 mg/m^2/d p.o.	1–28, then taper down; D/C on d 36	
	Vincristine	1.5 mg/m^2/d (to max 2 mg) I.V. bolus	1,8,15,22	
	Daunorubicin	45 mg/m^2/d I.V. bolus	1,8,15,22 *or* 1,2,3	
	Methotrexate	12 mg/m^2 (max 15 mg) i. thec.	30,32,37,39,44 or early if CNS is involved	
	Cranial irradiation	15 fractions to total 2,400 cGy for >2 yr old 2,000 cGy for 1–2 yr old 1,500 cGy for <1 yr old	29–33 36–40 43–47	
2. For Poor-Prognosis Childhood ALL (L-1), Adult ALL (L-2), and Burkitt's-like ALL (L-3)				
CALBG (VDPAM)	Vincristine	1.4 mg/m^2 (max 2 mg) I.V. bolus	1,8,15	
	Daunorubicin	45 mg/m^2/d I.V. bolus	1,2,3	
	Prednisone	40 mg/m^2/d p.o.	1–22, then taper down; D/C on d 29	
	Asparaginase	500 IU/kg/d (max 10,000) I.V. 1-h inf	22–31	
	Methotrexate	6.25 mg/m^2 i.thec. or Omaya reserv	8,15,22,29	The admin in CSF should continue 2 × after CSF becomes normal in case of CNS leukemia
Consolidation or Remission Reinduction Regimen				
H.DAC ASNase	Cytosine arabinoside (ara-C)	3 gm/m^2 I.V. 3-h inf q. 12 h	1,2,8,9	
	Asparaginase	6,000 IU/m^2 3 h after last ara-C dose	2 & 9	
AVDP	Asparaginase	15,000 IU/m^2 I.V.Sh.I.	1–5;8–12;15–19,22–26.	
	Vincristine	2 mg/m^2 (max 2 mg) I.V. bolus	8,15,22	
	Daunorubicin	30–60 mg/m^2 I.V. bolus	8,15,22	
	Prednisone	40 mg/m^2 p.o. q.d.	8–12;15–19;22–26	
Maintenance Regimens				
MVP Met	6-Mercaptopurine	50 mg/m^2 p.o.	q.d. × 10 wk	q. 12 wk × 3
	Methotrexate	15 mg/m^2 p.o. *and* 12 mg/m^2 (max 15 mg) i. thec. or Omaya reserv	q.d. on day 1 of wk 1–10 q.d. on d 1 of wk 11 & 12	
	Prednisone	40 mg/m^2 p.o.	q.d. of wk 11 & 12	
	Vincristine	1.5 mg/m^2 (max 2 mg)	q.d. on d 1 of wk 11 & 12	

Chronic Lymphocytic Leukemia

Regimen	Drugs	Dose & admin. rte.	Days of treatment	Frequency & comments
ChP	Chlorambucil	0.4–0.6 mg/kg p.o.	1	q. 3–4 wk
	Prednisone	60 mg/m^2 p.o. q.d.	1–4	until WBC nadir is 5,000/μl
CVP	Cyclophosphamide	300 mg/m^2 p.o. q.d. or 1,000 mg/m^2 I.V.	1–5 1	q. 4 wk until WBC nadir is 3,000/μl or
	Vincristine	1 mg/m^2 I.V. bolus	1 1	q. 4 wk × 6, then q. 12 wk × 6
	Prednisone	40 mg/m^2 p.o.	1–5	
CHOP	Cyclophosphamide	300 mg/m^2 p.o.	1–5	q. 4 wk × 6,
	Adriamycin (hydroxydaunorubicin)	25 mg/m^2 I.V. bolus	1	then q. 12 wk × 6 Recommended
	Vincristine (Oncovin)	1 mg/m^2 I.V. bolus	1	only for pts in
	Prednisone	40 mg/m^2 p.o.	1–5	stage C (Binet) or stages III & IV (Rai)
Fludarabine	Fludarabine	20 mg/m^2 I.V.	1–5	q. 4 wk until WBC nadir is 3000/μl or progression occurs

Hairy Cell Leukemia

Regimen	Drugs	Dose & admin. rte.	Days of treatment	Frequency & comments
INF	Alpha 2a or b interferon	3 × 10^6 U/d s.c. or I.M.	t.i.w.	q. wk × 26–52
PENT	2'-Deoxycoformicin (Pentostatin)	4 mg/m^2 I.V.	q. wk × 3	q. 8 wk × 6

Multiple Myeloma

Regimen	Drugs	Dose & admin. rte.	Days of treatment	Frequency & comments
VMCP	Vincristine	1 mg/m^2 (max 2 mg) I.V. bolus	1	q. 21 d
	Melphalan	5 mg/m^2/d p.o.	1–4	
	Cyclophosphamide	100 mg/m^2/d p.o.	1–4	
	Prednisone	40 mg/m^2/d p.o.	1–4	
MP	Melphalan	0.15 mg/kg/d p.o., then when CBC rises, 0.05 mg/kg/d p.o.	1–7 daily	Continuously
	Prednisone	0.8 mg/kg/d p.o. (max 100 mg/d)	1–14, then taper down for 6 wk	

Regimen	Drugs	Dose & admin. rte.	Days of treatment	Frequency & comments
VMCP-VCAP	Vincristine	1 mg/m^2 (max 2 mg) I.V. bolus	1 & 22	q. 42 d
	Melphalan	5 mg/m^2/d p.o.	1–4	
	Cyclophosphamide	100 mg/m^2/d p.o.	1–4;22–25	
	Prednisone	60 mg/m^2/d p.o.	1–4;22–25	
	Doxorubicin (Adriamycin)	25 mg/m^2 I.V. bolus	22	
M2	Melphalan	0.25 mg/kg/d p.o.	1–4	q. 28 d
	Prednisone	1 mg/kg/d p.o.	1–7	
	Vincristine	0.03 mg/kg I.V. bolus	1	
	Carmustine	1 mg/kg I.V.Sh.I.	1	
	Cyclophosphamide	10 mg/kg I.V.Sh.I.	1	
BCP	Carmustine (BCNU)	75 mg/m^2 I.V.Sh.I.	1	q. 28 d
	Cyclophosphamide	400 mg/m^2 I.V.Sh.I.	1	
	Prednisone	75 mg. p.o.	1–7	
VAD	Vincristine	0.4 mg/d (mixed in same I.V. solution with ADR) I.V.C.I. through central vein indwelling cath	1–4	q. 28 d
	Doxorubicin (Adriamycin)	9 mg/m^2		
	Dexamethasone	40 mg p.o.	1–4 9–12 17–20	
VBAP	Vincristine	2 mg I.V. bolus	1	q. 3–4 wk
	Carmustine (BCNU)	30 mg/m^2 I.V.Sh.I.	1	
	Doxorubicin (Adriamycin)	30 mg/m^2 I.V. bolus	1	
	Prednisone	20 mg t.i.d. p.o.	1–5	

DOSE ADJUSTMENTS—MULTIPLE MYELOMA

1. For all multiple myeloma combination chemotherapy regimens, dose attenuations due to bone marrow suppression are recommended for the following drugs: melphalan, cyclophosphamide, Adriamycin, and carmustine:

Granulocytes/μl	Platelets/μl	Doses administered
≥3,000	130,000	Full doses
2,000–2,990	100,000–129,000	50% of calc dose
1,500–2,000	75,000–99,990	25% of calc dose
<1,500	<75,000	Hold therapy & reevaluate within 1 wk × 2

2. Vincristine dose should be adjusted in relation to the development of peripheral neuropathy as follows:
—Dose should be reduced by 50% in case of markedly diminished deep tendon reflexes (DTRs) or persistent constipation despite adequate administration of catharics.
—Administration should be withheld if patient starts walking with a shuffling gait, if DTRs are absent, or if paralytic ileus develops.

3. Vincristine dose should also be reduced when serum direct bilirubin is rising:
—by 25% for >1.2 ≤1.5 mg/dl direct bilirubin
—by 50% for <2.5 ≤1.5 mg/dl
—by 75% for >2.5 mg/dl

Hodgkin's Disease

Regimen	Drugs	Dose & admin. rte.	Days of treatment	Frequency & comments
MOPP	Mechlorethamine (HN2) (Mustargen)	6 mg/m^2 I.V. bolus in a running inf	1 & 8	q. 28 d × 6
	Vincristine (Oncovin)	1.4 mg/m^2 I.V. bolus (max 2 mg)	1 & 8	
	Procarbazine	100 mg/m^2 p.o.	1–14	Diet without ripe cheese, avocado, nuts
	Prednisone	40 mg/m^2 p.o.	1–14	Only on 1st & 4th cyc
C-MOPP (same as MOPP but HN2 replaced by C if nausea and vomiting are intolerable)	Cyclophosphanide	650 mg/m^2 I.V.Sh.I.	1 & 8	
MVPP (same as MOPP but O replaced by V)	Vinblastine	6 mg/m^2 I.V. bolus	1 & 8	
ABVD	Doxorubicin (Adriamycin)	25 mg/m^2 I.V. bolus	1 & 15	q. 28 d × 6
	Bleomycin	2 U/d s.c.	4–10;18–24	
	Vinblastine	6 mg/m^2 I.V. bolus (max 10 mg)	1 & 15	
	Dacarbazine	250 mg/m^2 I.V.Sh.I. (200 cc D5%/W)	1 & 15	
MOPP/ABVD	MOPP		1–28	q. 56 d × 3
	ABVD		29–56	
MOPP/ABV Hybrid	Mechlorethamine (Mustargen)	6 mg/m^2 I.V. in a running inf	1	q. 28 d × 6
	Vincristine (Oncovin)	1.4 mg/m^2 I.V. bolus (max 2 mg)	1	
	Procarbazine	100 mg/m^2/d p.o.	1–7	Same diet restrictions
	Prednisone	40 mg/m^2/d p.o.	1–14	
	Doxorubicin (Adriamycin)	35 mg/m^2/d I.V. bolus	8	
	Bleomycin	10 U/m^2 I.V. inf after test dose	8	Should be preceded by hydrocortisone 100 mg I.V.
	Vinblastine	6 mg/m^2 I.V. bolus	8	
CVPD	Lomustine (CCNU)	75 mg/m^2 p.o.	1	q. 28 d
	Vinblastine	4 mg/m^2 I.V. bolus	1 & 8	
	Procarbazine	100 mg/m^2 p.o.	1–14	Same diet restrictions
	Prednisone	30 mg/m^2 p.o.	1–14	Only on 1st & 4th cyc
ACOPP (used in children)	Doxorubicin (Adriamycin)	60 mg/m^2 I.V. bolus	1	q. 42 d × 6
	Cyclophosphamide	300 mg/m^2 I.V.Sh.I.	14 & 20	
	Vincristine (Oncovin)	1.5 mg/m^2 (max 2 mg) I.V. bolus	14 & 20	
	Procarbazine	100 mg/m^2 p.o.	14–20	
	Prednisone	40 mg/m^2 p.o.	1–27 in cyc 1 & 4; 14–27 in cyc 2,3,5 & 6	

Regimen	Drugs	Dose & admin. rte.	Days of treatment	Frequency & comments
Salvage Regimens				
CAV	Lomustine (CCNU)	100 mg/m^2 p.o.	1	q. 42 d × 6
	Melphalan (Alkeran)	6 mg/m^2 p.o.	1–4;22–26	
	Vinblastine	4 mg/m^2 I.V. bolus	1 & 22	
CEM	Lomustine (CCNU)	120 mg/m^2 p.o.	1	q. 42 d
	Etoposide	100 mg/m^2 I.V.Sh.I.	1,2,3, & 22,23, 24	
		or		
		200 mg/m^2 p.o.	1,2,3 and 22,23,24	
	Methotrexate	200 mg/m^2 I.V.Sh.I.	1 & 22	
	Leucovorin	25 mg p.o. q. 6 h × 8	2,3, & 23, 24	

Non-Hodgkin's Lymphoma

Regimen	Drugs	Dose (mg/m^2) & admin. rte.	Days of treatment	Frequency & comments
C-MOPP	Cyclophosphamide	650 I.V.	1 & 8	q. 28 d × 6–12 cyc
	Vincristine (Oncovin)	1.4 I.V. (max 2 mg)	1 & 8	
	Procarbazine	100 p.o.	1–14	
	Prednisone	40 p.o.	1–14	
CHOP	Cyclophosphamide	750 I.V.	1	q. 21 d × 8–10 cyc (max doxorubicin dose 450 mg/m^2; for >300 mg/m^2 total dose, monitor ventric ejec fraction)
	Doxorubicin (hydroxydaunomycin)	50 I.V.	1	
	Vincristine (Oncovin)	1.4 I.V. (max 2 mg)	1 & 5	
	Prednisone	100 p.o.	1–5	
CHOP-Bleo	Cyclophosphamide	750 I.V.	1	q. 21 d × 8 (same restrictions as above for doxorubicin)
	Doxorubicin (hydroxydaunomycin)	50 I.V.	1	
	Vincristine (Oncovin)	1.4 I.V. (max 2 mg)	1	
	Prednisone	100 p.o.	1–5	
	Bleomycin	4 I.V.	1	
BCVP	Carmustine (BCNU)	60 I.V.	1	q. 21 d × 6–12 cyc
	Cyclophosphamide	1,000 I.V.	1	
	Vincristine (Oncovin)	1.4 I.V. (max 2 mg)	1	
	Prednisone	100 p.o.	1 & 15	
BACOP	Bleomycin	5 I.V.	15 & 21	q. 28 d × 5–10 cyc
	Doxorubicin (Adriamycin)	25 I.V.	1 & 8	
	Cyclophosphamide	650 I.V.	1 & 8	
	Vincristine (Oncovin)	1.4 I.V. (max 2 mg)	1 & 8	
	Prednisone	60 p.o.	15–28	
COMLA	Cyclophosphamide	1,500 I.V.	1	q. 12 wk × 3
	Vincristine (Oncovin)	1.5 I.V. (max 2 mg)	1,8 & 15	
	Methotrexate	120 I.V.	22, then weekly × 7	
	Leucovorin	15 p.o. q. 6 h × 8	23,24 (24 h after MTX) then weekly × 7	
	Cytosine arabinoside	300 I.V.	22, then weekly × 7	

Regimen	Drugs	Dose (mg/m^2) & admin. rte.	Days of treatment	Frequency & comments
m-BACOD	Methotrexate	200 I.V.	8 & 15	q. 21–28 d × 6–10 cyc
	Leucovorin	15 p.o. q. 6 h × 8	9,10; 16,17 (start 24 h after beginning MTX inf)	
	Bleomycin	4 I.V.	1	
	Doxorubicin (Adriamycin)	45 I.V.	1	
	Cyclophosphamide	600 I.V.	1	
	Vincristine (Oncovin)	1.0 I.V. (max 2 mg)	1	
	Dexamethasone	6 p.o.	1–5	
ProMACE	Prednisone	60 p.o.	1–14	q. 28 d × 6–10 cyc
	Methotrexate	1,500 I.V.	14	
	Leucovorin	15 p.o. q. 6 h × 8	15,16	
	Doxorubicin (Adriamycin)	25 I.V.	1 & 8	
	Cyclophosphamide	650 I.V.	1 & 8	
	Etoposide	120 I.V.	1 & 8	
ProMace-MOPP (flexi-therapy)	ProMace		1–14	q. 56 d × 6
	Standard MOPP		29–43	
ACOMLA	Doxorubicin (Adriamycin)	40 I.V.	1	q. 3 mo × 3
	Cyclophosphamide	1,000 I.V.	1	
	Vincristine (Oncovin)	2 I.V. (total)	1,8,15	
	Methotrexate	120 I.V.	22,29,35,43,50, 57,64,71	
	Leucovorin	25 p.o. (total)	24 h after MTX, q. 6 h × 6	
	Cytosine arabinoside (ara-C)	300 I.V.	1 hr after MTX on same days	
Pro-MACE (S Mtx)	Prednisone	60 p.o.	1–14	q. 21 d × 6–12 cyc
CYTABOM	Doxorubicin (Adriamycin)	25 I.V. bolus	1	
	Cyclophosphamide	650 I.V.Sh.I.	1	
	Etoposide	120 I.V.Sh.I.	1	
	Cytarabine	300 I.V.	8	
	Bleomycin	5 I.V.	8	
	Methotrexate	120 I.V.	8	
	Leucovorin	25 p.o. (total)	9 q. 6 h × 8 (24 h after MTX)	
COP-BLAM-III	Cyclophosphamide	350 I.V. (escalate to 500)	1 & 22	q. 6 wk × 6–8 cyc
	Vincristine (Oncovin)	1 I.V.C.I.	1–2	
		1.4 (max 2) I.V. bolus	22	
	Prednisone	40 p.o. q.d.	1–5; 22–27	
	Bleomycin	7.5 I.V. bolus *and*	1 & 22	
		7.5/d I.V.C.I.	1–5	
	Doxorubicin (Adriamycin)	35 I.V. bolus (escalate to 50)	1 & 22	
	Procarbazine (Matulane)	100 p.o	1–5; 22–27	

Regimen	Drugs	Dose (mg/m^2) & admin. rte.	Days of treatment	Frequency & comments
MACOP-B	Methotrexate	400 I.V.Sh.I. (hydration, alkalization of urine)	1 of wk 2,6,10	
	Doxorubicin (Adriamycin)	50 I.V. bolus	1 of wk 1,3,5,7,9,11	
	Cyclophosphamide	350 I.V.Sh.I.	1 of wk 1,3,5,7,9,11	
	Vincristine (Oncovin)	1.4 I.V. bolus	1 of wk 2,4,6,8,10,12	
	Bleomycin	10 U I.V. bolus	1 of wk 4,8,12	
	Prednisone	45 p.o.	q.d.; dose tapered over last 15 d	
	Co-trimoxazole	1 double-strength tab p.o.	b.i.d. throughout cyc	
VACOP-B	Etoposide (VP-16)	50 I.V.Sh.I. 100 p.o.	1 of wk 3,7,11 2,3 of wk 3,7,11	
	Doxorubicin (Adriamycin)	50 I.V. bolus	1 of wk 1,3,5,7,9,11	
	Cyclophosphamide	350 I.V.Sh.I.	1 of wk 1,3,5,7,9,11	
	Vincristine (Oncovin)	1.2 I.V. bolus	1 of wk 2,4,6,8,10,12	
	Bleomycin	10 I.V. bolus	1 of wk 2,4,6,8,10,12	
	Prednisone	45 p.o.	q.d. × 1 wk, then q.o.d. × 11 wk	
	Ketoconazole	200 p.o.	daily × 1 wk, then q.o.d. × 11 wk	
	Cimetidine	600 p.o.	b.i.d. × 1 wk, then q.o.d. × 11 wk	
	Co-trimoxazole	1 double-strength tab p.o.	b.i.d. throughout cyc	
MINE	MESNA (uroprotector)	1.33 g/m^2/d I.V.C.I.	1–4 1–4 q. 28 d × 6 cyc	
	Ifosfamide	1.33 g/m^2/d I.V.C.I.	1–3	
	Mitoxantrone (Novantrone)	8 I.V. bolus	1	
	Etoposide	65 I.V.Sh.I.	1–3	
IMVP-16	Ifosfamide	4g/m^2/d I.V.C.I.	1	q. 21–28 d × 6–8 cyc
	MESNA	4g/m^2/d I.V.C.I.	1 & 2	
	Etoposide (VP-16)	100 I.V.	1–3	
LSA2-L2 (pediatric cases; induction and consolidation phase)	Cyclophosphamide	1,200 I.V. bolus	1	
	Vincristine	1.5 (max) I.V. bolus	3,10,17,24	
	Prednisone	60 p.o. in 3 divided doses	3–31	
	Methotrexate	6.25 i.thec.	5,27,30,85,88	
	Daunorubicin	60 I.V. bolus	12,13	
	XRT (concomitantly to bulky disease)			
	Cytosine arabinoside	150 I.V. bolus	36–40; 43–47	
	Thioguanine	75 p.o. (8–12 h after cytosine arabinoside)	36–40; 43–47	
	Asparaginase	6,000 U/m^2	70–81	
	Carmustine	60 I.V. inf over 1 h	90	

Regimen	Drugs	Dose (mg/m^2) & admin. rte.	Days of treatment	Frequency & comments
LSA2-L2 (maintenance phase; start on day 94 of induction and consolidation phase)	Thioguanine	300 p.o.	1–4	q. 10 wk for total of 2–3 yr
	Cyclophosphamide	600 I.V.	5	
	Hydroxyurea	500 p.o.	15–18	
	Daunorubicin	45 I.V. bolus	19	
	Methotrexate	10 p.o.	30–33	
	Carmustine	60 I.V. (1-hr inf)	34	
	Cytosine arabinoside	150 I.V. bolus	44–47	
	Vincristine	1.5 (max 2) I.V. bolus	48	
	Methotrexate	6.25 i.thec.	58 & 61	
COMP (pediatric cases; induction phase)	Cyclophosphamide	1,200 I.V. 250 ml D5%/W	1	
	Vincristine (Oncovin)	2 (max) I.V. push	3,10,17,24	
	Methorexate	300 I.V. (60% of dose as I.V. push and 40% as 4-h inf in D5%/W)	12	
	Methotrexate	6.25 i.thec.	5,31,34	
	Prednisone	60 (max) p.o. q.d. in 4 divided doses	3–30	
COMP (maintenance phase; starts 7–21 d after last i.thec. MTX of induction)	Cyclophosphamide	1,000 I.V. inf in 250 ml D5%/W	1	q. 28 d × 18 mo
	Vincristine (Oncovin)	1.5 (max 2) I.V. bolus	1 & 14	
	Methotrexate	6.25 i.thec.	29 (1 of 2nd cycle)	
	Methotrexate	300 I.V. (60% of dose as I.V. push and 40% as 4-h inf in D5%/W	15	
	Prednisone	60 (max) p.o. q.d.	29 (1 of 2nd cyc) to 33 (5 of 2nd cyc)	
ACE	Cytosine arabinoside (ara-C)	150–300 24 h I.V.C.I.	1 & 8	q. 28 d × 4–6 cyc
	Cisplatin	80 I.V.Sh.I. with hydration, mannitol, antiemetics	1	
	Etoposide	100 I.V.Sh.I. or 200 p.o.	1 & 8	
HEIM	Hydroxyurea	1 g/m^2 p.o. q. 6 h	1 & 2	q. 21 d × 6 cyc
	Etoposide	80 I.V.Sh.I. then 160 p.o.	4 & 5 / 6	
	Ifosfamide	3 g/m^2 I.V.C.I.	4	
	MESNA	3 g/m^2 I.V.C.I.	4 & 5	

DOSE ADJUSTMENTS—ALL LYMPHOMA REGIMENS (HODGKIN'S DISEASE AND NON-HODGKIN'S LYMPHOMAS)

The following general recommendations can be made:

1. In case of bone marrow suppression reflected by low granulocyte and platelet counts, the dosage of these drugs should be decreased: cyclophosphamide, mechlorethamine, procarbazine, doxorubicin, carmustine, lomustine, cytosine arabinoside, methotrexate, etoposide, ifosfamide, dacarbazine, and vinblastine.

Granulocytes/µl	Platelets/µl	Doses administered
>3,000	130,000	Full doses
3,000–2,990	100,000–129,000	75% of calc dose
1,500–1,990	75,000–99,000	50% of calc dose
<1,500	75,000	Hold therapy

2. Vinblastine, vincristine, and doxorubicin should also be adjusted for cholestasis as follows:

Direct bilirubin level	Doses administered
<1.2 mg	Full dose
1.2–1.5	75% of calc dose
1.5–2.5	50% of calc dose
>2.5	Hold therapy

3. Bleomycin should not be administered beyond a total dose of 150 U/m^2 or whenever a drop by >20% of patient's diffusion capacity is noted or "interstitial streaking" develops on plain chest x-ray not explained by other pathologic process.

4. Vincristine and vinblastine doses should be decreased by 50% if DTRs are diminished or severe constipation develops. The drug should be discontinued when DTRs are completely suppressed.

Malignant Tumors of the Brain

Regimen	Drugs	Dose & admin. rte.	Days of treatment	Frequency & comments
Glioblastoma Multiforme				
BCNU-XRT	Carmustine (BCNU)	100 mg/m^2 I.V. 1-h inf _or_ 80 mg/m^2 I.V. 1-h inf	1,2 1,2,3	q. 6–8 wk × 6–10 cyc (1st cyc starts at same time as XRT & dexamethasone)
CCNU-XRT	Lomustine (CCNU)	120 mg/m^2 p.o. q.d.	1,2	q. 6 wk × 6–10 cyc (1st cyc starts at same time as XRT & dexamethasone)
BP-XRT	Lomustine (BCNU) Cisplatin (Platinol)	100 mg/m^2 I.V. 1-h inf 80 mg/m^2 I.V. with mannitol, hydration, antiemetics	1 1,22	q. 6 wk × 6 cyc (1st cyc starts at same time as XRT & dexamethasone)
Meduloblastoma				
CVP	Lomustine (CCNU) Vincristine Cisplatin (Platinol)	75 mg/m^2 p.o. 1.5 mg/m^2 (max 2 mg) I.V. 75 mg/m^2 I.V. in short NS inf with hydration, antiemetics, mannitiol	1 1,8,15,22 29,36,43,50 1,22	q. 42 × 8 cyc (except for vincristine, to be D/C after 8 wk) (1st cyc accompanies XRT & dexamthasone)

DOSE ADJUSTMENTS—MALIGNANT TUMORS OF THE BRAIN

1. For carmustine and lomustine, doses are related to the degree of bone marrow suppression:

Granulocytes/μl	Platelets/μl	Dose administered
≥ 3,000	≥ 130,000	Full dose
2,000–2,990	100,000–129,000	75% of calc dose
1,500–1,990	75,000–99,000	50% of calc dose
< 1,500	< 75,000	Hold therapy

2. For vincristine, dose should be decreased by 50% if deep tendon reflexes are decreased, if severe constipation persists, or serum direct bilirubin is 1.5–2.5 mg/dl. The drug should be withheld when DTRs are absent or serum direct bilirubin is > 2.5 mg/dl.
3. Administration of cisplatin should be postponed when serum creatinine is 1.5 mg/dl or creatinine clearance is < 60 ml/hr.

Head and Neck Cancer

For patients with unresectable or recurrent or metastatic lesions, no known standard chemotherapy regimens can prolong survival significantly. Regimens listed below are among those suggested for patients not eligible for clinical trials.

Regimen	Drugs	Dosage (mg/m^2) & admin. rte.	Days of treatment	Frequency & comments
PF	Cisplatin (Platinol)	100 I.V.Sh.I. with mannitol, I.V. hydration, antiemetics *or*	1	q. 3 wk × 10–12 cyc
		20 I.V. bolus c̄ same support	1–5	
	5-Fluorouracil	1,000/24 h. I.V.C.I.	1–5 *or* 2–6	
MBP	Methotrexate	40 I.M.	1 & 15	q. 3 wk × 6
	Bleomycin	10 (total dose) I.M.	1 & 15	
	Cisplatin (Platinol)	50 I.V. bolus c̄ supp. meas.	day 4	
PBML	Cisplatin (Platinol)	20 I.V. bolus c̄ supp. meas.	1–6	q. 3 wk × 4–6 cyc
	Bleomycin	10 I.V. 24-h inf	3–7	
	Methotrexate (high-dose)	240–700 I.V. Inf in D5%/½ NS	1	
	Leucovorin	50 I.V.	2	
		15 p.o.	q. 6 hr days 2,3,4	
MLF	Methotrexate	240 I.V. in 500 ml NS over 4 h	1	q. 3 wk
	Leucovorin	50 I.V. in 50 ml D5%/½ NS over 2 h	2 (24 h after MTX is started)	
		15 p.o.	q. 6 h days 2, 3	
	5-Fluorouracil	600 I.V. bolus 1 h after leucovorin is started	2	
COB	Cisplatin	100 I.V. c̄ supp. meas.	1	q. 21 d × 6 cyc
	Vincristine (Oncovin)	1 I.V.	1 & 5	
	Bleomycin	30/day I.V.C.I.	2–5	Only in first 3 cyc
MBC	Methotrexate	40 I.V. bolus or I.M.	1 & 15	q. 21 d × 3
	Bleomycin	10 I.V. or I.M.	1,8,15	
	Cisplatin	50 I.V. c̄ supp. meas.	4	
BPVM	Bleomycin	5 U/m^2/24 h I.V.C.I. in 1,000 ml NS alone or admixed c̄ DDP	1–5	× 28 d × 6 cyc
	Cisplatin (Platinol)	20 I.V. push *or* admixed c̄ BLM in 1,000 ml NS (hydration, mannitol, antiemetics)	1–5	
	Vinblastine *or*	6 I.V. bolus	1	
	Etoposide (VP-16)	50 I.V.Sh.I.	1,3,5	
	Methotrexate	40 I.V. bolus (before DDP)	1	

Lung Cancer

Small-Cell Lung Cancer

Regimen	Drugs	Dosage (mg/m^2) & admin. rte.	Days of treatment	Frequency & comments
CAV	Cyclophosphamide	1,000 I.V.Sh.I.	1	q. 3 wk × 6
	Doxorubicin (Adriamycin)	50 I.V. bolus	1	
	Vincristine	1.4 (max 2) I.V. bolus	1	
CAE	Cyclophosphamide	1,000 I.V.Sh.I.	1	q. 3 wk × 6
	Doxorubicin (Adriamycin)	50 I.V. bolus	1	
	Etoposide	50 I.V.Sh.I.	1–4	
		or		
		100 p.o.	1–4	
EP	Etoposide	50 I.V.Sh.I.	1–5	q. 3 wk × 4
		or		
		100 I.V.Sh.I.	1,3,5	
	Cisplatin (Platinol)	75–100 I.V.Sh.I. with mannitol, hydration, antiemetics	1	
EC	Etoposide	100 I.V.Sh.I.	1,2,3	q. 4 wk × 4
	Carboplatin	300 I.V.Sh.I.	1	
CAVEP (MSKCC)	Cyclophosphamide	1,200 I.V.Sh.I.	1	q. 4–5 wk × 4 cyc
	Doxorubicin (Adriamycin)	50 I.V. bolus	1	
	Vincristine	1.4 (max 2) I.V. bolus	1	
	Etoposide	120 I.V.Sh.I.	18,20,22	
	Cisplatin (Platinol)	60 I.V.Sh.I. c̄ antiemetics & mannitol	15	
CAVEP (NCI)	Cyclophosphamide	1,000 I.V.Sh.I.	1	q. 6 wk × 6
	Doxorubicin (Adriamycin)	50 I.V. bolus	1	
	Vincristine	1.4 (max 2) I.V. bolus	1	
	Etoposide	100 I.V.Sh.I.	22,23,24	
	Cisplatin (Platinol)	25 I.V.Sh.I. c̄ AE & M	22,23,24	
M-CAVEP	Cisplatin (Platinol)	50 I.V.Sh.I. c̄ AE & M	1,8	
	Etoposide	50 I.V.Sh.I.	1,2,3	
	Vincristine	1.4 (max 2) I.V. bolus	8	
	Cyclophosphamide	450 I.V.Sh.I.	15	
	Doxorubicin (Adriamycin)	50 I.V. bolus	15	
	Methotrexate	200 I.V.Sh.I.	22	
	Leucovorin	25 p.o. (total) q. 6 h × 8	23, 24	

Nonsmall-Cell Lung Cancer

In nonsmall-cell lung cancer, no known standard chemotherapy regimens can prolong survival significantly. Some suggested regimens for patients not eligible for clinical trials are listed below.

Regimen	Drugs	Dose (mg/m^2) & admin. rte.	Days of treatment	Frequency & comments
CAP	Cyclosphosphamide	500 I.V.Sh.I.	1	q. 3 wk × 6
	Doxorubicin (Adriamycin)	50 I.V. bolus	1	
	Cisplatin (Platinol)	80 I.V. NS Sh.I. with I.V. hydration, mannitol, antiemetics	1	
MVP	Mitomycin-C	10 I.V. bolus	1	q. 8 wk × 3
	Vinblastine	6 I.V. bolus	1,15,29,43	
	Cisplatin (Platinol)	100 I.V. as above	1 & 29	
EP	Etoposide	125 I.V.	1	
		125 I.V.	2,3	
		or		
		250 p.o.	2,3	
	Cisplatin	60 I.V.	1	
		or		
		20 I.V. with I.V. hydration, mannitol, antiemetics	1,2,3	
EC	Etoposide	100 I.V.	1	
		200 p.o.	2,3	
	Carboplatin	200 I.V.	1	
MEP	Mitomycin-C	10 I.V. bolus	1	q. 6 wk × 3
	Etoposide	120 I.V.Sh.I.	1 & 22	
	Cisplatin (Platinol)	80 I.V. c̄ supp. meas.	1 & 22	
MEP (5d)	Mitomycin-C	10 I.V. bolus	1	q. 8 wk × 3
	Etoposide	50 I.V.Sh.I. NS	1–5; 29–33	
	Cisplatin (Platinol)	20 I.V.Sh.I. NS c̄ supp. meas.	1–5; 29–33	
MACC	Methotrexate	40 I.V. bolus	1	q. 3 wk × 6–10 cyc
	Doxorubicin (Adriamycin)	40 I.V. bolus	1	
	Cyclosphosphamide	400 I.V.Sh.I.	1	
	Lomustine (CCNU)	30 p.o.	1	
COB	Cisplatin	100 I.V. c̄ supp. meas.	1	q. 21 d × 6
	Vincristine (Oncovin)	1 I.V.	1 & 5	
	Bleomycin	30/day I.V.C.I.	2–5	Only in the first 3 cyc
MBC	Methotrexate	40 I.V. bolus or I.M.	1 & 15	q. 21 d
	Bleomycin	10 I.V. or I.M.	1,8,15	
	Cisplatin	50 I.V. c̄ supp. meas.	4	
BPVM	Bleomycin	5 U/m^2/24 h I.V.C.I. in 1,000 ml NS alone or admixed c̄ DDP	1–5	q. 21–28 d × 5–6 cyc
	Cisplatin (Platinol)	20 I.V. push or admixed c̄ BLM in 1,000 ml NS (hydration, mannitol, antiemetics)	1–5	
	Vinblastine	6 I.V. bolus	1	q. 28 d × 6
	or			
	Etoposide	50 I.V.Sh.I.	1,3,5	
	Methotrexate	40 I.V. bolus (before DDP)	1	

Digestive System Malignancies

Esophageal Carcinoma

For recurrent or metastatic squamous cell carcinoma of the esophagus, the regimens below can be administered to patients who are not eligible for clinical trials.

For unresectable squamous cell carcinoma of the esophagus, combined modality therapy is used, with XRT given 5 days/wk (180–200 cGy/day) up to a total of 6,000–6,500 cGy; combination chemotherapy is administered every 3 wk, usually alternating chemotherapy agents as shown below.

Regimen	Drugs	Dose (mg/m^2) & admin. rte.	Days of treatment	Frequency & comments
PF	Cisplatin (Platinol)	100 I.V. NS Sh.I. or 24-h inf	1	c̄ supp. meas.
	5-Fluorouracil	1,000 I.V. D5%/½ NS I.V.C.I.	2–4	
MF	Mitomycin-C	10 I.V. bolus	22	
	5-Fluorouracil	1,000 I.V. D5%/½ NS	23–26	
MLF	Methotrexate	200 I.V.Sh.I.	43	
	Leucovorin	50 I.V. 2-h inf	44 (24 h after start of MTX)	
		then 15 p.o. q. 6 h × 8	44,45	
	5-Fluorouracil	500 I.V. bolus 1 h (after LCV is started)	44	

For recurrent or metastatic adenocarcinoma of the esophagus, regimens administered to patients with advanced gastric carcinoma (see below) can be used in patients not eligible for investigational protocols.

Gastric Carcinoma (Advanced Unresectable or Metastatic)

Regimen	Drugs	Dose (mg/m^2) & admin. rte.	Days of treatment	Frequency & comments
FAM	5-Fluourouracil	600 I.V. bolus	1,8,29,36	q. 56 d × 6
	Doxorubicin (Adriamycin)	30 I.V. bolus	1,29	
	Mitomycin-C	10 I.V. bolus	1	
APE(EAP)	Doxorubicin (Adriamycin)	20 I.V. bolus	1 & 7	q. 3–4 wk × 6
	Cisplatin (Platinol)	40 I.V. bolus c̄ supp. meas.	2 & 8	
	Etoposide	120 I.V.Sh.I.	4,5,6	
		(100 for pts >60 yr old)		
LF	Leucovorin	200 I.V. bolus or 2-h inf	1–5	q. 28 d × 12
	5-Fluorouracil	400 I.V. bolus 1 h after starting LCV	1–5	
FCE	5-Fluorouracil	900/d I.V.C.I.	1–5	q. 21 d × 6
	Cisplatin	20 I.V. bolus with hydration, antiemetics	1–5	
	Etoposide	90 I.V.Sh.I	1,3,5	

Pancreatic Carcinoma (Advanced Unresectable, Recurrent or Metastatic)

Regimen	Drugs	Dose (mg/m^2) & admin. rte.	Days of treatment	Frequency & comments
FAM-S	5-Fluorouracil	600 I.V. bolus	1,8,29,36	q. 56 d × 6
	Doxorubicin (Adriamycin)	30 I.V. bolus	1 & 29	
	Mitomycin-C	10 I.V. bolus	1	
	Streptozotocin	400 I.V.Sh.I.	1,8,29,36	Monitor blood glucose
SMF	Streptozotocin	500 I.V.Sh.I.	1,8,29,36	q. 56 d
	Mitomycin-C	10 I.V. bolus		
	5-Fluorouracil	600 I.V. bolus	1,8,29,36	
SD	Streptozotocin	500 I.V.Sh.I.	1–5	q. 42 d
	Doxorubicin	50 I.V. bolus	1 & 22	

Apudomas of the G.I. Tract

Regimen	Drugs	Dose (mg/m^2) & admin. rte.	Days of treatment	Frequency & comments
SF	Streptozotocin	500 I.V.Sh.I.	1–5	q. 4–6 wk × 6 cyc
	5-Fluorouracil	400 I.V. bolus	1–5	
SA	Streptozotocin	500 I.V.Sh.I.	1–5	q. 6 wk × 6 cyc
	Doxorubicin (Adriamycin)	50 I.V. bolus	1 & 22	Monitor blood sugar

Colorectal Carcinoma

Regimen	Drugs	Dose (mg/m^2) & admin. rte.	Days of treatment	Frequency & comments
Advanced Metastatic Disease				
LF (weekly)	Leucovorin	500 I.V. 2-h inf	1 wk of 1–6	q. 8 wk × 2
	5-Fluorouracil	600 I.V. bolus 1 h after LCV is started	1 of wk 1–6	
LF (monthly)	Leucovorin	200 I.V. bolus	1–5	q. 4 wk × 12
	5-Fluorouracil	370–400 I.V. bolus 1 h after LCV is started	1–5	
MF	Mitomycin-C	10 I.V. bolus	1	q. 56 d × 6
	5-Fluourouracil	400 I.V. bolus	1–5 & 29–33	
F-INF	5-Fluorouracil	750 I.V. bolus	1–5, then on d 29	q. wk × 48
	Alpha interferon	9 million U s.c.	1,3,5	q. wk × 52
Surgical Adjuvant Therapy (for Stages C and B$_3$)				
F-Lev	5-Fluorouracil	450 I.V. bolus	1–5	
		then 450 I.V. bolus	1 each wk	× 48 doses
	Levamisole	150 (total dose/day) p.o.	1–3 q. 2 wk	× 26 doses

Carcinoma of the Rectum and Anus (Loco-Regional Disease)

MF + XRT Regimen
1. XRT to the lesion or residual tumor postoperatively; usually 5,000 cGy (200 cGy/d × 5 d/wk × 5 wk).
2. Mitomycin-C: 10 mg/m^2 I.V. bolus day 1 of XRT.
3. 5-Fluorouracil: 1,000 mg/m^2/d by I.V. C.I. × 5 in first and fourth week of XRT.

Carcinoma of the Biliary Tract (Loco-Regional Disease)

The same MF + XRT regimen as for carcinoma of the rectum and anus should be used. For metastatic disease, the LF and MF regimens used for advanced metastatic colorectal carcinoma should be used.

DOSE ADUSTMENTS—ALL REGIMENS USED IN G.I. MALIGNANCIES

1. For 5-fluorouracil, doxorubicin, mitomycin-C, and etoposide, the dose should be reduced to the degree of bone marrow suppression represented by the level of granulocyte and platelet count:

Granulocytes/µl	Platelets/µl	Dose administered
≥ 3,000	≥ 130,000	Full dose
2,000–2,990	100,000–129,900	75% of calc dose
1,500–1,990	75,000– 99,900	50% of calc dose
< 1,500	< 75,000	Hold therapy

2. For streptozotocin, the dose should be adjusted to serum glucose level (SGL):

SGL (fasting)	Dose administered
< 120 mg/dl	Full dose
120–150 mg/dl	75% of calc dose
150–200 mg/dl	50% of calc dose
> 200 mg	Administer only with insulin coverage

Malignancies of the Genitourinary System

Metastatic Testicular Cancer and other Germ Cell Tumors

Regimen	Drugs	Dose and admin. rte.	Days of treatment	Frequency & comments
PVB	Cisplatin (Platinol)	20 mg/m^2 I.V. 15 min with hydration NS inf + antiemetics	1–5	q. 3 wk × 3
	Vinblastine	0.15 mg/kg I.V. bolus (preferably 6 h before bleomycin)	1 & 2	A 4th cycle (without bleomycin) is
	Bleomycin	30 U I.V.Sh.I. D5%/½ NS after testing for allergy	1,8,15	given if no CR achieved
BEP	Cisplatin (Platinol)	20 mg/m^2 I.V. as above	1–5	q. 3 wk × 4
	Etoposide	100 mg/m^2 I.V. 1-h NS inf	1–5	(omit bleomycin
	Bleomycin	30 U I.V.Sh.I. D5%/½ NS inf	1,8,15	in last cyc)
VAB-6	Vinblastine	4 mg/m^2 I.V. bolus	1	q. 28 d × 3
(induction)	Cyclophosphamide	600 mg/m^2 I.V. bolus	1	(omit bleomycin
	Actinomycin D	1 mg/m^2 I.V. bolus	1	in last cyc)
	Bleomycin	30 U I.V. bolus, then 20 U/m^2 by C.I.	1 1–3	
	Cisplatin	120 mg/m^2 I.V.Sh.I. NS c̄ mannitol, antiemetics	4	
VAB-6	Vinblastine	4 mg/m^2 I.V. bolus	1	q. 3 wk × 24
(maintenance)	Actinomycin D	1 mg/m^2 I.V. bolus	1	
	Chlorambucil	4 mg/m^2/d p.o.	1–14	
EP	Etoposide	100 mg/m^2 I.V.Sh.I. NS	1–5	q. 21 d × 6 (only
(induction)	Cisplatinum (Platinol)	20 mg/m^2 I.V. in 15-min NS inf with mannitol, antiemetics	1–5	for low-risk patients)
EP (maintenance)	Etoposide	200 mg/m^2/d p.o.	1–5	q. 28 d × 24 (this adjuvant regimen recommended for high-risk pts)
Salvage Regimen				
VIMP	Vinblastine	0.22 mg/kg I.V. bolus	1	
	Ifosfamide	1.2 g/m^2 I.V.C.I.	1–5	q. 21 d × 4
	MESNA	120 mg I.V. bolus, then 1.2 g/m^2 I.V.C.I.	1–5	
	Cisplatin (Platinol)	20 mg/m^2 I.V.Sh.I.	1–5	
CVEB	Cisplatin	40 mg/m^2 I.V.Sh.I. with mannitol, hydration, antiemetics	1–5	q. 3 wk × 4 (D/C bleomycin after
	Vinblastine	7.5 mg/m^2 I.V. bolus	1	90 U)
	Etoposide	100 mg/m^2 I.V.Sh.I.	1–5	
	Bleomycin	30 U I.V.Sh.I.	1 of wk 1–3	

Wilms' Tumor

Regimen	Drugs	Dose & admin. rte.	Days of treatment	Frequency & comments
AV	Actinomycin D	15 μg/kg I.V.Sh.I.	1–5 of wks 0,6,13,26—stg I plus in wks 40,49,58—stg II	In infants, dose is decreased to 7.5 μg/kg; this regimen is only for favorable histology stage I or II
	Vincristine	1.5 mg/m^2 (max 2 mg) I.V. bolus	1 of wk 1–10, then 1 of wk 13,26 for stg I; 1 of wk 15,24,33,42, 51,60 for stg II	
AVADR	Actinomycin D	15 μg/kg I.V.Sh.I.	1–5 of wk 0,6,13,26,39,52,65	For stage I or II (unfavorable histology) and for all stage III or IV cases
	Vincristine	1.5 mg/m^2 (max 2 mg) I.V. bolus	1 of wk 1–10; 1 & 5 of wk 13,26,39,52,65	
	Doxorubicin (Adriamycin)	20 mg/m^2 I.V. bolus	1,2,3 of wk 3,19,32,45,58	

Cancer of the Bladder and Urothelial Tract

Regimen	Drugs	Dose & admin. rte.	Days of treatment	Frequency & comments
M-VAC	Methotrexate	30 mg/m^2 I.V. bolus	1,15,22	q. 28 d × 4 (pts. who had prior XRT start doxorubicin at 15 mg/m^2)
	Vinblastine	3 mg/m^2 I.V. bolus	2,15,22	
	Doxorubicin (Adriamycin)	30 mg/m^2 I.V. bolus	2	
	Cisplatin	70 mg/m^2 I.V.Sh.I. with mannitol, hydration, antiemetics	2	
CISCA	Cisplatin	70–100 mg/m^2 I.V.Sh.I. with mannitol, hydration, antiemetics	2	q. 21–28 d × 4
	Cyclophosphamide	650 mg/m^2 I.V.Sh.I.	1	
	Doxorubicin (Adriamycin)	50 mg/m^2 I.V. bolus	1	
CAP	Cyclophosphamide	400 mg/m^2 I.V.Sh.I. $\bar{c}$ hydration	1	q. 21 d × 6
	Doxorubicin (Adriamycin)	40 mg/m^2 I.V. bolus	1	
	Cisplatin	60 mg/m^2 I.V. bolus $\bar{c}$ mannitol, hydration, antiemetics	1	

Prostatic Cancer (Stage D$_2$—Hormonal Therapy Failure)

Regimen	Drugs	Dose & admin. rte.	Days of treatment	Frequency & comments
DMF	Doxorubicin	50 mg/m^2 I.V. bolus	1	q. 3 wk × 6
	Mitomycin-C	10 mg/m^2 I.V. bolus		
	5-Fluorouracil	750 mg/m^2 I.V. bolus	1 & 2	

DOSE ADJUSTMENTS—ALL REGIMENS USED IN THERAPY OF G.U. MALIGNANCIES

1. For vinblastine, etoposide, cyclosphosphamide, dactinomycin, doxorubicin, methotrexate, mitomycin-C, 5-fluorouracil, and chlorambucil, the dose should be adjusted to the degree of bone marrow suppression:

Granulocytes	Platelets	Dose administered
>3,000	>130,000	Full dose
2,000–2,990	100,000–129,900	75% of calc dose
1,500–1,990	75,000–99,000	50% of calc dose
<1,500	<75,000	Hold therapy

2. Dosage of cisplatin should be reduced in case of renal insufficiency:

Serum creat.	Creat. clearance	Dose administered
<1.5	>60 ml/min	Full dose
1.5–1.7	45–60 ml/min	50% of calc dose
>1.7	<45 ml/min	Hold therapy

3. For bleomycin, therapy should be discontinued if fibrotic changes appear on chest x-ray or if abnormalities of diffusion capacity or allergic reactions are manifested.

Gynecological Malignant Neoplasms

Metastatic Epithelial Ovarian Carcinoma

Regimen	Drugs	Dose & admin. rte.	Days of treatment	Frequency & comments
PAC (CAP)	Cisplatin (Platinol)	50 mg/m^2 I.V.Sh.I. $\bar{c}$ mannitol, antiemetics, I.V. hydration	1	q. 3 wk × 8
	Doxorubicin (Adriamycin)	50 mg/m^2 I.V. bolus	1	
	Cyclophosphamide	500 mg/m^2 I.V.Sh.I.	1	
CP	Cyclophosphamide	1,000 mg/m^2 I.V.Sh.I.	1	q. 3 wk × 10
	Cisplatin (Platinol)	50–60 mg/m^2 I.V.Sh.I. $\bar{c}$ mannitol, hydration, antiemetics	1	
CDC	Carboplatin	300 mg/m^2 I.V. bolus	1	q. 4 wk × 6
	Doxorubicin	40 mg/m^2 I.V. bolus	1	
	Cyclophosphamide	500 mg/m^2 I.V.Sh.I	1	
CC	Carboplatin	300 mg/m^2 I.V. bolus	1	q. 3–4 wk × 12
	Cyclophosphamide	1,000 mg/m^2 I.V.Sh.I.	1	
AP	Doxorubicin (Adriamycin)	50–60 mg/m^2 I.V. bolus	1	q. 3 wk × 6–8 cyc
	Cisplatin (Platinol)	50–60 mg/m^2 I.V.Sh.I. $\bar{c}$ mannitol, hydration, antiemetics	1	
CHAP (or CHAD)	Cyclophosphamide	300–500 mg/m^2 I.V.Sh.I.	1	q. 4 wk × 6–8 cyc
	Hexamethylmelamine	150 mg/m^2 p.o.	1–7	
	Adriamycin	30–50 mg/m^2 I.V. bolus	1	
	Cisplatin (Platinol, cis-diamminedichloroplatinum)	50 mg/m^2 I.V.Sh.I. $\bar{c}$ mannitol, antiemetics, I.V. hydration	1	

Metastatic Germ Cell Ovarian Carcinoma*

Regimen	Drugs	Dose & admin. rte.	Days of treatment	Frequency & comments
VAC	Vincristine	1.2–1.5 mg/m^2 I.V. bolus (max 2 mg)	1	q. wk × 12
	Actinomycin D	0.3–0.4 mg/m^2 I.V.Sh.I.	1–5	q. 28 d
	Cyclosphosphamide	150 mg/m^2 I.V.Sh.I.	1–5	q. 28 d

*All regimens recommended for testicular germ cell carcinoma could also be used.

Gestational Trophoblastic Disease

Regimen	Drugs	Dose & admin. rte.	Days of treatment	Frequency & comments
DMC	Dactinomycin	0.30 mg/m^2 I.V.Sh.I.	1–5	q. 21 d × 8–10 cyc
	Methotrexate	11 mg/m^2 I.V. bolus	1–5	
	Cyclophosphamide	110 mg/m^2 I.V.Sh.I.	1–5	

Metastatic Carcinoma of the Uterine Corpus (Endometrial Carcinoma)

There is no standard regimen. The one given here is the most widely used.

Regimen	Drugs	Dose & admin. rte.	Days of treatment	Frequency & comments
AC(Meg)	Doxorubicin (Adriamycin)	60 mg/m² I.V. bolus		q. 31 d × 6–10 cyc
	Cisplatin	100 mg/m² Sh.I. NS c̄ mannitol, hydration, antiemetics	1	
	Megesterone acetate (Megace)	40 mg/ q.i.d. p.o.	1–21	If drug was not used while disease was progressing

Metastatic Squamous Cell Carcinoma of the Cervix, Vagina, and Vulva

There is no standard chemotherapy regimen for these neoplasms; however, some of the regimens used for the advanced squamous cell carcinoma of the head and neck can also be administered to these patients if they are not eligible for ongoing clinical trials. Other regimens that have been used with limited results are given below.

Regimen	Drugs	Dose & admin. rte.	Days of treatment	Frequency & comments
AM	Doxorubicin (Adriamycin)	50 mg/m² I.V. bolus	1	q. 3–4 wk × 6–8 cyc
	Methotrexate	20 mg/m² I.V. bolus	1 & 8	
BVMC	Bleomycin	7.5 U/m² I.V.C.I. NS	1–4 & 22–26	q. 56 d × 3
	Vincristine	0.5 mg I.V.C.I. NS or bolus (can be admixed c̄ BLM)	1–4 & 22–26	
	Mitomycin-C	20 mg/m² I.V. bolus	1	
BPVM	Bleomycin	5 U/m² I.V. 6-h or 24-h NS inf	1–5	q. 21 d × 6 (except D/C bleomycin after 4 cyc or if x-ray fibrosis develops)
	Cisplatin (Platinol)	25 mg/m² I.V. 6-h or 24-h NS inf (can be admixed c̄ BLM)	1–5	
	Vincristine	2 mg I.V. bolus	1	
	Methotrexate	200 mg/m² I.V. 1-h inf (with LCV 25 mg p.o. q. 6 h × 12 starting 24 h after start of MTX) *or* 40 mg/m² I.V. bolus	1 1	

NOTE: *Dose adjustments for gynecologic malignancies are similar to those recommended for gentourinary malignancies.*

Metastatic Carcinoma of the Breast

Regimen	Drugs	Dose & admin. rte.	Days of treatment	Frequency & comments
CMF	Cyclosphosphamide	100 mg/m^2/d p.o.	1–14	q. 28 d × 6 as
	Methotrexate	40 mg/m^2 I.V. bolus (30 mg/m^2 for pts >60 yr old)	1 & 8	adjuvant chemo-therapy or as necessary for metastatic disease
	5-Fluorouracil	500 mg/m^2 I.V. bolus	1 & 8	
CMFP	Cyclophosphamide	100 mg/m^2 I.V. bolus	1–14	q. 28 d × 6+ cyc
	Methotrexate	40 mg/m^2 I.V. bolus (same medication as for CMF)	1 & 8	
	5-Fluourouracil	500 mg/m^2 I.V. bolus	1 & 8	
	Prednisone	40 mg/m^2 p.o., then taper over 5 d	1–14	In 1st 3 cyc only
CAF	Cyclophosphamide	600 mg/m^2 I.V. bolus	1	q. 21–28 d × 6–15 cyc
	Doxorubicin (Adriamycin)	45 mg/m^2 I.V. bolus	1	Substitute MTX 30 mg/m^2 for ADR
	5-Fluorouracil	600 mg/m^2 I.V. bolus	1	when ADR cumula-tive dose of 450 mg/m^2 is reached
CMFVP (Cooper's regimen)	Cyclophosphamide	2.0–2.5 mg/kg p.o.	1–270	q.d.
	Methotrexate	0.7 mg/kg/wk I.V.	1	q. wk × 8
			then 1	q. 2 wk × 14
	5-Fluorouracil	12 mg/kg/wk I.V.	1	q. wk × 8
			then 1	q. 2 wk × 14
	Vincristine	0.035 mg/kg/wk I.V.	1	q. wk × 5
	Prednisone	0.75 mg/kg/d p.o.	1–10, then taper over 40 d	q.d.
VATH	Vinblastine	4.5 mg/m^2 I.V.	1	q. 21 d × 6
	Doxorubicin (Adriamycin)	45 mg/m^2 I.V.	1	
	Thio-tepa	12 mg/m^2 I.V.	1	
	Fluoxymesterone (Halotestin)	30 mg p.o.	1–21	
IMF	Ifosfamide	1.5 g/m^2 I.V.	1 & 8	
	MESNA	300 mg/m^2 I.V. before & at 4 & 8 h after IFX	1 & 8	
	Methotrexate	40 mg/m^2 I.V.	1 & 8	
	5-Fluorouracil	600 mg/m^2 I.V.	1 & 8	

Salvage Regimens

Regimen	Drugs	Dose & admin. rte.	Days of treatment	Frequency & comments
MiVb	Mitomycin-C	10 mg/m^2 I.V. push	1	q. 6 wk × 3–6 cyc
	Vinblastine	1.2 mg/m^2/d × 5 I.V.C.I.	1–5; 22–27	
MiVb	Mitomycin-C	10 mg/m^2 I.V. bolus	1	q. 6 wk × 3–6 cyc
	Vinblastine	6 mg/m^2 I.V. bolus	1 & 22	
MiVbC	Mitomycin-C	4 mg/m^2 I.V. bolus	1	q. 6 wk × 3–6 cyc
	Vinblastine	3 mg/m^2 I.V. bolus	1,15,29	
	Carmustine (BCNU)	50 mg/m^2 I.V.Sh.I.	1	
NoV	Mitoxantrone (Novantrone)	12 mg/m^2 I.V. bolus	1	q. 3 wk × 6 cyc
	Vincristine	1.5 mg/m^2 (max 2 mg) I.V. bolus	1	

Regimen	Drugs	Dose & admin. rte.	Days of treatment	Frequency & comments
NoVE	Mitoxantrone (Novantrone)	10 mg/m^2 I.V. bolus	1	q. 3–4 wk × 6
	Vincristine	1.5 mg/m^2 (max 2 mg) I.V. bolus	1	
	Etoposide	80 mg/m^2 I.V.Sh.I.	1–3	
		or		
		160 mg/m^2 p.o.	1–3	

DOSE ADJUSTMENTS—ALL REGIMENS FOR METASTATIC BREAST CARCINOMA

1. For bone marrow suppressing agents (e.g., methotrexate, 5-fluorouracil, doxorubicin, mitomycin-C, mitoxantrone, thio-tepa), dose reductions are related to the WBC and platelet count level:

Granulocytes/µl	Platelets/µl	Dose administered
>3,000	>130,000	Full dose
2,000–3,000	100,000–129,000	75% of calc dose
1,500–1,990	75,000–99,900	50% of calc dose
<1,500	<75,000	Hold therapy

2. For vincristine and vinblastine, the dose should be decreased by 50% if DTRs are decreased, and/or severe constipation persists or direct serum bilirubin is >2mg/dl. Medication should be withheld when DTRs are abolished or direct serum bilirubin is >2.5 mg/dl.

Medullary and Anaplastic Thyroid Carcinoma and Undifferentiated Nonsecretory Adrenal Cortical Carcinoma

Regimen	Drugs	Dose & admin. rte.	Days of treatment	Frequency & comments
DP	Doxorubicin (Adriamycin)	40–60 mg/m^2 I.V. bolus	1	q. 21 d × 6–10 cyc
	Cisplatin (Platinol)	60 mg/m^2 I.V. Sh.I. NS c̄ mannitol, hydration, antiemetics	1	

Sarcomas

Soft-Tissue Sarcomas

Regimen	Drugs	Dose & admin. rte.	Days of treatment	Frequency & comments
Unresectable High-Grade or Metastatic in Adults				
ADIC	Doxorubicin (Adriamycin)	60 mg/m^2 I.V. bolus	1	q. 21 d × 6–8 cyc
	Dacarbazine (DIC)	250 mg/m^2 I.V.Sh.I.	1–5	
CYVADIC	Cyclophosphamide	500 mg/m^2 I.V. push	2	q. 28 d × 6–8 cyc
	Vincristine (Oncovin)	1.5 mg/m^2 (max 2 mg) I.V. push	1	
	Doxorubicin (Adriamycin)	50 mg/m^2 I.V. push	2	
	Dacarbazine (DIC)	250 mg/m^2 I.V.Sh.I.	1–5	
CYVADACT	Cyclophosphamide	500 mg/m^2 I.V. push	2	q. 28 d × 6–8 cyc
	Vincristine	1.5 mg/m^2 (max 2 mg) I.V. push	1	
	Doxorubicin (Adriamycin)	50 mg/m^2 I.V. push	2	
	Dactinomycin (Actinomycin-D)	0.3 mg/m^2/d (max 0.5 mg) I.V.Sh.I.	3–5	
ID	Ifosfamide	5 g/m^2 I.V.C.I. × 24 h	1	q. 21 d × 6–8 cyc
	Doxorubicin	40 mg/m^2 I.V. bolus	1	
	MESNA	1 g/m^2 I.V. bolus prior to ifosfamide, then 4 g/m^2 × 32 h	1	
MAID	MESNA	2,500 mg/m^2 I.V.C.I.	1–4	q. 3 wk for 6–8 cyc (Adriamycin & dacarbazine admin only through central I.V. line)
	Doxorubicin (Adriamycin)	20 mg/m^2 I.V.C.I.	1–3	
	Ifosfamide	2,500 mg/m^2 I.V.C.I. admixed with MESNA	1–3	
	Dacarbazine	300 mg/m^2 I.V.C.I. admixed with ADR	1–3	
Unresectable High-Grade or Metastatic in Children				
VAC	Vincristine	1.5 mg/m^2 (max 2 mg)	1	q. 21 d × 12
	Dactinomycin (Actinomycin-D)	0.3 mg/m^2/d (max 0.5 mg) I.V.Sh.I.	1–3	
	Cyclophosphamide	500 mg/m^2 I.V. push	2	
VADRC	Vincristine	1.5 mg/m^2 (max 2mg) I.V. bolus	1	q. 21 d × 12
	Doxorubicin (Adriamycin)	30 mg/m^2 I.V. bolus	1,2	
	Cyclophosphamide	500 mg/m^2 I.V.Sh.I.	2	
VADRC/VAC	VADRC regimen		wk. 0,3,12,20,28 3,6,44,52	
	VAC regimen		wk 6,9,16,24,32,40,48; after wk 52, q. 4 wk. for another yr	
VAC (protracted)	Vincristine	2 mg/m^2 (max 2 mg)	1 of wk 1–12	
	Dactinomycin (Actinomycin D)	0.015 mg/kg (max 0.5 mg) I.V.Sh.I.	1–5	q. 3 mo × 6
	Cyclophosphamide	2.5 mg/kg/d p.o.		q.d. × 2 yr

Osteosarcomas (Metastatic or Residual Disease)

Regimen	Drugs	Dose & admin. rte.	Days of treatment	Frequency & comments
HDMTX/VCR	Methotrexate (high-dose)	100–750 mg/kg (children) 8–12 g/m^2 (adults) I.V. inf 4–6 h preceded by urine alkalization & I.V. hydration		q. 14–21 d × 12 (monitor serum MTX level)
	Leucovorin	15 mg p.o. (start 6–12 h after MTX is started; then q. 6 h × 12)	1–3	
	Vincristine	1.4 mg/m^2 (max 2 mg) I.V. bolus	1	
HDMTX/ADR	Methotrexate (high-dose)	100–750 mg/kg (children) 8–12 g/m^2 (adults) I.V. inf over 4 h	1	q. 28 d × 6 with same pre- cautions for I.V.
	Leucovorin	15 mg p.o. (start 2 h after MTX) q. 6 h × 12	1–3	hydration, urine alkalinization,
	Doxorubicin (Adriamycin)	0.80 mg/kg/d (children) I.V. bolus 45 mg/m^2/day (adults) I.V. bolus	15–17 15,16	and serum MTX monitoring
HDMTX/A/C	Methotrexate (high-dose)	100–750 mg/kg (children) 1–7 g/m^2 (adults) I.V. inf over 4 h	1	q. 28 d × 6 (same precautions as above)
	Leucovorin	15 mg p.o. (start 2 h after MTX) q. 6 h × 12	1–3	
	Doxorubicin (Adriamycin)	50 mg/m^2 I.V. bolus	15	
	Cyclosphosphamide	500 mg/m^2 I.V. bolus	15	
BCD	Bleomycin	12 U/m^2 I.V.Sh.I.	1 & 2	q. 14 d × 5, then continue s̄ BLM
	Cyclosphosphamide	600 mg/m^2 I.V.Sh.I.	1	
	Dactinomycin (Actinomycin D)	0.45 mg/m^2 I.V.Sh.I.	1 & 2	

*Osteosarcomas—Adjuvant Therapy**

Regimen	Drugs	Dose & admin. rte.	Days/weeks of treatment	Frequency & comments
Preoperative Induction Phase (Neoadjuvant Therapy)				
	Surgery:			
	Amputation		1 of 4th wk	
	Endoprosthesis		1 of 16th wk	
MV/BCD/A	Methotrexate (high-dose)	8–12 g/m^2 I.V. inf 1,000 U D5%/½ NS over 4 h (in children max 450 mg/kg)	1 of wk 1,2, 3,4,9,10,14,15	
	Leucovorin	25 mg p.o. q. 6 h × 12 (start 6 h after MTX inf onset)	1,2,3, of wk 1–4,9,10,14,15	
	Vincristine	1.4 mg/m^2 (max 2 mg) before MTX	1 of wk 1–4,9,10,14,15	
	Bleomycin	12 U/m^2 I.V.Sh.I.	1 of 6th wk	
	Cyclophosphamide	600 mg/m^2 I.V.	1 of 6th wk	
	Dactinomycin (Actinomycin D)	0.60 mg/m^2 I.V.Sh.I.	1 of 6th wk	
	Doxorubicin (Adriamycin)	30 mg/m^2 I.V. bolus × 3 d	1 of 11th wk	

*Pre- and postoperation—T-10 MSKCC

Regimen	Drugs	Dose & admin. rte.	Days/weeks of treatment	Frequency & comments
Postoperative Adjuvant Therapy				
1. For Poor Responders to Preoperative Chemotherapy:				
AC/BCD	Doxorubicin (Adriamycin)	30 mg/m^2 I.V. bolus × 2 d	1 of 1st & 4th wk	q. 10 wk × 3
	Cisplatin	120 mg/m^2 I.V. in NS 250 cc inf c̄ mannitol, antiemetics	1 of 1st & 4th wk	
	Bleomycin	12 U/m^2 I.V.Sh.I.	1 of 7th wk	
	Cyclophosphamide	600 mg/m^2 I.V.	1 of 7th wk	
	Dactinomycin	0.60 mg/m^2 I.V.Sh.I.	1 of 7th wk	
2. For Patients with Good Response to Preoperative Chemotherapy:				
MVA	Methotrexate (high-dose)	8–12 g/m^2 I.V. in 1,000 cc D5%/½ NS over 4 h	1 of wk 4,5,9,10	q. 12 wk q. 12 wk
	Leucovorin	25 mg p.o. q. 6 h × 12 (starting 6 h after MTX inf onset)		
	Vincristine	1.4 mg/m^2 (max 2 mg) I.V.	1 of wk 4,5,9,10	
	Doxorubicin (Adriamycin)	30 mg/m^2 × 3 d I.V.	1 of 6th wk	

Neuroblastoma (Stages III and IV)

Regimen	Drugs	Dose & admin. rte.	Days of treatment	Frequency & comments
CVD	Cyclophosphamide	750 mg/m^2 I.V.Sh.I.	1	q. 21 d × 6–10 cyc
	Vincristine	1.5 mg/m^2 (max 2 mg) I.V. bolus	5	
	Dacarbazine	250 mg/m^2 I.V.Sh.I.	1–5	
CA	Cyclophosphamide	150 mg/m^2/d p.o.	1–7	q. 21–28 d × 6–10
	Doxorubicin (Adriamycin)	35 mg/m^2 I.V. bolus	8	cyc

Malignant Melanoma

Regimen	Drugs	Dose & admin. rte.	Days of treatment	Frequency & comments
BHD	Carmustine (BCNU)	100–150 mg/m^2 I.V.Sh.I.	1	q 6 wk × 6
	Hydroxyurea	1,480 mg/m^2/d p.o.	1–5; 22–26	
	Dacarbazine	100–150 mg/m^2 I.V.Sh.I.	1–5; 22,26	
D-Act	Dacarbazine	750 mg/m^2 I.V.Sh.I.	1	q. 4 wk × 6
	Dactinomycin (Actinomycin D)	1 mg/m^2 I.V.Sh.I.	1	
VBD	Vinblastine	6 mg/m^2 I.V. bolus	1 & 2	q. 28 d × 4–6
	Bleomycin	15 U/m^2/d I.V.C.I.	1–5	cyc
	Cis-diamminedichloroplatinum (Platinol)	50 mg/m^2 I.V.Sh.I. c̄ hydration, mannitol, antiemetics	5	
VDP	Vinblastine	5 mg/m^2 I.V. bolus	1 & 2	q. 21–28 d ×
	Dacarbazine	150 mg/m^2 I.V.Sh.I.	1–5	4–6 cyc
	Cisplatin (Platinol)	75 mg/m^2 I.V.Sh.I. c̄ hydration, mannitol, antiemetics	5	
DBTC	Dacarbazine	220 mg/m^2/d I.V.Sh.I.	1–3; 22–24	q 6 wk × 4
	Carmustine (BCNU)	150 mg/m^2 I.V.Sh.I.	1	
	Tamoxifen	10 mg p.o. b.i.d.	daily	
	Cisplatin	25 mg/m^2/d I.V.Sh.I.	1–3; 22–24	
CBC	Lomustine (CCNU)	80 mg/m^2 p.o.	1	q 6 wk × 6
	Bleomycin	15 U/m^2/d I.V.Sh.I.	3–7	
	Cisplatin	40 mg/m^2/d I.V.Sh.I.	8	
BELD	Bleomycin	15 mg s.c.	1–4	q 4–6 wk × 6
	Vindesine (Eldisine)	3 mg/m^2 I.V.	1 & 5	
	Lomustine	80 mg/m^2 p.o.	1	
	Dacarbazine	200 mg/m^2 I.V.Sh.I.	1–5	
DVC	Dacarbazine	250 mg/m^2 I.V.Sh.I.	1–5	q 4–6 wk × 6
	Vindesine	3 mg/m^2 I.V. bolus	1	
	Cisplatin	100 mg/m^2 in 500 ml NS c̄ antiemetics & heavy hydration	1	
POC	Procarbazine	100 mg/m^2 (max 150 mg) p.o.	1–10	q. 4–6 wk × 6
	Vincristine (Oncovin)	1.4 mg/m^2 (max 2 mg) I.V. bolus	1 & 8	
	Lomustine (CCNU)	150 mg/m^2 (max 200 mg) p.o.	1	

Supportive Therapy

Antiemetic Therapy: Current Dosage and Scheduling Recommendations

Class/drug	Recommended dosage and schedule	Comments
Phenothiazenes		
Prochlorperazine	5–10 mg I.V. or orally q. 4–6 h; 25 mg q. 6 h	Diphenhydramine 25–50 mg may be given with each dose
Perphenazine	Loading dose of 2–5 mg over 60 min; then 2–4 mg I.V. or orally q. 4 h (or 0.5 mg/h C.I.)	Diphenhydramine 25–50 mg may be given with each dose
Thiethylperazine	10 mg q. 4–6 h	Available in oral, I.M., and rectal forms
Benzquinamides		
Benzquinamide	50 mg q. 4 h or 25 mg q. 2–4 h I.M.	
Trimethobenzamide	250 mg p.o. or 200 mg supp. q. 4 h	
Butyrophenones		
Haloperidol	0.5–1 mg orally or I.M. q. 8 h	
Droperidol	Loading dose of 10 mg I.V.; then 2 mg/h by C.I. during chemotherapy admin.	
Substituted benzamides		
Metoclopramide	1–2 mg/kg I.V. 30 min before chemotherapy and repeated every 2 h for 2 doses, then every 3 h for 3 doses	0.75 mg/kg/dose may be given for less emetogenic regimens. Diphenhydramine 50 mg may be given with the first dose
Corticosteroids		
Dexamethasone	8–10 mg I.V. q. 6 h for 4 doses	
Cannabinoids		
Tetrahydro-cannabinol	10 mg orally (max 15 mg) 4–5 h before chemotherapy; then q. 4 h during chemotherapy admin.	
Hypnotics and sedatives		
Lorazepam	1.5–2 mg/kg I.V. or sublingually (max 4 mg) q. 12 h	
$5HT_3$ receptor antagonists		
Ondansetron (GR38032F)	0.15 mg/kg I.V. piggyback in 50 ml NS over 15 min before chemotherapy, then q 3–4 hr × 2 doses or 1 mg/hr × 24 hr C.I. if needed	Occasional constipation and headaches may occur

Narcotic Analgesics Widely Used for Severe Pain

Name	Route	Dose (mg)	Peak (h)	Duration (h)	Plasma half-life (h)	Comments
Morphinelike agonists						
Morphine	I.M.	10	0.5–1	4–6	2–3.5	Standard of comparison for narcotic-type analgesics
	p.o.	60	1.5–2	4–7		
Morphine (long-acting) (MS Contin or Roxanol)	p.o.	60	6	8–12		
Codeine	I.M.	130	0.5–1	4–6	3	Like morphine; excellent oral potency
	p.o.	200				
Hydromorphone (Dilaudid)	I.M.	1.5	0.5–1	4–5	2–3	
	p.o.	7.5	1.5–2	4–7		
Levorphanol (Levo-Dromoran)	I.M.	2	0.5–1	4–6	12–16	
	p.o.	4	1.5–2	4–7		
Meperidine (Demerol)	I.M.	75	0.5–1	4–5	3–4	Slightly shorter acting; poor oral potency
	p.o.	300	1.2	4–6		
Methadone (Dolophine)	I.M.	10	0.5–1	4–6	15–30	Good oral potency
	p.o.	20	1.5–2	4–7		
Oxycodone	p.o.	30	1	4–6	na	Available only (5-mg doses) in combination with acetaminophen or aspirin
Oxymorphone	I.M.	1	0.5–1	4–6	na	
Mixed agonist/antagonists						
Pentazocine	I.M.	60	0.5–1	4–6	2–3	Mixed agonist/antagonist; less abuse liability than morphine; included in schedule IV of Controlled Substances Act
	p.o.	180	1.5–2	4–7		
Butorphanol	I.M.	2	0.5–1	4–6	2.5–3.5	
Nalbuphine	I.M.	10	0.5–1	4–6	5	
Partial agonists						
Buprenorphine (Buprenex)	I.M.	0.4	0.5–1	4–6	na	Partial agonist of the morphine type; less abuse liability than morphine; does not produce psychotomimetic effects
	s.c.	0.8	2–3	5–6		

Current Antidepressant Medications

Generic name	Trade names (U.S.)	Dose range/day	Plasma levels (ng/ml)
Heterocyclics			
Amitriptyline HCl	Elavil, Etraphon Endep, Limbitrol Triavil	175–300	100–250
Amoxapine HCl	Asendin	100–600	–
Desipramine HCl	Norpramin, Pertofrane	100–300	100–300
Doxepin HCl	Adapin, Sinequan	25–300	100–200
Fluoxetine HCl	Prozac	20–80	–
Imipramine HCl	Tofranil, Janimine	30–300	150–300
Maprotiline HCl	Ludiomil	225–300	200–500
Nortriptyline HCl	Aventyl, Pamelor	20–150	50–150
Protriptyline HCl	Vivactyl	25–300	100–200
Trimipramine maleate	Surmontil	25–300	–
Other classes			
Alprazolam	Xanax	1.5–4.5	–
Trazodone HCl	Desyrel	50–600	–

Supportive Treatment Orders for High-Dose Chemotherapy

SUPPORTIVE TREATMENT DURING INTERMEDIATE AND HIGH-DOSE THERAPY ($>$20 MG/M^2/DOSE) WITH CISPLATIN

Treatment should not be instituted if patient has creatinine clearance $\leq$ 60 ml/24 hr or a platelet count of $\leq$ 75,000/μl.

The following orders are recommended for the first administration of cisplatin (DDP) dissolved in 250 cc NS and infused (usually over 1-hr period). They can be adjusted for the second cycle in accordance with the intensity of the side effects or lack thereof generated by the first administration.

1. Cisplatin (_________)* I.V. in 250 cc NS over 1–2 hr.

2. Oral hydration during the 16 hr preceding DDP administration (at least 2,000 ml liquids).

3. Mannitol 12.5 g I.V. bolus before DDP or added to the DDP infusion.

4. Prochlorperazine 10 mg I.V. piggyback before DDP, then q. 6 hr I.V. piggyback or p.o. $\times$ 8.

5. Dexamethasone 10 mg I.V. PB before DDP, then q. 6 hr I.V. PB or p.o. $\times$ 4.

6. Ranetidine 150 mg p.o. b.i.d. $\times$ 3 days.

7. Lorazepam 1 mg p.o. b.i.d. $\times$ 3 days.

8. Metoclopromide 75–100 mg I.V. piggyback before DDP, then q. 2 hr $\times$ 2.

9. Diphenhydramine hydrochloride 25 mg I.V. piggyback before first and third dose of metoclopromide.

10. I.V. hydration: 1,000 ml D5%/½ NS with KCl 20 mEq over 4–6 hr following DDP administration.

11. Magnesium oxide 400 mg or magnesium gluconate 500 mg p.o. t.i.d. following DDP $\times$ 7 days.

12. Dronabinol 5 mg p.o. q. 4 hr $\times$ 6 doses can be added to previous orders if patient still has had nausea and vomiting (first dose 3 hr before chemotherapy).

---

*Space is left for addition of the indicated dose of DDP in various regimens.

SUPPORTIVE TREATMENT DURING INTERMEDIATE AND HIGH-DOSE THERAPY (>100 MG/M²/DOSE) WITH METHOTREXATE (MTX)

Treatment should not be instituted if patient has creatinine clearance of ≤ 60 mg/24 hr, platelet count of $\leq 100,000/\mu l$, granulocyte count of $\leq 3000/\mu l$, and/or urine pH of ≤ 6.

The following orders are recommended for the first MTX infusion. They can be adjusted for the second cycle in accordance with the intensity of side effects or lack thereof generated by the first administration.

1. MTX (preservative free) (_________)* mg I.V. in D 5%/½ NS at a concentration of 2 mg/ml up to maximum dilution of 1,000 ml to be administered at a rate of 250 cc/hr.

2. Oral hydration during the 16 hr preceding the MTX administration (at least 2,000 ml liquids) and continuing for 48 hr after MTX (3,000 ml/24 hr).

3. Sodium bicarbonate 500–1,000 mg p.o. t.i.d. 24 hr prior and 72 hr after MTX administration (to keep urine pH > 6 < 7.5). If patient cannot take p.o. medication it can be administered I.V.

4. Prochlorperazine 10 mg I.V. piggyback before MTX then p.o. q.i.d. × 2 days.

5. Leucovorin:
   —15 mg p.o. starting 24 hr after start of MTX infusion of maximum 1,000 mg/m², then q. 6 hr × 7 or until serum MTX level is $< 10^{-11}$ mEq/L.
   —25 mg I.V. in 100 ml D5%/½ NS 6 hr after starting MTX dose of >1 g/m², then p.o. q. 6 hr × 11 or until serum MTX level is $< 10^{-11}$ mEq/L.

---

*Space is left for addition of the indicated dose of MTX in various regimens.

SUPPORTIVE TREATMENT DURING HIGH-DOSE I.V. THERAPY (>1 G/M²/DOSE) WITH CYTARABINE (ARA-C)

The following orders are recommended for administration of high-dose ara-C:

1. Cytosine arabinoside (_________)* mg I.V. in 500 ml D5%/½ NS over 3 hr, usually q. 12 hr × 3–7 days.

2. Steroid ophthalmic solution (Cortisporin) 2 drops each eye q. 6 hr × 10 days.

3. Prochlorperazine 10 mg I.V. piggyback q. 6–8 hr throughout duration of ara-C infusion.

4. Lorazepam p.o. b.i.d. × 7–10 days.

5. I.V. hydration with D5%/½ NS 84–126 cc/126 cc/hr as tolerated.

6. Add KCl 40–80 mEq/L of fluids as needed.

---

*Space is left for addition of the indicated dose of ara-C in various regimens.

Dose Adjustments of Chemotherapy Drugs Related to Abnormalities of Various Systems and Organs

The following composite table lists the adjustments that should be made in the calculated dosage of various chemotherapy agents in relation to various tissue or organ abnormalities that develop and are still present at the time the drug is scheduled to be administered again. Dose reductions recommended should be regarded only as general guidelines to be corroborated with other factors such as previous treatment with XRT at sites containing a significant proportion of body's bone marrow; nutritional status; nadir of blood count; and age if over 75. Various combination regimens may have specific dose attenuation requirements derived from long-term experience with these regimens.

It is important to mention that it is generally advisable before reducing the dose of various drugs to postpone the administration of the whole combination regimen for 1 wk (maximum 2) when the dose reduction may not be necessary; this in view of the fact that maintaining the intensity of the dose of most chemotherapeutic regimens has been found to be the most important factor contributing to their full efficacy. It is also likely that these recommendations, especially those concerning the adjustments due to bone marrow suppression, may need to be drastically changed in the future, when the concomitant administration of colony-stimulating factors with cytotoxic agents could become common practice.

Drug	Platelet counts ($10^{-3}/\mu$l)			Granulocyte counts ($10^{-3}/\mu$l)			Creatinine clearance (ml/min)		Direct bilirubin (mg/dl)			DTRs		Comments
	<130 ≥100	<100 ≥75	<75	<3.0 ≥2.0	<2.0 ≥1.5	<1.5	<60 ≥45	<45	>1.2 ≤1.5	>1.5 ≤2.5	>2.5	±	Absent	
m-AMSA	—	—	—	—	—	—	—	—	—	50	75	—	—	
Bleomycin	—	—	—	—	—	—	—	50	—	—	—	—	—	D/C† in case of pulmon. fibrosis on x-ray or ↓ pulmon. diffus. cap.
Carmustine (BCNU)	25*	50	hold	25	50	hold	—	—	—	—	—	—	—	
Cisplatin	—	25	50	—	—	—	50**	hold	—	—	—	—	—	D/C if hearing loss (by audiometry) develops; give Mg suppl if serum Mg <1.5 mEq/L or <2 mg/dl
Cyclophosphamide	25	50	hold	25	50	hold	—	50	—	—	—	—	—	Hold if proper fluid intake cannot be provided; D/C in case of cystitis
Cytarabine	25	50	hold	25	50	hold	—	—	—	—	—	—	—	Dose reductions do not apply to treatment of leukemia
Dacarbazine	25	50	hold	25	50	hold	—	—	—	—	—	—	—	
Dactinomycin	25	50	hold	25	50	hold	—	—	—	—	—	—	—	
Daunorubicin	25	50	hold	25	50	hold	—	—	25	50	75	—	—	Dose reductions do not apply for acute leukemias; D/C if LVEF§ <40%
Doxorubicin	25	50	hold	25	50	hold	—	—	25	50	75	—	—	
Etoposide	25	50	hold	25	50	hold	—	—	25	50	75			
Fludarabine	25	50	hold	25	50	hold	—	—	—	—	—	—	—	
Fluorouracil	25	50	hold	25	50	hold	—	25	—	—	—	—	—	
Hexamethylmelamine	25	50	hold	25	50	hold	—	—	—	—	—	—	—	
Hydroxyurea	25	50	hold	25	50	hold	—	—	—	—	—	—	—	In CML dose reductions, follow a specific schedule
Lomustine (CCNU)	25	50	hold	25	50	hold	—	—	—	—	—	—	—	
Mechlorethamine	25	50	hold	25	50	hold	—	—	—	—	—	—	—	
Melphalan														
Mecaptopurine														

Drug	Platelet counts (10⁻³/µl)			Granulocyte counts (10⁻³/µl)			Creatinine clearance (ml/min)		Direct bilirubin (mg/dl)			DTRs		Comments
	<130 ≥100	<100 ≥75	<75	<3.0 ≥2.0	<2.0 ≥1.5	<1.5	<60 ≥45	<45	>1.2 ≤1.5	>1.5 ≤2.5	>2.5	$\pm$	Absent	
Methotrexate	25	50	hold	25	50	hold	50	hold	—	50	hold	—	—	Hold if liver enzymes deteriorate, if proper hydration is not possible, or if urine pH is not >6; reduce dose or hold if 3rd space fluid is present
Mitomycin-C	25	50	hold	25	50	hold	—	50	—	—	—	—	—	D/C if fibrosis develops on chest x-ray or any unexplained deterioration of renal function or hemolysis occurs
Mitoxantrone	25	50	hold	25	50	hold	—	—	25	50	75	—	—	D/C in case of cardiac arrhythmia
Procarbazine	25	50	hold	25	50	hold	—	—	—	—	—	—	—	
Streptozotocin	—	—	—	—	—	—	—	50	—	—	—	—	—	
Thioguanine	25	50	hold	25	50	hold	—	—	—	—	—	—	—	
Triethylene-thiophospheramide	25	50	hold	25	50	hold	—	—	—	—	—	—	—	
Vinblastine	—	25	hold	25	50	hold	—	—	25	50	75	50	hold	D/C in case of paralytic ileus
Vincristine	—	—	—	—	25	hold	—	—	25	50	75	50	hold	

*Dose reduction given in % to be subtracted from original calculated dose
**Cisplatin dose adjusted only during course of ongoing treatment; no patient should initially receive drug if creatinine clearance is <60 ml/min
†Discontinue
§LVEF = left ventricular ejection fraction

Table A-1. Abbreviations and Symbols Used in this Appendix

Note: In specifying the days of a treatment cycle on which a drug is administered, a hyphen between 2 numbers indicates that drug is to be administered daily during the period of time defined by the 2 numbers, inclusive of the second number. An ampersand (&) between 2 numbers indicates that the drug is to be administered on the specified days of the treatment cycle.

ADR	doxorubicin
b.i.d.	twice a day
c̄	with
calc dose	calculated dose
CALGB	Cancer and Acute Leukemia Group B
cGy	centigray (1 cGy = 1 rad)
CR	complete response
CSF	cerebrospinal fluid
cyc	cycle
D5%/½ NS	5% dextrose/half normal saline solution
D5%/W	5% dextrose/water solution
D/C	discontinue
DDP	cisplatin
DTR	deep tendon reflex
d	day
h	hour
inf	infusion
I.M.	intramuscular
I.V.C.I.	intravenous continuous infusion
I.V.Sh.I.	intravenous short infusion
IFX	ifosfamide
i.thec.	intrathecally
IU	international unit
kg	kilogram
LCV	leucovorin
max	maximum
m²	meter squared
MSKCC	Memorial Sloan-Kettering Cancer Center
Mg	magnesium
mg	milligram
MTX	methotrexate
mo	month
NCI	National Cancer Insitute
ng	nanogram (= millimicrogram)
NS	normal saline solution
p.o.	orally
q.	every
q.d.	once daily
q. 5 d, etc.	every 5 days, etc.
q. 2 wk, etc.	every 2 weeks, etc.
q. 2 d × 6, etc.	every 2 days until 6 doses have been given, etc.
s̄	without
s.c.	subcutaneous(ly)
supp. meas.	supportive measures
t.i.d.	3 times a day
U	unit
WBC	white blood cell (count)
wk	week
XRT	radiation therapy
yr	year
/	per
>	more than
<	less than

INDEX